MW00635417

PRINCIPLES *of* CARDIAC AND VASCULAR COMPUTED TOMOGRAPHY

PRINCIPLES *of* CARDIAC AND VASCULAR COMPUTED TOMOGRAPHY

Stuart J. Hutchison, MD, FRCP(C), FACC, FAHA, FSCCT

Clinical Professor of Medicine
Departments of Cardiac Sciences, Medicine, and Radiology
University of Calgary;
Director of Echocardiography
Foothills Medicine Centre and Libin Cardiovascular Institute
Calgary, Alberta, Canada

Naeem Merchant, MD, FRCP(C)

Clinical Professor of Medicine
Departments of Cardiac Sciences, Medicine, and Radiology
University of Calgary
Calgary, Alberta, Canada

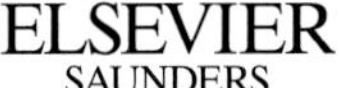

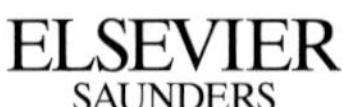

1600 John F. Kennedy Blvd.
Ste 1800
Philadelphia, PA 19103-2899

PRINCIPLES OF CARDIAC AND VASCULAR
COMPUTED TOMOGRAPHY ISBN: 978-1-4377-0407-5

Library of Congress Cataloging-in-Publication Data

Hutchison, Stuart J., author.
Principles of cardiac and vascular computed tomography / Stuart J. Hutchison, Naeem Merchant.
p. ; cm.
Includes bibliographical references and index.
ISBN 978-1-4377-0407-5 (hardcover : alk. paper)
I. Merchant, Naeem, author. II. Title.
[DNLM: 1. Cardiovascular Diseases–radiography. 2. Tomography, X-Ray Computed–methods.
3. Diagnostic Techniques, Cardiovascular. WG 141.5.T6]
RC683.5.I42
616.1'075722–dc23 2014016976

Content Strategist: Dolores Meloni
Content Development Specialist: Marybeth Thiel
Publishing Services Manager: Pat Joiner
Design Direction: Steven Stave
Illustrations Manager: Lesley Frazier

Printed in China

Last digit is the print number: 9 8 7 6 5 4 3 2 1

To my Noel Keith, Liam James, and Cindy, for the truly immeasurable gifts of love, belief, and time.

To my coauthor, Naeem Merchant, simply the best cardiac imager I have ever had the pleasure to work with. For your extraordinary generosity, astonishing acuity and breadth of knowledge, affable and inspired intellect and integrity, and, in no way less as well, for the gift of friendship.

To Kanu Chatterjee, MBBS, the best mentor a physician could ever hope to have. Never exceeded, you inspired legions to grow to become their best and make the greatest contribution to medicine that they could.

SJH

To Laurie, Adam, and Hannah, my loves, and whose love means the most. Thank you for your gifts of patience, trust, and time.

To Stuart, my friend, and the best physician I know. Thank you for your gifts of inspiration, commitment, and perseverance.

To Leon, who first planted a seed so many years ago. Thank you for your gifts of guidance, perspective, and your own gentle wisdom.

NM

ACKNOWLEDGMENTS

Our sincere appreciation to the following individuals: Natasha Andjelkovic, PhD; Jehangir Appoo, MD; Eike Bohme, MD; Patrice Bret, MD; Jagdish Butany, MBBS; Ian Chan, MD; Martin Channdonet, MD; Kanu Chatterjee, MBBS; Andrew Common, MD; Victor Davis; Sybo Dijkstra; Kim Eagle, MD; Tracy Eliot, MD; Behram Engineer, MSC; Lee Errett, MD; Paul Fedak, MD; James Froelich, MD; Ralph Haberl, MD; Mark Hansen, MD; James Hare, MBBS (Hons), PhD; Eric Herget, MD; Christian Holtzheuter, MD; Bill Kent, MD; Bill Kidd, MD; Terry Kieser, MD; David Latter, MD; Jonathan Leipsic, MD; Anne Lenehan; John H. MacGregor, MD; Andrew Maitland, MD; Danny Marcuzzi, MD; Brent Mitchell, MD; Narinder Paul, MD; Visal Pen, MD; Susan Pioli; Philip Prather; Yves Provost, MD; Greg Prystai, MD; Paolo Raggi, MD; Mike Regan; Rob Sevick, MD; Glen Sumner, MD; Yon Mi Sung, MD; Inga Tomas; Chris Vrettos, PhD; Leon de Vries, PhD; Howard Walton; Jason Wong, MD; Sayeh Zielke, MD, MBA.

CONTENTS

VIDEO CONTENTS

1 Introduction

Cardiac computed tomography (CT), the most highly developed application of x-ray imaging, is currently experiencing more advancement per year than ever in its history—probably more than any other imaging modality in the history of x-ray–based medical imaging.

THE ROAD TO THE PRESENT

X-Rays

Wilhelm Conrad Roentgen was awarded the first Nobel Prize in Physics in 1901 for the first intentional generation and use of x-rays, in 1895. He was a firm academic traditionalist, and, intending to preserve his scientific integrity, he signed away all commercial rights to his invention. His name lives on as one of many units of (medical) radiation. His descriptions of the physics of his novel form of "rays" were so definitive that they still constitute a large proportion of the theory of x-ray radiation.

Angiography and Catheterization

The first cardiac catheterization performed may be the one done by Claude Bernard in 1844 on a horse.[1,2] The first human cardiac catheterization was performed in 1929 by a surgery resident, Werner Forssmann, on himself. Using his right hand, Forssmann blindly passed a urethral catheter up the basilar vein in his left arm. He then walked down to the floor below and used, by himself, an x-ray fluoroscopy unit, which enabled him to determine that the catheter was not within the heart. He then advanced the catheter further until he confirmed that it was indeed within the right ventricle, thereby affirming Law Number Six from Samuel Shem's *The House of God* that "there is no body cavity that cannot be reached with a #14G needle and a good strong arm." Forssmann then documented the position of the tip of the catheter using radiographs. He was rewarded for his feat by being fired from the training program, but he ultimately was awarded a Nobel Prize in Medicine, nearly three decades later, in 1956.[3,4]

The first human angiogram probably was performed on the excised hand of a cadaver, with injection of an empiric contrast-enhancing formula of heavy metals and petroleum jelly into the hand vessels.

The first coronary angiogram was inadvertent. In 1958, Mason Sones, the great pioneer of coronary angiography, was performing a cardiac catheterization on a 26-year-old man with rheumatic aortic and mitral valve disease. The aortic root catheter inadvertently fell into the right coronary ostium, resulting in a powered injection of 50 mL of contrast dye, intended for the aortic root, into the right coronary artery. The patient was asystolic for 5 seconds, but recovered with bradycardia. Purely by chance, angiography was shown to be feasible and tolerable and to yield clinically useful images (Fig. 1-1).[5]

Sones, Seldinger, Judkins, and others pioneered many developments to enable peripheral arterial access, selective angiography, adequate image intensifiers, and development of rotating gantries that allowed first left-right rotation and later craniocaudal rotation.

In 2012, approximately 600,000 angiograms were performed in Germany, approximately 150,000 in Canada, and nearly 2 million in the United States, with an overall complication rate of 3.6% and a mortality rate of 0.1%. The average annual cost of coronary angiography in the United States exceeds $9 billion.[6] The yearly worldwide number of coronary angiograms performed is unknown. Angiography remains the current standard for imaging of coronary artery stenosis, delivery of percutaneous coronary intervention, and determination of surgical bypass amenability. Cardiac CT is vying to offer accurate noninvasive angiography; it is a bold prerogative.

Cross-Sectional Imaging and Computed Tomography

Conventional x-ray imaging, planar or angiographic, is superimposition-based imaging and often provides a challenge to the interpretation of radiographs and the performance of angiograms.

The development of cross-sectional two-dimensional imaging began more than four decades ago. The first CT scanner, the brainchild of Sir Godfrey

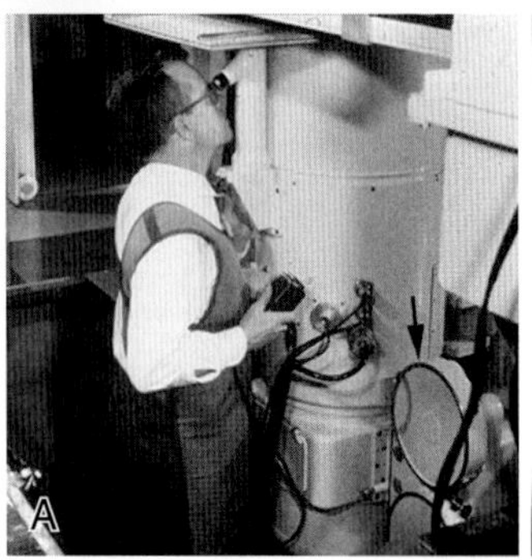

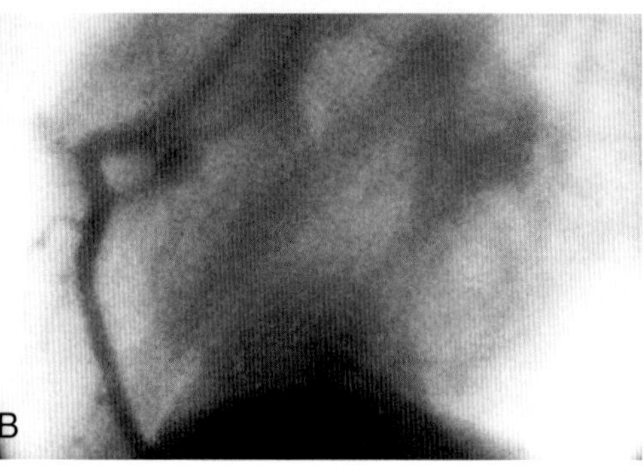

Figure 1-1. A, Mason Sones and the 11-inch image intensifier used for the first coronary arteriogram. The image intensifier is placed below the catheterization table. The arrow points to the 35-mm Arriflex cine camera. **B,** Right coronary artery, left anterior oblique position frame from the first coronary arteriogram, October 30, 1958. (Reprinted with permission from Bruschke AVG, Sheldon WC, Shirey EK, Proudfit WL: A half century of selective coronary arteriography. *J Am Coll Cardiol* 54(23):2139-2144, 2009.)

Hounsfield, became available in 1971. The first patient was scanned during the following year. This CT scanner system was able to scan only a small structure, such as a head, but within a decade, enlargement of the scanner gantry would allow whole-body scanning. Limited by the computer processing speed available at that time, generation of an image after scanning required almost an entire day. Within a year commercial development of the device began. The system launched a new era in cross-sectional diagnostic imaging that has helped in the management of innumerable patients with medical and surgical diseases and trauma. Hounsfield was awarded the Nobel Prize in medicine in 1972. His name lives on in the field of CT as a unit of attenuation of CT scanning—the Hounsfield unit (HU).

In 1973, at the Mayo Clinic, Erik L. Ritman developed the dynamic spatial reconstructor (DSR), a device that could generate a large number of image slices with improved temporal resolution.[7] Standing more than a story tall and using 14 x-ray tubes that took 3 seconds to rotate all the way around the patient, the DSR's enormous size is often cited as a turning point in the development of engineering advances of CT technology, not the least of which was achieving economies of space and radiation.

Early development wrestled with both the basics of the engineering suitable to this novel form of imaging and the processing of the data obtained to generate images. CT scanner designs have gone through four generations thus far, with each generation obtaining images by different positioning and sequencing of the beam-forming and beam-detecting units.

Electron beam CT (EBCT) scanning is heavily represented in medical literature, but it has largely outlived its clinical use. EBCT systems did not use any parts that moved around the patient. An electron beam from an x-ray source ("gun") was focused by coils, then deflected by magnetic fields generated by other coils, and deflected again off a crescentic array that directed the beam across the patient's body at different angles, resulting in "slices," typically 3 mm thick. The system was unique for having no moving parts (no gantry), in contrast to current mechanical CT systems, which have an enormous amount of sophisticated equipment rotating at high speed around the patient during scanning. Few companies manufactured EBCT systems, and few systems have been produced in the last decade, but many machines are still operational. Despite its outdated qualities, EBCT had relatively good temporal resolution and very good spatial resolution and constituted a notable development and advancement in image quality. EBCT is most significant for its contribution to the medical research in noninvasive imaging and cardiac disease by coronary artery calcium scoring. However, EBCT yielded large slices (1.5–3 mm), was quite susceptible to image noise and artifacts, and could acquire only one (or two at the most) slices per breath-hold. Scan times were problematically long, taking 40 to 50 cardiac cycles. Although it briefly offered imaging superior to that of mechanical scanning, which was in its infancy at the time, EBCT soon was technologically surpassed for cardiac imaging by mechanical scanners. The ongoing representation of EBCT in the medical literature (generally in the form of well-performed clinical series at one to two decades of follow-up to calcium studies performed in the early 1990s) has led to some confusion about its current standing.

By the early 1990s, CT scanners had evolved from acquiring a sequence of scan slices through the field of interest (i.e., sequential scanners) to rotating around the patient while he or she was simultaneously passed through the scanner. CT systems defined as rotational, spiral, or helical became, and remain, the norm.

The basic components of CT systems developed steadily over three decades. Single-detector single-slice CT (SSCT) evolved to multiple-detector CT (MDCT) and multislice CT (MSCT) by 2000 or, simply, cardiac CT (CCT). Other key developments include:

- **X-ray tubes** that could produce large volumes of optimal uniform quality output with very good temporal responsiveness

TABLE 1-1 Spatial and Temporal Resolution of Conventional Angiography, IVUS, and CTA

	CONVENTIONAL ANGIOGRAPHY	IVUS	CT CORONARY ANGIOGRAPHY
Spatial resolution (μm)	200	125	350
Temporal resolution (msec)	5–10	—	40–100

CTA, computed tomographic angiography; IVUS, intravascular ultrasound.

- **Collimeters** to adequately control beam width and reduce the radiation emission to the minimum essential for image acquisition
- A **gantry** housing the x-ray tube and the detectors that could be moved with sufficient control and variable speed and had the means to offload the large and progressively increasing amount of information from the gantry at extreme speed
- **Tables** that could feed the patient into the gantry at precisely controllable speeds, thereby rendering image acquisition **helical** or **spiral** as a **Z-plane** was added to the X- and Y-planes of images to render acquisition **volumetric**
- **Detectors** of sufficient width to enable imaging of the heart in one rotation (256- and 320-MDCT) and detectors of superior quality (garnet-based rather than gadolinium-based)
- Software advances made it possible to:
  - ECG "**gate**" image acquisition to the cardiac cycle
  - Allow image display along non-planar lines to follow curving cardiovascular structures along their own long axis
  - Generate different perspectives on structures by means such as 3D volume rendering and endoluminal displays
  - Process hundreds to thousands of images for morphologic and functional evaluation of cardiac chambers and valves
- **Workstations** to facilitate the interface of all of this new technology.

Although much CT technology developed steadily, the last decade has seen markedly accelerated development. Within a period of just 5 years, CT developed from single-slice to 2-, 4-, 8-, 16-, 32-, 40-, and then 64-slice imaging, which is the current standard. Subsequent development yielded 128- (briefly), 256- (128 × 2) and 320- (128 × 2 + 64 to give 10 cm of coverage) slice scanners, to begin an era of single cardiac cycle acquisition (in optimal circumstances).

Numerous improvements have lowered radiation exposure by more than a logarithm. Now that MDCT has acquired greater spatial and temporal resolution, it has become capable of cardiac imaging and more capable of coronary imaging. Interest and involvement by cardiologists in participation and partnership with radiology in cardiovascular CT (CVCT) in the last half decade has increased significantly, and CVCT also has resonated with the media and population at large as a noninvasive means to identify coronary disease.

The novelty of the field of cardiac and coronary CT and its attraction for cardiologists have led to the following, all since 2005:

- Formalization and standardization of training requirements[8] and examination certification[9]
- CT training within the context of multimodality imaging,[10] clinical competence,[11,12] and laboratory operational standards
- Appropriateness of use of cardiac CT[13] and of integration of structured reporting across cardiovascular imaging[14]

Given the inherent challenges of imaging coronary arteries, because of their small size, considerable motion, tendency to develop atherosclerosis and to attract calcium, and stents—both of which produce problematic artifacts—coronary evaluation is understandably one of the last applications of MDCT to reach fruition. It is not there yet, in terms of having anything nearly equal to conventional coronary angiography across the breadth of clinical permutations of coronary disease, comorbidities, cardiac rhythm, heart rate, body size, and provision of a platform for intervention (Table 1-1).

THE PRESENT

Noncoronary and noncardiac applications of cardiovascular imaging are by comparison far better established. In fact, CT pulmonary angiography has become the de facto replacement for conventional pulmonary angiography, and CT aortography now dominates aortic imaging. With the focus of attention on cardiac CT split somewhere between the quest to replace conventional coronary angiography and concerns regarding its radiation risks, advances in noncoronary aspects of cardiac imaging have been somewhat eclipsed. Cardiac CT yields morphological imaging of cardiac structures of superb quality; is developing promising perfusion and late enhancement capabilities, as well as some aspects of tissue characterization; and is developing far beyond just improvements of coronary imaging, which may provide more enduring future roles should the gambit to replace coronary imaging not succeed.

The summary statement from the Society of Cardiovascular Computed Tomography on training, competency, and certification in cardiac CT, including ACCF/AHA cardiac CT categories, fellowship and physician-in-training initial training criteria for Level 1, Level 2, and Level 3, and ACCF/AHA requirements for maintenance of competency can be found in Pelberg et al.[15]

The ACCF 2008 Training Statement on Multimodality Noninvasive Cardiovascular Imaging can be found in Thomas et al.[10]

THE FUTURE

For coronary computed tomographic angiography (CTA) to develop toward maturity, the following are needed:

- Studies that establish that CTA improves clinical outcomes within defined patient groups or subgroups
- Studies that establish cost-effectiveness
- Studies that report accuracy on a per-patient rather than per-segment basis
- Recognition that the performance of CTA is not predicated on high degrees of patient selection and exclusion
- Radiation exposure does not exceed that of conventional angiography, and image quality is similar to conventional angiography across all cases, including, for example, those with irregular heart rhythms.
- Development of the ability to suppress artifacts from calcium and stents without losing image quality of soft tissues
- Development of the ability to obtain adequate imaging of small coronary vessels, which have largely been excluded from analysis
- Optimal integration of cardiac CT assessment into a multimodality approach to cardiac imaging

References

1. Cournand A. Cardiac catheterization; development of the technique, its contributions to experimental medicine, and its initial applications in man. *Acta Med Scand Suppl.* 1975;579:3-32.
2. Silverman BD. Claude Bernard. *Clin Cardiol.* 1996;19(11):916-918.
3. Forssmann-Falck R. Werner Forssmann: a pioneer of cardiology. *Am J Cardiol.* 1997;79(5):651-660.
4. Forssmann W. Die Sondierung des rechten Herzens. *Klinishe Wochenschrift.* 1929;8:2085-2087.
5. Bruschke AV, Sheldon WC, Shirey EK, Proudfit WL. A half century of selective coronary arteriography. *J Am Coll Cardiol.* 2009;54(23):2139-2144.
6. Kalra MK, Brady TJ. Current status and future directions in technical developments of cardiac computed tomography. *J Cardiovasc Comput Tomogr.* 2008;2:71-80.
7. Jorgensen SM, Whitlock SV, Thomas PJ, et al. Dynamic spatial reconstructor: a high-speed, stop-action, 3-D, digital radiographic imager of moving internal organs and blood. *Proc SPIE.* 1991:1346:doi:10:1117/12.23346.
8. Budhoff MJ, Achenbach S, Berman D, et al. Task Force 13: Training in advanced cardiovascular imaging (computed tomography). *J Cardiovasc Comput Tomogr.* 2008;2:130-115.
9. Min JK, Abbara S, Berman D, et al. Blueprint of the certification examination in cardiovascular computed tomography. *J Cardiovas Comput Tomogr.* 2008;2(4):263-271.
10. Thomas JD, Zoghbi WA, Beller GA, et al. ACCF 2008 Training Statement on Multimodality Noninvasive Cardiovascular Imaging: A Report of the American College of Cardiology Foundation/American Heart Association/American College of Physicians Task Force on Clinical Competence and Training Developed in Collaboration With the American Society of Echocardiography, the American Society of Nuclear Cardiology, the Society of Cardiovascular Computed Tomography, the Society for Cardiovascular Magnetic Resonance, and the Society for Vascular Medicine. *J Am Coll Cardiol.* 2009;53(1):125-146.
11. Kramer CM, Budoff MJ, Fayad ZA, et al. ACCF/AHA 2007 clinical competence statement on vascular imaging with computed tomography and magnetic resonance. A report of the American College of Cardiology Foundation/American Heart Association/American College of Physicians Task Force on Clinical Competence and Training. *J Am Coll Cardiol.* 2007;50(11):1097-1114.
12. Budoff MJ, Cohen MC, Garcia MJ, et al. ACCF/AHA clinical competence statement on cardiac imaging with computed tomography and magnetic resonance: a report of the American College of Cardiology Foundation/American Heart Association/American College of Physicians Task Force on Clinical Competence and Training. *J Am Coll Cardiol.* 2005;46(2):383-402.
13. Hendel RC, Manesh PR, Kramer CM, Poon M. ACCF/ACR/SCCT/SCMR/ASNC/NASCI/SCAI/SIR Appropriateness Criteria for Cardiac Computed Tomography and Cardiac Magnetic Resonance Imaging. *J Am Col Cardiol.* 2006;48(7):1475-1497.
14. Douglas PS, Hendel RC, Cummings JE, et al. ACCF/ACR/AHA/ASE/ASNC/HRS/NASCI/RSNA/SAIP/SCAI/SCCT/SCMR 2008 Health Policy Statement on Structured Reporting in Cardiovascular Imaging. *J Am Coll Cardiol.* 2009;53(1):76-90.
15. Pelberg R, Budoff M, Goraya T, et al. Training, competency, and certification in cardiac CT: a summary statement from the Society of Cardiovascular Computed Tomography. *J Cardiovasc Comput Tomogr.* 2011;5(5):279-285.

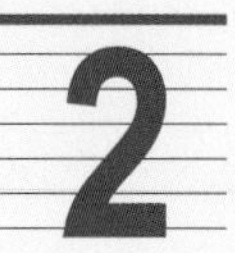

2 Overview of the Process, Exclusions and Risks, and Preparation

Key Points

- Review of patient and study issues, planning, and preparation are required before the scan is performed. The degree of planning and preparation has a direct impact on the adequacy of the obtained images.
- Attention to technical factors and selection of optimal scanning settings is essential to acquiring a complete data set of optimal quality.
- Following the scan:
  - Review the quality of the study and identify artifacts (some artifacts can be eliminated by changing reconstruction parameters).
  - Select reconstruction parameters and verify that the reconstructions are optimal for the referring question.
  - Review the study to address the cardiac (cardiovascular) indication.
  - Review the study to address noncardiac pathologies.
  - Archive the scan.
- Much of the potential quality of a study can be forfeited by poor preparation; conversely, many motion artifacts, electrocardiographic (ECG) artifacts, contrast artifacts, and field of view (FOV) errors can be avoided by sufficient preparation.
- Prepare the patient for the study (e.g., describe sensations to expect, explain the need for no movement).
- Have the patient practice breath-holding until it is being reliably performed.
- Establish a good ECG signal.
- Establish reliable IV access in the right arm.
- Consider β-blocker use and monitor accordingly.

OVERVIEW OF THE PROCESS

Pre-Scanning Issues

Study Issues

- ❐ Review the case history.
- ❐ Establish:
  - The primary indication for the study
    - Other indications for the study
  - Contraindications to the study
  - The appropriateness of CT versus other alternative modalities for the indication and for the patient
- ❐ Select:
  - The optimal scanning protocol
  - The optimal radiation-lowering features
  - The optimal contrast injection technique

Patient Issues

- ❐ Appropriate patient exclusion and selection
- ❐ Appropriate preparation:
  - To ensure predictable contrast delivery, via the right side:
    - IV location: right antecubital vein
    - IV size: sufficient size (≥18G) to allow for the needed high flow rate (4–5 mL/sec)
  - To avoid problematic increase in heart rate during the study:
    - Ensure that the patient understands that there will be noise during the scanning.
    - Confirm that the patient understands that there will be a warm sensation during the study.
    - Consider β-blocker use; evaluate for risk-benefit ratio.
      - Short-term oral use
      - Use with or without IV supplementation
  - Administer sublingual nitroglycerin for coronary studies.
  - To achieve predictable position of the heart during the scan:
    - The patient must understand and practice consistent breath-holding for the study.
  - To avoid motion artifacts, the patient must understand that he or she must not:
    - Move during the scan
    - Take a second breath during the scan
    - Release the breath during the scan
    - Swallow during the scan

Scanning Issues to Resolve

- ❐ Verification of protocol selection:
  - Decide whether or not to perform:
    - A noncontrast scan first
    - Calcium scoring
    - A delayed scan
  - Select gating mode:
    - Prospective gating
    - Retrospective gating

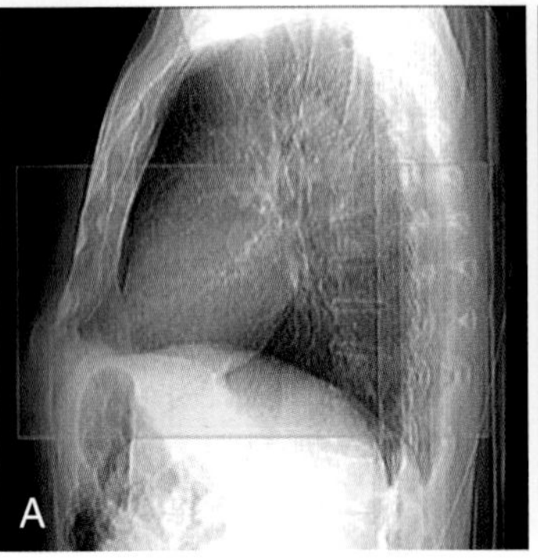

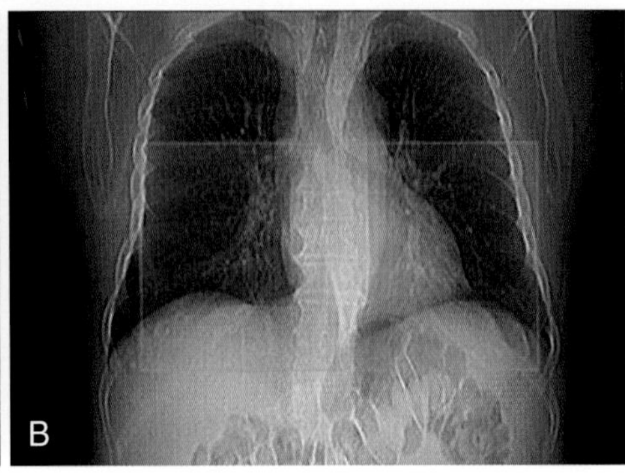

Figure 2-1. Scout images obtained before a CT angiogram. The scout makes it possible to determine the appropriate field of view for the cardiac CT study.

- ❒ Verify contrast injection:
  - Technique
    - Injection technique:
      - Single injection
      - Dual injection
      - Triple injection
    - Bolus technique
      - "Test bolus" method
      - "Bolus tracking" method
  - Rate, duration, and amount of injection
  - Site of injection
- ❒ Selection of an FOV that is suitable to capture both the superior and inferior extent of the region of interest (e.g., coronary tree). Recall that the breath taken during the study may not be of the same depth as the one taken for the topographic view that the FOV was selected on.
- ❒ The greater the needed anatomic coverage, the greater the FOV, but the greater the FOV:
  - The greater the radiation dosage
  - The larger the voxel size
- ❒ In order of increasing FOV size (Fig. 2-1):
  - CTA of the coronary tree only
  - CTA with saphenous vein graft coverage
  - CTA with internal mammary arterial graft imaging
  - Pulmonary embolism (PE) protocol
  - Aorta protocol
  - Lower extremity vasculature
- ❒ Selection of technical factors appropriate for the patient's body habitus (e.g., milliamps)

Post-Scanning

Quality Assurance Analysis

- ❒ Verification that the achieved anatomic coverage is complete:
  - Did the upper limit of the scan capture the upper extent of anatomic interest?
  - Did the lower limit of the scan capture the lower extent of anatomic interest?
- ❒ Verification of quality of the scan
  - Quality check:
    - Artifacts
    - Signal-to-noise ratio (SNR)
  - Quality assurance (QA) of the ECG:
    - Minimal heart rate change during the study
    - No arrhythmias
  - QA of the contrast technique:
    - Contrast opacification quality
    - If coronary CTA:
      - Left heart chambers and aorta: excellent contrast effect
      - Right heart: mild residual contrast effect

Image Reconstruction

- ❒ Reconstruction of images from the data set as needed to address the referring question (Fig. 2-2)
  - Standard: axial, sagittal, coronal
  - With or without the following views:
    - Cardiac-specific
    - 3D
    - Maximum intensity projection
    - Curved multiplanar reconstruction
    - Straightened
    - Cross-sectional perpendicular view to the centerline (intravascular ultrasound view)
    - Other
- ❒ If there is reason to be concerned that:
  - Image reconstruction did not depict the heart without motion in diastole:
    - Reconstruct the images at another phase of the cardiac cycle (e.g., 70%, 75%, 80%)
  - Image reconstruction did not depict the heart at end-systole:
    - Reconstruct the images at another phase of the cardiac cycle (e.g., 35%, 40%).

Image Review

- ❒ Cardiac pathology review
  - Review axial images
  - Use additional modalities as suited to the case
- ❒ Noncardiac pathology review
- ❒ Comparison to previous studies
- ❒ Are further reconstructions needed?

Study Archiving

- ❒ Images to be archived must be selected.
  - Selected image sequences will be archived; the data set seldom is archived.
- ❒ Site of archiving must be selected.

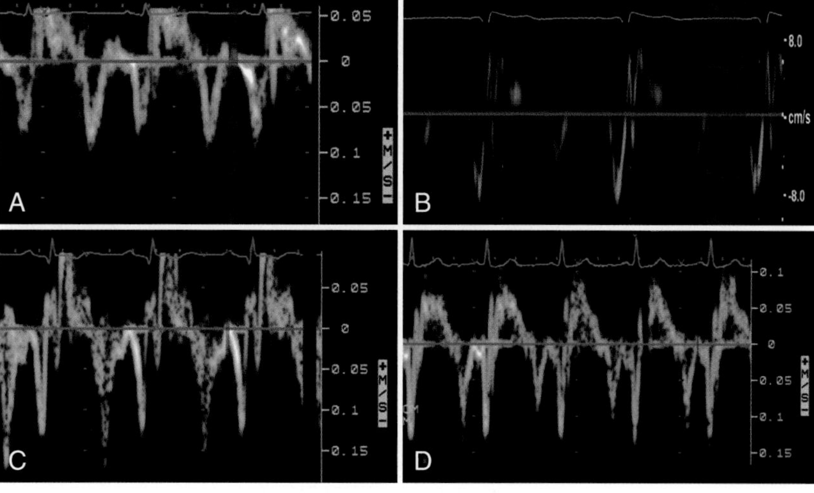

Figure 2-2. Tissue Doppler recording at the mitral annulus level in four different patients, all with corresponding ECG tracings. In each case the motion-free interval, the ideal phase for CCT image acquisition, is indicated on the last cardiac cycle of the tracing by a vertical red line. It can be seen that the motion-free interval is generally very short. The tracings in panel B reveal that lower heart rate is associated with a longer "diastasis" motion-free phase between early and late diastolic filling/motion, which allows for better quality CCT image acquisition.

EXCLUSIONS TO CT ANGIOGRAPHY

Critical steps to achieve safe studies of optimal quality include:

- Correct selection of patients
- Correct exclusion of patients who will have poor quality studies
- Correct exclusion of patients who will be exposed to higher risk
- Best preparation of the patient
- Best preparation of the ECG signal
- Heavy coronary calcium predictably impairs interpretation of coronary CTA.
    - Calcium above a certain level observed on a calcium scoring protocol before CTA may preclude the utility of performing the CTA (e.g., Agatston score ≥ 750 or ≥ 1000).
    - Calcium scoring may reduce overall radiation exposure, if used to select for CTA, which may be the most practical use of calcium scoring.
- Temporal resolution issues
    - Tachycardia
    - Arrhythmia, if very irregular
    - Heart rate variability
- Contrast dye intolerance
    - Renal insufficiency (creatinine clearance < 30 mL/min)
    - Decompensated heart failure
    - Severe allergy
- Dyspnea: i.e., the patient is not expected to be able to breath-hold for 20 to 30 seconds.
- Claustrophobia
- β-Blocker intolerance (if β-blockers are expected to be needed)
- Morbid obesity
- Stents (probably). Large stents less so; small stents more so.
- Intracardiac devices (e.g., pacemakers or implantable cardioverter defibrillators may limit the evaluation of the right coronary artery)

OPTIMAL SELECTION AND PREPARATION

The patient must be prepared well for what to expect. Although scanning proceeds automatically once initiated, *any* movement during the scanning or substantial heart rate acceleration will compromise the quality of the acquired images. Therefore, the patient must completely understand what to do and what not to do. If, for example, a patient is aware of the sensation to expect from dye injection, his or her anxiety and subsequent increase in heart rate during the study will be less.

Patient Review

Patient review is discussed in detail in Abbara et al.[1]

Initial Screening

- Initial screening is described in Box 2-1.

Pretest Instructions

- Pretest instructions are presented in Box 2-2.

Patient Instructions

- Have the patient assume a comfortable position.
- Have the patient place his or her arms behind the head or up on the scanner to avoid artifact and to reduce radiation absorption.
- Have the patient practice taking single inspirations of equal size to avoid variations in the size or rhythm of inspirations during the scan. Breath-holding should be practiced several times.
- Avoid body motion.
    - The patient must not move during the examination.
    - The patient must not swallow during the examination.

BOX 2-1 Initial Screening

1. History taking to evaluate for:
   a. Pregnancy or potential pregnancy: According to ACR recommendations "All imaging facilities should have policies and procedures to identify pregnant patients prior to imaging, and to consider any possible risks to the fetus of any planned administration of contrast material, taking into consideration the potential clinical benefits of the examination."
   b. Contraindication to contrast media or other medications including β-blockers and nitroglycerin
   c. Renal insufficiency and risk of contrast-induced nephrotoxicity (CIN)
   d. Prior allergic reactions to any allergens
   e. Active bronchospastic disease, hypertrophic cardiomyopathy, severe aortic valve stenosis, or other precautions or contraindications to β-blockers
   f. Current medications (especially sildenafil, vardenafil, tadalafil, or metformin)
   g. Any other pertinent medical history
2. Assessment of the ability to follow breath-hold commands and perform inspiratory breath-hold
3. Assessment of body weight
4. Assessment of heart rate (preferably after inspiration) and arrhythmia
5. Assessment of blood pressure

Reprinted with permission from Abbara S, Arbab-Zadeh A, Callister TQ, et al. SCCT guidelines for performance of coronary computed tomographic angiography: a report of the Society of Cardiovascular Computed Tomography Guidelines Committee. J Cardiovasc Comp Tomogr. *2009;3:190-204.*

BOX 2-2 Pretest Instructions

1. No food for 3–4 hours before examination.
2. May drink water or clear fluids up until time of examination (patient should be well hydrated for renal protection, for ease of establishing venous access, and to avoid postprocedure hypotension).
3. No caffeine products for 12 hours before examination, because they might hinder efforts to reduce the heart rate before scanning. This includes coffee, tea, energy drinks, energy pills, diet pills, and most soda.
4. Take all regular medications the day of examination, especially blood pressure medicine.
5. Take pre-medications for contrast allergy as prescribed by the ordering physician. As an example, the standard Greenberger regimen is prednisone, 50 mg by mouth, 13, 7, and 1 hour before contrast exposure, in addition to diphenhydramine 50 mg by mouth 1 hour before contrast exposure.[2]
6. Metformin use must be discontinued for at least 48 hours after the contrast administration. Metformin itself is not nephrotoxic, but it is exclusively renally cleared. If renal failure is precipitated by iodinated contrast, a toxic accumulation of metformin may result, which can induce lactic acidosis. There is no evidence that withholding metformin *before* a contrast procedure is protective, although this approach has been adopted by some.

Reprinted with permission from Abbara S, Arbab-Zadeh A, Callister TQ, et al. SCCT guidelines for performance of coronary computed tomographic angiography: a report of the Society of Cardiovascular Computed Tomography Guidelines Committee. J Cardiovasc Comput Tomogr. *2009;3:190-204.*

Patient Information

❒ Patients should be informed that:
- They will hear the sound of the scanning (gantry rotation).
- They will feel the (cold) injection of dye and saline moving up their arm.
- They will then feel warm shortly after the contrast injection.

Breath-Holding

Rationale for breath-holding: Acquisition of cardiac CT image data sets will take 2 to 20 seconds, depending on the scanner and parameters of the scan.

16-slice CT	20 seconds
40-slice CT	14 seconds
64-slice CT	10 seconds
320-slice CT	2 seconds

The heart must be in a stable position in the chest throughout the duration of acquisition. The heart is in a stable position within the chest at only two points during the respiratory cycle: end-inspiration and end-expiration. Either end-expiration or end-inspiration is suitable, because each is fairly reproducible. By convention, end-inspiration is used for cardiac CT, although end-expiration is probably more reproducible. The lack of reproducibility of the inspiratory volume (which determines the position of the heart in the chest) is a problem that may haunt a coronary CTA study: the FOV is chosen based on the surview/topographic images obtained by a first inspiration/breath-hold. The actual scan is acquired shortly after, during a second inspiration/breath-hold. If the two inspiratory volumes are different, and if the FOV was cropped tight, then the FOV may fail to capture the desired region. This is why it is necessary to walk the patient through the inspiration maneuvers carefully.

β-Blockers

Optimal heart rate is 50 to 65 beats per minute.

β-Blockers are generally advisable for CTA studies unless the resting heart rate is nearly, or frankly, bradycardic. β-Blockers increase the diastasis period of diastole to facilitate acquisition (unless

TABLE 2-1 β-Blockers

ADMINISTRATION	DRUG	DOSE	ONSET	HALF-LIFE
Oral	Metoprolol tartrate	50–100 mg	1 hr	3–7 hr Metabolites: 8 hr
	Atenolol	50–100 mg	2 hr	6–10 hr
Intravenous	Metoprolol tartrate	2.5–5.0 mg Up to 15 mg Use caution >15 mg; can go to 30 mg	1 min	3–4 hr Metabolites: 8 hr
	Atenolol	2.5–5.0 mg Up to 10 mg	1 min	6–10 hr
	Esmolol	0.5 mg/kg 25–50 mg	1–2 min	9 min

they disproportionally increase the PR interval), and reduce heart rate increment, R–R (R-wave to R-wave) variation, and ectopy, all of which may induce artifacts. β-Blockers have been shown to improve image quality (on 16-slice MDCT).[3] Nonetheless, a slow resting heart rate does not ensure that there is no problematic increase in heart rate increment during the study.

Factors that tend to raise heart rate during the study include:

- ❐ Anxiety
- ❐ Stimulation from sound
- ❐ Contrast dye injection sensation
- ❐ Breath-holding
- ❐ Contrast dye load

It is fortuitous if the patient is already on chronic β-blocker therapy, because this likely confers better blockade, and, therefore, image quality.

Short-term β-blocker therapy (Table 2-1) often is employed to reduce the heart rate and attenuate the tendency for the heart rate to increase during the study. Monitoring during and after the study is advisable. β-Blockers may be given orally or intravenously in the setting of coronary CTA. There is probably a tendency to underdose in this setting. Intravenous β-blockers require observation after the scan.

Other Medications

- ❐ **Anxiolytics:** Short-acting anxiolytics may be of use for some patients.
- ❐ **Nitroglycerine** (400–800 μg sublingually), in the absence of contraindications such as resting hypotension, impaired cardiac output, hypertrophic obstructive cardiomyopathy, or recent use of sildenafil achieves coronary vasodilation and improves image quality.[1]
- ❐ **Oxygen supplementation:** Consider whether the patient is dyspneic or hypoxic.

Intravenous Access

- ❐ The IV access must be of adequate size (e.g., 18G) to ensure good contrast dye flow.
- ❐ The IV access must be in the right antecubital vein.
- ❐ The IV flow must be verified before any injection.
- ❐ Access sites to be avoided:
  - **Left arm:** The left subclavian artery and internal thoracic artery ostium often are obscured by streak artifact from the left subclavian or brachiocephalic vein when contrast is injected via access in the left arm.
  - **Central lines:** The timing of the contrast arrival will be off; it will arrive early. Any use of central lines should first have the safety of power injection through them verified.
  - **Hand veins** are more likely to render the arrival of dye late, and are more likely to "blow" and infiltrate.

ECG Recording

Cardiac gating is essential for cardiac CT and coronary CTA, and is increasingly advisable for most cardiovascular CT applications. Streak artifacts may be generated by the ECG lead, and from noise or wander of the recording. A clear ECG signal is a prerequisite, as is correct lead placement. Proper ECG electrode preparation is intended to maximize signal and minimize noise.

- ❐ Clean skin.
- ❐ Consider cleansing with alcohol to optimize recording.
- ❐ Shave hair, if present.
- ❐ Ensure connections are secure.
- ❐ The ECG leads should not be placed over the precordium, because:
  - The metal contact will result in streak artifacts in the vicinity of the heart.
  - Pectoral muscle activity may generate electrical artifact.

Verification of a good quality and reliable ECG signal is well worth the time and effort (Table 2-2).

TABLE 2-2 ECG Signal Trouble-Shooting

PROBLEM	CAUSE	SOLUTION
Low-amplitude signal	Poor vector alignment	Change lead orientation
	Low gain setting	Increase gain
	Poor preparation	Reapply electrodes
Artifact	Loose ECG leads	Reapply the patches
	Loose connections	Verify the contact of the patches and cables
	Loose cables	Reconnect or change cables
	Static or ambient electricity	
	Patient movement	Instruct
	Patient tremors	Warm patient with blankets
Wandering signal	Loose connections	Verify connections

CREATININE CLEARANCE

Creatinine clearance (CrCl) is used clinically as an approximation of the glomerular filtration rate (GFR). However, because creatinine also is secreted by the renal tubules, CrCl overestimates the GFR by 10% to 20% at lower filtration levels characteristic of the more advanced stages (stage 5 and possibly stage 4) of chronic renal insufficiency. The GFR is the volume of fluid filtered from the renal (kidney) glomerular capillaries into Bowman's capsule per unit time.

Cockroft and Gault Formula

The Cockroft and Gault formula is used to estimate the CrCl rate:

$$[(140 - \text{age}) \times \text{weight (kg)} \times F]/(\text{plasma creatinine} \times 0.81356)$$

Normal values:

SEX	AVERAGE	RANGE
Male	70 ± 14 mL/min/m^2 120 ± 25 mL/min/1.73 m^2 (or 175 L/day)	97–137 mL/min/1.73 m^2 (0.93–1.32 mL/sec/m^2 IU) 55–146 mL/min/1.73 m^2
Female	60 ± 10 mL/min/m^2 95 ± 0 mL/min/1.73 m^2 (or 135 L/day)	88–128 mL/min/1.73 m^2 (0.85–1.23 mL/sec/m^2 IU) 52–134 mL/min/1.73 m^2

- ❐ Therefore, the needed variables are:
  - Age (years)
  - Height (centimeters)
  - Gender (male or female)
- ❐ Note:[4]
  - $F = 1$ if male or 0.85 if female
  - Plasma creatinine is expressed in µmol/L units.
  - Weight (in kilograms):
    - Actual weight is not used, given its poor relation to lean body mass. Estimated lean body mass is calculated from the patient's height.
      - Male (kg): 50 kg + 0.9 kg for each cm of height > 152 cm
      - Female (kg): 45.5 kg + 0.9 kg for each cm of height > 152 cm
    - This estimation of lean body mass from height applies only to adults.
  - Extremes of body habitus and composition are not well served by this equation.
  - There are significant assumptions made in the calculation of creatinine clearance, many of which are not valid in clinical practice:
    - That there is a stable equilibrium of both creatinine production and elimination; hence, the equation does not lend itself to changes in status in renal function, which is extremely common among the inpatient population.
  - GFR is age-related:
    - Normal GFR at 30 years of age is 125 ± 25 mL/min/1.73 m^2
    - GFR normally falls at a rate of 1 mL/min/1.73 m^2/year
  - Some cardiac medications (e.g., quinidine and procainamide) as well as cimetidine and some antibiotics reduce creatinine clearance.
  - Check the calculation twice.

The severity of chronic kidney disease (CKD) is described by six stages. The three most severe stages are defined by the Modification of Diet in Renal Disease estimated GFR (MDRD-eGFR) value, whereas the first three also depend on whether there is other evidence of kidney disease (e.g., proteinuria).

- ❐ CKD
  - Normal kidney function

- GFR > 90 mL/min/1.73 m^2
- No proteinuria

❒ CKD Stage 1
- GFR > 90 mL/min/1.73 m^2
- Evidence of kidney damage

❒ CKD Stage 2 (mild)
- GFR 60–89 mL/min/1.73 m^2
- Evidence of kidney damage

❒ CKD Stage 3 (moderate)
- GFR 30–59 mL/min/ 1.73 m^2

❒ CKD Stage 4 (severe)
- GFR 15–29 mL/min/1.73 m^2

❒ CKD Stage 5
- Kidney failure (dialysis or kidney transplant needed)
- GFR <15 mL/min/1.73 m^2

References

1. Abbara S, Arbab-Zadeh A, Callister TQ, et al. SCCT guidelines for performance of coronary computed tomographic angiography: a report of the Society of Cardiovascular Computed Tomography Guidelines Committee. *J Cardiovasc Comput Tomogr.* 2009;3(3): 190-204.
2. Greenberger P, Patterson R. Prednisone-diphenhydramine regimen prior to use of radiographic contrast media. *J Allergy Clin Immunol.* 1979;63(4):295.
3. Shim SS, Kim Y, Lim SM. Improvement of image quality with beta-blocker premedication on ECG-gated 16-MDCT coronary angiography. *AJR Am J Roentgenol.* 2005;184(2):649-654.
4. Min JK, Abbara S, Berman D, et al. Blueprint of the certification examination in cardiovascular computed tomography. *J Cardiovasc Comput Tomogr.* 2008;2(4):263-271.

3 Radiation and Radiation Risk

Key Points

- Radiation exposure is an inherent and undeniable risk of cardiac CT.
- The favored unit to express radiation exposure per CT scan is the millisievert (mSv).
- Radiation risk relates linearly to exposure.
- Strategies to minimize radiation exposure should always be undertaken, and consideration should be given to alternatives that do not involve radiation (e.g., echocardiography or MRI).
- The risk of the scan must be weighed against the benefit of the procurable information, in the context of other means that may be available to garner the same information.
- Conversely, the risk of failing to identify or diagnose significant lesions must be considered in the context of concern about radiation-associated risk.
- Younger women represent the single highest risk group from cardiac CT scanning, because:
  - Younger patients are more susceptible to malignancy.
  - The radiation dose is higher in women because greater doses are needed to image the heart deep to breast-attenuating soft tissue.
  - Breast cancer is a risk.
  - The latent interval to develop malignancy is offset several-fold by expected years of life.
- Radiation exposure inherent in cardiac CT scanning has fallen by more than a logarithm within the past 10 years, and submillisievert (<1 mSv) exposure is feasible with the newest generation of equipment.

CONTEXT AND PERSPECTIVE

Although the risk per single CT scan is small, given the enormous numbers of CT scans performed, this risk is neither small nor dismissible. Approximately 60 to 65 million CT scans of all types were performed in the United States in 2006[1]—one per five citizens. The rate is increasing at 10% to 25% per year. Approximately two thirds of a billion CT scans have been performed in the United States alone since 1980. It has been established that over the last several decades, the amount of radiation exposure per person per year has increased conspicuously (600% in 3 decades), due mainly to the proliferation of CT scanning.[2] Medical imaging procedures, especially tomographic imaging and nuclear medicine, are important sources of exposure to ionizing radiation.[3]

Thus, even if the risks of CT scanning are small per scan, given the sheer volume of scans, the risk does translate into events.[4] It is estimated, although not yet proved, that approximately 0.4% of all cancer in the United States may be attributed to CT scanning.[4,5] Radiation risk should be responsibly and knowledgeably addressed whenever cardiac CT (CCT), coronary computed tomographic angiography (CTA), electron beam CT (EBCT), or other type of CT scanning is being considered or when nuclear testing or any form of imaging that entails radiation exposure to patients is an option.

The actual risks of medical radiation are neither tabulated nor known; currently, they have been estimated only by models that understandably engender some controversy.[6,7] The models are based on data from nuclear blasts over Hiroshima and Nagasaki, from the Chernobyl nuclear reactor leak, and from exposure of individuals engaged in nuclear testing for medical purposes,[5] as well as from patients exposed to radiation. Unfortunately, more real data pertaining to emerged cancer risks in patients undergoing CT scanning for reasons other than cancer have never been gathered. It is a sobering fact that much medical diagnostic testing entails radiation exposure equivalent to what occurred at the periphery of Hiroshima and Nagasaki, whose populations, followed for half a century, did exhibit excessive rates of cancer.[8,9]

Tubiana[6] has understandably stated that overestimation of risk "may deprive patients of beneficial examinations." Some of the controversy itself is controversial, such as objection to the linear no-threshold risk of radiation.[10,11]

Few data have been tabulated to substantiate so many statements about CT scanning and the manner and the matter of its use. The net effect of CT scanning is simply the summation of the reduction of morbidity and mortality of lives by useful clinical diagnosis guiding successful therapy, and the incurred morbidity and mortality from radiation, contrast media, and other complications attributable to its use.

RADIATION AND RISK OVERVIEW

Biological Effects of Ionizing Radiation VII (2005)

The Biological Effects of Ionizing Radiation (BEIR) VII conference changed the paradigm of medical radiation risk modeling from a "threshold" to a "linear" risk model:

> *A comprehensive review of available and biophysical data supports a linear-no-threshold risk model—that the risk of cancer proceeds in a linear fashion at lower doses without a threshold and that the smallest dose has the potential to cause a small increase in risks to humans.*

This landmark conference and its published proceedings are notable for advancing constructive discussion on radiation risk, which directed the discussion toward responsible management of the risk. This discussion then prompted enormous research and development and introduction of hardware and software upgrades and developments in CT scanner design and function that have brought about significant reductions in radiation exposure. The controversy regarding threshold versus linear risk simmers, based on radiotherapy data.

Organizations with Positions on the Linear No-Threshold Model

Organizations have taken a variety of positions on the linear no-threshold (LNT) model at <100 mSv[10]:

- ❒ Basically supportive
  - US National Research Council Biological Effects of Ionizing Radiation (BEIR) VII Phase 2 (2006)
  - International Commission on Radiological Protection (2005)
  - US National Council on Radiation Protection and Measurements (2001)
  - United Nations Scientific Committee on the Effects of Atomic Radiation (2000)
  - UK National Radiological Protection Board (1995)
- ❒ LNT is oversimplication: risk estimates should not be used at <50 mSv:
  - Health Physics Society (2004)
- ❒ LNT overestimates risk:
  - French Academy of Sciences/National Academy of Medicine (2004)
  - American Nuclear Society (2001)

Metrics of Radiation Dose

The subject of radiation dosage is highly complex; accordingly, radiation dosage can be expressed in a variety of metrics. The "effective dose" is widely quoted because it reflects biologic risk, although effective dose estimates do not apply to any individual patient. It is, however, far easier to determine the amount of emitted radiation than to determine the absorbed radiation, let alone the real biologic risk (Table 3-1).

In its *Clinical Policy Statement for Noninvasive Cardiac Imaging*, the American College of Radiology has recommended that cardiac imaging be restricted to no more than 13 mSv.[12] The goal of medical diagnostic imaging is for radiation exposure to be as low as reasonably achievable and still be effective.

Units of Radiation

- ❒ 1 Sv = 100 rem
- ❒ 1 mSv = 0.1 rem = 100 mrem
- ❒ 1 Sv = 1 Gr ("grey"), when dealing with photons

Factors Affecting Radiosensitivity

- ❒ **Linear energy transfer (LET):** the propensity of energy to transfer from ionizing radiation

TABLE 3-1 Metrics of Radiation Dose

Metric	Volume CT dose index (CTDI)	Dose-length product (DLP) (required in Europe)	Effective dose (E)
Unit	mGy	MGy*cm	mSv
Description	Average volume within the scan volume	DLP = $CTDI_{vol}$ (mGy) × scan length (cm)	Represents biologic risk
Notes	A per-scan rotation metric Local dose (affected by kV, mAs) intensity Dose from the beam and its scatter	A per-exam metric Integrates the CTDI over the scan length (which is affected by pitch) Integral of intensity and coverage	A per-exam metric Intensity + coverage + sensitivity $Dose_{effective}$ = DLP × 0.017

CTDI, CT dose index; DLP, dose-length product; E, effective dose.

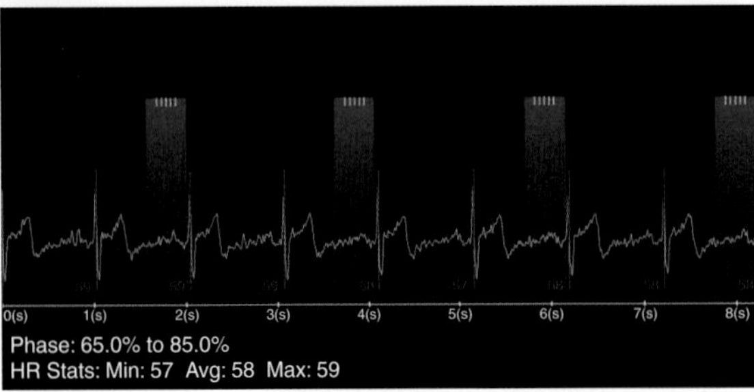

Figure 3-1. ECG-gated prospective "pulsed" acquisition, acquired between the 65th and 85th percentiles of the cardiac cycle.

TABLE 3-2 Other Lifetime Risks of Death as Benchmarks to the Risk of CT Scanning

DEATH FROM	ODDS
Cardiovascular disease	1:2.6
Cancer	1:4
Car accident	1:4,000
Plane crash	1:100,000
Lightning	1:2,320,000

to tissue. X-rays have a small linear energy transfer.

- **Relative biologic effectiveness (RBE):** As the LET of radiation increases, the ability to produce biologic damage increases. This is quantitatively described as the RBE. The RBE of CT x-ray is 1. X-rays have a small biologic effectiveness.
- **Age:** Humans are most radiosensitive before birth and become progressively less sensitive with age. X-ray exposure should be assiduously avoided or—if absolutely essential— minimized during pregnancy.

Tube Voltage

Tube voltage is a major determinant of radiation exposure, and body size is the main determinant of voltage requirement. In most patients 100 to 120 kV tube voltage is sufficient for cardiac imaging. The radiation variation is the square of the variation of the tube voltage. Therefore, the occasional use of 140 kV to image very large patients prominently increases radiation exposure, and, conversely, reducing tube voltage to 100 or 80 kV in very small adults diminishes the radiation exposure by 30% to 50% while preserving contrast-to-noise ratio.[13] Tube voltage should be reduced to 100 kV when body weight is less than 85 kg and BMI is less than 30 kg/m^2 (Fig. 3-1).[14]

Lifetime Adjusted Risk

The lifetime adjusted risk (LAR) of cancer attributable to prior CT scanning is debated, with estimates ranging from 1:2000 to 1:10,000. With an estimated latency of 12 years between exposure and development of cancer, the risk is lower in older populations and greater in younger populations.

Radiation Risk in Cardiac CT

It is easier to quantify the amount of exposed or absorbed radiation than to estimate the risk of the radiation. The attributed risk depends largely on the model used to project the risk, and all models have engendered some controversy. Most of the data on radiation risks are extrapolated from nuclear blast radiation exposure, and some originate from nuclear power generation station mishaps.

Animal data obtained in dogs suggest that there is a threshold of 200 mSv to the risk of radiation, but current recommendations (BEIR VII) articulate that there is no threshold and that risk is proportional to exposure.

In the following example of a model/calculation of risk for cardiac CT scanning, note all of the assumptions and that a range of numbers rather than a number is more appropriate (Table 3-2).

Assume the following:

- 10 mSv per CT scan
- CT after age 45 years, half of lifetime remaining
- Lifetime risk of cancer is relatively high: 1:1000 per 10 mSv over 70 years lifespan
- 1 person in 4 dies of cancer each year
- cancer/(100 persons × 10 mSv × lifetime) × 1 death/cancer × lifetime/2 = 15 deaths/ (100,000 person cardiac CT)

The highest single proportion of the total effective dose of radiation that patients are exposed to is from myocardial perfusion imaging (11%), although CT scanning cumulatively (CT abdomen, pelvis, chest, CT angiography, non-chest, CT head/brain, cervical spine, lumbar spine, neck) accounts for nearly half (45%). Diagnostic cardiac catheterization accounts for 5% and PCI for 2%. Chest radiography accounts for less than 1% (0.7%).[15]

Radiation Dose from Cardiac CT Scanning and Lifetime Risks

Einstein et al.[16] examined the radiation dose and lifetime risk of cancer from older 16-slice CTA and later from 64-slice CT scanners. The authors presented their estimation of radiation effective doses by different cardiac imaging modalities.

From 16-slice CT scanners, the average of the examined radiation dose was 9 mSv, increasing by 2.5 mSv to 11.5 mSv when calcium scoring was

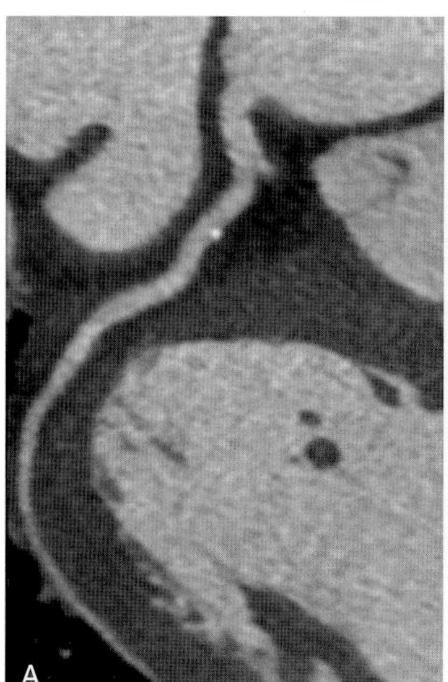

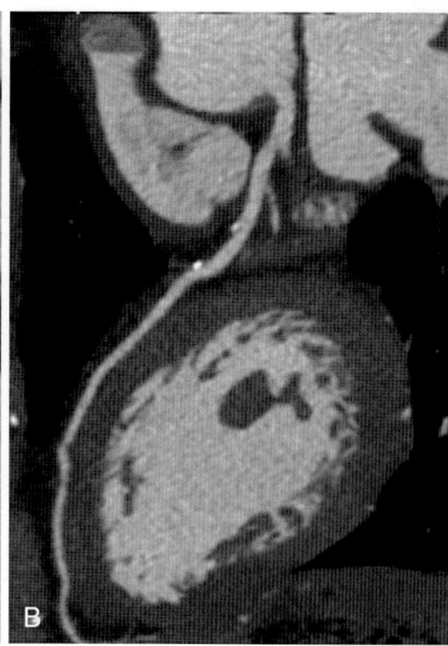

Figure 3-2. Low-dose coronary CTA (<1 mSv): high-quality images. Mild atherosclerotic disease.

included. Women were exposed to more radiation than were men (13.5 mSv versus 11 mSv). The authors estimated the lifetime risk of cancer from 16-slice CT scanners to be 1:1600 (worst-case scenario: 1:500). The expected increase in cancers was in lung cancer and breast cancer. The radiation dose from 64-slice CT is estimated to be 50% higher.[17]

In a different publication, Einstein et al.[10] presented their calculation of lifetime attributable/adjusted risk (LAR) from 64-sclice CT scanners in an article cautioning against the overly aggressive use of coronary CT angiography. Their calculations of risk suggest that there is a non-negligible (as per BEIR VII) lifetime adjusted risk of malignancy associated with coronary and cardiac CT. This risk was age dependent because of (1) the latency of 12 or more years to development of radiation-induced malignancy and (2) the greater susceptibility to malignancy in younger patients. CT scanning of both the heart and aorta entailed greater radiation exposure and risk. The highest LARs were of lung cancer and of breast cancer in younger women. X-ray tube modulation significantly reduced calculated risk[10] (Fig. 3-2; Tables 3-3 through 3-5).

Cardiac CTA entails a range of radiation exposure depending on hardware, software, protocols, and selected dose reduction modalities. The amount of soft tissue encountered by x-rays influences the radiation dosage. For example:

- Radiation dosage is 1.5 times higher in women versus men because of greater breast soft tissue attenuation and absorption.
- Large variations in patient dose absorption during the CT examination occur depending on the angle of incidence of x-rays (e.g., greater chest width and bony structures encountered on lateral angle of incidence).
- Large patients will always be exposed to more radiation because increased energy output is required to penetrate their greater amount of soft tissue.

Factors in CT Scanning That Influence Radiation and Risk

- The decision to scan:
  - Decide whether to refer for or perform CT scanning rather than an alternative and non–radiation-entailing test (e.g., echocardiography or cardiac MRI)
  - Weigh the information expected to be gained from the study against the risks.
  - Avoid multiple or repeat scans unless strictly necessary.
  - Avoid scans under conditions that will predictably produce low-quality results (e.g., presence of irregular cardiac rhythms, calcium, small coronary stents).
- CT scan technique and modalities employed:
  - Minimize scan time.
  - Minimize field of view to the area of interest (e.g., heart versus thorax).
  - Use the minimum effective current and voltage.
  - Use dose-modulation techniques to lessen radiation.
  - Prospective gating, in general, decreases radiation.
  - Avoid LV function assessment, which entails irradiation through the cardiac cycle.

TABLE 3-3 Amount of Radiation in Cardiac CT Versus Other Cardiac Investigations (Baseline Exposures)

EXPOSURE	AVERAGE RADIATION (mSv)	APPROXIMATE RANGE (mSv)	NOTES
Radiation Exposures, by Way of Comparison			
Yearly background radiation	3.6		
Exposure/hr in an airplane	0.02		
Echocardiography			
Transthoracic	0.0		
TEE	0.0		
ICE	0.0		The fluoroscopy to deliver the wires entails some radiation.
Cardiac MRI	0.0		
Chest Radiography			
Posteroanterior and lateral[17]	0.1	[0.05–0.24]	Mainly from the lateral
Posteroanterior	0.01–0.02[3]		
Lateral	0.15		
Nuclear Cardiology			
MUGA scan	5–8[3]		
Sestamibi scan	9[18]–13		
Thallium-201 scan			
Scan	19		
Stress / rest	41[18]		
PET			
18F FDG	14[18]		
Rubidium-82	5[18]		
Coronary Angiography / PCI / Cardiac Fluoroscopy			
			4- to 6-fold variation in fluoroscopic radiation exposure in cardiac catheterization laboratories[19]
Coronary angiography	7[3,18] 5.6 ± 3.6[20]	[2–16][18]	
PCI	5–20[3]	[7–75][18]	
Radiofrequency ablation	15[18]	[7–75][18]	
Computed Tomography			
Noncardiac			
Head	1–2[3]		
Cervical spine	6[3]		
Neck	3[3]		
Chest	5–7[3,18]	[4–18][18]	
Abdomen	3–8[3,18]	[4–25][18]	
Abdominal/pelvis	8–11		
Lumbar spine	6[3]		

TABLE 3-3 Amount of Radiation in Cardiac CT Versus Other Cardiac Investigations (Baseline Exposures)—cont'd

EXPOSURE		AVERAGE RADIATION (mSv)	APPROXIMATE RANGE (mSv)	NOTES
Computed Tomography—cont'd				
Pelvis		3–6[3,18]	[3–10][18]	
PE Protocol				
AAD protocol		15[3]		
AAA protocol		12		
CT fluoroscopy		74 mSv[21]		CT fluoroscopy generates a radiation dose up to 20 times the dose of CT scanning.[21]
Cardiac				
Calcium scoring		0.8–3[18]	[1–12][18]	
Coronary CTA		10–15	[2.5–40]	
16-CT		14.7±2.2[20]		
		6.4±1.9[13]		
64-CT	***Non-Dual Source***	11.0±4.1[13]		
	Without tube modulation	15[18]	[12–18][18]	
	With tube modulation	9[18]	[8–18][18]	
	Retrospective gating	21.1±6.7[22]		
	Prospective triggering	3[18]	[2–4][18]	
		4.3±1.3[22]		
	Dual Source	7.8[23]		
	DS "step-and-shoot"	2.5±0.8[24]	[1.2–4.4][24]	
	DS prospective gating 70%	2.2±0.8[25]		
	DS tube modulation	13[18]	[6–17][18]	
		4.3±1.3[22]		
		1.2[26]		
64-CT, 256-CT, 320-CT	Prospective Triggering / low kV / iterative reconstruction of raw data	<1 mSv[27]		

AAA, abdominal aortic aneurysm; AAD, acute aortic dissection; CTA, CT angiography; DS, dual source; FDG, fluorodeoxyglucose; ICE, intracardiac echocardiography; MUGA, multigated acquisition scan; PCI, percutaneous coronary intervention; PET, positron emission tomography; TEE, transesophageal echocardiography.

- Use state-of-the-art equipment to lessen radiation.
- Take steps to achieve a low heart rate (<60 bpm) for large detector scanners such as 320-CT.[28]

❒ Patient selection:
- In addition to the issues already listed, general avoidance of scanning young patients who are more susceptible to the risk of radiation is prudent.
- Because cardiac CT scanning of females involves greater radiation, and because cancer risk models predict breast cancer as a risk, the general avoidance of scanning younger patients should be maximal in young females.

CT Scanning Developments That May Reduce Radiation

❒ Automated cardiac cycle phase identification

❒ Detector improvements:
- More efficient detectors
- Ultrafast detectors

❒ More efficient collimation, for 5% to 30% reduction[29]

❒ Dose based on body size:
- BMI 25–30: 120 kV
- BMI < 25: 100 kV

❒ Dose modulation ("tube pulsing"), 30% to 50% reduction (depends on heart rate):
- More efficient/responsive dose modulation, 10% reduction

- Lower dosing (<5%) outside of tube pulsing, 10% to 15% reduction
- "Step and shoot" prospective gating, 79% reduction[22]

❒ "Adaptive" dosing to the registered signal, 20 to 70%[30-32]

TABLE 3-4 Radiation Dose and Risk

PROCEDURE	RADIATION DOSE
Typical background radiation	
North America	3 mSv/year
Australia	1.5 mSv/year
Exposure by airline crew flying New York to Tokyo polar route	9 mSv/year
Current limit (averaged) for nuclear industry employees	20 mSv/year
Former routine limit for nuclear industry employees. It is also the dose rate that arises from natural background levels in several places in Iran, India, and Europe.	50 mSv/year
Lowest level at which any increase in cancer is clearly evident	100 mSv/year
Criterion for relocating people after Chernobyl accident	350 mSv/lifetime
The level recorded at the Japanese nuclear site, March 15, 2011	400 mSv/hour
Causes temporary radiation sickness such as nausea, decreased WBC count, but not single-dose death. Above this, severity of illness increases with dose.	1000 mSv (single dose)
Would kill about half of those receiving it within a month.	5000 mSv (single dose)

From BBC News–Health, http://www.bbc.co.uk/news/health-12722435, based on data from World Nuclear Association.
WBC, white blood cell.

❒ Dual source scanning

❒ Automated dose variation depending on the angle of the beam vis-à-vis the body

❒ Prospective gating, 79% reduction of radiation[22]

❒ Faster scanning

❒ Alternative reconstruction algorithm that reduces noise and allows for administration of less radiation to obtain a given level of signal to noise (30–50%).

❒ Minimization of the pre- and post-scan fields, 5% to 25% reduction of radiation

❒ Single cardiac cycle acquisition

A logarithmic (or greater) variation in radiation exposure can occur depending on which radiation economizing modalities are available or selected. Some modalities, although desirable for their radiation economy, increase the chance of image acquisition problems. The most successful modalities offer radiation economy without jeopardizing study quality.

AMERICAN HEART ASSOCIATION SCIENCE ADVISORY RECOMMENDATIONS[18*]

❒ Medical imaging is the largest controllable source of radiation exposure to the U.S. population, and its most important determinant is the ordering health care provider. Therefore:
- Physician education should emphasize that cardiac imaging studies that expose patients to ionizing radiation should be ordered only after thoughtful consideration of the potential benefit to the patient and in keeping with established appropriateness criteria (*Class I, Level of Evidence C*).

*Reprinted with permission from *Circulation.* 2009;119(7):1056-1065. © 2009, American Heart Association, Inc.

TABLE 3-5 Estimated Relative Risks of Attributable Cancer Incidence Associated with a Single Computed Tomography Coronary Angiography Scan*

		HEART SCANNED		HEART AND AORTA SCANNED	
AGE (YR)	SEX	STANDARD	TUBE CURRENT MODULATION	STANDARD	TUBE CURRENT MODULATION
80	Male	1.0	0.7	1.4	0.9
60	Male	2.6	1.7	3.8	2.4
40	Male	3.2	2.1	4.7	3.0
20	Male	4.8	3.1	6.9	4.5
80	Female	2.4	1.6	3.1	2.0
60	Female	7.0	4.6	8.9	5.8
40	Female	11.5	7.5	14.2	9.3
20	Female	22.9	14.9	28.6	18.6

*Comparison to an 80-year-old man receiving a standard cardiac scan. Standard indicates tube current modulation not used.
Reprinted with permission from Einstein AJ, Henzlova MJ, Rajagopalan S. Estimating risk of cancer associated with radiation exposure from 64-slice computed tomography coronary angiography. *JAMA.* 2007;298(3):317–323.

- The risks that an important diagnosis may be missed if appropriate diagnostic imaging studies are not performed because of radiation dose concerns should be considered (*Class IIa, Level of Evidence C*).
- Health care providers should diligently review patient records, including those from other medical institutions, to ensure that imaging studies that use ionizing radiation are not repeated needlessly (*Class I, Level of Evidence C*).
- Health care providers should discuss the risks and benefits of planned imaging procedures with patients whenever practical and appropriate (*Class I, Level of Evidence C*).

❒ Routine surveillance radionuclide stress tests or cardiac CTs in asymptomatic patients at low risk for ischemic heart disease are not recommended (*Class III, Level of Evidence B*).

❒ Once it has been established that a cardiac imaging study that uses ionizing radiation is needed, every effort should be made to reduce patient dose while balancing image noise and quality sufficient for confident interpretation (*Class I, Level of Evidence C*). The procedural details for minimizing radiation dose in various imaging modalities are beyond the scope of this chapter but have been detailed elsewhere.

❒ Longitudinal tracking of individual cumulative lifetime dose for patients currently is not practical. The modeling required to individualize dose is very complex and difficult to achieve, and the necessary tools and information systems to accomplish this for different imaging modalities are currently not available. The usefulness and societal value of such an undertaking are uncertain (*Class III, Level of Evidence B*).

- Imaging experts and manufacturers should continue working on developing consistent radiation output metrics for each diagnostic modality and on making such information automatically part of the imaging record (*Class I, Level of Evidence C*). This will facilitate efficient and reliable analysis of dose reference levels and trends.
- The imaging community should actively participate in the voluntary determination of diagnostic reference levels for radiation doses from cardiac radiographic imaging procedures to establish radiation doses as benchmarks for comparisons between practices on a national level (*Class I, Level of Evidence B*).

References

1. *CT Market Summary Report.* Des Plaines, Illinois 2006.
2. Schauer DA, Linton OW. NCRP Report No. 160, Ionizing radiation exposure of the population of the United States, medical exposure—are we doing less with more, and is there a role for health physicists? *Health Phys.* 2009;97(1):1-5.
3. Fazel R, Krumholz HM, Wang Y, et al. Exposure to low-dose ionizing radiation from medical imaging procedures. *N Engl J Med.* 2009;361(9):849-857.
4. Brenner DJ, Hall EJ. Computed tomography—an increasing source of radiation exposure. *New Engl J Med.* 2007;357(22): 2277-2284.
5. Berrington de Gonzalez A, Darby S. Risk of cancer from diagnostic X-rays: estimates for the UK and 14 other countries. *Lancet.* 2004;363(9406):345-351.
6. Tubiana M. Computed tomography and radiation exposure. *N Engl J Med.* 2008;358(8):850, author reply 852-853.
7. Cardis E, Vrijheid M, Blettner M, et al. The 15-Country Collaborative Study of Cancer Risk among Radiation Workers in the Nuclear Industry: estimates of radiation-related cancer risks. *Radiat Res.* 2007;167(4):396-416.
8. Pierce DA, Preston DL. Radiation-related cancer risks at low doses among atomic bomb survivors. *Radiat Res.* 2000;154(2): 178-186.
9. Preston DL, Ron E, Tokuoka S, et al. Solid cancer incidence in atomic bomb survivors: 1958-1998. *Radiat Res.* 2007;168(1):1-64.
10. Einstein AJ, Henzlova MJ, Rajagopalan S. Estimating risk of cancer associated with radiation exposure from 64-slice computed tomography coronary angiography. *JAMA.* 2007;298(3):317-323.
11. Health effects of low-level radiation. *Position Statement 41.* American Nuclear Society, June 2001.
12. Weinreb JC, Larson PA, Woodard PK, et al. American College of Radiology clinical statement on noninvasive cardiac imaging. *Radiology.* 2005;235(3):723-727.
13. Hausleiter J, Meyer T, Hadamitzky M, et al. Radiation dose estimates from cardiac multislice computed tomography in daily practice: impact of different scanning protocols on effective dose estimates. *Circulation.* 2006;113(10):1305-1310.
14. Abbara S, Arbab-Zadeh A, Callister TQ, et al. SCCT guidelines for performance of coronary computed tomographic angiography: a report of the Society of Cardiovascular Computed Tomography Guidelines Committee. *J Cardiovasc Comput Tomogr.* 2009; 3(3):190-204.
15. Fazel R, Krumholz HM, Wang Y, et al. Exposure to low-dose ionizing radiation from medical imaging procedures. *N Engl J Med.* 2009;361(9):849-857.
16. Einstein AJ, Sanz J, Dellegrottaglie S, Nilite M, Henzlova MJ, Rajagopalan S. Radiation dose and predictable cancer risk in multidetector-row computed tomography coronary angiography (CTCA). *J Am Coll Cardiol.* 2006;47(Suppl A):114A.
17. Kim RJ. Diagnostic testing. *J Am Coll Cardiol.* 2006;47(Suppl 11): D23-D27.
18. Gerber TC, Carr JJ, Arai AE, et al. Ionizing radiation in cardiac imaging: a science advisory from the American Heart Association Committee on Cardiac Imaging of the Council on Clinical Cardiology and Committee on Cardiovascular Imaging and Intervention of the Council on Cardiovascular Radiology and Intervention. *Circulation.* 2009;119(7):1056-1065.
19. Laskey WK, Wondrow M, Holmes Jr DR. Variability in fluoroscopic X-ray exposure in contemporary cardiac catheterization laboratories. *J Am Coll Cardiol.* 2006;48(7):1361-1364.
20. Coles DR, Smail MA, Negus IS, et al. Comparison of radiation doses from multislice computed tomography coronary angiography and conventional diagnostic angiography. *J Am Coll Cardiol.* 2006;47(9):1840-1845.
21. Silverman SG, Tuncali K, Adams DF, Nawfel RD, Zou KH, Judy PF. CT fluoroscopy-guided abdominal interventions: techniques, results, and radiation exposure. *Radiology.* 1999;212(3): 673-681.
22. Maruyama T, Takada M, Hasuike T, Yoshikawa A, Namimatsu E, Yoshizumi T. Radiation dose reduction and coronary assessability of prospective electrocardiogram-gated computed tomography coronary angiography: comparison with retrospective electrocardiogram-gated helical scan. *J Am Coll Cardiol.* 2008;52(18): 1450-1455.
23. Stolzmann P, Scheffel H, Schertler T, et al. Radiation dose estimates in dual-source computed tomography coronary angiography. *Eur Radiol.* 2008;18(3):592-599.
24. Scheffel H, Alkadhi H, Leschka S, et al. Low-dose CT coronary angiography in the step-and-shoot mode: diagnostic performance. *Heart.* 2008;94(9):1132-1137.
25. Gutstein A, Dey D, Cheng V, et al. Algorithm for radiation dose reduction with helical dual source coronary computed tomography angiography in clinical practice. *J Cardiovasc Comput Tomogr.* 2008;2(5):311-322.
26. Stolzmann P, Leschka S, Scheffel H, et al. Dual-source CT in step-and-shoot mode: noninvasive coronary angiography with low radiation dose. *Radiology.* 2008;249(1):71-80.
27. Heilbron BG, Leipsic J, Submillisievert coronary computed tomography angiography using adaptive statistical iterative reconstruction—a new reality. *Can J Cardiol.* 2010;26(1):35-36.

28. Hoe J, Toh KH. First experience with 320-row multidetector CT coronary angiography scanning with prospective electrocardiogram gating to reduce radiation dose. *J Cardiovasc Comput Tomogr.* 2009;3(4):257-261.
29. McCollough CH, Primak AN, Saba O, et al. Dose performance of a 64-channel dual-source CT scanner. *Radiology.* 2007;243:775-784.
30. Greess H, Wolf H, Suess C, Kalender WA, Bautz W, Baum U. [Automatic exposure control to reduce the dose in subsecond multislice spiral CT: phantom measurements and clinical results]. *Rofo.* 2004;176(6):862-869.
31. Mulkens TH, Bellinck P, Baeyaert M, et al. Use of an automatic exposure control mechanism for dose optimization in multidetector row CT examinations: clinical evaluation. *Radiology.* 2005;237(1):213-223.
32. Maher MM, Kalra MK, Toth TL, Wittram C, Saini S, Shepard J. Application of rational practice and technical advances for optimizing radiation dose for chest CT. *J Thorac Imaging.* 2004;19(1): 16-23.

4 Contrast Enhancement

Key Points

- Contrast enhancement is crucial to optimal CT angiography and to most applications of cardiovascular CT.
- Synchronizing contrast delivery to image acquisition for CT angiography requires that the contrast be present within the left heart and aorta but diminished or diluted within the right heart cavities by a part-saline/part-contrast bolus.
- For dissection protocols and pulmonary embolism protocols, no saline "chaser" is needed.
- Few good alternatives to iodinated contrast are currently available.
- Pre-contrast images are useful to:
  - Identify vascular calcification
  - Identify acute intramural hematoma
- Delayed (30- to 120-second) images are useful to characterize:
  - The filling of the left atrial appendage
  - The false lumen of a chronic aortic dissection
- Contrast enhancement is essential for all forms of cardiovascular CT other than:
  - Calcium scoring
  - Identification of:
    - Pericardial or other calcification
    - Intramural hematomas of the aorta
    - Intramyocardial fat
  - Cardiac tumor assessment

OPTIMAL ENHANCEMENT

Vascular and cardiac blood pool contrast enhancement is determined by the interaction of iodine administration and blood flow. The goals of contrast administration are:

- ❐ Adequate opacification of cavities and vessel lumen
- ❐ Avoidance of both under- and over-opacification. It is important to recognize that excessive contrast concentration generates high attenuation artifact.
  - Starburst high-attenuation artifacts from the superior vena cava (SVC) are among the most common of all annoying and frustrating artifacts.
  - CT angiography (CTA) requires high left heart/aortic contrast and low right heart contrast (high right heart opacification confounds assessment of the right coronary artery and the right ventricular contours).
- ❐ Optimal enhancement depends on the purposes of the study.
  - The optimum contrast effect for vascular enhancement is 300 to 500 HU.
  - The optimal contrast effect for coronary plaque characterization is less: 250 to 350 HU.
- ❐ Optimal opacification requires a near-steady level of contrast throughout the entire duration of the study.
- ❐ Synchronization of opacification to image acquisition phase is crucial. For CTA, the principal challenge is to synchronize these three variables:
  - The arrival of the contrast medium in the left heart
  - Washout from the right heart with the saline push
  - Acquisition phase

ACQUISITION TIME AND CONTRAST NEED

As scanners are developed that can use larger numbers of slices and provide greater breadth of scanning, acquisition time is falling, as is the needed duration of contrast effect, and, therefore, the volume of contrast needed. In comparison to 10-slice scanners, 64-slice scanners need only half the volume of contrast. In comparison to 16-slice scanners, 64-slice scanners need one third less contrast.

Factors That Increase the Amount of Contrast Needed

- ❐ Larger field of view: e.g., post-aortocoronary bypass studies where the field of view along the Z-axis is from the subclavian arteries to the base of the heart (to visualize internal thoracic arteries as well as the heart)
- ❐ Slower (fewer detectors) scanners
- ❐ Lesser pitch

Factors That Reduce the Amount of Contrast Needed

- ❒ Faster (more detectors) scanners
- ❒ Smaller scan length
- ❒ Greater pitch

Issues of Practicality

- ❒ A robust protocol is wiser than an ambitious protocol.
- ❒ A dual-head injector is preferable (for contrast and for saline).
- ❒ The greater the kV, the greater the penetration and the lesser the contrast effect.

Injection

- ❒ Site
  - **Right antecubital vein.** Use of the left antecubital vein is likely to result in high-attenuation artifact in the left subclavian vein, which may "bloom" or generate streak artifacts that cross the left subclavian artery/internal thoracic/mammary artery ostium and obscure it.
  - Hand veins should be avoided.
  - Central lines, unless labeled for IV injection, should be avoided.
- ❒ Size
  - A short 20-gauge IV catheter may be used for smaller patients.
  - An 18-gauge IV catheter is more appropriate for larger patients.

Dilute Contrast "Chaser"

It is becoming increasingly common to follow the contrast bolus with a "chaser" of dilute contrast (20–30% contrast with 70–80% saline) of the same volume as the injected saline so that there is diminished right heart cavitary attenuation but a smoother rendering of the blood-pool attenuation.

Saline "Chaser"

Otherwise, the same volume (as the contrast volume) of saline typically is injected to avoid excess concentration of contrast within the right heart chambers so that the right coronary artery imaging is devoid of high-attenuation artifacts arising from the right heart chambers.

Occasionally, small bubbles of air from the IV tubing can be seen within the right heart. These are generally inconsequential; however, if there is a history of congenital heart disease or suspicion of Eisenmenger syndrome physiology, an IV air bubble filter should be used. Because this may decrease the overall rate of contrast injection (approximately 3 mL/sec), administration of a larger volume of contrast or dual injection into both arms should be considered (Figs. 4-1 and 4-2).

Scan Delay Modes

Two methods of scan delay are available: the test bolus method and bolus tracking.

Test Bolus Method

A standard test bolus is 10 to 20 mL of contrast medium with a 50-mL chaser of saline. Many prefer this method because it reliably times contrast transit from the site of injection, wherever and whatever that may be, to the left-sided circulation.

Automatic Bolus Tracking/Monitoring Method

The automatic bolus method is one of several automated scan-assist modalities to facilitate and standardize scanning. A region-of-interest (ROI) cursor is placed on any chamber or vessel as seen on a scout view. When the ROI senses a predetermined attenuation number (usually 110 HU), the acquisition initiates automatically. For coronary CTA, the ROI typically is placed over either the ascending or descending aorta. ROI placement over the ascending aorta entails some risk that the acquisition will be prematurely initiated by high-attenuation artifacts emanating from the adjacent SVC well before the contrast has entered the left circulation. A pacemaker or implantable cardioverter defibrillator (ICD) lead in the SVC may have the same inadvertent effect. The automatic bolus method obviates the need for 20 mL of contrast for a test dose. (Tables 4-1 through 4-3).

Potential Contrast-Related Problems

- ❒ Excess contrast concentration
- ❒ Inadequate contrast concentration
- ❒ Scan acquired ahead of the contrast medium
- ❒ Scan acquired behind the contrast medium
- ❒ Streak artifacts from contrast material in the SVC or right heart
- ❒ Excessive contrast within the right heart
- ❒ Nephrotoxicity
- ❒ Allergy
- ❒ Interstitial injection/"blown" peripheral IV
- ❒ Cost
- ❒ Need for IV access

Pre-Contrast Imaging

- ❒ For calcification
- ❒ For detection of intramural hematoma of the aorta
- ❒ For assessment of cardiac masses and tumors

Post-Contrast Imaging

- ❒ Delayed/late scan of aortic dissection, to better contrast opacify the false lumen (120–150 seconds delay)
- ❒ "Delayed enhancement" of myocardium (5- to 10-minute delay)

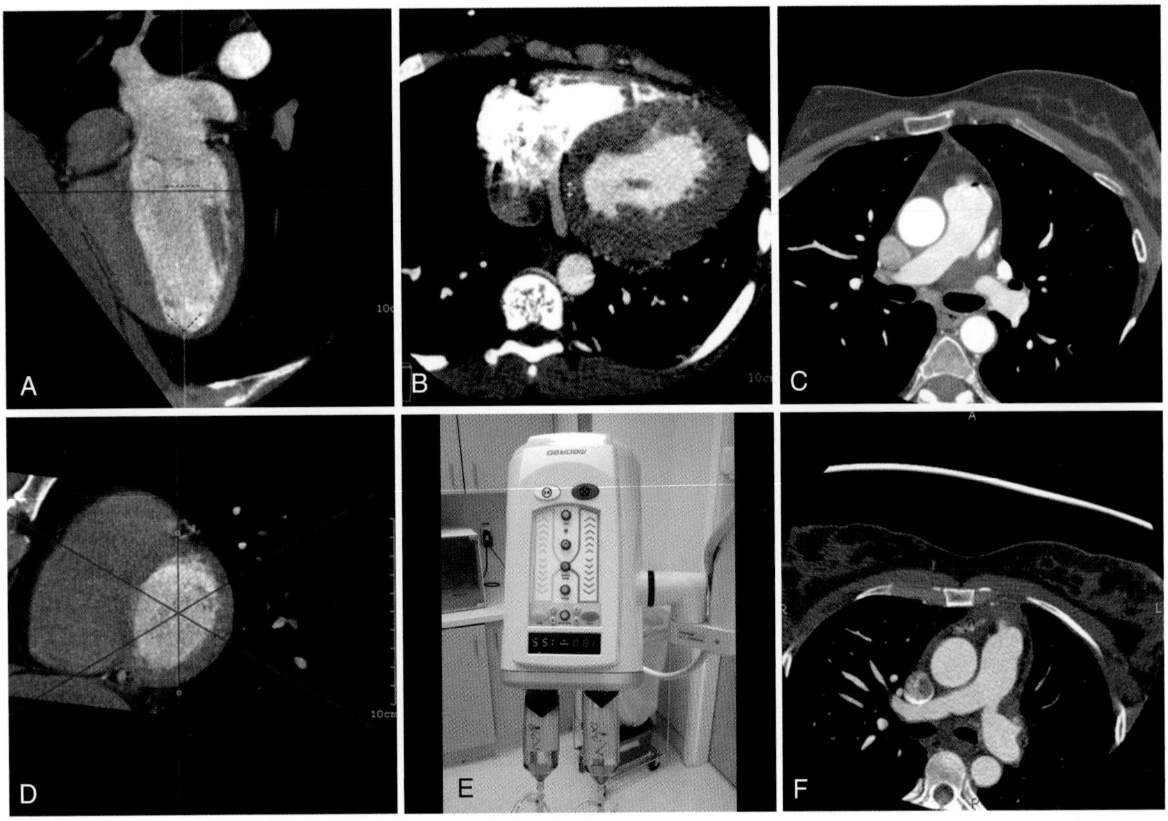

Figure 4-1. For the purposes of coronary CT angiography (CTA), there is optimal contrast enhancement of the left heart chambers and aorta (from the contrast injection) and optimal "washout" of contrast on the right heart chambers (from subsequent saline chaser injection), as seen on these two cardiac views. **A–C,** Dual-headed injector capable of serially injecting a selected volume and rate of iodinated contrast injection and, subsequently, a volume and rate of saline "chaser" injection, with control console. **D–F,** Two axial images from a cardiac CTA demonstrating a small bubble of gas within the right ventricle. Tiny bubbles of air are seen within the right atrial appendage. An air bubble is seen floating against the anterior wall of the main pulmonary artery, due to injection of a small volume of air with the contrast injection. For the purposes of coronary CTA, there is suboptimal/poor contrast enhancement timing. The high contrast concentration in the right heart will render analysis of the right coronary artery difficult.

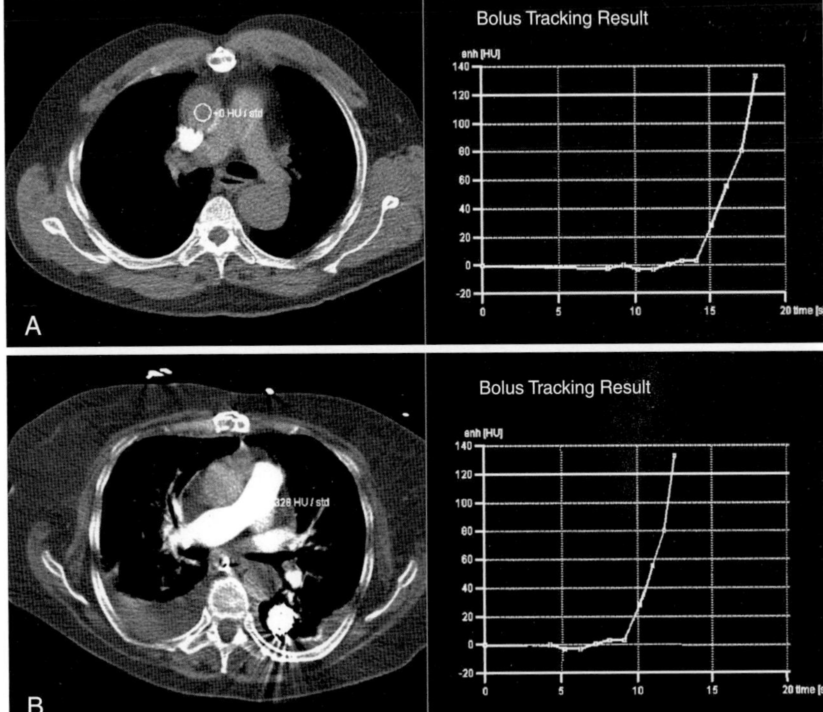

Figure 4-2. Automated bolus tracking scan assist methods for coronary and aortic imaging (**A**) and for pulmonary artery imaging (**B**). The region of interest (ROI) usually is placed over the ascending aorta for coronary CT angiography, although, as can be seen, streak artifact from dye within the superior vena cava is in close proximity. The attenuation/enhancement versus time curve reveals 18 seconds before the 130 HU threshold is achieved. The ROI is placed over the main pulmonary artery for pulmonary embolism protocol, and the threshold is achieved sooner.

TABLE 4-1 Test Bolus versus Bolus-Tracking Methods

Test Bolus Methods

SOURCE	CONTRAST MEDIA	TEST BOLUS (CONTRAST/SALINE)	DIAGNOSTIC INJECTION (CONTRAST/SALINE)	INJECTION RATE	TRIGGER REGION OF INTEREST	ADDITIONAL DELAY
Ferencik et al.[1]	Iopamidol, 300 mg/mL	15/40 mL	60–70/40 mL	5 mL/sec	Proximal ascending aorta	Unreported
Achenbach et al.[2]	Iomeprol, 400 mg/mL	10/50 mL	80/50 mL	Unreported	Proximal ascending aorta above coronary ostia	2 sec
Raff et al.[3]	Iohexol, 350 mg/mL	10/40 mL	100/40 mL	5 mL/sec	Unstated	Unreported

Bolus-Tracking Methods

SOURCE	CONTRAST MEDIA	DIAGNOSTIC INJECTION (CONTRAST/SALINE)	INJECTION RATE	TRIGGER ROI	THRESHOLD	DELAY POST-THRESHOLD
Leber et al.[4]	Iopamidol, 300 mg/mL	80 mL/no saline	5 mL/sec	Ascending aorta	100 HU	Unreported
Husmann et al.[5]	Idixanol, 320 mg/mL	80/30 mL	5 mL/sec	Ascending aorta	140 HU	5 sec
Pugliese et al.[6]	Iomeprol, 400 mg/mL	100 mL/no saline	5 mL/sec	Unreported	Unreported	Unreported
Penn	Iohexol, 350 mg/mL	Triphasic injection (80 mL contrast at 4.5 mL/sec) followed by 40% contrast: 60% saline (40 mL at 4 mL/sec), followed by 100% saline (40 mL at 4 mL/sec)	Triphasic injecton	Descending thoracic aorta	120 HU	8 sec

Penn, unpublished data from The Hospital of the University of Pennsylvania.
ROI, region of interest.
From Boonn WW, Litt HL, Charagundla SR. Optimizing contrast injection for coronary CT angiography and functional cardiac CT. *Suppl Appl Radiol.* 2007:51-57.

IS THERE AN ALTERNATIVE TO IODINATED CONTRAST?

For the purposes of cardiovascular CT (CVCT), there are no standard alternatives to iodinated contrast medium. Gadolinium, the contrast agent used in MRI and magnetic resonance angiography scanning, has sometimes been proposed. Gadolinium is only one fifth as concentrated as iodine, but is twice as "bright" per concentration. Therefore, because it is a weaker contrast agent, the amount needed for CT purposes is large (often 2 ampules). Because a quantity of more than 60 mL is nephrotoxic, as with iodinated contrast, and because the images are not as uniformly of good quality as they are with iodine, gadolinium has not gained favor in CVCT as an alternative to iodinated contrast. In addition, gadolinium is extremely expensive, and nephrogenic sclerosis is a concern in renal insufficiency.

In limited series, gadolinium has been used as an alternative to iodine for CVCT,[8] achieving lesser density in coronary arteries than iodinated contrast (135 HU versus 253 HU).[9] Newer-generation scanners may have more success with gadolinium enhancement than has been yet achieved.

TABLE 4-2 ROI Location for Different Study Indications

CT SCAN PURPOSE	AUTOMATED BOLUS TRACKING/ROI SITE
Coronary angiography	Ascending aorta ± 5-second delay
Left heart structures	Ascending aorta ± 5-second delay
Left-to-right intracardiac shunting	Left atrium
Right-to-left intracardiac shunting	Right atrium
Pulmonary angiography	Main pulmonary artery
Right heart structures	Right ventricle or main pulmonary artery
Thoracic aorta	Ascending aorta ± 5-second delay
Abdominal aorta	Descending aorta

ROI, region of interest.

Calcium Scoring as a Gatekeeper to CTA

- ❒ Review any previous calcium score studies before the patient's appointment and decide whether or not to perform CTA.
- ❒ Administer β-blockade and sublingual nitroglycerin as per CTA protocol.
- ❒ Follow calcium score protocol.
- ❒ Calculation of calcium score
- ❒ Gatekeeping by calcium score
  - CTA is performed if the calcium score is less than 400.
  - CTA is not performed if the calcium score is greater than 1000.
  - If the calcium score is greater than 400 but less than 1000, CTA is performed at the discretion of the responsible physician, taking into account the distribution of mural calcification along coronary arteries.

TABLE 4-3 Contrast-Related Artifacts and Their Causes

STUDY GOAL	PROBLEM	CAUSE
LV geometry	Inadequate right-sided delineation of the septum	Excessive dye washout of the right ventricular chambers, diminishing or eliminating attenuation difference of the septum and the RV blood pool (scan acquisition too late)
RV geometry	Inadequate right-sided delineation of the right heart chambers	Excessive dye washout of the right ventricular chambers
Coronary arteries	Streak artifact arising in the right heart obscuring the RCA	Excessive dye concentration in the right heart cavities (scan too early, insufficient saline chaser)
PE	Inadequate pulmonary artery contrast	Inadequate dye concentration in the pulmonary arteries: 1. Scan too early. Note that in PE with right ventricular failure, cardiac output is reduced, increasing the interval between injection and time to acquisition. 2. Scan too late. Injection through a central line leads to early right heart and pulmonary artery opacification, and washout.
Aorta	Streak artifact arising from the SVC	Excessive dye concentration in the SVC (insufficient saline chaser)
	Inadequate aortic contrast	Scan too early

LV, left ventricle; PE, pulmonary embolism; RCA, right coronary artery; RV, right ventricle; SVC, superior vena cava.

References

1. Ferencik M, Nomura CH, Maurovich-Horvat P, et al. Quantitative parameters of image quality in 64-slice computed tomography angiography of the coronary arteries. *Eur J Radiol.* 2006;57(3):373-379.
2. Achenbach S, Ropers D, Kuettner A, et al. Contrast-enhanced coronary artery visualization by dual-source computed tomography—initial experience. *Eur J Radiol.* 2006;57(3):331-335.
3. Raff GL, Gallagher MJ, O'Neill WW, Goldstein JA. Diagnostic accuracy of noninvasive coronary angiography using 64-slice spiral computed tomography. *J Am Coll Cardiol.* 2005;46(3):552-557.
4. Leber AW, Knez A, von Ziegler F, et al. Quantification of obstructive and nonobstructive coronary lesions by 64-slice computed tomography: a comparative study with quantitative coronary angiography and intravascular ultrasound. *J Am Coll Cardiol.* 2005; 46(1):147-154.
5. Husmann L, Alkadhi H, Boehm T, et al. Influence of cardiac hemodynamic parameters on coronary artery opacification with 64-slice computed tomography. *Eur Radiol.* 2006;16(5):1111-1116.
6. Pugliese F, Mollet NR, Runza G, et al. Diagnostic accuracy of non-invasive 64-slice CT coronary angiography in patients with stable angina pectoris. *Eur Radiol.* 2006;16(3):575-582.
7. Boonn WW, Litt HL, Charagundla SR. Optimizing contrast injection for coronary CT angiography and functional cardiac CT. *Suppl Appl Radiol.* 2007:51–57.
8. Coche EE, Hammer FD, Goffette PP. Demonstration of pulmonary embolism with gadolinium-enhanced spiral CT. *Eur Radiol.* 2001; 11(11):2306–2309.
9. Carrascosa P, Capunay C, Bettinotti M, et al. Feasibility of gadolinium-diethylene triamine pentaacetic acid enhanced multidetector computed tomography for the evaluation of coronary artery disease. *J Cardiovasc Comput Tomogr.* 2007;1(2):86–94.

5 Noise and Artifacts

Key Points

- Artifacts are so common as to be universal.
- Prevention is the best cure.
- Review the study for artifacts before reading it, so as not to be "tricked."
- Use retrospective gating reconstructions and different phase reconstructions liberally to obviate whatever artifacts may be present.

All forms of imaging are subject to artifacts, and proficiency with artifact recognition and suppression is critical for best practice of any form of imaging, including cardiovascular CT (CVCT).[1] In terms of diagnostic imaging, what sets the heart apart from all other organs is the rapidity of its motion. Motion of any sort remains one of the most common causes of artifacts for all modalities of cardiac imaging.

Temporal resolution is, therefore, a crucial aspect of cardiac imaging. The temporal resolution of current 64-slice cardiac CT (CCT) is 140 msec, which is sufficient to image most small cardiac structures at any given phase of the cardiac cycle[2]; therefore, imaging, especially CT coronary angiography, is intentionally gathered in the quiescent phase of diastole[3]-diastasis.

Other regularly encountered causes of artifacts or suboptimal CT scan quality include suboptimal settings, inadequate electrocardiographic (ECG) gating, and high-attenuation artifacts.

Optimal examinations with great clarity are feasible.

Prevention of artifacts should be the preferred approach, because there are limited means to edit away artifacts.

PREVENTION OF ARTIFACT

- To reduce patient motion:
  - Prepare the patient before the scan.
  - Eliminate any communication barriers so patient can follow instructions. The services of a translator may be necessary.
  - Prepare the patient to anticipate the warm sensation of contrast dye injection and not be alarmed by it (to attempt to avoid heart rate [HR] increase during the scan).
  - Have the patient practice breath-holding until successful.
  - Instruct the patient not to swallow during scanning.
- Use β-blockers to avoid HR acceleration during the scan.
- To avoid excessive R-R variation:
  - Exclude patients with frank arrhythmias.
  - Use β-blockers to suppress HR acceleration.
- Use optimal kilovolts and milliamps.
- To optimize sampling during diastasis:
  - Although use of retrospective gating increases radiation exposure, it provides more versatility and robustness in reconstructing images from different phases (e.g., 70%, 75%, and 80% phases of the cardiac cycle) to find one without motion-related artifacts.

Each study should be assessed for noise level and artifacts before image interpretation is initiated because this establishes a baseline sense of image adequacy and may justify the exclusion of ectopic cardiac cycles.

Many studies will have more than one form of artifact.

NOISE

With CT scanning, multiple mechanisms can affect image quality. One of these is image noise. Noise can be defined or measured as the standard deviation of Hounsfield unit voxel values within a homogeneous phantom, usually a water phantom. Usually, the lower the noise, the higher the signal-to-noise ratio (SNR), and the better the image quality is. A number of factors affect the amount of noise, including technical parameters, patient factors, and image reconstruction and post-processing. Technical parameters of kilovoltage potential (KvP), milliamps, and exposure time influence the amount of noise within the image. Patient size—for example, morbid obesity—can attenuate the number of x-ray photons reaching the detector and increase the

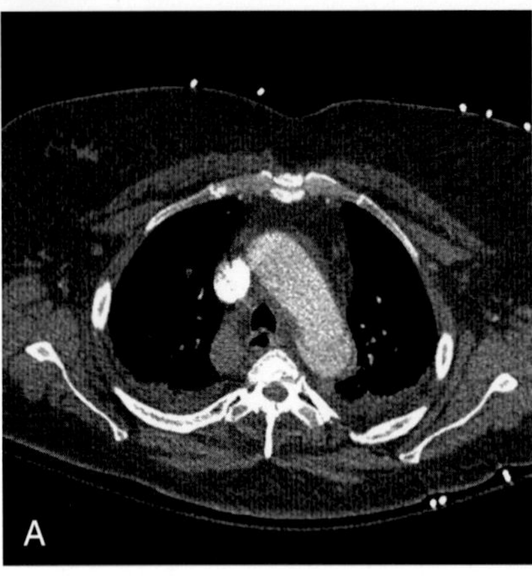

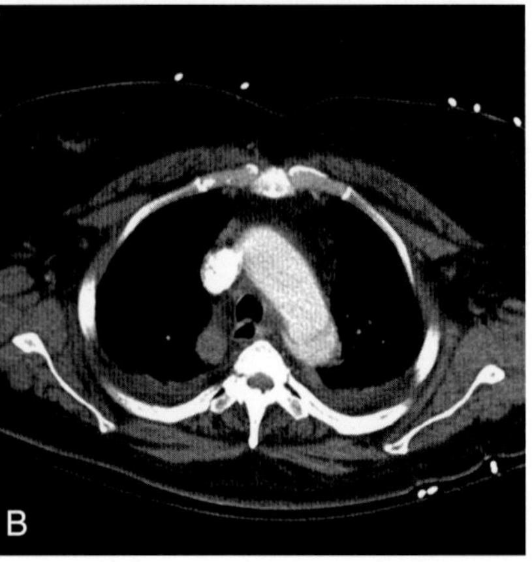

Figure 5-1. Contrast-enhanced axial CT scan views at the aortic arch level demonstrating the effective noise reduction with thicker slices. **A,** 0.75-mm thickness. **B,** 5-mm thickness.

amount of noise, therefore often requiring an increase to the standard parameters of kVp and mA. Noise also can be modulated after image acquisition by altering the reconstruction kernel, with sharper kernels generating noisier images, as well as by increasing the slice thickness, which generally increases the SNR of an image (Fig. 5-1).

Causes of Prominent Noise

- Large patient
- Increased kilovolts
- Thin slices
- Random fluctuations in x-ray numbers being detected, and electric noise in the system (noise is not affected by pitch)

Noise Banding

- Appearance: wormy look
- ECG triggering problem—ECG noise or sensing problem

TYPES OF ARTIFACTS

Slab or Band Artifacts (Figs. 5-2 and 5-3)

- **Appearance**: equal-sized slabs with different brightness (HU) due to different contrast concentration or with different SNR. Image acquisition for coronary CTA deliberately washes out the contrast from the right heart; this occurs during acquisition and is essentially a normal effect of the saline chaser.
- Slab artifacts may be seen in three-dimensional virtual reality (3DVR) images or sagittal images.
- **Causes**:
  - Commonly, a normal byproduct of prospective acquisition
  - Incorrect use of contrast
    - Excessive contrast present
    - Injection too early
  - Possible solution: Avoid excessive contrast effect
- Solution: Seldom affects image quality, virtually a normal finding as dye washes through the right heart

Stair-Step Artifacts (Fig. 5-4)

- **Appearance**: 10- to 12-mm high vertical steps (along the Z-plane; therefore best seen in sagittal and coronal images); anatomic structures of one plane are offset with respect to the next plane.
- Stair-step artifacts usually occur on the heart.
- Stair-step artifacts also may occur on adjacent structures.
- **Problem**: Review of axial images may lead to the impression of a pseudostenosis at the level of the step; therefore, the presence of a step must be recognized.
- **Cause**: motion of either the heart or the patient
  - **Cardiac motion.** Steps may be single (e.g., due to a single ventricular ectopic beat) or multiple. Causes of step artifacts as a result of nondiastolic phase acquisition include:
    - Irregular heart rhythm of any cause
    - Irregular heart rate
    - Inadequate ECG signal
    - Incorrect reconstruction parameters
  - **Non-cardiac motion** (e.g., respiration, swallowing, limb motion). Steps due to noncardiac motion generally are apparent across intrathoracic structures. Step artifacts due to patient motion also may be present in reformatted maximum intensity projection and multiplanar reconstruction images.
    - To establish that nonrespiratory motion is responsible for the step, one must confirm that:
      - A double dome of diaphragm is present.
      - Block artifacts are present over the diaphragm.
      - The stair-step is present over the sternum but not over the spine on sagittal view.
      - Motion blurring due to breathing can be identified by reviewing lung windows

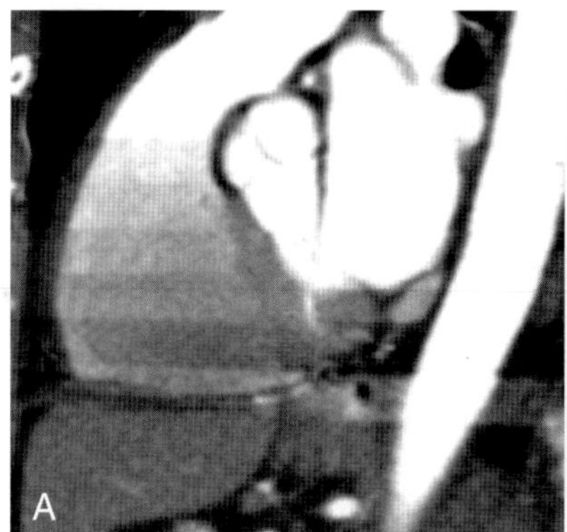

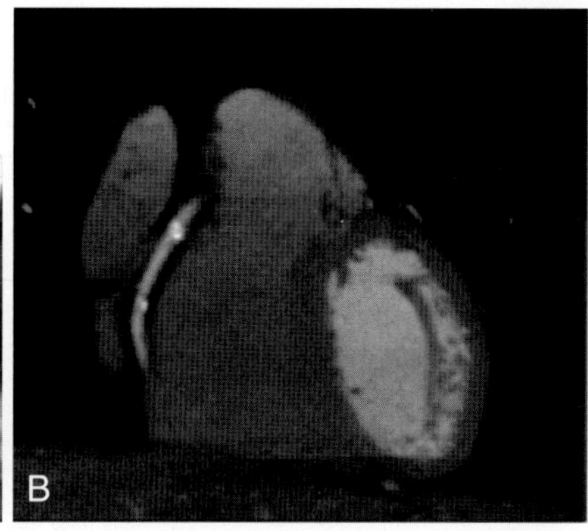

Figure 5-2. **A,** Banding artifacts from differential contrast effect in the right ventricle (RV) as the contrast enhancement encountered on progressive scans in the caudal direction lessens due to saline chaser infusion. **B,** Banding artifacts from differential contrast effect in the RV as the contrast enhancement encountered on progressive scans in the caudal direction lessens due to saline chaser infusion.

that demonstrate blurriness of the lung parenchyma.

- Possible solutions:
  - There is little to do for the affected study.
  - If steps are limited to the heart and the heart rate had accelerated excessively, β-blockers would help.
  - A retrospectively acquired study may allow a piecemeal approach to coronary artery reconstruction, with different segments of a vessel being reconstructed at different phases, ultimately allowing for incremental but near-complete evaluation of a coronary artery.

Streak /Beam-hardening Artifacts (Figs. 5-5 through 5-8)

- **Appearance**: thin straight bands and (white and dark) radiating lines, often with a starburst appearance, due to excessive attenuation differences in the image. Scrolling down the axial images, they appear to "windmill."
- The encountering of dense material by the incident x-ray beams may increase the mean energy of the beam and the selective attenuation of the lower-energy x-rays, resulting in the heterogeneous artifact of bright and dark lines.
- Streak artifacts usually are caused by metallic objects, calcified objects, or excess contrast concentration.
- **Causes:**
  - Reflection of radiation off of:
    - Metallic objects (e.g., pacers, wires, clips, prosthetic valves, leads, coils, stents, and electrodes)
    - Calcified objects
    - Excessive contrast concentration
    - Clothes
    - Contrast material
  - Slice reconstruction too thin (<0.75 mm)
- Possible solutions:
  - Streaking artifacts caused by metallic implants: no real solutions available, but such artifacts do not usually preclude diagnosis

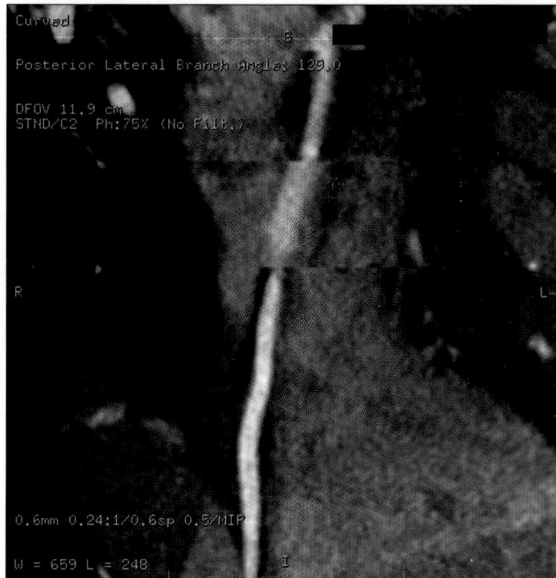

Figure 5-3. Banding artifact is a type of motion artifact, but it usually occurs as a result of an increase in heart rate during the scan. In this case, the proximal portion of the right coronary artery is blurred and not assessable.

  - Streaking from excessive contrast effect in the right heart: use a saline chaser with optimal timing
  - Thicker slice
  - Possible improvement with different phase reconstruction
  - Axial (prospective imaging) may decrease blurring of beam-hardening artifacts.
- Streak artifacts may obscure an area of interest, or may corrupt it. If, for example, a dark streak artifact from an atrial pacer lead in the right atrium darkens the right coronary artery, it may result in the appearance of a stenosis.

Blurring Artifacts (Fig. 5-9)

- **Appearance**: nonsharp appearance, blurring, or suffusing of areas of image detail
- Blur artifacts may be local or generalized throughout the image.
- Blur artifact may result in slab artifacts in 3DVR, sagittal, and coronal images.

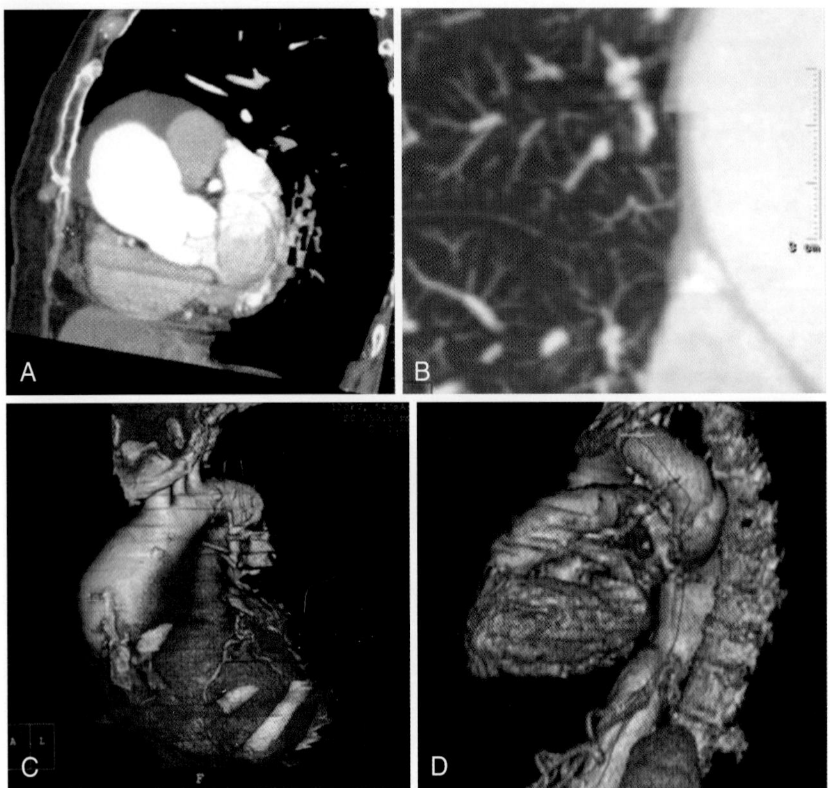

Figure 5-4. **A,** Stair-step artifact resulting from respiration. There is an abrupt step seen over the sternum due to respiration, which typically moves the sternum more than the spine. **B,** Stair-step artifact from respiration. There is an abrupt step seen over the ascending aorta due to respiratory motion. **C,** Severe stair-step artifact from respiration on a 3D volume-rendered view. **D,** Stair-step artifact on a 3D volume-rendered view.

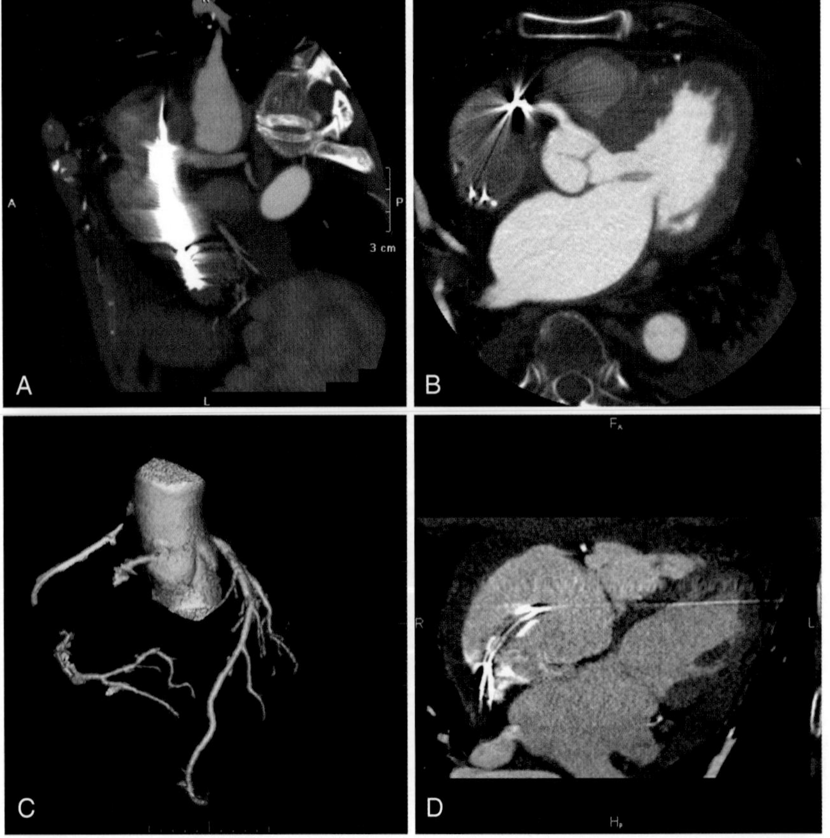

Figure 5-5. **A,** Long-axis maximum intensity projection (MIP) image through the right ventricle demonstrates marked beam-hardening artifact from a reformatted implantable cardioverter defibrillator. This artifact is augmented due to the MIP projection. **B,** Axial image from a cardiac CT study demonstrates extensive beam-hardening artifact from a pacemaker within the right atrial appendage. **C,** Volume-rendered image demonstrates pacer artifact projecting above the right coronary artery (RCA), and causing an extensive artifact obscuring evaluation of the proximal RCA. **D,** A single axial image from a cardiac CT angiogram demonstrates a combination artifact on beam-hardening and motion secondary to movement of pacemaker device within the right atrium. There is also an associated streak artifact seen coursing through the image from right to left.

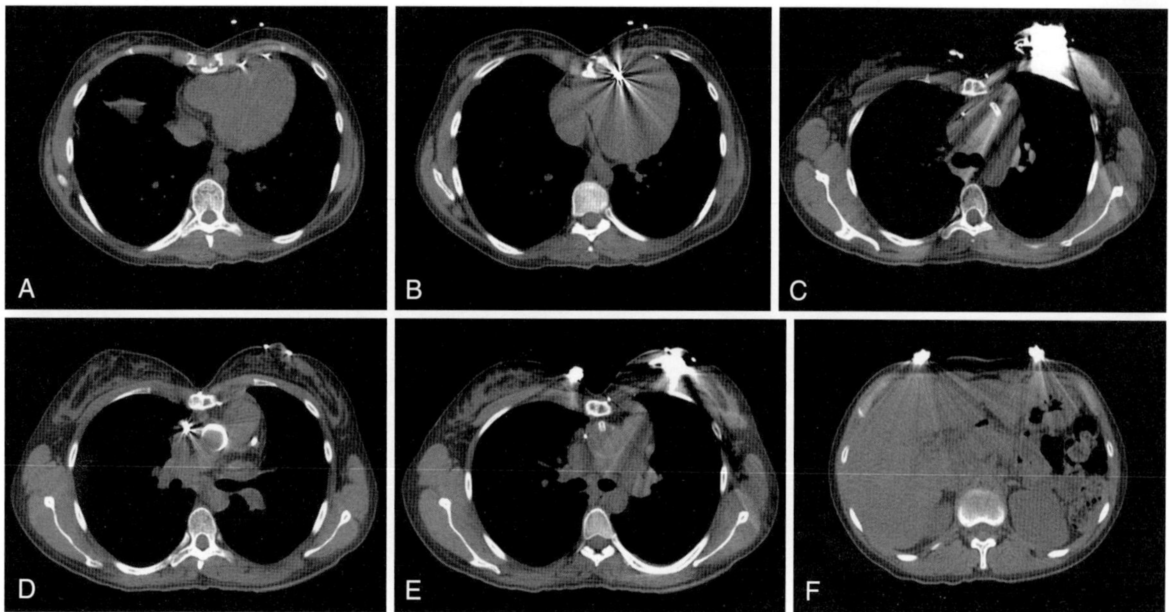

Figure 5-6. **A,** Streak artifacts over the anterior surface of the heart are present, caused by an epicardial pacemaker wire. There has been a prior sternotomy (actually three). **B,** Prominent streaks are caused by the epicardial corkscrew pacemaker lead. **C,** Extensive streak artifact is present, caused by the (left infraclavicular) pacemaker pack. **D,** Streak artifact from a right coronary stent is present. The same size and type of stent is present in a vein graft to the left coronary artery, but is not causing the same degree of artifact. **E,** Streak artifact from the pacemaker pack is present. A stent into the ostium of a left coronary graft is nearly perfectly seen along its long axis, and is without any artifact. **F,** Streak artifact from two surface ECG electrodes is present.

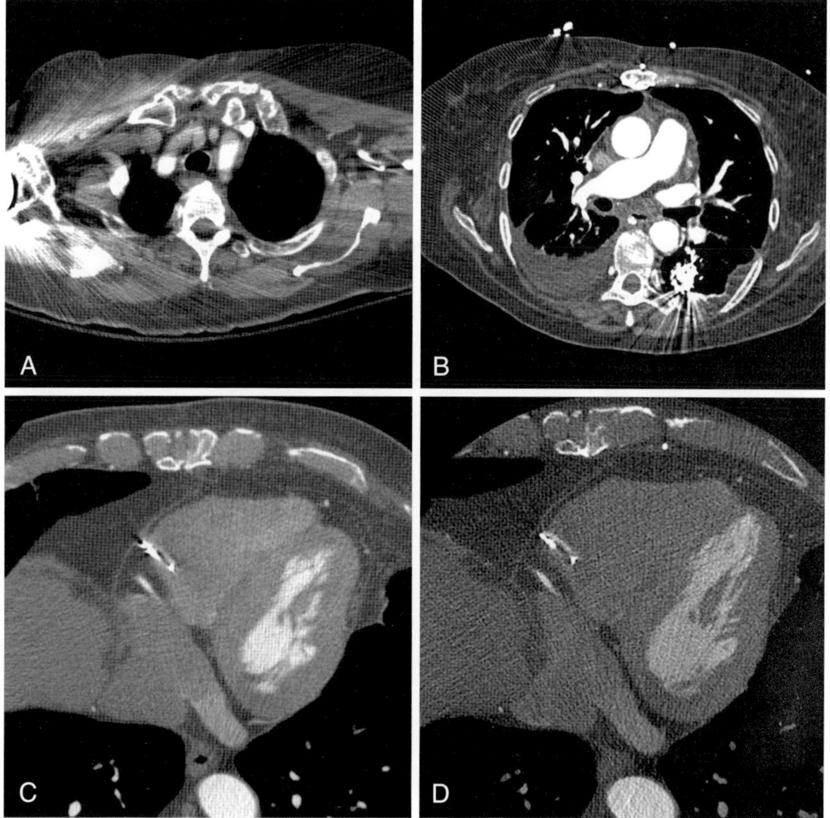

Figure 5-7. **A,** Beam-hardening streak artifacts from a shoulder prosthesis cross and contaminate the visualization of the arch branch vessels and the aorta. **B,** Severe beam-hardening streak artifacts from a large collection of wire coils in the left posterior chest. **C** and **D,** Two cardiac CT images obtained in the same patient 1 year apart. Studies were done for evaluation of bypass graft patency. **C,** Image obtained in the standard fashion. **D,** Image obtained using a high-definition CT scanner, with improved in-plane spatial resolution. Multiple surgical clips are seen adjacent to an RCA bypass graft. On the standard acquisition on the left, the underlying bypass graft is difficult to visualize due to extensive beam-hardening artifact. The high-definition acquisition has significantly less beam-hardening artifact associated with it, allowing for better visualization of the underlying vessel.

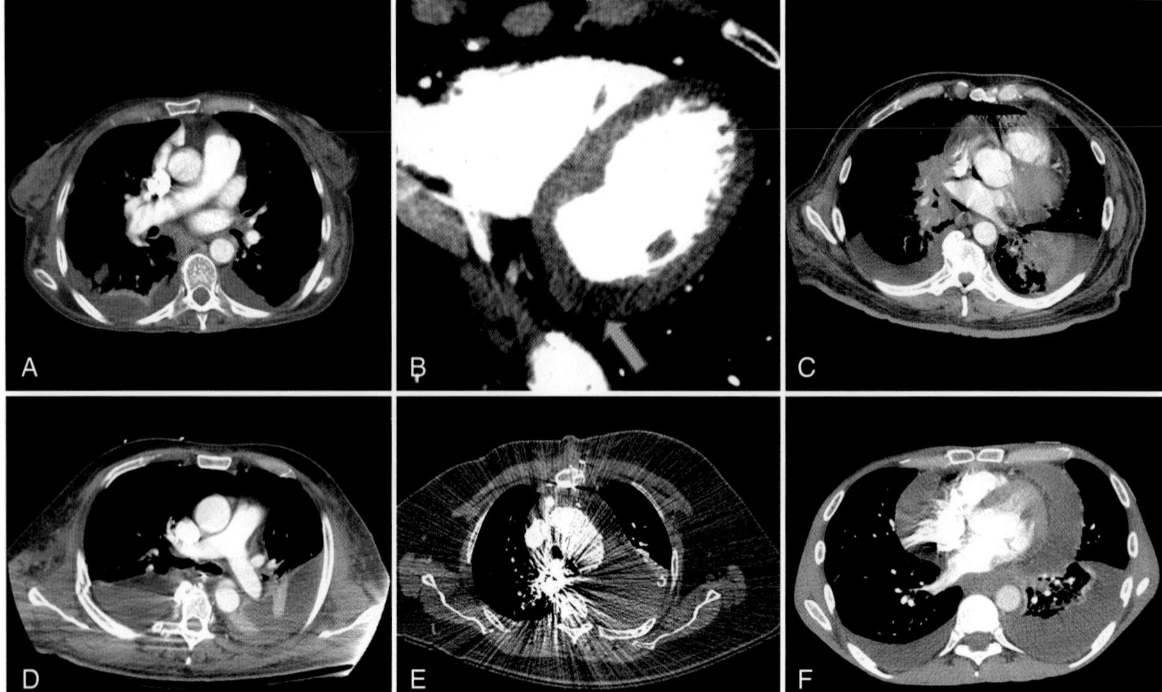

Figure 5-8. **A,** Streaking or beam-hardening artifact, usually caused by excess attenuation from dye in the superior vena cava (SVC), is seen radiating from the SVC. **B,** Beam-hardening artifact of the myocardium arising from the descending aorta. **C,** Beam-hardening artifacts emanating from the anterior surface of a pneumopericardial-pericardial effusion. **D,** Beam-hardening streak artifacts off the spine, that cross numerous structures, including the aorta, and complicate its assessment. It can still be seen, though, that there is a false aneurysm off the anterior wall of the aorta, due to traumatic disruption. **E,** Severe beam-hardening streak artifacts crossing the chest and obfuscating the assessment of the aorta. The artifact is due to a large collection of wire coils. The large aortic stent, by way of comparison, is not responsible for artifact. **F,** Streak artifact arising from the right heart due to excess dye concentration within the right heart. The right ventricular and right atrial free walls are extensively obscured by the artifact. A large pericardial effusion and bilateral pleural effusions are present.

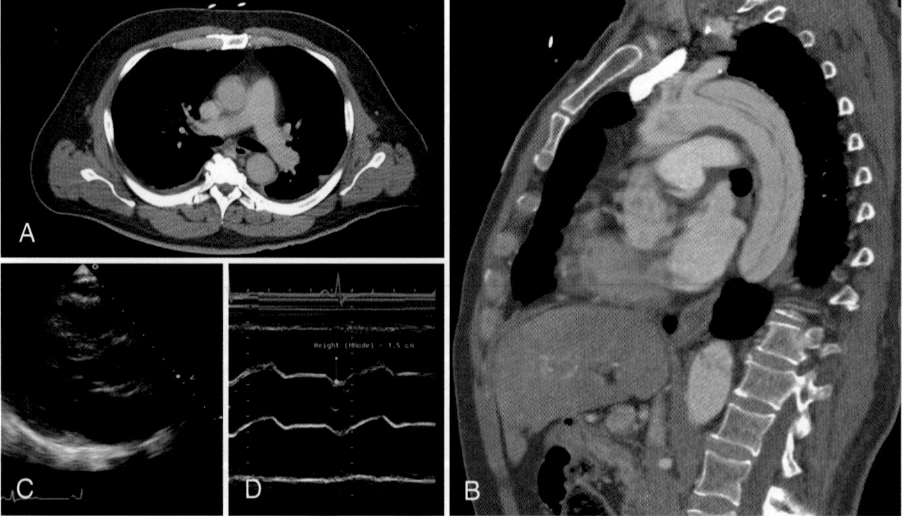

Figure 5-9. **A,** Contrast-enhanced sagittal plane view of the aortic arch and descending thoracic aorta revealing a type B aortic dissection. Over several centimeters, at the proximal aortic arch level, either the flap is seen in two positions due to motion artifact, or there is a second intimal flap. In this case, there was only one intimal flap. **B,** Non–ECG-gated chest CT scan with prominent motion artifact of the aortic root, but not of the descending aorta, due to the motion imparted by the heart on the aortic root and ascending aorta. During acquisition, the aortic root was in both systolic and at least one of two diastolic positions. **C,** Parasternal long-axis view at the aortic root level with superimposition of diastolic and systolic frames. The position of the aortic valve and aortic root may be seen to vary in systole, in terms of both its anteroposterior and long-axis locations. **D,** M-mode recording at the aortic root level reveals 1.5 cm of total anteroposterior motion during the cardiac cycle of a normal heart. In systole, the aortic root is pulled anteriorly, whereas in early diastole, the aortic root moves posteriorly, and, in late diastole following atrial contraction, moves further posteriorly.

❐ **Causes**:
- Motion
  - Wrong phase (review reconstruction at different phases)
  - Breathing
  - Rhythm
- Poor SNR
- Insufficient mA
- Patient too obese
- Slice too thick
- Poor contrast opacification
- Calcification
- Stents

❐ Possible solutions:
- Use more milliamps if patient was too large and milliamperage was too low
- Use another (harder) kernel

Blooming Artifact

Dense, highly attenuating material has the tendency to result in widening of its image, with the widening proportional to the density. Objects are thus not visualized at their true size. This artifact is less apparent on thinner-detector 64-slice scanners but is still a problem for both calcium and stents.

❐ Increasing spatial resolution by use of a sharper kernel will help sharpen the dense structure, but may diminish the depiction of soft structures.

❐ Dual energy (80 kVp and 140 kVp) CCT appears to reduce overestimation of calcium volume by more than 40%.

❐ High-spatial-resolution technologies show promise in reducing blooming artifacts.

Other Artifacts

Some artifact patterns are unusual and unusually prominent, often are seen in the presence of prosthetic material, and may appear differently depending on the plane of image orientation (Fig. 5-10).

Mirror Artifact

A mirror artifact is a post-processing artifact that is seen when a curved multiplanar reconstruction is generated. An explanation of this artifact is as follows:

❐ Curved reformatted views have an axis (horizontal or vertical), which depends on the general shape of the vessel.

❐ Curved reformations have the ability to rotate the angle of view around the center line of a given curve.

A rotational angle view of the curve corresponds to rotating the rays which composed the image around this central line axis. In some geometries, for example, if the vessel makes a small horizontal "S" at some place in the course of a primarily vertical vessel, there will be angles where

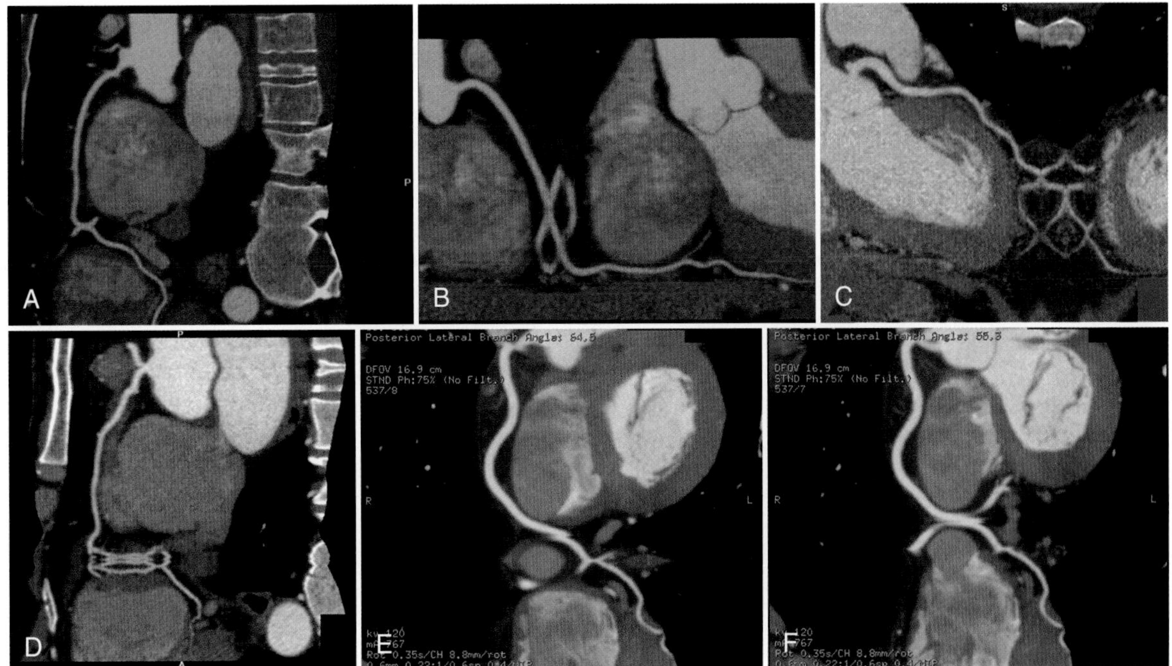

Figure 5-10. Multiple curved reformatted images of an obtuse marginal branch (**A**) and a right coronary artery (**B**). These images demonstrate a mirror artifact of the coronary arteries. This post-processing type of artifact usually is seen only with curved multiplanar reformats and occurs when the vessel is tortuous or curves back on itself. This causes a misrepresentation of the spatial localization of the vessel at its point of curvature. **C** and **D**, Two curved reformatted images of an obtuse marginal branch on the left and RCA on the right. These images demonstrate a mirror lattice-like artifact of the coronary arteries. This artifact occurs when the vessel is tortuous or curves back on itself slightly. This causes a misrepresentation of the spatial localization of the vessel at its point of curvature. **E** and **F**, Misregistration artifact of the distal right coronary artery.

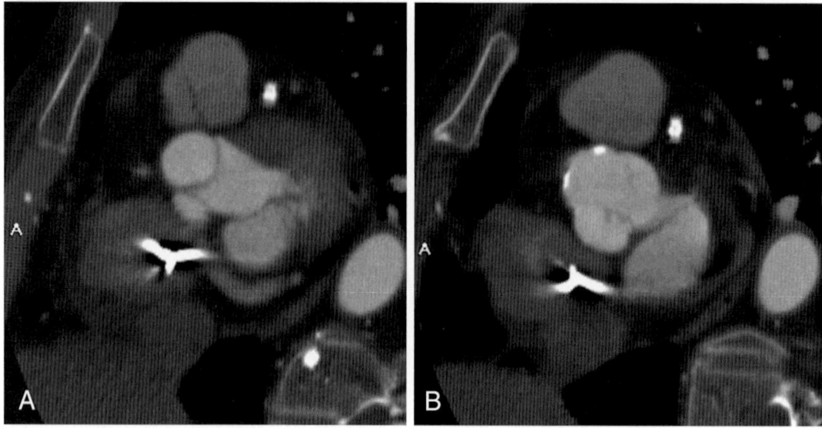

Figure 5-11. Short-axis oblique images from a helically acquired cardiac CT study. An implantable cardioverter defibrillator (ICD) lead is seen projecting from the right atrium. These images demonstrate an unusual type of beam-hardening artifact that occurs due in part to the metallic artifact, in this case from the ICD, and in part to motion from cardiac pulsation, which confers to the beam-hardening artifact a "windmilling" rotational appearance. **See Video 5-1.**

a ray will hit the same vessel twice (in each extremity of the S). This means that there will be two locations in the vessel generating the exact same ray, and therefore creating a mirror-like duplication for some angles close to this S shape.

Artifacts That Replicate Pathologies

The main consequence of the types of artifacts just discussed is that their presence may obscure detection of a significant lesion. Artifacts that are similarity to actual pathologies are the most worrisome and may be very difficult to disprove or prove, short of extensive alternative forms of imaging or exploration. Distinguishing linear artifacts that replicate the appearance of intimal flaps from true flaps presents a regular challenge.

Windmilling

"Windmilling" is a descriptive term for a motion artifact that usually results when a beam-hardening artifact occurs in a circular fashion due to an intracardiac device. This is commonly seen in patients who have intraventricular pacemaker leads or implantable cardioverter defibrillator leads during helical cardiac acquisition (Fig. 5-11; **Video 5-1**).

NOTES

- **Early start.** An early start to image acquisition may occur if regionally high contrast in the SVC generates high-attenuation artifact that is sampled by the ROI in the ascending aorta.
- Suggestions:
  - Use tracking software.
  - Use a test bolus.
  - Place the ROI in the descending aorta.
- Learn to recognize ECG gating artifacts. Most single-step artifacts are from single premature beats.
- **Problem:** Acquisition is missing the quiescent motionless phase of the cardiac cycle.
  - Solution: Choose the best phase for reconstruction, but if a given vessel or vessel segment is blurred, review other phases of reconstruction that may demonstrate the given segment better. This approach works primarily for retrospective imaging, and can be used with prospectively acquired studies that have a moderate amount of padding (~20%) around the acquisition trigger.
- **Partial volume averaging effect**. If a high-attenuation object is smaller than the voxel within which it was imaged, and the surrounding tissue was of low attenuation, then the average attenuation in the voxel will be lower than that of the object and the item of interest will not be represented. Similarly, if a dark streak artifact extends into an area of interest, the image of the area of interest will suffer from partial volume averaging effect. Conversely, if a bright streak artifact extends into an area of interest, its appearance also will be affected by partial averaging effects.

References

1. Nakanishi T, Kayashima Y, Inoue R, Sumii K, Gomyo Y. Pitfalls in 16-detector row CT of the coronary arteries. *Radiographics.* 2005;25(2):425-438.
2. Hoffmann MH, Shi H, Schmitz BL, et al. Noninvasive coronary angiography with multislice computed tomography. *JAMA.* 2005;293(20):2471-2478.
3. Hoffmann MH, Shi H, Manzke R, et al. Noninvasive coronary angiography with 16-detector row CT: effect of heart rate. *Radiology.* 2005;234(1):86-97.

6 CT Coronary Angiography

Key Points

- CT coronary angiography (CTA) has been the principal goal of development of cardiac CT (CCT). The momentum of cardiac CT development has been toward both improving image quality and reducing radiation exposure.
- CT coronary angiography is able to provide high negative predictive value of significant coronary artery disease.
- CT coronary angiography is able to quantify coronary artery disease, although with limitations.
- Current limitations of coronary CT angiography include patient exclusions, coronary calcium, poor ability to characterize small (<2 mm diameter) arteries and branches, and limited outcomes data.

ACC/AHA 17-SEGMENT CORONARY MODEL

Comparative studies of coronary CT angiography (CTA) versus angiographic quantitative coronary analysis (QCA) assessment of coronary anatomy usually are performed comparing the presence or absence of angiographically significant stenosis (>50%) among the "17-segment model" of coronary anatomy.

IMAGING CORONARY ARTERIES: LUMINAL ASSESSMENT

Imaging of the coronary artery lumen is a particular challenge for CT scanning, given:

- The small luminal size (especially when diseased)
- The rapid motion (up to 150 mm/sec, particularly for the arteries in the atrioventricular grooves) through several phases of the cardiac cycle (early systole, early diastole and late diastole—if in sinus rhythm)
- The potential of rhythm or rate irregularity during scanning/acquisition
- The need for the patient to hold his or her breath during the procedure
- The presence of stents and the tendency of diseased coronary arteries to attract calcification—both of which confer problematic signal "blooming" (partial volume averaging) artifacts.
- The combination of motion, blooming artifact, and partial signal averaging effect that substantially reduces the depiction of the lumen within calcified and stented coronary arteries

Attaining equivalence in accuracy between CTA and catheter angiography is a challenge that has not been met as of 2014. Catheter angiography has substantially greater imaging resolution (spatial and especially temporal) and hugely greater versatility, yielding clinically adequate images despite calcification and stents, irregular cardiac rhythms, variable cardiac heart rates, and spontaneous or mechanical ventilation, on stable ambulatory patients and patients in cardiogenic shock (Table 6-1).

Thus, catheter-based angiography has logarithmically greater temporal resolution and several-fold better spatial resolution than contemporary CTA. CTA technology is developing in terms of both spatial and, more importantly, temporal resolution, but the technology gap is notable, and the clinical performance gap is broad in real life. Patients undergoing catheter-based coronary angiography are extremely heterogeneous with respect to many parameters that are relevant to CTA imaging:

- Variable heart rates:
  - Low (due to physiologic, pathologic or pharmacologic reasons) to tachycardic
  - β-blocker tolerant to β-blocker intolerant
  - Unstable heart rates
- Heart rhythm: normal sinus rhythm to arrhythmia of all forms
- Variable potential for artifact:
  - No calcification or minor calcification to heavy calcification
  - No stents
  - Multiple stents, including stenting within stenting
  - Stenting within calcified areas

Given the inherent lesser spatial resolution of CTA, its best coronary application, and probably its earliest, will be to establish that the lumens of large coronary vessels and bypass grafts are not stenotic.

Magnetic resonance angiography (MRA) is becoming increasingly capable[2] and exhibits

TABLE 6-1 Catheter versus CT Angiography and MR Angiography

	CATHETER ANGIOGRAPHY		CT ANGIOGRAPHY		MRI ANGIOGRAPHY
Resolution					
Spatial (mm)	0.2		0.4–0.75		0.7–1.0 mm
Temporal (ms)	4–7		165–330 Dual source: 60–100		0
3D rendering	—		Excellent		Limited
Experience	Huge		Modest		Limited
Radiation (mSv)	3–4		Newer scanners (mSv)	Older scanners (mSv)	None
		Prospective	0.5–4	4–10	
		Retrospective	4–8	12–20	
Ability to image/ characterize the wall	Poor (only dense and thick calcium is apparent)		Good		Poor

TABLE 6-2 Accuracy of 64-Slice CT to Detect Coronary Lesions Compared with IVUS

	SENSITIVITY (%)	SPECIFICITY (%)
Left mainstem	100	100
Right coronary artery	83	100
Left anterior descending coronary artery	87	93
Left circumflex coronary artery	71	77
Total	84	91

IVUS, intravascular ultrasound.
From Leber AW et al. Quantification of obstructive and nonobstructive coronary lesions by 64-slice computed tomography: a comparative study with quantitative coronary angiography and intravascular ultrtasound. *J Am Coll Cardiol.* 2005;46(1):147.

comparable sensitivity and specificity and accuracy to coronary CTA (at least the older 16-CT) when compared to QCA for vessels 1.5 mm or larger in very highly selected patients and select centers.[1] Comparison of cardiac magnetic resonance (CMR) with current state-of-the-art equipment does not confirm contemporary equivalence of CMR and CTA. A 3-tesla system with increased signal-to-noise ratio (SNR) allows for increased spatial resolution in whole-heart MRA techniques.

Because the motion, size, and orientation of coronary arteries are different, the accuracy of 64-slice multislice CT (64-MSCT) for the detection of coronary stenoses depends on which vessel is being investigated, due to differences in vessel size and the amount of motion through diastole. The right coronary artery and the left circumflex artery are subject to more motion than the left anterior descending (LAD) artery due to the mechanical effect or motion imparted by atrial contraction[2] (Table 6-2).

In patients with normal heart rates, multisegment reconstruction algorithms tend to have superior diagnostic accuracy and image quality compared with half-scan reconstruction algorithms.[3] Automatic selective phase acquisition software in large detector platforms (≥256 slice) and single cardiac cycle acquisition are expected to optimize acquisition with respect to avoidance of diastolic motion and image reconstruction artifacts resulting from multicycle reconstructions.

CALCIUM, CALCIUM SCORING, AND CALCIUM ARTIFACT

The presence of calcium, while useful for calcium scoring, is a problem for coronary CTA. The presence of calcium leads to false-positive determination of stenosis[4] as well as overestimation of stenosis. It is more difficult to visualize the lumen in the presence of calcium, due to the "blooming artifact" (i.e., partial volume averaging) of calcium, which is responsible for overestimation of plaque size and stenosis severity. Any motion encountered during acquisition further compounds the blooming and increases the overestimation of stenosis and underestimation of lumen. Blooming artifact is seen less frequently with 64-CCT but remains a significant problem.

The addition of calcium scoring to coronary CTA does not add significantly to the determination of disease.[5] A high calcium score should be seen as a reason not to proceed with CTA, however.

EVIDENCE-BASED REVIEW OF CORONARY CTA

Since about 2005, an accelerating body of evidence has been developing that establishes that coronary CTA is feasible, but within limits that require careful patient selection and preparation. The many limits are represented by the numerous patient exclusions seen in published studies. As the technology has developed, the list of limitation, particularly in terms of patient selection and preparation, has diminished, but exclusions remain numerous and define the nature of use of CTA.

To date, CTA studies have been most useful in excluding disease or classifying disease, if it is present, rather than in performing the vital task of providing a roadmap to plan revascularization procedures in patients with significant disease.

The earliest series using 4-slice CCT equipment, entirely as expected, yielded results inferior to 16-CCT, which currently is considered the bare minimum technology to use for coronary CTA. Today the current standard is 64-CCT or >64-CCT, as presented in the tables in this chapter. Significantly, 64-CCT has not been proven equivalent to conventional angiography. The recent arrival of 256- and 320-CCT, which enable whole heart acquisition in a single cardiac cycle, is expected to provide further imaging benefits, and results of these techniques are eagerly anticipated. Whether they are not just improvements but improvements that render CCT comparable to conventional catheter angiography remains to be seen.

All studies published to date reflect a high degree of selection of patients, establishing that although CTA is feasible, it is not universally feasible, unlike catheter-based techniques. As the temporal resolution of coronary CTA improves, the possibility of including patients with heart rates greater than 75 bpm (who currently are excluded) is emerging, as is the possibility of including patients with irregular heart rhythms. As temporal resolution improves, false-negative CTA studies due to motion artifacts may become less common.[6]

Most comparative studies performed before the introduction of 64-CCT in 2005 are notable for:

- ❒ Use of a segment-by-segment comparison, which predictably increases the power of the study
- ❒ Comparison of only vessels ≥1.5 (or ≥2.0) mm in luminal size versus all segments, which is not realistic in excluding CAD or in planning revascularization techniques
- ❒ Comparison of assessable vessels

More recent studies have strived to include:

- ❒ All segments, regardless of size
- ❒ Vessel comparison (single-, double-, triple-vessel disease)
- ❒ Patient comparison (disease vs. no disease)

To achieve the greatest plausibility and comparative power for conventional coronary angiography, the ideal and most credible studies of coronary CTA will entail no more exclusions than those of coronary angiography and will validate that the use of coronary CTA in the context of potential use of conventional angiography provides a significant outcome or cost benefit.

Summary of CTA for the Detection of CAD

The use of CTA for the detection of CAD is summarized in Figure 6-1 and Tables 6-3 through 6-10.

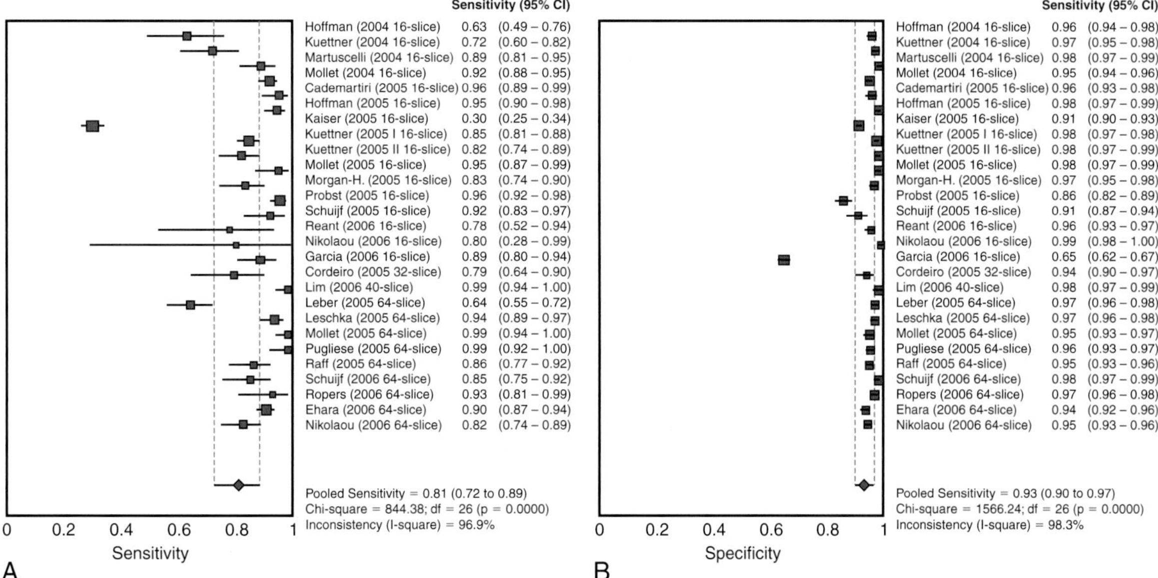

Figure 6-1. **A,** Plot and table of per-segment sensitivity of multislice computed tomography–coronary angiography (MSCT-CA) compared with coronary angiography (CA). **B,** Plot and table of per-segment specificity of MSCT-CA compared with CA. CI, confidence interval; df, degrees of freedom. (Reprinted with permission from Hamon M, Biondi-Zoccai GG, Malagutti P, et al. Diagnostic performance of multislice spiral computed tomography of coronary arteries as compared with conventional invasive coronary angiography: a meta-analysis. *J Am Coll Cardiol.* 2006;48(9):1896-1910.)

TABLE 6-3 4-CCT Assessment of Native Coronaries

AUTHOR	JOURNAL	YEAR	*n*	NONASSESS. (%)	SENSITIVITY (%)	SPECIFICITY (%)	PPV (%)	NPV (%)
Achenbach et al.[7]	Circ	2001	64	32	85	76	59	98
Becker et al.[8]	JCAT	2002	28	5	81	90	97	89
Knez et al.[9]	Am J Card	2001	42	6	78	98	—	—
Kopp et al.[10]	Eur Heart J	2002	102	16	86	96	—	—
Lau et al.[5]	Radiology	2005	50	—	79	95	—	—
Nieman et al.[11]	Lancet	2001	31	27	56	97	—	—
Nieman et al.[11]	Lancet	2001	31	27	81	97	—	—
Nieman et al.[12]	Circ	2002	59	7	95	86	—	—
Nieman et al.[13]	Heart	2002	53	30	58	76	—	—
Nieman et al.[14]	Radiology	2003	24	33	85	73	—	—
Vogl et al.[15]	Radiology	2002	64	—	75	91	—	—
Kuettner et al.[16]	JACC	2004	66	—	37	99	—	—

CCT, cardiac CT; nonassess., nonassessable; NPV, negative predictive value; PPV, positive predictive value.

TABLE 6-4 12-CCT Assessment of Native Coronaries

AUTHOR	JOURNAL	YEAR	*n*	NONASSESS. (%)	SENSITIVITY (%)	SPECIFICITY (%)	PPV (%)	NPV (%)
Ropers et al.[17]	Circ	2003	77	12	93	92	79	97

CCT, cardiac CT; nonassess., nonassessable; NPV, negative predictive value; PPV, positive predictive value.

TABLE 6-5 16-CCT Assessment of Native Coronaries

AUTHOR	JOURNAL	YEAR	*n*	NONASSESS. (%)	SENSITIVITY (%)	SPECIFICITY (%)	PPV (%)	NPV (%)
Achenbach et al.[18]	Eur Heart J	2005	57	5	94	97	—	99
Achenbach et al.[19]	Circ	2004	22	—	82	88	—	—
Heuschmid et al.[20]	Am J Roent	2005	37	0	59	87	—	—
				CAC < 1000	93	94	68	99
Hoffmann M et al.[21]	JAMA	2005	103	6	95	98	—	99
Hoffmann U et al.[4]	Circ	2004	33	—	63	96	64	96
				(good image quality)	82	93	—	—
Kefer et al.[1]	JACC	2005	52	—	82	79	—	—
Kuettner et al.[22]	JACC	2004	58	16	72	97	—	—
				(Agatston <1000)	98	98	—	—
Kuettner et al.[23]	Heart	2005	72	7	85	98	—	96

TABLE 6-5 16-CCT Assessment of Native Coronaries—cont'd

AUTHOR	JOURNAL	YEAR	*n*	NONASSESS. (%)	SENSITIVITY (%)	SPECIFICITY (%)	PPV (%)	NPV (%)
Kuettner et al.[24]	JACC	2005	72	0	82	98	87	97
Martuscelli et al.[25]	Eur Heart J	2004	64	16	89	98	90	98
Mollet et al.[26]	JACC	2004	128	7	92	95	79	98
Mollet et al.[27]	JACC	2005	51	n/a	95	98	87	99
Morgan-Hughes et al.[28]	Heart	2005	58	2	83	97	—	97
Romeo et al.[29]	JACC	2005	53	12% transplant pt	83	95	71	95
Schuijf et al.[30]	Am J Cardiol	2005	45	6	83	97	—	97
Cademartiri et al.[31]	Radiol Med (Torino)	2005	60	2	93	97	99	86
Cademartiri et al.[32]	Am J Roentgenol	2006	38	0	92	96	87	97
Cademartiri et al.[33]	Radiol Med (Torino)	2005	40	0	96	96	86	99
Dewey et al.[34]	Invest Radiol	2005	129	9	83	86	—	96
Fine et al.[35]	Int J Cardiac Imaging	2004	50	2	87	97	—	98
Kaiser et al.[36]	Eur Heart J	2005	149	23	30	91	—	83
Aviram et al.[37]	Int J Cardiovasc Intervent	2005	22	—	86	98	—	98
Garcia et al.[38]	JAMA	2006	187	29	85	91	—	99
Gulati et al.[39]	Natl Med J India	2005	31	14	85	94	76	96

CCT, cardiac CT; nonassess., nonassessable; NPV, negative predictive value; PPV, positive predictive value.

TABLE 6-6 32-CCT

AUTHOR	JOURNAL	YEAR	*n*	NONASSESS. (%)	SENSITIVITY (%)	SPECIFICITY (%)	PPV (%)	NPV (%)
Cordeiro et al.[40]	Heart	2005	30	20	76	94	—	96

CCT, cardiac CT; nonassess., nonassessable; NPV, negative predictive value; PPV, positive predictive value.

TABLE 6-7 40-CCT

AUTHOR	JOURNAL	YEAR	*n*	NONASSESS. (%)	SENSITIVITY (%)	SPECIFICITY (%)	PPV (%)	NPV (%)
Lim et al.[41]	Clin Radiol	2005	30	0	99	98	94	99

CCT, cardiac CT; nonassess., nonassessable; NPV, negative predictive value; PPV, positive predictive value.

TABLE 6-8 64-CCT Assessment of Native Coronaries

AUTHOR	JOURNAL	YEAR	*n*	NONASSESS. (%)	SENSITIVITY (%)	SPECIFICITY (%)	PPV (%)	NPV (%)
Leber et al.[2]	JACC	2005	59		64	97		
				No severe calcium	87	98		
Leschka et al.[42]	Eur Heart J	2005	57	n/a	94	97		99
Mollet et al.[43]	Circ	2005	52	2	99	95	76	99
Raff et al.[44]	JACC	2005	70	12	86	95	66	98
Pugliese et al.[45]	Eur Radiol	2005	35	6	99	96	78	99
Ropers et al.[46]	Am J Cardiol	2006	84	4	93	97		100
Fine et al.[47]	Am J Cardiol	2006	66	6	95	96	97	92
Nikolaou et al.[48]	AJR	2006	72	6	97	79		96
Weustink et al.[49]	JACC	2007	100					
	Per segment		1489		95 [90–97]	95 [90–97]	95 [90–97]	95 [90–97]
	Per patient		100		95 [90–97]	95 [90–97]	95 [90–97]	95 [90–97]
Schuijf et al.[50]	Am J Cardiol	2006	61	1	85	98		
Ehara et al.[51]	Circ	2006	99	8	90	94		
					Pre-test probability	Post-test negative	Post-test positive	
Meijboom et al.[52]	JACC	2007	254					
			105	High probability	87	17	96	
			83	Intermediate probability	53	0	88	
			66	Low probability	13	0	68	
Shabestari et al.[53]	Am J Cardiol	2007	35		92	97	77	99
				Agatston <100		83		
				Agatston >400		60		
Meijboom et al.[54]	Heart	2007	104		92	91	60	99
Miller et al.[55]	NEJM	2008	291	Agatston <600, >1.5 mm	85 [79–90]	90 [83–94]	91 [85–95]	83 [75–89]
Budoff et al.[56]	JACC	2008	230	1%				
		≥50% stenosis	55		95	83	64	99
		≥70% stenosis	31		94	83	48	99
Meijboom et al.[57]	JACC	2008	360	Per patient	99 [98–100]	64 [55–73]	86 [82–90]	97 [94–100]
				Per segment	88 [85–91]	90 [89–92]	47 [44–51]	99 [98–99]

CCT, cardiac CT; nonassess., nonassessable; NPV, negative predictive value; PPV, positive predictive value.

TABLE 6-9 64-CCT Assessment of Native Coronaries

PATIENTS (NO.)	NOT EVALUABLE (%)	SENSITIVITY (%)	SPECIFICITY (%)	PPV (%)	NPV (%)
701	3.8 (27/701) (95% CI: 2.6–5.6)	98 (398/404) (95% CI: 95–99)	90 (263/293) (95% CI: 86–93)	93 (394/4240) (95% CI: 90–95)	95 (263/273) (95% CI: 93–98)

CCT, cardiac CT; NPV, negative predictive value; PPV, positive predictive value.
Data from Schroeder S, Achenbach S, Bengel F, et al. Cardiac computed tomography: indications, applications, limitations, and training requirements: report of a Writing Group deployed by the Working Group Nuclear Cardiology and Cardiac CT of the European Society of Cardiology and the European Council of Nuclear Cardiology. *Eur Heart J.* 2008;29(4):531-556.

TABLE 6-10 64-CCT Assessment of Native Coronaries

ANALYSIS	NO.	SENSITIVITY (95% CI)	SPECIFICITY (95% CI)
Per segment	22,798	0.81 (0.72-0.89)	0.93 (0.90-0.97)
Per vessel	2,726	0.82 (0.80-0.85)	0.91 (0.90-0.92)
Per patient	1,570	0.96 (0.94-0.98)	0.74 (0.65-0.84)

CCT, cardiac CT.
Data from Hamon M, Biondi-Zoccai GG, Malagutti P, et al. Diagnostic performance of multislice spiral computed tomography of coronary arteries as compared with conventional invasive coronary angiography: a meta-analysis. *J Am Coll Cardiol.* 2006;48(9):1896-1910.

CORONARY CTA

Review of coronary CTA usually begins with a review of axial images and then moves on to maximum intensity projection (MIP) images and reformats (e.g., multiplanar reconstructions and cross-sectional multiplanar reconstructions) to follow the course of the coronary arteries. Workstation software has increasingly included features to assist with coronary (or other) vessel extraction and then depiction. "Seed" markers are placed by the origin of the vessel of interest and distally along its course. Using edge detection algorithms, the vessel is "extracted" and depicted. As the images of the extracted vessel become, to some extent, abstract (for example, a curved artery is depicted in a straightened fashion), reference MIP and 3D images often are displayed concurrently to depict the course of the vessel. These images are usually shown as curved reformations with a single-pixel-thick line coursing down the center of the vessel. Edge detection algorithms allow for maintenance of the center line positioning as the vessel curves. The curve can be represented in any degree of rotation around the center line, which can aid in visualizing eccentric lesions. In addition, cross-sectional "cuts" or planes perpendicular to the long axis of the curved reformations allow for circumferential evaluation of any segment of the analyzed coronary artery (Figs. 6-2 through 6-23; **Videos 6-1 through 6-21**).

COMPARISON OF CORONARY CTA AND QCA FOR QUANTIFICATION OF STENOSIS

To date, only a few studies have published direct comparisons of degree of luminal narrowing by coronary CTA versus catheter angiography QCA or intravenous ultrasound (IVUS). The following observations are common to these studies:

- Coronary CTA correlates (imperfectly) with catheter-based angiographic determination of luminal narrowing.
- Limitations of spatial resolution, calcium, and blurring are seen.
- Coronary CTA is not able to accurately offer "percent stenosis" per case that agrees closely with catheter measurements.
- Older CCT coronary CTA systems tend to systematically overestimate luminal narrowing, especially because of their lower spatial and temporal resolution. This may be compounded by the greater blurring/blooming artifact from calcium. Newer systems exhibit less of this tendency due to improvements in spatial resolution and less of a tendency to exhibit blurring/blooming.
- The presence of calcium tends to increase the "positivity" of stenosis on CTA (it may confer false positives and overestimate coronary CTA assessment of severity,[60]) and may "overcall" complete occlusions.
- Coronary CTA may systematically underestimate percent area narrowing compared with IVUS.[3]

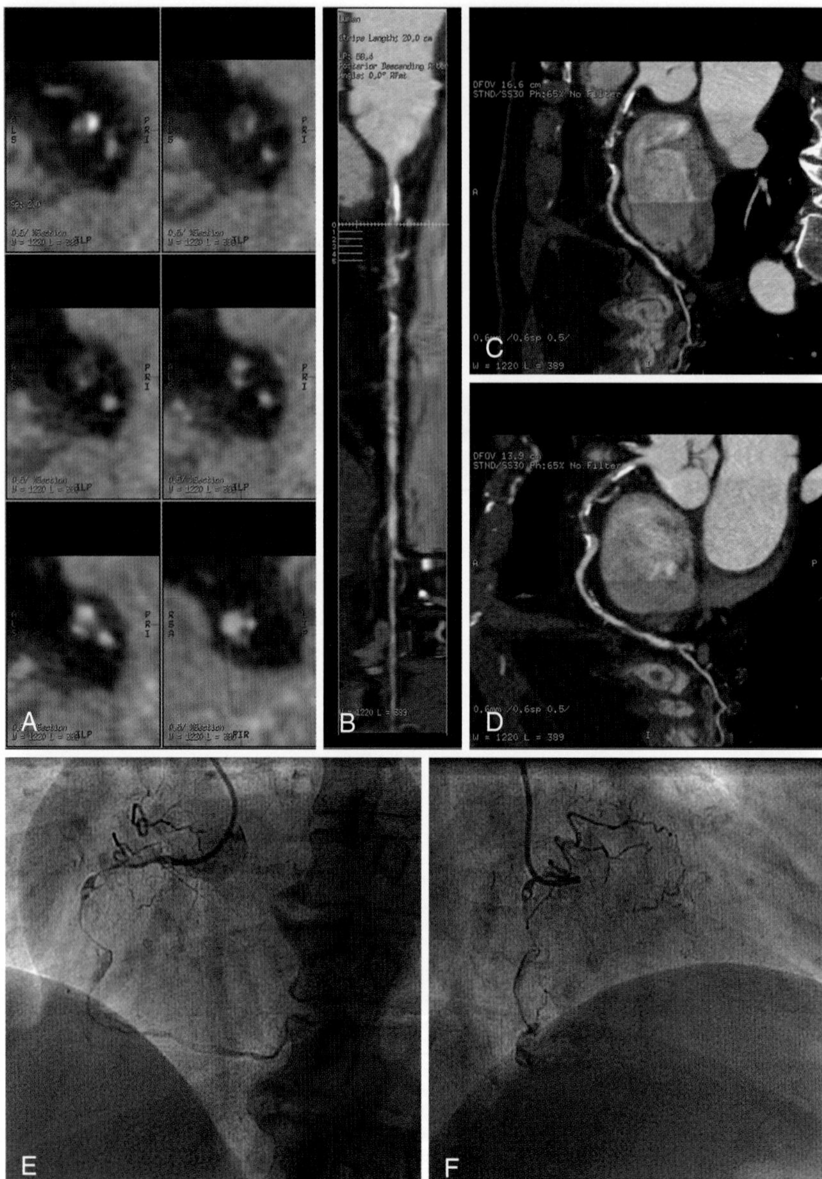

Figure 6-2. Multiple reconstructions from a cardiac CT study in a 58-year-old woman with a history of angina and an indeterminant myocardial perfusion imaging (MPI) study. The straight and curved reconstructions demonstrate two complex, severe lesions within the proximal right coronary artery (RCA). Cross-sectional evaluation across the more proximal lesion demonstrates mixed plaque, and near-total occlusion. The distal RCA has an approximately 50% soft plaque lesion proximal to the crux. A patent ductus arteriosus (PDA), however is free of disease and is a good-sized vessel. The patient went on to angiography, which demonstrated high-grade stenosis in the proximal RCA, and multiple proximal RCA collaterals. Faint contrast is seen coursing through the remainder of the RCA, but with poor visualization of the other lesions and the non-stenosed PDA. See **Videos 6-1 and 6-2.**

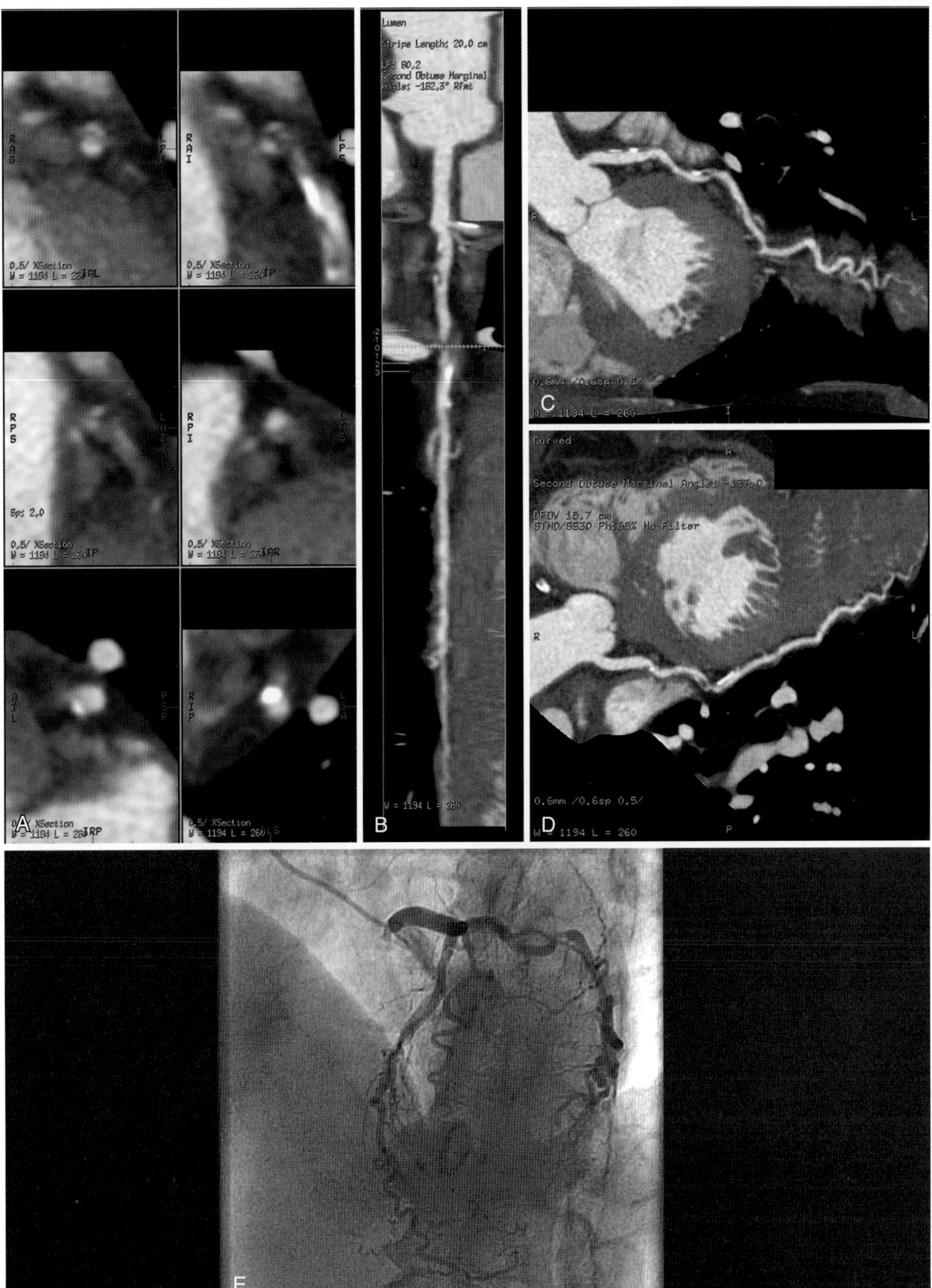

Figure 6-3. Same patient as Figure 6-2. Multiple cardiac CT reconstructions through a large obtuse marginal branch in a 58-year-old woman with a history of angina and indeterminate myocardial perfusion imaging study. These images demonstrate mild proximal circumflex and obtuse marginal disease. The proximal portion of the large obtuse marginal branch has a severe 70% stenosis. Cross-sectional images demonstrate this to be a mixed plaque stenosis. Conventional coronary angiography (left anterior oblique projection) demonstrates a 70% proximal obtuse marginal branch stenosis. See Figures 6-1 and 6-2 and **Videos 6-1 and 6-2.**

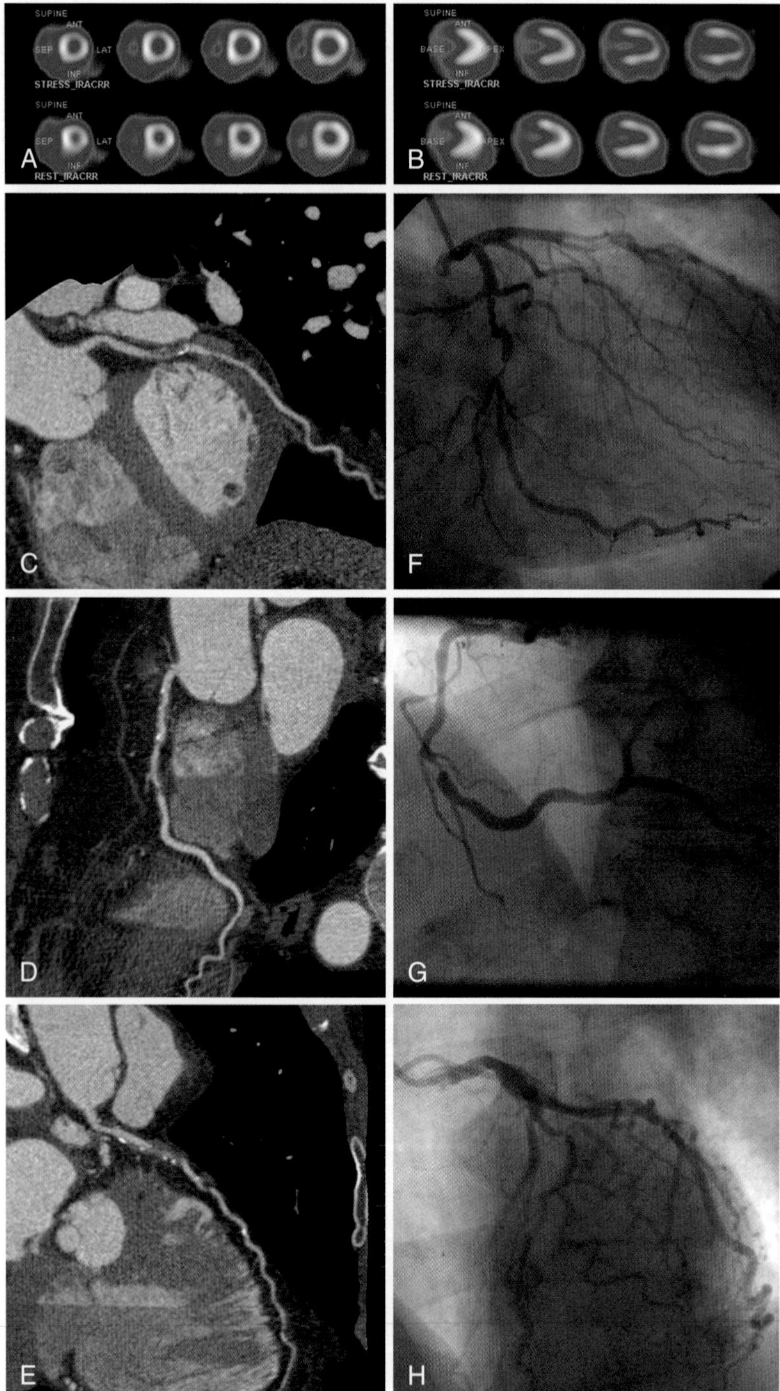

Figure 6-4. A 57-year-old man with typical angina. The patient underwent a nuclear medicine stress perfusion study (**A** and **B**). Stress views are located superiorly, and the resting views are located inferiorly, with short-axis views on the left and long-axis views on the right. No evidence of a resting or stress perfusion defect is seen. The patient, however, subsequently was referred for a cardiac CT study. Images from that study follow (**C–E**), and corresponding conventional angiographic images are shown in parts **F–H. C** and **F,** There is a mixed 50% stenosis in the proximal left circumflex artery and a severe 70% stenosis in the mid-left circumflex artery, imaged on both the CCT and the coronary angiogram. **D** and **G,** A tight 80% to 90% mid-right coronary artery stenosis is present, imaged on both the CCT and the coronary angiogram. **E** and **H,** A complex 70% to 80% proximal-to-mid left anterior descending artery stenosis is present, imaged on both the CCT and the coronary angiogram. Severe triple-vessel disease was present. The lack of any corresponding regions of perfusion abnormality on the myocardial perfusion imaging study is plausibly due to the occurrence of balanced ischemia, a known challenge/pitfall of nuclear medicine imaging. **See Videos 6-3 through 6-5.**

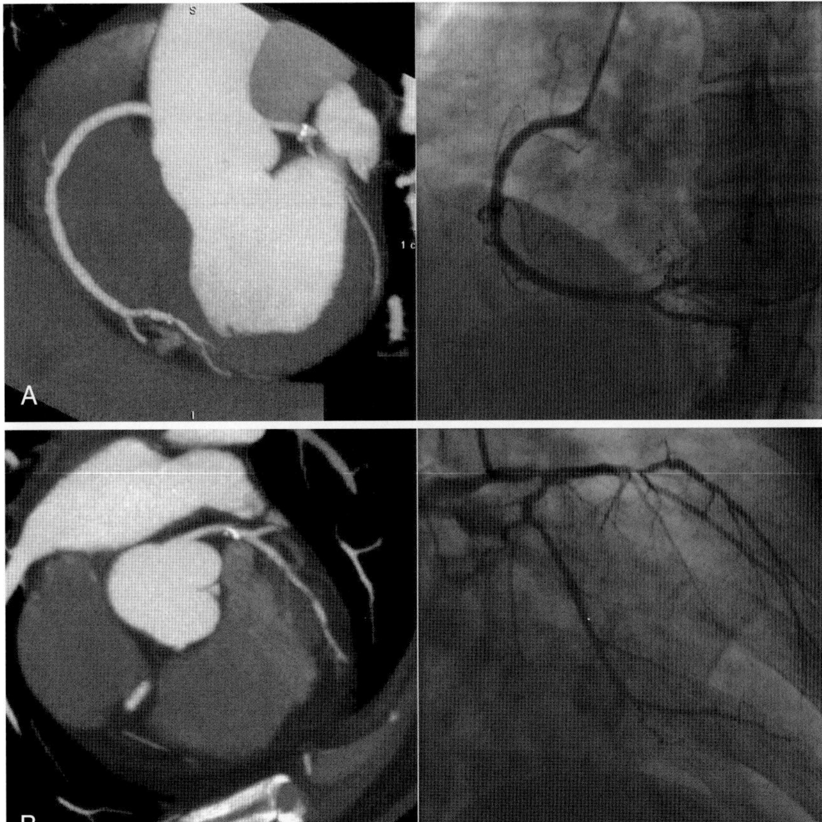

Figure 6-5. A 57-year-old man with chest pain, and an equivocal myocardial perfusion imaging (MPI) study. **A,** A mild (<30%) stenosis within the mid-right coronary artery. **B,** MIP reconstruction of the left main coronary artery demonstrates a moderate amount of mixed plaque in the distal left main coronary artery causing a 50% to 60% left main stenosis. These findings were confirmed on the patient's conventional angiogram to the right. The patient was referred for surgical consultation. **See Videos 6-6 and 6-7.**

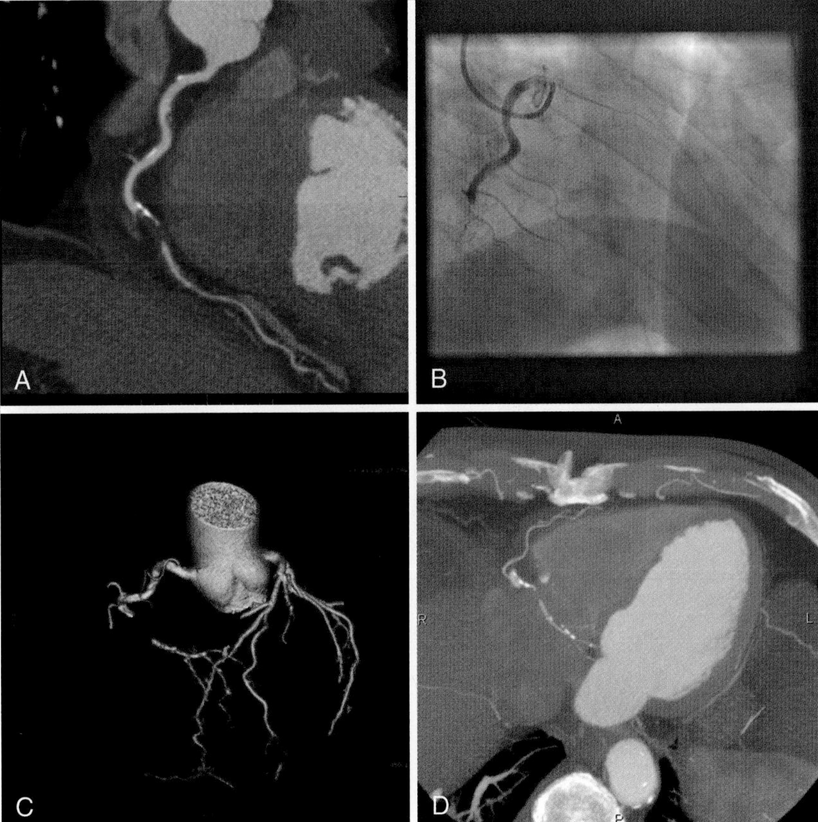

Figure 6-6. A 74-year-old man presents with an acute coronary syndrome. **A,** Coronary CTA reveals a complete occlusion of the right coronary artery (RCA) due to mixed plaque that is mostly "soft." **B,** Corresponding angiogram image corroborates the occlusion of the RCA. **C,** 3D volume-rendered image depicts the RCA occlusion and collaterals from the distal left anterior descending artery toward acute marginal territory. **D,** Maximum intensity projection image reveals the acute marginal branches by which (some of the) reconstitution of the ongoing RCA occurs. **See Video 6-8.**

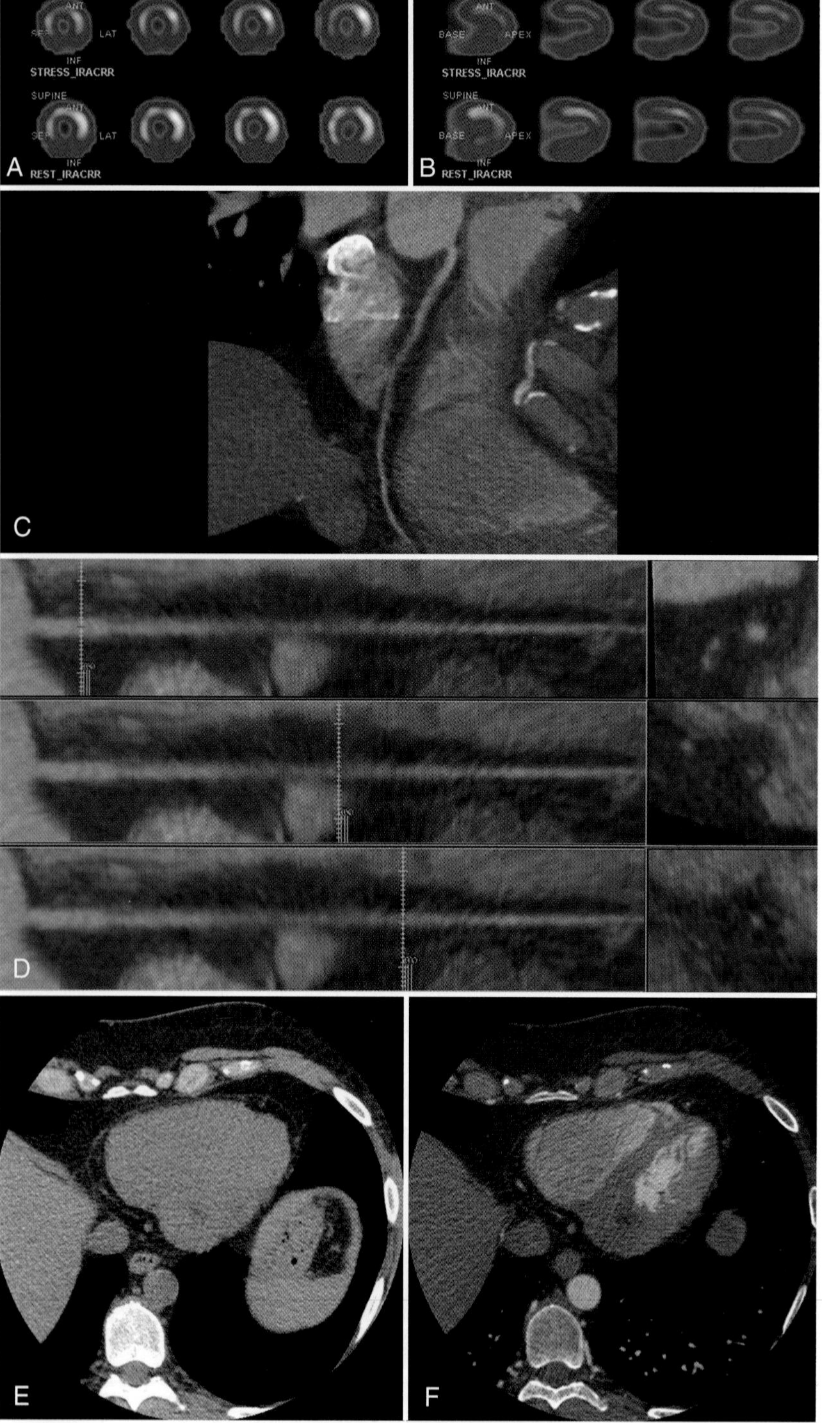

Figure 6-7. Multiple images from a 47-year-old man with chest pain. **A** and **B,** Nuclear medicine myocardial perfusion imaging study demonstrated a moderate-sized, partially reversible inferior wall defect. Stress images are placed superiorly with rest images inferiorly. The patient went on to have coronary CT angiography (**C**). A second panel demonstrates a curved multiplanar reconstruction of the right coronary artery (RCA) (**D**). A severe soft plaque stenosis is seen in the mid-RCA. Stretched views of the RCA had been obtained with corresponding cross-sectional views in the proximal RCA, through the mid-RCA lesion, and just distal to the mid-RCA lesion. The cross-sectional views (**E** and **F**) confirm the severe stenosis and the soft plaque component to the stenosis. The bottom left images show a noncontrast calcium score study. The patient's overall calcium score was zero. There is a moderate-sized area of low attenuation seen in the basal inferior wall. This is also identified on the axial source CTA image (**F**). This area of low attenuation represents fatty metaplasia, and a prior chronic infarct, corresponding with the nuclear medicine study. These CT images, however, are limited in their ability to determine how much residual viability is associated with the region of the prior infarct.

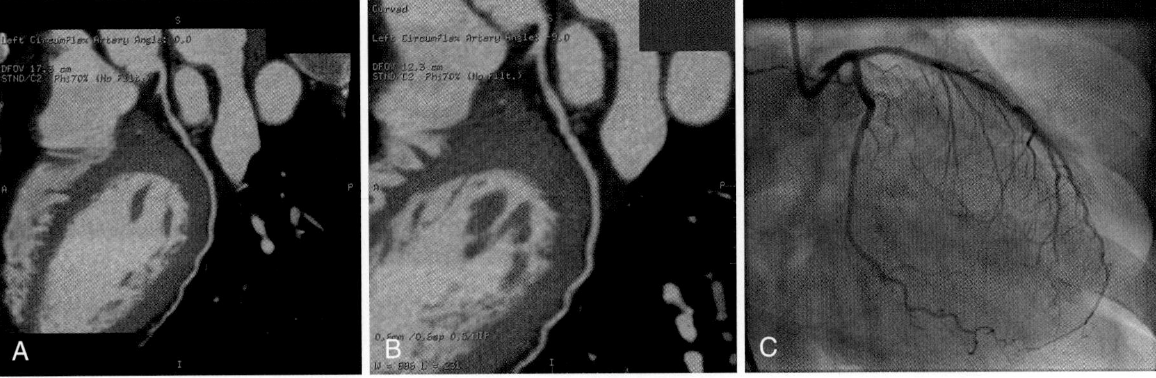

Figure 6-8. A 52-year-old man presented with typical angina and an indeterminant myocardial perfusion study. Curved reformatted images through the circumflex and obtuse marginal branch do not demonstrate any evidence of a circumflex system stenosis. The corresponding conventional angiogram confirms no obstructive circumflex lesion. See Figures 6-9 and 6-10 and **Videos 6-9 through 6-12.**

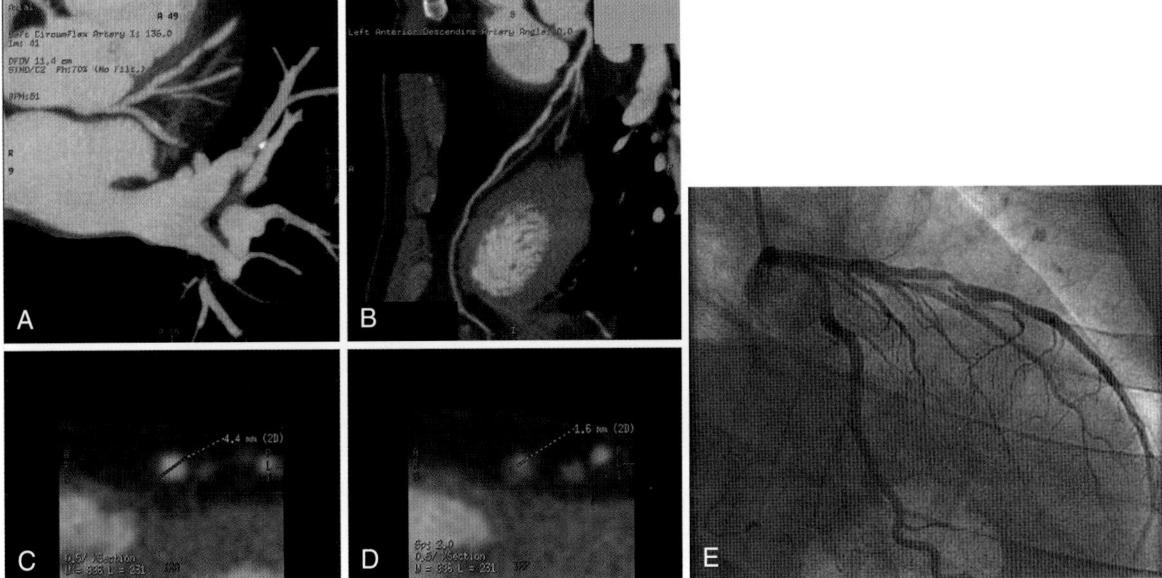

Figure 6-9. Same patient as Figure 6-8. A maximum intensity projection image (**A**) and a curved multiplanar reformatted image (**B**) demonstrate a moderate to severe soft plaque lesion within the mid-left anterior descending artery (LAD). Cross-sectional evaluation of the lesion is seen in **C** and **D**. Quantitative analysis suggests an intermediate severity lesion at 60% to 70%. Selective angiography (**E**) of the left coronary artery confirms the 60% to 70% mid-LAD lesion. A fractional flow or reserve (FFR) evaluation across the lesion demonstrated an FFR of 0.90, not significant. See Figures 6-8 and 6-10 and **Videos 6-9 through 6-12.**

- There is no correlation between stenosis difference and stenosis severity.[44]
- Lack of temporal resolution seems to be responsible for some cases in which coronary CTA is not sensitive to angiographic stenosis.[6]
- Use of segment comparison versus vessel comparison (one-, two-, or three-vessel disease) or patient comparison (diseased or not) provides an increase of the data that improves the significance of correlations but that does translate on a per patient basis.[60]
- Small vessels tend to be underrepresented due to partial volume averaging effects[61] and their common exclusion from studies.

The use of IVUS as a standard is understandable, but IVUS is not without imaging challenges. Determining the inner margin of the stenosis is usually straightforward, but determination of the outer margin of a plaque may be very difficult if the plaque is thick or dense with calcium. Establishing the outer elastic lamina by IVUS so as to determine plaque area or volume becomes

Text continued on page 56

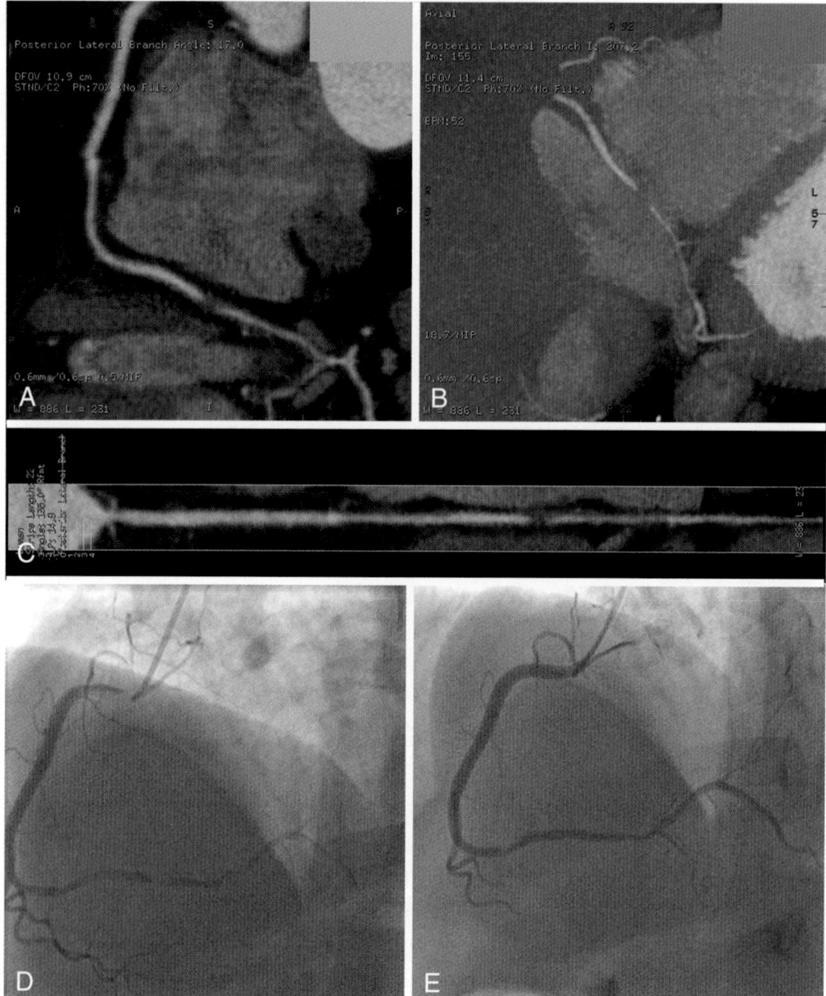

Figure 6-10. Same patient as Figure 6-8. Reformatted multiplanar (**A** and **B**) and vessel extraction (**C**) images through the right coronary artery (RCA) demonstrate a severe soft plaque stenosis with subtotal occlusion of the distal RCA. The patient went on to have conventional angiography. Selective injection of the RCA demonstrated a corresponding severe stenosis of the distal RCA (**D**). The patient went on to have successful percutaneous transluminal coronary angioplasty of the lesion (**E**). See Figures 6-8 and 6-9 and **Videos 6-9 through 6-12.**

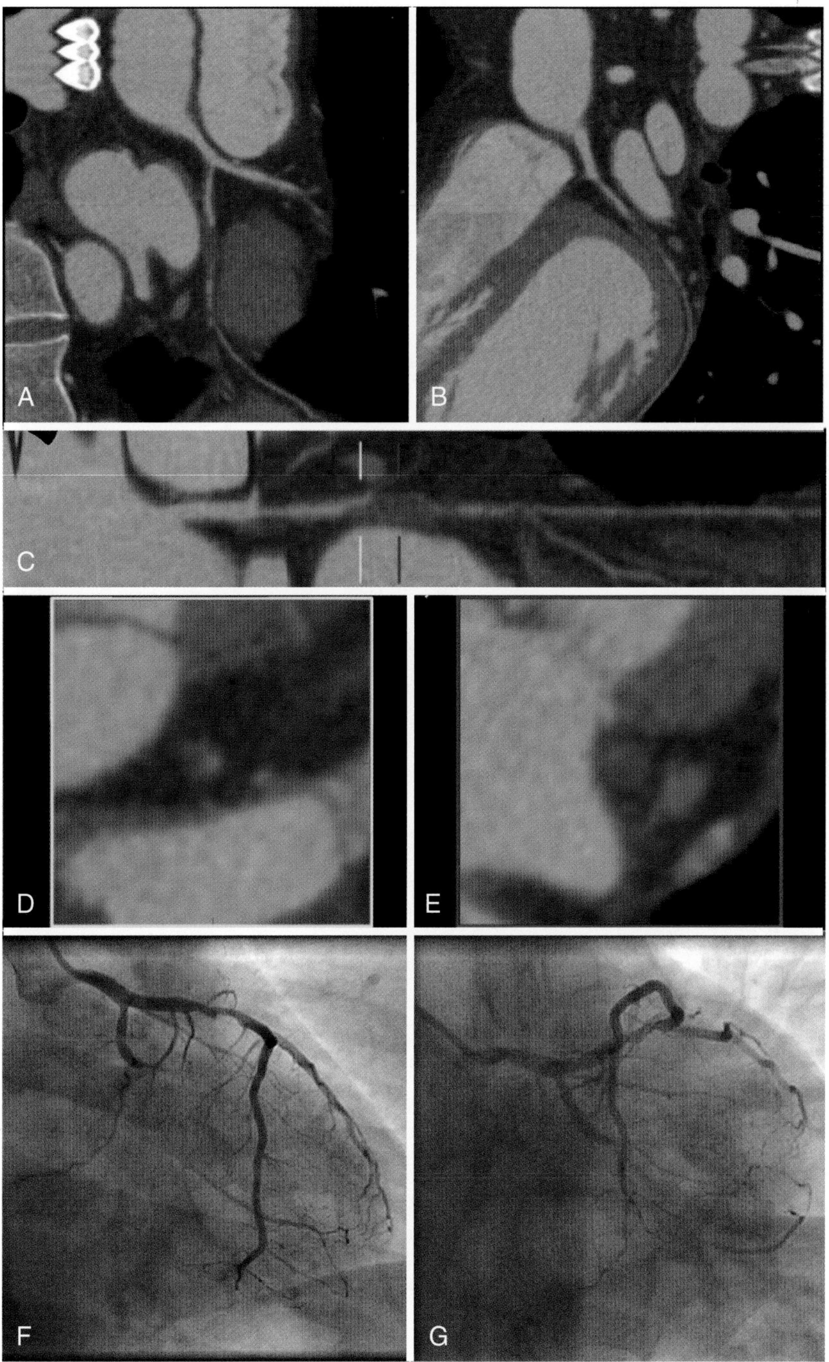

Figure 6-11. A 52-year-old man presented to the emergency department with chest pain, nonspecific ECG changes, and a mild increase in serum troponin levels. **A** and **B,** Curved multiplanar reconstruction images demonstrate an occlusion or high-grade stenosis in the proximal circumflex artery. The straightened view (**C**), with corresponding cross-sectional views (**D** and **E**) demonstrate partial and then no contrast within the lumen, more in keeping with an occlusion. The patient underwent emergent coronary angiography (**F** and **G**), confirming the finding of an occluded circumflex artery. He also has mild left anterior descending artery disease. **See Videos 6-13 and 6-14.**

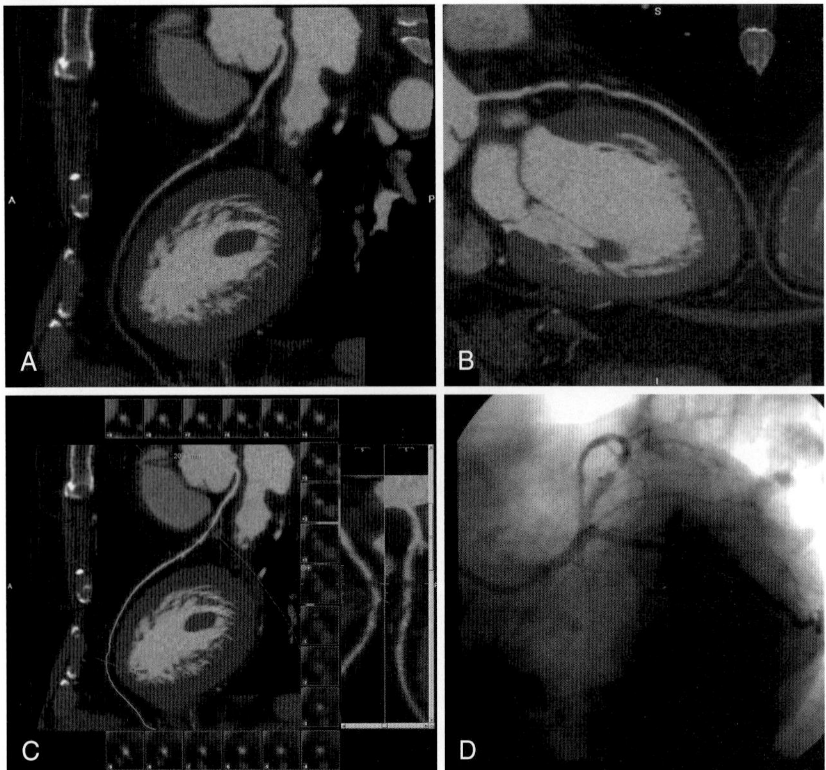

Figure 6-12. Curved mutliplanar reconstructions and intravenous ultrasound (IVUS) views of the left anterior descending (LAD) artery demonstrate a severe lesion in the mid-LAD. On the curved multiplanar reconstructions (**A** and **B**) it appears to be 100%. By the IVUS views (**C**) there is a spot of contrast, indicating a small lumen. The angiographic view (**D**) reveals the lesion to be 95%.

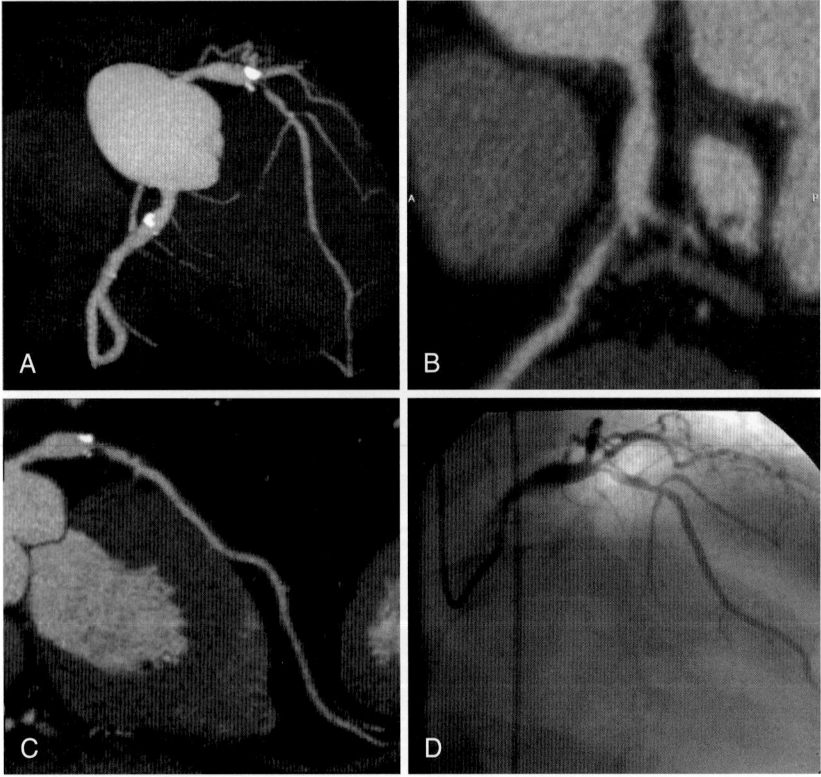

Figure 6-13. A 62-year-old man with chest pain. His cardiac CT images demonstrate mild to moderate narrowing of the proximal left main coronary artery followed by moderate ectasia of the mid-to distal left main coronary artery. The distal left main coronary artery has a moderate amount of calcification. There is a severe ostial stenosis, which is primarily soft plaque in etiology, of the left anterior descending (LAD) artery that is 70% to 80% in severity. The corresponding conventional angiogram (**D**) demonstrates selective catheterization of the left coronary artery and confirms the findings seen on cardiac CT, with ectasia of the distal left main coronary artery, and a severe 80% ostial LAD stenosis. See Figure 6-14 and **Videos 6-15 and 6-16.**

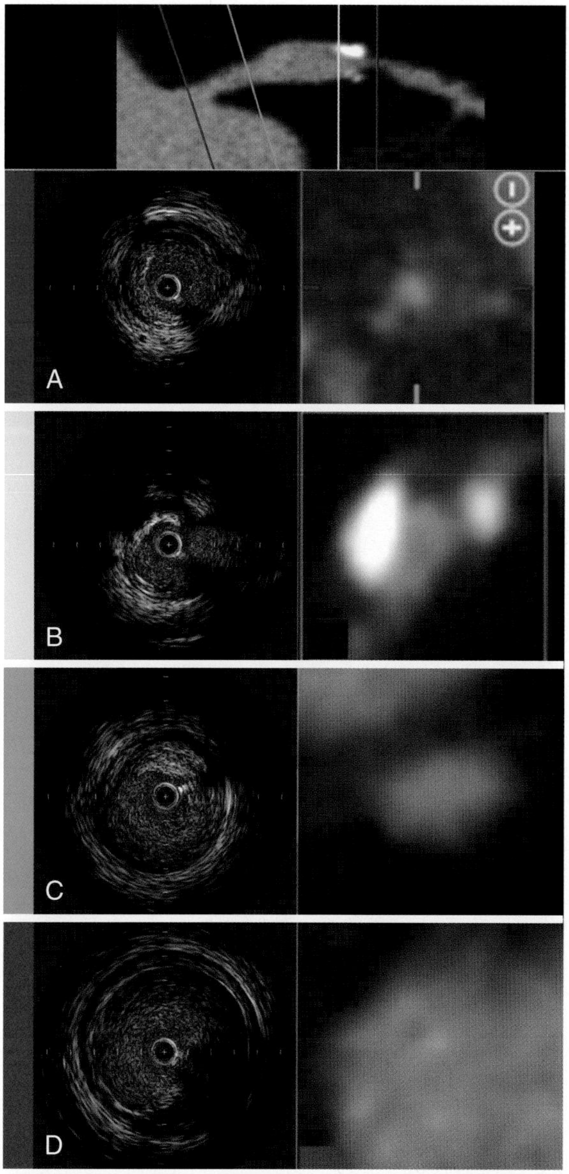

Figure 6-14. Same patient as Figure 6-13. This figure attempts to correlate cross-sectional views from a cardiac CT study with an intravenous ultrasound (IVUS) study performed at the time of conventional angiography. The paired IVUS and cross-sectional CT images are color-coded, and correspond with the points of acquisition marked on the curve multiplanar reformation at the top of the figure. **A,** Severe ostial LAD stenosis, which is almost completely soft plaque in etiology. **B,** Moderate calcium within the distal left main coronary artery, seen as peripheral curvilinear echogenicity with posterior shadowing on the IVUS image. **C,** Image obtained in the mid-left main coronary artery demonstrates mild eccentric soft plaque. **D,** Image obtained at the left main ostium/ascending aorta demonstrates no plaque. See Figure 6-13 and **Videos 6-15 and 6-16.**

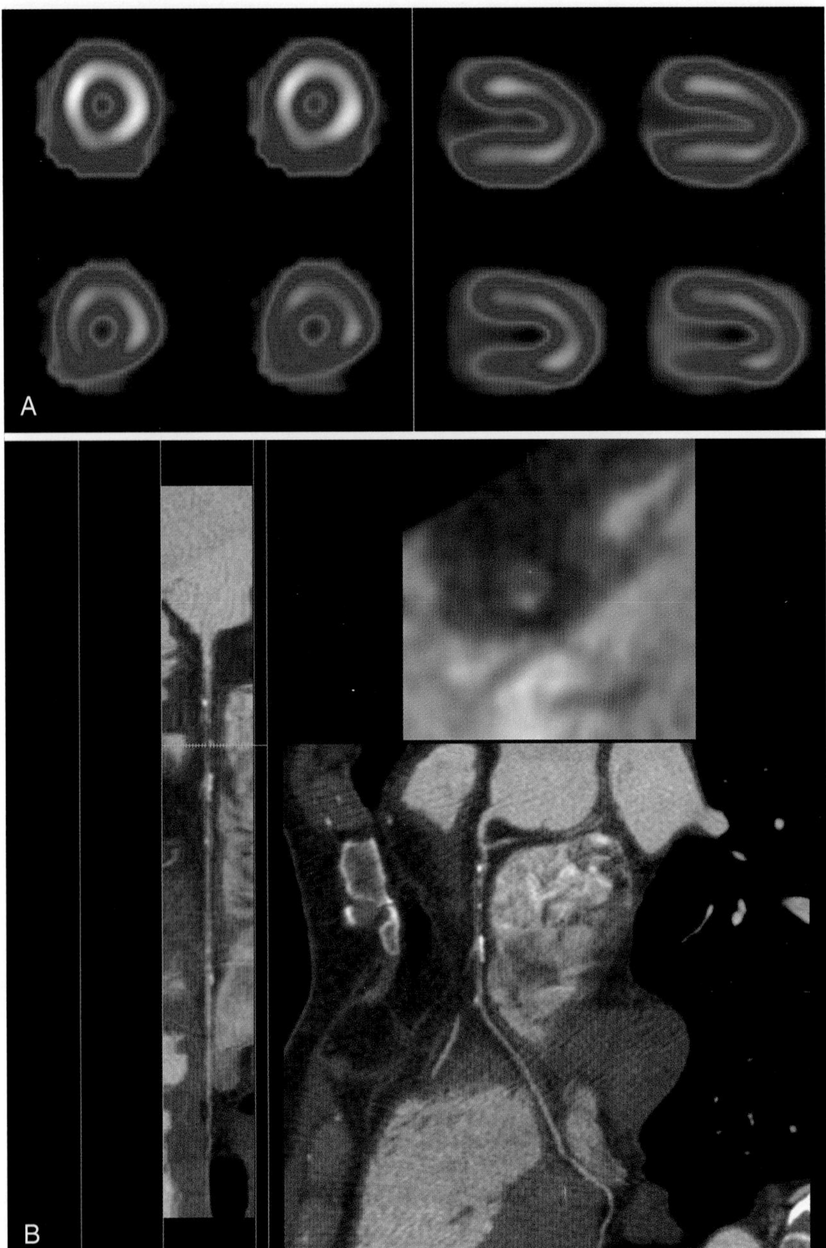

Figure 6-15. A 68-year-old man presented with typical angina and shortness of breath on exertion. A nuclear medicine perfusion study (**A**) demonstrated a moderate-sized reversible defect involving the basal to mid-inferior wall. The patient was referred for CT angiography (**B**), which demonstrated proximal occlusion of the right coronary artery by an elongated complex lesion made up of soft and calcified plaque.

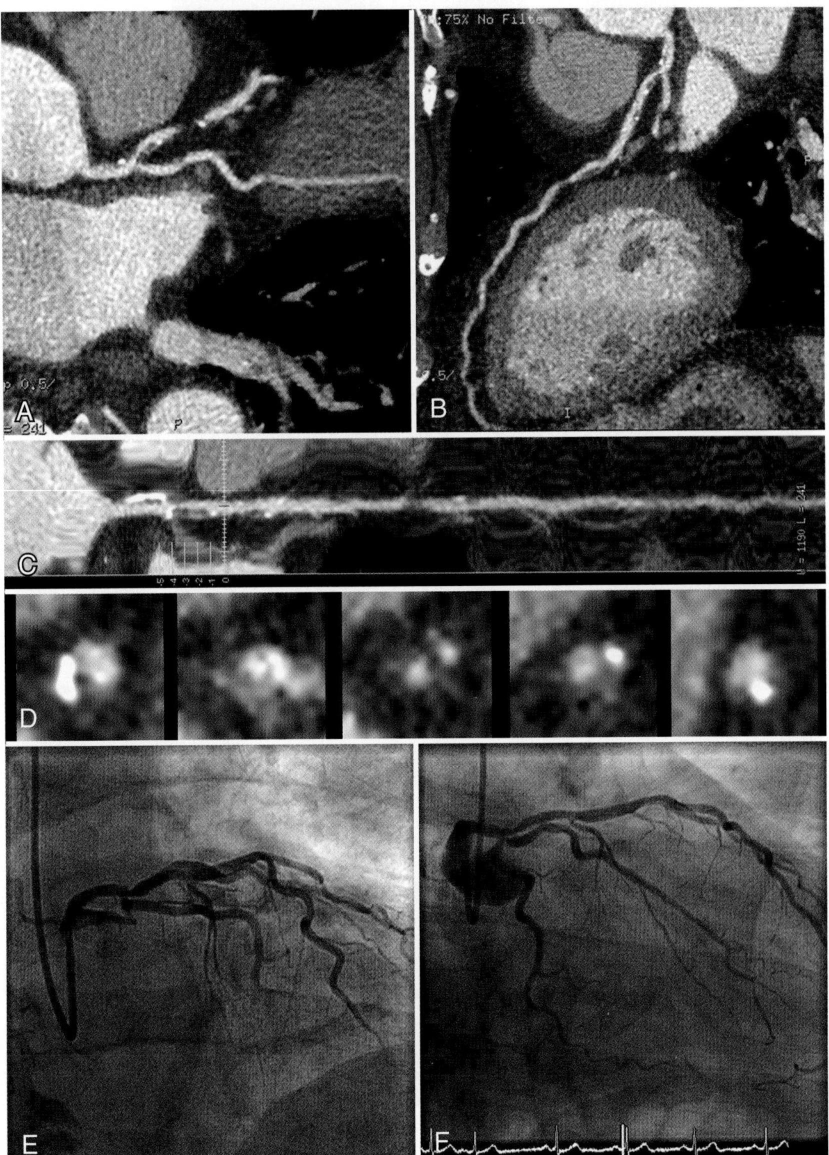

Figure 6-16. A 69-year-old man with a history of chest pain. **A** and **B,** CPR views of the left anterior descending artery (LAD) demonstrate a severe 70% ostial LAD stenosis. The mid-LAD lesion (**B**) represents misregistration artifact. A clean straight line is seen extending through the coronary artery, and into the adjacent soft tissues. **C** and **D**, Straightened view and corresponding cross-sections below it demonstrate mixed plaque extending from the distal left main coronary artery to the LAD. The linear demarcation on the straightened view (**C**) corresponds with the cross-sectional views (**D**). **E** and **F,** The patient went on to conventional angiography. Selective injection of the left coronary artery confirms the severe ostial LAD stenosis. **See Videos 6-17 and 6-18.**

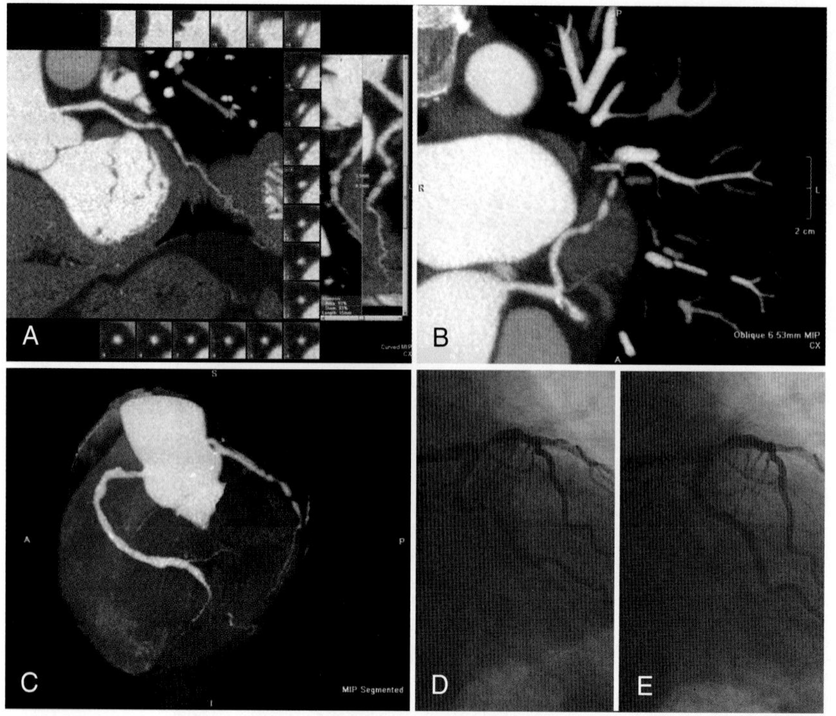

Figure 6-17. A 55-year-old man presented to the emergency department with atypical chest pain and nonspecific ECG changes. CT angiographic maximum intensity projection and curved reformatted images (**A**, **B**, **C**) demonstrate multiple lesions within a large obtuse marginal branch. The proximal-most lesion is moderate, at 50%. The subsequent two lesions are severe, one at 80% and the other greater than 90%. The two severe lesions in the midportion of this obtuse marginal branch demonstrate an interposing segment of dilatation, and are constituted entirely by soft plaque. The patient was sent for coronary angiography. **D** demonstrates these two severe tandem lesions within the obtuse marginal branch, correlating well with the CTA. Angioplasty and stenting of the obtuse marginal branch were then carried out with a good result (**E**). See Figure 6-18.

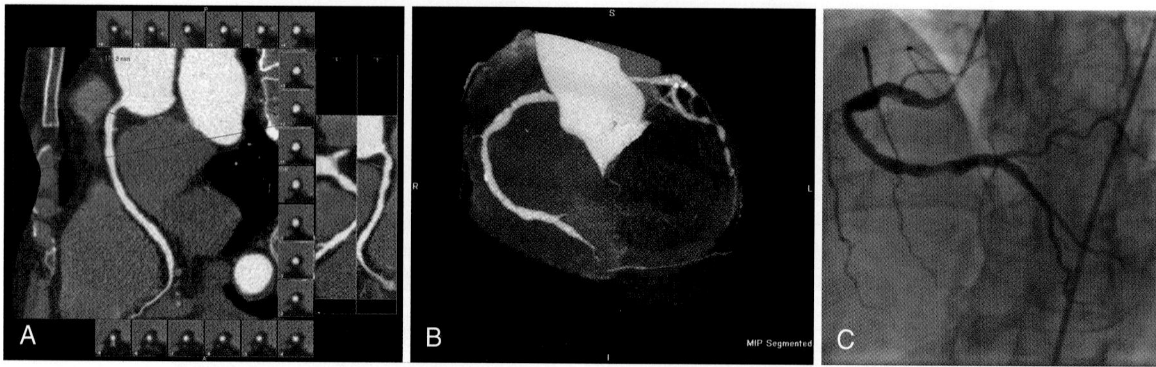

Figure 6-18. Same patient as Figure 6-17. The CT angiographic maximum intensity projection (**B**) and curved reformatted images (**A**) demonstrate mild to moderate atherosclerotic ectasia of the proximal to mid-right coronary artery (RCA), but no evidence of a significant RCA stenosis. Severe OM1 stenoses were identified.

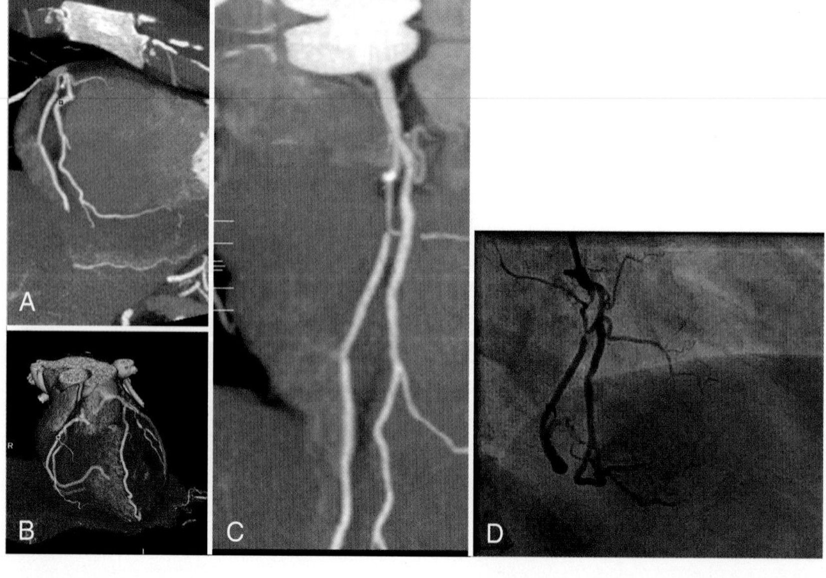

Figure 6-19. A 53-year-old man presented with atypical chest pain and multiple risk factors. A myocardial perfusion study demonstrated a possible mild anterior defect. Multiple reconstructed images through the right coronary artery (RCA) from a cardiac CT study demonstrate an unusual variant of RCA anatomy (**A**–**C**). The posterolateral branch arises from the proximal RCA and extends into the intraventricular groove. There is a severe (>70%) stenosis in the proximal portion of this posterolateral branch. The RCA demonstrates mild irregularity, but no evidence of a stenosis. These findings are confirmed on the left anterior oblique projection of the patient's conventional coronary angiogram (**D**). See Figures 6-20 and 6-21 and **Videos 6-19 through 6-21.**

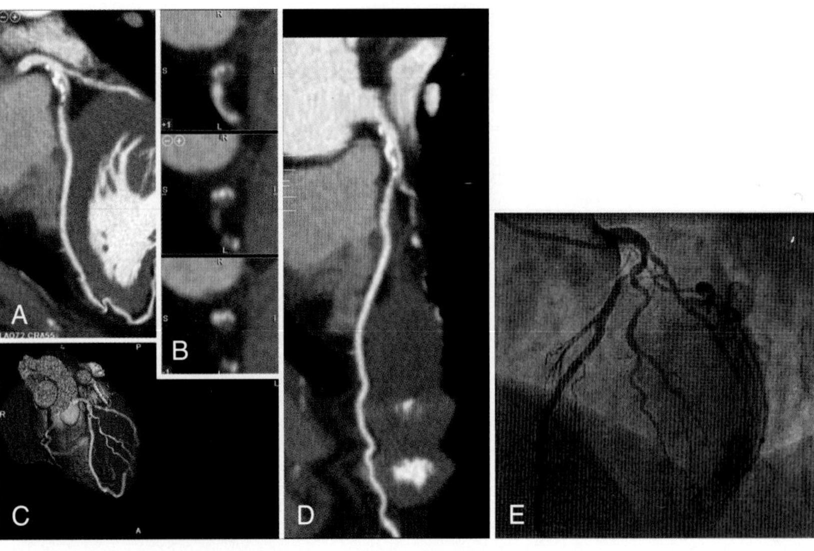

Figure 6-20. Same patient as Figure 6-19. A myocardial perfusion imaging study demonstrated a possible mild anterior defect. Multiple reconstructed images through the left anterior descending (LAD) artery demonstrate complex plaque within the proximal LAD. (**A–D**). At the level of the first diagonal branch takeoff there is a severe mixed plaque stenosis greater than 70%. The LAD is a large type III vessel (**A**), coursing well around the apex of the left ventricle. The severe proximal to mid-LAD stenosis is confirmed on the conventional angiogram (**E**). See Figures 6-19 and 6-21 and **Videos 6-19 through 6-21.**

Figure 6-21. Same patient as Figure 6-19. A myocardial perfusion imaging study demonstrated a possible mild anterior defect. Multiple reconstructed images through the proximal circumflex artery demonstrate mixed plaque in the ostial/proximal circumflex artery causing a 50% stenosis. The corresponding conventional angiogram at the bottom of this figure confirms a 50% ostial circumflex artery stenosis. See Figures 6-19 and 6-20 and **Videos 6-19 through 6-21.**

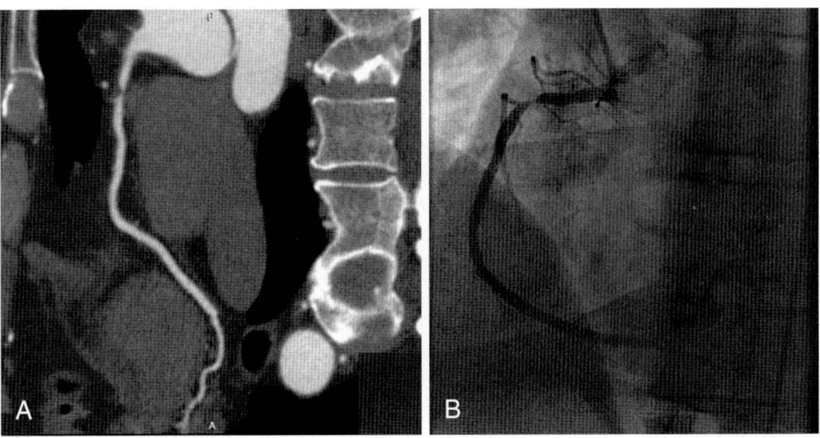

Figure 6-22. CTA (**A**) and matching conventional angiography (**B**) of a patient with a severe stenosis of the proximal right coronary artery.

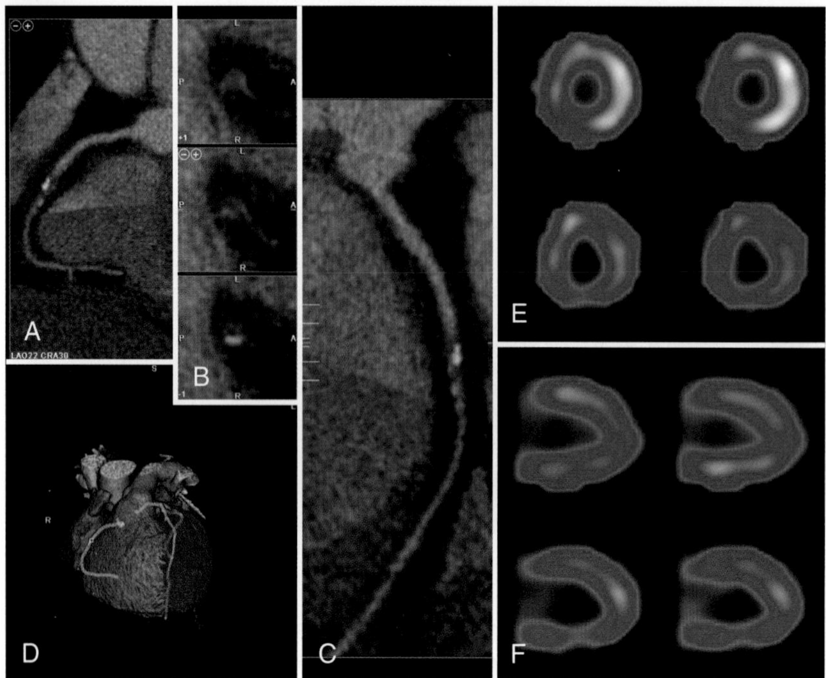

Figure 6-23. **A** through **D,** Contrast-enhanced cardiac CT curved multiplanar reformatted and intravenous ultrasound images demonstrating occlusion of the mid-right coronary artery due to mixed plaque. **E** through **F,** Myocardial perfusion scanning revealing an associated reversible inferior defect.

increasingly difficult as the artery is increasingly diseased with plaque. Hence, some of the lack of correlation of CTA observations with IVUS is intrinsic to the limitations of CTA, but some is intrinsic to the limitations of IVUS (Fig. 6-24). In one case, an unusual cause of coronary stenosis—a surgical suture—was detected by CCT (Fig. 6-25).

REPORTING OF CORONARY ARTERY STENOSIS SEVERITY

Numerous reporting schemes have been employed to convey the severity of coronary artery stenosis.

❒ Visual estimate of the percent of stenosis:
- The lack of highly reliable correlation with conventional angiography percent stenosis estimates dampens enthusiasm for reporting by percent stenosis.
- However, supporters advocate use of percent stenosis on the basis of anticipation of better correlation with newer scanners, of intention to achieve good correlation, and of recognition of the clinical implications of potential for miscategorization if categories are used.

❒ There are variations in quartile description of stenoses (Table 6-11).

"Significant" is often defined as stenosis of more than 50% of the diameter and "severe" as stenosis of 70% to 75% of the diameter. This differs, however, from general coronary angiography, where "significant" is applied to lesions greater than 70%, except for the left main stem coronary artery, where "significant" means stenosis of more than 50%.

Issues with Catheter Estimates of Coronary Stenosis Severity

It is important to recall how imperfectly catheter-based angiography correlates with itself: interobserver laboratory variability: 10.4%[64]; interobserver variability: 11.2%[64]; and intraobserver correlation of visual assessment of catheter-based angiography and of QCA (percent stenosis: ±5%,[64] minimal luminal diameter: ±0.15–0.28 mm).[64] Furthermore, the visual angiographic estimate of coronary stenosis severity and QCA estimate of coronary stenosis severity do not necessarily correlate with fractional flow reserve determination of flow limitation, especially for lesions of moderate severity.[65] Interobserver concordance tends to be poor (Spearman 0.36). For moderate lesions, visual estimate achieves good sensitivity (80%) and negative predictive value (91%) but poorer specificity (47%) and even less positive predictive value (25%) when compared with fractional flow reserve.[65] "Frame bias" has been shown to significantly affect the variability of QCA coronary stenosis severity estimate in PCI.[66] The use of different catheters (8F versus 6F) as the reference diameter confers variability to the QCA estimate of coronary stenosis severity (coefficient of variation 18.5% for minimal luminal diameter, 10.4% for percent stenosis).[65] Contrary to expectation, experience in angiographic assessment does not necessarily continue to improve observer accuracy.[67]

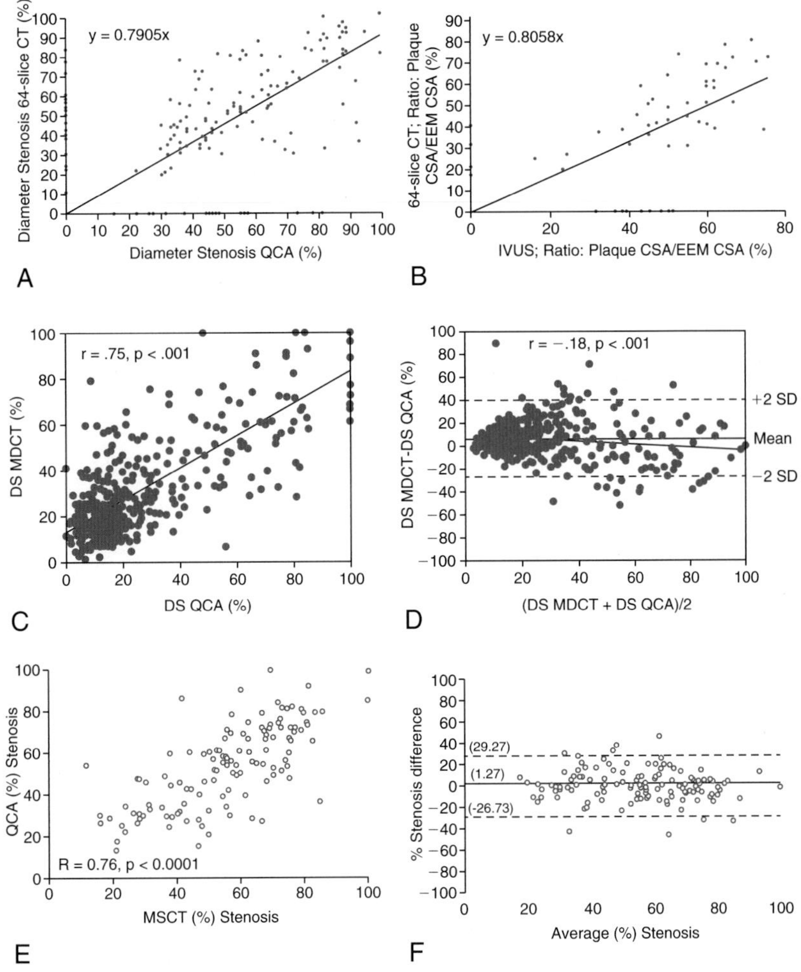

Figure 6-24. **A** and **B,** 64-slice CT angiography (CTA). **A,** The diameter stenosis by multidetector CT (MDCT) correlates with those obtained by catheter-based quantitative coronary analysis (QCA) assessment ($r = 0.54$), but tend to be 20% less. **B,** CTA plaque versus intravenous ultrasound (IVUS) plaque ($r = 0.61$). CTA estimates the plaque area to be, on average, 9% less than by IVUS. **C** and **D,** 16-slice CTA. Quantitative coronary CTA correlates with QCA (0.75; $P < .001$), and significantly improves the diagnostic accuracy (receiver operator characteristic area under the curve [AUC] 0.81 versus 0.92; $P < .001$). **E** and **F,** 64-Slice CTA. Plaque volumes by MDCT correlate with those by catheter-based QCA assessment ($r = 0.76$; $P < .0001$), but coronary CTA systematically underestimates volume. Lower right plot: Bland-Altman analysis, where the solid line indicates systematic error (the mean difference is 1.3 ± 14.2%) and the hatched lines indicate 95% agreement. There is no correlation between stenosis difference and stenosis severity. 92% of observations are within 25% error. CSA, cross-sectional area; DS MDCT, diameter stenosis MDCT; DS QCA, diameter stenosis quantitative coronary angiography; EEM, external elastic lamina; MSCT, multislice computed tomography. (**A** and **B** reprinted with permission from Leber AW, Knez A, von Ziegler F, et al. Quantification of obstructive and nonobstructive coronary lesions by 64-slice computed tomography: a comparative study with quantitative coronary angiography and intravascular ultrasound. *J Am Coll Cardiol.* 2005;46(1):147-154; **C** and **D** reprinted with permission from Kefer J, Coche E, Legros G, et al. Head-to-head comparison of three-dimensional navigator-gated magnetic resonance imaging and 16-slice computed tomography to detect coronary artery stenosis in patients. *J Am Coll Cardiol.* 2005;46(1):92-100; **E** and **F** reprinted with permission from Raff GL, Gallagher MJ, O'Neill WW, Goldstein JA. Diagnostic accuracy of noninvasive coronary angiography using 64-slice spiral computed tomography. *J Am Coll Cardiol.* 2005;46(3):552-557.)

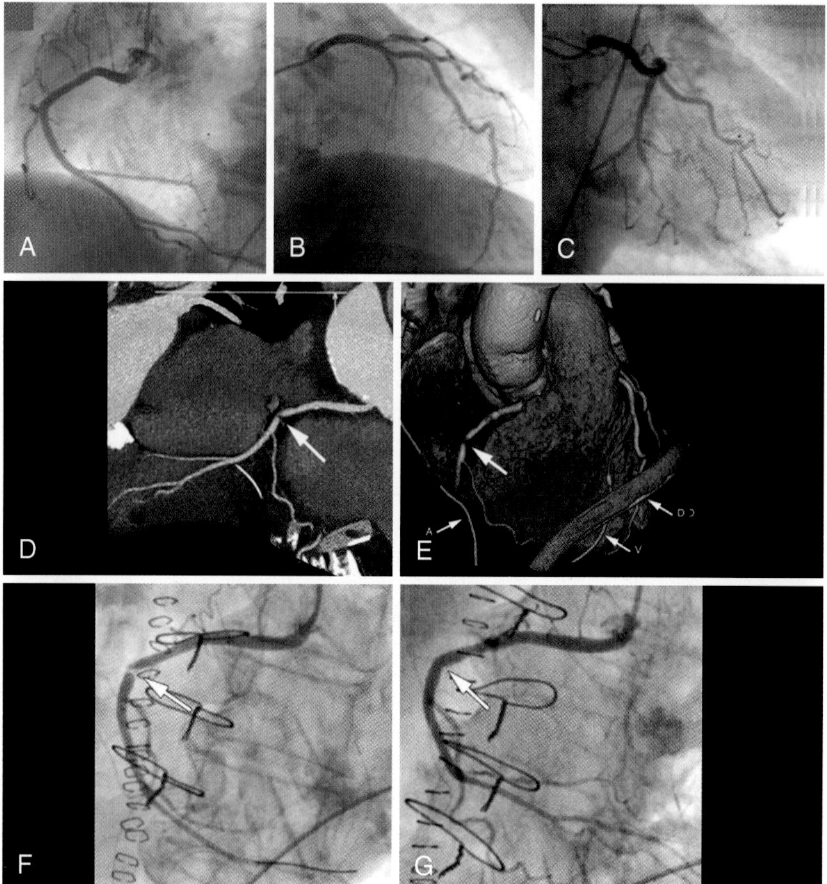

Figure 6-25. **A** through **C,** Presurgical coronary angiogram that showed the absence of coronary artery stenoses. **A,** Right coronary artery. **B,** Left anterior descending coronary artery. **C,** Left circumflex coronary artery. **D** and **E,** Stenosis of the right coronary artery in coronary CT angiography performed on the fifth postoperative day. **D,** Multiplanar curved reconstruction of the right coronary artery in a coronary CT angiogram shows a high-grade, eccentric coronary artery stenosis *(arrow)* proximal to the right ventricular branch. **E,** Three-dimensional visualization of the right coronary artery stenosis (*large arrow*). Atrial temporary epicardial pacing lead (A); ventricular temporary epicardial pacing lead (V); pericardial drain (D). **F** and **G:** Invasive coronary angiography and percutaneous intervention performed after the CT angiogram. The right coronary artery stenosis is confirmed (**F,** *arrow*) and successfully treated by stent implantation (**G**). The suture had been placed to close an atrial cannulation site. (Reprinted with permission from Seltmann M, Achenbach S, Muschiol G, Feyrer R. Suture-induced right coronary artery stenosis. *J Cardiovasc Comput Tomogr.* 2010;4(3):215-217.)

TABLE 6-11 Quartile Descriptors of Stenosis Severity

BASIC QUARTILES (%)	ADAPTED QUARTILES (%)	OTHER[62] (%)	2008 KEY DATA ELEMENTS AND DEFINITIONS FOR CARDIAC IMAGING REPORT[63] (%)
<25	<25	Normal appearing: 0–24	Normal
26–50	26–50	Mild: 25–49	<50
51–75	51–70	Moderate: 50–74	50–70
76–100	71–100	Severe: ≥75	>70–99
			Occluded

Visual estimates may achieve better correlation than caliper estimates.[68] Agreement tends to be better for proximal coronary segments than distal coronary segments[68] and worse for moderate lesions.

Humblingly, there is poor correlation between the physiologic assessment of intermediate coronary stenoses (determined by fractional flow reserve) and the anatomic assessment by both visual and quantitative assessment of both coronary angiography and coronary CTA. The diagnostic accuracy in detecting a hemodynamically significant lesion (FFR < 0.75) for the different modalities and modes of interpretation is presented in Table 6-12.[69]

There is poor correlation of the physiologic assessment of intermediate coronary stenoses (determined by fractional flow reserve) with

TABLE 6-12 Diagnostic Accuracy to Detect a Hemodynamically Significant Coronary Lesion by Modality

MODALITY/TECHNIQUE	DIAGNOSTIC ACCURACY (%)
CTCA visual estimate	49
Quantitative CTCA	71
Coronary angiography—visual estimate	61
Quantitative coronary angiography	67

CTCA, CT coronary angiography.

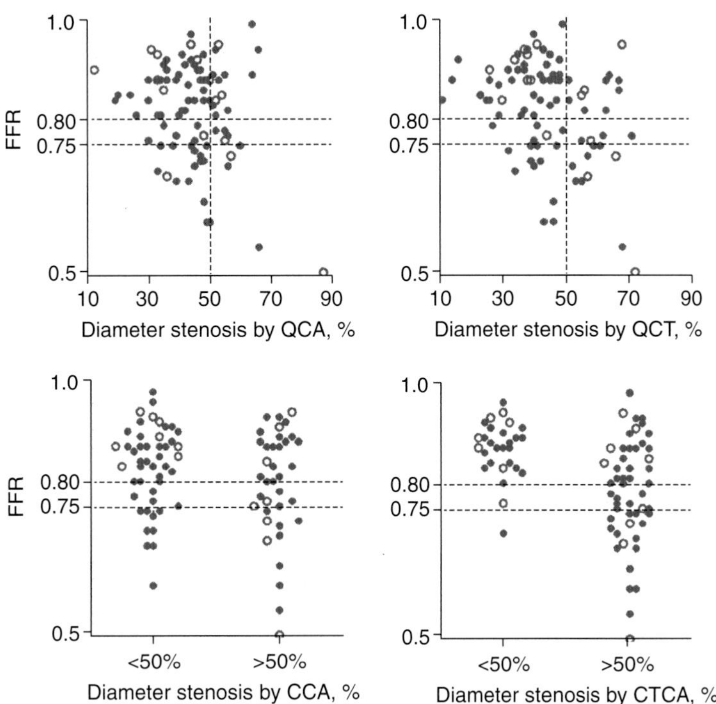

Figure 6-26. Scatter plots of fractional flow or reserve (FFR) versus quantitative coronary angiography (QCA), quantitative computed tomography (QCT), conventional coronary angiography (CCA), and CT coronary angiography (CTCA). QCA, coronary angiography CCA, and CTCA are plotted versus FFR. There was a weak, but significant, negative correlation between QCA and FFR ($r = -0.30$) and between QCT and FFR ($r = -0.32$). Coronary arteries smaller than 3.5 mm are depicted as solid circles; coronary arteries larger than 3.5 mm are indicated as open circles. (Reprinted with permission from Meijboom WB, Van Mieghem CA, van Pelt N, et al. Comprehensive assessment of coronary artery stenoses: computed tomography coronary angiography versus conventional coronary angiography and correlation with fractional flow reserve in patients with stable angina. *J Am Coll Cardiol.* 2008;52(8):636-643.)

anatomic assessment by both visual and quantitative assessment of both coronary angiography and coronary CTA. The diagnostic accuracies in detecting a hemodynamically significant lesion (FFR < 0.75) for the different modalities and modes of interpretation are as follows:

- Coronary angiography—visual estimate: 61%
- Coronary angiography—quantitative: 67%
- Coronary CT angiography—visual estimate: 49%
- Coronary CT angiography—quantitative: 71%

Ultimately, image analysis of coronary stenosis severity by catheter technique, CTA, or MRI inevitably entails degrees of variability (Figs. 6-26 and 6-27). The variability of catheter-based determinations of coronary stenosis severity must be remembered when considering CTA correlation with catheter-based angiography used as the "gold" or reference standard.

CHARACTERIZATION OF CORONARY LESION AND ARTERIES

Coronary Plaque Volume (Fig. 6-28)

- When compared with IVUS, 64-CCT is able to quantify coronary arterial plaque volume with good correlation ($r^2 = 0.69$) and fair-to-moderate interobserver variability (37%) in patients subjected to the usual exclusions and inclusions. 16-CCT studies demonstrate substantial underestimation of plaque volume by CCT (24 ± 35 mm^3 versus 43 ± 60 mm^3, $P < .001$).[19]

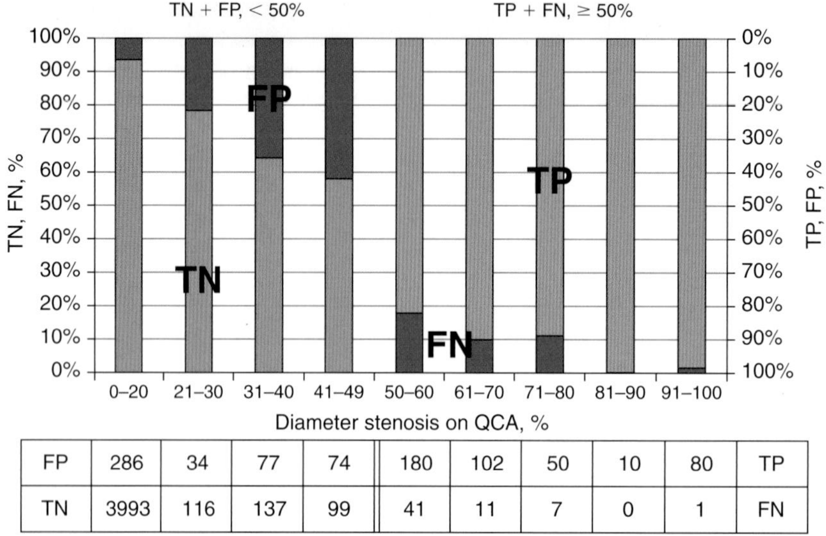

FP	286	34	77	74	180	102	50	10	80	TP
TN	3993	116	137	99	41	11	7	0	1	FN

Figure 6-27. Diagnostic performance of CT coronary angiography (CTCA) per segmental analysis categorized by diameter stenoses on quantitative coronary angiography (QCA). In the graph, the diagnostic performance of CTCA is shown according to various diameter stenoses as measured by QCA in a per-segment analysis. The absolute number of segments per stenosis category is shown in the table. The highest frequency of overestimated (FF) and underestimated (FN) coronary stenoses by CTCA was clustered around the cutoff value of 50% diameter reduction (significant coronary stenosis). FN, false negative; FP, false positive; TN, true negative; TP, true positive. (Reprinted with permission from Meijboom WB, Meijs MF, Schuijf JD, et al. Diagnostic accuracy of 64-slice computed tomography coronary angiography: a prospective, multicenter, multivendor study. *J Am Coll Cardiol.* 2008;52(25):2135-2144.)

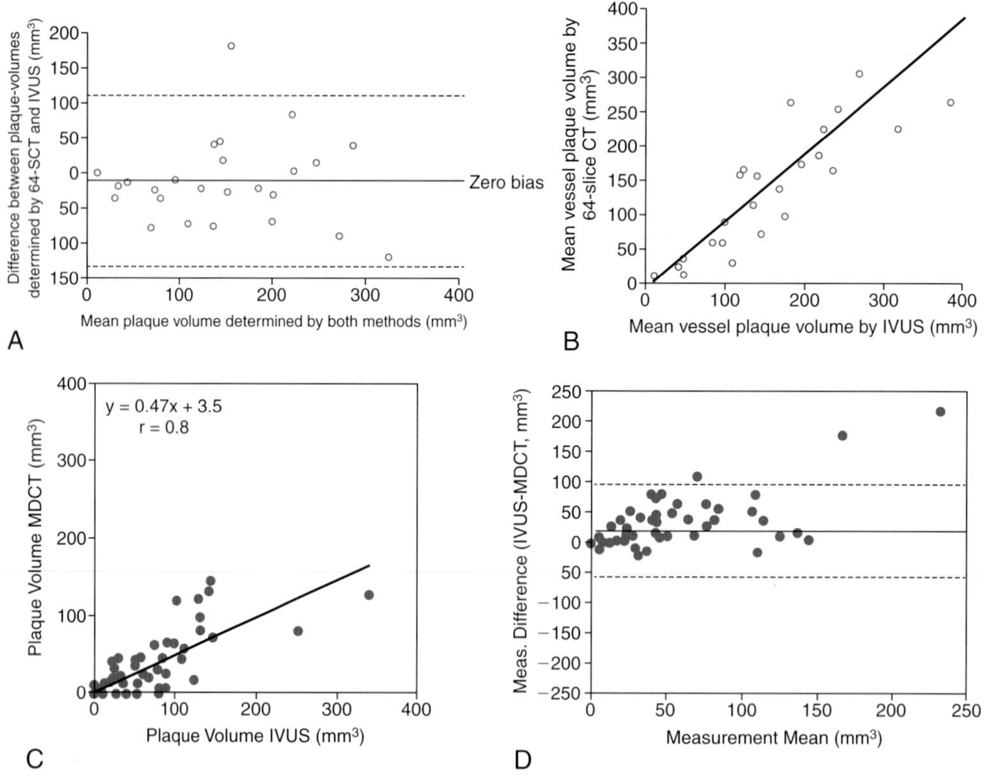

Figure 6-28. Bland-Altman (**A**) and correlation graph (**B**) for plaque volumes per vessel determined by intravascular ultrasound (IVUS) versus 64-slice computed tomography (SCT). Vessel plaque volume is underestimated systematically by 64-slice computed tomography ($P < .05$), and correlation is moderate (Spearman correlation coefficient $r^2 = 0.69$). **C** and **D,** Plaque volumes by multidetector CT correlate with those by intravenous ultrasound assessment ($r = 0.8$; $P < .001$), but coronary CT angiography systematically underestimates volume. **D,** Bland-Altman analysis. The solid line represents systematic error (the mean difference is 19 mm^3); the hatched lines indicate 95% agreement. (**A** and **B** reprinted with permission from Leber AW, Knez A, von Ziegler F, et al. Quantification of obstructive and nonobstructive coronary lesions by 64-slice computed tomography: a comparative study with quantitative coronary angiography and intravascular ultrasound. *J Am Coll Cardiol.* 2005;46(1):147-154; **C** and **D** reprinted with permission from Achenbach S, Moselewski F, Ropers D, et al. Detection of calcified and noncalcified coronary atherosclerotic plaque by contrast-enhanced, submillimeter multidetector spiral computed tomography: a segment-based comparison with intravascular ultrasound. *Circulation.* 2004;109(1):14-17.)

Coronary Arterial Remodeling

- The earliest reports on plaque differences in acute infarction versus stable angina patients were generated from electron beam CT (EBCT) technology[70] but have been corroborated by CCT.[71]
- A remodeling ratio great than 1.05 (Glagovian remodeling) at the site of a lesion is more than twice as likely to be seen in unstable lesions, whereas a remodeling ratio of less than 0.9 is nearly twice as likely to be seen in stable lesions.[72]
- By virtue of imaging lumen, plaque, and outer wall, CCT is able to image arterial remodeling (and "negative" remodeling) in stenotic and nonstenotic vessel segments.[73]
- CCT findings correlate with angiographic[74] and IVUS findings.[73,75] Lesions responsible for acute coronary syndrome (ACS), when imaged by CCT, appear to have larger cross-sectional areas and greater remodeling indices than other lesions in patients with ACS, and also are greater than those of lesions in patients with stable CSD.[71]

Ability to Exclude Atheromatous Plaque

- The ability of coronary CTA to exclude the presence of atheromatous plaque, compared with the standard of IVUS, is good in selected patients and at selected centers. It is more difficult to exclude noncalcified plaque.
  - 16-CCT
    - 92% of segments correctly excluded[76,77]
      - Sensitivity to detect coronary calcified plaque: 94%[77]
      - Sensitivity to detect exclusively noncalcified plaque: 53%[77]
  - 64-CCT
    - 94% of segments correctly excluded[78]

Coronary Plaque Tissue Characterization

- Image characterization of plaque detail, particularly of plaque calcification, is confounded by high luminal contrast enhancement. Optimal luminal enhancement for plaque characterization is lower than usual (200–250 HU) to permit discrimination of lumen from plaque calcium (Fig. 6-29).
- Characterization of plaque tissue, according to attenuation characteristics (Table 6-13), originally dichotomized plaque as hard versus soft, equating this with calcified and noncalcified. Subsequently, plaque characterization evolved to soft, hard, and calcified. More recently, characterization has attempted to identify scattered micropatterns of calcification as well as gross calcification, and also lipid core areas. The evolution of coronary CT technology from 16-CCT to 64-CCT has enabled more accurate plaque identification and characterization. However, identification still depends on the same technology and still struggles with high signal problems from calcification, such as detector "afterglow," partial volume averaging effect, and the wide range of attenuation characteristics of tissue calcium. The characterization of highly heterogeneous plaque composition generates another category: "mixed."[78] The use of IVUS as a standard engenders some questions about the accuracy of the standard for detecting lipid.

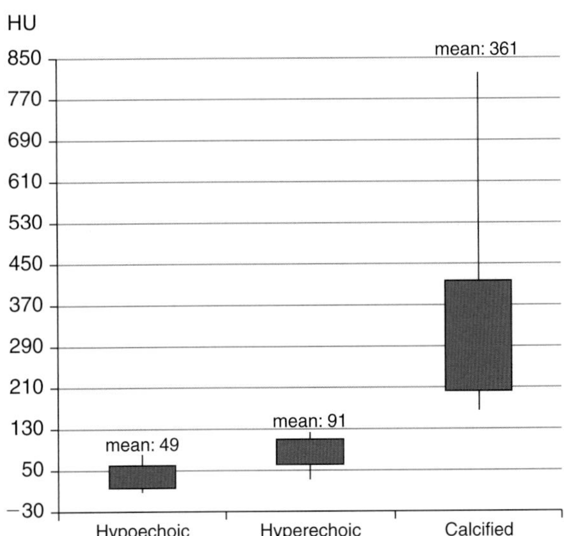

Figure 6-29. CT density values for hypoechoic, hyperechoic, and calcified plaques. Each box describes the distribution of density values within a standard deviation. The "whiskers" above and below each box indicate the range between the lowest and highest observed density value. The differences of the mean CT density values among hypoechoic, hyperechoic, and calcified plaques were significant, with a P value <.02. (Reprinted with permission from Leber AW, Knez A, Becker A, et al. Accuracy of multidetector spiral computed tomography in identifying and differentiating the composition of coronary atherosclerotic plaques: a comparative study with intracoronary ultrasound. *J Am Coll Cardiol.* 2004;43(7):1241-1247.)

TABLE 6-13 Plaque Characterization

	"SOFT" PLAQUE	"HARD" PLAQUE	CALCIFIED PLAQUE	"MIXED" PLAQUE
Other names		Intermediate plaque		
Purported histology and composition	Contains lipid and collagen tissue	Contains collagen tissue	Micro and macro deposits of calcium crystals	
CCT attenuation– "Rule-of-thumb"	<60 HU	60–120 HU	≥120 HU	
16-CCT[79]	14 ± 26 HU	91 ± 21 HU	419 ± 194 HU	
16-CCT[80]	49 ± 22 HU	91 ± 22 HU	391 ± 156 HU	
IVUS, ICUS characterization[79]	Hypoechoic: >80% of the plaque area is composed of tissue with echogenicity less than that of the adventitia	Hypoechoic: >80% of the plaque area is composed of tissue with echogenicity as bright as or brighter than that of the adventita	Calcified plaque involving bright echogenicity with acoustic shadowing accompanying >90° of the vessel wall circumference	
16-CCT visualization and coronary segment characterization versus IVUS[80]	78%	78%	95%	
16-CCT visualization and coronary segment characterization versus IVUS[19]	"Non-calcified" segments 1. Containing noncalcified plaque: sensitivity: 78%, specificity: 87% 2. Exclusively noncalcified: sensitivity: 53%		Non-calcified: sensitivity: 94%, specificity: 94%	
64-CCT visualization and coronary segment characterization versus IVUS[78]	70%	83%	95%	94%

CCT, cardiac CT; ICUS, International Contrast Ultrasound Society; IVUS, intravascular ultrasound.

Plaque Characteristics

- ❒ Calcified ("hard")
- ❒ Fibrous versus noncalcified "soft"
- ❒ Mixed (both calcified and noncalcified)

Coronary Thrombosis

- ❒ Intracoronary thrombus has been imaged by CCT.[81]

Coronary Dissection

- ❒ Spontaneous coronary dissection has been recognized by 16-CCT.[82]

Characterization of Unstable Versus Stable Lesions

- ❒ Characterization of coronary ACS culprit plaques versus stable angina pectoris plaques by 64-CCT reveals differences, particularly in the presence of positive remodeling, in plaque "softness" and the presence of only spotty calcification rather than large calcification in ACS culprit plaques (Figs. 6-30 through 6-37).[83]

CLINICAL APPLICATIONS OF CORONARY CTA

The role(s) of coronary CTA remain undefined. In particular, more prognostic information is needed. Most studies have been small, single center in origin, and more encouraging of ongoing investigation than of establishing a role. Furthermore, the usual exclusions of irregular rhythm, renal insufficiency, and other such variables substantially limit its applicability. The highly limited information on the utility of coronary CTA has lead to the publication of appropriateness criteria, because it is still early for guidelines.

Coronary CTA as a Gatekeeper to Conventional Angiography

It has been proposed, although only with very limited validation, that coronary CTA may be a cost-effective gatekeeper to coronary catheter angiography in patients with mildly abnormal or equivocal myocardial perfusion scans.[84]

Percent	Positive remodeling	NCP <30HU	30HU<NCP <150HU	Spotty calcification	Large calcification
ACS	87	79	100	63	22
SAP	12	9	100	21	55
	p < .0001	p < .0001		P = .0005	P = .004

Figure 6-30. Plaque characteristics of culprit lesions in acute coronary syndrome (ACS) and target lesions in stable angina pectoris (SAP) patient groups. Noncalcified plaques (NCP) <30 HU and spotty calcification were more frequently observed in the culprit ACS lesions. (Reprinted with permission from Motoyama S, Kondo T, Sarai M, et al. Multislice computed tomographic characteristics of coronary lesions in acute coronary syndromes. *J Am Coll Cardiol.* 2007;50(4):319-326.)

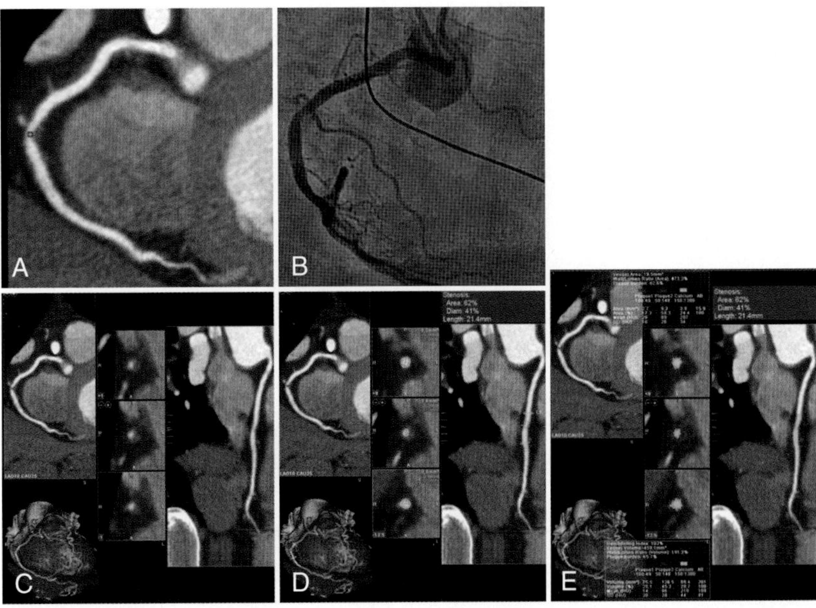

Figure 6-31. A 48-year-old man with atypical chest pain, increased risk factors for coronary artery disease, and left bundle branch block abnormality on an ECG. **A,** A curved reformatted image through the right coronary artery (RCA). Visually, this demonstrated a 30% to 40% mid-RCA stenosis. **B,** A conventional coronary angiogram demonstrates a similar finding. The potential of more quantitative evaluation of the coronary arteries is illustrated in **C** through **E**. **C,** Curved multiplanar reformat and cross-sectional evaluation through the mid-RCA lesion. **D,** An automated quantitative coronary analysis evaluation of the lesion, generating 41% stenosis. **E,** A semiautomated analysis of soft plaque, and plaque burden in this patient. Plaque components are broken down on the basis of their attenuation.

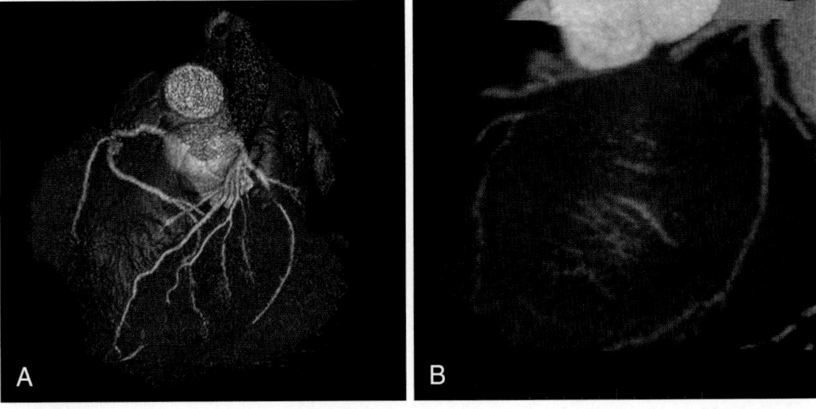

Figure 6-32. Cardiac CT images from a 54-year-old woman with atypical angina and equivocal myocardial perfusion imaging study. **A,** Volume-rendered image of the coronary artery tree. **B,** Maximal intensity projection image. Both these images demonstrate a severe stenosis/near occlusion of the proximal OM1 branch, which is a large vessel.

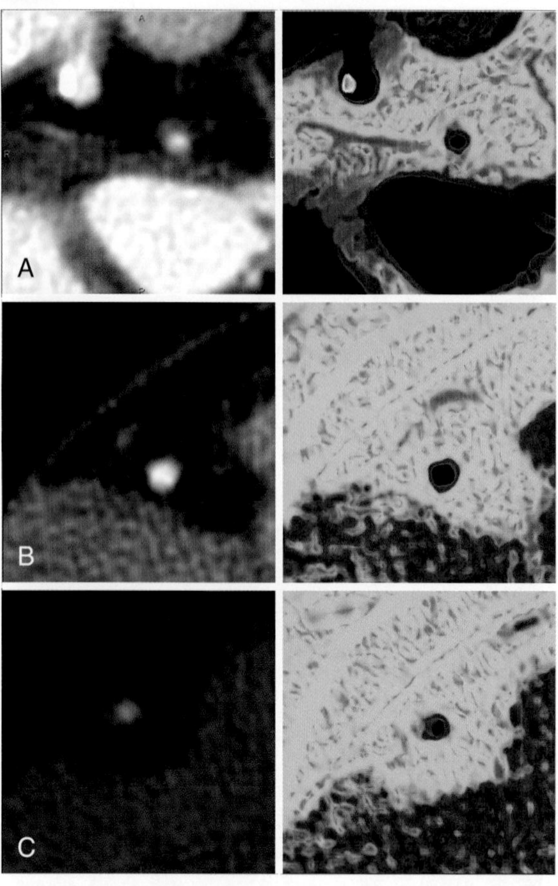

Figure 6-33. Cross-sectional images of the coronary arteries with corresponding intravenous ultrasound type reformations. **A,** A cross section through the left main stem demonstrating a focus of calcified plaque and the proximal left circumflex artery demonstrating a peripheral rim of low-attenuation soft plaque. **B,** A cross section of the mid-right coronary artery (RCA) demonstrating a normal-appearing vessel. **C,** A cross section of the RCA immediately distal to the image of the middle images revealing a mild (30%) stenosis and a moderate-sized peripheral low-attenuation (soft) plaque. The vessel appears to have undergone Glagovian remodeling.

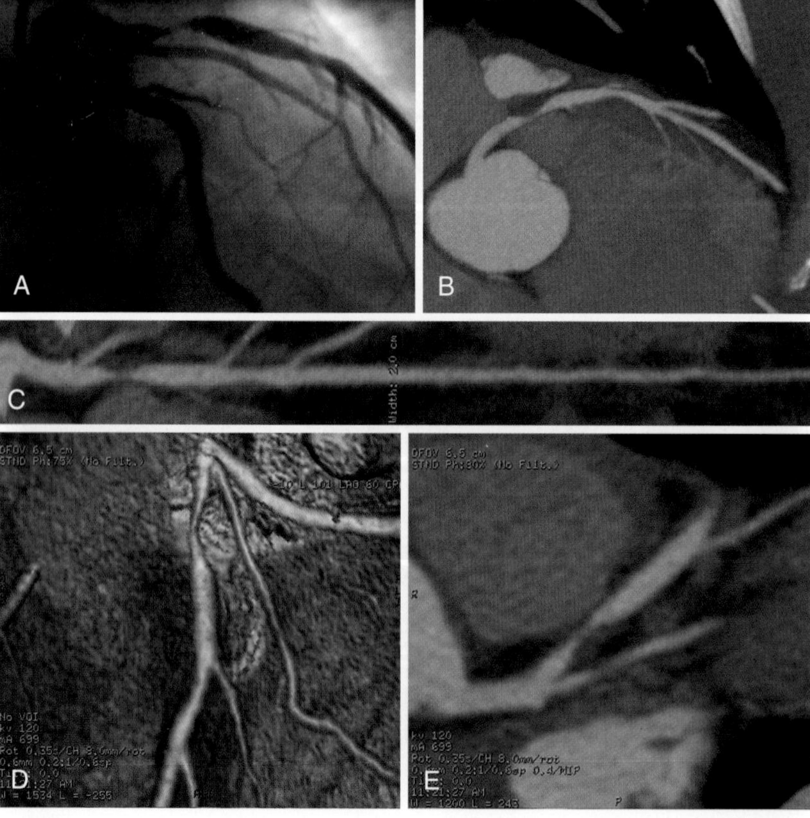

Figure 6-34. Coronary CT angiography (CCTA) of a 38-year-old man with angina on high-level athletic effort. The myocardial perfusion scan was negative, and he had a calcium score of zero. By CCTA, a significant noncalcified plaque is imaged in the proximal left anterior descending artery, which was corroborated by conventional angiography. Stenting eliminated the symptoms.

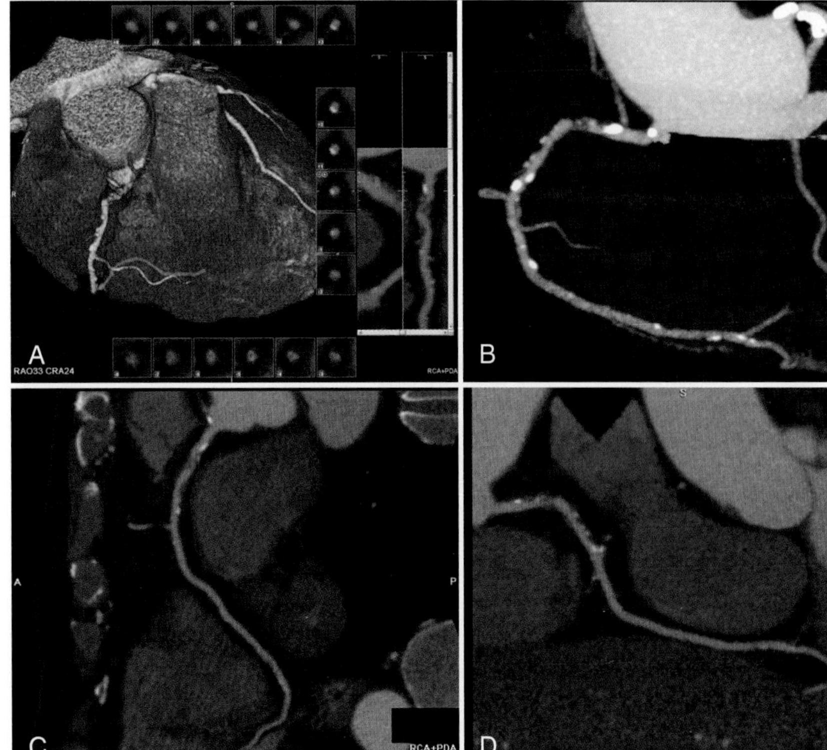

Figure 6-35. Complex disease of the right coronary artery with calcified/hard plaque, soft plaque, and mixed plaque. The most severe stenosis in the proximal portion is very eccentric and affords a very oblique lumen. As is usually the case, the mutiplanar reformatted image provides a more helpful rendering of the lumen and the plaques than did the 3D reconstructions and the maximum intensity projections.

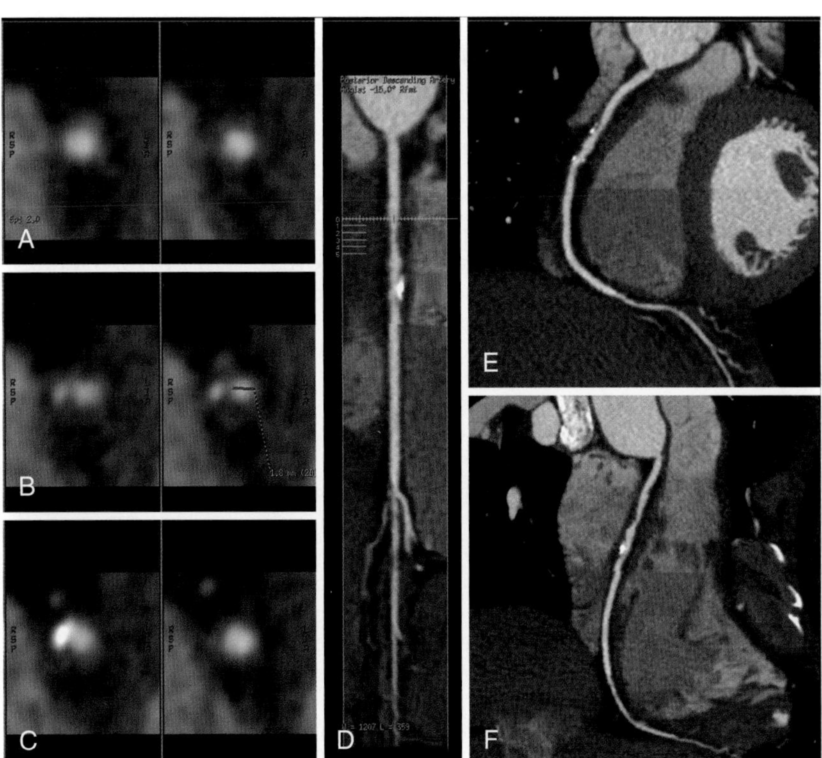

Figure 6-36. A 42-year-old man presented with typical angina and an indeterminant MPI study. Multiple reformatted images from a cardiac CT study demonstrate a mild amount of mixed plaque within the proximal right coronary artery, which causes a 30% to 40% stenosis.

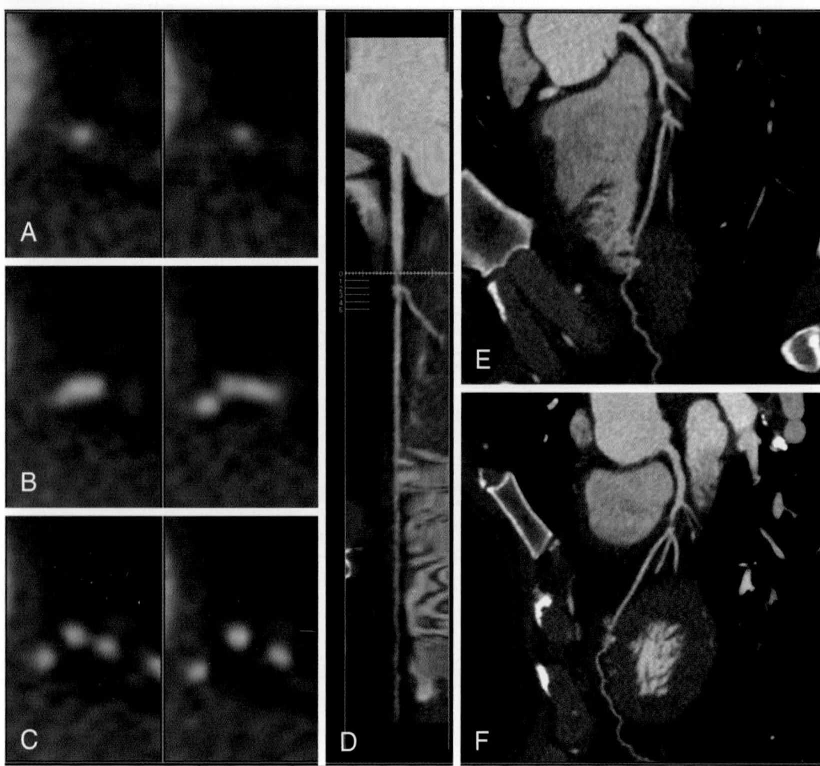

Figure 6-37. Same patient as Figure 6-36. Multiple reformatted images from a cardiac CT study demonstrate a moderate to severe, 60% to 70% proximal left anterior descending stenosis that is composed entirely of soft plaque.

Further Stratification in Symptomatic Patients

Among symptomatic patients, coronary CTA results reclassify the probability of CAD (Table 6-14).[52] In a series of 181 patients presenting with chest pain who underwent both myocardial perfusion imaging and 64-CT, where 97 of the patients had normal myocardial perfusion scans and coronary CTA studies of adequate quality to interpret, a wide range of underlying CAD was encountered in the normal scans.[85]

Prognostication in Symptomatic Patients

Two single-center studies of symptomatic patients have demonstrated that coronary CTA affords some prognostication of all-cause mortality. Both studies identified similar findings:

- Very low mortality rate associated with findings of mild stenoses or absence of stenosis
  - Mild (<50%) or no stenosis: 0.3%[86] (all-cause) mortality over an average of 15 months follow-up[87]
  - No stenosis: 0% 1-year cardiac event rate[88]
- Higher 1-year cardiac event rates in patients with obstructive versus nonobstructive disease:[88] 30% versus 8%
- Higher 1-year cardiac event rate in the presence of nonobstructive disease than in absence of disease, if these profiles were distinguished:[88] 8% versus 0%
- Graded mortality and cardiac event rates according to the number of vessels involved[87, 88]

A two-center study of 2076 consecutive patients followed for a mean of 16 ± 8 months demonstrated with multivariate analysis that CAD severity was a predictor of adverse cardiac events (hazard ratio 3.02 [1.17 to 1.86]) and that left ventricular ejection fraction had incremental predictive value over CAD severity (hazard ratio 1.47 [1.06 to 1.29]).[89]

One meta-analysis of 11 articles including 7335 participants (age 59.1 ± 2.6 years, 62.8% male) with suspected CAD determined that the presence of one or more significant coronary stenoses was associated with an annualized event rate of 11.9% inclusive of revascularization and 6.4% excluding revascularization, and conferred a hazard ratio of 10.74 for studies excluding revascularization. Adjustment on the basis of coronary calcification did not alter the prognostic significance.[90]

Another meta-analysis evaluated 18 studies including 9592 patients and determined that the presence of obstructive (>50% luminal stenosis) versus normal was associated with an 8.8% versus 0.17% rate of major adverse cardiac event (MACE). The pooled negative likelihood ratio for MACE after normal cardiac CT findings was 0.008 (0.0004–0.17; $P < .001$). The positive likelihood ratio was 1.70 (1.42–2.02; $P < .001$); sensitivity was 0.99 (0.93–1.00), and specificity was 0.41 (0.31–0.52; $P < .001$). Incremental risk was associated with stratification by no cardiac CT-detectable CAD, nonobstructive stenosis (<50% diameter), or obstructive stenosis (>50% luminal diameter).

TABLE 6-14 Reclassification of Probability of CAD by CTA in Symptomatic Patients

RISK	*n*	PRE-TEST PROBABILITY (%)	POST-TEST (CTA) PROBABILITY (%) AFTER NEGATIVE CTA	POST-TEST (CTA) PROBABILITY (%) AFTER POSITIVE CTA
High	105	87	17	96
Intermediate	83	53	0	88
Low	66	13	0	68

CAD, coronary artery disease; CTA, CT angiography.
Data from Meijboom WB, van Mieghem CA, Mollet NR, et al. 64-slice computed tomography coronary angiography in patients with high, intermediate, or low pretest probability of significant coronary artery disease. *J Am Coll Cardiol.* 2007;50(15):1469-1475.

The PROspective Multicenter Imaging Study for Evaluation of Chest Pain (PROMISE) trial is a randomized trial of cardiac CTA performed with 64 channels, or more, versus initial functional stress testing in 10,000 low- to intermediate-risk patients. The trial is intended to assess "in the real world" whether cardiac CT will reduce death and myocardial function by 20% compared to an initial function testing–guided strategy.[91]

The international registry CONFIRM trial (Coronary CT Angiography Evaluation for Clinical Outcomes: An International Multicenter Registry) of 23,854 patients without known CAD demonstrated that nonobstructive and obstructive CAD diagonosed by cardiac CT scanning are associated with higher rates of mortality and that risk profiles differed according to gender and age.[92]

In the ER setting:

- In the CT-STAT (Caronary Computed Tomographic Angiography for Systematic Triage of Acute Chest Pain Patients to Treatment) trial, the use of cardiac CT scanning versus MPI resulted in less time to diagnosis (median time of 2.9 hours versus 6.3 hours; $P < .0001$), lesser lost cost(−38%, $P < .0001$), but no difference in cardiac events ($P = .29$).[93]
- The ROMICAT (Rule Out Myocardial Infarction Using Computer Assisted Tomography) trial followed 368 patients (mean age 53 ± 12 years; 61% male) who had presented to the emergency department with chest pain and an initially negative troponin and "non-ischemic" ECG for 2 years (median follow-up of 23 months). The probability of MACE increased across the following categories:
  - No cardiac CT depicted CAD (0%)
  - Nonobstructive (<50%) CAD (4.6%)
  - Obstructive (>50%) CAD (30.3%; $P < .0001$).
- The ROMICAT II trial of 1000 patients who had presented to the emergency department with chest pain and an initially negative troponin and who were randomized to standard evaluation versus CCT evaluation demonstrated that CCT evaluation led to 18 fewer hours in hospital, with 50% of the CCT-evaluated patients being discharged within 9 hours versus only 15% of patients undergoing standard care. The reduced time in the ED was associated with ED cost reductions of 10% to 20%.[94]
- The ACRIN PA trial of 1370 low-risk patients presenting to the ED with chest pain/potential ACS randomized in a 1:2 ratio to standard triage or to CCT evaluation at five centers demonstrated that CCT evaluation led to more patients being discharged directly from the ED (50% versus 23%) and earlier discharge (18 hours versus 25 hours; $P < .001$) than did standard evaluation. CCT evaluation also was superior in detecting CAD (9% versus 3%).[95]

Coronary CTA to Assess for CAD in Patients with Left Bundle Branch Block

Left bundle branch block (LBBB) presents significant technical challenges for both stress echocardiography and nuclear perfusion techniques to accurately detect underlying CAD. Early studies suggest that coronary CTA appears to be able to discriminate the presence or absence of significant CAD among patients with LBBB in sinus rhythm (Table 6-15).[96]

Coronary CTA to Assess for CAD in Patients Referred for Aortic Valve Replacement

Many patients undergoing aortic valve replacement have a fairly low likelihood of having significant CAD—for example, the young to middle-aged population with a bicuspid aortic valve. In patients with active endocarditis of the aortic valve, coronary CTA is attractive to avoid catheterization-related risks (Table 6-16).

Coronary CTA for Transplanted Hearts

The need for yearly coronary angiography surveillance for transplant-related coronary disease may be an avenue for coronary CTA to keep patients from accruing catheterization risks (Table 6-17).

Coronary CTA for Patients with Dilated Cardiomyopathy

Many patients with dilated cardiomyopathy (DCM) have a low risk of underlying CAD, and the potential negative predictive value of CTA appears useful (Table 6-18).

TABLE 6-15 CTA for the Assessment of CAD in Patients with LBBB

	CT	*n*	SENSITIVITY (%)	SPECIFICITY (%)	PPV (%)	NPV (%)	ACCURACY (%)
Patients with LBBB[96]	64-CT	66					
Per segment			97	95	93	97	95
Per patient			72	99	91	97	97

CAD, coronary artery disease; CTA, CT angiography; LBBB, left bundle branch block; NPV, negative predictive value; PPV, positive predictive value.

TABLE 6-16 CTA for the Assessment of CAD in Patients Referred for Aortic Valve Replacement

	CT	*n*	SENSITIVITY (%)	SPECIFICITY (%)	PPV (%)	NPV (%)	ACCURACY (%)
Gilard et al.[97]	16-CT	55	100	80	55	100	—
Agatston <1000	All cases without CAD detected. Avoidance of angiography in 80% of cases.						
Agatston >1000	Avoidance of angiography in only 6% of cases.						
Meijboom et al.[98]	64-CT	145	92 [81–98]	82 [52–94]	82 [59–94]	100 [91–100]	100 [78–100]
Reant et al.[99]	16-CT	40	78	98	42	99	—
Manghat et al.[100]	16-CT	35	81	95	58	98	—
	Excluding Agatston >1000		90	98	60	100	—
Scheffel et al.[101]	64-CT	63	100	95	87	100	—

AVR, aortic value replacement; CAD, coronary artery disease; CTA, CT angiography; NPV, negative predictive value; PPV, positive predictive value.

TABLE 6-17 Coronary CTA for Transplanted Hearts

	CT	*n*	SENSITIVITY (%)	SPECIFICITY (%)	PPV (%)	NPV (%)	ACCURACY (%)
Sigurdsson et al.[102]	16	54 pts; 791 segments	86	99	81	99	—
Romeo et al.[103]	16	53 pts; 450 segments	83	95	71	95	93

NPV, negative predictive value; PPV, positive predictive value.

TABLE 6-18 CTA for the Assessment of Dilated Cardiomyopathy and Ischemic Dilated Cardiomyopathy

	CT	*n*	SENSITIVITY (%)	SPECIFICITY (%)	PPV (%)	NPV (%)	ACCURACY (%)
Andreini et al.[104]							
DCM		44	99	96	81	100	
Ischemic cardiomyopathy		17					
Controls (normal LV function + CAD)		139	86	96	86	96	

CAD, coronary artery disease; CTA, CT angiography; DCM, dilated cardiomyopathy; LV, left ventricle; NPV, negative predictive value; PPV, positive predictive value.

Coronary CTA for Assessment of Acute Chest Pain

Among 98 patients presenting to an ED, 16-CCT encountered significant problems with patient BMI and heart rate and was not sufficiently diagnostic.[105] 64-CT offered improved triage, establishing the absence or presence of significant CAD in 75% of cases. The remaining 25% of cases had intermediate disease or unclear CT scans and required subsequent stress testing (Table 6-19).[106]

Coronary CTA for Patients with Non–ST-Segment Elevation Myocardial Infarction ACS

Diagnostic and not prognostic studies of coronary CTA for patients with non–ST-segment elevation myocardial infarction (NSTEMI) ACS have been presented (Table 6-20).

Coronary CTA as a Screening Tool for CAD in Asymptomatic Individuals

Among 1000 consecutively enrolled asymptomatic middle-aged individuals (50 ± 9 years, range, 35–74 years; 63% male; NCEP guideline risk factors per patient: 1 ± 1, range 0–4; two or more risk factors in 41%) who underwent 64-CT:[62]

- Atheroscelerotic plaques (>25% diameter stenosis) were identified in 22%.
- Significant (>50%) lesions were present in 5%.
- Severe lesions (>75% stenosis) were present in 2%.
- By 17 ± 2 months of follow-up, there were only 15 (1.5%) events, all in patients with CAD:
  - Unstable angina: $n = 1$
  - Revascularization: $n = 14$
- Most (87%) events (notably revascularizations prompted by CTA results) occurred within 90 days of CTA.

The basis for recommending CTA for routine screening of asymptomatic individuals is poorly supported (Tables 6-21 and 6-22).

CCT PROTOCOL POINTS

- **Coverage:** Heart only
- **Landmark:** Scout topogram: Carina to below cardiac silhouette for calcium score, or low-dose localizer if a calcium score study is not performed. For CTA, choose a location 2 cm above the left main ostium and 2 cm below the last image with the heart on it.
- **Contrast:**
  - 70 mL contrast at 5 mL/sec for BMI < 30
  - 80 mL contrast at 6 mL/sec for BMI > 30
- **Automated trigger set:** Ascending aorta 1 cm above the left main ostium: 180 HU
- **Test bolus technique:** Ascending aorta 1 cm above the left main ostium. Inject 10 to 20 mL of contrast at either 5 or 6 mL/sec depending on BMI, followed by 30 to 50 mL of saline at 5 mL/sec. To minimize dose, begin image acquisition 10 sec after contrast injection, with test bolus image acquisition occurring every other heart beat and ending when contrast density within the ascending aorta begins to diminish. An ROI in the ascending aorta will determine the peak enhancement and the appropriate delay.
- **Additional scan:** A pre-contrast scan enables calcium scoring, which may be used as a "gatekeeper" for determining whether or not to proceed, depending on the calcium score observed.
- **Post-processing:**
  - **Prospective acquisition**: Reconstruct the data for the full thickness of the "pad" at intervals of 3% to 5%. For example, if the pad thickness is 10% on either side of 75% of the R-R interval, then data is reconstructed from 60% to 80% at intervals of 3% to 5%. Lung reconstructions usually are generated from the calcium score, which may be able to better assess the presence of calcium within a nodule over lung reconstructions from the CTA data set.
  - **Retrospective acquisition**: For the CTA data set, three reconstruction schemes are available:
    - Reconstruct the data at 3% to 5% intervals on either side of 75% of the R-R interval, or elsewhere in the cardiac cycle if moderate motion artifact is present. Reconstruction at 30% to 40% of the R-R interval may allow for better visualization of the RCA if motion artifact or a higher heart rate is present.
    - Select one slice from default 75% reconstructed images that show the three coronary arteries in cross section. Reconstruct that single slice each 20 msec for the entire R-R interval. Difficult cases may need reconstruction of two slices for proper identification of best cardiac phase to freeze the motion of the coronary arteries.
    - Choose the best cardiac phase (msec) to freeze the motion of the three coronary arteries. Reconstruct the entire volume data set at best cardiac phase + 20 msec before and after the best cardiac phase, with a total of three cardiac phases to be reconstructed. If heart rate is low and there is no cardiac motion, one best phase may be sufficient.
  - Reconstruct the entire volume data set at 2 mm each 10% of the R-R interval from 0% to 90% for functional evaluation. Lung reconstructions usually are generated from the calcium score, which may offer a better assessment of the presence of calcium within a nodule over lung reconstructions from the CTA data set.

TABLE 6-19 CTA for the Assessment of Chest Pain

STUDY	CT	*n*	SENSITIVITY (%)	SPECIFICITY (%)	PPV (%)	NPV (%)	ACCURACY (%)
Rubinshtein et al.[107] ED patients presenting with chest pain and negative ECGs and biomarkers, prediction re death/ MI/revascularization in hospital and over 15 months	64-slice	58	92	76	52	97	
ROMICAT Trial[108] Normal initial troponin, nondiagnostic ECG. Endpoint: ACS during admission or major adverse event within 6 months	64-slice	368					
For ACS presentation: absence of CAD			100 [98–100]			100 [89–100]	
For ACS presentation: presence of CAD			77 [59–90]			98 [95–99]	
				Of plaque for ACS: 54 [49–60] Of stenosis for ACS: 87 [83–90]			
Goldstein et al.[109] MSCT cases discharged if minimal disease, stress tested if intermediate disease, coronary angio if >70% stenosis. End point = safety, diagnostic efficacy, time and cost of care	64-slice	197 MSCT = 99, SOC = 98		Both strategies 100% safe. MSCT immediately excluded or identified CAD in 75% (67 normals, 8 severe disease). 25% underwent stress testing for intermediate disease or nondiagnostic MSCT scans.			
				MSCT	**SOC**		
	Diagnostic time			3.4 hr	15 hr	$P < .001$	
	Costs			$1586	$1872	$P < .001$	
	Repeat CP evaluations			2%	7%	$P = .10$	
Rubinshtein et al.[110] Impact on decision-making in patients with intermediate probability of ACS *n* = 58, 38% previously diagnosed with CAD	Prior to the CCT exam, clinical diagnosis of ACS made in 71%. Diagnosis altered in 31%, including 10/22 without known CAD and 8/19 with known CAD.						
				PRE-CCT	**POST-CCT**		
Patients without known CAD	Considered to have ACS			22	12	$P = .002$	
	Recommended for hospitalization			28	14	$P = .002$	
Patients with known CAD	Considered to have ACS			19	11	$P = .005$	
	Recommended for hospitalization			22	19	$P = .008$	

ACS, acute coronary syndrome; CAD, coronary artery disease; CCT, cardiac CT; CP, cardiopulmonary; CTA, CT angiography; ED, emergency department; MI, myocardial infarction; MSCT, multislice CT; NPV, negative predictive value; PPV, positive predictive value; SOC, standard of core.

TABLE 6-20 CTA for the Diagnosis of Coronary Artery Disease in Patients with Acute Coronary Syndrome

ED PATIENTS WITH NON-STEMI ACS	CT	*n*	SENSITIVITY (%)	SPECIFICITY (%)	PPV (%)	NPV (%)	ACCURACY (%)
Meijboom et al.[54]	64-slice	104	100 [95–100]	75 [47–92]	96 [89–99]	100 [70–100]	

ACS, acute coronary syndrome; CTA, CT angiography; ED, emergency department; NPV, negative predictive value; PPV, positive predictive value; STEMI, ST segment elevation myocardial infarction.

TABLE 6-21 Detection of Coronary Artery Disease in Symptomatic Patients Without Known Heart Disease

		APPROPRIATE USE SCORE (1–9)		
INDICATION	**PRETEST PROBABILITY OF CAD**	**LOW**	**INTERMEDIATE**	**HIGH**
Nonacute Symptoms Possibly Representing an Ischemic Equivalent				
1	ECG interpretable AND Able to exercise	U (5)	A (7)	I (3)
2	ECG interpretable OR Unable to exercise	A (7)	A (8)	U (4)
Acute Symptoms with Suspicion of ACS (Urgent Presentation)				
3	Definite MI		I (1)	
4	Persistent ECG ST-segment elevation following exclusion of MI		U (6)	
5	Acute chest pain of uncertain cause (differential diagnosis includes pulmonary embolism, aortic dissection, and ACS ["triple rule out"])		U (6)	
6	Normal ECG and cardiac biomarkers	A (7)	A (7)	U (4)
7	ECG uninterpretable	A (7)	A (7)	U (4)
8	Nondiagnostic ECG OR Equivocal cardiac biomarkers	A (7)	A (7)	U (4)

ACS, acute coronary syndrome; CAD, coronary artery disease; MI, myocardial infarction.
All indications are for CTA unless otherwise noted. A indicates appropriate; I, inappropriate; and U, uncertain.
Reprinted with permission from Taylor AJ, Cerqueira M, Hodgson JM, et al. ACCF/SCCT/ACR/AHA/ASE/ASNC/NASCI/SCAI/SCMR 2010 appropriate use criteria for cardiac computed tomography. *J Am Coll Cardiol.* 2010;56(22):1864-1894.

TABLE 6-22 Detection of Coronary Artery Disease/Risk Assessment in Asymptomatic Patients Without Known Coronary Artery Disease

		APPROPRIATE USE SCORE (1–9)		
INDICATION	**GLOBAL CHD RISK ESTIMATE**	**LOW**	**INTERMEDIATE**	**HIGH**
Noncontrast CT for CCS				
9	Family history of premature CHD	A (7)		
10	Asymptomatic No known CAD	I (2)	A (7)	U (4)
Coronary CTA				
11	Asymptomatic No known CAD	I (2)	I (2)	U (4)

CAD, coronary artery disease; CCS, coronary calcium score; CHD, coronary heart disease; CTA, CT angiography.
Reprinted with permission from Taylor AJ, Cerqueira M, Hodgson JM, et al. ACCF/SCCT/ACR/AHA/ASE/ASNC/NASCI/SCAI/SCMR 2010 appropriate use criteria for cardiac computed tomography. *J Am Coll Cardiol.* 2010;56(22):1864-1894.

References

1. Kefer J, Coche E, Legros G, et al. Head-to-head comparison of three-dimensional navigator-gated magnetic resonance imaging and 16-slice computed tomography to detect coronary artery stenosis in patients. *J Am Coll Cardiol.* 2005;46(1):92-100.
2. Leber AW, Knez A, von Ziegler F, et al. Quantification of obstructive and nonobstructive coronary lesions by 64-slice computed tomography: a comparative study with quantitative coronary angiography and intravascular ultrasound. *J Am Coll Cardiol.* 2005;46(1): 147-154.
3. Dewey M, Laule M, Krug L, et al. Multisegment and halfscan reconstruction of 16-slice computed tomography for detection of coronary artery stenoses. *Invest Radiol.* 2004;39(4):223-229.
4. Hoffmann U, Moselewski F, Cury RC, et al. Predictive value of 16-slice multidetector spiral computed tomography to detect significant obstructive coronary artery disease in patients at high risk for coronary artery disease: patient-versus segment-based analysis. *Circulation.* 2004;110(17):2638-2643.
5. Lau GT, Ridley LJ, Schieb MC, et al. Coronary artery stenoses: detection with calcium scoring, CT angiography, and both methods combined. *Radiology.* 2005;235(2):415-422.
6. Achenbach S, Daniel WG. Computed tomography of the coronary arteries: more than meets the (angiographic) eye. *J Am Coll Cardiol.* 2005;46(1):155-157.
7. Achenbach S, Giesler T, Ropers D, et al. Detection of coronary artery stenoses by contrast-enhanced, retrospectively electrocardiographically-gated, multislice spiral computed tomography. *Circulation.* 2001;103(21):2535-2538.
8. Becker CR, Knez A, Leber A, et al. Detection of coronary artery stenoses with multislice helical CT angiography. *J Comput Assist Tomogr.* 2002;26(5):750-755.
9. Knez A, Becker CR, Leber A, et al. Usefulness of multislice spiral computed tomography angiography for determination of coronary artery stenoses. *Am J Cardiol.* 2001;88(10):1191-1194.
10. Kopp AF, Schroeder S, Kuettner A, et al. Non-invasive coronary angiography with high resolution multidetector-row computed tomography. Results in 102 patients. *Eur Heart J.* 2002;23(21): 1714-1725.
11. Nieman K, Oudkerk M, Rensing BJ, et al. Coronary angiography with multi-slice computed tomography. *Lancet.* 2001;357(9256): 599-603.
12. Nieman K, Cademartiri F, Lemos PA, Raaijmakers R, Pattynama PM, De Feyter PJ. Reliable noninvasive coronary angiography with fast submillimeter multislice spiral computed tomography. *Circulation.* 2002;106(16):2051-2054.
13. Nieman K, Rensing BJ, Van Geuns RJ, et al. Non-invasive coronary angiography with multislice spiral computed tomography: impact of heart rate. *Heart.* 2002;88(5):470-474.
14. Nieman K, Pattynama PM, Rensing BJ, Van Geuns RJ, De Feyter PJ. Evaluation of patients after coronary artery bypass surgery: CT angiographic assessment of grafts and coronary arteries. *Radiology.* 2003;229(3):749-756.
15. Vogl TJ, Abolmaali ND, Diebold T, et al. Techniques for the detection of coronary atherosclerosis: multi-detector row CT coronary angiography. *Radiology.* 2002;223(1):212-220.
16. Kuettner A, Kopp AF, Schroeder S, et al. Diagnostic accuracy of multidetector computed tomography coronary angiography in patients with angiographically proven coronary artery disease. *J Am Coll Cardiol.* 2004;43(5):831-839.
17. Ropers D, Baum U, Pohle K, et al. Detection of coronary artery stenoses with thin-slice multi-detector row spiral computed tomography and multiplanar reconstruction. *Circulation.* 2003;107(5): 664-666.
18. Achenbach S, Ropers D, Pohle FK, et al. Detection of coronary artery stenoses using multi-detector CT with 16x0.75 collimation and 375 ms rotation. *Eur Heart J.* 2005;26(19):1978-1986.
19. Achenbach S, Moselewski F, Ropers D, et al. Detection of calcified and noncalcified coronary atherosclerotic plaque by contrast-enhanced, submillimeter multidetector spiral computed tomography: a segment-based comparison with intravascular ultrasound. *Circulation.* 2004;109(1):14-17.
20. Heuschmid M, Kuettner A, Schroeder S, et al. ECG-gated 16-MDCT of the coronary arteries: assessment of image quality and accuracy in detecting stenoses. *AJR Am J Roentgenol.* 2005; 184(5):1413-1419.
21. Hoffmann MH, Shi H, Schmitz BL, et al. Noninvasive coronary angiography with multislice computed tomography. *JAMA.* 2005;293(20):2471-2478.
22. Kuettner A, Trabold T, Schroeder S, et al. Noninvasive detection of coronary lesions using 16-detector multislice spiral computed tomography technology: initial clinical results. *J Am Coll Cardiol.* 2004;44(6):1230-1237.
23. Kuettner A, Beck T, Drosch T, et al. Image quality and diagnostic accuracy of non-invasive coronary imaging with 16 detector slice spiral computed tomography with 188 ms temporal resolution. *Heart.* 2005;91(7):938-941.
24. Kuettner A, Beck T, Drosch T, et al. Diagnostic accuracy of non-invasive coronary imaging using 16-detector slice spiral computed tomography with 188 ms temporal resolution. *J Am Coll Cardiol.* 2005;45(1):123-127.
25. Martuscelli E, Romagnoli A, D'Eliseo A, et al. Accuracy of thin-slice computed tomography in the detection of coronary stenoses. *Eur Heart J.* 2004;25(12):1043-1048.
26. Mollet NR, Cademartiri F, Nieman K, et al. Multislice spiral computed tomography coronary angiography in patients with stable angina pectoris. *J Am Coll Cardiol.* 2004;43(12):2265-2270.
27. Mollet NR, Cademartiri F, Krestin GP, et al. Improved diagnostic accuracy with 16-row multi-slice computed tomography coronary angiography. *J Am Coll Cardiol.* 2005;45(1):128-132.
28. Morgan-Hughes GJ, Roobottom CA, Owens PE, Marshall AJ. Highly accurate coronary angiography with submillimetre, 16 slice computed tomography. *Heart.* 2005;91(3):308-313.
29. Romeo G, Houyel L, Angel CY, Brenot P, Riou JY, Paul JF. Coronary stenosis detection by 16-slice computed tomography in heart transplant patients: comparison with conventional angiography and impact on clinical management. *J Am Coll Cardiol.* 2005;45(11):1826-1831.
30. Schuijf JD, Bax JJ, Salm LP, et al. Noninvasive coronary imaging and assessment of left ventricular function using 16-slice computed tomography. *Am J Cardiol.* 2005;95(5):571-574.
31. Cademartiri F, Marano R, Luccichenti G, et al. Image assessment with multislice CT coronary angiography. *Radiol Med (Torino).* 2005;109(3):198-207.
32. Cademartiri F, Mollet NR, Runza G, et al. Improving diagnostic accuracy of MDCT coronary angiography in patients with mild heart rhythm irregularities using ECG editing. *AJR Am J Roentgenol.* 2006;186(3):634-638.
33. Cademartiri F, Runza G, Marano R, et al. Diagnostic accuracy of 16-row multislice CT angiography in the evaluation of coronary segments. *Radiol Med (Torino).* 2005;109(1-2):91-97.
34. Dewey M, Kaufels N, Laule M, et al. Magnetic resonance imaging of myocardial perfusion and viability using a blood pool contrast agent. *Invest Radiol.* 2004;39(8):498-505.
35. Fine JJ, Hopkins CB, Hall PA, Delphia RE, Attebery TW, Newton FC. Noninvasive coronary angiography: agreement of multi-slice spiral computed tomography and selective catheter angiography. *Int J Cardiovasc Imaging.* 2004;20(6):549-552.
36. Kaiser C, Bremerich J, Haller S, et al. Limited diagnostic yield of non-invasive coronary angiography by 16-slice multi-detector spiral computed tomography in routine patients referred for evaluation of coronary artery disease. *Eur Heart J.* 2005;26(19): 1987-1992.
37. Aviram G, Finkelstein A, Herz I, et al. Clinical value of 16-slice multi-detector CT compared to invasive coronary angiography. *Int J Cardiovasc Intervent.* 2005;7(1):21-28.
38. Garcia MJ, Lessick J, Hoffmann MH. Accuracy of 16-row multidetector computed tomography for the assessment of coronary artery stenosis. *JAMA.* 2006;296(4):403-411.
39. Gulati GS, Seth S, Kurian S, Jagia P, Sharma S. Non-invasive diagnosis of coronary artery disease with 16-slice computed tomography. *Natl Med J India.* 2005;18(5):236-241.
40. Cordeiro MA, Miller JM, Schmidt A, et al. Non-invasive half millimetre 32 detector row computed tomography angiography accurately excludes significant stenoses in patients with advanced coronary artery disease and high calcium scores. *Heart.* 2006;92(5):589-597.
41. Lim MC, Wong TW, Yaneza LO, De Larrazabal C, Lau JK, Boey HK. Non-invasive detection of significant coronary artery disease with multi-section computed tomography angiography in patients with suspected coronary artery disease. *Clin Radiol.* 2006;61(2): 174-180.
42. Leschka S, Alkadhi H, Plass A, et al. Accuracy of MSCT coronary angiography with 64-slice technology: first experience. *Eur Heart J.* 2005;26(15):1482-1487.
43. Mollet NR, Cademartiri F, van Mieghem CA, et al. High-resolution spiral computed tomography coronary angiography in patients referred for diagnostic conventional coronary angiography. *Circulation.* 2005;112(15):2318-2323.
44. Raff GL, Gallagher MJ, O'Neill WW, Goldstein JA. Diagnostic accuracy of noninvasive coronary angiography using 64-slice spiral computed tomography. *J Am Coll Cardiol.* 2005;46(3):552-557.
45. Pugliese F, Mollet NR, Runza G, et al. Diagnostic accuracy of non-invasive 64-slice CT coronary angiography in patients with stable angina pectoris. *Eur Radiol.* 2006;16(3):575-582.

46. Ropers D, Rixe J, Anders K, et al. Usefulness of multidetector row spiral computed tomography with 64- × 0.6-mm collimation and 330-ms rotation for the noninvasive detection of significant coronary artery stenoses. *Am J Cardiol.* 2006;97(3):343-348.
47. Fine JJ, Hopkins CB, Ruff N, Newton FC. Comparison of accuracy of 64-slice cardiovascular computed tomography with coronary angiography in patients with suspected coronary artery disease. *Am J Cardiol.* 2006;97(2):173-174.
48. Nikolaou K, Knez A, Rist C, et al. Accuracy of 64-MDCT in the diagnosis of ischemic heart disease. *AJR Am J Roentgenol.* 2006; 187(1):111-117.
49. Weustink AC, Meijboom WB, Mollet NR, et al. Reliable high-speed coronary computed tomography in symptomatic patients. *J Am Coll Cardiol.* 2007;50(8):786-794.
50. Schuijf JD, Pundziute G, Jukema JW, et al. Diagnostic accuracy of 64-slice multislice computed tomography in the noninvasive evaluation of significant coronary artery disease. *Am J Cardiol.* 2006; 98(2):145-148.
51. Ehara M, Surmely JF, Kawai M, et al. Diagnostic accuracy of 64-slice computed tomography for detecting angiographically significant coronary artery stenosis in an unselected consecutive patient population: comparison with conventional invasive angiography. *Circ J.* 2006;70(5):564-571.
52. Meijboom WB, van Mieghem CA, Mollet NR, et al. 64-slice computed tomography coronary angiography in patients with high, intermediate, or low pretest probability of significant coronary artery disease. *J Am Coll Cardiol.* 2007;50(15):1469-1475.
53. Shabestari AA, Abdi S, Akhlaghpoor S, et al. Diagnostic performance of 64-channel multislice computed tomography in assessment of significant coronary artery disease in symptomatic subjects. *Am J Cardiol.* 2007;99(12):1656-1661.
54. Meijboom WB, Mollet NR, Van Mieghem CA, et al. 64-Slice CT coronary angiography in patients with non-ST elevation acute coronary syndrome. *Heart.* 2007;93(11):1386-1392.
55. Miller JM, Rochitte CE, Dewey M, et al. Diagnostic performance of coronary angiography by 64-row CT. *N Engl J Med.* 2008;359(22): 2324-2336.
56. Budoff MJ, Dowe D, Jollis JG, et al. Diagnostic performance of 64-multidetector row coronary computed tomographic angiography for evaluation of coronary artery stenosis in individuals without known coronary artery disease. *J Am Coll Cardiol.* 2008; 52(21):1724-1732.
57. Meijboom WB, Meijs MF, Schuijf JD, et al. Diagnostic accuracy of 64-slice computed tomography coronary angiography: a prospective, multicenter, multivendor study. *J Am Coll Cardiol.* 2008; 52(25):2135-2144.
58. Schroeder S, Achenbach S, Bengel F, et al. Cardiac computed tomography: indications, applications, limitations, and training requirements: report of a Writing Group deployed by the Working Group Nuclear Cardiology and Cardiac CT of the European Society of Cardiology and the European Council of Nuclear Cardiology. *Eur Heart J.* 2008;29(4):531-556.
59. Hamon M, Biondi-Zoccai GG, Malagutti P, Agostoni P, Morello R, Valgimigli M. Diagnostic performance of multislice spiral computed tomography of coronary arteries as compared with conventional invasive coronary angiography: a meta-analysis. *J Am Coll Cardiol.* 2006;48(9):1896-1910.
60. Christian TF. Anatomy of an emerging diagnostic test: computed tomographic coronary angiography. *Circulation.* 2005;112(15): 2222-2225.
61. Achenbach S, Moshage W, Ropers D, Bachmann K. Comparison of vessel diameters in electron beam tomography and quantitative coronary angiography. *Int J Card Imaging.* 1998;14(1):1-7.
62. Choi EK, Choi SI, Rivera JJ, et al. Coronary computed tomography angiography as a screening tool for the detection of occult coronary artery disease in asymptomatic individuals. *J Am Coll Cardiol.* 2008;52(5):357-365.
63. Hendel RC, Budoff MJ, Cardella JF, et al. ACC/AHA/ACR/ASE/ASNC/HRS/NASCI/RSNA/SAIP/SCAI/SCCT/SCMR/SIR 2008 Key data elements and definitions for cardiac imaging: a report of the American College of Cardiology/American Heart Association Task Force on Clinical Data Standards (Writing Committee to Develop Clinical Data Standards for Cardiac Imaging). *J Am Coll Cardiol.* 2009;53(1):91-124.
64. Sirnes PA, Myreng Y, Molstad P, Golf S. Reproducibility of quantitative coronary analysis, assessment of variability due to frame selection, different observers, and different cinefilmless laboratories. *Int J Card Imaging.* 1996;12(3):197-203.
65. Fischer JJ, Samady H, McPherson JA, et al. Comparison between visual assessment and quantitative angiography versus fractional flow reserve for native coronary narrowings of moderate severity. *Am J Cardiol.* 2002;90(3):210-215.
66. Fischell TA, Maheshwari A, Mirza RA, Haller S, Carter AJ, Popma JJ. Impact of frame selection on quantitative coronary angiographic analysis after coronary stenting. *Catheter Cardiovasc Interv.* 2005;64(4):460-467.
67. Beauman GJ, Vogel RA. Accuracy of individual and panel visual interpretations of coronary arteriograms: implications for clinical decisions. *J Am Coll Cardiol.* 1990;16(1):108-113.
68. Holder DA, Johnson AL, Stolberg HO, et al. Inability of caliper measurement to enhance observer agreement in the interpretation of coronary cineangiograms. *Can J Cardiol.* 1985;1(1):24-29.
69. Meijboom WB, Van Mieghem CA, van Pelt N, et al. Comprehensive assessment of coronary artery stenoses: computed tomography coronary angiography versus conventional coronary angiography and correlation with fractional flow reserve in patients with stable angina. *J Am Coll Cardiol.* 2008;52(8):636-643.
70. Leber AW, Knez A, White CW, et al. Composition of coronary atherosclerotic plaques in patients with acute myocardial infarction and stable angina pectoris determined by contrast-enhanced multislice computed tomography. *Am J Cardiol.* 2003;91(6): 714-718.
71. Hoffmann U, Moselewski F, Nieman K, et al. Noninvasive assessment of plaque morphology and composition in culprit and stable lesions in acute coronary syndrome and stable lesions in stable angina by multidetector computed tomography. *J Am Coll Cardiol.* 2006;47(8):1655-1662.
72. Schoenhagen P, Ziada KM, Kapadia SR, Crowe TD, Nissen SE, Tuzcu EM. Extent and direction of arterial remodeling in stable versus unstable coronary syndromes: an intravascular ultrasound study. *Circulation.* 2000;101(6):598-603.
73. Achenbach S, Ropers D, Hoffmann U, et al. Assessment of coronary remodeling in stenotic and nonstenotic coronary atherosclerotic lesions by multidetector spiral computed tomography. *J Am Coll Cardiol.* 2004;43(5):842-847.
74. Motoyama S, Kondo T, Sarai M, et al. Multislice computed tomographic characteristics of coronary lesions in acute coronary syndromes. *J Am Coll Cardiol.* 2007;50(4):319-326.
75. Schoenhagen P, Tuzcu EM, Stillman AE, et al. Non-invasive assessment of plaque morphology and remodeling in mildly stenotic coronary segments: comparison of 16-slice computed tomography and intravascular ultrasound. *Coron Artery Dis.* 2003;14(6): 459-462.
76. Leber AW, Knez A, Becker A, et al. Accuracy of multidetector spiral computed tomography in identifying and differentiating the composition of coronary atherosclerotic plaques: a comparative study with intracoronary ultrasound. *J Am Coll Cardiol.* 2004;43(7):1241-1247.
77. Achenbach S, Moselewski F, Ropers D, et al. Detection of calcified and noncalcified coronary atherosclerotic plaque by contrast-enhanced, submillimeter multidetector spiral computed tomography: a segment-based comparison with intravascular ultrasound. *Circulation.* 2004;109(1):14-17.
78. Leber AW, Becker A, Knez A, et al. Accuracy of 64-slice computed tomography to classify and quantify plaque volumes in the proximal coronary system: a comparative study using intravascular ultrasound. *J Am Coll Cardiol.* 2006;47(3):672-677.
79. Schroeder S, Kopp AF, Baumbach A, et al. Noninvasive detection and evaluation of atherosclerotic coronary plaques with multislice computed tomography. *J Am Coll Cardiol.* 2001;37(5): 1430-1435.
80. Leber AW, Knez A, Becker A, et al. Accuracy of multidetector spiral computed tomography in identifying and differentiating the composition of coronary atherosclerotic plaques: a comparative study with intracoronary ultrasound. *J Am Coll Cardiol.* 2004;43(7):1241-1247.
81. Von Dem Bussche N, Isaacs DL, Goodman ET, Hassankhani A, Mahmud E. Imaging of intracoronary thrombus by multidetector helical computed tomography angiography. *Circulation.* 2004; 109(3):432.
82. Chang SM, Huh A, Bianco JA, Wann LS. Spontaneous coronary dissection on multiple detector computed tomography (MDCT). *J Cardiovasc Comput Tomogr.* 2007;1:60-61.
83. Motoyama S, Kondo T, Sarai M, et al. Multislice computed tomographic characteristics of coronary lesions in acute coronary syndromes. *J Am Coll Cardiol.* 2007;50(4):319-326.
84. Cole JH, Chunn VM, Morrow A, Buckley RS, Phillips GM. Cost implications of initial computed tomography angiography as opposed to catheterization in patients with mildly abnormal or equivocal myocardial perfusion scans. *J Cardiovasc Comput Tomogr.* 2007;1:21-26.
85. van Werkhoven JM, Schuijf JD, Jukema JW, et al. Anatomic correlates of a normal perfusion scan using 64-slice computed tomographic coronary angiography. *Am J Cardiol.* 2008;101(1):40-45.

86. Min JK, Shaw LJ, Devereux RB, et al. Prognostic value of multidetector coronary computed tomographic angiography for prediction of all-cause mortality. *J Am Coll Cardiol.* 2007;50(12):1161-1170.
87. Min JK, Shaw LJ, Devereux RB, et al. Prognostic value of multidetector coronary computed tomographic angiography for prediction of all-cause mortality. *J Am Coll Cardiol.* 2007;50(12):1161-1170.
88. Pundziute G, Schuijf JD, Jukema JW, et al. Prognostic value of multislice computed tomography coronary angiography in patients with known or suspected coronary artery disease. *J Am Coll Cardiol.* 2007;49(1):62-70.
89. Chow BJ, Wells GA, Chen L, et al. Prognostic value of 64-slice cardiac computed tomography severity of coronary artery disease, coronary atherosclerosis, and left ventricular ejection fraction. *J Am Coll Cardiol.* 2010;55(10):1017-1028.
90. Bamberg F, Sommer WH, Hoffmann V, et al. Meta-analysis and systematic review of the long-term predictive value of assessment of coronary atherosclerosis by contrast-enhanced coronary computed tomography angiography. *J Am Coll Cardiol.* 2011;57(24):2426-2436.
91. Mark DB, Kong DF. Cardiac computed tomographic angiography: what's the prognosis? *J Am Coll Cardiol.* 2010;55(10):1029-1031.
92. Min JK, Dunning A, Lin FY, et al. Age- and sex-related differences in all-cause mortality risk based on coronary computed tomography angiography findings results from the International Multicenter CONFIRM (Coronary CT Angiography Evaluation for Clinical Outcomes: An International Multicenter Registry) of 23,854 patients without known coronary artery disease. *J Am Coll Cardiol.* 2011;58(8):849-860.
93. Goldstein JA, Chinnaiyan KM, Abidov A, et al. The CT-STAT (Coronary Computed Tomographic Angiography for Systematic Triage of Acute Chest Pain Patients to Treatment) trial. *J Am Coll Cardiol.* 2011;58(14):1414-1422.
94. Hoffmann U, Truong QA, Schoenfeld DA, et al. Coronary CT angiography versus standard evaluation in acute chest pain. *N Engl J Med.* 2012;367(4):299-308.
95. Litt H, Miller C, Gatsonis C, et al. ACRIN PA 4005: Multicenter Randomized Controlled Study of a Rapid "Rule Out" Strategy Using CT Coronary Angiogram Versus Traditional Care for Low-Risk ED Patients with Potential Acute Coronary Syndromes. *N Engl J Med.* 2012.
96. Ghostine S, Caussin C, Daoud B, et al. Non-invasive detection of coronary artery disease in patients with left bundle branch block using 64-slice computed tomography. *J Am Coll Cardiol.* 2006;48(10):1929-1934.
97. Gilard M, Cornily JC, Pennec PY, et al. Accuracy of multislice computed tomography in the preoperative assessment of coronary disease in patients with aortic valve stenosis. *J Am Coll Cardiol.* 2006;47(10):2020-2024.
98. Meijboom WB, Mollet NR, van Mieghem CA, et al. Pre-operative computed tomography coronary angiography to detect significant coronary artery disease in patients referred for cardiac valve surgery. *J Am Coll Cardiol.* 2006;48(8):1658-1665.
99. Reant P, Brunot S, Lafitte S, et al. Predictive value of noninvasive coronary angiography with multidetector computed tomography to detect significant coronary stenosis before valve surgery. *Am J Cardiol.* 2006;97(10):1506-1510.
100. Manghat NE, Morgan-Hughes GJ, Broadley AJ, et al. 16-detector row computed tomographic coronary angiography in patients undergoing evaluation for aortic valve replacement: comparison with catheter angiography. *Clin Radiol.* 2006;61(9):749-757.
101. Scheffel H, Leschka S, Plass A, et al. Accuracy of 64-slice computed tomography for the preoperative detection of coronary artery disease in patients with chronic aortic regurgitation. *Am J Cardiol.* 2007;100(4):701-706.
102. Sigurdsson G, Carrascosa P, Yamani MH, et al. Detection of transplant coronary artery disease using multidetector computed tomography with adaptative multisegment reconstruction. *J Am Coll Cardiol.* 2006;48(4):772-778.
103. Romeo G, Houyel L, Angel CY, Brenot P, Riou JY, Paul JF. Coronary stenosis detection by 16-slice computed tomography in heart transplant patients: comparison with conventional angiography and impact on clinical management. *J Am Coll Cardiol.* 2005;45(11):1826-1831.
104. Andreini D, Pontone G, Pepi M, et al. Diagnostic accuracy of multidetector computed tomography coronary angiography in patients with dilated cardiomyopathy. *J Am Coll Cardiol.* 2007;49(20):2044-2050.
105. Huber S, Huber M, Dees D, Redmond FA, Wilson JM, Flamm SD. Usefulness of multislice spiral computed tomography coronary angiography in patients with acute chest pain in the emergency department. *J Cardiovasc Comput Tomogr.* 2007;1:29-37.
106. Ghostine S, Caussin C, Daoud B, et al. Non-invasive detection of coronary artery disease in patients with left bundle branch block using 64-slice computed tomography. *J Am Coll Cardiol.* 2006;48(10):1929-1934.
107. Rubinshtein R, Halon DA, Gaspar T, et al. Usefulness of 64-slice cardiac computed tomographic angiography for diagnosing acute coronary syndromes and predicting clinical outcome in emergency department patients with chest pain of uncertain origin. *Circulation.* 2007;115(13):1762-1768.
108. Hoffmann U, Bamberg F, Chae CU, et al. Coronary computed tomography angiography for early triage of patients with acute chest pain: the ROMICAT (Rule Out Myocardial Infarction using Computer Assisted Tomography) trial. *J Am Coll Cardiol.* 2009;53(18):1642-1650.
109. Goldstein JA, Gallagher MJ, O'Neill WW, Ross MA, O'Neil BJ, Raff GL. A randomized controlled trial of multi-slice coronary computed tomography for evaluation of acute chest pain. *J Am Coll Cardiol.* 2007;49(8):863-871.
110. Rubinshtein R, Halon DA, Gaspar T, et al. Impact of 64-slice cardiac computed tomographic angiography on clinical decision-making in emergency department patients with chest pain of possible myocardial ischemic origin. *Am J Cardiol.* 2007;100(10):1522-1526.

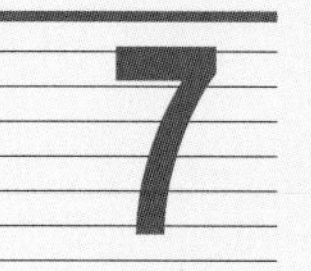

CTA Assessment of Coronary Artery Stents

Key Points

- Although stents are easy to visualize by cardiac CT (CCT), their lumen is difficult to assess. The assessment of patency or restenosis of coronary stents is a challenge for CCT angiography, but one that is increasingly being met.
- Assessment of larger stented arteries is far more successful than that of smaller stented arteries.
- The potential "blooming" artifacts from the metal mesh of coronary stents is greatly compounded by motion.
- Use of different "windowing" and filters is needed to minimize the intrusion of blooming artifact.
- Background atherosclerotic coronary artery calcification only compounds stented coronary artery assessment.
- In larger stents with better imaging, visualization of the lumen is feasible, but in smaller stents and in lower-quality studies, luminal assessment is still challenging. Hence, a priori knowledge of the stent size and its location should be obtained to ascertain whether coronary computed tomographic angiography has a reasonable chance of imaging the stented artery accurately.
- Stent gaps and stent fracture are well imaged by CCT, as is stent overhang into the left main coronary artery.

CCT IMAGING OF CORONARY STENTS

The accurate assessment of coronary stents remains a major challenge for cardiac CT (CCT), and although the stent itself is readily imaged, the lumen within it is not, because the stent material confers "blooming" artifact. Stents with a denser "weave" are harder to image. A stent deployed within a stent for restenosis leaves little chance of accurately depicting the lumen. Small amounts of motion during acquisition disperse the partial volume averaging effect over more voxels, increasing the depiction of the stent and further reducing the luminal depiction. Thicker struts confer greater artifact. As would be expected, the patency of large vessels or stents is easier to assess, as the blooming artifact is less likely to obscure the whole lumen.[1] False positives occur in 5% to 10% of cases, reducing the positive predictive value. Bifurcation lesions are difficult to assess. Although CCT and intravascular ultrasound (IVUS) data generally correlate, CCT tends to overestimate stent diameter.[2] Only studies that are either small, single-center, or select have been presented thus far, and almost always of stents of 2.5 mm or larger, which remains the lower limit of reasonable size to assess by CCT.[3] Few series have been published with 64-CCT systems. The generally pessimistic data[7] that were obtained in studies of older systems, such as those using 16-CCT, still are considered the norm, so that it is still thought that, in most cases, the presence or absence or extent of in-stent restenosis cannot be determined (Tables 7-1 through 7-3).[4]

The detail of the stent is variably, but usually fairly, defined by CCT.[7] The metallic composition of the stent has a major effect on the brightness of the stent—for example, that of the ACS RX Multilink (Abbott Vascular, Abbott Park, IL) is 269 ± 19 HU, whereas that of the Sirius Carbostent (Sorin Biomedica Cardio, Saluggia, Italy) is 437 ± 29 HU. The metallic composition also affects the ability to image the detail of the stent. A sharp or detail reconstruction kernel often is used to minimize the blooming artifact caused by the metallic struts of a stent. This modulation of the technique is felt to increase the conspicuity of subtle neo-intimal hyperplasia within the stent. Use of a wide window (width 1500 HU; center 300 HU) is also recommended, as this, in conjunction with a sharper kernel, will minimize blooming artifact.[5]

Restenosis or thrombosis is apparent as lower-attenuation material within the stent; visually or quantitatively, this can be referred to elsewhere in the vessel or better yet, to the ascending aorta: a reading of 0.81 predicts patency with a sensitivity of 91% and a specificity of 95%.[3]

Expected severe artifact problems associated with imaging stents include:

- ❐ Small vessels or small stents[3]
- ❐ Multiple stents at one site (overlap)
- ❐ Stents with more metal

TABLE 7-1 CCT for the Evaluation of Coronary Artery Stents

AUTHOR	JOURNAL	YEAR	CT	NO. PATIENTS/ STENTS	NONASSESS. (%)	LESION	SENSITIVITY (%)	SPECIFICITY FOR ISR (%)	PPV (%)	NPV (%)
Schuijf et al.[24]	Am J Cardiol	2004	16	22	1		78	100	—	—
Van Mieghem et al.[2]	Circ	2007	—	—	—	70 LMCA only	100	91	67	100
Cademartiri et al.[6]	JACC	2007	64	182	7%	192 stents all ≥2.5 mm	95	93	63	99
Gaspar et al.[7]	JACC	2005	40	65	—		72	93	65	95
Oncel et al.[8]	Radiol	2007	—	30/39	0		89	95	94	90
Oncel et al.[9]	Am J Radiol	2008	Dual source	30/39	—	Stenosis and occlusion	100	94	89	100
Pugliese et al.[10]	Heart	2008	—	100/178	5		94	92	77	98
Ehara et al.[11]	JACC	2007	—	81/125	12		91	93	77	98
Rixe et al.[12]	Eur Heart J	2006	64	64/102	42%		86	98	86	98
Rist et al.[13]	Acad Radiol	2006	64	75	8%		75	92	67	94
Abdelkarim et al.[3]	JCCT	2010	64	55/122	4%		91	95	96	91

ISR, in-stent restenosis; LMCA, left main coronary artery; nonassess, nonassessable; NPV, negative predictive value; PPV, positive predictive value.

TABLE 7-2 CCT for the Evaluation of Left Mainstem Coronary Artery Stenting

AUTHOR	JOURNAL	YEAR	CT	NO. PATIENTS/ STENTS	SENSITIVITY (%)	SPECIFICITY (%)	PPV (%)	NPV (%)
Van Mieghem et al.[2]	Circ	2007	16/64	74	100	91	67	10

NPV, negative predictive value; PPV, positive predictive value.

TABLE 7-3 CCT for the Evaluation of Coronary Artery Stents

NO. PATIENTS/ STENTS	NOT EVALUABLE (%)	SENSITIVITY (%)	SPECIFICITY (%)	PPV (%)	NPV (%)
482/682	12 (82/682) 95% CI: 9.7–15	91 (105/115) 95 CI: 85–96	93 (461/494) 95 CI: 91–95	76 (105/138)	98 (461/471)

NPV, negative predictive value; PPV, positive predictive value.
Data from Schroeder S, Achenbach S, Bengel F, et al. Cardiac computed tomography: indications, applications, limitations, and training requirements: report of a Writing Group deployed by the Working Group Nuclear Cardiology and Cardiac CT of the European Society of Cardiology and the European Council of Nuclear Cardiology. *Eur Heart J.* 2008;29(4):531-556.

- ❒ Calcium in underlying plaque
- ❒ Artifacts from sternal wires, clips, pacemakers
- ❒ Hypodense restenosis material in proximity to high-attenuation stent material

Some unusual stent-related problems, such as stent-induced coronary aneurysm formation, have been imaged by CCT.[15]

Adequate CCT Imaging of Patent Stents

Figures 7-1 through 7-7 show adequate CCT imaging of patent stents.

Inadequate CCT Imaging of Patent Stents

Figure 7-8 illustrates inadequate CCT imaging of patent stents.

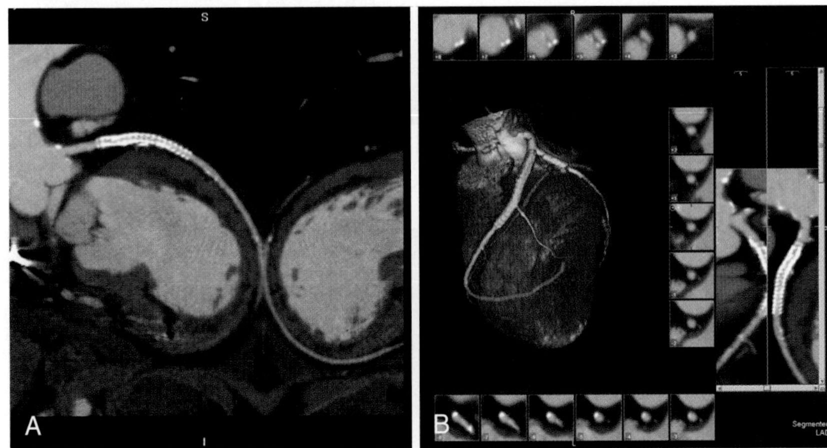

Figure 7-1. Multiple images from a cardiac CT study in a patient with prior coronary artery stenting within the left anterior descending (LAD) coronary artery. Despite a high-quality study, the lack of any motion artifact, and high contrast density within the coronary arteries, the proximal to mid-LAD stent is virtually unassessable, due primarily to the size of the stent and its strut structure. There is no evidence of an LAD stenosis at either the proximal or the distal ends of the stent.

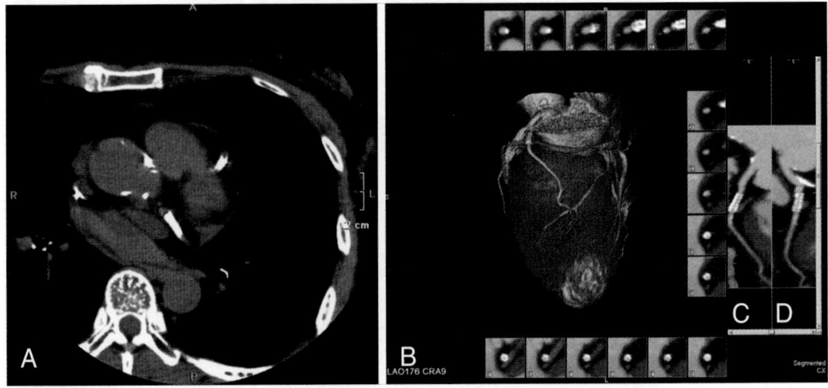

Figure 7-2. A 62-year-old woman with known coronary artery disease. The patient has a history of prior stent placement. Stents can be difficult to distinguish from underlying coronary artery calcification. Multiple cross-sectional images through the stent within the proximal circumflex artery demonstrate too much blooming artifact for proper evaluation.

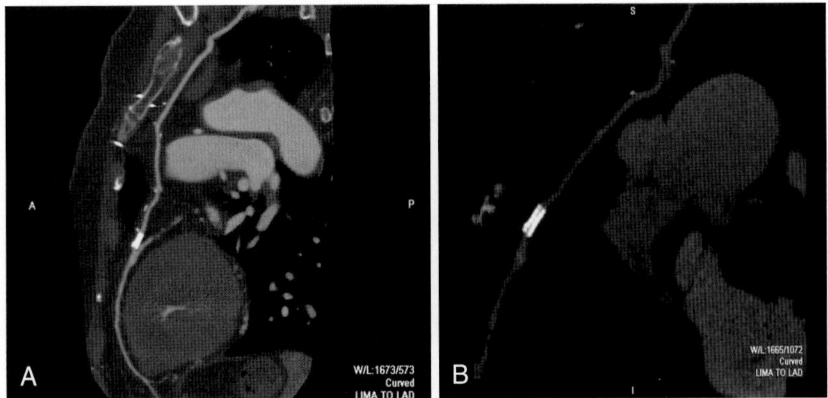

Figure 7-3. Two images from a cardiac CT study performed to evaluate bypass graft patency demonstrate a patent left internal mammary artery (LIMA) graft with a stent just above the anastomosis of the LIMA and the left anterior descending artery (LAD). Altering the window and width levels (**B**) allows better visualization through the stent.

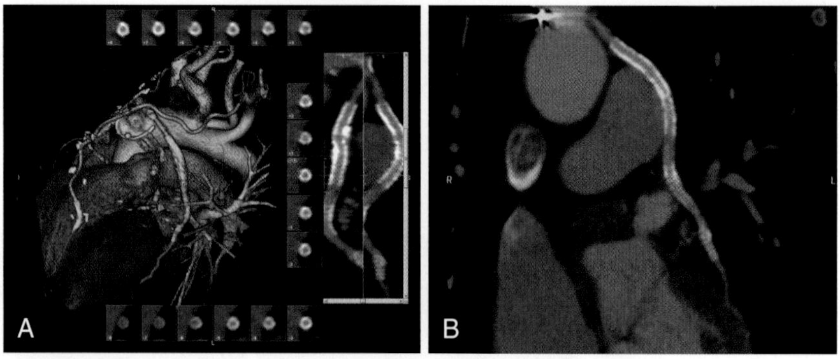

Figure 7-4. A graft from the saphenous vein to the second obtuse marginal branch (SVG-0M2) demonstrates moderate (50%) ostial stenosis, with five stents seen in the ongoing graft. There is no evidence of in-stent stenosis or thrombosis.

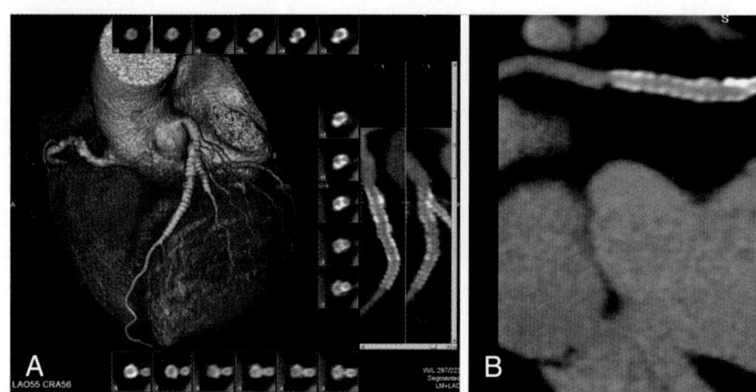

Figure 7-5. Multiple curved reformations from a cardiac CT study demonstrate no evidence of in-stent stenosis or thrombosis within a stented left anterior descending (LAD) artery or in a stented first diagonal branch. There is a mild amount of soft plaque seen proximal to the LAD stent, causing a stenosis of less than 20%.

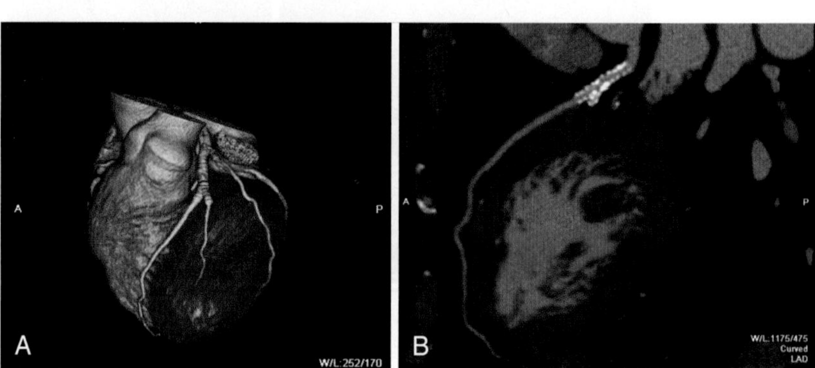

Figure 7-6. Curved images from a cardiac CT study for stent evaluation. The proximal left anterior descending (LAD) artery with a second stent extending into the D1 branch demonstrates patency with no evidence of incident stenosis. The ongoing LAD is normal.

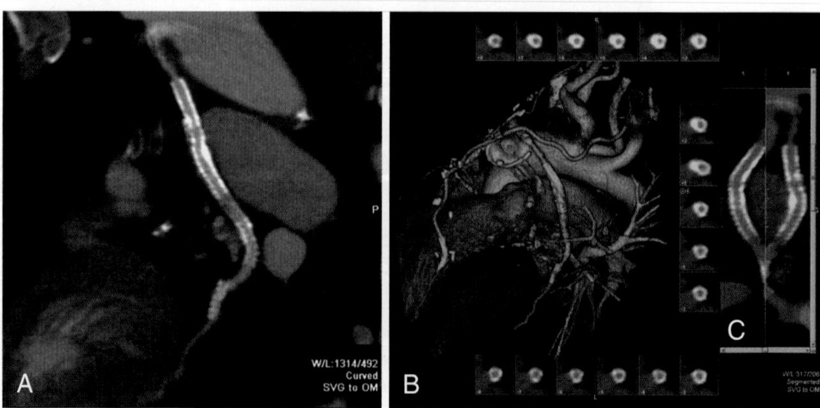

Figure 7-7. **A,** Curved reformatted view of a patent multiply-stented saphenous vein graft to the obtuse marginal branch of the left circumflex artery. **B,** Three-dimensional reconstruction and vessel extraction cross-sectional views of a patent multiply-stented saphenous vein graft to the obtuse marginal branch of the left circumflex artery.

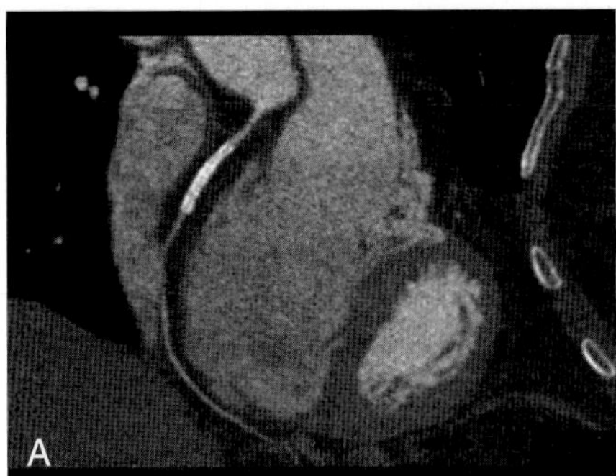

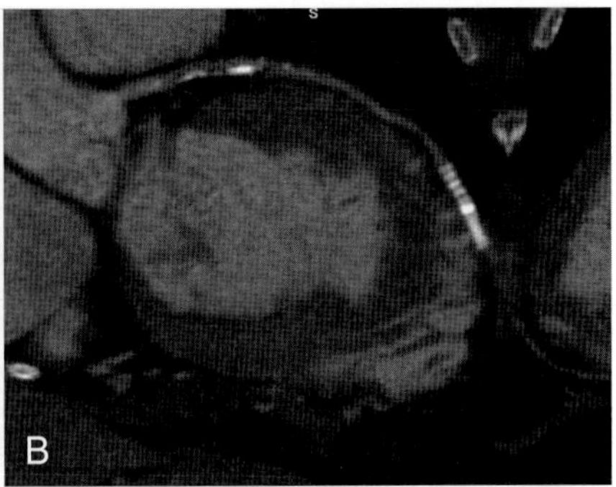

Figure 7-8. Curved reformations from cardiac CT studies in two different patients demonstrate nonassessable stents. Strut thickness precludes evaluation of the underlying coronary artery lumen due to blooming artifact.

STENT FRACTURE, STENT GAP, AND IN-STENT RESTENOSIS

Insertion of multiple stents has become common. Stent gap is readily detected by 64-CT, more so than by conventional angiography. As would be expected, stent gap sets the stage for in-stent/between stent stenosis; stent gap seen on CTA is associated with 28% of in-stent restenosis (ISR), and ISR is found in nearly half (46%) of stent gaps. Stent gap in the setting of a single stent likely represents stent fracture, and in the setting of multiple stents, may represent stent fracture or overlap failure.[16-18]

POTENTIAL STENT-RELATED COMPLICATIONS DETECTABLE BY CCT

- In-stent restenosis[15] (Figs. 7-9 to 7-19; **Videos 7-1** through **7-4**)
- Stent gaps and restenosis[15,16] (Fig. 7-20)
- Stent fracture and restenosis[17,18] (Fig. 7-21)
- Drug-eluting stent-related aneurysms[19–21] (Fig. 7-22)
- Mycotic stent-related pseudoaneurysms and pseudoaneurysm-associated fistula[22,23]
- Stent migration or dislodgement[15]
- Stent protrusion from a coronary ostia (Fig. 7-23; **Video 7-5)**
- Stent collapse due to excessive angulation

CT ANGIOGRAPHY PROTOCOL FOR THE EVALUATION OF CORONARY STENTS—DIFFERENCES FROM STANDARD CORONARY CTA PROTOCOL

- Use sharp or high-detail kernels.
- Select optimal (wider) window width (1500 HU) and center (300 HU).
- Consider using a higher concentration of iodine (370 mg I/mL).

The influence of thinner slices, different filters, and special reconstruction techniques is seen in Figures 7-24 and 7-25.

CCT Protocol Points (Table 7-4)

- **Coverage**: Standard, unless there are bypass grafts to interrogate as well as the coronary arteries
- **Contrast**: A higher density of iodine is preferable (350–400 mg/mL), in part to compensate for increased noise from the edge-enhancing convolution kernels
- **Post-processing**: Because of beam-hardening and blooming artifacts from stent material, kernels of higher spatial resolution are used to minimize these artifacts. Window width (~200 HU) and level optimization (~1500 HU) improve delineation of the stented lumen.

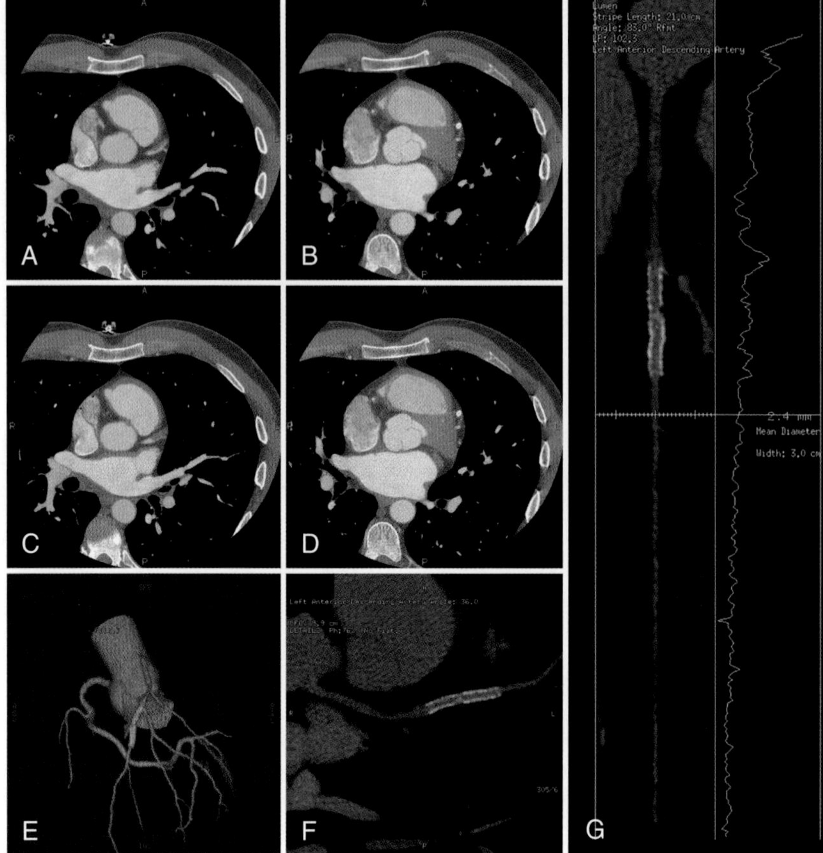

Figure 7-9. Multiple axial volume-rendered and curved reformatted images through the left main and left anterior descending (LAD) arteries using a high-detail reconstruction kernel. These images demonstrate two stents within the mid-LAD. The stents are patent. A tiny amount of new intimal hyperplasia is seen in the distal aspect of the proximal stent. The proximal LAD demonstrates a moderate amount of soft plaque causing a 50% proximal LAD stenosis.

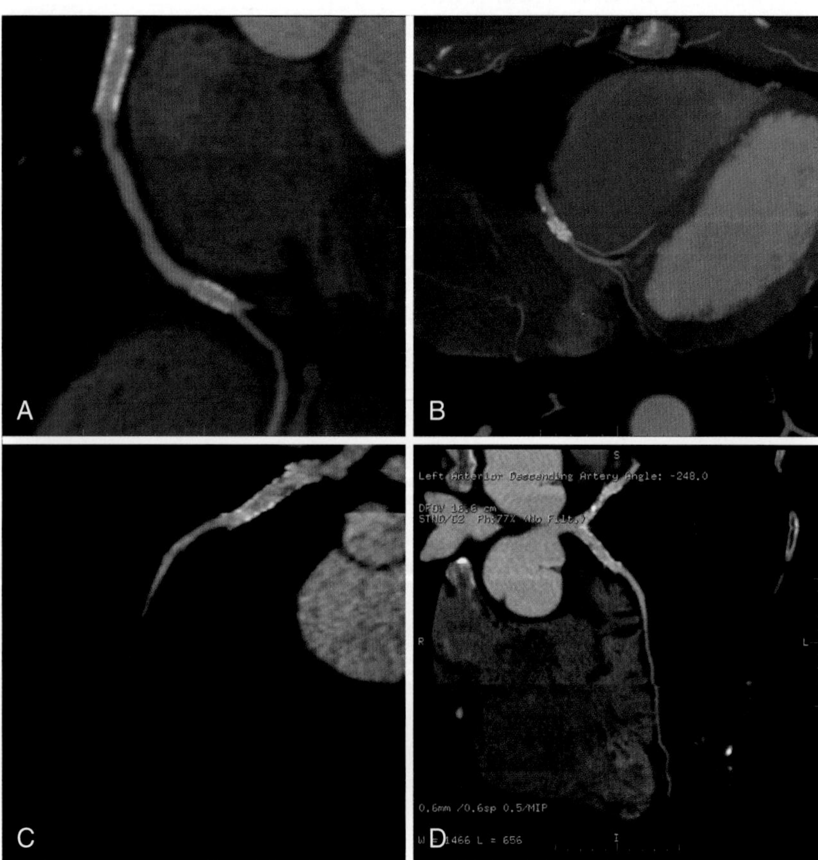

Figure 7-10. Multiple curved reformats and maximum intensity projection (MIP) images in a patient with three coronary stents: two in the right coronary artery (RCA) and one in the mid-left anterior descending artery. **A** and **B**, Normal-appearing stents with no evidence of in-stent stenosis or thrombus. A mild amount of soft plaque is seen distal to the proximal RCA stent (**B**) as well as a mild stenosis of mixed plaque proximal to the distal stent (**A**). **C** and **D** demonstrate a mild in-stent stenosis proximally within a left anterior descending (LAD) stent.

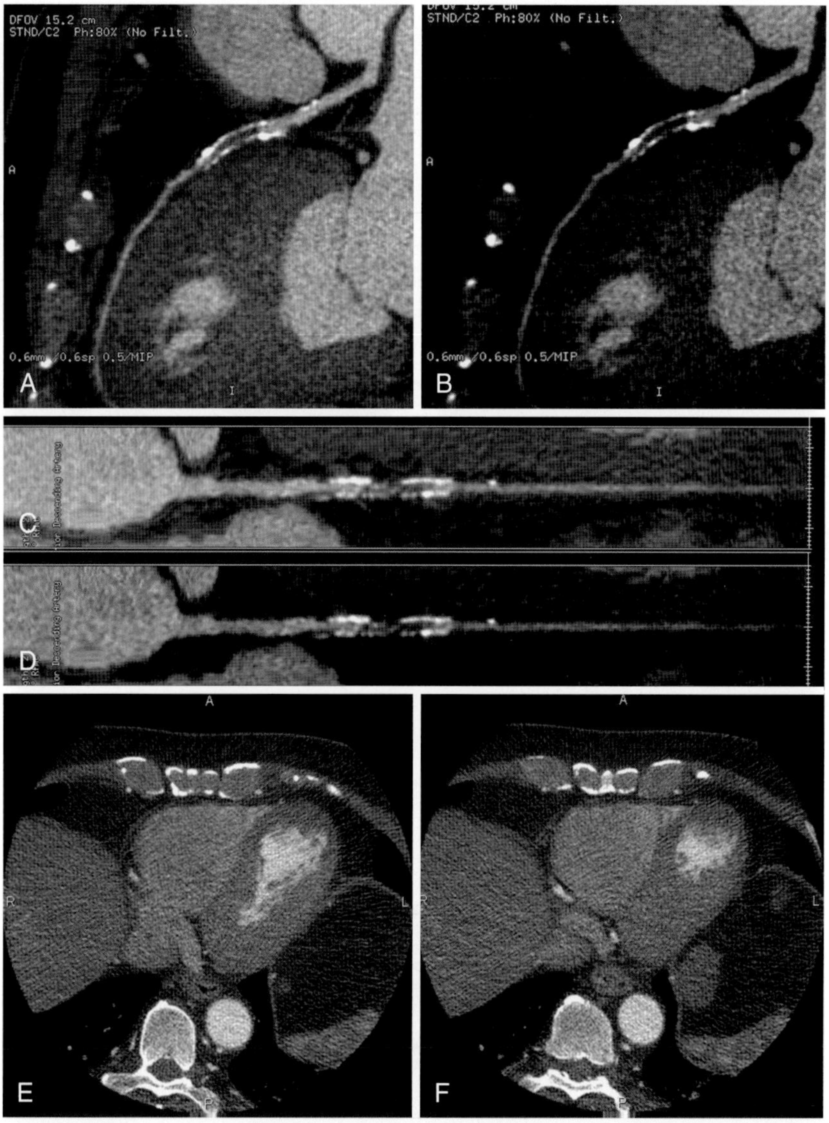

Figure 7-11. Multiple curved reformats demonstrate severe in-stent stenosis within the second of two left anterior descending stents. Window width and level optimization allow for better visualization of the in-stent disease. Axial source images demonstrate poor contrast opacification of the apex of the left ventricle (LV), likely related to slow flow and poor contrast enhancement in a poorly contracting LV apex.

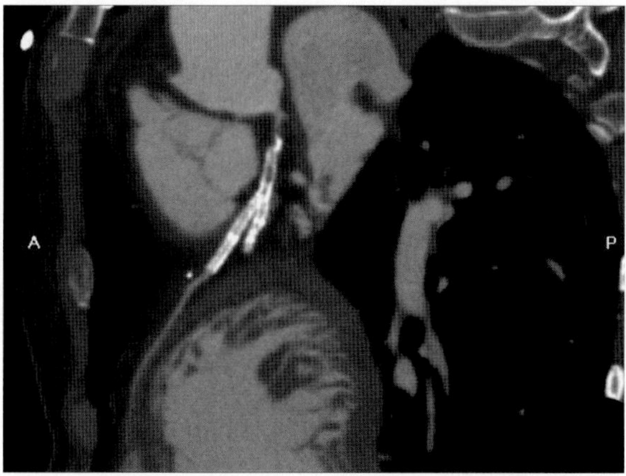

Figure 7-12. Multiple stents inserted with a Y technique. Severe left main stenosis with in-stent thrombosis/restenosis is seen in the proximal left anterior descending artery. A, anterior; P, posterior.

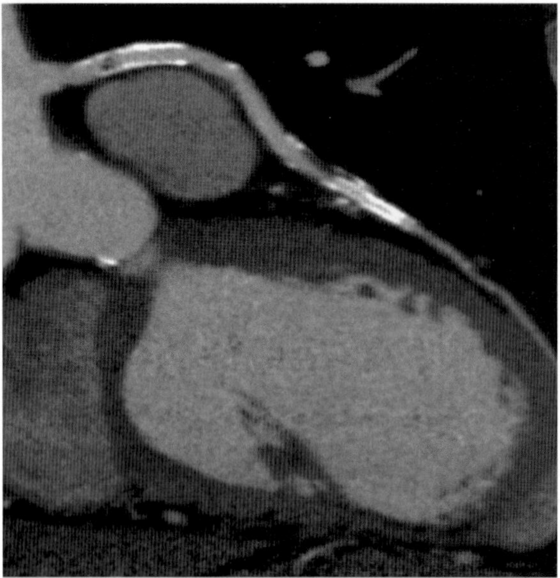

Figure 7-13. Curved reformat of a saphenous vein graft to the left anterior descending (LAD) artery demonstrating moderate in-stent stenosis in a proximal stent, with a mild amount of disease seen distally at the level of the graft. A stent within the proximal LAD is patent with no evidence of in-stent stenosis or thrombosis.

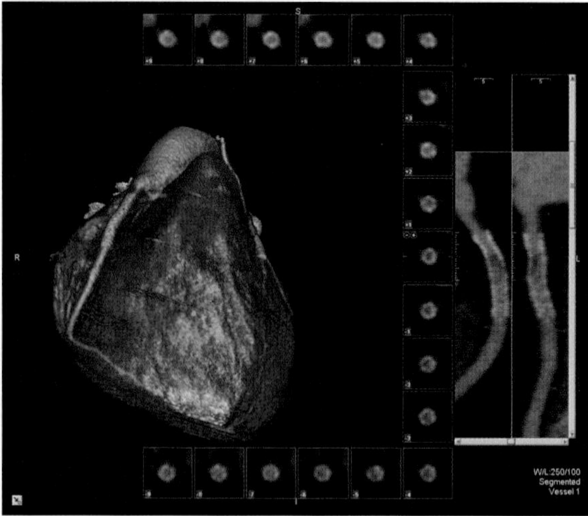

Figure 7-14. Multiple cross-sectional and curved reformatted images from a cardiac CT study in a patient with recurrent angina 14 months post-stenting of the proximal right coronal artery (RCA). The proximal portion of the stent demonstrates a moderate amount of low-attenuation material within the stent, consistent with in-stent restenosis of the proximal RCA stent.

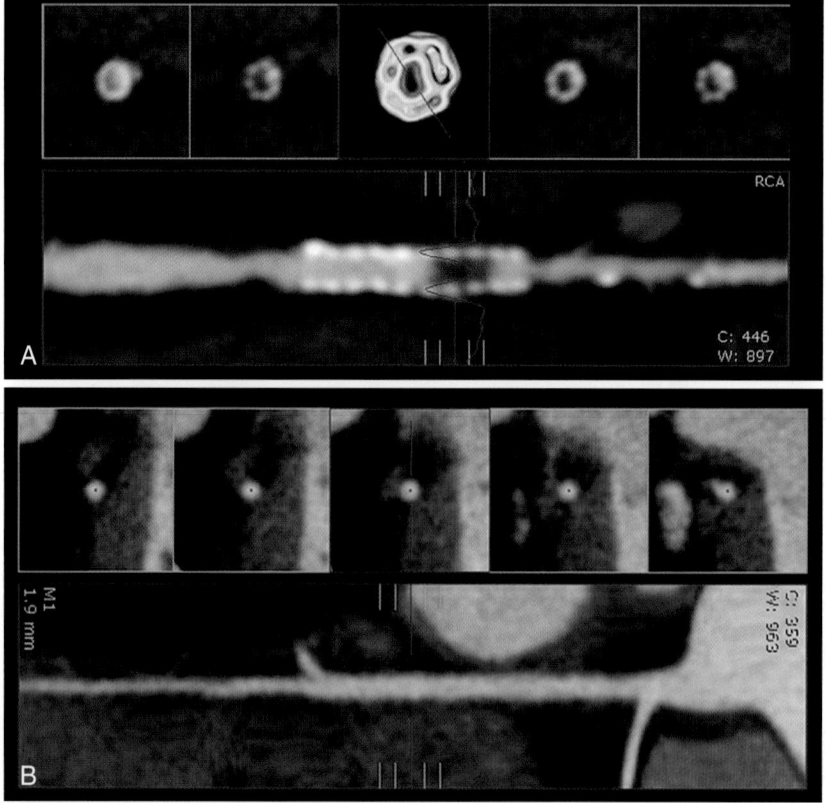

Figure 7-15. CT coronary angiography vessel extraction views of in-stent stenosis (**A**) and a nondiseased vessel (**B**).

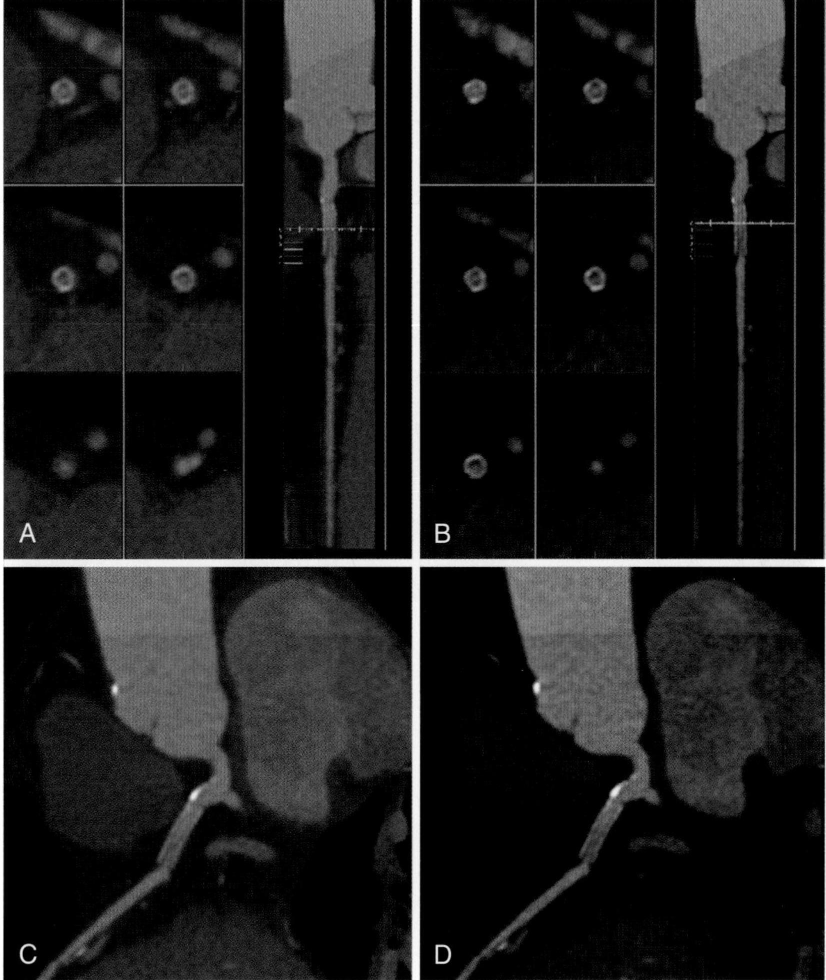

Figure 7-16. **A** and **C,** Suboptimal windowing and right image–optimal windowing of a patient with prior left anterior descending (LAD) stenting and suspected in-stent restenosis. **B** and **D,** Window-optimized images reveal more than 50% in-stent restenosis.

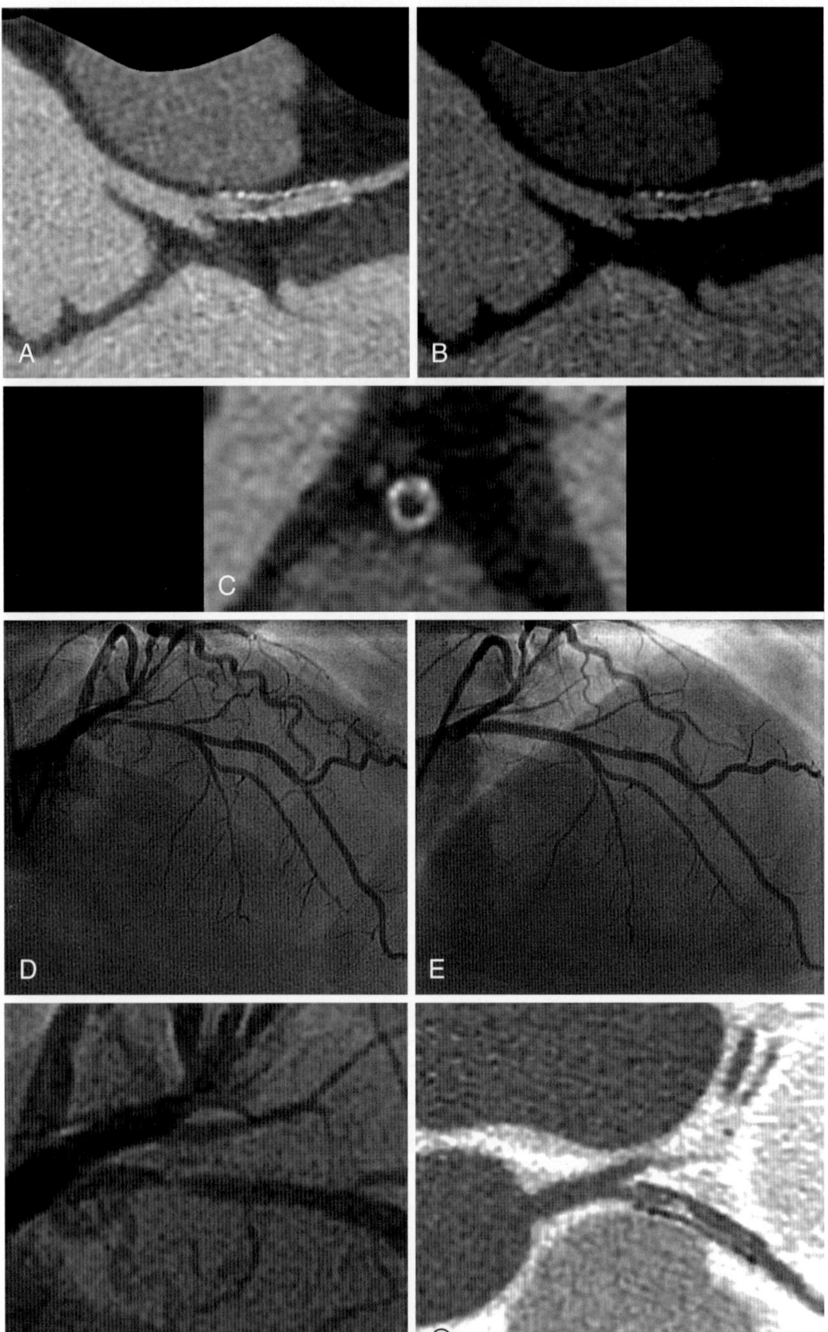

Figure 7-17. A 55-year-old man with a prior history of an anterior myocardial infarction and placement of a bare metal stent 2 years prior who was experiencing increasing exertional shortness of breath and chest pain. Multiple cardiac CT images using a high-resolution protocol demonstrate a moderate amount of low attenuation within the proximal to midportion of the left anterior descending (LAD) artery stent. **A** and **B** have been reconstructed using a dedicated edge-enhancing kernel. As these higher spatial frequency convolution filters tend to increased noise, it is preferable to use a higher contrast density of iodine (350 mg/mL was used in this case). **B** was obtained at wide window settings (window with 1500 HU, window level 300 HU), which helped to set a favorable balance between signal and noise. The cross-section view (**C**) of the proximal portion of the stent demonstrates almost entire filling of the lumen with low-attenuation material, consistent with a high-grade in-stent restenosis. A conventional angiogram confirms severe in-stent restenosis (**D**), with subsequent reangioplasty (**E**). **F,** A zoomed-in version of the conventional angiogram (shown in **D**) demonstrates high-grade in-stent restenosis. **G,** Inverted CT image demonstrates the region of in-stent restenosis. **See Videos 7-1 and 7-2.**

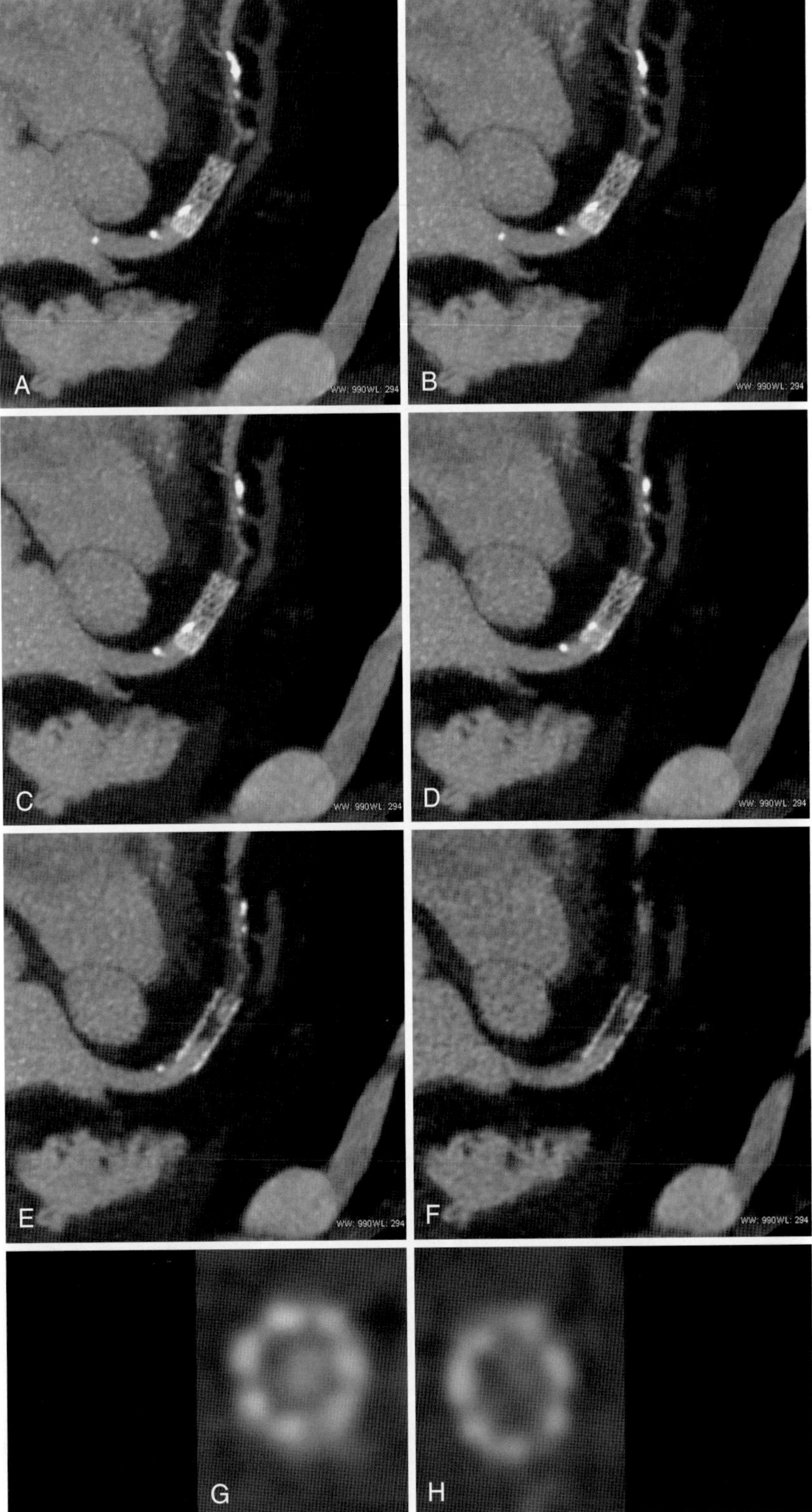

Figure 7-18. Sequential maximum intensity projection images through a stent demonstrate a large bulk of low-attenuation material within the stent. Cross-sectional images before (**G**) and at the site of (**H**) occlusion.

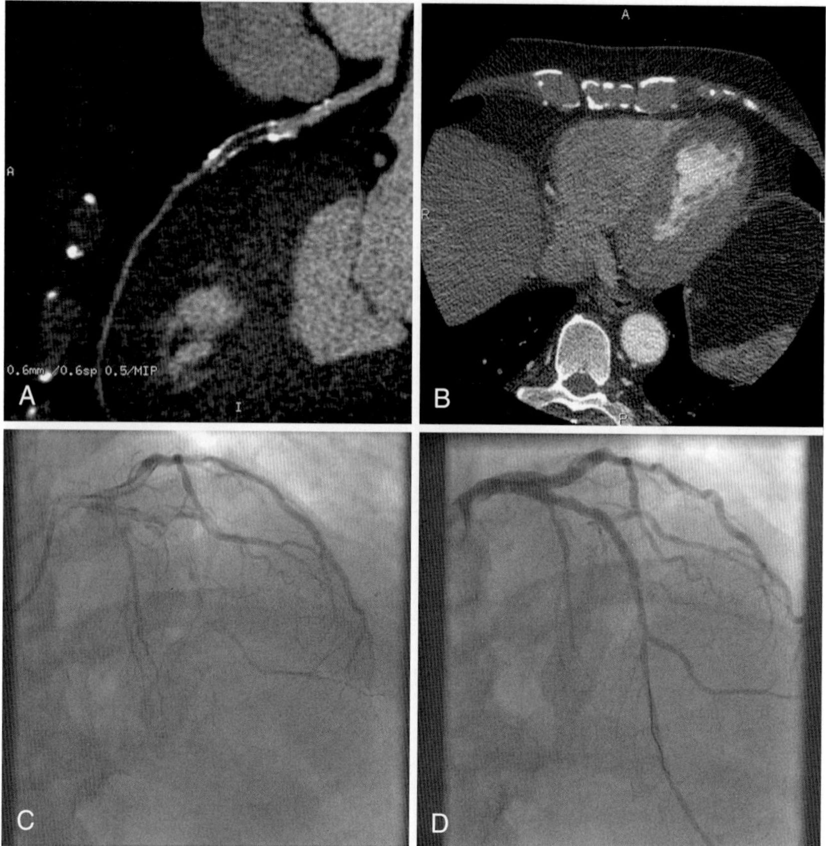

Figure 7-19. A 62-year-old man with known coronary artery disease and prior placement of a mid-left anterior descending (LAD) artery stent presents with worsening angina. A cardiac CT study was performed. **A,** A curved reformatted image demonstrates extensive low attenuation throughout the course of the LAD stent, raising concern for extensive in-stent restenosis. Contrast does fill the ongoing LAD. **B,** A small to moderate area of low attenuation within the LV apex, which may represent slow flow or an evolving thrombus. The patient proceeded to conventional coronary angiography. **C,** Occlusion of the LAD was found. **D,** The patient went on to have successful re-angioplasty and stenting of the LAD lesion. **See Videos 7-3 and 7-4.**

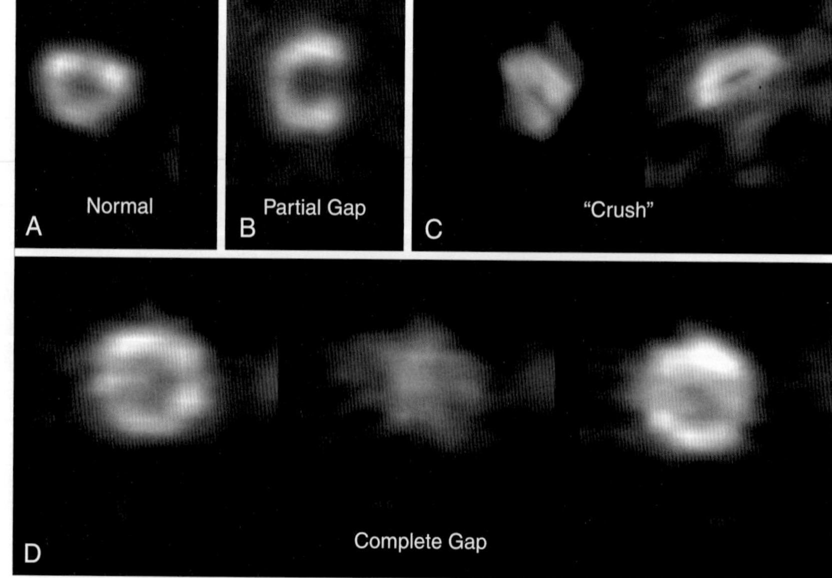

Figure 7-20. Stent gap patterns. **A,** Normal; **B,** partial; **C,** crush; and **D,** complete. The center image in **D** shows a complete gap; the images on the left and right show normal areas. (Reprinted with permission from Hecht HS, Polena S, Jelnin V, et al. Stent gap by 64-detector computed tomographic angiography relationship to in-stent restenosis, fracture, and overlap failure. *J Am Coll Cardiol.* 2009;54(21):1949-1959.)

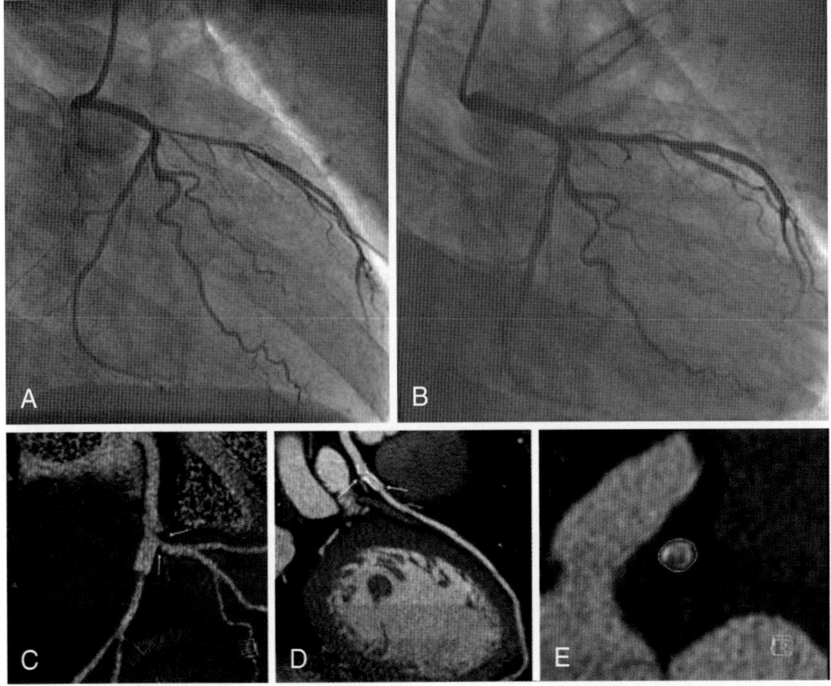

Figure 7-21. A 43-year-old man presented with acute anterior myocardial infarction. A critical ostial stenosis of the left anterior descending coronary artery and moderate distal left main lesion were visualized at primary coronary angiography (**A**) and successfully treated with stent implantation (**B**). Four weeks later the patient reported angina pectoris at rest. A dual-source CT scan was performed. Stent-induced arterial stretch, stent fracture, in-stent restenosis, and ostial circumflex stenosis were precisely visualized. Coronary angiography confirmed in-stent restenosis and circumflex stenosis but was unable to show stent fracture (**C–E**). Coronary CT depicts stent fractures even in those cases that are not clearly depicted by conventional angiography. (Reprinted with permission from Sozzi FB, Civaia F, Rossi P, et al. Coronary stent fracture and in-stent restenosis at coronary computed tomography. *J Am Coll Cardiol.* 2009;54(23):2199.)

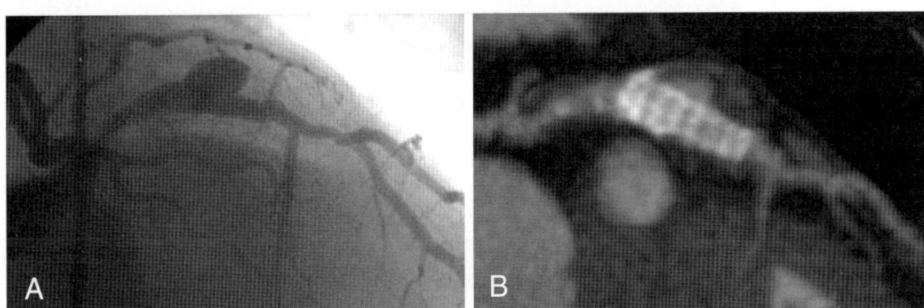

Figure 7-22. Angiographic (**A**) and CT angiographic (**B**) images of coronary artery aneurysm after drug-eluting stent implantation. A coronary artery aneurysm was discovered 18 months after drug-eluting stent implantation. (Reprinted with permission from Aoki J, Kirtane A, Leon MB, Dangas G. Coronary artery aneurysms after drug-eluting stent implantation. *JACC Cardiovasc Interv.* 2008;1(1):14-21.)

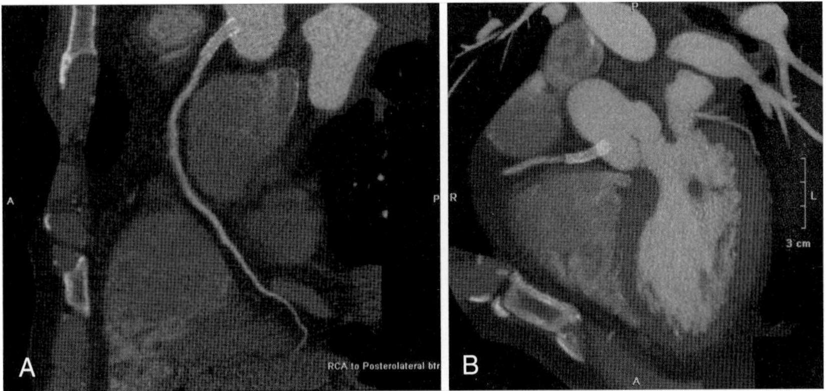

Figure 7-23. Chest pain post–percutaneous intervention prompted CT angiography. The stent was large and proximal and is plausible without thrombus or restenosis. The proximal margin of the stent protrudes 6 mm into the aorta. **See Video 7-5.**

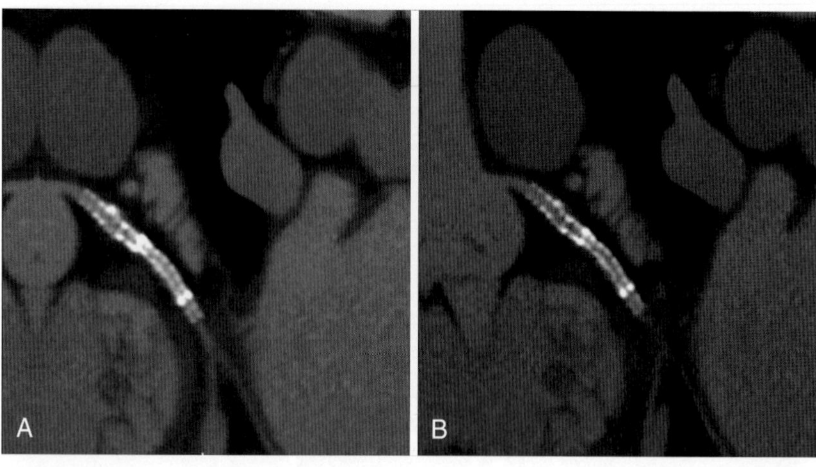

Figure 7-24. Two curved multiplanar reformatted images from a cardiac CT stent in a patient with prior circumflex artery stenting. **A,** Image obtained in a standard reconstruction algorithm. **B,** Image obtained using a higher spatial frequency reconstruction kernel. A subtle amount of low attenuation seen in the proximal portion of the stented circumflex artery representing a small amount of in-stent restenosis is better appreciated on the higher-spatial-frequency reconstruction shown in **B**.

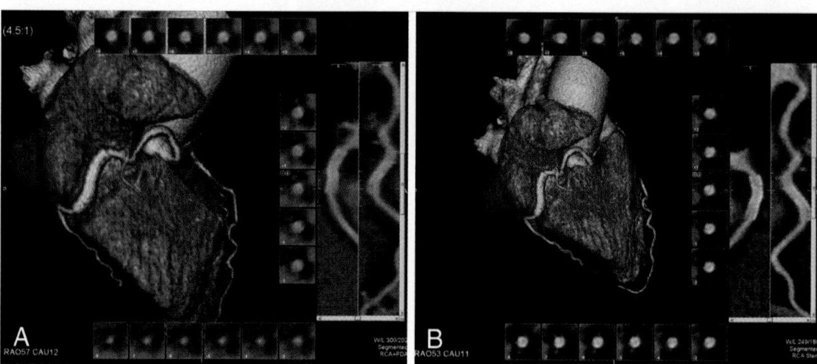

Figure 7-25. Curved reformations through a right coronary artery (RCA) with a mid-RCA stent. **A,** Normal soft tissue reconstruction. **B,** A high-detail kernel was used for reconstruction. This allows better visualization through the stented region with a resultant decrease in blooming artifact. No evidence of in-stent stenosis or thrombosis was found.

TABLE 7-4 ACCF 2010 Appropriateness Criteria for the Use of Cardiac CT to Evaluate Risk Assessment Post–Coronary Artery Bypass Revascularization

	APPROPRIATENESS RATING	INDICATION	MEDIAN SCORE
Symptomatic ischemic equivalent	Appropriate	None listed	—
	Uncertain	Prior coronary stent with stent diameter ≥ 3 mm	6
	Inappropriate	Prior coronary stent with stent diameter < 3 mm or not known	3
Asymptomatic — prior coronary stenting	Appropriate	Prior left main coronary stent Stent diameter ≥ 3 mm	7
	Uncertain	Stent diameter ≥ 3 mm Time since PCI: ≥2 years	4
	Inappropriate	Stent diameter < 3 mm or not known Time since PCI: <2 years	2
		Stent diameter < 3 mm or not known Time since PCI: ≥2 years	2
		Stent diameter ≥ 3 mm Time since PCI: <2 years	3

PCI, percutaneous intervention.

Data from Taylor AJ, Cerqueira M, Hodgson JM, et al. ACCF/SCCT/ACR/AHA/ASE/ASNC/NASCI/SCAI/SCMR 2010 appropriate use criteria for cardiac computed tomography. A report of the American College of Cardiology Foundation Appropriate Use Criteria Task Force, the Society of Cardiovascular Computed Tomography, the American College of Radiology, the American Heart Association, the American Society of Echocardiography, the American Society of Nuclear Cardiology, the North American Society for Cardiovascular Imaging, the Society for Cardiovascular Angiography and Interventions, and the Society for Cardiovascular Magnetic Resonance. *J Am Coll Cardiol.* 2010;56(22):1864-1894.

References

1. Nieman K, Ligthart JM, Serruys PW, De Feyter PJ. Images in cardiovascular medicine. Left main rapamycin-coated stent: invasive versus noninvasive angiographic follow-up. *Circulation.* 2002; 105(18):e130-e131.
2. van Mieghem CA, Cademartiri F, Mollet NR, et al. Multislice spiral computed tomography for the evaluation of stent patency after left main coronary artery stenting: a comparison with conventional coronary angiography and intravascular ultrasound. *Circulation.* 2006;114(7):645-653.
3. Abdelkarim MJ, Ahmadi N, Gopal A, Hamirani Y, Karlsberg RP, Budoff MJ. Noninvasive quantitative evaluation of coronary artery stent patency using 64-row multidetector computed tomography. *J Cardiovasc Comput Tomogr.* 2010;4(1):29-37.
4. Romeo G, Houyel L, Angel CY, Brenot P, Riou JY, Paul JF. Coronary stenosis detection by 16-slice computed tomography in heart transplant patients: comparison with conventional angiography and impact on clinical management. *J Am Coll Cardiol.* 2005; 45(11):1826-1831.
5. Pugliese F, Cademartiri F, van Mieghem C, et al. Multidetector CT for visualization of coronary stents. *Radiographics.* 2006;26(3): 887-904.
6. Cademartiri F, Schuijf JD, Pugliese F, et al. Usefulness of 64-slice multislice computed tomography coronary angiography to assess in-stent restenosis. *J Am Coll Cardiol.* 2007;49(22):2204-2210.
7. Gaspar T, Halon DA, Lewis BS, et al. Diagnosis of coronary in-stent restenosis with multidetector row spiral computed tomography. *J Am Coll Cardiol.* 2005;46(8):1573-1579.
8. Oncel D, Oncel G, Karaca M. Coronary stent patency and in-stent restenosis: determination with 64-section multidetector CT coronary angiography—initial experience. *Radiology.* 2007;242(2): 403-409.
9. Oncel D, Oncel G, Tastan A, Tamci B. Evaluation of coronary stent patency and in-stent restenosis with dual-source CT coronary angiography without heart rate control. *AJR Am J Roentgenol.* 2008;191(1):56-63.
10. Pugliese F, Weustink AC, Van Mieghem C, et al. Dual source coronary computed tomography angiography for detecting in-stent restenosis. *Heart.* 2008;94(7):848-854.
11. Ehara M, Kawai M, Surmely JF, et al. Diagnostic accuracy of coronary in-stent restenosis using 64-slice computed tomography: comparison with invasive coronary angiography. *J Am Coll Cardiol.* 2007;49(9):951-959.
12. Rixe J, Achenbach S, Ropers D, et al. Assessment of coronary artery stent restenosis by 64-slice multi-detector computed tomography. *Eur Heart J.* 2006;27(21):2567-2572.
13. Rist C, von Ziegler F, Nikolaou K, et al. Assessment of coronary artery stent patency and restenosis using 64-slice computed tomography. *Acad Radiol.* 2006;13(12):1465-1473.
14. Schroeder S, Achenbach S, Bengel F, et al. Cardiac computed tomography: indications, applications, limitations, and training requirements: report of a Writing Group deployed by the Working Group Nuclear Cardiology and Cardiac CT of the European Society of Cardiology and the European Council of Nuclear Cardiology. *Eur Heart J.* 2008;29(4):531-556.
15. Gade CL, Lin F, Feldman DN, Weinsaft JW, Min JK. Assessment of coronary artery aneurysm after stent placement for myocardial infarction: evaluation by multidetector computed tomography. *J Cardiovasc Comput Tomogr.* 2008;2(2):117-119.
16. Hecht HS, Polena S, Jelnin V, et al. Stent gap by 64-detector computed tomographic angiography relationship to in-stent restenosis, fracture, and overlap failure. *J Am Coll Cardiol.* 2009;54(21): 1949-1959.
17. Sozzi FB, Civaia F, Rossi P, Rusek S, Dor V. Coronary stent fracture and in-stent restenosis at coronary computed tomography. *J Am Coll Cardiol.* 2009;54(23):2199.
18. Lim HB, Hur G, Kim SY, et al. Coronary stent fracture: detection with 64-section multidetector CT angiography in patients and in vitro. *Radiology.* 2008;249(3):810-819.
19. Alfonso F, Perez-Vizcayno MJ, Ruiz M, et al. Coronary aneurysms after drug-eluting stent implantation: clinical, angiographic, and intravascular ultrasound findings. *J Am Coll Cardiol.* 2009;53(22): 2053-2060.
20. Levisay JP, Roth RM, Schatz RA. Coronary artery aneurysm formation after drug-eluting stent implantation. *Cardiovasc Revasc Med.* 2008;9(4):284-287.
21. Li SS, Cheng BC, Lee SH. Images in cardiovascular medicine. Giant coronary aneurysm formation after sirolimus-eluting stent implantation in Kawasaki disease. *Circulation.* 2005;112(8): e105-e107.
22. Jang JJ, Krishnaswami A, Fang J, Go M, Ben VC. Images in cardiovascular medicine. Pseudoaneurysm and intracardiac fistula caused by an infected paclitaxel-eluting coronary stent. *Circulation.* 2007; 116(14):e364-e365.
23. Le MQ, Narins CR. Mycotic pseudoaneurysm of the left circumflex coronary artery: a fatal complication following drug-eluting stent implantation. *Catheter Cardiovasc Interv.* 2007;69(4):508-512.
24. Schuijf JD, Bax JJ, Jukema JW, et al. Feasibility of assessment of coronary stent patency using 16-slice computed tomography. *Am J Cardiol.* 2004;94:427-430.

CTA Assessment of Saphenous Vein Grafts and Internal Thoracic (Mammary) Arteries

Key Points

- Coronary artery bypass grafts are amenable to cardiac CT angiography assessment because they are larger in size than native arteries and are subject to little motion artifact and little calcification, factors that otherwise present major limitations to CCT.
- The abundance of surgical clips on internal thoracic and mammary grafts is an impediment to adequate CCT angiography.
- Unfortunately, the need to assess native coronary artery disease, which is always advanced in patients who have had a prior bypass, renders coronary graft assessment only a portion of the necessary evaluation.
- However, CCT coronary graft angiography may be useful in well-chosen cases, such as mapping graft course in cases where reoperation is anticipated.

CORONARY BYPASS GRAFT ASSESSMENT

Coronary bypass grafts, both venous and arterial, are more readily evaluated by CT angiography (CTA) than are coronary arteries, because of:

- Their large diameter (more so for venous than arterial conduits)
- Their minimal motion, when compared with coronary arteries, because they are largely extracardiac
- Their general lack of calcification, versus the common and often extensive calcification of native coronary arteries
- Simpler courses (but not always) with little overlap. Some exceptions:
  - Posterior transverse sinus course of a venous graft or right internal mammary artery (RIMA) graft to the circumflex
  - Twisted course of vein grafts if multiple and adjacent
  - The presence of jump-grafts (sequential graft insertions; usually saphenous)
  - Internal thoracic artery positioned tightly against the chest wall, in which case the use of bone extraction software when post-processing may eliminate depiction of the internal mammary artery (IMA) graft

Potential Uses of Coronary CTA in Patients with Coronary Artery Bypass Grafts

- Nonvisualization of a coronary artery bypass graft (CABG) at the time of catheter angiography
- Chest pain in a patient with CABG
- Prior to repeat open heart surgery (CABG or valve surgery), to localize the bypass grafts relative to the sternum and intended sternotomy

Problems with Bypass Graft Assessment

- The large field of view. This is especially true if there is an internal thoracic artery to be imaged, because the field of view will extend from above the subclavian artery down to the diaphragm. This requires:
  - Longer breath-hold and greater chance for motion artifact
  - Greater radiation exposure
- Surgical clips abound around mammary arteries and may present a challenge and sometimes a problem when the adjacent lumen is being imaged.
- Sternal wires also may cause artifacts, as may ECG electrodes, which can confound assessment of anterior bypass grafts.
- The direction of flow within a graft cannot be established by its opacification. It is tempting to view opacification as indicative of anterograde flow. This becomes a problem, however, when there is a proximal severe-appearing lesion: assumption of anterograde filling implies nonocclusion, whereas retrograde filling of a proximally occluded graft may have been the case.

- If a left internal thoracic artery graft is present, the contrast will have to be injected via the right arm to avoid high-attenuation artifacts in the left subclavian artery; such artifacts may confound imaging of the ostium of the internal thoracic artery.
- If both the left and right internal thoracic arteries are used as conduits, then the ostium of one of the two will be obscured by subclavian vein overattenuation artifacts.
- Often a larger concentration of metallic clips is seen at the graft-native vessel anastomosis, resulting in a beam-hardening artifact and obscuring the depiction of the anastomosis.
- Cardiac CT (CCT) is better at assessing bypass grafts than native vessels, which are, of course, always diseased in the scenario of bypass grafting, often extensively, and may be calcified. Adequate and complete visualization of the native vessels distal to the bypass graft anastomosis may be (often is) problematic, because the native coronary arteries at this level tend to be smaller.
- Stenting within bypass grafts is still a challenge; however, stents within grafts often are better assessed than native stented vessels due to the larger size of the grafts and less cardiac motion.
- Interobserver agreement of quantification of lesions is poor: less than 50%.[1]
- For more information, see Tables 8-1 and 8-2.

Other suggested applications of coronary CTA include "trouble-shooting" of bypass cases. Coronary CTA has detected the inadvertent surgical complication of insertion of a saphenous vein graft into the anterior cardiac vein.[2]

CTA images of normal saphenous and arterial bypass grafts are seen in Figures 8-1 through 8-5 and in **Video 8-1**).

CTA images of arterial bypass grafts with stenoses, obstructions, stents, complicated courses or design, or advanced distal native vessel disease are seen in Figures 8-6 through 8-10.

CTA images of saphenous bypass grafts with stenoses, obstructions, stents, complicated courses or design, inadvertent anastomosis, or advanced distal native vessel disease are seen in Figures 8-11 through 8-19.

Unusual complications of coronary artery bypass grafting sometimes may be seen:

- Tenting of the pericardium and right ventricular outflow tract to the sternum (Fig. 8-20)
- Sternal dehiscence (Fig. 8-21)
- False aneurysm development at the proximal anastomosis (Figs. 8-22 and 8-23)
- Saphenous vein bypass graft aneurysm development (see Chapter 11)
- Dissection of a bypass graft

Complications of coronary artery bypass grafts include:

- Stenosis
- Occlusion
- Aneurysm[18-20]
- Dissection[21]
- Disruption of a proximal anastamosis[22]
- Dehiscence[23]
- Rupture of a saphenous bypass aneurysm[24]
- Mycotic aneurysm with rupture[25]
- Aneurysm with hemoptysis[26]
- Aneurysm with emboli[27]
- Aneurysm with anterior mediastinal mass[28]
- Spasm
- Bypass graft insertion into a cardiac vein[2]

CARDIAC CT PROTOCOL POINTS

- No calcium scoring—low-dose scout imaging only to verify that there is adequate field of view to include the entire left and right internal mammary territory.
- If there is a left internal mammary artery (LIMA) graft but no RIMA graft, injection should be done via the right antecubital vein, rather than the left, to avoid left subclavian vein dye-related artifacts compromising imaging of the proximal left internal mammary artery.
- Landmark: 1 cm above lung apices if LIMA or RIMA is to be evaluated, to below the level of the heart
- For more information, see Table 8-3.

TABLE 8-1 Cardiac CT Assessment of Coronary Artery Bypass Grafts

AUTHOR	JOURNAL	YEAR	CT	NO. PTS/NO. GRAFTS	NONASSESS. (%)	GRAFT TYPES (SVG:IMA)	LESION	SENSITIVITY (%)	SPECIFICITY (%)	PPV (%)	NPV (%)
Achenbach et al.[3]	Am J Cardiol	1997	EBCT	25	4	55:1	Occlusion	100	100		
					16		Stenosis	100	97		
Chiurlia et al.[4]	Am J Cardiol	2005	16-CT	52	99	117:47	Occlusion	100	100		
							Stenosis	96	100		
Martuscelli et al.[5]	Circulation	2004	16-CT	96		166:85	Occlusion	100	100		
							Stenosis	90	100		
				84			Anastomosis	97	100		
Nieman et al.[6]	Radiology	2003	4-CT	109	16			93	42	70	81
Ropers et al.[7]	Am J Cardiol	2001	MSCT	65	0	162:20	Occlusion	97	98	97	98
					38		Stenosis	75	92	71	93
Schlosser et al.[8]	JACC	2004	16-CT	51	0	91:40		96	95	81	99
Anders et al.[9]	Eur J Radiol	2006	16-CT	32	18	74:19	Occlusion	100	98		
							Stenosis	81	87		
Salm et al.[10]	Am Heart J	2005	16-CT	25	8	53:14	Occlusion	100	100	100	100
					8	53:14	Stenosis	100	94	50	100
Moore et al.[1]	Clin Radiol	2005		50		0%	Occlusion	100	100		
						0%	Stenosis	100	99		
Burgstahler et al.[11]	Int J Cardiol	2006	16-CT		0	43 g	Occlusion	100	100		100
					5		Stenosis	100	93		100
Schuijf et al.[12]	Am J Cardiol	2004	16-CT		1	43 g	Occlusion	96	100		99
					15		Stenosis	100	96		100
Pache et al.[13]	Eur Heart J	2006	64-CT		0	93 g	Occlusion	100	100		100
					6		Stenosis	100	100		100

Stauder et al.[14]	Eur Radiol	2006	16-CT	20							
					22.5	80 art	Stenosis	96	97	96	97
					7.3	180 svg	Stenosis	99	94	92	99
					31	Native	Stenosis	92	77	88	85
Malagutti et al.[15]				52/109		Grafts		99	96		
						Native		89	93	50	
Ropers et al.[16]				Graft occlusion	0			100	100	100	100
				Graft stenosis							
				Native arteries	0			100	94	92	100
					9			86	76	44	96

art, arterial grafts; EBCT, electron beam CT; MSCT, multislice CT; nonassess., nonassessable; NPV, negative predictive value; PPV, positive predictive value; svg, saphenous vein graft.

TABLE 8-2 CCT for the Detection of Bypass Graft Occlusion, Bypass Graft Stenoses, and of the Native Coronary Artery Tree

	NOT EVALUABLE (%)	SENSITIVITY (%)	SPECIFICITY (%)	PPV (%)	NPV (%)
Graft occlusion	0.7 (3/418) (95% CI: 0.15–2.1)	100 (130/130) (95% CI: 97–100)	100 (494/495) (95% CI: 99–100)	99 (130/131) (95% CI: 96–100)	100 (494/494) (95% CI: 99–100)
Graft stenosis	6.4 (39/611) (95% CI: 4.6–8.6)	97 (184/1889) (95% CI: 94–99)	95 (337/354) (95% CI: 92–97)	92 (184/201) (95% CI: 87–95)	99 (337/342) (95% CI: 97–100)
Native arteries	19.6 (333/1697) (95% CI: 18–22)	95 (524/545) (95% CI: 93–97)	75 (608/813) (95% CI: 72–78)	67 (424/629) (95% CI: 64–71)	97 (608/629) (95% CI: 95–98)

NPV, negative predictive value; PPV, positive predictive value.
From Schroeder S, Achenbach S, Bengel F, et al: Cardiac computed tomography: indications, applications, limitations, and training requirements: report of a Writing Group deployed by the Working Group Nuclear Cardiology and Cardiac CT of the European Society of Cardiology and the European Council of Nuclear Cardiology. *Eur Heart J.* 2008;29(4):531-556.

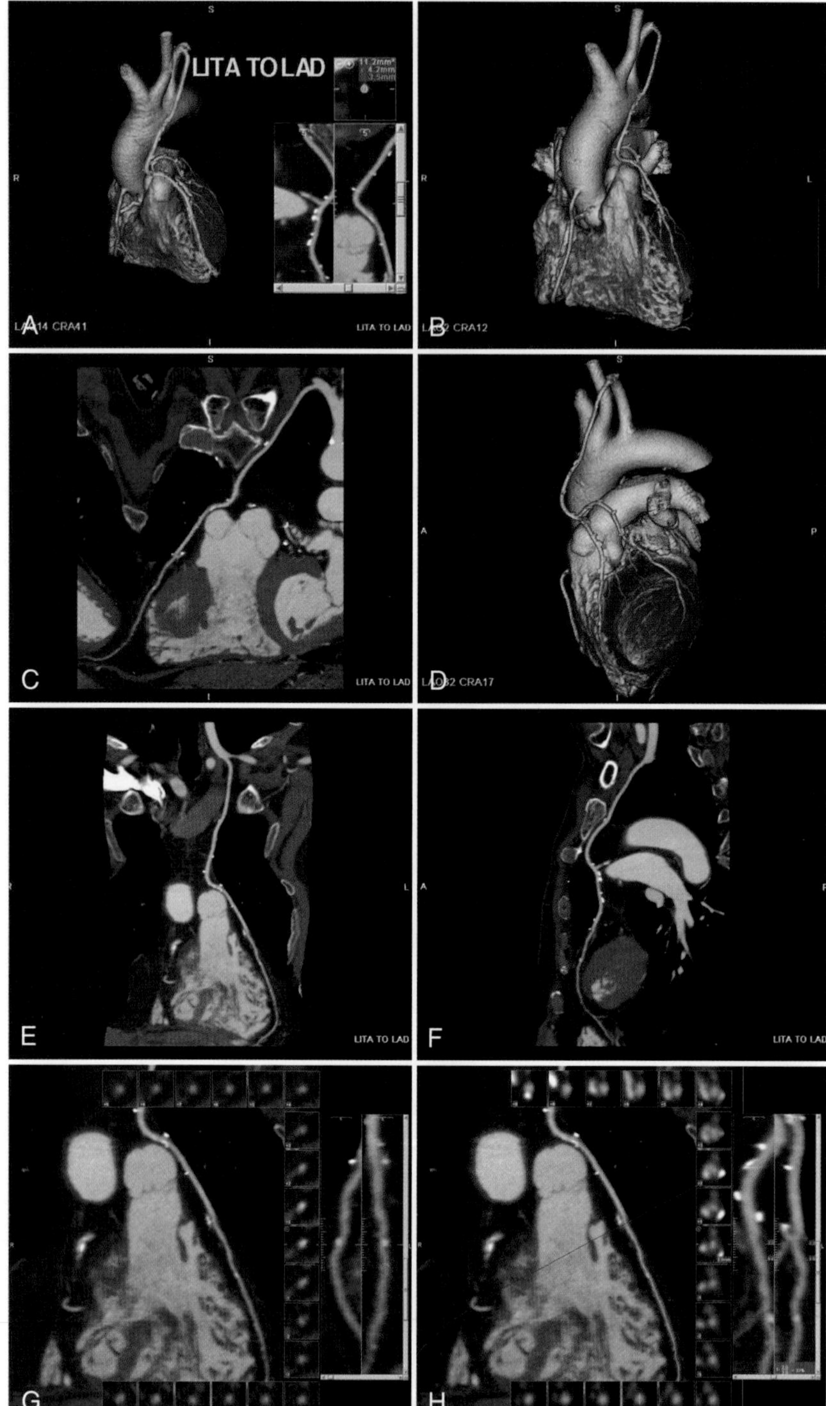

Figure 8-1. Multiple curved reformatted images and volume-rendered images demonstrate a patent left internal thoracic artery (LITA)–left anterior descending artery (LAD) graft, with no evidence of an anastomotic stenosis. No significant ongoing LAD disease is seen. See Figures 8-2 to 8-4 and **Video 8-1**.

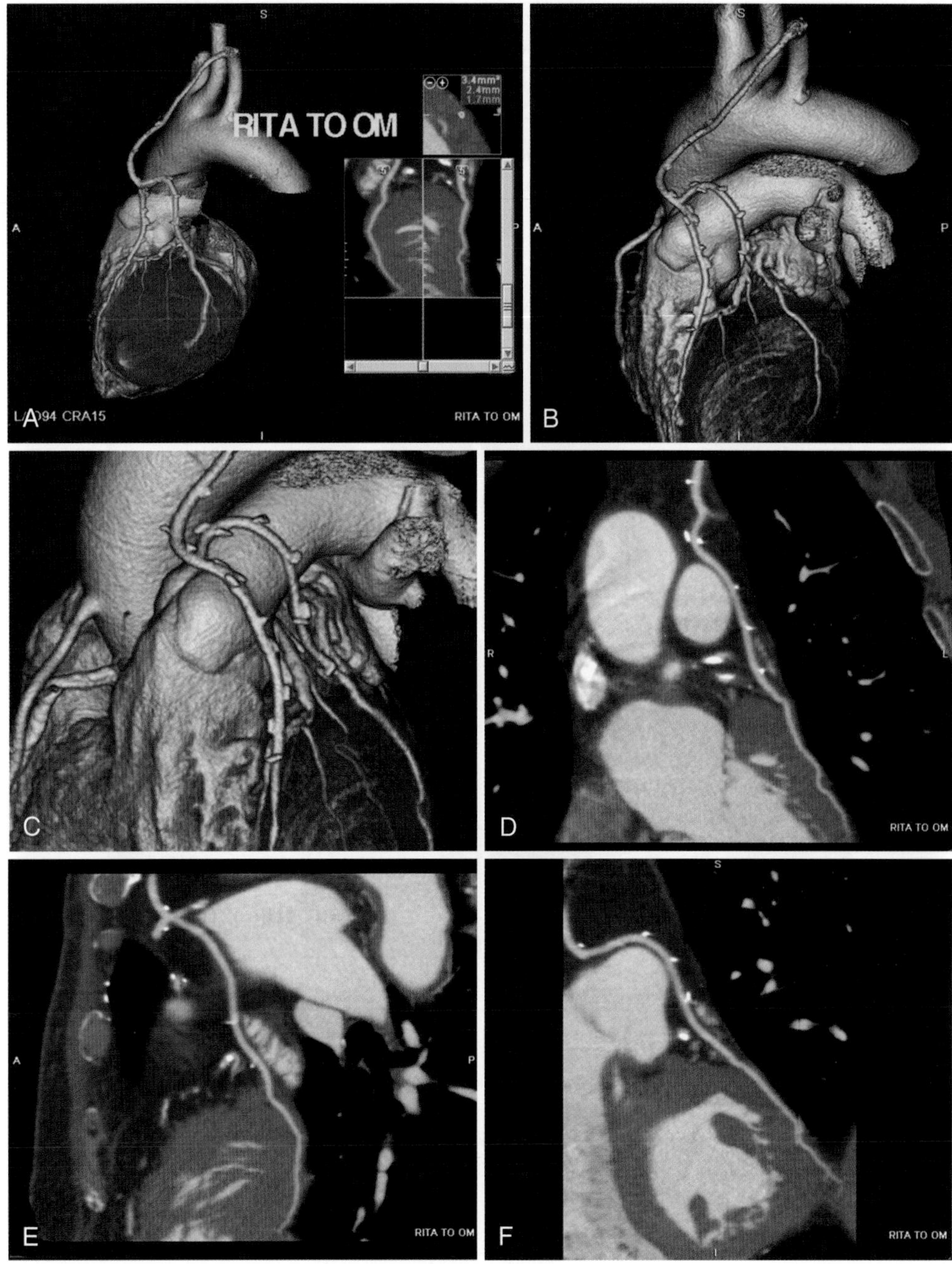

Figure 8-2. Multiple curved and volume-rendered images demonstrate a patent right internal thoracic artery (RITA) to obtuse marginal artery (OM) graft with no evidence of an anastomotic stenosis. See Figures 8-1, 8-3, and 8-4 and **Video 8-1.**

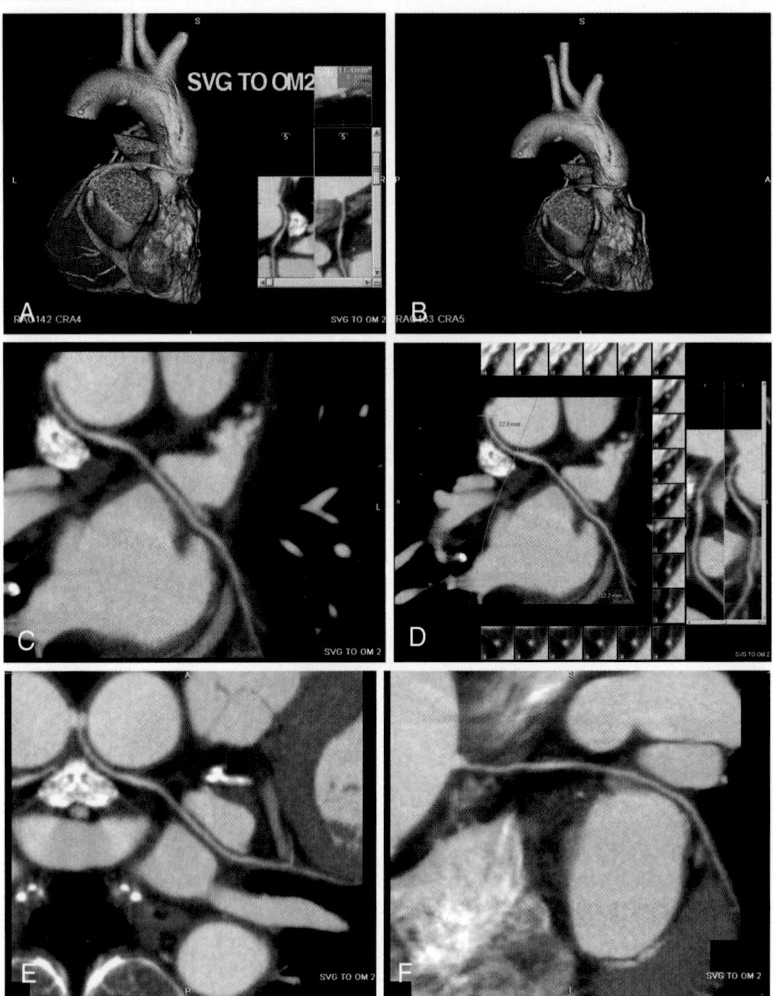

Figure 8-3. Multiple volume-rendered and curved reformatted images demonstrate a saphenous vein graft (SVG) extending to the second branch of the obtuse marginal artery (OM2). This demonstrates a mild 30% to 40% proximal stenosis within the graft. No evidence of an anastomotic stenosis is seen. See Figures 8-1, 8-2, and 8-4 and **Video 8-1.**

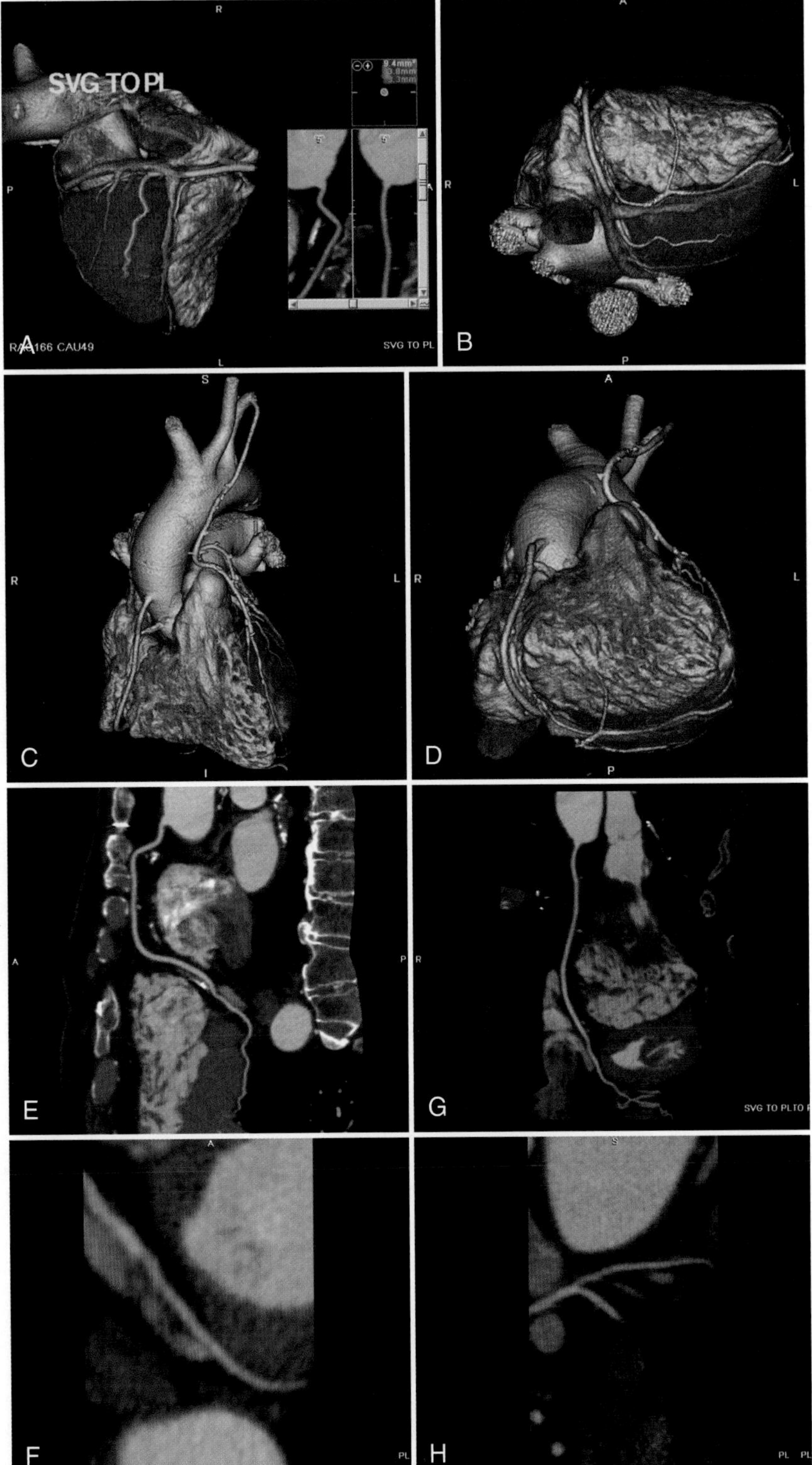

Figure 8-4. Multiple volumetric and curved reformatted images demonstrate a patent saphenous vein graft (SVG) extending to the posterolateral (PL) artery. There is no evidence of an anastomotic stenosis or ongoing disease within the posterolateral branch. See Figures 8-1, 8-2, and 8-3 and **Video 8-1.**

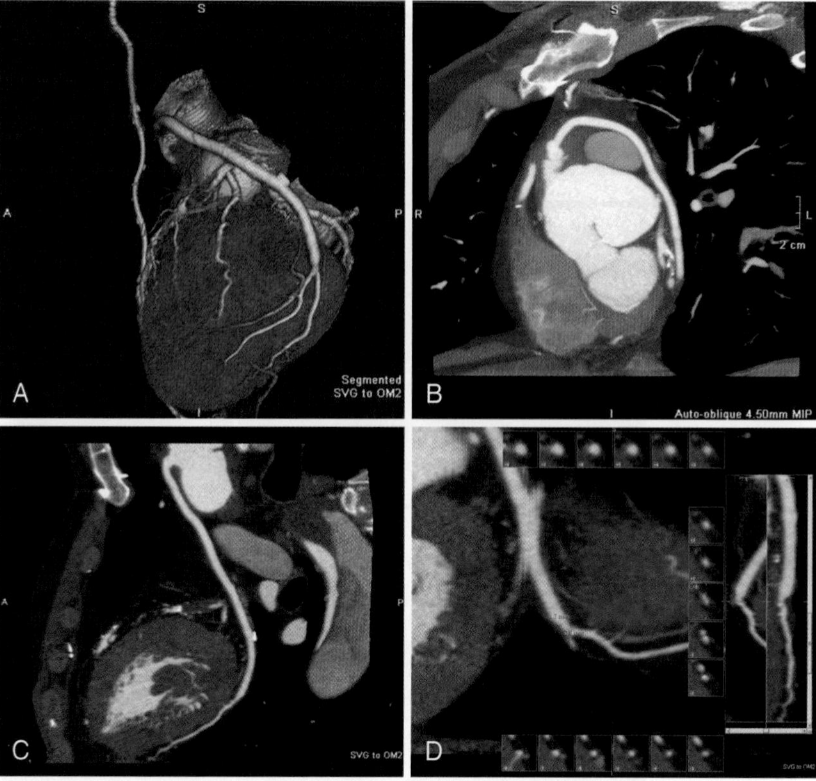

Figure 8-5. Multiple images from a cardiac CT study in a patient with prior coronary artery bypass grafting (left anterior descending artery [LAD] to left internal mammary artery [LIMA]/not shown, and saphenous vein graft [SVG] to the second branch of the obtuse marginal artery [OM2]) who has worsening angina. These images demonstrate different approaches to evaluation of a bypass graft. In this case, volume-rendered imaging of the left upper quarter demonstrates a patent, large SVG anastomosing to the second obtuse marginal branch. A minute image in the right upper quadrant shows the same vessel. Curved reformatted images also nicely demonstrate a patent SVG to OM to graft. No evidence of graft stenosis was seen.

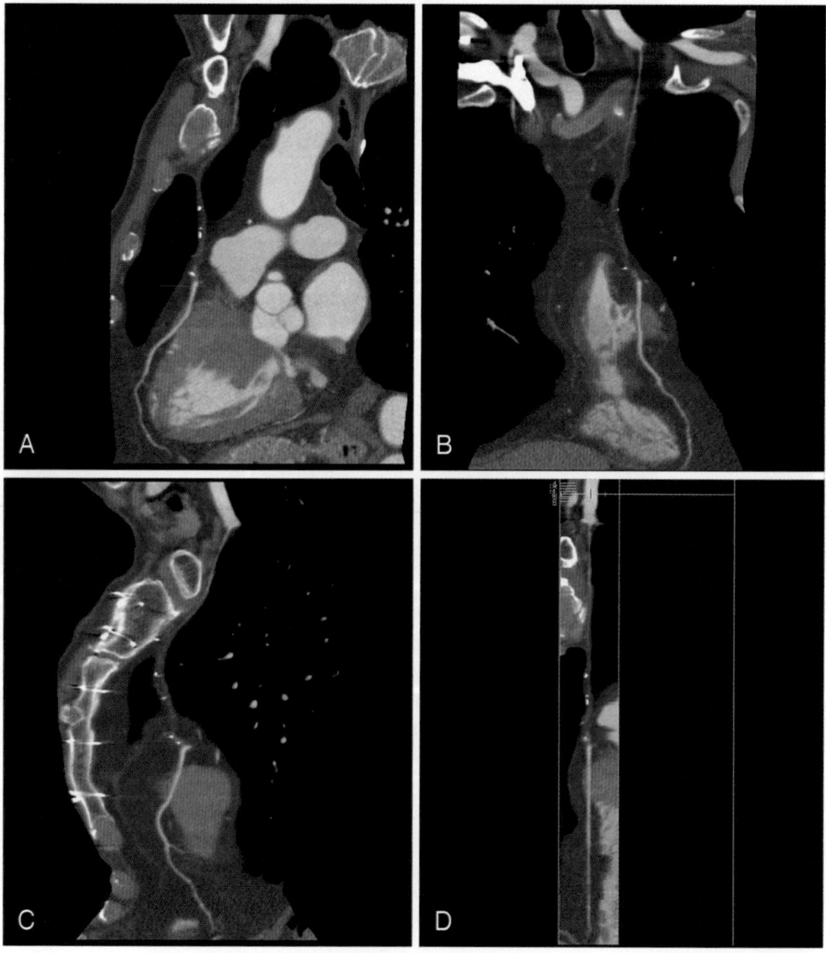

Figure 8-6. Multiple curved reformatted images demonstrate an occluded left internal mammary artery graft within its mid-portion. The ongoing left anterior descending artery does reconstitute from antegrade flow and collateral flow.

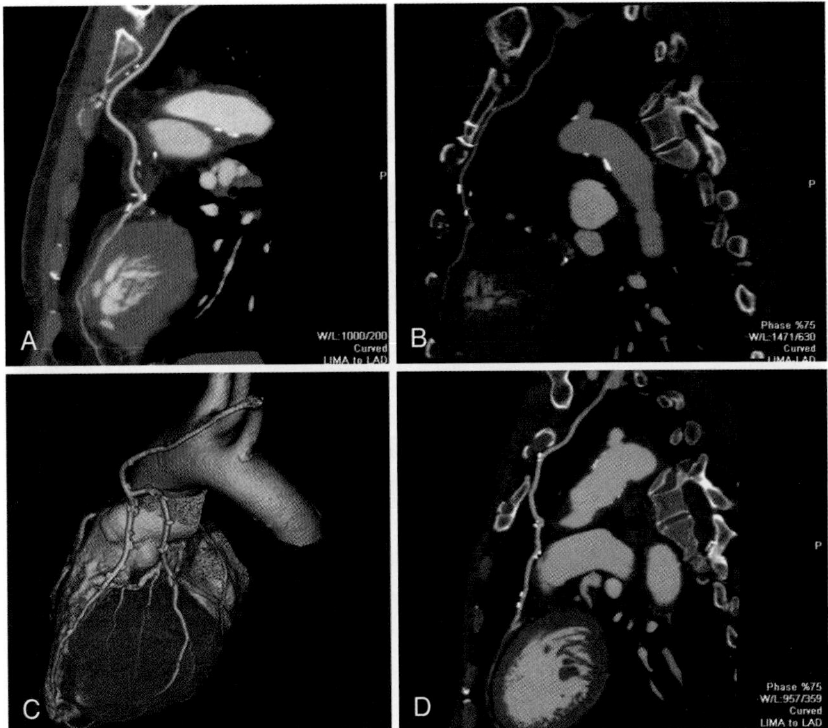

Figure 8-7. **A,** Cardiac CT angiography (CTA) demonstrates a patent left internal mammary artery (LIMA) graft with no evidence of an anastomotic stenosis. The ongoing left anterior descending artery (LAD) has a long, deep intramyocardial segment distal to the anastomosis, and then reenters the epicardial space in the fashion of a type II LAD. **B,** Curved reformat through a patent LIMA graft demonstrates its intimal retrosternal course prior to a normal anastomosis with the mid-LAD. It would be important to be aware of this course if re-sternotomy is required in the future. **C,** A single volume-rendered image demonstrating a LIMA graft to the LAD with a jump graft to a large obtuse marginal branch. Both grafts are patent. **D,** Curved reformation through the LIMA demonstrates a patent LIMA graft with no anastomotic stenosis, but severe disease within the ongoing LAD.

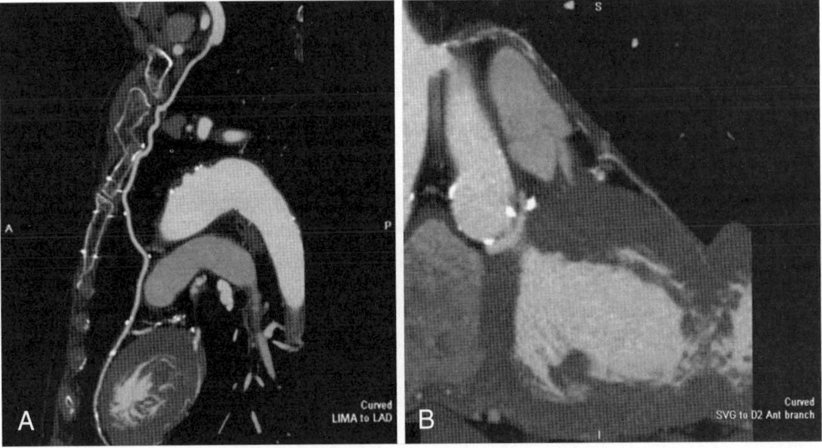

Figure 8-8. A 67-year-old man with angina post–aortocoronary bypass grafting. **A,** The left internal mammary artery (LIMA) graft is patent without anastomotic narrowings or the interval development of a distal left anterior descending artery (LAD) stenosis. **B,** The saphenous bypass graft to the obtuse marginal branch has occluded. SVG, saphenous vein graft.

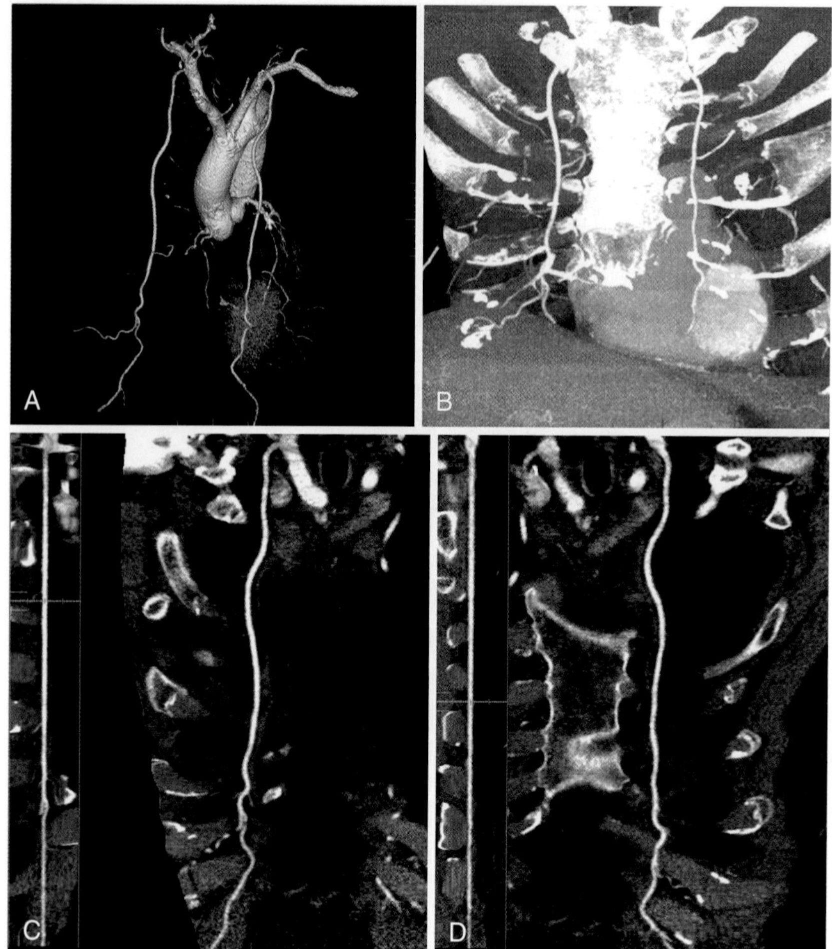

Figure 8-9. Multiple images from a gated thoracic aortic study in a 72-year-old woman pre–coronary artery bypass grafting. The study was performed to evaluate the subclavian arteries, right internal mammary artery, and left internal mammary artery. This image set demonstrates volume-rendered maximum intensity projections and curved reformat and screw through the right and left internal mammary arteries. These demonstrate normal caliber, with no evidence of disease within the internal mammary arteries, or involving their origins from the subclavian arteries on either side.

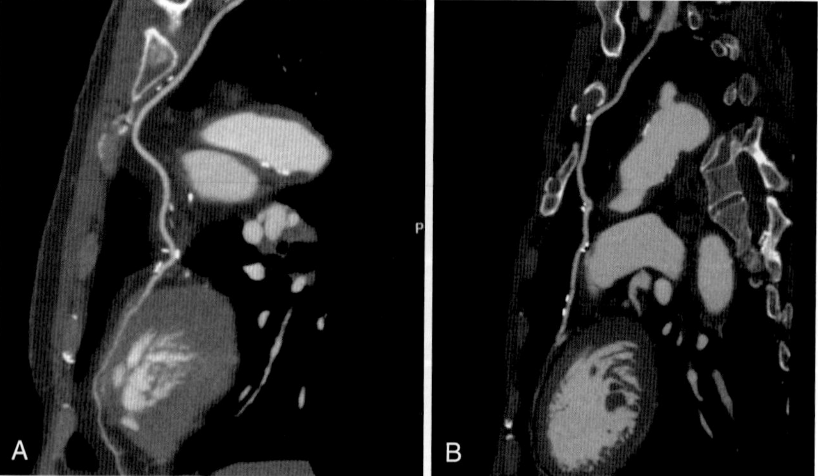

Figure 8-10. Two different patients with patent left internal mammary artery (LIMA) grafts. Although numerous surgical clips are seen along the course of the LIMA grafts, it usually is possible to find projections that enable depiction of the lumen without interference from the clips.

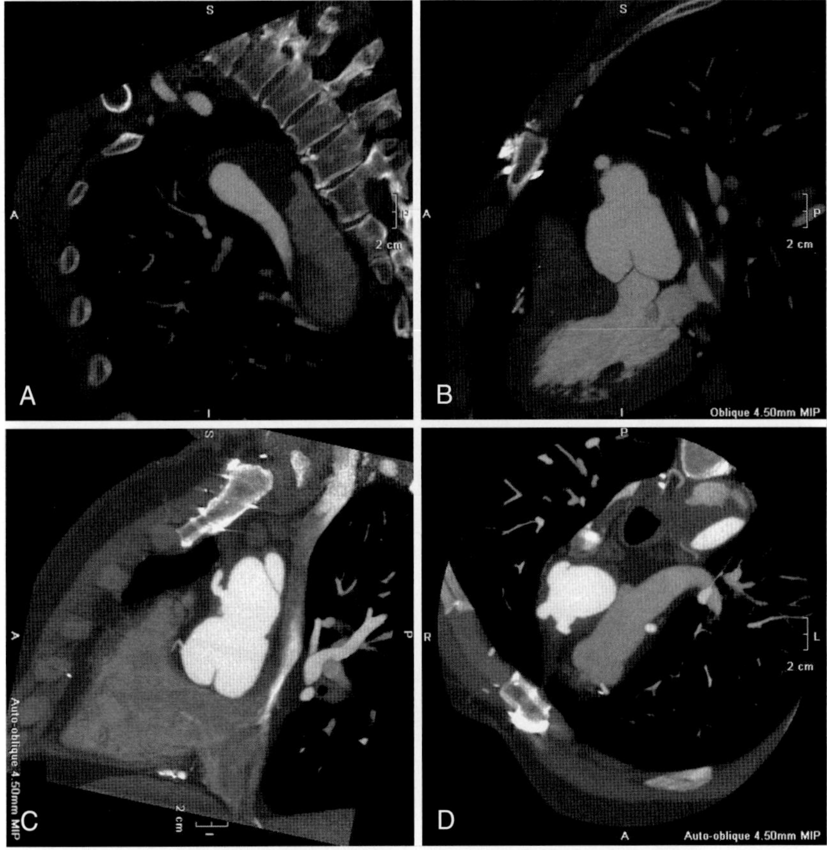

Figure 8-11. Multiple ECG gated images through the thoracic aorta in a patient with prior type A dissection, and a graft within the ascending aorta, with sparing of the aortic root. Prior coronary artery bypass grafting was performed at the time of emergent surgery. **A,** An intimal flap within the descending thoracic aorta, with partial thrombosis of the false lumen. **B,** An enlarged aortic root. The origin of the right coronary artery (RCA) graft also is seen. **C,** A slightly irregular RCA graft origin. An intimal flap is seen in the mid-descending aorta. **D,** The origin of two bypass grafts arising from the ascending aorta. MIP, maximal intensity projection.

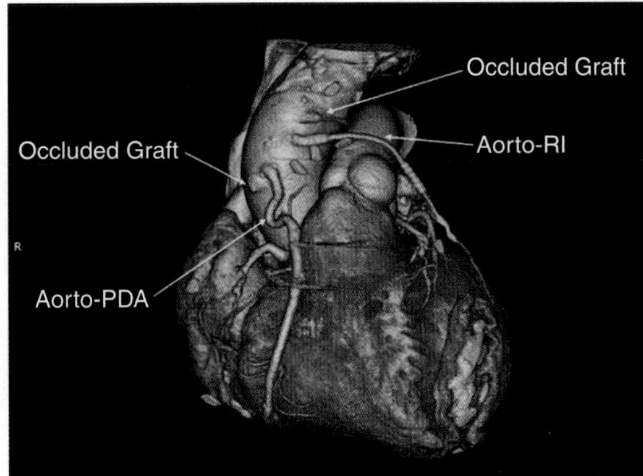

Figure 8-12. A single volume-rendered image in a patient with multiple bypass grafts. There are two saphenous bypass graft stumps. The saphenous vein graft to the patent ductus arteriosus (PDA) is patent. The saphenous vein graft to the ramus branch is patent and has proximal and mid-graft stents. RI, ramus intermedius.

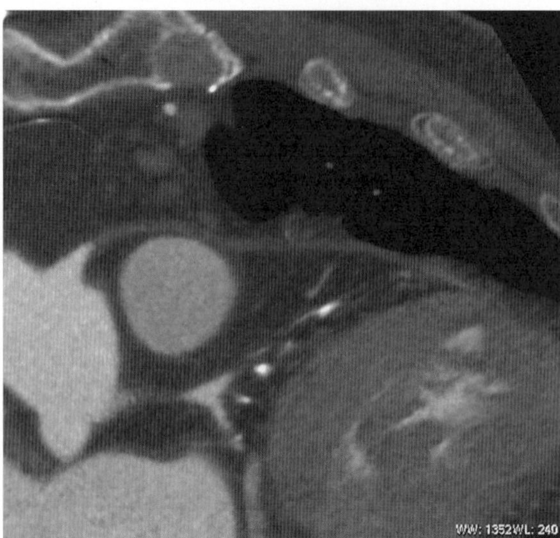

Figure 8-13. Curved reformation demonstrates an occluded saphenous vein graft to the first diagonal branch.

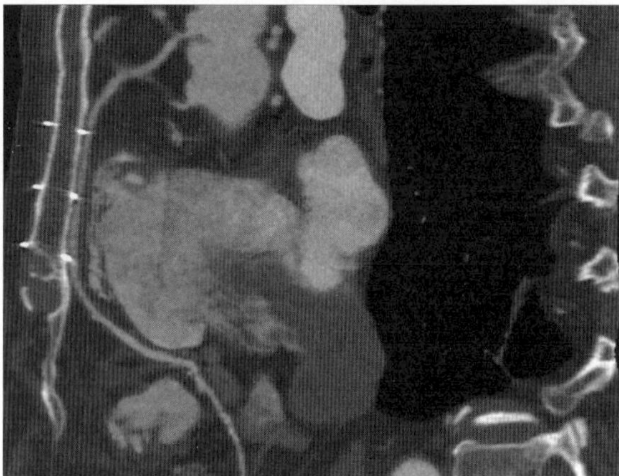

Figure 8-14. Curved reformation of a saphenous vein to distal right coronary artery graft demonstrates a moderate ostial stenosis and marked close apposition of the mid-portion of the graft with the retrosternal space.

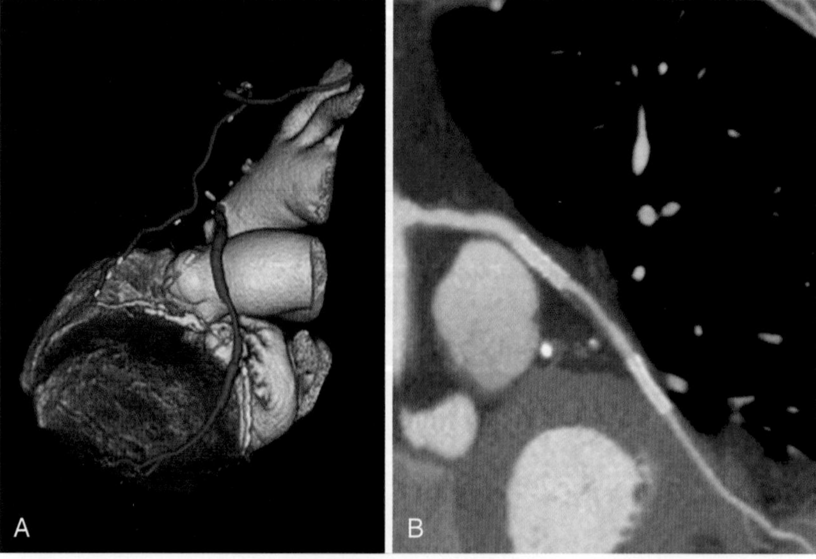

Figure 8-15. A 68-year-old man post–aortocoronary bypass grafting and stenting of a saphenous bypass graft to a distal obtuse marginal branch of the left circumflex artery. **A,** The left internal mammary artery was patent and there was no development of distal disease within the left anterior descending artery. **B,** Moderate disease has developed between two stents in the saphenous graft to the obtuse marginal branch.

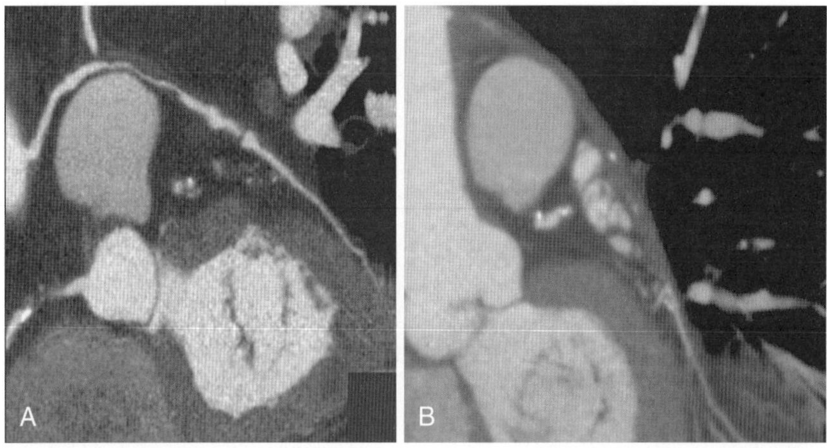

Figure 8-16. Images from two different patients with significant stenotic disease (**A**) and occlusion (**B**) of saphenous bypass grafts.

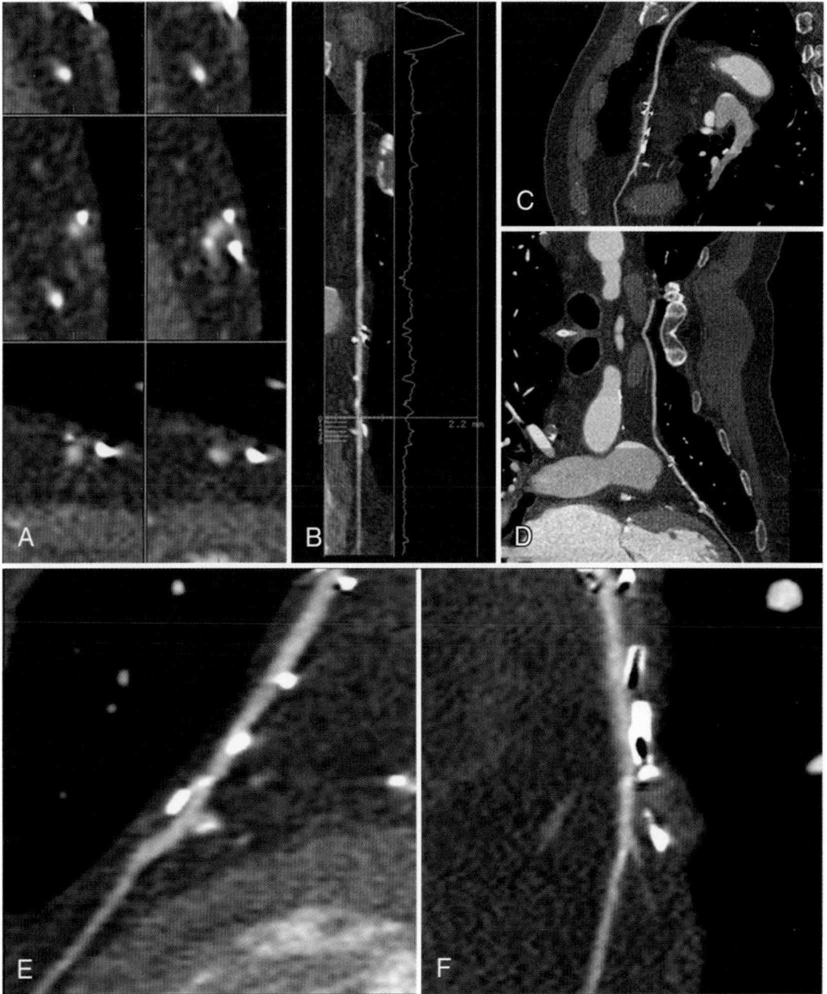

Figure 8-17. Multiple reformatted images from a cardiac CT study in a patient with prior left internal mammary artery (LIMA) grafting, and recurrent angina. **A–D,** Cross-sectional and curved reformatted images demonstrate a patent LIMA graft. **E** and **F,** The distal anastomosis of the LIMA graft to the left anterior descending artery (LAD). Despite the presence of multiple clips, the anastomosis is well identified, with no evidence of an anastomotic stenosis. No stenosis is seen in the ongoing LAD.

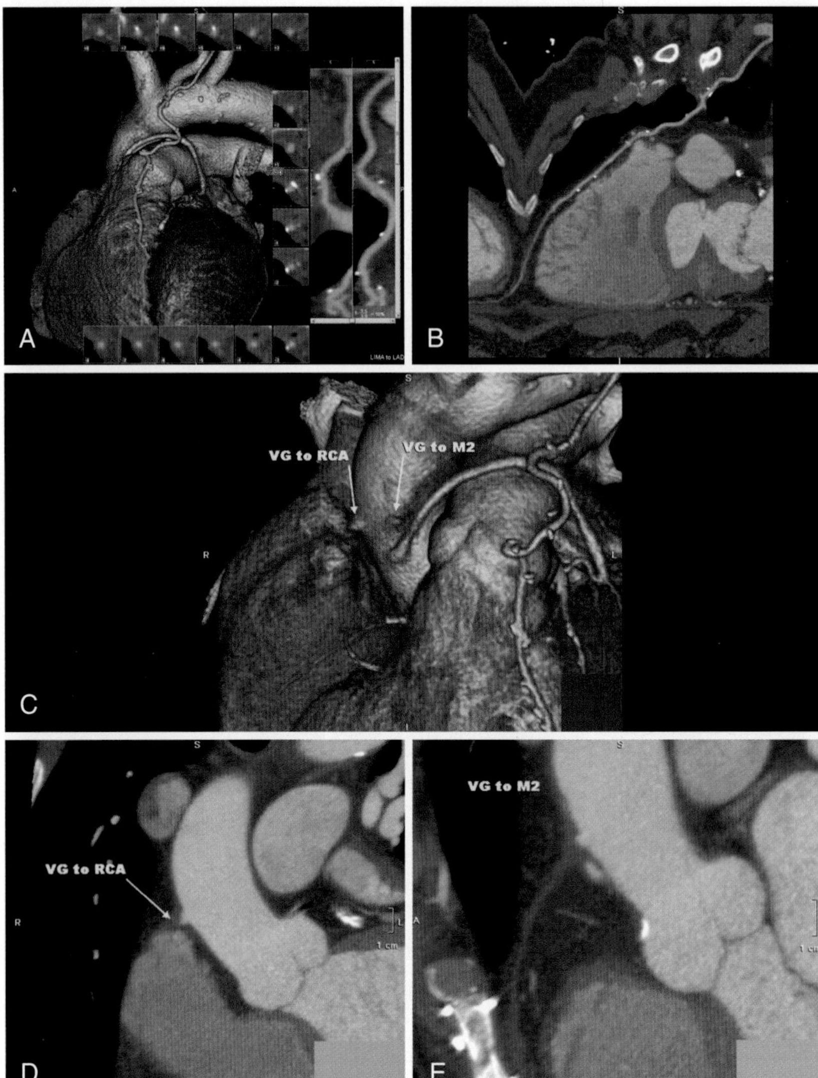

Figure 8-18. Multiple images from a cardiac CT study in a patient with recurrent angina post–quadruple bypass graft surgery. The patient was sent for conventional angiography. A patent left internal mammary artery (LIMA) and saphenous vein graft (SVG) to the first diagonal branch were noted. The right coronary artery (RCA) and obtuse marginal branch graphs are not identified. The patient came for cardiac CT evaluation of the remaining two bypass grafts. **A** and **B,** A patent, normal-appearing LIMA graft and patent ongoing left anterior descending artery (LAD). **C,** Volume-rendered image demonstrates two nipple-like extensions from the anterior aspect of the descending aorta representing occluded grafts to the RCA. These are once again demonstrated in short thickness maximum intensity projection images in **D** and **E**. M2, second obtuse marginal; VG, vein graft.

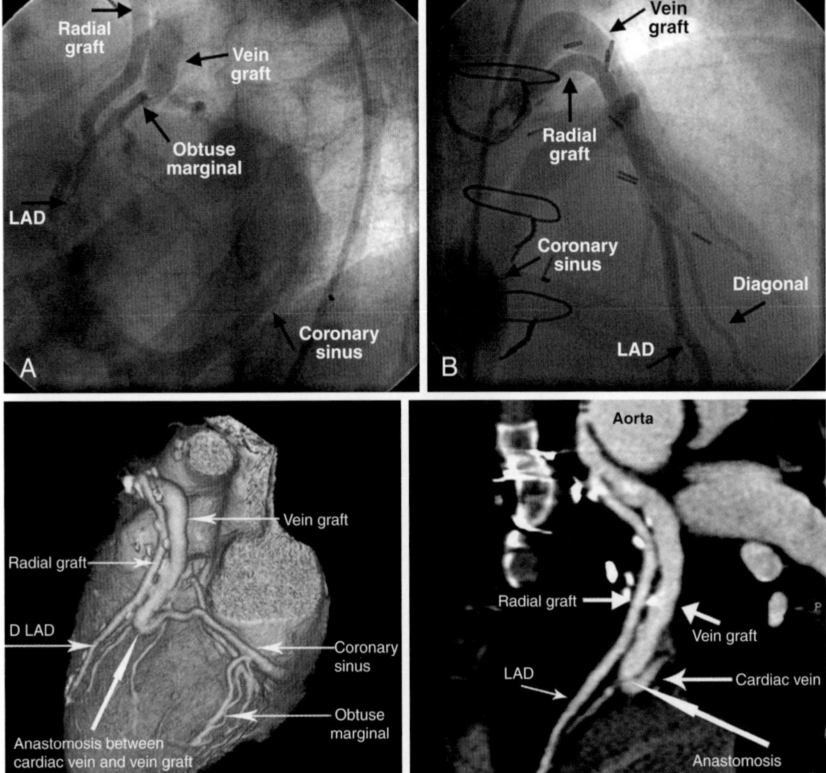

Figure 8-19. Saphenous vein graft to the anterior cardiac vein. **A** and **B,** Invasive angiography with selective injection in the left circumflex saphenous vein graft (SVG). The coronary sinus fills before the coronary arteries (**A**). The simultaneous filling in the left anterior descending (LAD) artery and the coronary sinus is shown (**B**). **C,** Three-dimensional CT reconstruction shows the attachment of the SVG to a cardiac vein, which subsequently drains into the coronary sinus. **D,** Multiplanar reconstruction of the left circumflex SVG shows its anastomosis to the cardiac vein. (Reprinted with permission from Al-Mallah M, Mohyi J, Ananthasubramaniam K. Inadvertent anastomosis of saphenous vein graft to a cardiac vein detected with coronary computed tomographic angiography. *J Cardiovasc Comput Tomogr.* 2008;2(1):61-63.)

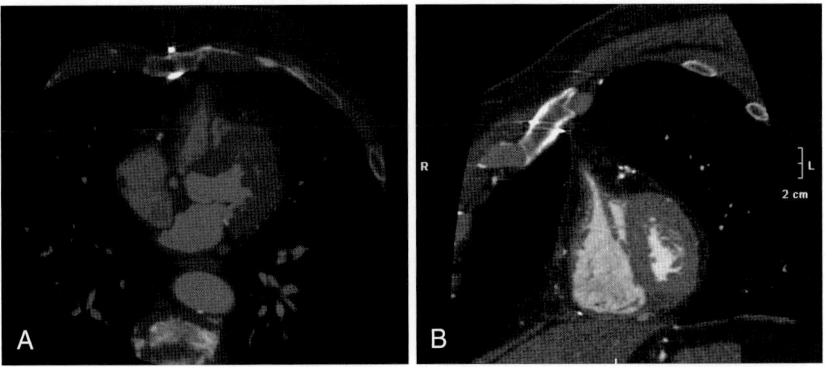

Figure 8-20. Two images from a cardiac CT study demonstrate marked tenting and peaking of the right ventricular outflow tract with the localized adhesion of the pericardium to the substernal region post–coronary artery bypass grafting.

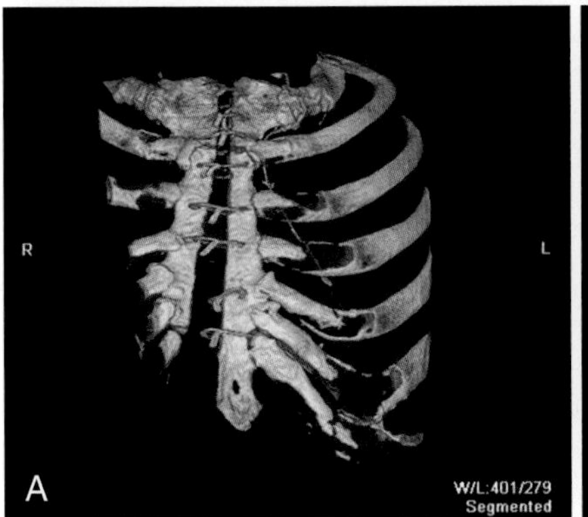

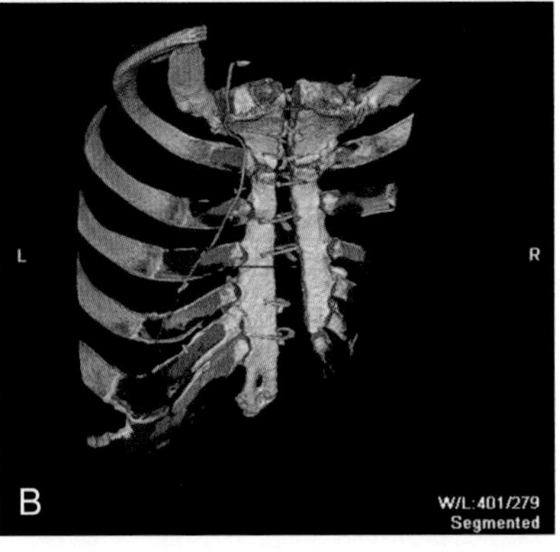

Figure 8-21. Two volume-rendered images from a cardiac CT study demonstrate dehiscence of the median sternotomy.

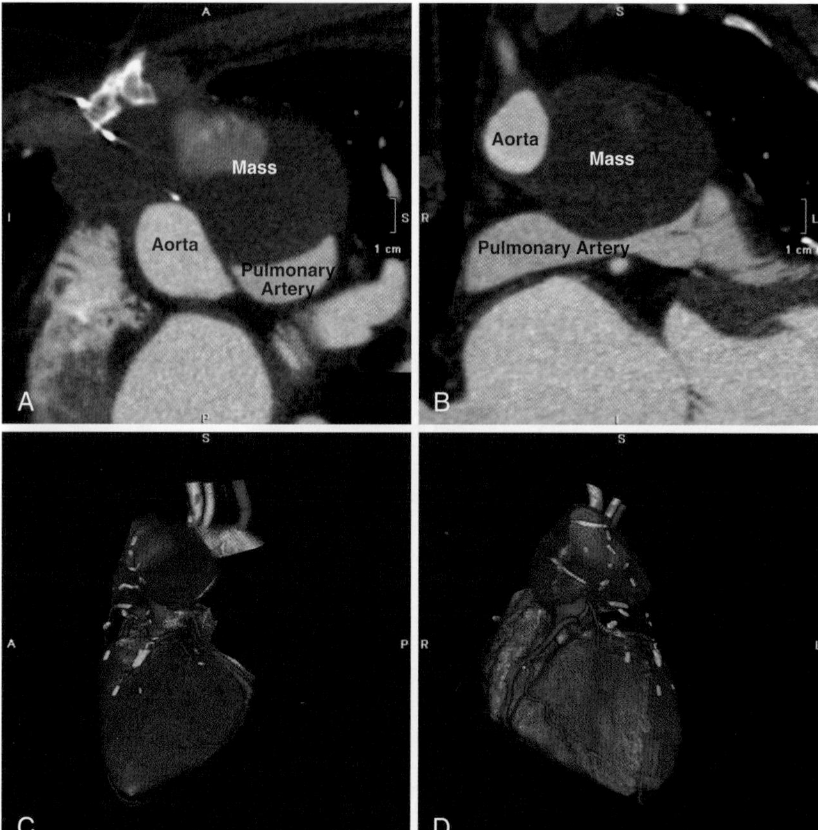

Figure 8-22. A 45-year-old woman, post–aortocoronary bypass complicated by sternal infection and recurrent angina 3 months after the procedure. **A** and **B,** Multiplanar reformations from a cardiac CTA study demonstrate a large complex mediastinal collection with marked compression of the main and right pulmonary arteries and the ascending aorta. **C** and **D,** Two volume-rendered images demonstrate this mediastinal mass. The left internal mammary artery to left anterior descending artery graft is occluded. A saphenous vein graft to the obtuse marginal artery is not visualized, and is presumed to be occluded as well.

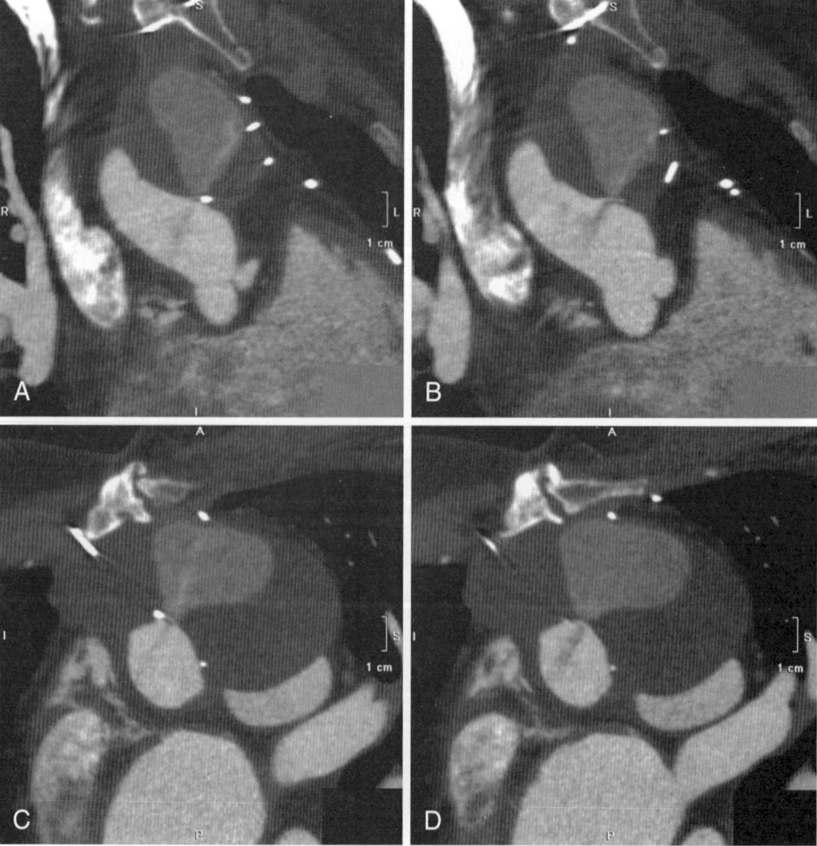

Figure 8-23. Arising off the aorta at the site of a vein graft–associated surgical clip is a complex cavity that demonstrates mixed attenuation. The more central enhancing component represents admixture of contrast and blood within the cavity, defining the cavity as a false aneurysm. A large amount of surrounding mural thrombus is present. A jet of more concentrated contrast material is seen extending from the aorta into the false aneurysm from the saphenous vein graft anastomotic clip site. A corresponding jet of lower attenuation is seen in the ascending aorta, extending from the adjacent false aneurysm. The jets into the false aneurysm and back out of it into the aorta represent the typical reciprocating flow of a false aneurysm. This suggests that the false aneurysm in under high pressure.

TABLE 8-3 ACCF 2010 Appropriateness Criteria for the Use of Cardiac Computed Tomography to Evaluate Risk Assessment Postrevascularization

	APPROPRIATENESS RATING	INDICATION	MEDIAN SCORE
Symptomatic (ischemic equivalent)	Appropriate	Evaluation of graft patency after CABG	8
		Localization of coronary bypass grafts and other retrosternal anatomy Prior to reoperative chest or cardiac surgery	8
Asymptomatic	Appropriate	None	
	Uncertain	Prior CABG Time since CABG: ≥5 years ago	5
	Inappropriate	Prior CABG Time since CABG: <5 years ago	2

Data from Taylor AJ, Cerqueira M, Hodgson JM, et al. ACCF/SCCT/ACR/AHA/ASE/ASNC/NASCI/SCAI/SCMR 2010 appropriate use criteria for cardiac computed tomography. A report of the American College of Cardiology Foundation Appropriate Use Criteria Task Force, the Society of Cardiovascular Computed Tomography, the American College of Radiology, the American Heart Association, the American Society of Echocardiography, the American Society of Nuclear Cardiology, the North American Society for Cardiovascular Imaging, the Society for Cardiovascular Angiography and Interventions, and the Society for Cardiovascular Magnetic Resonance. *J Am Coll Cardiol.* 2010;56(22):1864-1894.

References

1. Moore RK, Sampson C, MacDonald S, Moynahan C, Groves D, Chester MR. Coronary artery bypass graft imaging using ECG-gated multislice computed tomography: comparison with catheter angiography. *Clin Radiol.* 2005;60(9):990-998.
2. Al-Mallah M, Mohyi J, Ananthasubramaniam K. Inadvertent anastomosis of saphenous vein graft to a cardiac vein detected with coronary computed tomographic angiography. *J Cardiovasc Comput Tomogr.* 2008;2:61-63.
3. Achenbach S, Moshage W, Ropers D, Nossen J, Bachmann K. Noninvasive, three-dimensional visualization of coronary artery bypass grafts by electron beam tomography. *Am J Cardiol.* 1997;79(7):856-861.
4. Chiurlia E, Menozzi M, Ratti C, Romagnoli R, Modena MG. Follow-up of coronary artery bypass graft patency by multislice computed tomography. *Am J Cardiol.* 2005;95(9):1094-1097.
5. Martuscelli E, Romagnoli A, D'Eliseo A, et al. Evaluation of venous and arterial conduit patency by 16-slice spiral computed tomography. *Circulation.* 2004;110(20):3234-3238.
6. Nieman K, Pattynama PM, Rensing BJ, Van Geuns RJ, De Feyter PJ. Evaluation of patients after coronary artery bypass surgery: CT angiographic assessment of grafts and coronary arteries. *Radiology.* 2003;229(3):749-756.
7. Ropers D, Ulzheimer S, Wenkel E, et al. Investigation of aortocoronary artery bypass grafts by multislice spiral computed tomography with electrocardiographic-gated image reconstruction. *Am J Cardiol.* 2001;88(7):792-795.
8. Schlosser T, Konorza T, Hunold P, Kuhl H, Schmermund A, Barkhausen J. Noninvasive visualization of coronary artery bypass grafts using 16-detector row computed tomography. *J Am Coll Cardiol.* 2004;44(6):1224-1229.
9. Anders K, Baum U, Schmid M, et al. Coronary artery bypass graft (CABG) patency: assessment with high-resolution submillimeter 16-slice multidetector-row computed tomography (MDCT) versus coronary angiography. *Eur J Radiol.* 2006;57(3):336-344.
10. Salm LP, Bax JJ, Jukema JW, et al. Comprehensive assessment of patients after coronary artery bypass grafting by 16-detector-row computed tomography. *Am Heart J.* 2005;150(4):775-781.
11. Burgstahler C, Beck T, Kuettner A, et al. Non-invasive evaluation of coronary artery bypass grafts using 16-row multi-slice computed tomography with 188 ms temporal resolution. *Int J Cardiol.* 2006;106(2):244-249.
12. Schuijf JD, Bax JJ, Jukema JW, et al. Feasibility of assessment of coronary stent patency using 16-slice computed tomography. *Am J Cardiol.* 2004;94(4):427-430.
13. Pache G, Saueressig U, Frydrychowicz A, et al. Initial experience with 64-slice cardiac CT: non-invasive visualization of coronary artery bypass grafts. *Eur Heart J.* 2006;27(8):976-980.
14. Stauder NI, Kuttner A, Schroder S, et al. Coronary artery bypass grafts: assessment of graft patency and native coronary artery lesions using 16-slice MDCT. *Eur Radiol.* 2006;16(11):2512-2520.
15. Malagutti P, Nieman K, Meijboom WB, et al. Use of 64-slice CT in symptomatic patients after coronary bypass surgery: evaluation of grafts and coronary arteries. *Eur Heart J.* 2007;28(15):1879-1885.
16. Ropers D, Ulzheimer S, Wenkel E, et al. Investigation of aortocoronary artery bypass grafts by multislice spiral computed tomography with electrocardiographic-gated image reconstruction. *Am J Cardiol.* 2001;88(7):792-795.
17. Schroeder S, Achenbach S, Bengel F, et al. Cardiac computed tomography: indications, applications, limitations, and training requirements: report of a Writing Group deployed by the Working Group Nuclear Cardiology and Cardiac CT of the European Society of Cardiology and the European Council of Nuclear Cardiology. *Eur Heart J.* 2008;29(4):531-556.
18. Zahn R, Jessl J, Achenbach S, Ropers D, Schwab J, Daniel WG. Treatment of a large coronary saphenous bypass graft aneurysm by implantation of covered stents. *Clin Res Cardiol.* 2006;95(6):313-315.
19. Yousem D, Scott Jr W, Fishman EK, Watson AJ, Traill T, Gimenez L. Saphenous vein graft aneurysms demonstrated by computed tomography. *J Comput Assist Tomogr.* 1986;10(3):526-528.
20. Breuckmann F, Nassenstein K, Barkhausen J, Erbel R. Giant aneurysm of an aortocoronary saphenous bypass graft. *Eur J Cardiothorac Surg.* 2006;29(3):410.
21. Saito T, Saito N, Komatsu Y, Sekiguchi Y, Asajima H. Chronic dissection of internal mammary artery graft. *Int J Cardiol.* 2008;127(3):e124-e125.
22. Stone IM, Aranda JM, Thurer RJ, Clark R, Befeler B. Disruption of proximal aortosaphenous vein anastomosis. Late complication of aortocoronary bypass surgery. *Chest.* 1977;71(4):544-546.
23. Cujec B, Bharadwaj B, Chait P, Hayton R. Dehiscence of the proximal anastomosis of aortocoronary bypass graft. *Am Heart J.* 1990;120(5):1217-1220.
24. Shapeero LG, Guthaner DF, Swerdlow CD, Wexler L. Rupture of a coronary bypass graft aneurysm: CT evaluation and coil occlusion therapy. *AJR Am J Roentgenol.* 1983;141(5):1060-1062.
25. Douglas BP, Bulkley BH, Hutchins GM. Infected saphenous vein coronary artery bypass graft with mycotic aneurysm. Fatal dehiscence of the proximal anastomosis. *Chest.* 1979;75(1):76-77.
26. Nielsen JF, Stentoft J, Aunsholt NA. Haemoptysis caused by aneurysm of saphenous bypass graft to a coronary artery. *Scand J Thorac Cardiovasc Surg.* 1988;22(2):189-191.
27. Taliercio CP, Smith HC, Pluth JR, Gibbons RJ. Coronary artery venous bypass graft aneurysm with symptomatic coronary artery emboli. *J Am Coll Cardiol.* 1986;7(2):435-437.
28. Lopez-Velarde P, Hallman GL, Treistman B. Aneurysm of an aortocoronary saphenous vein bypass graft presenting as an anterior mediastinal mass. *Ann Thorac Surg.* 1988;46(3):349-350.

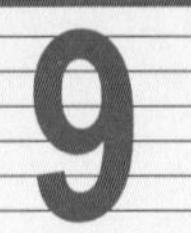

Coronary Artery Anomalies of Origin and Course

Key Points

- Anomalies of coronary ostia and course are more common than appreciated.
- Cardiac CT angiography is the preferred test to characterize anomalies of the coronary ostia and course. The ability to anatomically depict both the structure and course of the coronary artery and the immediately adjacent structures provides comprehensive assessment of coronary anomalies.
- Cardiac CT is able to provide more extensive (distal) characterization of coronary anomalies than can cardiac MRI.

A wide range of coronary artery anomalies have been described, reflecting the many permutations of abnormalities of the following anatomic details:

- The location of the ostium:
  - Which sinus of Valsalva
  - Where in the sinus of Valsalva
  - Ascending aorta
  - The aortic arch
  - The descending aorta
  - The innominate artery
  - The common carotid artery
  - The internal thoracic artery
  - The pulmonary artery
  - A bronchial artery
  - The left ventricle
- Common versus separate ostium with other coronary arteries
- The shape of the ostia (slit-like or not)
- Congenital ostial stenosis
- Congenital ostial atresia
- The initial course of the artery—within the wall of the aorta (i.e., intramural) or not
- The angulation of the initial course—tangential or not
- The ongoing course of the artery:
  - Anterior to the pulmonary artery
  - Intra-arterial (between the aorta and the pulmonary artery)
  - Through the crista supraventricularis portion of the septum
  - Dorsal/retroaortic (posterior to the aorta)
- Epicardial or intramyocardial course

Understandably, many classifications have been proposed to describe anomalies of the coronary ostia and their course, and the terminology they use often varies. For example, most series would describe "separate ostia of the LCX and LAD," whereas some describe an "absent left main stem." Many series and classifications are very detailed, whereas others, particularly the smaller series, are less detailed. Merging the data from different series to arrive at an overall picture is a challenge.

Anomalies of the coronary ostia and their course are the most common anomalies observed at angiography, accounting for 90% of such cases. The remaining 10% are anomalies of termination—i.e., coronary fistulae. Anomalies of the coronary ostia and their course most commonly involve the left coronary artery, especially the left circumflex coronary artery, which accounts for about 60% of observed anomalies of origin and course.

THE MOST COMMON CORONARY ANOMALIES

- Left circumflex artery (LCX) arising from:
  - A separate ostia in the right sinus of Valsalva (69%)
  - LCX arising from the proximal right coronary artery (RCA; 31%)
- Single coronary artery from the left sinus of Valsalva
- Both coronary arteries arising from the right sinus of Valsalva
- Left anterior descending artery (LAD) arising from the right sinus of Valsalva

Overall, the most common course of an anomalous artery is anterior or posterior to the great vessels, rather than intra-arterial, although nearly half of anomalous right coronary arteries have an intra-arterial course.[1]

TERMINOLOGY OF ANOMALIES OF COURSE

Anomalies of course may be described using the following terminology[2,3]:

- Type A: **A**nterior to the pulmonary artery, or pre-pulmonic course
- Type B: **B**etween the aorta and pulmonary artery, or intra-arterial course
- Type C: Through the **c**rista supraventricularis; also known as intraseptal, septal, subpulmonary course, or "tunneled"
- Through the right ventricular (RV) infundubulum
- Type D: **D**orsal pathway, or posterior" or retro-aortic course
- Mixed

Torres et al.[3] reported on 6000 consecutive cardiac CT (CCT) cases. Of 15 anomalous left coronary arteries arising from the right sinus of Valsalva and anomalous right coronary arteries arising from the left sinus of Valsalva, and coursing between the aorta and the pulmonary artery, the following patterns were seen: two were intra-arterial, four were intraseptal, eight had a mixed intra-arterial/intraseptal course, and one coursed through the right ventricular infundibulum. These findings challenge the traditional classification of the course of anomalous coronary arteries (Fig. 9-1).

INCIDENCE OF CORONARY ARTERY ANOMALIES

The true incidence of coronary anomalies is unknown; furthermore, despite a considerable number of papers describing coronary anomalies in depth,[4] the true range of anomalies is incompletely mapped out. The reported incidence varies depending on the definition,[2,5] the methodology used, and the patient profile (the pretest probability) assessed.

Incidence by Modality

- Echocardiography: 0.1%
- Angiography[6,7]: 1.0%
- Autopsy: 0.12%

Incidence by Patient Profile

- Asymptomatic individuals: unknown
- High school athletes with sudden death: 11%
- Competitive athletes (<35 years) with sudden death[8]: 13%
- Military recruits with nontraumatic sudden death[9]: 33%
- Angiography/bypass surgery (CAD) Coronary Artery Surgery Study (CASS): 0.3%

DETERMINING THE CLINICAL RELEVANCE OF CORONARY ARTERY ANOMALIES[10]

Most patients with coronary anomalies are asymptomatic throughout life, and most coronary anomaly patterns are believed to be benign (~70–80%). Only about 20% to 30% of those recognized are considered potentially serious or lethal.

Coronary anomalies that do not commonly have clinical risk include those with high ostia, multiple ostia, or "split" courses, and those that do not plausibly impair coronary flow (i.e., do not

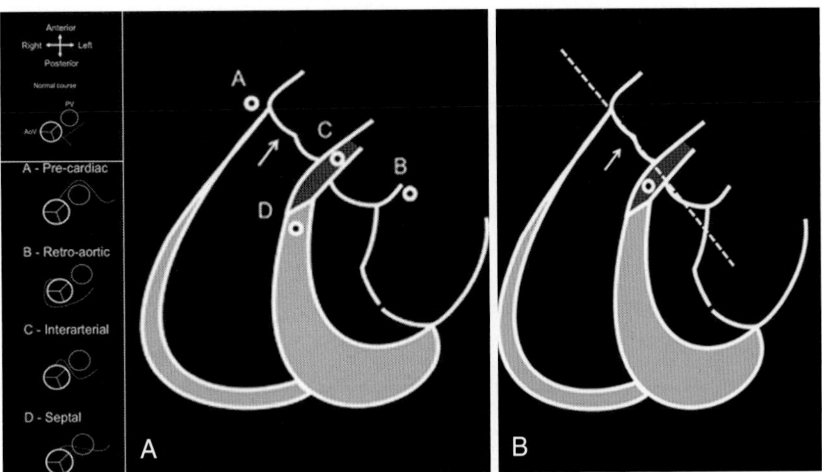

Figure 9-1. A, Traditional classification of the proximal course of an anomalous left coronary artery from the opposite coronary sinus of Valsalva or right coronary artery. Diagram of aortic and pulmonary valves seen en face (*left*) showing the normal course of the left main coronary artery with its main branches and the proximal course of the four subtypes (A to D) of anomalous left coronary arteries (*middle*). Position C marks the classic interarterial course. Diagram in oblique sagittal reformation (*right*) showing the proximal course of the 4 subtypes (*open circles,* A to D) in relation to the pulmonary valve (*arrow*). Aov, aortic valve; PV, pulmonary valve. **B,** Right ventricular infundibulum (RVI) subtype of the proximal course of an anomalous left coronary artery from the opposite coronary sinus of Valsalva or right coronary artery (RCA). On the basis of traditional criteria derived from conventional coronary angiography (CCA), the proximal course of this vessel would have been classified as septal once it travels below the level of the pulmonary valve (*dashed line*). The vessel, however, does not penetrate the interventricular septum and is surrounded by epicardial fat (*light gray*). (Reprinted with permission from Torres FS, Nguyen ET, Dennie CJ, et al. Role of MDCT coronary angiography in the evaluation of septal vs interarterial course of anomalous left coronary arteries. *J Cardiovasc Comput Tomogr.* 2010;4(4):246-254.)

have congenital stenosis or atresia, do not have a tangential take-off, do not have an intramural course, do not have an intra-arterial course) or supply with desaturated blood (i.e., do not arise from the pulmonary artery).

Establishing that a coronary anomaly is the cause of clinical symptoms or presentation requires that alternative explanations and plausible associations be excluded.

Occasional clinical manifestations include sudden death, ventricular fibrillation, myocardial infarction, cardiomyopathy, syncope, and chest pain.

Major clinical presentations appear to be more common with certain patterns of anomalies and with certain patient groups. Among high school athletes who experience sudden nontraumatic death, coronary anomalies are the second most common cause of death. Similarly, it has been reported that coronary artery anomalies may be the second most common cause of sudden death in competitive athletes less than 35 years of age (second only to hypertrophic cardiomyopathy).[11,12] In an autopsy series of military recruits, coronary artery anomalies were the most common cause of sudden nontraumatic death.[13]

A given anomaly, though, may have disparate clinical profiles: it may be found in a young patient who is symptomatic and who is being assessed for the these symptoms, or it may be "incidentally" detected well into adult life when angiography for coronary artery disease (CAD) evaluation or CT scanning for other purposes is performed. Many notable cases have been documented where, for example, longevity was achieved by a patient who had an anomaly generally thought to be "potentially serious" or "lethal."

The many permutations of anomalies lessen their overall clinical relevance; however, several recurrent themes have emerged.[14-18] Among young athletes with anomalous coronary arteries who experience sudden death, over three quarters of the anomalies have an intra-arterial course. The intra-arterial course of the left main coronary artery (LMCA) is associated with higher risk than a retro-aortic course, although the retro-aortic course may be associated with risk.[19,20] Although the classic intra-arterial anomaly associated with increased clinical risk is the intra-arterial LMCA, intra-arterial LAD and RCA anomalies also are associated with increased risk.[11]

An "intramural" course (Fig. 9-2), completely within the wall of the aorta, appears to be a serious anomaly, associated with sudden death during athletic exertion.[21] An anomalous intramural course often is associated with an angulated initial course. Anatomically, the initial segment of the coronary artery is entirely within the wall of the aorta, and there is one adventitia. Identification of an intramural course requires high-resolution imaging or surgical inspection.

Initially, the intra-arterial course of an anomaly itself was thought to be responsible for the clinical risk, with hypotheses such as compression of the anomalous course by the pulmonary artery trunk and aorta during dilation associated with exercise resulting in myocardial ischemia and clinical risk. It is increasingly being recognized, however, that it is the abnormal ostium or initial course of the coronary artery associated with the intra-arterial course that confers the risk. Abrupt ("tangential") angulation of the initial course (take-off) may be associated with "kinking" of the artery and a slit-like ostium. It also has been hypothesized that spasm of the anomalous intra-arterial coronary artery contributes to myocardial ischemia and clinical risk.[19,22-26]

At the same time, the surgical approach to intra-arterial coronary artery anomalies has evolved beyond aortocoronary bypass grafting to an increased focus on "un-roofing" or "marsupializing" the narrowed ostium/initial course.

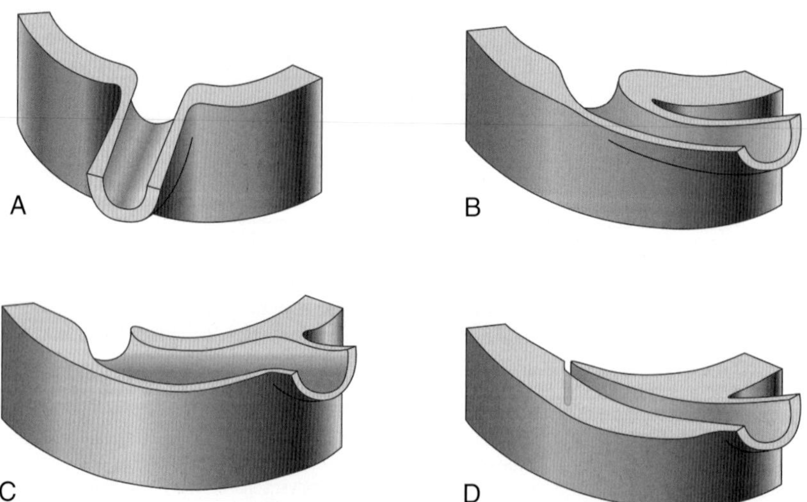

Figure 9-2. Normal (**A**), tangential (**B**), and intramural (**C**) "take-off" (origins) of a coronary artery. **D**, An intramural origin with a slitlike initial portion.

ASSOCIATIONS OF CORONARY ANOMALIES

Most coronary anomalies occur in isolation, i.e., without associated congenital cardiac or vascular anomalies. However, some forms of congenital heart disease are commonly associated with coronary artery anomalies.

Tetralogy of Fallot

Tetralogy of Fallot (ToF) is the prototypical disorder of associated congenital heart disease and coronary anomalies. The anomalies are critically relevant to corrective surgery for ToF, because the coronary artery anomalies render the coronary circulation vulnerable to damage by surgery. The incidence of associated coronary anomalies is 1% to 10%. The most common associated anomalies are:

- A large conus artery
- An LAD with an anomalous course (LAD arising from the proximal RCA or off the right sinus of Valsalva) that crosses the right ventricular outflow tract (RVOT; 37%). This is more common when the aortic root is more anterior, rightward, or lateral.[27,28]
- A single coronary artery

Delineation of the origin and course of coronary arteries should be achieved before any intervention on the RVOT.[28] CCT is able to detect LAD anomalies associated with ToF.[29]

Transposition of the Great Arteries (TGA)

Transposition of the great arteries (TGA) is often associated with coronary artery anomalies that confer risk of injury to the coronary circulation at the time of surgery. The most common associated anomalies are:

- Anomalous origin of the RCA from the posterior right sinus or off the left main from the posterior left sinus, seen in 60% of cases
- Anomalous origin of the LCX off the RCA, seen in 16% to 20% of cases
- More complex anomalies also seen with TGA.[30,31]
  - The LCX arises from the RCA
  - The LAD arises from the RCA
  - The LCA arises from the right sinus
  - Solitary coronary arteries
  - Intramyocardial courses
- Following successful arterial switch operation, intrinsic thickening and extrinsic compression or torsion may occur.[28]

Truncus Arteriosus

Truncus arteriosus infrequently may be associated with coronary anomalies.

ANOMALIES OF CORONARY OSTIA AND COURSE

See Box 9-1 and Figures 9-3 through 9-7.

Box 9-1 Anomalies of Coronary Ostia and Course

LMCA
High origin (above STJ)
  CCT incidence: 0.20%
  Angiography incidence: 0.13%
Ectopic origin within the LSV (Fig. 9-3)
  CCT incidence: 0.59%
  Angiography incidence: 0.41%
Absent = separate LAD and LCx ostia (Figs. 9-3, 9-8)
  CCT incidence: 0.59%
  Angiography incidence: 0.02%
RCS: arising from a separate ostium, a common ostium, or a common solitary coronary artery with any of the following courses:
  Intra-arterial (± a slitlike ostium, ± an intramural course) (Figs. 9-3, 9-9, 9-11)
  RV infundibuum (Figs. 9-3, 9-12, 9-13)
  Septal (Figs. 9-3, 9-14)
  Retroaortic (Figs. 9-3, 9-15)
  Anterior to the RVOT (Fig. 9-3)
  Mixed
NCS
Arising from the PA (ALCAPA / BWG syndrome) (Figs. 9-3, 9-16 to 9-19; **Videos 9-1 and 9-2**)
  Angiography incidence: 0.01%
Arising from the innominate artery

LAD
High origin (above the STJ)
Separate ostium from the LCx (Fig. 9-3)
Separate ostium from the LCx abnormal location within the LSV
RCS: arising from a separate ostium, a common ostium, or a common solitary coronary artery with any of the following courses:
  Intra-arterial (± a slitlike ostium, ± an intramural course) (Figs. 9-4, 9-20, 9-21)
  RV infundibuum (Fig. 9-4)
  Septal (Fig. 9-4)
  Anterior to the RVOT (Fig. 9-4)
RCS: arising from the RCA (may run with an intra-arterial, septal, RV infundibular, retroaortic, or anterior course) (Fig. 9-4)
Split LAD: first half from the LMCA continuation and the second half from a large AM branch (Fig. 9-4)
Arising from the PA (Fig. 9-4)
Dual/bifid LAD:
  Type 1: early bifurcation into a short (terminating high within the anterior interventricular groove) and a long LAD parallel to the AIV groove on the left side
  Type 2: early bifurcation into a short (terminating high within the anterior interventricular groove)

Continued

Box 9-1 Anomalies of Coronary Ostia and Course—cont'd

and a long LAD parallel to the AIV groove on the right side
Type 3: early bifurcation into a short (terminating high within the anterior interventricular groove) and a long LAD with an intramyocardial course
Type 4: early bifurcation into a short (terminating high within the anterior interventricular groove) and a long LAD arising from the RCA Intramyocardial courses ("myocardial bridging")

LCx
Separate ostium from the LAD
Separate ostium from the LCx abnormal location within the LSV
RCS: arising from a separate ostium, a common ostium, or a common solitary coronary artery with any of the following courses:
Intra-arterial (± a slitlike ostium, ± an intramural course)
Septal
Retroaortic (Figs. 9-22, 9-23; **Video 9-3**)
Anterior to the RVOT
Mixed
RCS: arising frm the RCA (may run with an intra-arterial, septal, RV infundibular, retroaortic, or anterior course)
Arising from the LVOT/subaortic
Arising from a diagonal branch
CCT incidence: 0.20%
LCx: RCA interconnection
Angiography incidence: 0.00%
Intramyocardial courses ("myocardial bridging")

RCA
High origin (above STJ)
Angiography incidence: 0.15%
Ectopic origin within the RSV
CCT incidence: 0.79%
LCS: arising from a separate ostium, a common ostium, or a common solitary coronary artery with any of the following courses:
Intra-arterial (± a slitlike ostium, ± an intramural course) (Figs. 9-24 to 09-33; **Videos 9-4 to 9-13)**
Retroaortic
Mixed
Arising from the LVOT / subaortic
Arising from the PA (RCAPA)[15] (Fig. 9-34)
Angiography incidence: 0.00%
Split RCA (first half of the PDA from the RCA and the second half from an AM)
CCT incidence: 0.98%
Arising from the innominate artery (Fig. 9-35)
Intra-atrial course
Superdominant RCA (no LCx)
Arising from the NCS
RCA Tunnel
Intramyocardial courses ("myocardial bridging")

SINGLE CORONARY ARTERY
Arising from the RSV:
R1: Follows the normal course of an RCA (Fig. 9-36)
R2: LCA crosses at base of heart (Figs. 9-37, 9-38)
R3: LAD and LCx arise separately/absent LMCA
Arsing from the LSV:
L1: Follows the normal course of an LCA
L2: RCA crosses at base of heart
Arising from the NCS

AIV, anterior interventricular vein; ALCAPA, anomalous left coronary artery from the pulmonary artery; AM, acute marginal; CCT, cardiac CT; LAD, left anterior descending; LCA, left coronary artery; LCS, left coronary sinus; LCX, left circumflex coronary artery; LMCA, left main coronary artery; LSV, left sinus of valsalva; LVOT, left ventricular outflow tract; NCS, noncoronary sinus; PA, pulmonary artery; PDA, posterior descending coronary artery; RCA, right coronary artery; RCAPA, right coronary artery arising from the pulmonary artery; RCS, right coronary sinus; RSV, right sinus of valsalva; RV, right ventricle; RVOT, right ventricular outflow tract; STJ, sinotubular junction.
Incidence data from ref. 10. Angiography incidence data from ref. 7.

Solitary Coronary Artery

A common ostium to the left and right coronary arteries (i.e., a solitary coronary artery) may be seen. It may arise off the left or the right sinus and may occur in several patterns and courses. Nearly two dozen variants of solitary coronary arteries have been described.

The Lipton classification,[32] which is angiographically based and practical, categorizes solitary coronary arteries as left- or right-sinus based. The solitary coronary artery is first described by "L" or "R" according to whether it arises from the left or right sinus of Valsalva, respectively. The classification then subcategorizes solitary coronary arteries as group I, II, or III. Group I represents the extension of the normal course of the right or left coronary artery to arborize into a complete coronary tree. Group II represents solitary arteries that arise from proximal aspects of left or right coronary arteries and that cross the base of the heart and then continue within the orientations of normal coronary arteries. Group III represents separate origins of the LAD and LCX from the origin/proximal aspect of a right coronary artery.

In cases in which the left coronary artery arises off the proximal RCA, the left coronary artery may course to the left heart as a single LMCA before dividing on the left side into the LAD and LCX, or the separate LAD and LCX may pursue different courses. The LAD typically runs anterior to the pulmonary artery, between the aorta and pulmonary artery (intra-arterial course), or through the crista supraventricularis of the septum. The left circumflex artery typically runs with either a type B ("between") or D ("dorsal") pathway.

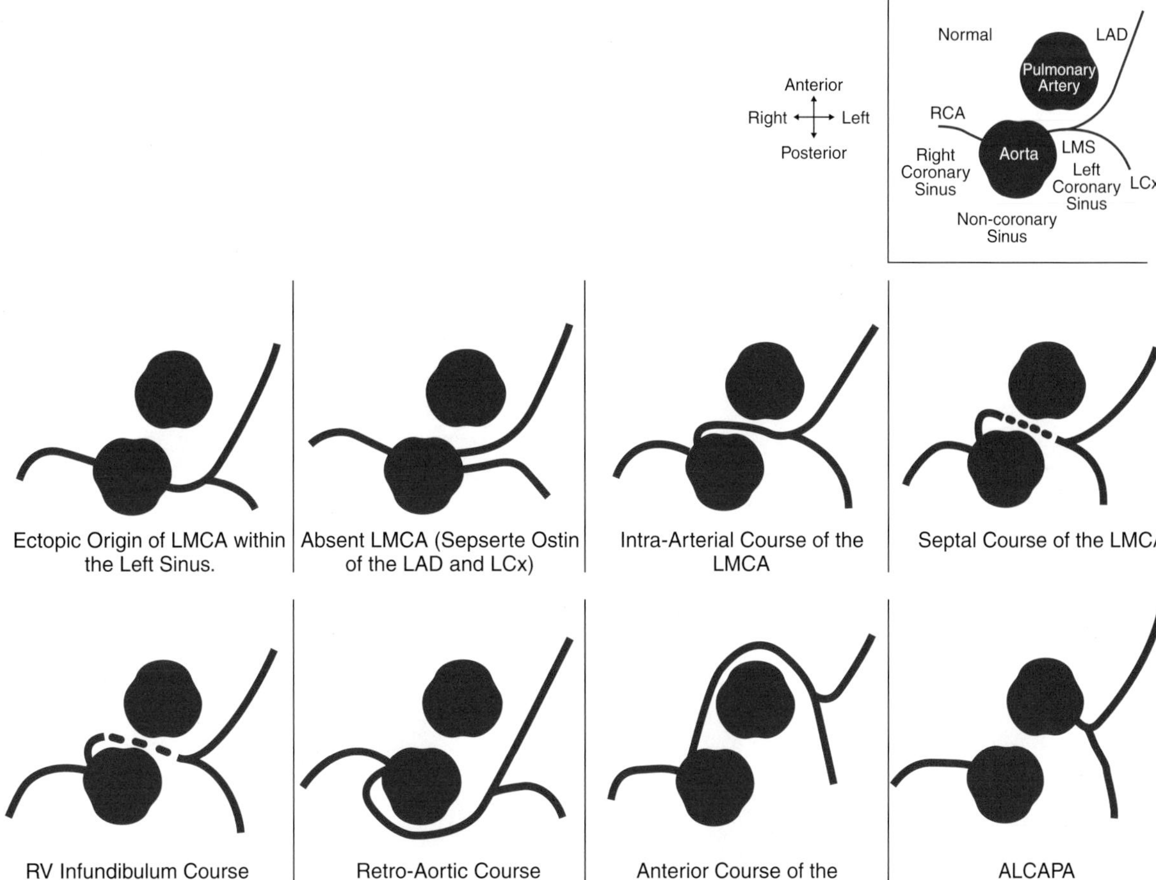

Figure 9-3. Anomalies of the left main coronary artery (LMCA). ALCAPA, anomalous left coronary artery from the pulmonary artery; LAD, left anterior descending artery; LCx, left circumflex artery; LMS, left main stem; RCA, right coronary artery.

A single coronary artery with the left main stem arising from the RCA off the right sinus and an intra-arterial course may be a serious or lethal variant.

A single coronary artery arising off the pulmonary artery is a serious or lethal variant because the entire heart will be perfused with desaturated blood (see the section Anomalous Origin of Coronary Arteries from the Pulmonary Artery).

CONGENITAL ATRESIA OR STENOSIS OF A CORONARY ARTERY

Assessment of the clinical relevance of coronary artery anomalies in adulthood is complicated by the presence of precocious coronary atherosclerosis. In young patient populations, congenital anomalies can be identified with a low risk of CAD being involved in the observed anomalies.

Congenital stenosis of a coronary artery usually is produced by a membrane-like or tunnel-like maldevelopment, often with an oblique course, sometimes intramural before it exits the aortic root.[25] Congenital stenosis often is associated with an intramural segment (i.e., within the wall of the aorta).

Coronary artery atresia produces a dimple of the ostium of the coronary artery, forming a string-like structure without a patent lumen.

See Figures 9-8 through 9-10 for more information.

ANOMALOUS ORIGIN OF CORONARY ARTERIES FROM THE PULMONARY ARTERY

A left coronary artery arising from the pulmonary artery is an example of an anomalous origin of coronary arteries (ALCAPA; also known as Bland-White-Garland syndrome). This artery will perfuse the left ventricle with poorly oxygenated blood or will serve as an effluent fistula into the pulmonary artery. ALCAPA usually leads to ischemic cardiomyopathy (which may or may not cause ischemic mitral insufficiency) early in life, with the attendant risks of heart failure and arrhythmic death. Although it is serious in most cases, a few individuals have been reported to have lived well into

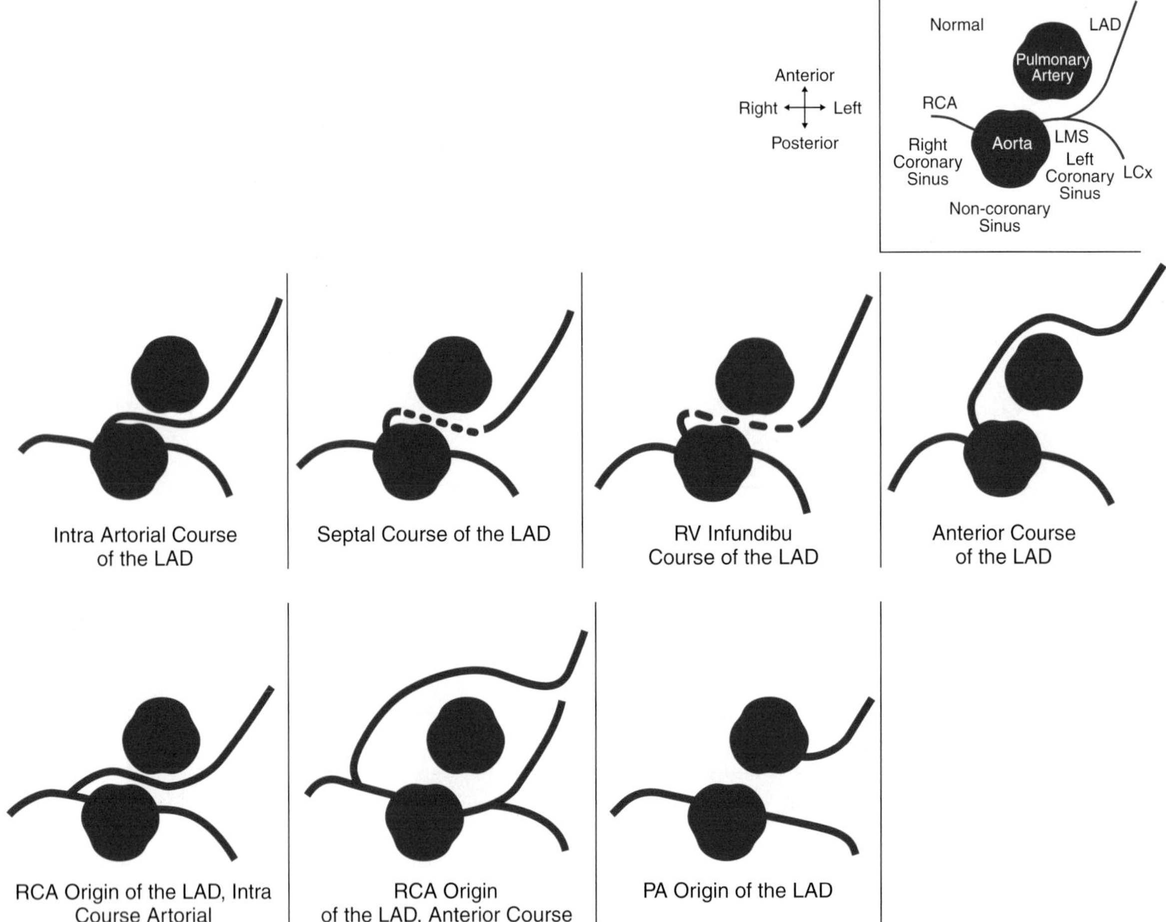

Figure 9-4. Anomalies of the left anterior descending (LAD) artery. LCx, left circumflex artery; LMS, left main stem; PA, pulmonary artery; RCA, right coronary artery.

adulthood with this anomaly. Collateralization from the RCA to the left coronary artery territory is critical for survival. Thus ALCAPA is considered a serious, even lethal, anomaly.[33]

Improvements in the medical and surgical management of hibernating myocardium have led to greater survival for persons with this anomaly.[28]

The incidence is approximately 1:300,000 live births.

See Figures 9-11 through 9-39; **Videos 9-1 through 9-13**.

ACC/AHA 2008 GUIDELINES FOR THE MANAGEMENT OF ADULTS WITH CONGENITAL HEART DISEASE: RECOMMENDATIONS FOR ANOMALOUS LEFT CORONARY ARTERY FROM THE PULMONARY ARTERY[28]

In 2008, the ACC/AHA presented guidelines for the management of adults with congenital heart disease who had an anomalous left coronary artery arising from the pulmonary artery.[28]

Class I*

1. In patients with an anomalous left coronary artery from the pulmonary artery (ALCAPA), reconstruction of a dual coronary artery supply should be performed. The surgery should be performed by surgeons with training and expertise in CHD at centers with expertise in the management of anomalous coronary artery origins. (*Level of Evidence: C*)
2. For adult survivors of ALCAPA repair, clinical evaluation with echocardiography and noninvasive stress testing is indicated every 3 to 5 years. (*Level of Evidence: C*)

Clinical Course

There has been no consistent correlation between long-term outcome and late symptoms, noninvasive ischemia and blood flow abnormality testing,

*Reprinted with permission from *Circulation*. 2008;118:2395-2451.

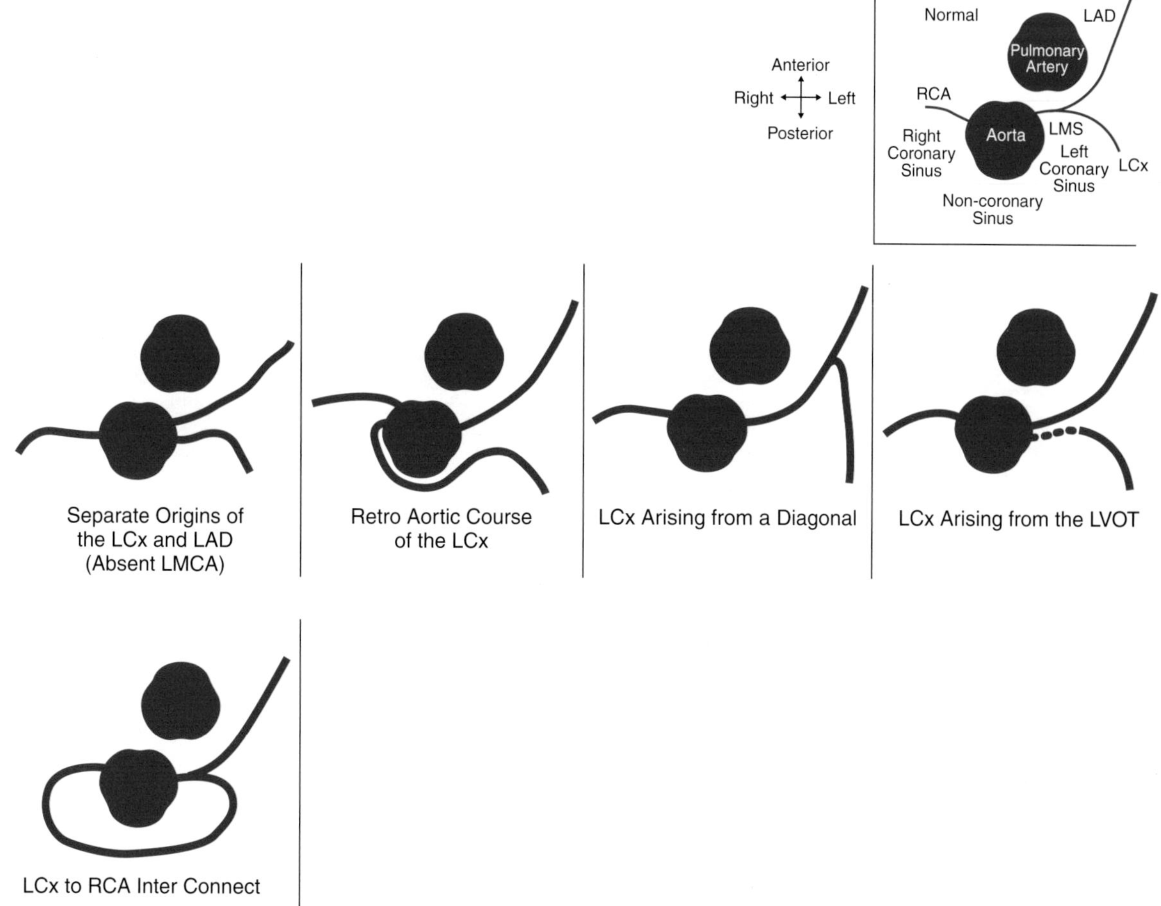

Figure 9-5. Left circumflex (LCx) anomalies. LAD, left anterior descending artery; LMCA, left main coronary artery; LMS, left main stem; LVOT, left ventricular outflow tract; RCA, right coronary artery.

residual coronary anatomic or flow abnormalities, or late interventions.

Management Strategies

Surgical Intervention. When patients present in adulthood with decreased systolic function and previously unrecognized ALCAPA, the committee suggests surgical myocardial revascularization to achieve a dual coronary supply, regardless of myocardial viability testing, given the lack of current data to correlate such testing with outcomes. Given the increasing awareness of residual coronary artery, myocardial, and valvular abnormalities, the committee suggests surveillance with echocardiography and noninvasive ischemia provocation testing every 3 to 5 years for patients after repair of ALCAPA. Coronary artery reimplantation or coronary bypass grafting has been used for repair.

Surgical and Catheterization-Based Intervention. Surgical repair by either arterial bypass or, more commonly, reimplantation of the anomalous coronary artery into the aorta is indicated because of the risk of sudden cardiac death.[34,35] If ischemia is demonstrated in patients after repair of ALCAPA with either concomitant symptomatology or echocardiographic changes, the committee recommends invasive catheterization with planned intervention determined by clinical findings.

ACC/AHA 2008 GUIDELINES FOR THE MANAGEMENT OF ADULTS WITH CONGENITAL HEART DISEASE: RECOMMENDATIONS FOR CONGENITAL CORONARY ANOMALIES OF ECTOPIC ARTERIAL ORIGIN

The ACC/AHA also published guidelines for the management of adults with congenital heart disease who had congenital coronary anomalies of ectopic arterial origin.[28]

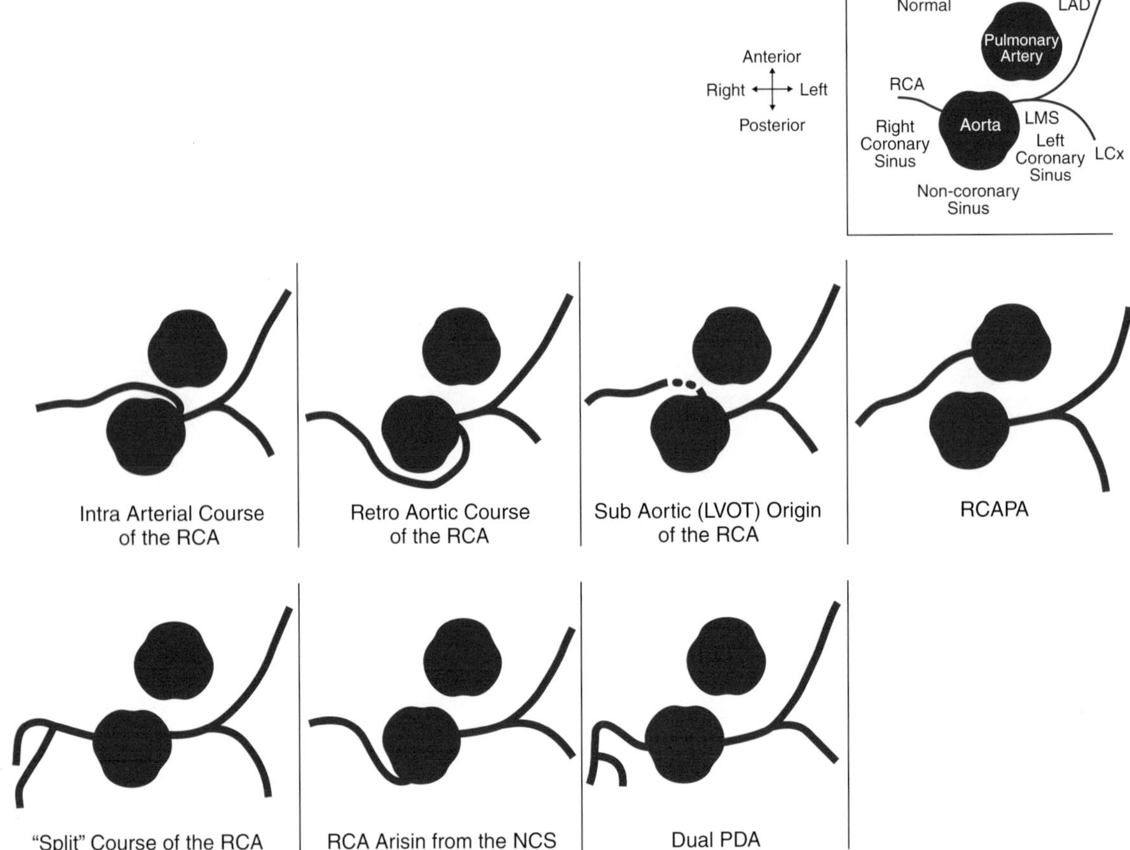

Figure 9-6. Right coronary artery (RCA) anomalies. LAD, left anterior descending artery; LCx, left circumflex artery; LMS, left main stem; LVOT, left ventricular outflow tract; PDA, patent ductus arteriosus; RCAPA, right coronary artery from the pulmonary artery.

Class I*

1. The evaluation of individuals who have survived unexplained aborted sudden cardiac death or with unexplained life-threatening arrhythmia, coronary ischemic symptoms, or LV (left ventricular) dysfunction should include assessment of coronary artery origins and course. (*Level of Evidence: B*)
2. CT or magnetic resonance angiography is useful as the initial screening method in centers with expertise in such imaging. (*Level of Evidence: B*)
3. Surgical coronary revascularization should be performed in patients with any of the following indications:
   a. Anomalous left main coronary artery coursing between the aorta and pulmonary artery. (*Level of Evidence: B*)
   b. Documented coronary ischemia due to coronary compression (when coursing between the great arteries or in intramural fashion). (*Level of Evidence: B*)
   c. Anomalous origin of the right coronary artery between aorta and pulmonary artery with evidence of ischemia. (*Level of Evidence: B*)

Class IIa

1. Surgical coronary revascularization can be beneficial in the setting of documented vascular wall hypoplasia, coronary compression, or documented obstruction to coronary flow, regardless of inability to document coronary ischemia. (*Level of Evidence: C*)
2. Delineation of potential mechanisms of flow restriction via intravascular ultrasound can be beneficial in patients with documented anomalous coronary artery origin from the opposite sinus. (*Level of Evidence: C*)

Class IIb

1. Surgical coronary revascularization may be reasonable in patients with anomalous left anterior descending coronary artery coursing between the aorta and pulmonary artery. (*Level of Evidence: C*)

*Reprinted with permission from *Circulation.* 2008;118:2395-2451.

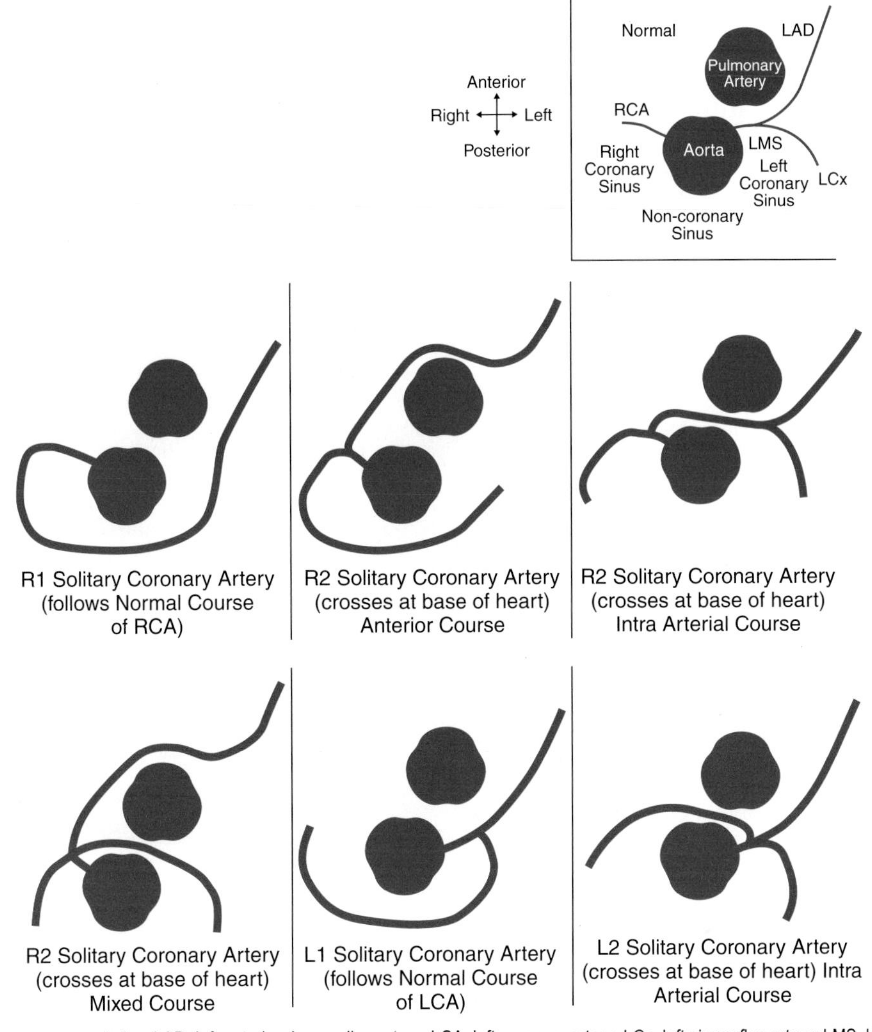

Figure 9-7. Solitary coronary arteries. LAD, left anterior descending artery; LCA, left coronary artery; LCx, left circumflex artery; LMS, left main stem; RCA, right coronary artery.

CLINICAL FEATURES AND EVALUATION OF THE UNOPERATED PATIENT[28]

Preintervention Evaluation

Patients may present with aborted sudden death, chest pain, arrhythmia, LV dysfunction, or exercise-induced presyncope or syncope. Recently, clinical ischemia provocation screening has been suggested to reduce the global risk of sudden cardiac events in athletes who participate in high-risk competitive sports; however, individual case reports in which such testing failed to reveal at-risk abnormalities in athletes who later succumbed to sudden coronary death due to anomalous coronary origins highlight the need for further improvement in screening strategies. Visualization of coronary artery course is achieved by CT or MRI.[36,37]

To date, anatomic delineation of a coronary artery course between the aorta and pulmonary artery in a young (<50 years) person remains the greatest known risk for an adverse event, with or without symptoms.[21] Catheter-based measurement of flow reserve and coronary intravascular ultrasonography have the potential to delineate mechanisms of potential flow obstruction and are increasingly part of diagnostic and therapeutic algorithms.[38,39] Currently, especially in patients younger than age 50 years, the committee recommends coronary CT or MRI for more definitive definition of coronary course in persons suspected of having anomalous coronary origins.

Management Strategies[28]

Surgical and Catheterization-Based Intervention

Both surgical revascularization (e.g., marsupialization, coronary bypass, or coronary reimplantation) and limited cases of transcatheter stenting have been reported to have short-term stability, without long-term follow-up.[40] Coronary bypass

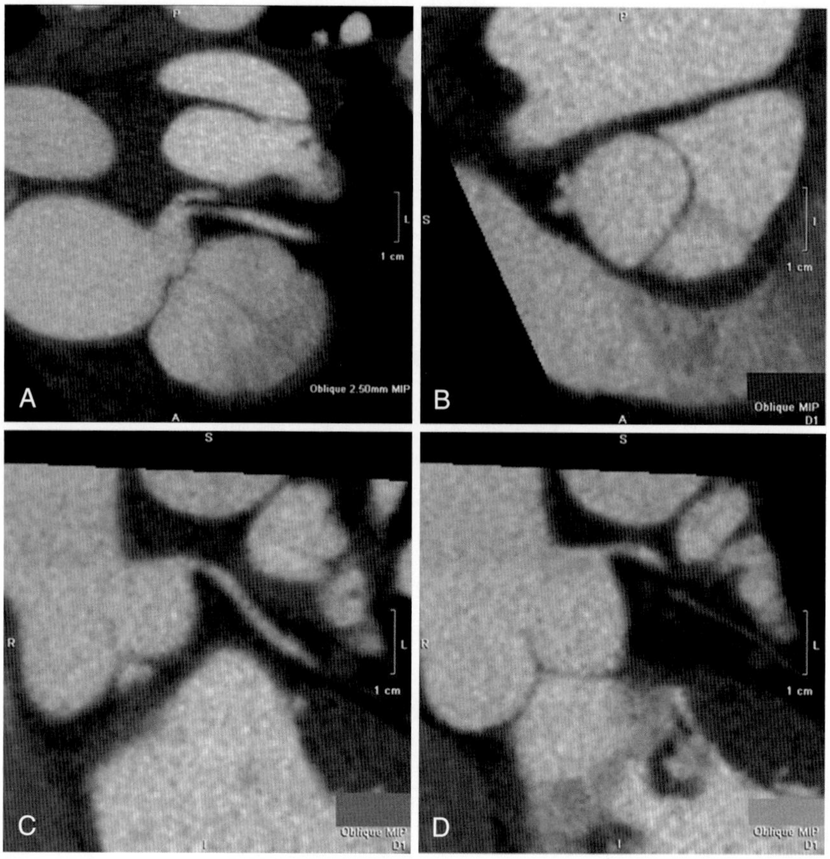

Figure 9-8. A 47-year-old man presenting with atypical chest pain and a strongly positive family history for coronary artery disease. Composite images from a cardiac CT scan demonstrate a variant of coronary artery anatomy, with the left anterior descending and circumflex arteries arising from the left sinus of Valsalva with separate individual ostia. No evidence of an ostial or coronary artery stenosis is seen.

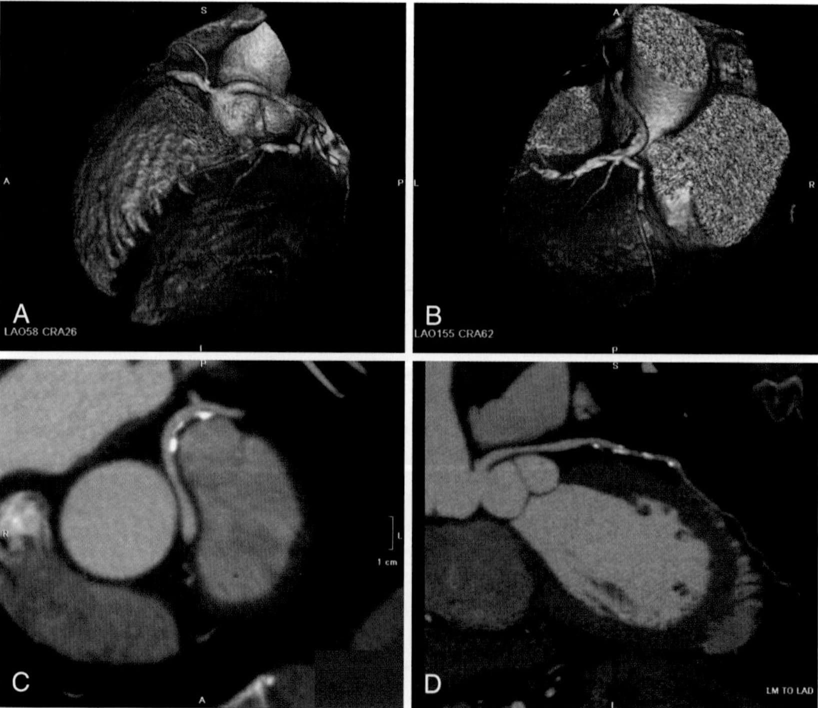

Figure 9-9. A 52-year-old man presenting with chest pain and an abnormal myocardial perfusion imaging study. Composite images from a cardiac CT study demonstrate anomalous origin of the left main coronary artery from the right coronary cusp. This arises from a separate ostium relative to the right coronary artery. The left main coronary artery (LMCA) courses between the aorta and right ventricular outflow tract. The LMCA is only mildly narrowed in its interarterial course. The LMCA then bifurcates into a left anterior descending (LAD) and a circumflex artery. The ongoing LAD demonstrates mild to moderate, primarily calcified plaque with a superficial intramyocardial course in its midportion.

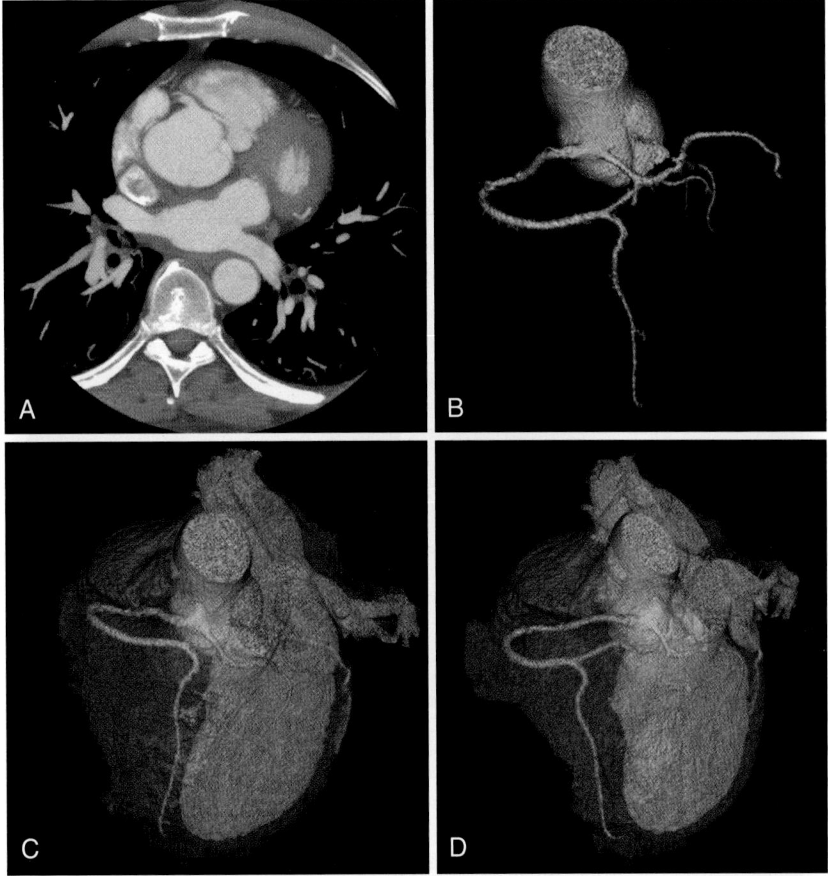

Figure 9-10. A 38-year-old with multiple cardiac risk factors, atypical chest pain, and an equivocal myocardial perfusion imaging study. **A,** An axial short-thickness maximum intensity projection demonstrates an anomalous origin of the left coronary artery from the right sinus of Valsalva. The left main coronary artery courses between the aorta and the right ventricular outflow tract/main pulmonary artery to enter the epicardial fat in the upper interventricular groove. It then bifurcates into a moderate-sized circumflex system, and a small type I left anterior descending artery (LAD) which ends intramyocardially within the mid-septum. The right coronary artery has a normal origin, and is a normal-appearing vessel giving off a very large patent ductus arteriosus, which extends around the apex of the left ventricle, compensating for the small type I LAD.

grafting is increasingly viewed less favorably in light of the potential for competitive flow.[41] Surgical revascularization in centers with expertise in the surgical management of anomalous coronary arteries is suggested.[21,42,43] Surgical repair is indicated when the left coronary arteries arise from the opposite sinus and course between the aorta and pulmonary artery. Surgical repair also is indicated when the right coronary artery arises from the opposite sinus or courses between the aorta and pulmonary artery in association with concomitant symptoms, or when there is evidence of otherwise unexplained inducible ischemia in these territories.[44-46] When the patient has an anomalous RCA and no evidence of ischemia, management is more controversial. A conservative approach in this situation may be reasonable. Given the not uncommon occurrence of anomalous coronary origins and their potential for a devastating outcome, it is imperative that improved data be obtained regarding diagnosis, follow-up, and longer-term outcomes.

2011 ACCF/AHA GUIDELINE FOR CORONARY ARTERY BYPASS GRAFT SURGERY[46]

Anomalous Coronary Artery Recommendations

Class I

1. Coronary revascularization should be performed in patients with:
   a. A left main coronary artery that arises anomalously and then courses between the aorta and pulmonary artery. (*Level of Evidence: B*)
   b. A right coronary artery that arises anomalously and then courses between the aorta and pulmonary artery with evidence of myocardial ischemia. (*Level of Evidence: B*)

Class IIb

1. Coronary revascularization may be reasonable in patients with a LAD coronary artery that arises anomalously and then courses between the aorta and pulmonary artery. (*Level of Evidence: C*)

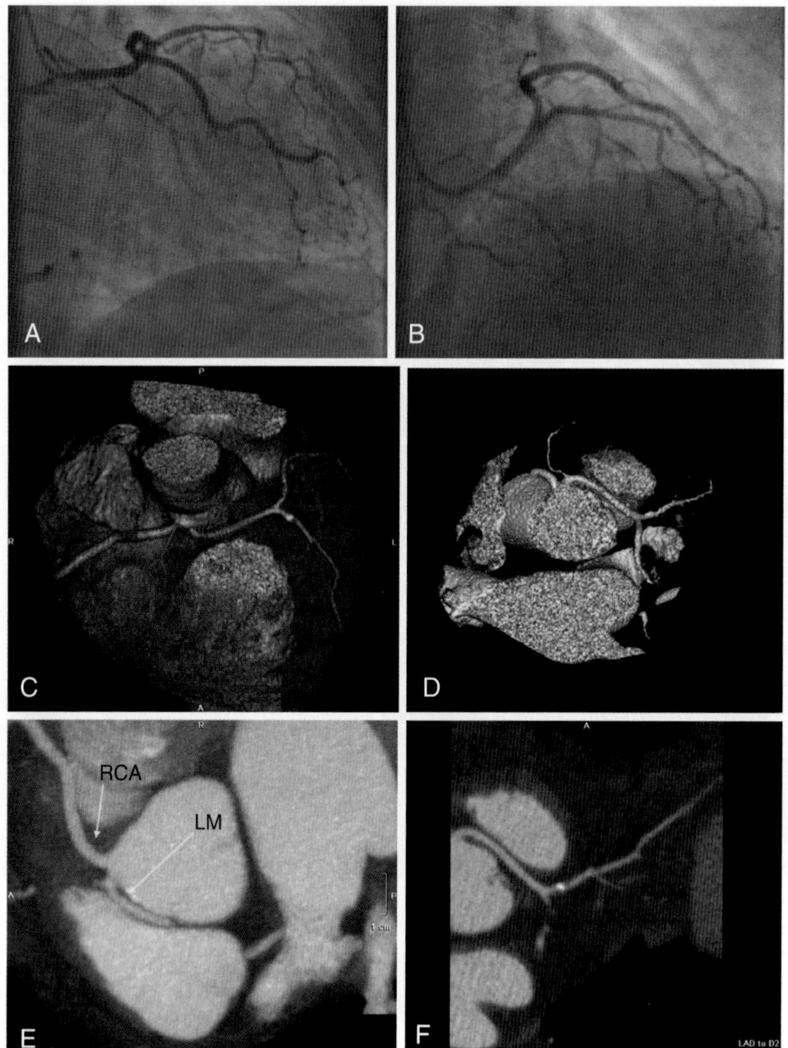

Figure 9-11. A 47-year-old man presenting with chest pain. **A** and **B,** The patient underwent coronary angiography. The left main (LM) stem coronary artery was found to have an unusual configuration, originating from the right sinus of Valsalva. It was uncertain at the time of angiography whether the LM course was anterior to the main pulmonary artery or interarterially between the aorta and main pulmonary artery (MPA). A cardiac CT study was subsequently performed. **C** and **D,** The volume-rendered images demonstrate the course of the LM to be interarterial. The MPA/right ventricular outflow tract has been removed in order to visualize the LM. **E** and **F,** A separate origin of the LM from the right sinus of Valsalva is seen. The caliber of the LM is maintained, with no evidence of stenosis at either the ostium of the LM or along its intra-arterial course. A small amount of calcification is seen in the proximal portion of the left anterior descending artery (LAD). The ongoing LAD is a small type I vessel. RCA, right coronary artery.

CCT IMAGING OF CORONARY ANOMALIES

CCT depicts the origin, the course, and the diameter of coronary arteries, as well as their relation to cardiac structures. Hence, CCT is ideally suited to identify coronary anomalies, particularly their origin and proximal course.[3] Even older 16-multidetector CT–based studies showed very good correlation with angiography; contemporary systems yield excellent depiction,[47,48] although CCT may fail to depict the smaller distal portions of coronary arteries and their branches, and the distal insertion of smaller fistulae.[48] CCT is useful to identify coronary anomaly patterns, evaluate suspected coronary anomalies (suspected from echocardiography or catheterization), and evaluate unclear findings from conventional coronary angiography.

Three-dimensional reconstructions are useful to depict the anatomic relations of an anomaly of coronary origin and course, as are maximum intensity projections and multiplanar reconstructions. Multiplanar and associated cross-sectional imaging (intravascular ultrasound [IVUS] views) are useful to identify eccentric, narrowed, compressed, or kinked lumens.

CCT Protocol Points

- The standard CCT protocol is utilized.[49]
- See Table 9-1 for more information.

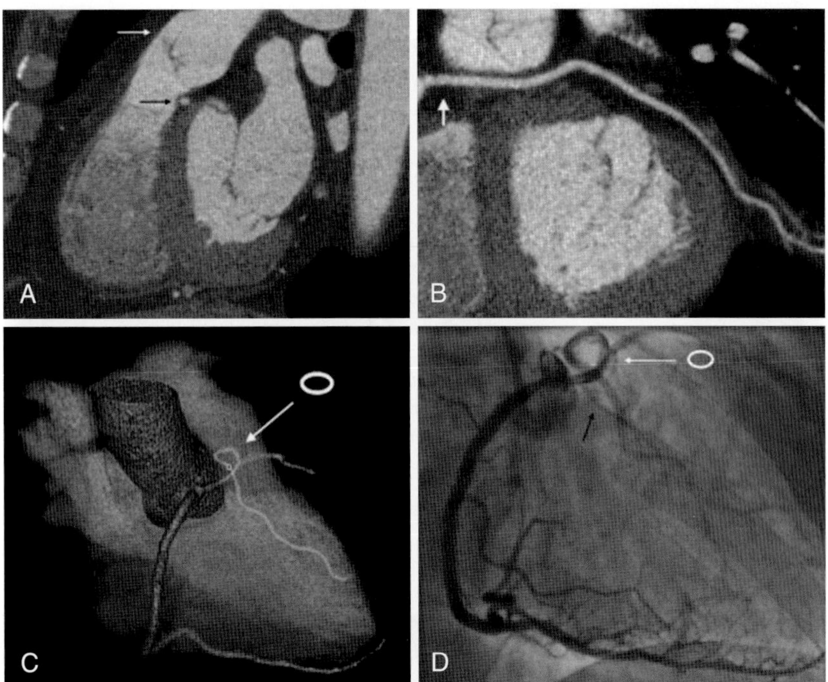

Figure 9-12. Discordant multidetector computed tomography coronary angiography (low interarterial) and conventional coronary angiography (CCA) (septal) classifications of an anomalous left main coronary artery (LMCA) from the right coronary sinus of Valsalva (RSV). **A,** Sagittal reformation showing the anomalous LMCA (*black arrow*) below the level of the pulmonary valve (*white arrow*). **B,** Curved reformation showing the epicardial position of the LMCA (*white arrow*), corresponding to a right ventricular infundibulum (RVI) course (type 4). Note that this anomalous LMCA does not penetrate the interventricular septum. **C,** 3D volume-rendering reconstruction in right anterior oblique (RAO) projection (CCA simulation) showing the LMCA and left circumflex coronary artery corresponding to the "eye sign" (*white arrow and circle*). **D,** CCA image in RAO projection showing the eye sign (*white arrow and circle*) and also septal branch arising from the LMCA (*black arrow*), findings that would indicate a septal course by traditional criteria. (Reprinted with permission from Torres FS, Nguyen ET, Dennie CJ, et al. Role of MDCT coronary angiography in the evaluation of septal vs interarterial course of anomalous left coronary arteries. *J Cardiovasc Comput Tomogr.* 2010;4(4):246-254.)

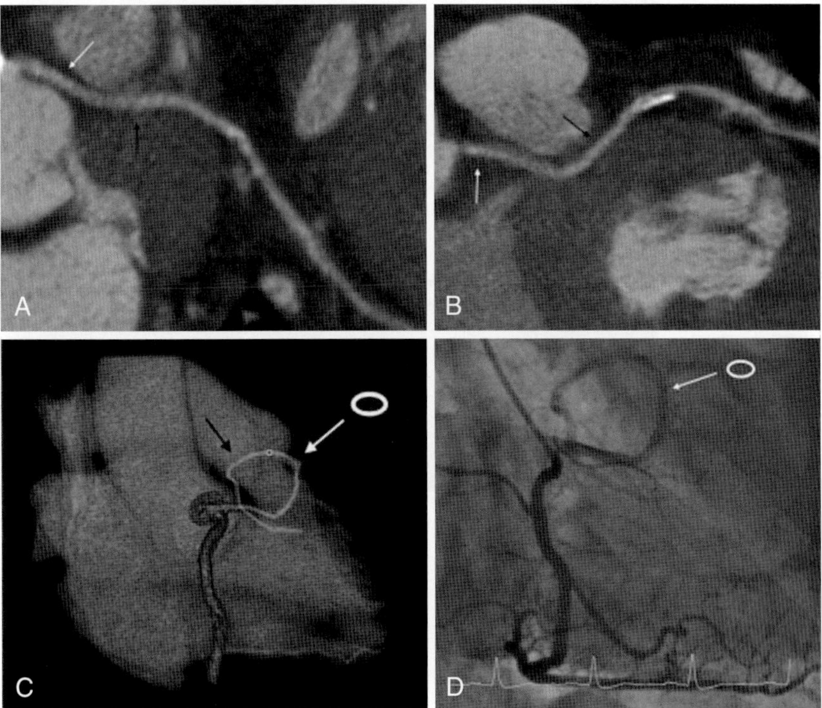

Figure 9-13. Discordant multidetector computed tomography coronary angiography (mixed course) and conventional coronary angiography (CCA) (septal) classifications of an anomalous left main coronary artery (LMCA) from the right coronary sinus of Valsalva. **A** and **B,** Curved reformations showing the proximal epicardial (*white arrows*) and intramyocardial (*black arrows*) segments of the anomalous coronary artery, indicating a mixed course (type 3). **C,** 3D volume-rendering reconstruction in right anterior oblique (RAO) projection (CCA simulation) showing the LMCA and left circumflex coronary artery (*black arrow*) corresponding to the "eye sign" (*white arrow* and *circle*). **D,** CCA in RAO projection showing the "eye sign" (*white arrow and circle*), a finding that would indicate a septal course by traditional criteria. (Reprinted with permission from Torres FS, Nguyen ET, Dennie CJ, et al. Role of MDCT coronary angiography in the evaluation of septal vs interarterial course of anomalous left coronary arteries. *J Cardiovasc Comput Tomogr.* 2010;4(4):246-254.)

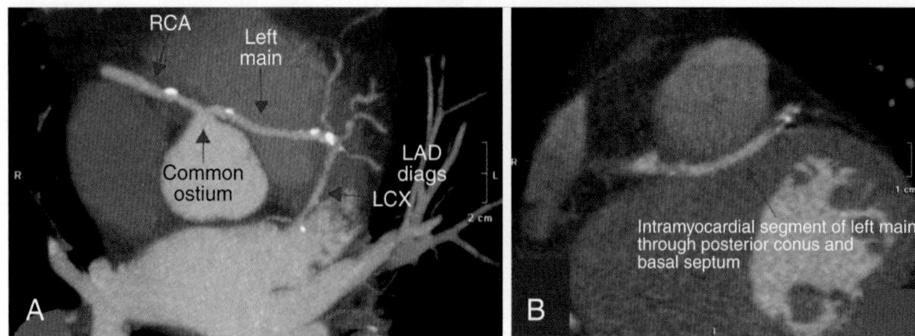

Figure 9-14. Contrast-enhanced curved multiplanar reformatted image. There is a common ostium to the left and right coronaries off of the right sinus. The left main coronary artery is not directly interarterial, but runs through the septum. Calcium is seen in a number of places, including the distal left main coronary artery. LAD, left anterior descending artery; LCX, left circumflex artery; RCA, right coronary artery.

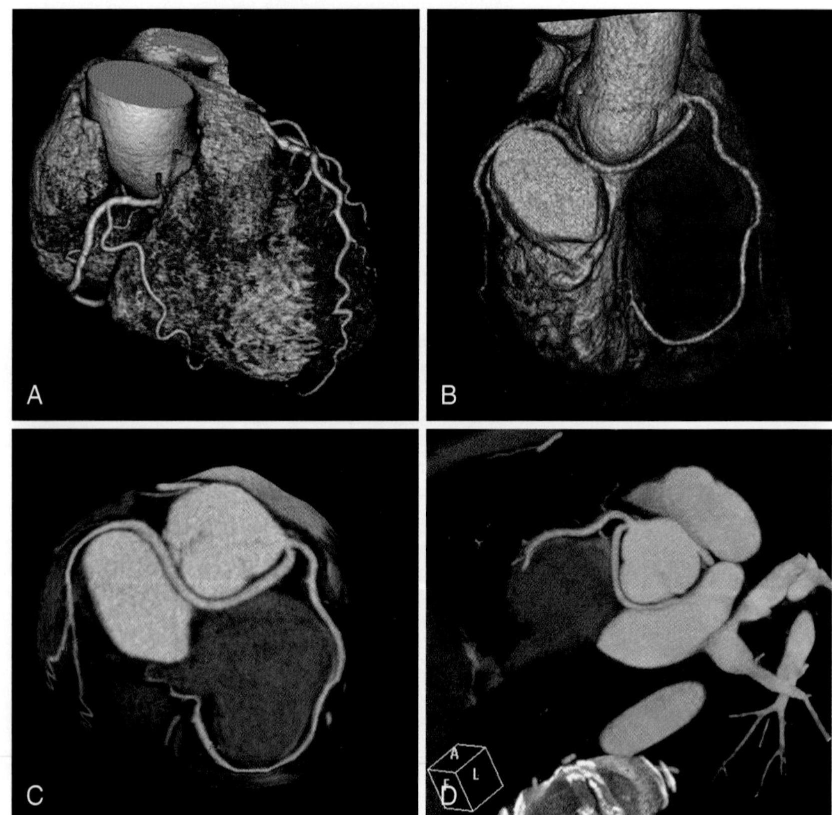

Figure 9-15. Volume-rendered globe and curved multiplanar reformatted images reveal the retro-aortic course of the left circumflex artery, which arises off of a common ostium with the right coronary artery. Also, the left anterior descending coronary artery arises off its own ostium and has an intra-arterial course.

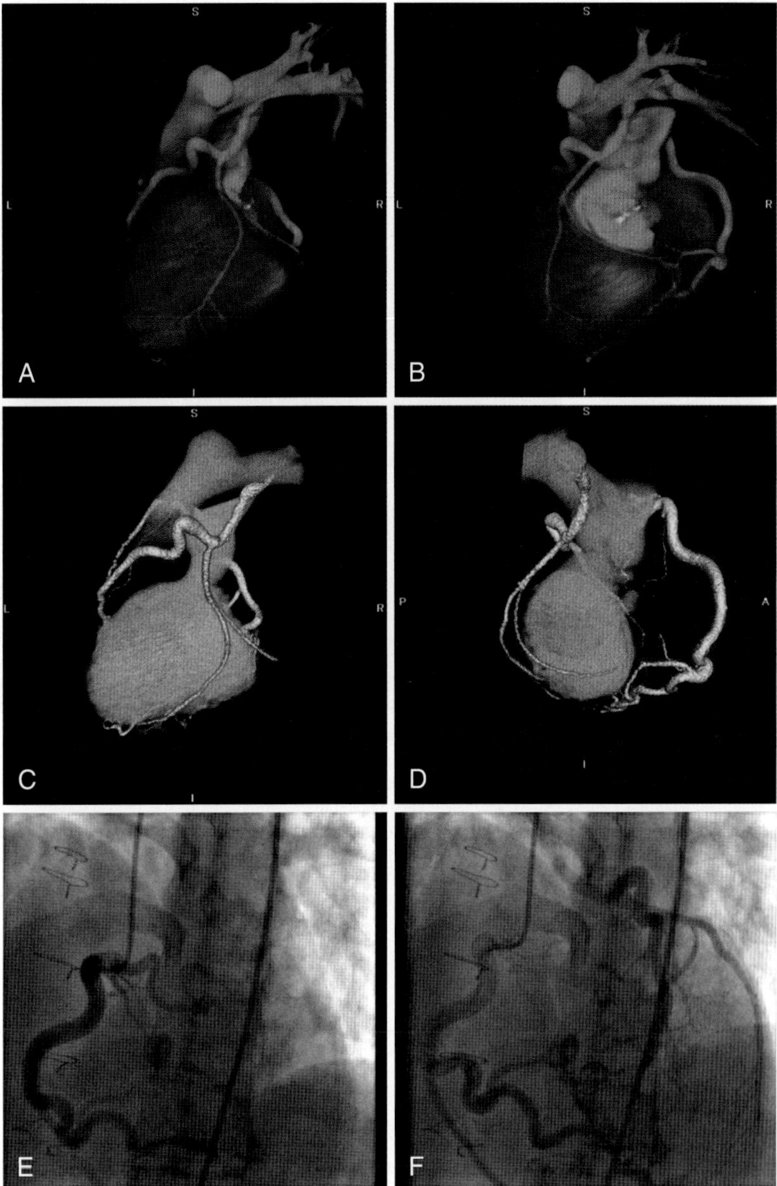

Figure 9-16. Multiple volume-rendered CT angiography images demonstrate an anomalous vessel arising from the right pulmonary artery extending to the left anterior intraventricular groove. Two spot images from a right coronary angiogram demonstrate filling of the right coronary artery, with retrograde filling of the left coronary arterial tree likely via collateral pathways, and filling of an anomalous vessel extending to the right pulmonary artery. This would fulfill the definition of an anomalous left coronary artery from the pulmonary artery. **See Videos 9-1 and 9-2.**

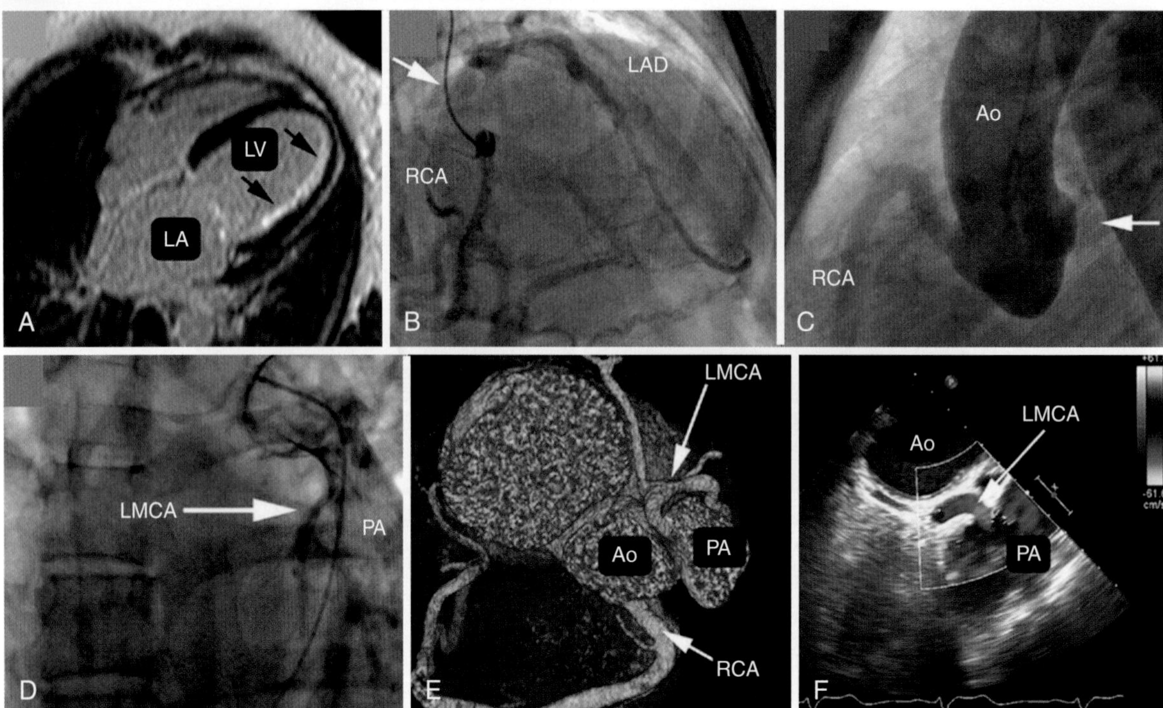

Figure 9-17. New-onset cardiomyopathy discovered in a 42-year-old woman presenting with moderate left ventricular (LV) dilation and systolic dysfunction (LV ejection fraction 46%), associated with diffuse hypokinesis. **A,** Gadolinium-enhanced cardiovascular MRI revealed subendocardial hyperenhancement of the anterior and lateral walls compatible with fibrosis or necrosis (*arrows*), a pattern not usually observed in common cardiomyopathies. Invasive coronary angiography showed a well-developed right coronary artery (RCA), with collaterals running to the left anterior descending coronary artery (LAD) (**B**), which did not arise from the left coronary sinus (**C,** *arrow*). **D,** Pulmonary angiography confirmed an anomalous left main coronary artery (LMCA) arising from the pulmonary artery (PA). **E,** Coronary multislice CT was performed to establish the three-dimensional course of the vessels, confirming the anomalous LMCA arising from the PA. **F,** Transesophageal Doppler echocardiography identified flow reversal at rest in the LMCA (*arrow*), explaining how chronic myocardial ischemia leading to subendocardial fibrosis could result in the present cardiomyopathy. Ao, aorta; LA, left atrium. (Reprinted with permission from Bagur R, Michaud N, Bergeron S, et al. Adult Bland-White-Garland syndrome presenting as cardiomyopathy characterized by subendocardial fibrosis. *J Am Coll Cardiol.* 2010;56(8):e15.)

Alternative Imaging of Coronary Arteries

- **Coronary angiography** (catheter-based) was the traditional diagnostic test, although whether or not it is the current gold-standard modality is unclear. Realistically, catheter angiography does generate some equivocal, ambiguous, or incorrect interpretations. The inability to directly image the extracoronary structures along the course of a coronary anomaly is the main drawback. However, the ability to perform high-resolution cross-sectional IVUS imaging is a strength.
- **MRI** was the original advanced imaging modality to assess proximal coronary anatomy and diameter, and has shown good agreement with conventional angiography,[50,51] although imperfect sensitivity (88%).[52] CCT and MRI appear roughly equivalent. The current use of cardiac MRI would be best limited to assessment of anomalies or suspected anomalies in a patient with renal insufficiency or other contraindication to iodinated contrast material.
- **Echocardiography** is a relatively poor test to identify and characterize coronary anomalies in adults, but is quite a good screening test in very young children. The more distal extent of coronary anatomy is not assessable by echocardiography. Echocardiography offers an excellent means to evaluate congenital heart disease, especially in children, and particularly when performed by pediatric cardiologists.

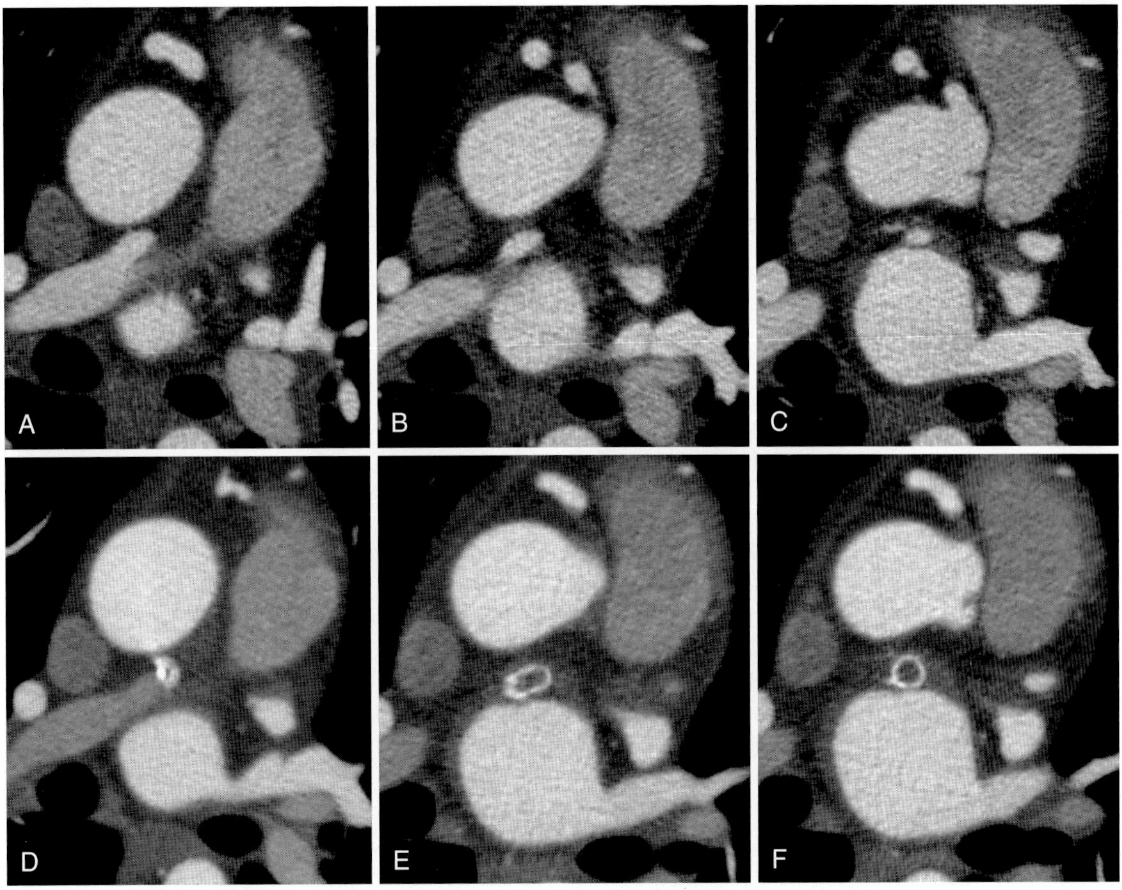

Figure 9-18. Multiple composite images in a patient with anomalous left coronary artery from the pulmonary artery (ALCAPA). **A** through **C**, Images from a cardiac CT study demonstrate the presence of an ALCAPA. **A** shows the communication point of the left anterior descending and right pulmonary arteries. Note a markedly enlarged right coronary artery, which acts as a collateral pathway for the left anterior descending (LAD) artery. **D** through **F**, Cardiac CT in the same patient post-placement of an Amplatzer occluding device. The occluding device is within the LAD, with subsequent thrombosis of the LAD.

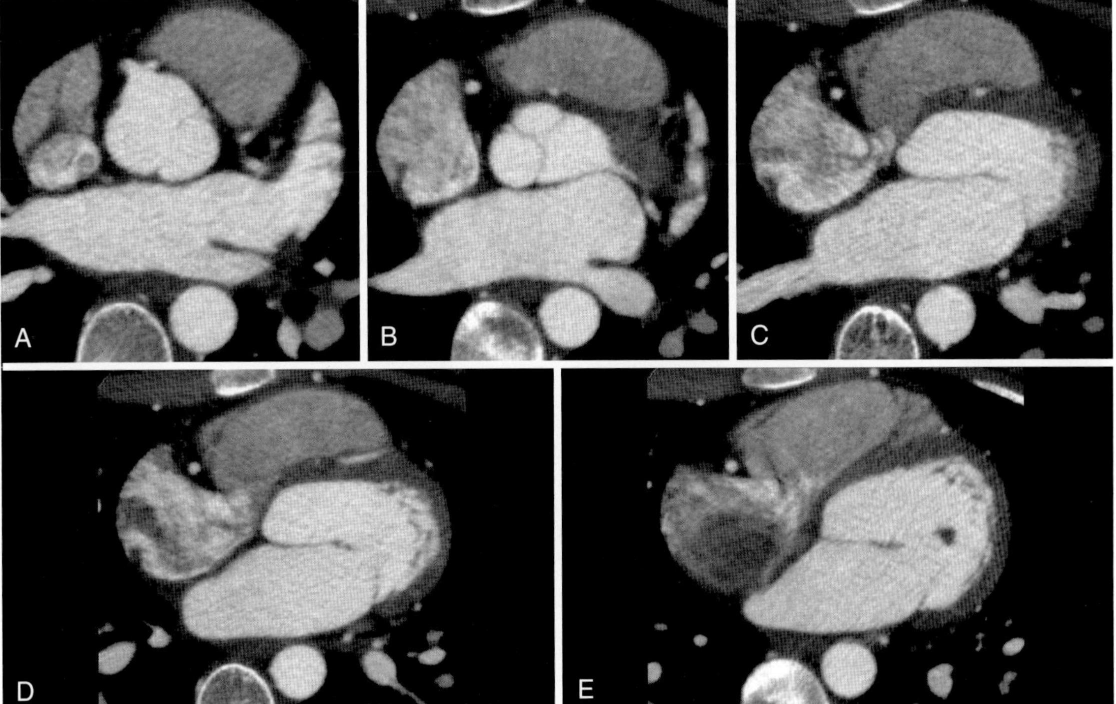

Figure 9-19. Composite images from a cardiac CT study demonstrate anomalous origin of the left coronary artery from the right sinus of Valsalva. This tunnels between the right ventricular outflow tract and the aorta and courses intramyocardially within the intraventricular septum.

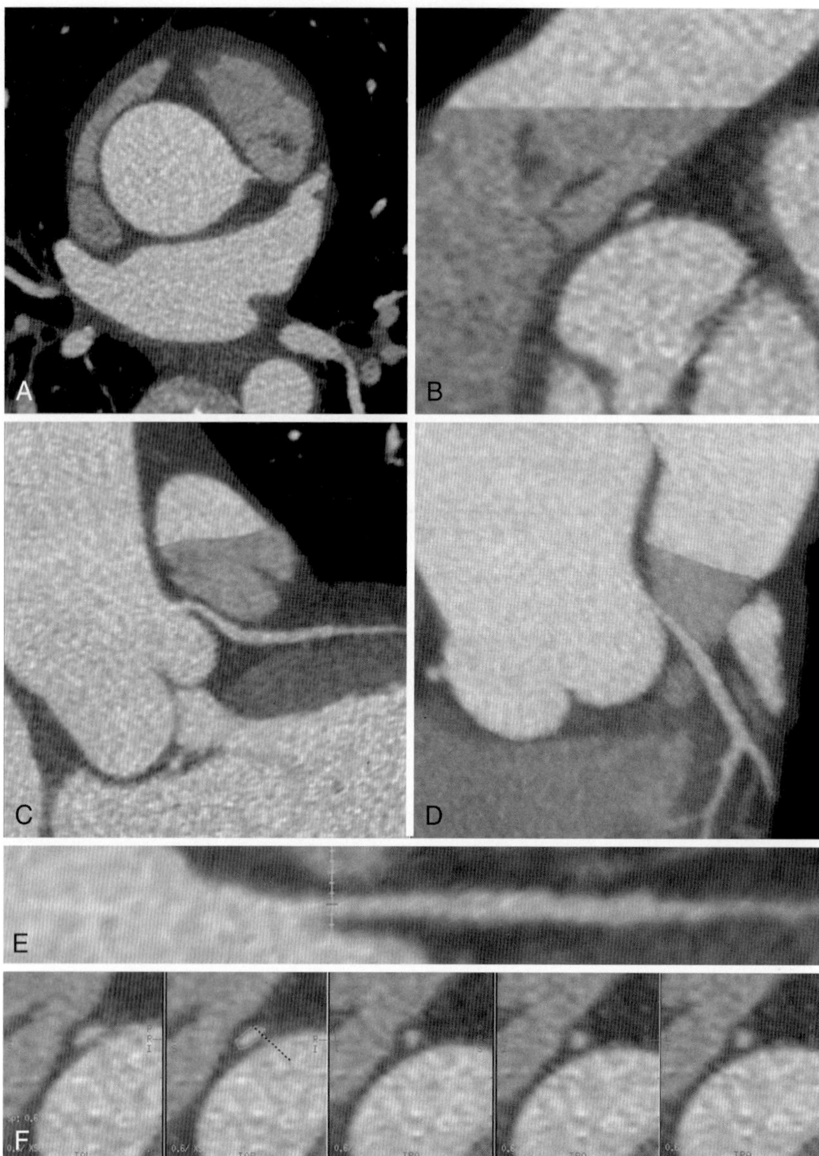

Figure 9-20. Multiple cardiac CT images obtained in a 44-year-old man with a history of atypical chest pain and multiple cardiac risk factors. The axial image (**A**) demonstrates two important findings. The first is the presence of a moderate ascending aortic aneurysm, which measured 4.7 cm. The second is an unusual origin of the left coronary artery. The left coronary artery arises from the left sinotubular junction, above the level of the left sinus of Valsalva. In this particular case, likely due in part to the dilatation of the ascending aorta, this high origin causes the proximal portion of the left coronary artery to be mildly to moderately narrowed in an oval fashion as it courses between the ascending aorta and the right ventricular outflow tract/main pulmonary artery.

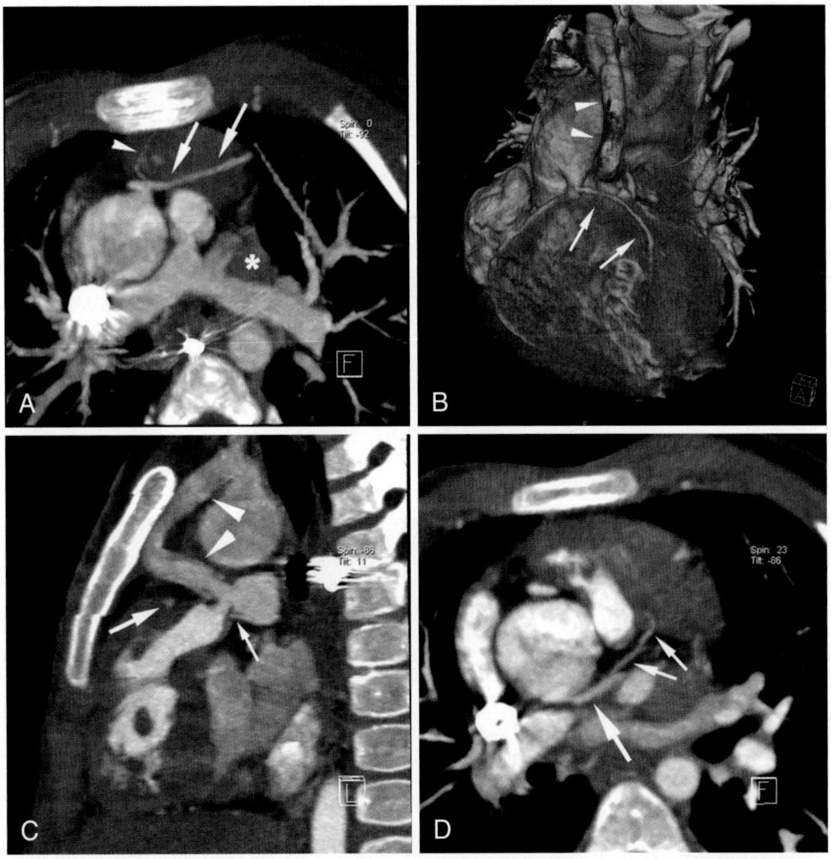

Figure 9-21. A, Two-dimensional maximum intensity projection (5-mm thickness) in transaxial orientation. The left anterior descending coronary artery can be seen to arise from a right coronary artery ostium that has an anterior position. The left anterior descending coronary artery crosses the right ventricular outflow tract (*arrows*). An *arrowhead* indicates a small side branch also extending across the right ventricular outflow tract. The *asterisk* denotes a left persistent superior vena cava. **B,** Three-dimensional reconstruction, volume-rendering technique seen from an anterior position. The anomalous left anterior descending coronary artery can be seen to course over the right ventricular outflow tract (*arrows*). The *arrowheads* point at the subclavian to pulmonary artery shunt. **C,** Two-dimensional multiplanar reconstruction (5-mm thick maximum intensity projection) along the right ventricular outflow tract. A cross-section of the anomalous left anterior descending coronary artery is seen (*large arrow*); approximately 2 mm of myocardium is between the vessel and the right ventricular outflow tract. The *arrowheads* point at the shunt that had been placed between the brachiocephalic trunk and the pulmonary artery. The *small arrow* points at the pulmonary stenosis. **D,** Two-dimensional maximum intensity projection (5-mm thickness) showing a small septal branch (*small arrows*) arising from the left main coronary artery (*large arrow*). Because of the clockwise rotation of the aortic root, the ostium of the left main coronary artery is displaced posteriorly. (Reprinted with permission from Achenbach S, Dittrich S, Kuettner A. Anomalous left anterior descending coronary artery in a pediatric patient with Fallot tetralogy. *J Cardiovasc Comput Tomogr*. 2008;2:55-56.)

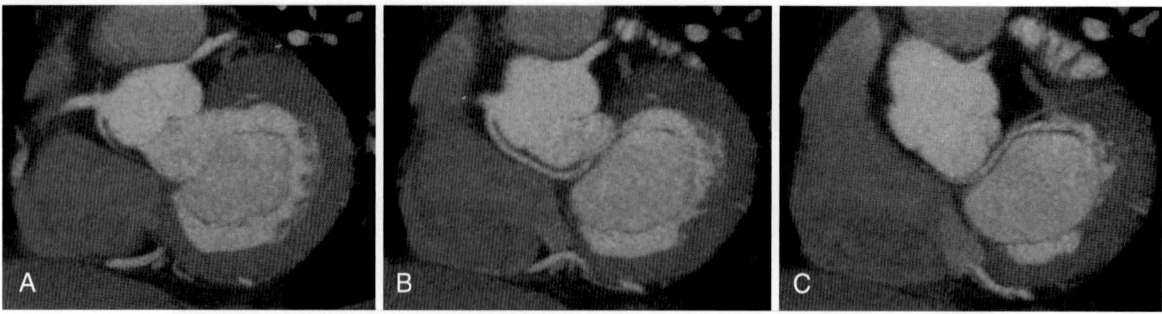

Figure 9-22. Multiple composite images from a cardiac CT study demonstrate anomalous origin of the circumflex artery, which arises in a conjoint fashion with the right coronary artery, from the right coronary cusp. This circumflex artery then extends inferior to the aortic root and out to the left atrioventricular groove.

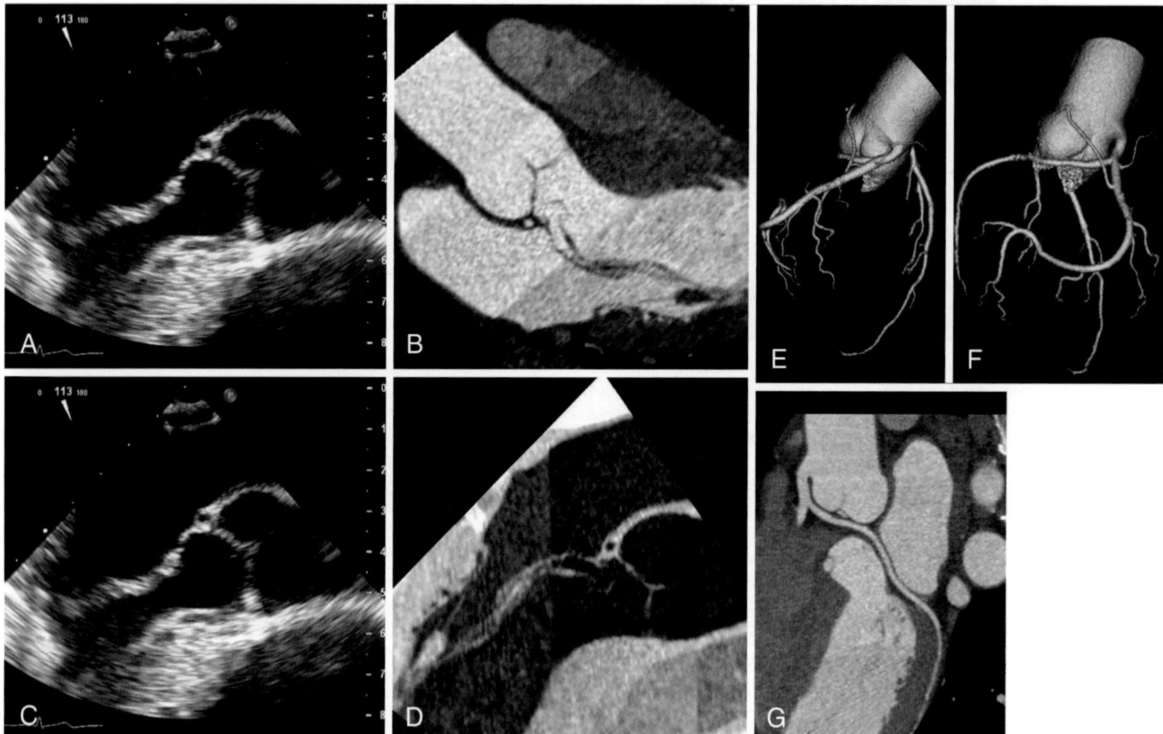

Figure 9-23. A 49-year-old woman presented with chest pain. An initial echocardiogram was performed. The echocardiographic images demonstrate a small rounded structure posterior to the aorta interposed between the aorta and the left atrium posteriorly. The possibility of an anomalous coronary artery was raised, and a cardiac CT scan was performed. The multiplanar reformatted images (**B** and **D,** gray scale inverted) demonstrates similar appearance to that seen on the echocardiogram. A contrast-filled, rounded structure is seen situated below the noncoronary cusp surrounded by epicardial fat. **E** and **F,** The volume-rendered and curved multiplanar reconstruction images demonstrate an anomalous circumflex coronary artery. This arises from the right coronary artery and courses behind the aorta and then into the left atrioventricular groove. No evidence is seen of an associated stenosis. **See Video 9-3.**

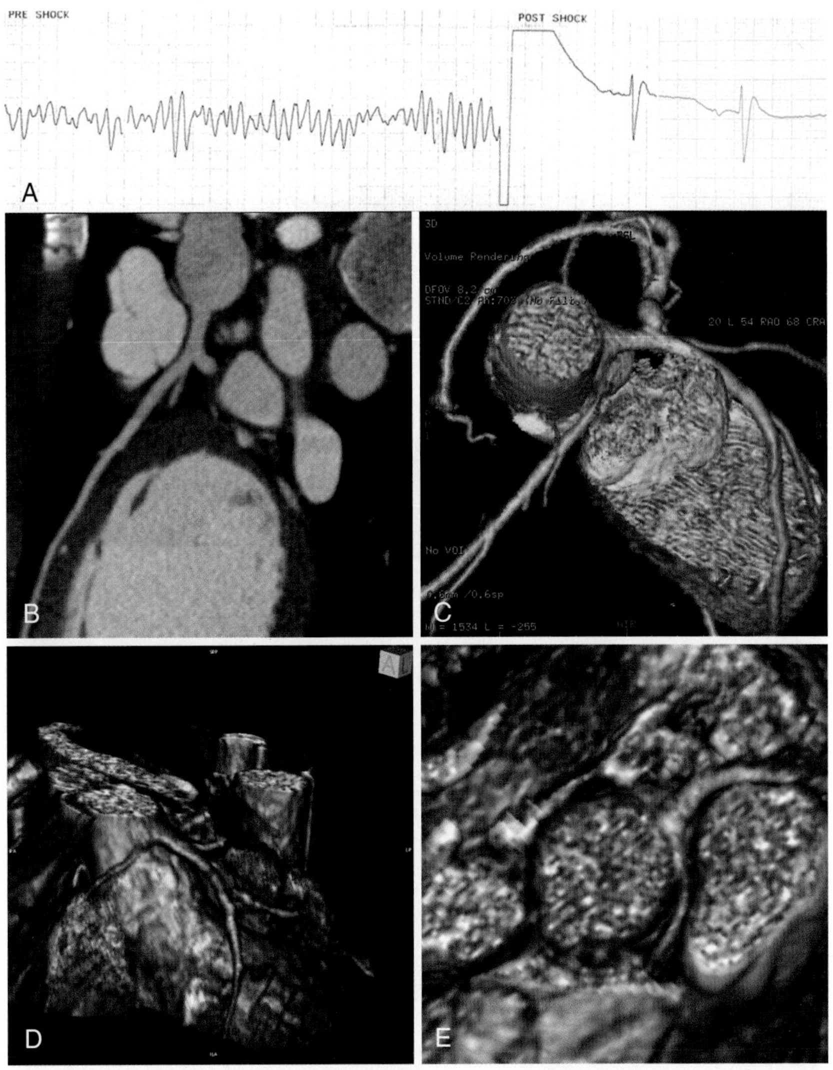

Figure 9-24. A 17-year-old boy presented in ventricular fibrillation (Vfib) arrest. **A,** ECG at presentation demonstrates ventricular fibrillation reverting to sinus rhythm post shock. **B** and **C,** CT angiography reformations demonstrate anomalous origin of the right coronary artery (RCA) from the left sinus of Valsalva, coursing between the aorta and the main pulmonary artery/right ventricular outflow tract. The RCA is slitlike in configuration in its intra-arterial course and then attains a normal caliber as it enters the right atrioventricular groove. **D** and **E,** Coronary magnetic resonance angiography depicting the anomalous course of the right coronary artery, and less well, the narrowing of the proximal segment.

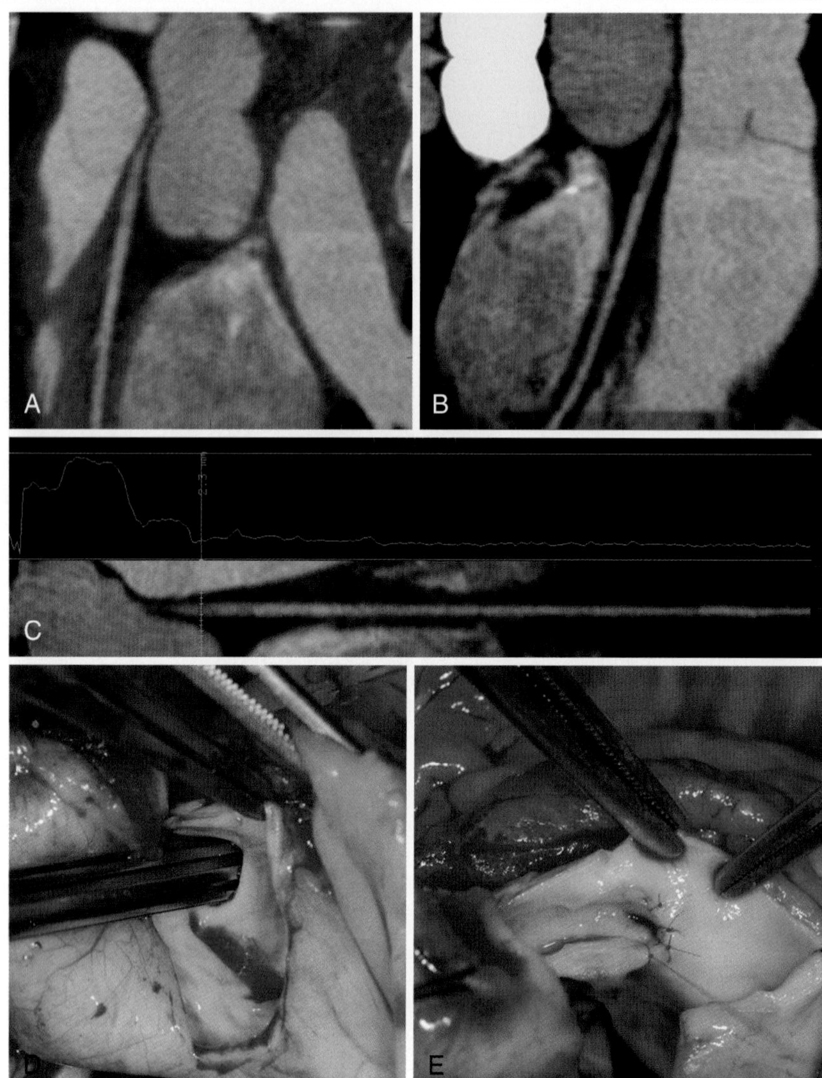

Figure 9-25. Some case as Figure 9-24. **A–C,** Reformatted images demonstrate an anomalous origin of the right coronary artery (RCA) from the left sinus of Valsalva, coursing between the aorta and the main pulmonary artery/right ventricular outflow tract. The RCA is slit-like in configuration in its intra-arterial course and then obtains a normal caliber as it enters the right atrioventricular groove. **D** and **E**, Intraoperative photos of the same case seen in Figures 9-35 and 9-36. Sucker is present in the left main stem coronary ostium. The ostium to the right coronary artery is a tiny dimple beneath it, slightly obscured by blood. Intraoperative photo reveals the "unroofed" RCA origin. (Image courtesy of David Ross MD, Edmonton, Alberta, Canada.)

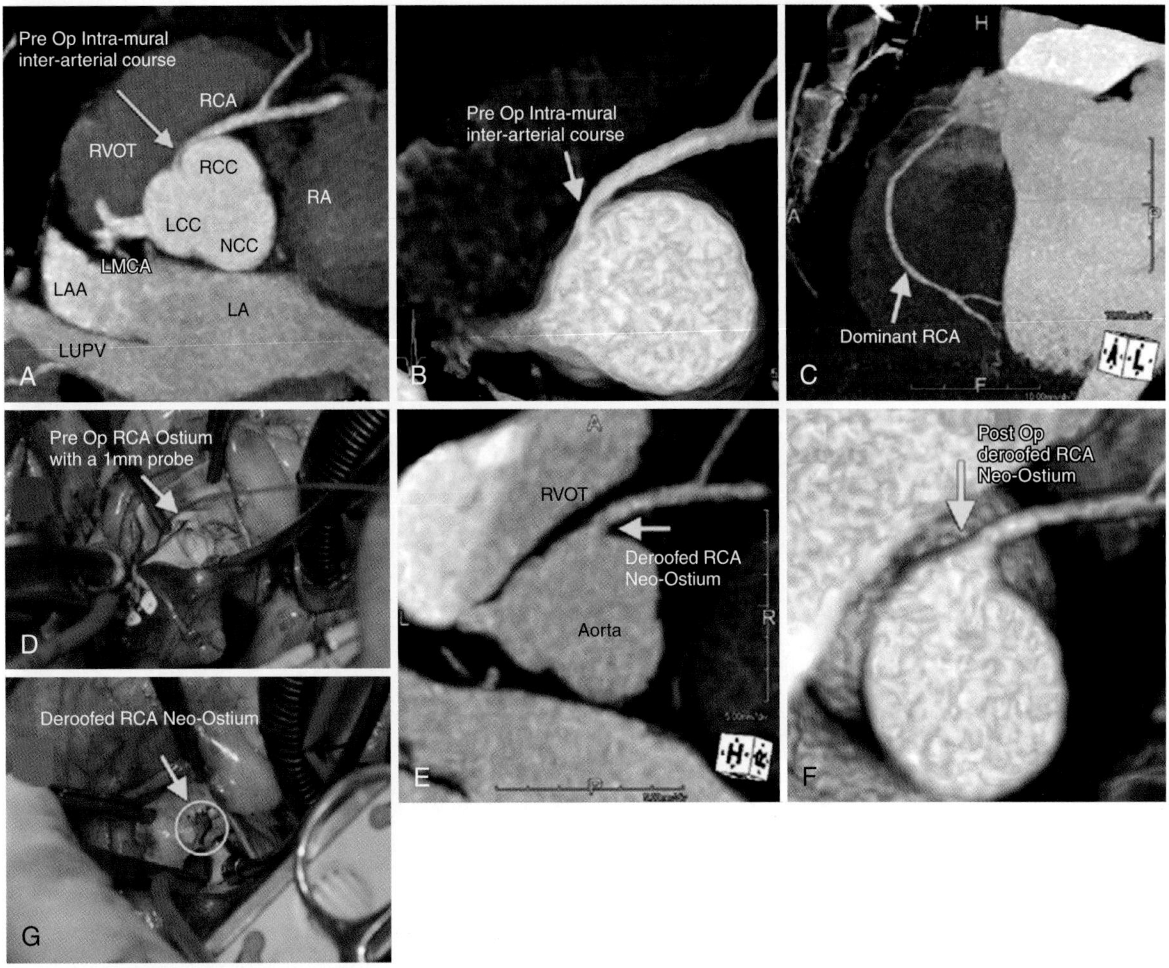

Figure 9-26. A 42-year-old woman had experienced chronic chest pain upon exertion for 5 years. The patient was able to exercise to 10 metabolic equivalents without symptoms or electrocardiographic abnormalities with an exercise echocardiography stress test; however, the echocardiography portion of the stress test revealed inferior wall hypokinesis at peak stress, which is indicative of inducible inferior wall myocardial ischemia. Therefore, multidetector dual source CT coronary angiography was performed, revealing a coronary artery calcium score of 0 with no evidence of atherosclerosis. However, the dominant right coronary artery (RCA) was found to originate from a narrow slitlike opening in the left coronary sinus of Valsalva coursing anteriorly and toward the right with a proximal intramural, interarterial course (**A–D**). This anomaly accounted for the abnormality on the exercise echocardiogram. The patient was referred for deroofing of the proximal RCA with creation of a neo-ostium (**E**). Surgery was successful with no unforeseen events, and the patient had complete resolution of symptoms. LA, left atrium; LAA, left atrial appendage; LCC, left common carotid artery; LMCA, left main coronary artery; LUPV, left upper pulmonary vein; NCC, noncoronary cusp; RA, right atrium; RCC, right common carotid artery; RVOT, right ventricular outflow tract. (Reprinted with permission from Ailiani R, De Oliveira N, Harbin D, et al. Successful treatment of an unusual cause of myocardial ischemia. *J Am Coll Cardiol.* 2009;54(3):277.)

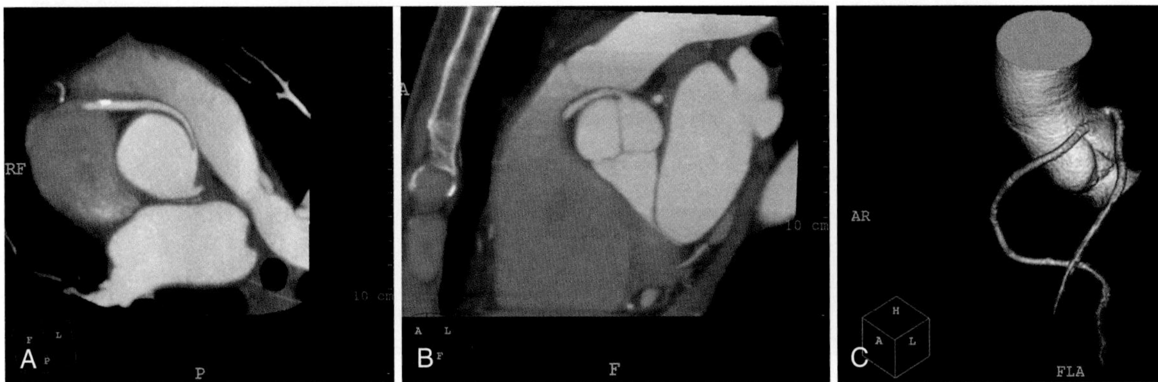

Figure 9-27. A, Maximum intensity projection (MIP). The origin of the right coronary artery (RCA) is ectopic and the course is anomalous. The RCA arises from the left coronary sinus and runs with an intra-arterial course. The ostium and very proximal left main coronary artery are seen separately and just posteriorly to it. **B,** MIP image. The anomalous origin and intra-arterial course of the RCA are depicted. The sinus architecture is more easily appreciated on this view. **C,** 3D reconstruction. The RCA is seen crossing in front of the aorta (the pulmonary artery is not seen). The left anterior descending coronary artery is depicted and runs anteriorly. The circumflex is not depicted.

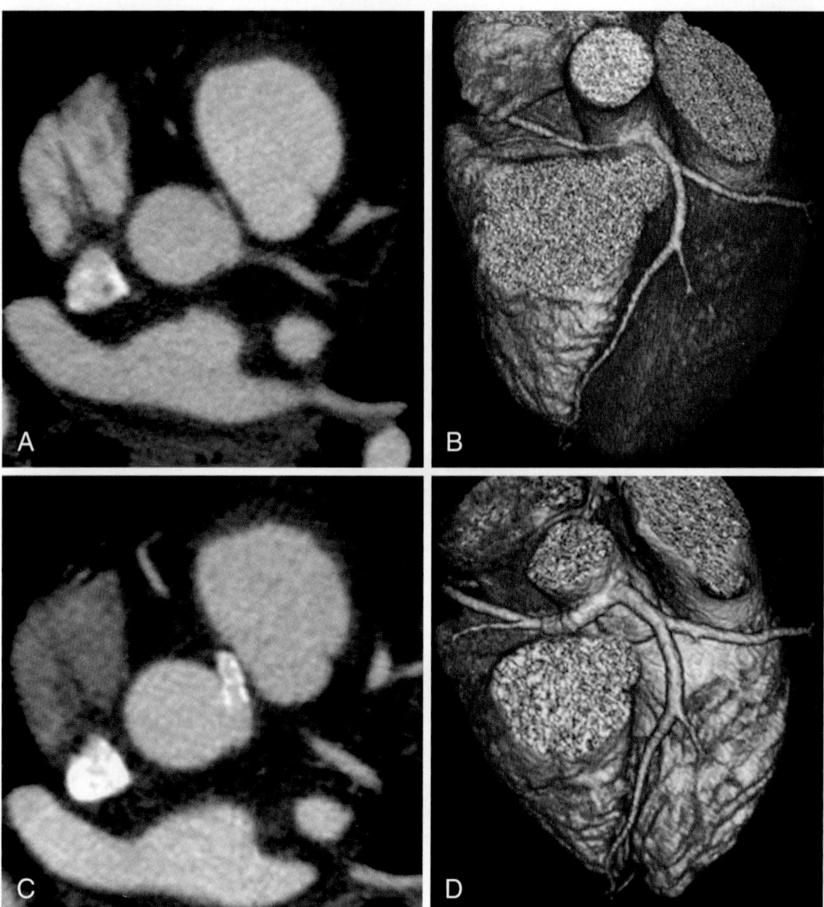

Figure 9-28. Multiple images from two separate cardiac CT studies on the same patient. **A** and **B,** The origin of the right coronary artery (RCA) from the left coronary on the left sinus of Valsalva with a proximal slit-like component. The patient had malignant ventricular dysrhythmia, and the decision was made to insert a stent. A stent is seen extending from the right sinus of Valsalva into the proximal RCA, with resolution of the slit-like configuration.

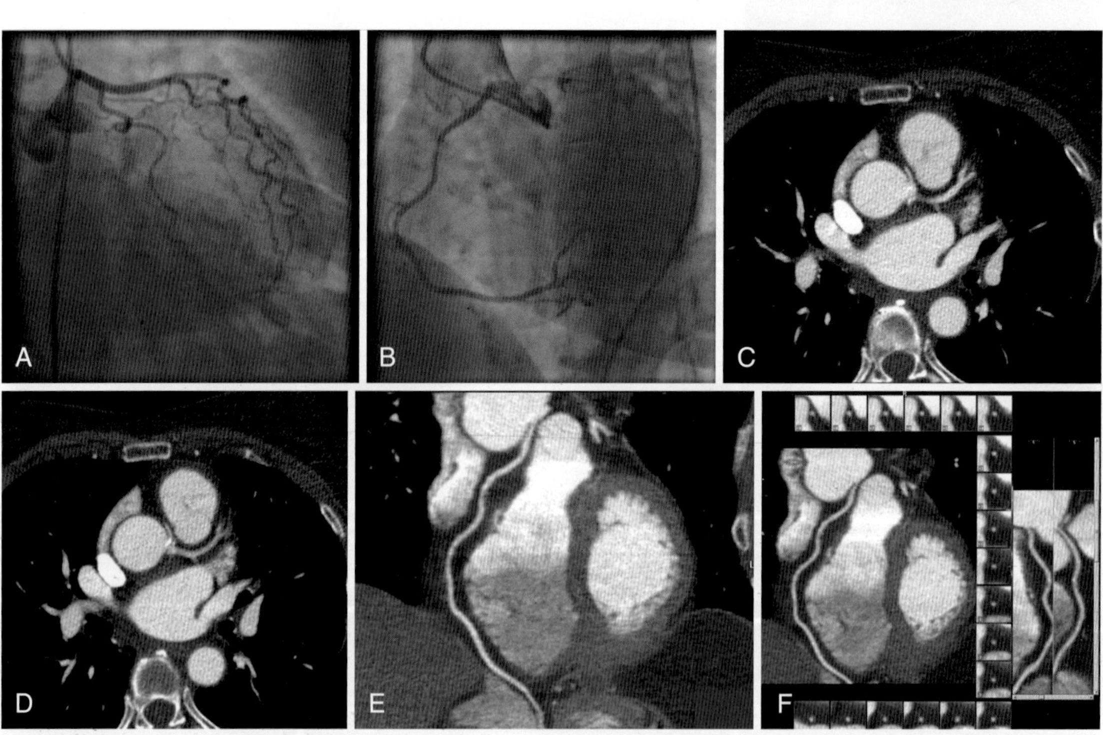

Figure 9-29. A 47-year-old woman with a history of nonsustained ventricular tachycardia presented for coronary angiography. **A** and **B,** Images from a coronary angiogram demonstrate a normal-appearing left coronary artery angiogram. The ostium of the right coronary artery is difficult to visualize. There is a mild 30% lesion in the proximal right coronary artery (RCA). **C–F,** Multiple axial and curved reformatted images in the same patient demonstrate an anomalous origin of the RCA from the left coronary cusp. This courses between the aorta and the right ventricular outflow tract and has a slit-like configuration. A small amount of calcification at the origin of the RCA is also noted. A primarily soft plaque 30% lesion in the proximal RCA is also seen, correlating well with the patient's coronary angiogram. **See Videos 9-4 and 9-5.**

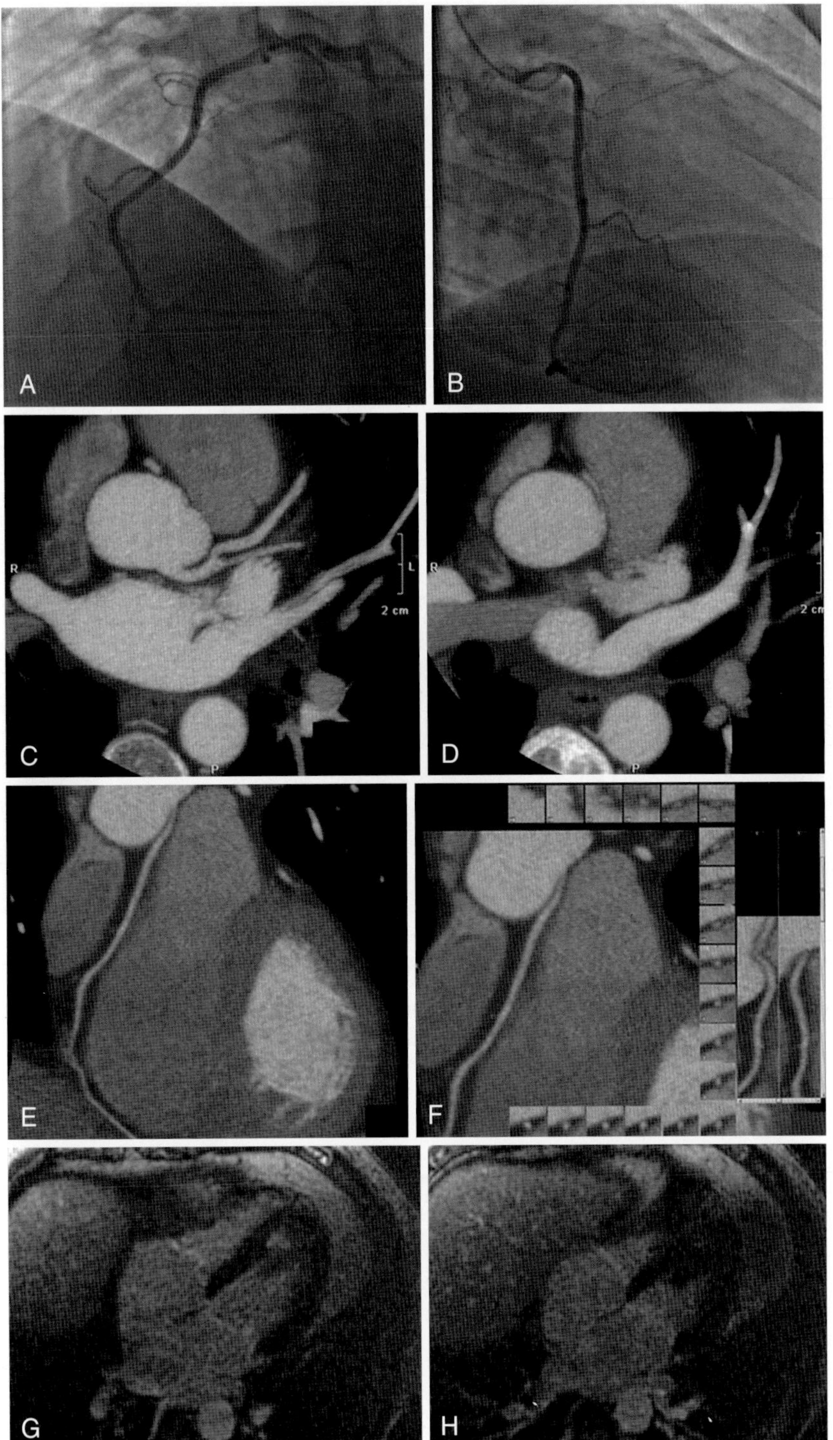

Figure 9-30. Composite images in a 34-year-old woman with syncopal episodes. Initial coronary angiography demonstrates poor visualization of the origin of the right coronary artery (RCA), raising the possibility of an anomalous coronary artery. Axial maximum intensity projection and curved reformatted images demonstrate an anomalous origin of the RCA from the left coronary sinus with a slit-like proximal RCA between the aorta and the right ventricular outflow tract. Two four-chamber delayed enhanced cardiac MR images demonstrate a focus of subendocardial delayed enhancement within the mid-inferoseptal region. This likely represents a small region of subendocardial infarction. **See Videos 9-6 through 9-8.**

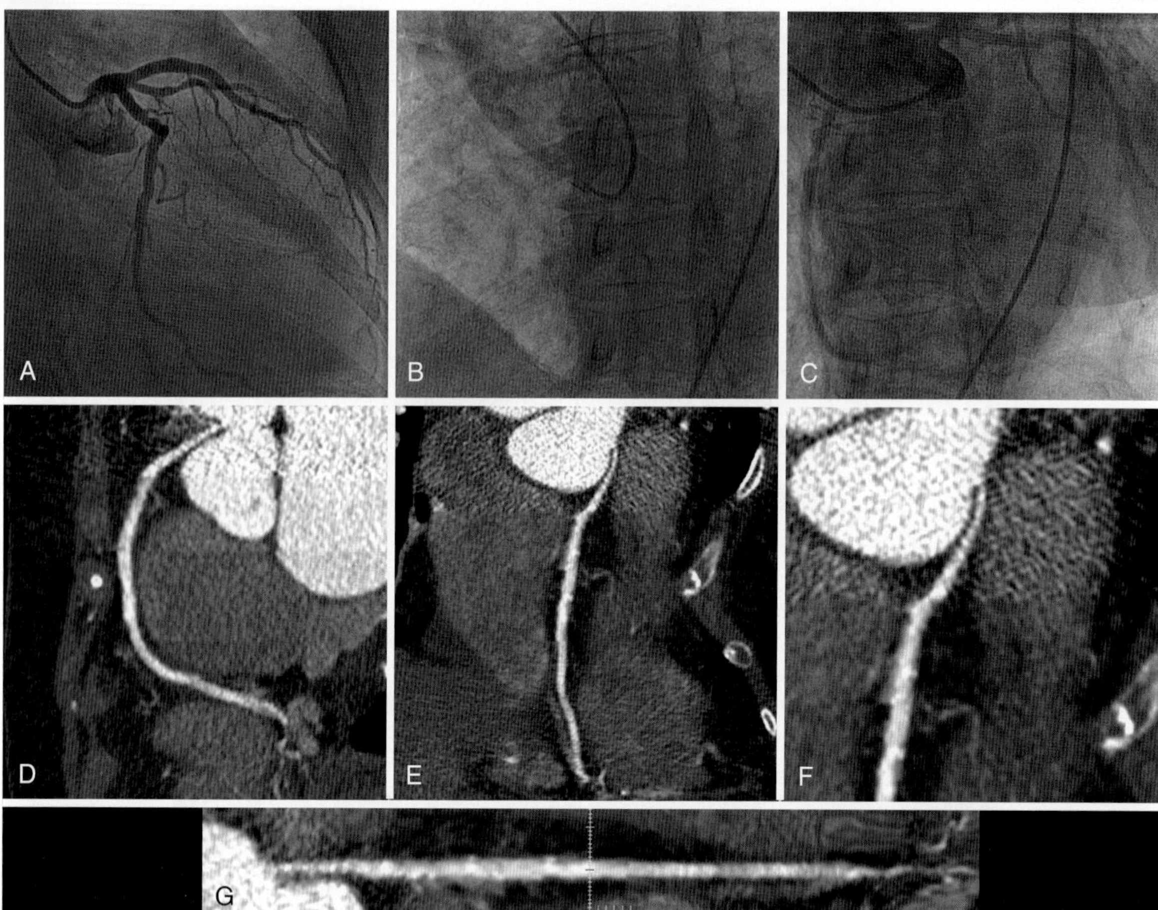

Figure 9-31. A 72-year-old woman with severe mitral regurgitation, atrial fibrillation, and chest pain. **A,** A conventional angiogram was initially performed. Selective catheterization of the left coronary artery (LCA) demonstrated a normal left anterior descending artery and circumflex system. **B,** An attempt to engage the right coronary artery (RCA), which was unsuccessful. **C,** Contrast within the RCA and proximal LCA from the aortic root injection. The origin of the RCA was difficult to assess, so cardiac CT was performed. The RCA was found to arise anomalously from the left coronary sinus. It courses interarterially between the aorta and the main pulmonary artery, where the RCA is at least moderately narrowed with a near slit-like configuration. The majority of the RCA is well visualized in this patient with atrial fibrillation, and shows no significant stenosis. **See Videos 9-9 through 9-11.**

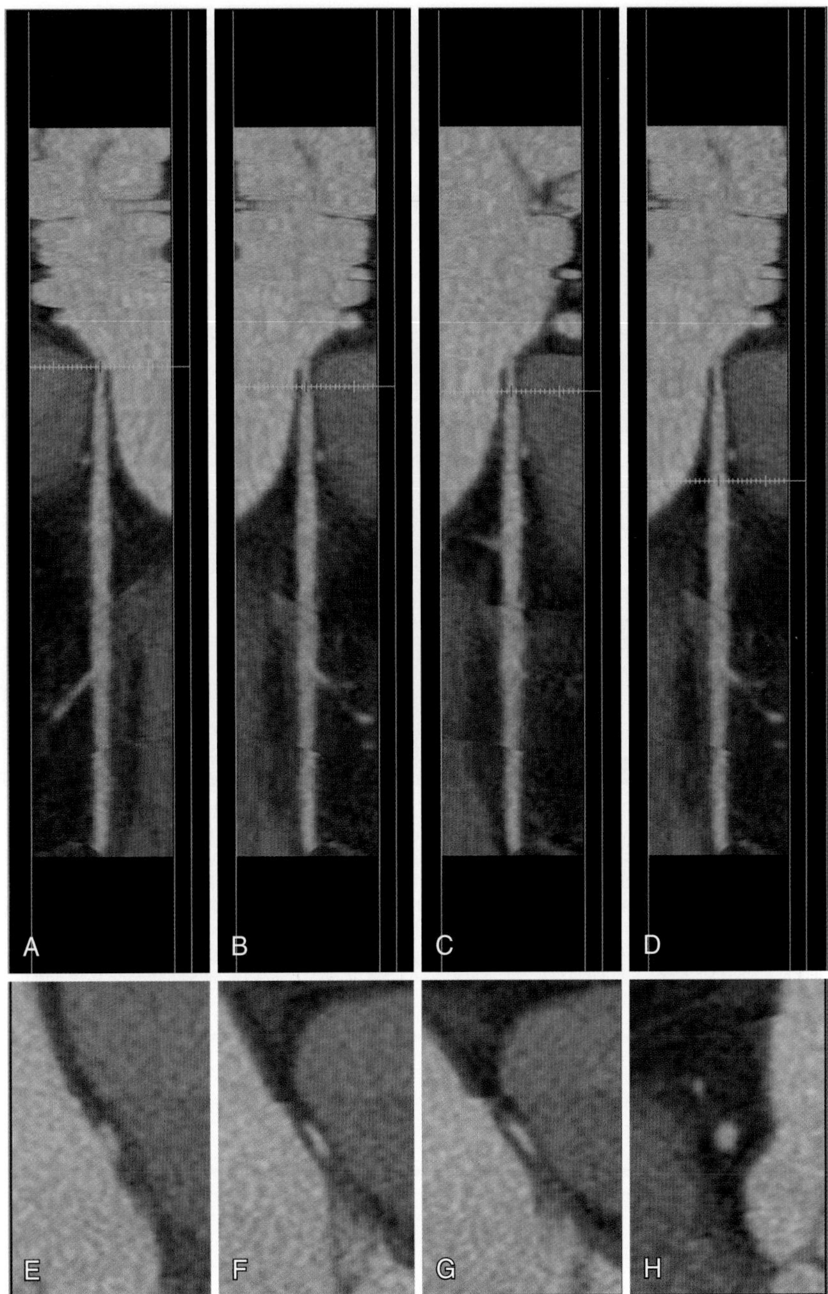

Figure 9-32. **A–D,** Straightened views through an anomalous right coronary artery (RCA), arising from the left sinus of Valsalva, and coursing between the aorta and the right ventricular outflow tract/main pulmonary artery. **E–H,** Representative cross sections through the intra-arterial course are seen below each straightened view, demonstrating the slit-like appearance of the anomalous coronary artery as it courses intra-arterially. **A** and **E** demonstrate the cross-sectional view at the origin of the RCA from the aorta. **B** and **F** demonstrate the proximal and mid-interarterial course of the RCA. **D** and **H** demonstrate a cross section through the proximal RCA in the upper right atrioventricular groove.

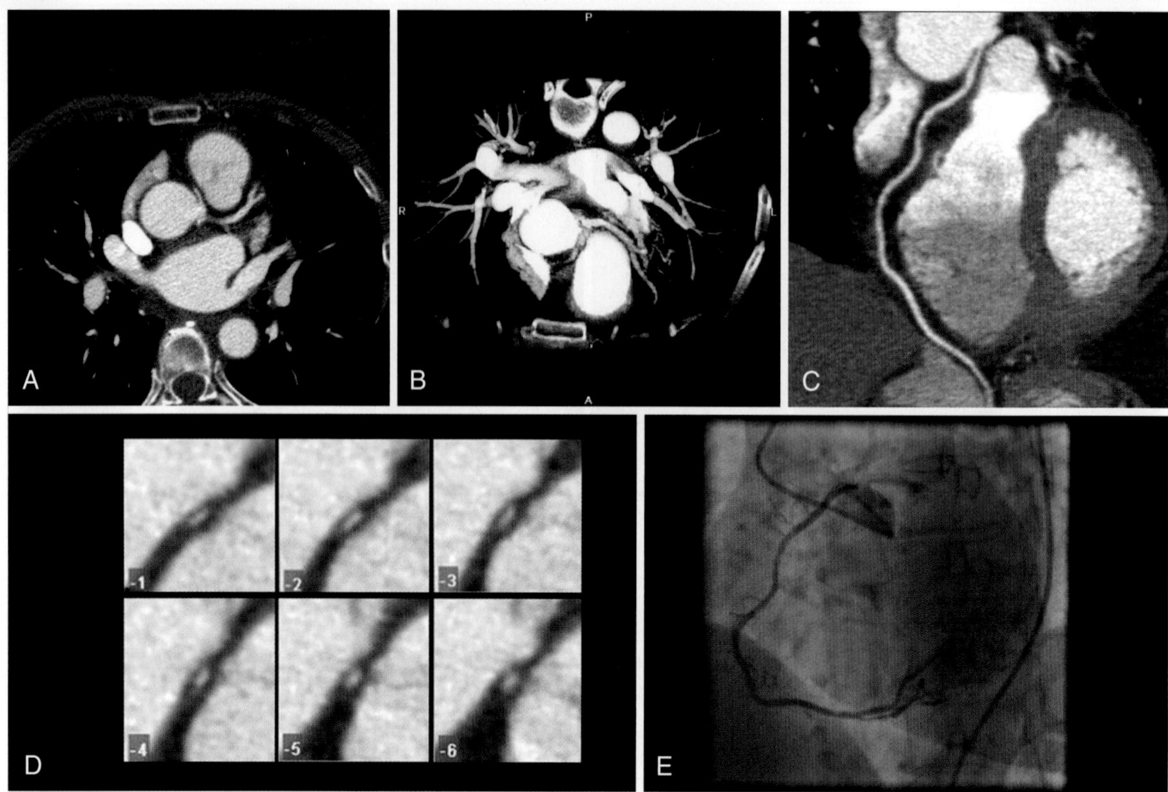

Figure 9-33. A 52-year-old woman presented with shortness of breath and presyncope. **A,** Anomalous origin of the right coronary artery (RCA) is seen arising from the left sinus of Valsalva. The RCA and the left main coronary artery appeared to arise from the same ostium. The proximal RCA is slit-like and narrowed. **B,** Volume-rendered image demonstrating the interarterial course of the anomalous RCA between the aorta and the main pulmonary artery. **C,** A curved multiplanar image through the RCA demonstrates a slit-like proximal interarterial course of the RCA. There is a mild 30% stenosis in the proximal RCA, but no evidence of a significant atherosclerotic stenosis in the remainder of the RCA. **D,** Multiple cross-section views through the interarterial course of the RCA demonstrate a slit-like RCA configuration proximally, with the RCA regaining a more normal caliber as it enters the right atrioventricular groove. **E,** The patient went on to conventional angiography. At conventional angiography, it was not possible to selectively cannulate the RCA. Injection into the aortic root was suggestive of an anomalous RCA origin, but this was not as well delineated as on CT angiogram. **See Videos 9-12 and 9-13.**

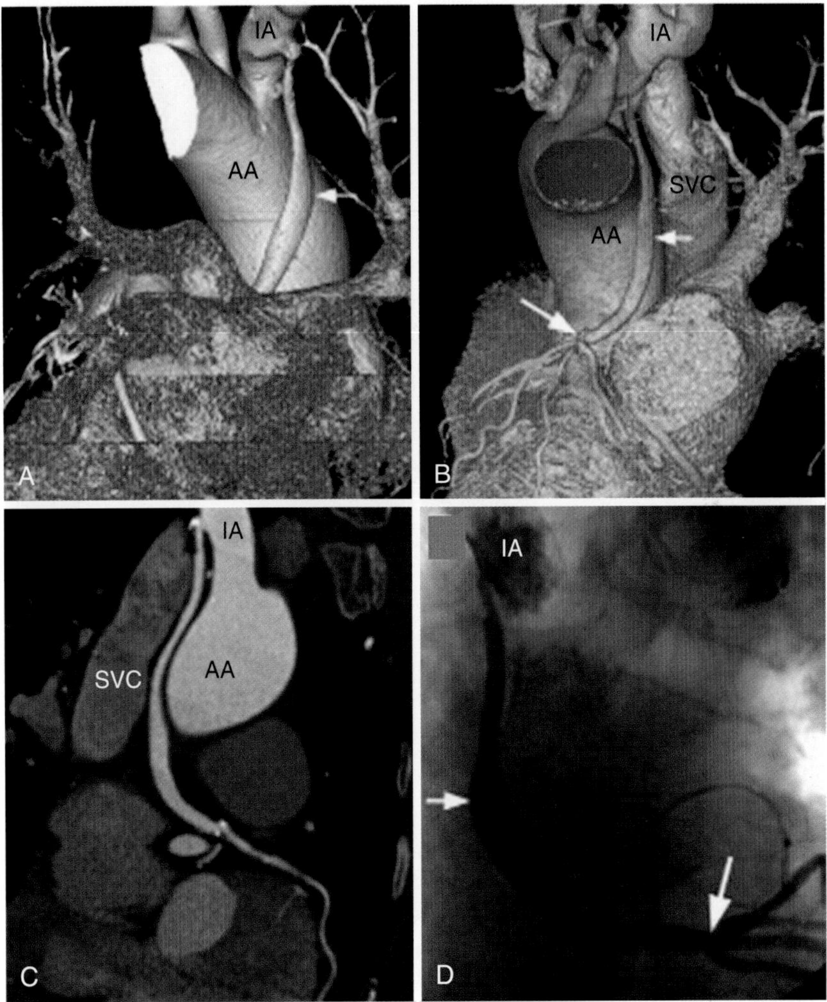

Figure 9-34. Anomalous origin of left coronary artery from innominate artery (IA). A 78-year-old woman was admitted with chest pain. Coronary angiography revealed a normal right coronary artery. The left coronary artery (LCA) could not be intubated and could not be demonstrated on right coronary angiography or root aortography. On electrocardiography-gated 64-slice CT coronary angiography, there was neither coronary artery nor any dimpling originating from the left sinus of Valsalva. The LCA *(arrows)* was seen arising from the right innominate artery (IA), going along with the ascending aorta (AA), and eventually reaching its normal position (**A–C**). On second coronary angiography, the anomalous origin of the LCA from the IA was confirmed (**D**). This patient had no history of previous thoracic surgery. SVC, superior vena cava. (Reprinted with permission from Kim YM, Choi RK, Lee CK. Anomalous origin of left coronary artery from innominate artery. *J Am Coll Cardiol.* 2009;54(2):176.)

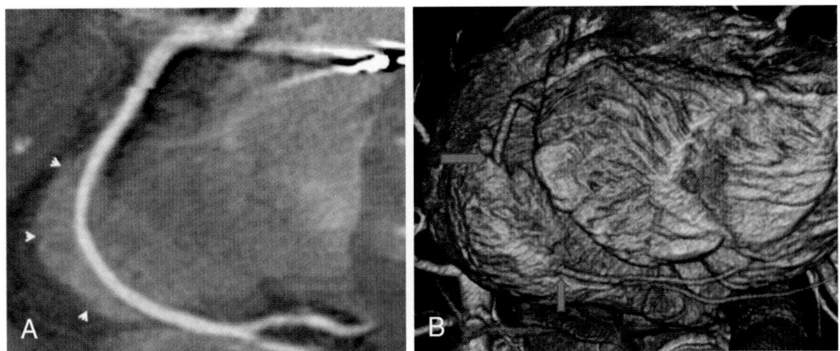

Figure 9-35. **A,** Curved planar reformat showing 4- to 5-cm intracavitary course of RCA. *Arrowheads* denote the lateral wall of the right atrium. **B,** Volume-rendered image of the right heart in the region of the atrioventricular groove, showing points of entry and exit of the intracavitary RCA. (Reprinted with permission from Zalamea RM, Entrikin DW, Wannenburg T, Carr JJ. Anomalous intracavitary right coronary artery shown by cardiac CT: a potential hazard to be aware of before various interventions. *J Cardiovasc Comput Tomogr.* 2009;3(1):57-61.)

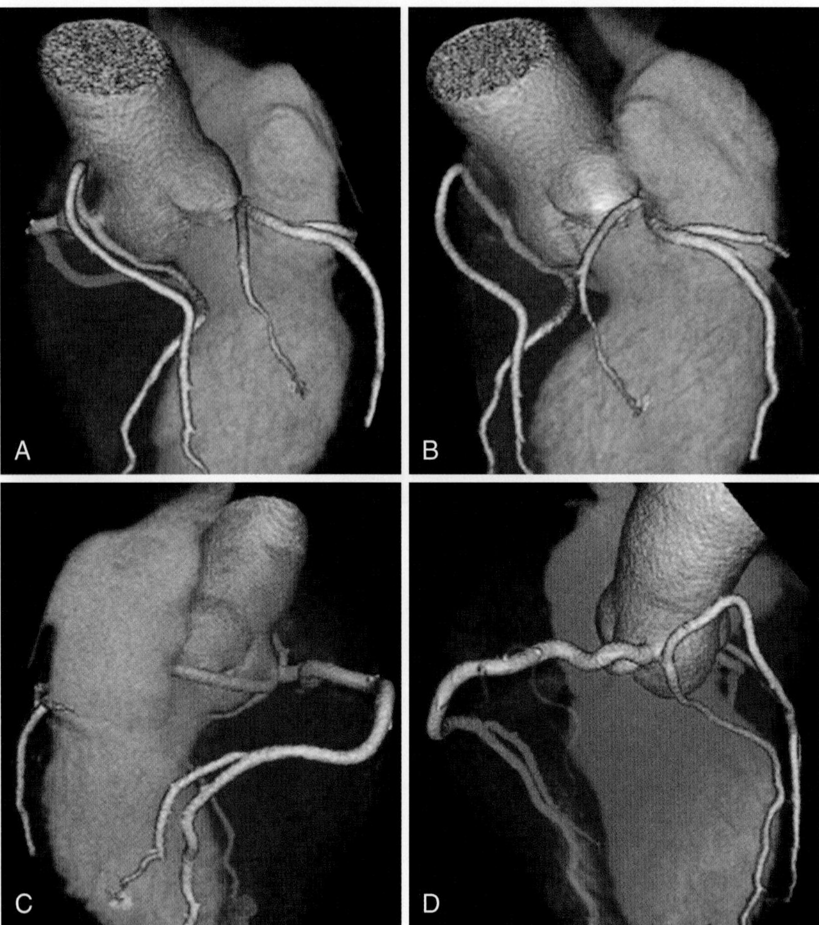

Figure 9-36. Anomalous origin of the left anterior descending artery (LAD) from the right coronary sinus, with an anterior course to the pulmonary artery. The left circumflex artery and a ramus intermedius have a common origin.

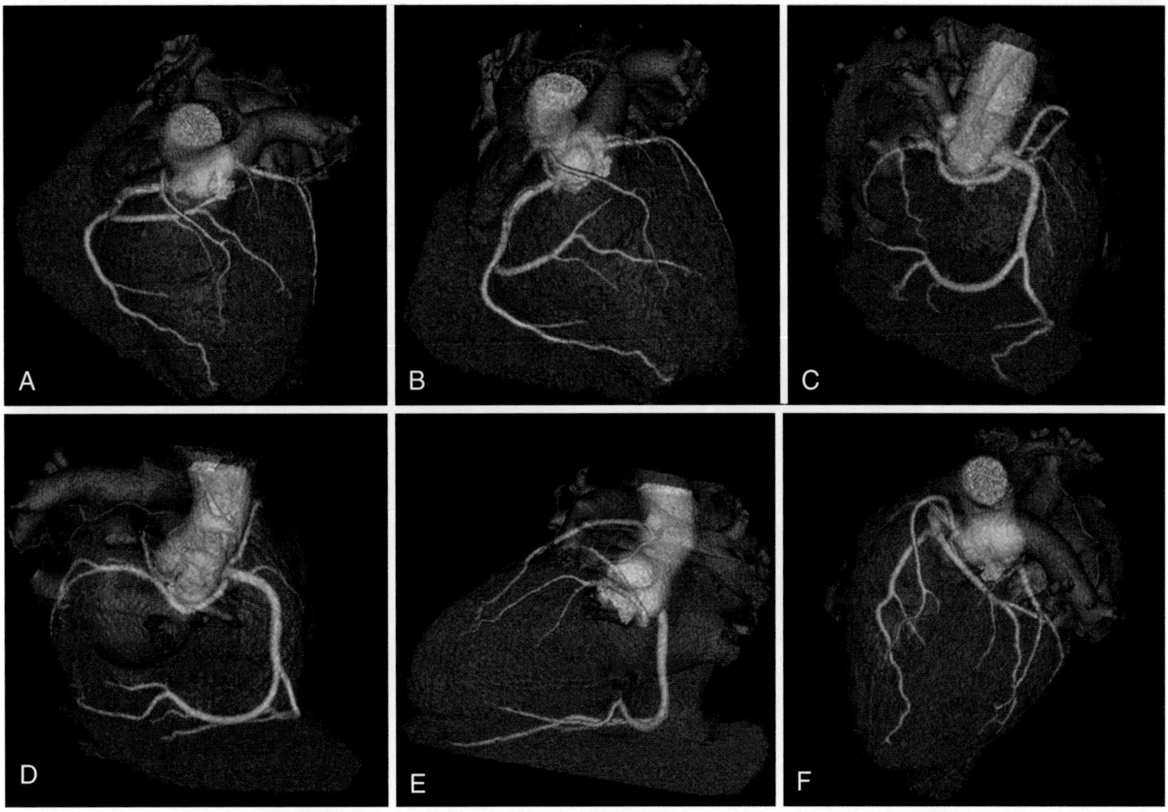

Figure 9-37. A 44-year-old woman presented with atypical chest pain and nonspecific ECG changes. Multiple volume-rendered images from cardiac CT study demonstrate an unusual, rare form of coronary artery anomaly. A solitary coronary artery is present. The coronary artery arises from the right sinus of Valsalva. An ongoing large dominant right coronary artery (RCA) is seen. There is a variant of normal anatomy involving the RCA, with the posterior descending coronary artery arising as an acute marginal branch from the mid-RCA. There is a large ongoing posterolateral trunk and posterolateral branches. The left coronary artery arising from this common origin courses posterior to the aorta to the superior portion of the intraventricular groove. There it bifurcates into the left anterior descending and circumflex arteries.

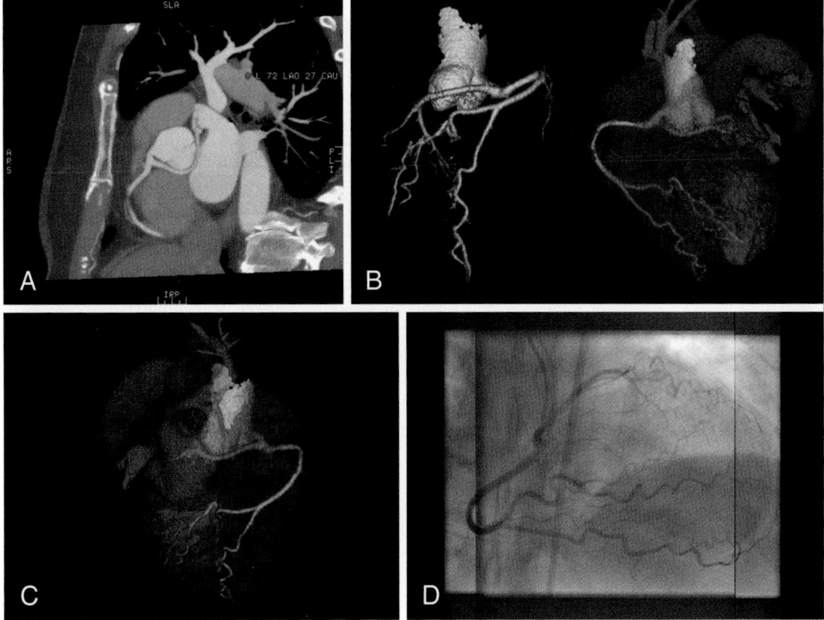

Figure 9-38. A 56-year-old woman presented with stress (Takotsubo) cardiomyopathy and incidentally was found to have a solitary coronary artery arising from the right sinus of Valsalva. The right coronary artery is large and dominant. The left coronary artery is small and has an intra-arterial course. The left anterior descending artery is very short. As can be seen on the CT images in comparison to the angiogram (composite image), the CT images allow ready depiction of origin and course with respect to other structures.

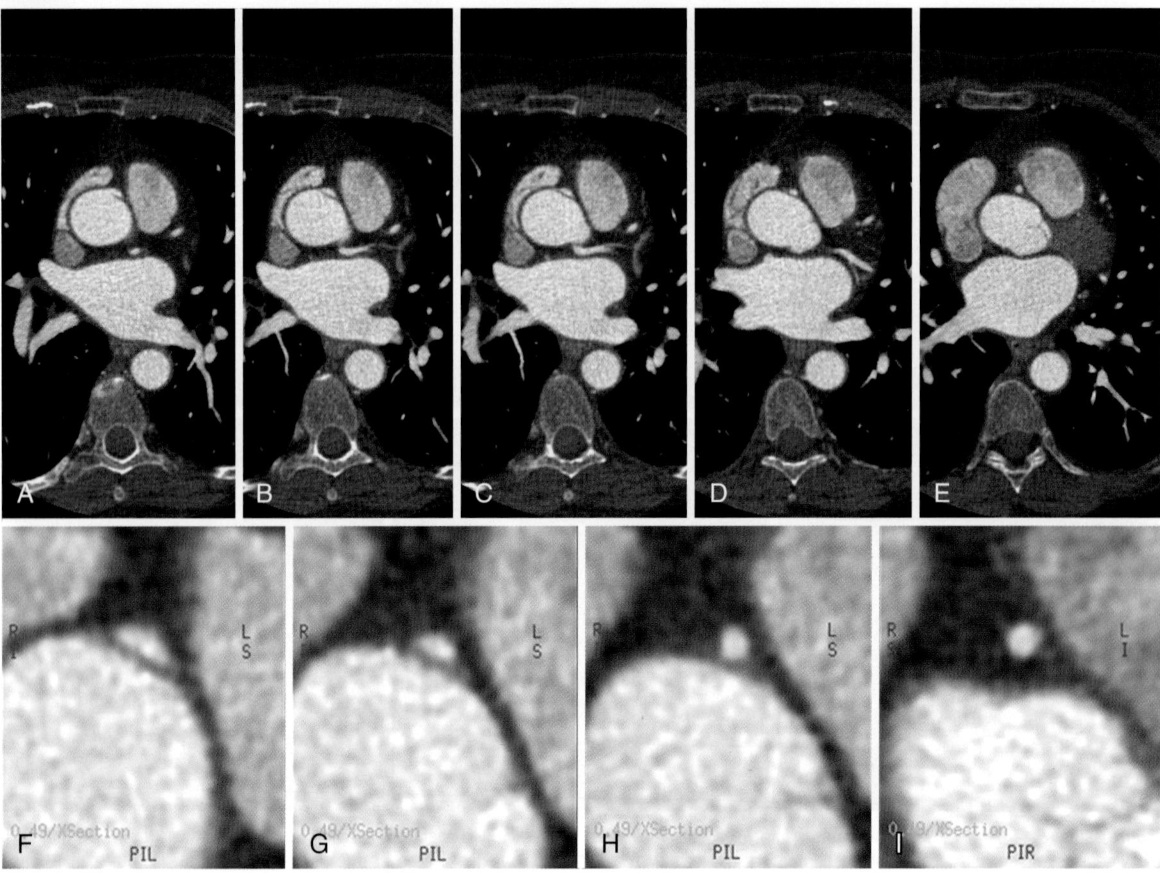

Figure 9-39. A 47-year-old man with atypical chest pain. **A–E,** multiple axial images from a coronary CT study demonstrate an unusual origin to the right coronary artery (RCA), which arises at the level of the sinotubular junction above the right sinus of Valsalva with an initially intramural course. **F–I,** Enlarged images demonstrate the deformity of the ostial RCA due to its intramural course, although without significant associated stenosis.

TABLE 9-1 ACCF 2010 Appropriateness Criteria for the Use of Cardiac Computed Tomography to Evaluate Coronary Fistulae

	APPROPRIATENESS RATING	INDICATION	MEDIAN SCORE
Evaluation of adult congenital heart disease	Appropriate	Assessment of anomalies of coronary arterial and other thoracic arteriovenous vessels	9

Data from Taylor AJ, Cerqueira M, Hodgson JM, et al. ACCF/SCCT/ACR/AHA/ASE/ASNC/NASCI/SCAI/SCMR 2010 appropriate use criteria for cardiac computed tomography. A report of the American College of Cardiology Foundation Appropriate Use Criteria Task Force, the Society of Cardiovascular Computed Tomography, the American College of Radiology, the American Heart Association, the American Society of Echocardiography, the American Society of Nuclear Cardiology, the North American Society for Cardiovascular Imaging, the Society for Cardiovascular Angiography and Interventions, and the Society for Cardiovascular Magnetic Resonance. *J Am Coll Cardiol.* 2010;56(22):1864-1894.

References

1. Click RL, Holmes Jr DR, Vlietstra RE, Kosinski AS, Kronmal RA. Anomalous coronary arteries: location, degree of atherosclerosis and effect on survival–a report from the Coronary Artery Surgery Study. *J Am Coll Cardiol.* 1989;13:331-537.
2. Ropers D, Ping DC, Achenbach S. Right-sided origin of the left main coronary artery: typical variants and their visualization by cardiac computerized tomography. *JACC Cardiovasc Imaging.* 2008;1:579-681.
3. Torres FS, Nguyen ET, Dennie CJ, et al. Role of MDCT coronary angiography in the evaluation of septal vs interarterial course of anomalous left coronary arteries. *J Cardiovasc Comput Tomogr.* 2010;4:246-254.
4. Reig J. Anatomical variations in the coronary arteries. II. Less prevalent variations: coronary anomalies. *Eur J Anat.* 2004;8:19-53.
5. Angelini P. Coronary artery anomalies–current clinical issues: definitions, classification, incidence, clinical relevance, and treatment guidelines. *Tex Heart Inst J.* 2002;29:271-278.
6. Wilkins CE, Betancourt B, Mathur VS, et al. Coronary artery anomalies: a review of more than 10,000 patients from the Clayton Cardiovascular Laboratories. *Tex Heart Inst J.* 1988;15:166-173.
7. Yamanaka O, Hobbs RE. Coronary artery anomalies in 126,595 patients undergoing coronary arteriography. *Cathet Cardiovasc Diagn.* 1990;21:18-40.
8. Maron BJ, Carney KP, Lever HM, et al. Relationship of race to sudden cardiac death in competitive athletes with hypertrophic cardiomyopathy. *J Am Coll Cardiol.* 2003;41:974-980.
9. Eckart RE, Scoville SL, Campbell CL, et al. Sudden death in young adults: a 25-year review of autopsies in military recruits. *Annals of Internal Medicine.* 2004;14(11):829-834.
10. Earls J, Berman E, Urban B, Curry C, Lane KL. The prevalence and appearance of anomalous coronary arteries on 16-detector row MDCT coronary angiography. *RSNA2004.* 2004.
11. Loewinger L, Gopal A, Budoff MJ. Right-sided origin of the left main coronary artery evaluated by cardiac computed tomography angiography. *Journal of Cardiovascular Computed Tomography.* 2007;1: 112-113.
12. Kim YM, Choi RK, Lee CK. Anomalous origin of left coronary artery from innominate artery. *J Am Coll Cardiol.* 2009;54:276.
13. Friedman ML, Makaryus AN, Henry S, Makaryus JN, Boxt LM. Subaortic origin of the left circumflex coronary artery. *J Cardiovasc Comput Tomogr.* 2008;2:112-154.
14. Bowden GY, De la Rosa Hernandez A, Vargas Torres MJ, et al. Severe ischemia in an elderly patient with anomalous origin of the right coronary artery from the left main. *J Am Coll Cardiol.* 2009;53:733.
15. Barker CM, Srichai MB, Meyer DB, Sedlis SP. Anomalous right coronary artery from the pulmonary artery. *J Cardiovasc Comput Tomogr.* 2007;1(3):166-167.
16. Rogers IS, Truong QA, Cury RC, Hoffmann U. Incidental discovery of a rare single coronary artery anomaly by cardiac multidetector computed tomography. *J Cardiovasc Comput Tomogr.* 2008;2(1): 59-60.
17. Yturralde F, Nesto R, Wald C. Congenital single coronary artery with an absent left main coronary artery. *J Cardiovasc Comput Tomogr.* 2008;2(1):50-51.
18. Van Camp SP, Bloor CM, Mueller FO, Cantu RC, Olson HG. Nontraumatic sports death in high school and college athletes. *Med Sci Sports Exerc.* 1995;27(5):641-647.
19. Shirani J, Roberts WC. Origin of the left main coronary artery from the right aortic sinus with retroaortic course of the anomalistically arising artery. *Am Heart J.* 1992;124(4):1077-1078.
20. Murphy DA, Roy DL, Sohal M, Chandler BM. Anomalous origin of left main coronary artery from anterior sinus of Valsalva with myocardial infarction. *J Thorac Cardiovasc Surg.* 1978;75(2): 282-285.
21. Basso C, Maron BJ, Corrado D, Thiene G. Clinical profile of congenital coronary artery anomalies with origin from the wrong aortic sinus leading to sudden death in young competitive athletes. *J Am Coll Cardiol.* 2000;35(6):1493-1501.
22. Cheitlin MD, De Castro CM, McAllister HA. Sudden death as a complication of anomalous left coronary origin from the anterior sinus of Valsalva, a not-so-minor congenital anomaly. *Circulation.* 1974;50(4):780-787.
23. Roberts WC. Major anomalies of coronary arterial origin seen in adulthood. *Am Heart J.* 1986;111(5):941-963.
24. Frescura C, Basso C, Thiene G, et al. Anomalous origin of coronary arteries and risk of sudden death: a study based on an autopsy population of congenital heart disease. *Hum Pathol.* 1998;29(7): 689-695.
25. Taylor AJ, Byers JP, Cheitlin MD, Virmani R. Anomalous right or left coronary artery from the contralateral coronary sinus: "high-risk" abnormalities in the initial coronary artery course and heterogeneous clinical outcomes. *Am Heart J.* 1997;133(4): 428-435.
26. Maddoux GL, Goss JE, Ramo BW, et al. Angina and vasospasm at rest in a patient with an anomalous left coronary system. *Cathet Cardiovasc Diagn.* 1989;16(2):95-98.
27. Gupta D, Saxena A, Kothari SS, et al. Detection of coronary artery anomalies in tetralogy of Fallot using a specific angiographic protocol. *Am J Cardiol.* 2001;87(2):241-244 A249.
28. Warnes CA, Williams RG, Bashore TM, et al. ACC/AHA 2008 guidelines for the management of adults with congenital heart disease: a report of the American College of Cardiology/American Heart Association Task Force on Practice Guidelines (Writing Committee to Develop Guidelines on the Management of Adults With Congenital Heart Disease). Developed in Collaboration With the American Society of Echocardiography, Heart Rhythm Society, International Society for Adult Congenital Heart Disease, Society for Cardiovascular Angiography and Interventions, and Society of Thoracic Surgeons. *J Am Coll Cardiol.* 2008;52(23):e1-e121.
29. Achenbach S, Dittrich S, Kuettner A. Anomalous left anterior descending coronary artery in a pediatric patient with Fallot tetralogy. *J Cardiovasc Comput Tomogr.* 2008;2:55-56.
30. Shaher RM, Puddu GC. Coronary arterial anatomy in complete transposition of the great vessels. *Am J Cardiol.* 1966;17(3): 355-361.
31. Elliott LP, Amplatz K, Edwards JE. Coronary arterial patterns in transposition complexes. Anatomic and angiocardiographic studies. *Am J Cardiol.* 1966;17(3):362-378.
32. Lipton MJ, Barry WH, Obrez I, Silverman JF, Wexler L. Isolated single coronary artery: diagnosis, angiographic classification, and clinical significance. *Radiology.* 1979;130(1):39-47.
33. Keith JD. The anomalous origin of the left coronary artery from the pulmonary artery. *Br Heart J.* 1959;21(2):149-161.
34. Purut CM, Sabiston Jr DC. Origin of the left coronary artery from the pulmonary artery in older adults. *J Thorac Cardiovasc Surg.* 1991;102(4):566-570.
35. Dodge-Khatami A, Mavroudis C, Backer CL. Anomalous origin of the left coronary artery from the pulmonary artery: collective review of surgical therapy. *Ann Thorac Surg.* 2002;74(3): 946-955.
36. Ropers D, Moshage W, Daniel WG, Jessl J, Gottwik M, Achenbach S. Visualization of coronary artery anomalies and their anatomic course by contrast-enhanced electron beam tomography and three-dimensional reconstruction. *Am J Cardiol.* 2001;87(2): 193-197.
37. McConnell MV, Ganz P, Selwyn AP, Li W, Edelman RR, Manning WJ. Identification of anomalous coronary arteries and their anatomic course by magnetic resonance coronary angiography. *Circulation.* 1995;92(11):3158-3162.
38. Angelini P. Coronary artery anomalies: an entity in search of an identity. *Circulation.* 2007;115(10):1296-1305.
39. Angelini P, Velasco JA, Ott D, Khoshnevis GR. Anomalous coronary artery arising from the opposite sinus: descriptive features and pathophysiologic mechanisms, as documented by intravascular ultrasonography. *J Invasive Cardiol.* 2003;15(9): 507-514.
40. Doorey AJ, Pasquale MJ, Lally JF, Mintz GS, Marshall E, Ramos DA. Six-month success of intracoronary stenting for anomalous coronary arteries associated with myocardial ischemia. *Am J Cardiol.* 2000;86(5):580-582 A510.
41. Fedoruk LM, Kern JA, Peeler BB, Kron IL. Anomalous origin of the right coronary artery: right internal thoracic artery to right coronary artery bypass is not the answer. *J Thorac Cardiovasc Surg.* 2007;133(2):456-460.
42. Taylor AJ, Rogan KM, Virmani R. Sudden cardiac death associated with isolated congenital coronary artery anomalies. *J Am Coll Cardiol.* 1992;20(3):640-647.
43. Davis JA, Cecchin F, Jones TK, Portman MA. Major coronary artery anomalies in a pediatric population: incidence and clinical importance. *J Am Coll Cardiol.* 2001;37(2):593-597.
44. Romp RL, Herlong JR, Landolfo CK, et al. Outcome of unroofing procedure for repair of anomalous aortic origin of left or right coronary artery. *Ann Thorac Surg.* 2003;76(2):589-595 discussion 595-586.
45. Frommelt PC, Frommelt MA, Tweddell JS, Jaquiss RD. Prospective echocardiographic diagnosis and surgical repair of anomalous origin of a coronary artery from the opposite sinus with an interarterial course. *J Am Coll Cardiol.* 2003;42(1):148-154.

46. Hillis LD, Smith PK, Anderson JL, et al. 2011 ACCF/AHA Guideline for Coronary Artery Bypass Graft Surgery: executive summary: a report of the American College of Cardiology Foundation/American Heart Association Task Force on Practice Guidelines. *J Am Coll Cardiol.* 2011;58(24):2583-2614.
47. Datta J, White CS, Gilkeson RC, et al. Anomalous coronary arteries in adults: depiction at multi-detector row CT angiography. *Radiology.* 2005;235(3):812-818.
48. Deibler AR, Kuzo RS, Vohringer M, et al. Imaging of congenital coronary anomalies with multislice computed tomography. *Mayo Clin Proc.* 2004;79(8):1017-1023.
49. Taylor AJ, Cerqueira M, Hodgson JM, et al. ACCF/SCCT/ACR/AHA/ASE/ASNC/NASCI/SCAI/SCMR 2010 appropriate use criteria for cardiac computed tomography. A report of the American College of Cardiology Foundation Appropriate Use Criteria Task Force, the Society of Cardiovascular Computed Tomography, the American College of Radiology, the American Heart Association, the American Society of Echocardiography, the American Society of Nuclear Cardiology, the North American Society for Cardiovascular Imaging, the Society for Cardiovascular Angiography and Interventions, and the Society for Cardiovascular Magnetic Resonance. *J Am Coll Cardiol.* 2010;56(22):1864-1894.
50. McConnell MV, Ganz P, Selwyn AP, Li W, Edelman RR, Manning WJ. Identification of anomalous coronary arteries and their anatomic course by magnetic resonance coronary angiography. *Circulation.* 1995;92(11):3158-3162.
51. Post JC, van Rossum AC, Bronzwaer JG, et al. Magnetic resonance angiography of anomalous coronary arteries. A new gold standard for delineating the proximal course? *Circulation.* 1995;92(11):3163-3171.
52. Taylor AM, Thorne SA, Rubens MB, et al. Coronary artery imaging in grown up congenital heart disease: complementary role of magnetic resonance and x-ray coronary angiography. *Circulation.* 2000;101(14):1670-1678.

Coronary Artery Anomalies of Termination: Fistulae and Arteriovenous Malformations

Key Point

- Cardiac CT angiography is the test of choice to depict the entire course of coronary artery anomalies of termination. The conduit portions of the dilated segments are easier to identify than are the site(s) of drainage if those sites are multiple and small. Differential contrast attenuation may help reveal sites of drainage.

CORONARY ARTERY FISTULAE

A coronary artery fistula (CAF) is a solitary communication between a coronary artery and one of any of the following: cardiac chambers or arterial venous, coronary venous, or pulmonary arterial conduits—that is, a disorder of coronary artery termination.[1] Coronary artery fistulae also may be of anomalous origin.[2]

The incidence of CAFs in the population is unknown. The incidence within angiographic series is 0.1% to 0.2%, second in frequency of all coronary artery congenital abnormalities, after anomalous origin of the coronary arteries.[3]

Coronary fistulae usually are congenital, but occasionally they may be posttraumatic or iatrogenic.

Most congenital coronary fistulae drain into adjacent cardiac chambers or vessels:

- The right heart atrium
- The right ventricle
- The pulmonary arteries[4]
- The coronary sinus
- The superior vena cave: right atrial junction[5]
- The hepatic veins[6]
- The bronchial arteries[7]

The incidence of multiple or large fistulae is approximately 0.05%, and the incidence of small fistulae is approximately 0.1% to 0.4% of angiographic series.[8]

The right heart receives the drainage of 90% of congenital coronary artery fistulae; however, some congenital coronary artery fistulae may drain into the left heart.[9]

Congenital fistulae may arise from:

- The left coronary artery: 50% to 60%, more commonly in the left anterior descending artery (LAD) than in the left circumflex artery (LCX)
- The right coronary artery (RCA): 30% to 40%
- Both coronary arteries: 2% to 5%

Although the RCA and LAD are the most commonly involved vessels, left circumflex coronary artery fistulae do occur, with drainage into sites such as the right atrium, the coronary sinus, and even the uncommon site of the left ventricle.[10]

Multiple microfistulae from the coronary artery to the left ventricle have been described, arising off the distal portion of the coronary arteries. These have a female preponderance.[11,12]

Typically, congenital coronary artery fistulae are conspicuously tortuous and have resulted in dilation ("flow-dependent dilation") of the coronary arteries that feed them.

Most coronary artery fistula are asymptomatic. Potential complications are listed in the next sections of this chapter. Ischemia within the territory of the fistula may be detected scintigraphically or by evidence of prior infarction within the territory. In the absence of angiographically evident disease within the artery or fistula, the findings of ischemia or infarction likely implicate the fistula. Although the diagnosis of coronary steal is not easy to establish, it has been demonstrated in the setting of coronary fistula.[13]

Spontaneous closure of congenital coronary fistulae has been reported.[14]

Visualization of the distal portions of fistulae by CCT, especially if small, may be incomplete.[15]

Etiologies of Coronary Artery Fistula

- Congenital
- Acquired
  - Iatrogenic
    - Aortocoronary bypass grafting[16]
      - Aortopulmonary artery[17]
      - Coronary artery-to-vein fistula[18]
    - Congenital heart surgery repair[19]
    - Post- myotomy or post-myectomy for hypertrophic obstructive cardiomyopathy [20]
    - Endomyocardial biopsy
    - Maze procedure[21]
  - Aortic dissection[22]
  - Penetrating trauma[23]
  - Coronary artery dissection with rupture into an adjacent structure
  - Coronary artery aneurysm with rupture into an adjacent structure
  - Atherosclerosis
  - Takayasu arteritis[24]
  - Neovascularization into a large left atrial thrombus[25]

Potential Complications

- Volume overload pathophysiology: congestive heart failure
- Infection: endovascular/endocarditis
- Coronary steal pathophysiology
  - Ischemia
  - Angina
- Arrhythmia
- Syncope[9]
- Aneurysm formation of the fistula[26,27]
- Fistula rupture
- Fistula dissection
- Effusion[28]
- Tamponade[29,30]
- Hemorrhage/hematoma within the pericardial space[31]
- Giant enlargement with compression of adjacent structures
- Coronary artery to left ventricular false aneurysm fistula[32]

Patterns of Coronary Artery Fistulae

Coronary artery fistulae may occur in one or more permutations of:

- Source artery or arteries
- Drainage chamber(s) or venous structure(s)
- Absence or concurrence of congenital heart disease[33]
- Absence or concurrence of acquired heart disease(s)

Hence, one fistula may drain into more than one low-pressure structure,[34,35] and more than one fistula may drain into a single low-pressure structure,[36,56] in the presence or absence of congenital or acquired heart disease.

Although the generalities of RCA and LAD source to right-sided or venous structures is the general rule, the range of permutations is vast and still incompletely known. A small sampling of infrequent but notably complex cases includes the following:

- Coronary artery to coronary sinus fistula (CACSF) may occur in association with congenital stenosis of the coronary sinus ostium and retrograde drainage via a persistent left superior vena cava.[37]
- A case with four coronary to pulmonary artery fistulae also has been detailed.[38]
- Coronary artery fistulae have been described in hypertrophic cardiomyopathy and mitral stenosis.[39]

Potential CTA Findings of Coronary Artery Fistula

- Generally enlarged feeder vessel size
- Tortuosity of the fistula
- Aneurysm of the fistula
- Calcification of the fistula, generally in its dilated or aneurysmal portions
- Differential contrast/attenuation marking the site(s) of return of the fistula into chambers or vessels with lower attenuation
- Visualization of the surrounding chambers and hence the path of the fistula. The ability of cardiac CT to image the surrounding anatomy directly is the principal advantage when compared with conventional angiography, as is the overall robustness to manipulate a volumetric data set to solve the details of:
  - Fistula source
  - Fistula course
  - Fistula site of termination
  - Fistula complications such as aneurysm, calcification, thrombosis, hemorrhage

Treatment

- Asymptomatic/small size: observation
- Asymptomatic/large size: intervention advocated by some
- Symptomatic/large size: consideration of intervention

Potential Interventions[40]

- Endovascular
  - Coiling (currently the most common catheter-based intervention)[41]
  - Otherwise: device closure, detachable balloons, plugs, various chemicals
- Surgical[42,43]
  - Ligation
  - Ligation with bypass

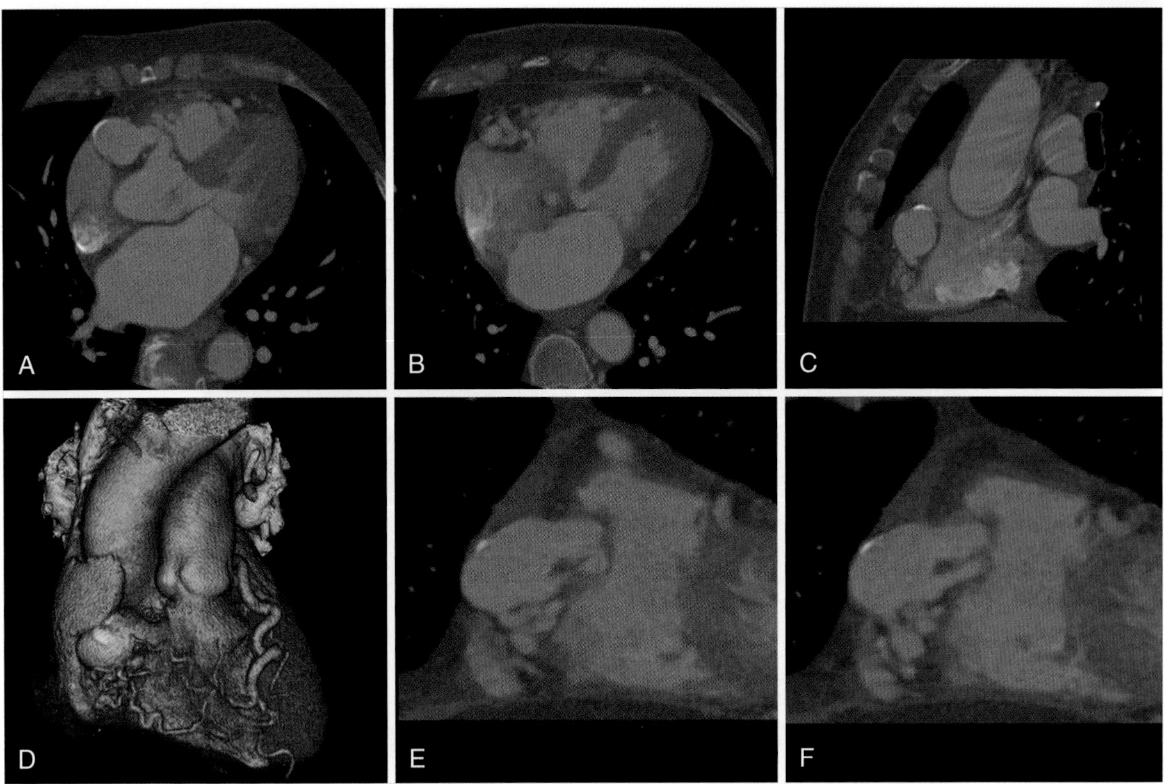

Figure 10-1. ECG-gated cardiac CT scan of a patient with a right coronary artery fistula. The feeder aspect of the fistula is the proximal right coronary artery, which is more dilated than the proximal left coronary artery. The proximal portion of the fistula is an aneurysm that gives rise to more than one exiting vessel. The aneurysmal portion is partially calcified. See Figure 10-2 and **Videos 10-1 and 10-2.**

Variants of CAF are illustrated as follows:

- CAF arising from the right coronary artery: Figures 10-1 and 10-2 and **Videos 10-1 and 10-2**
- CAF arising from the left circumflex coronary artery: Figures 10-3 through 10-6 and **Videos 10-3 through 10-7**
- CAF arising from the left main stem coronary artery: Figure 10-7 and **Videos 10-8 and 10-9**
- CAF draining into the pulmonary artery: Figures 10-8 through 10-14 and **Videos 10-10 and 10-11**
- Infected CAF: Figures 10-15 and 10-16 and **Video 10-12**.
- Iatrogenic CAF arising from septal branches of the LAD post-myotomy/myectomy: Figure 10-17
- Coronary artery to left ventricle fistulae: Figures 10-18 and 10-19.

CORONARY ARTERIOVENOUS MALFORMATIONS

Coronary arteriovenous malformation (CAVM) is a complex lesion with multiple feeding arteries and draining chambers with numerous intertricated fragile small vessels in between, forming a lattice or plexus of vessels. At surgery, CAVMs often are described as a "bag of worms."

The terms *coronary artery fistula* and *arteriovenous malformation* are used liberally and often interchangeably in the medical literature, although many cases have features of both. The CAF and CAVMs represent two ends of a spectrum, from single/solitary origin, tract, and termination to multiple origins, tracts, and terminations. Distinguishing between them is important, because their differences are significant in terms of amenability to percutaneous treatment, amenability to surgical treatment, success of surgical treatment, and risks of surgical treatment. The generally solitary target/tract of a coronary artery fistula is far more amenable to percutaneous or surgical treatment. Coronary artery arteriovenous malformations respond less successfully to either means of intervention, and surgically pose a higher risk of bleeding.

For images of CAVMs, see Figure 10-20 and **Video 10-13.**

CT Angiography Protocol for the Evaluation of Coronary Artery Fistula and Arteriovenous Malformations: Differences from Standard Coronary CTA Protocol

- The standard coronary CTA protocol usually suffices for the detection of coronary artery fistula and AVMs that are limited to the heart proper.

Text continued on page 153

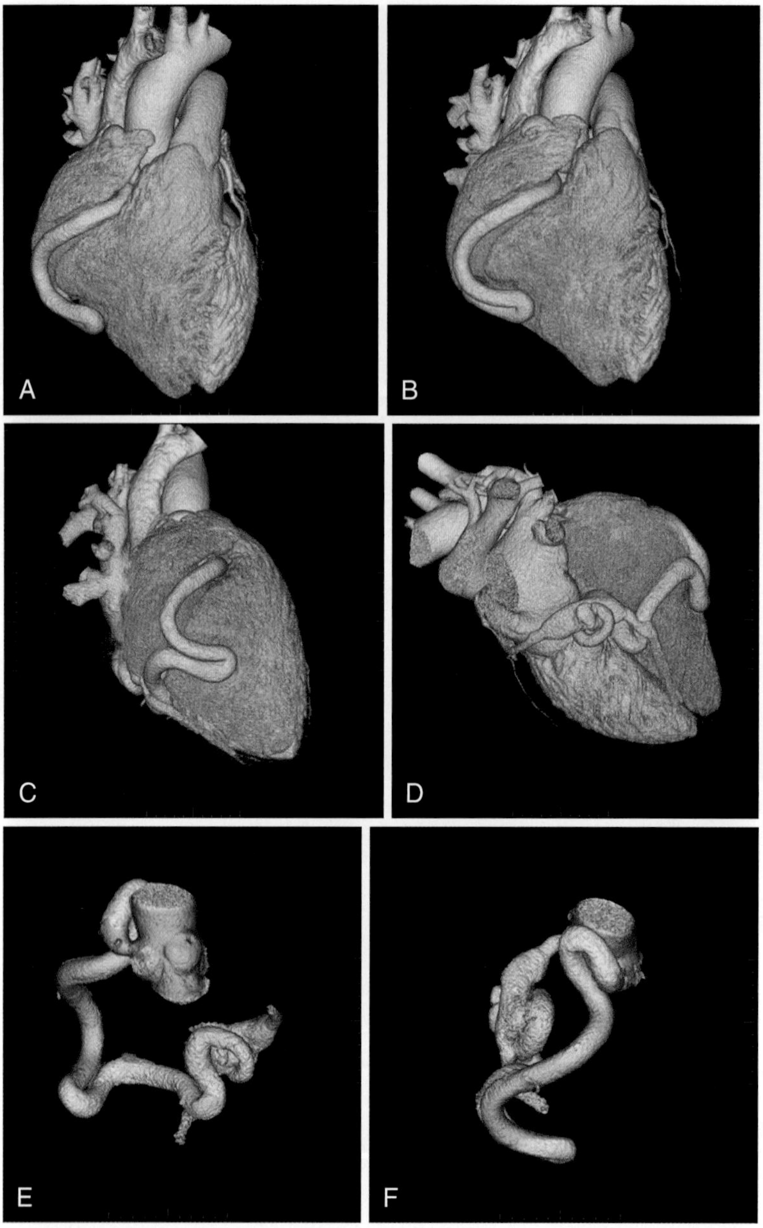

Figure 10-2. Multiple volume-rendered images demonstrating a large right coronary artery to coronary sinus fistula. Note the marked enlargement of the coronary sinus. See Figure 10-1 and **Videos 10-1** and **10-2.**

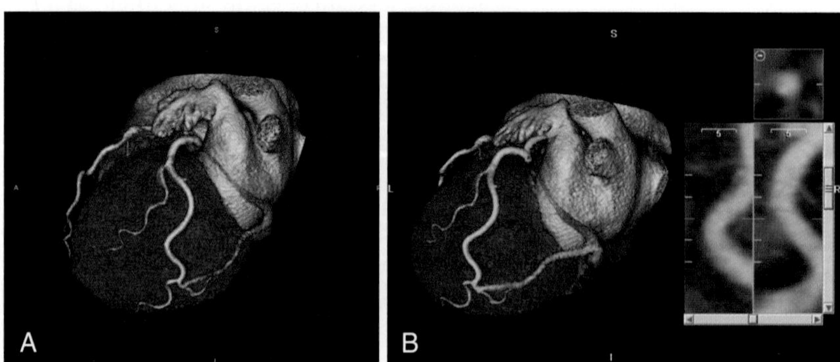

Figure 10-3. Volume-rendered images demonstrating a small coronary artery to coronary vein fistula extending from a second obtuse marginal branch to an inferior marginal coronary vein. See **Video 10-3.**

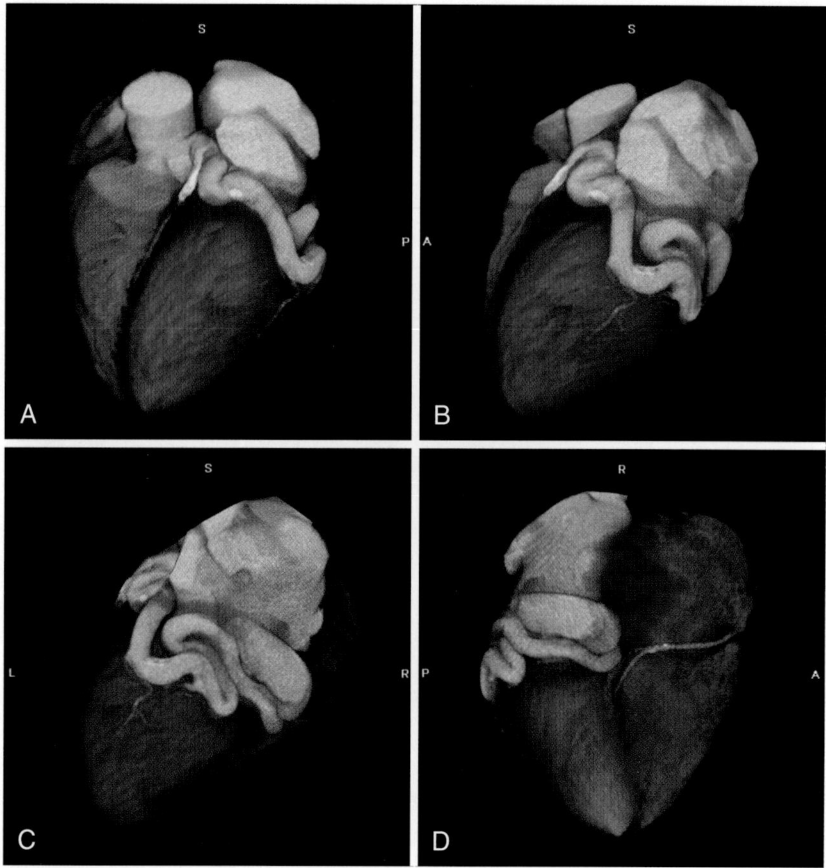

Figure 10-4. Volume-rendered images demonstrate a markedly enlarged and tortuous circumflex artery fistulizing into a dilated coronary sinus. See Figure 10-5 and **Videos 10-4 through 10-6.**

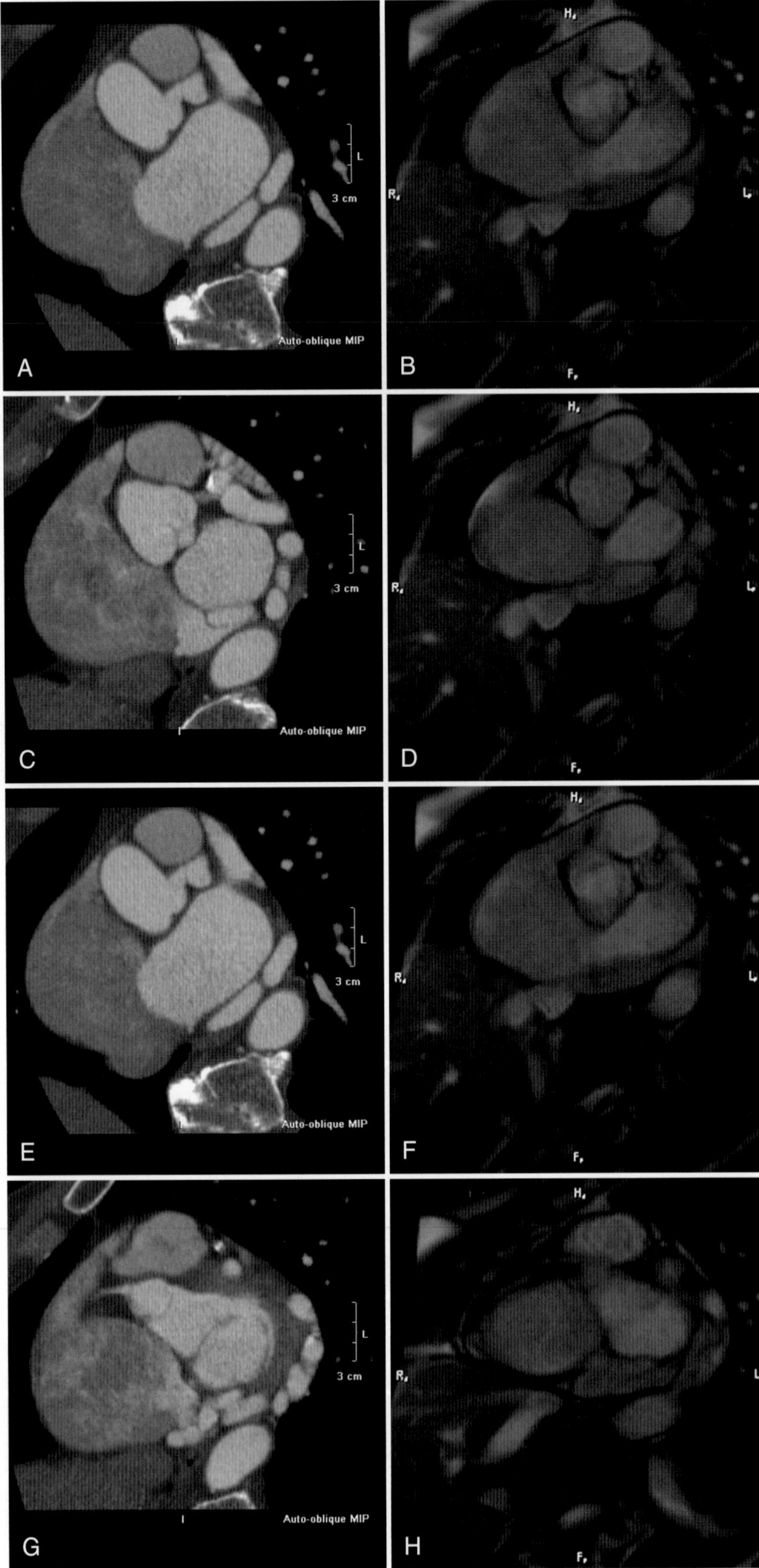

Figure 10-5. Short-axis oblique images of a coronary angiogram with corresponding MR images demonstrating the enlarged circumflex artery, which mimicked a vascular retroatrial mass on echocardiography. See Figure 10-4 and **Videos 10-4 through 10-6.**

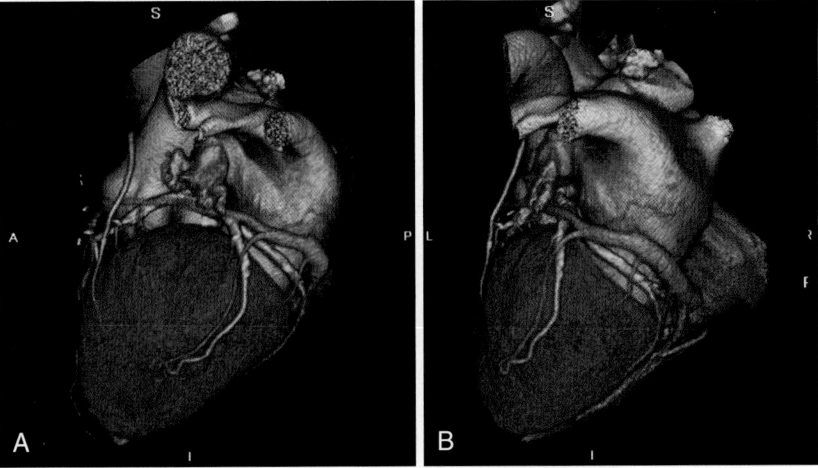

Figure 10-6. Two volume-rendered images demonstrate a small coronary artery to coronary vein fistula. The communication occurs between an obtuse marginal branch and marginal arterial branch and a small superolateral marginal vein, which is a tributary to the great cardiac vein. See **Video 10-7.**

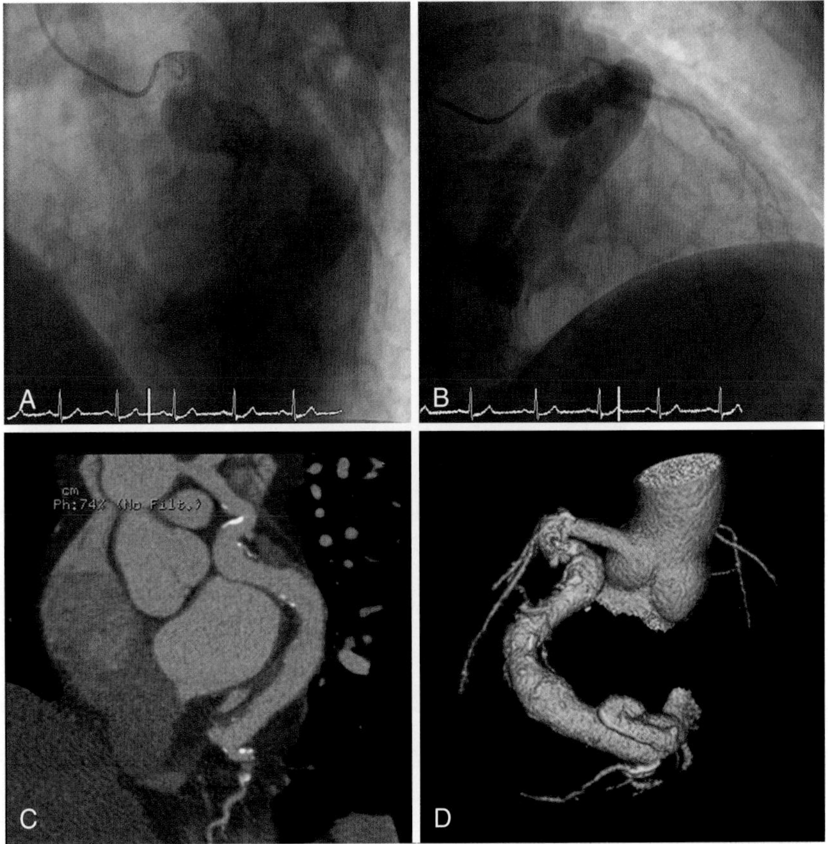

Figure 10-7. Left anterior oblique (**A**) and right anterior oblique (**B**) coronary angiography demonstrating a large fistula arising from the left coronary artery. **C**, Maximum intensity projection image revealing a fistula arising from the left main stem coronary artery and emptying into the distal coronary sinus. **D**, 3D reconstruction of the left main stem to coronary sinus fistula. See **Videos 10-8 and 10-9.**

Figure 10-8. Two volume-rendered images from a cardiac CT study demonstrating a moderate-sized arteriovenous fistula from the left anterior descending artery to the main pulmonary artery. A small aneurysm is also noted.

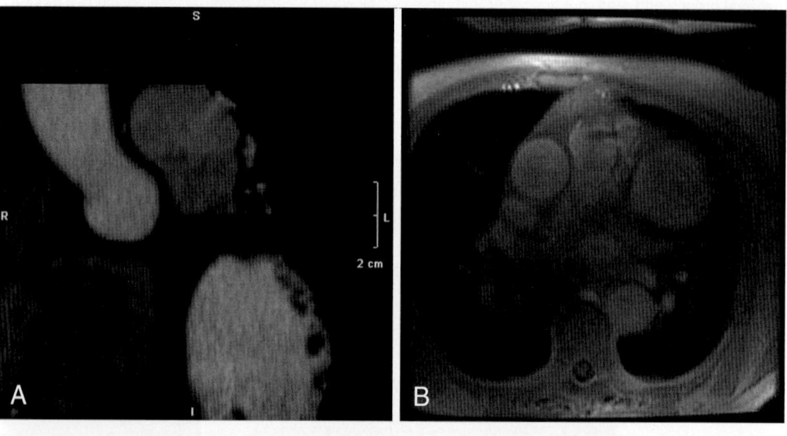

Figure 10-9. A, A coronal reformation of a CT angiogram demonstrating a jet extending into the main pulmonary artery from a left anterior descending artery (LAD) to main pulmonary artery fistula. **B,** Cine gradient echo image from an MR study demonstrates a large coronary artery aneurysm with an associated fistulous connection from the LAD into the main pulmonary artery. Note the signal void at the level of the jet. See **Video 10-10.**

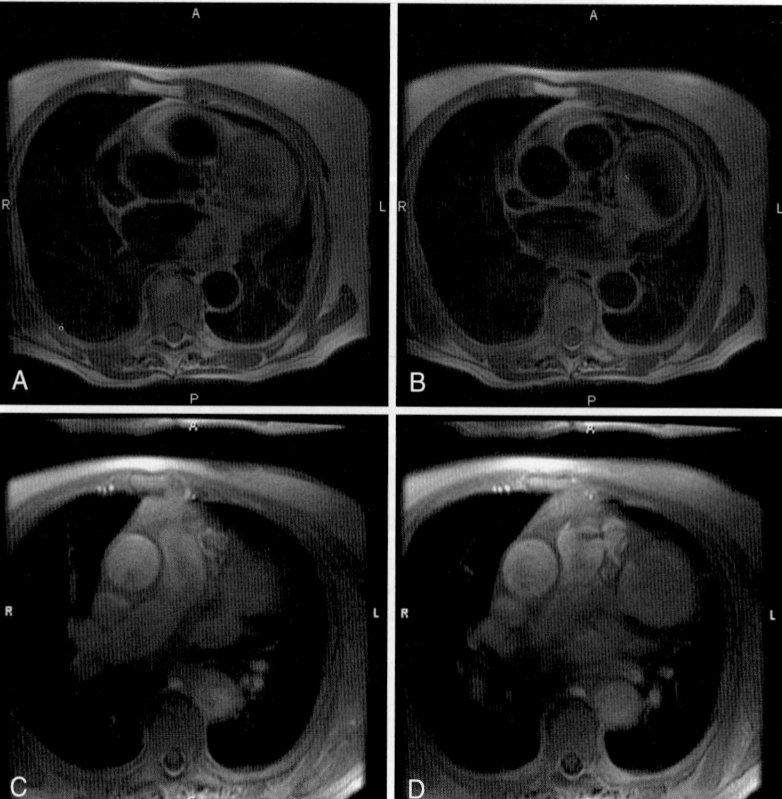

Figure 10-10. An 81-year-old woman presented with chest pain and an abnormal echocardiogram, raising suspicion for a possible patent ductus arteriosus. Multiple images from a cardiac MRI are shown. The upper two panels are gated fast spin-echo images showing multiple serpiginous signal voids in the region of the left main coronary artery as well a giant aneurysm with peripheral slow flow or thrombus, situated to the right of the main pulmonary artery. Cine gradient echo images confirm the large coronary aneurysm with an associated fistula into the main pulmonary artery. Note the plume of signal void in the main pulmonary artery (**D**) representing the fistula jet.

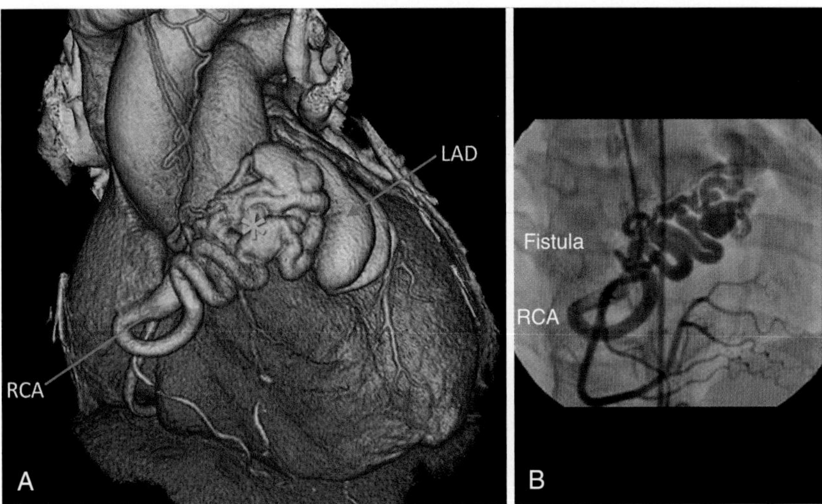

Figure 10-11. **A,** Three-dimensional volume-rendered reconstruction of the CT scan shows dilated branches of the right coronary artery (RCA) communicating with branches of the left anterior descending (LAD) artery, forming an aneurysmal Vieussens' arterial ring *(asterisk)*. **B,** Coronary angiography, left anterior oblique cranial projection. The RCA was free of epicardial disease and showed two fistulae originating from the proximal third of the vessel and emptying into a vascular pouch before entering into the main pulmonary artery. (Reprinted with permission from Hirzallah MI, Horlick E, Zelovitzky L. Coronary artery to main pulmonary artery fistulae via a Vieussens' arterial ring. *J Cardiovasc Comput Tomogr.* 2010;4(5):339-341.)

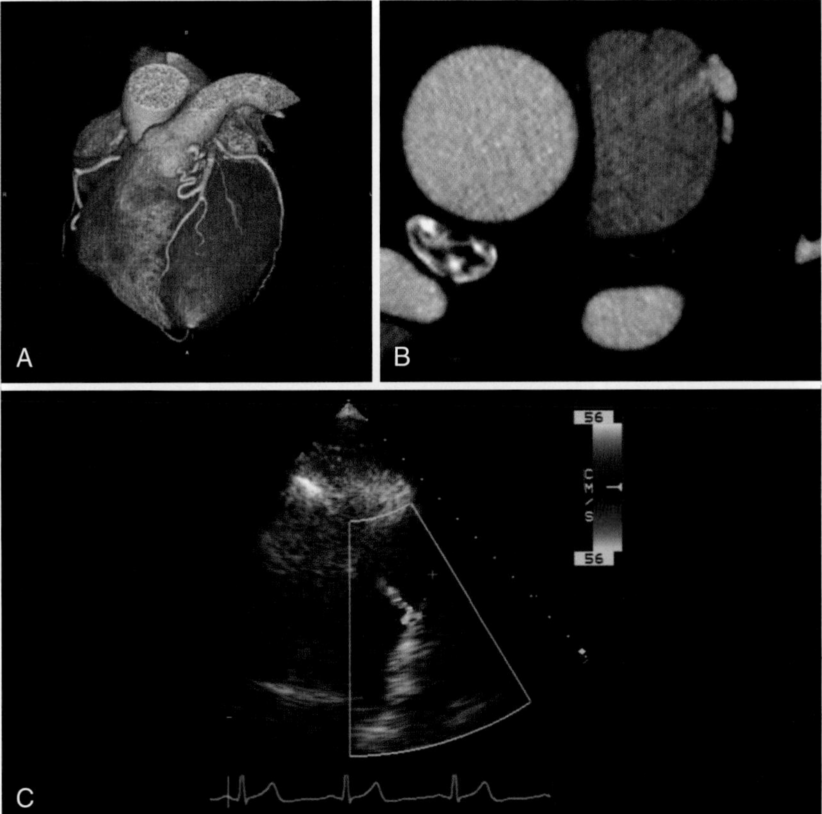

Figure 10-12. Composite image demonstrates a left anterior descending artery (LAD) to main pulmonary artery fistula. An axial source image demonstrates the fistulous connection into the main pulmonary artery above the level of the pulmonic valve. Corresponding color Doppler echo images demonstrate the diastolic jet extending from the LAD into the main pulmonary artery. See **Video 10-11.**

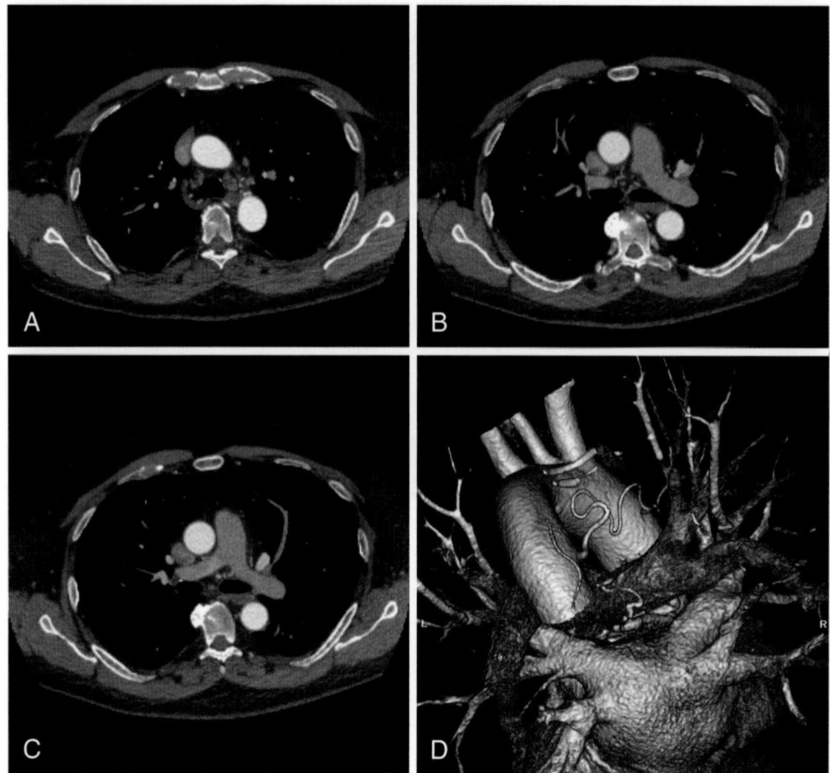

Figure 10-13. Note the multiple small filamentous and tortuous fistulae arising from the underside of the ascending aorta and terminating in the lungs.

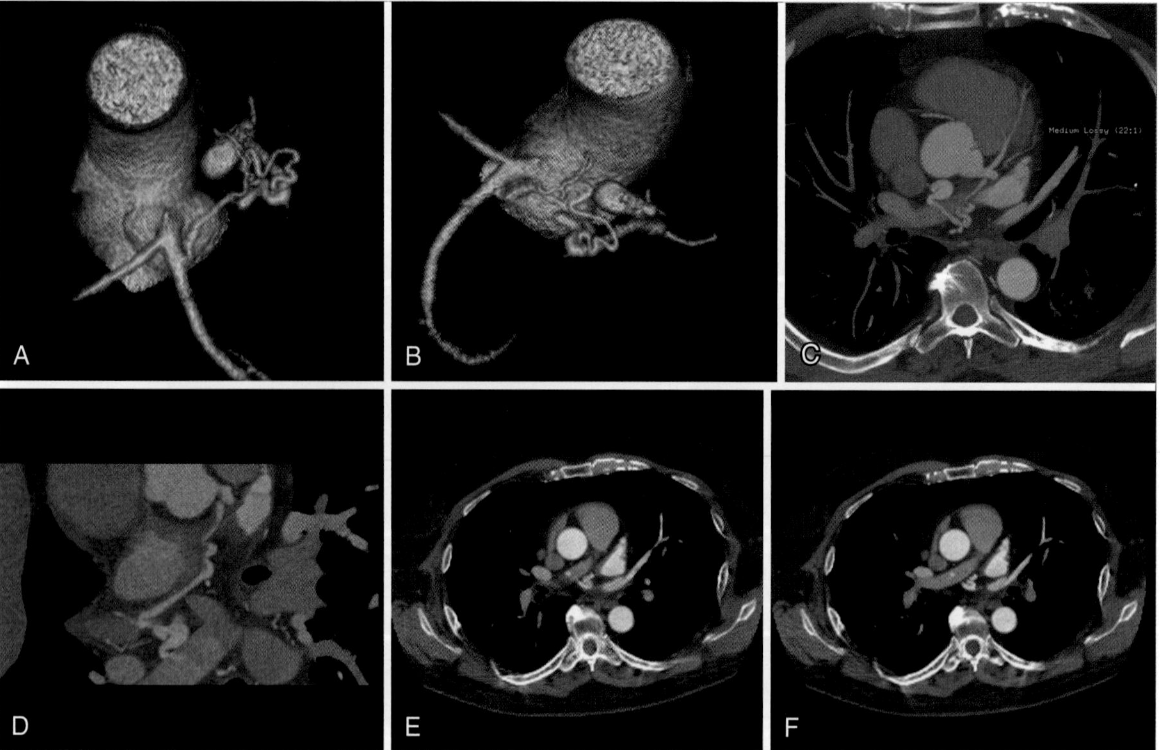

Figure 10-14. Note, in the same patient as in Figure 10-13, a tortuous fistula arising off the left circumflex artery and terminating in the main pulmonary artery. Note the return of higher-attenuation blood via the fistula in the proximal right pulmonary artery (**E** and **F**).

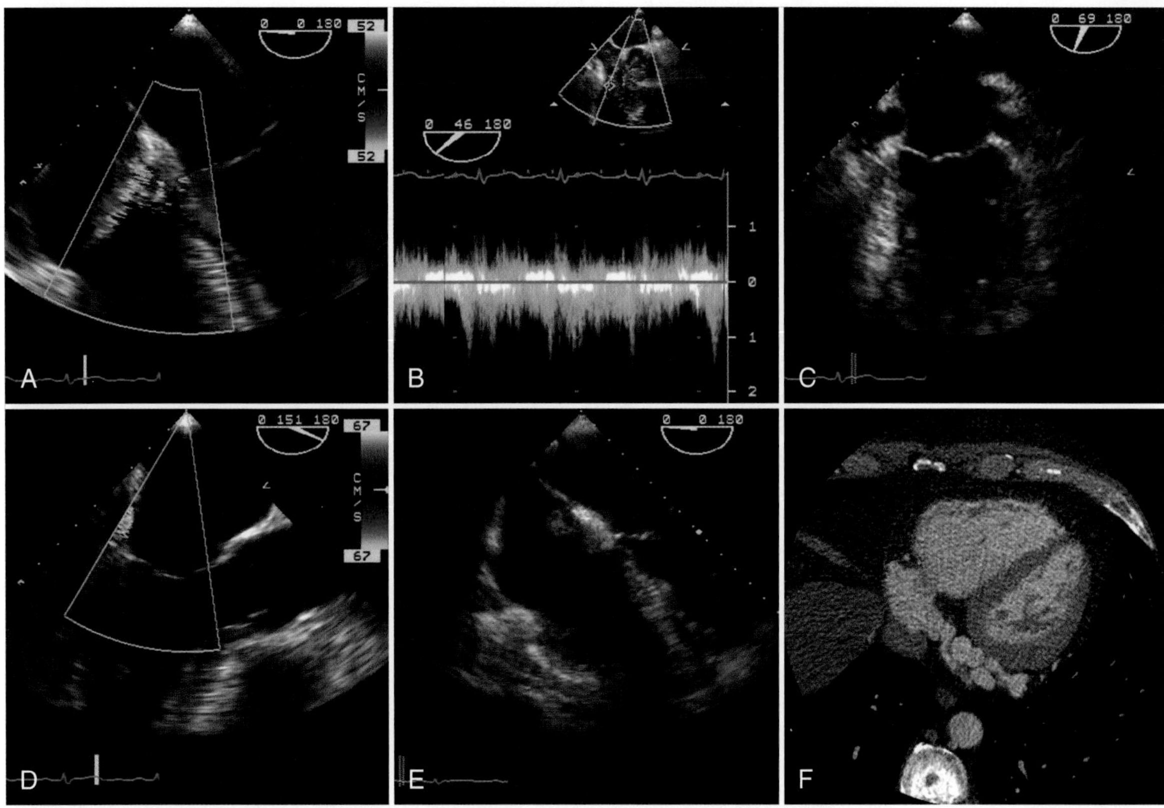

Figure 10-15. A 49-year-old man with *Streptococcus mitis* sepsis underwent a transesophageal echocardiogram (TEE) for evaluation of bacterial endocarditis. **A,** A four-chamber view TEE demonstrates an unusual jet of color flow with aliasing in the medial portion of the right. **B,** Spectral Doppler demonstrates continuous flow at this site. **C,** A two-chamber view demonstrates multiple unusual circular structures adjacent to the medial aspect of the left atrium. They appear extracardiac in location. Color Doppler flow mapping in this region in the left ventricular outflow tract (LVOT) projection demonstrates flow within these circular structures. **D,** An irregular soft tissue mass is present along the right atrial aspect of the interatrial septum consistent with a vegetation. The patient was treated for bacterial endocarditis and improved clinically. A follow-up CT scan (**F**) to evaluate the unusual vascular structures seen on the TEE demonstrates multiple large tortuous tubular contrast-filled structures of the left atrioventricular groove communicating with an enlarged coronary sinus, confirming the echocardiographer's suspicion of a large coronary artery to coronary sinus fistula—in this case, from the circumflex artery to the coronary sinus. The os of the coronary artery fistula had been the nidus of the prior infective endocarditis. See **Video 10-12.**

- ❒ Standard field of view will be adequate for coronary artery fistulae within the heart proper. The field of view may, however, have to be increased to follow the full course of a fistula to an extracardiac drainage site, such as the hepatic veins.
- ❒ Diminishing the right heart contrast by pushing pure saline rather than mixed contrast/saline is important to visualize the sites of return of the right heart of contrast-laden fistulae.

AORTA–RIGHT ATRIAL TUNNEL

An aorta–right atrial tunnel is a rare congenital abnormality in which an abnormal tubular extracardiac communication occurs between the ascending aorta and the right atrium. The aorta–right atrial tunnel is distinguished from a coronary artery fistula by having its origin separate from the coronary arteries. The origin of the aorta–right atrial tunnel usually is at the sinus level, but may be above the sinotubular junction. The probable cause for this condition appears to be a congenital deficiency of the elastic lamina in the aortic media. This abnormal communication can arise from any of the sinuses of Valsalva, but origin from the left sinus of Valsalva is most common (94%), with origin from the right sinus less common (5%) and from the noncoronary sinus rare (1%).[44] The aorta–right atrial communication/tunnel behaves like a left-to-right shunt. Its clinical relevance varies, from being an incidental finding in adults when small to resulting in CHF in infants when large. Also, aorta–right atrial tunnels may enlarge into aneurysms, rupture, or become infected.[45-49] Traditionally, the recommended treatment for this condition is surgical closure, but increasingly treatment is being done by percutaneous closure of the aorta–right atrial tunnel. Surgical closure allows for reconstruction of a sinus of Valsalva, if necessary, in addition to closure of the shunt.

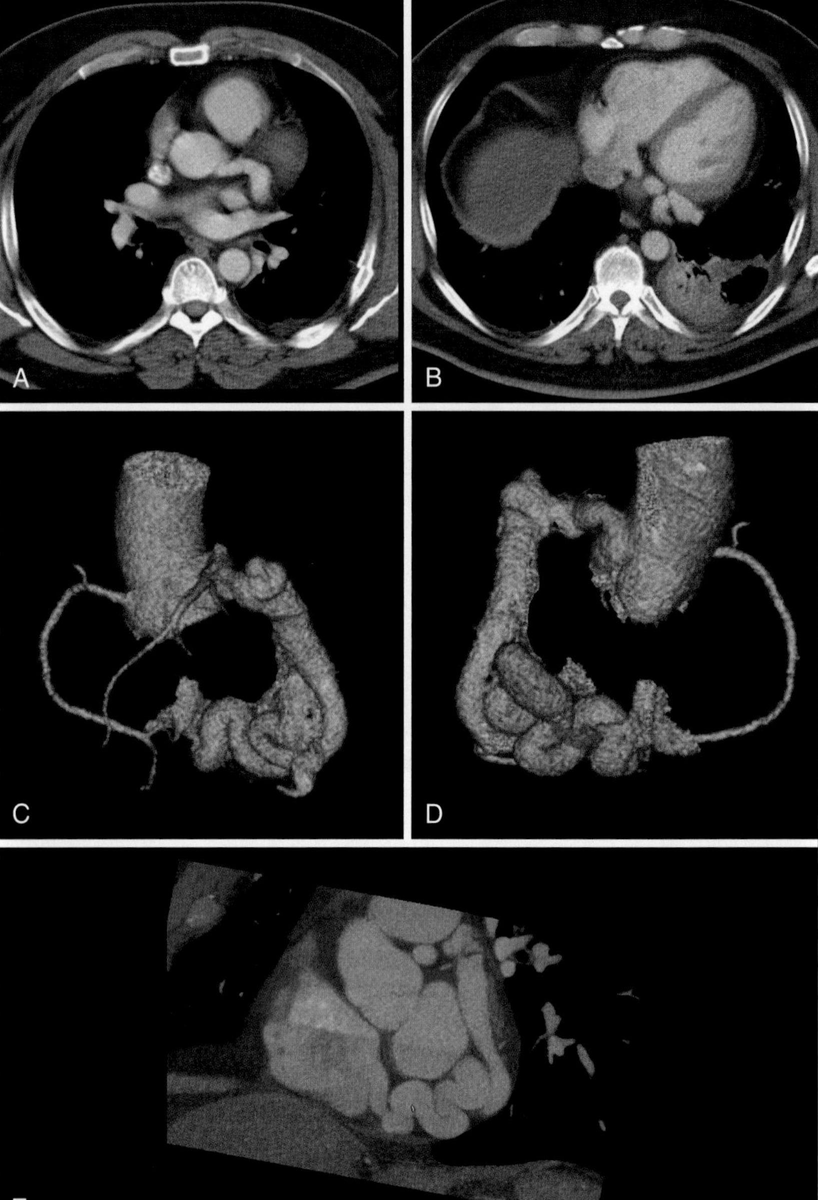

Figure 10-16. A 50-year-old man was involved in a high-speed motor vehicle accident. **A** and **B,** Axial CT images from a pan scan study done for trauma evaluation. An unusual-appearing curvilinear vascular structure was seen in the posterior aspect of the heart extending into the left atrioventricular groove. There was no evidence of a pericardial effusion or pericardial thickening. **A,** A transverse, minimally displaced rib fracture of one of the left mid ribs. A moderate-sized lung contusion is seen in the left lower lobe (**B**). Because of the uncertain etiology of the mediastinal vascular structure, a gated cardiac CT was performed. **C** and **D,** Volume-rendered images demonstrate a large tortuous vascular structure to be the circumflex coronary artery. **E,** The sagittal oblique maximum intensity projection image shows the tortuous circumflex artery confluence into the coronary sinus, confirming that this represents a congenital coronary artery to coronary sinus fistula, an incidental finding in this patient with thoracic trauma. See **Video 10-12.**

For images of aorta–right atrial tunnels, see Figure 10-21.

CCT Protocol Points

- The standard CCT protocol is followed.
- Contrast: A higher rate of injection of the saline push (6 mL/sec) helps to unopacify the right side of the heart and can aid in identifying the site(s) of fistulization within the right heart.

ACC/AHA 2008 Guidelines for Adults with Congenital Heart Disease: Recommendations for Coronary Arteriovenous Fistula[51]

See Table 10-1.

*Class I**

1. If a continuous murmur is present, its origin should be defined either by echocardiography, MRI, CT angiography, or cardiac catheterization. (*Level of Evidence: C*)
2. A large CAVF, regardless of symptomatology, should be closed via either a transcatheter or surgical route after delineation of its course and its potential to fully obliterate the fistula. (*Level of Evidence: C*)
3. A small to moderate CAVF in the presence of documented myocardial ischemia, arrhythmia,

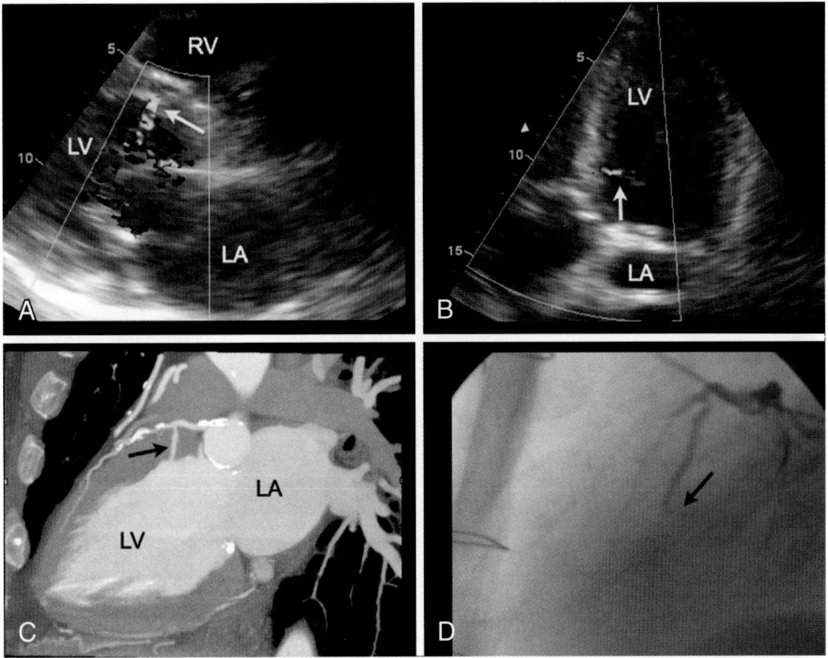

Figure 10-17. A 73-year-old man with a recent septal myomectomy and coronary artery revascularization for symptomatic hypertrophic obstructive cardiomyopathy presented with new-onset chest discomfort. On transthoracic echocardiography, diastolic blood flow was seen originating from the interventricular septum into the left ventricular (LV) cavity (*white arrows*), on both the parasternal long-axis and apical four-chamber views (**A** and **B**). A reformatted maximum-intensity projection of a retrospectively electrocardiographically gated cardiac CT scan demonstrated a coronary artery fistula between the first septal perforator branch of the left anterior descending coronary artery and the LV (**C**, *black arrow*), confirmed by coronary angiography (**D**). Acquired coronary artery to LV fistulas can occur after surgical septal myomectomy in patients with hypertrophic obstructive cardiomyopathy. Multimodality cardiac imaging using transthoracic echocardiography, CT, and catheterization is useful for diagnosis and follow-up. LA, left atrium; RV, right ventricle. (Reprinted with permission from Garber PJ, Hussain F, Koenig JK, et al. Multimodality imaging of a coronary artery fistula after septal myomectomy in hypertrophic cardiomyopathy. *J Am Coll Cardiol.* 2011;57(9):e95.)

otherwise unexplained ventricular systolic or diastolic dysfunction or enlargement, or endarteritis should be closed via either a transcatheter or surgical approach after delineation of its course and its potential to fully obliterate the fistula. (*Level of Evidence: C*)

Class IIa

1. Clinical follow-up with echocardiography every 3 to 5 years can be useful for patients with small, asymptomatic CAVF to exclude development of symptoms or arrhythmias or progression of size or chamber enlargement that might alter management. (*Level of Evidence: C*)

Class III

1. Patients with small, asymptomatic CAVF should not undergo closure of CAVF. (*Level of Evidence: C*)

Clinical Course

Although the potential for associated myocardial ischemia and infarction, endarteritis, dissection, and rupture has been documented, there are few data associating occurrence, shunt properties, anatomic features, and outcomes. Increasing fistula and shunt size may be associated with increased abnormalities of coronary flow and complications that include chest pain, decreased life expectancy, and risk of rupture.[52] Small fistulae may increase slowly in size with advancing age and changes in systemic blood pressure and aortic compliance. Periodic clinical evaluation with imaging such as echocardiography to assess both the size of the fistula and ventricular function is reasonable. Sometimes, small fistulae are detected as an incidental finding on echocardiography.

Preintervention Evaluation

Transcatheter delineation of the course of the CAVF and access to distal drainage should be performed in all patients with audible continuous murmur and recognized CAVF.

Recommendations for Management Strategies

Class I

1. Surgeons with training and expertise in CHD should perform operations for management of patients with CAVF. (*Level of Evidence: C*)
2. Transcatheter closure of CAVF should be performed only in centers with expertise in such procedures. (*Level of Evidence: C*)
3. Transcatheter delineation of CAVF course and access to distal drainage should be performed in all patients with audible continuous murmur and recognition of CAVF. (*Level of Evidence: C*)

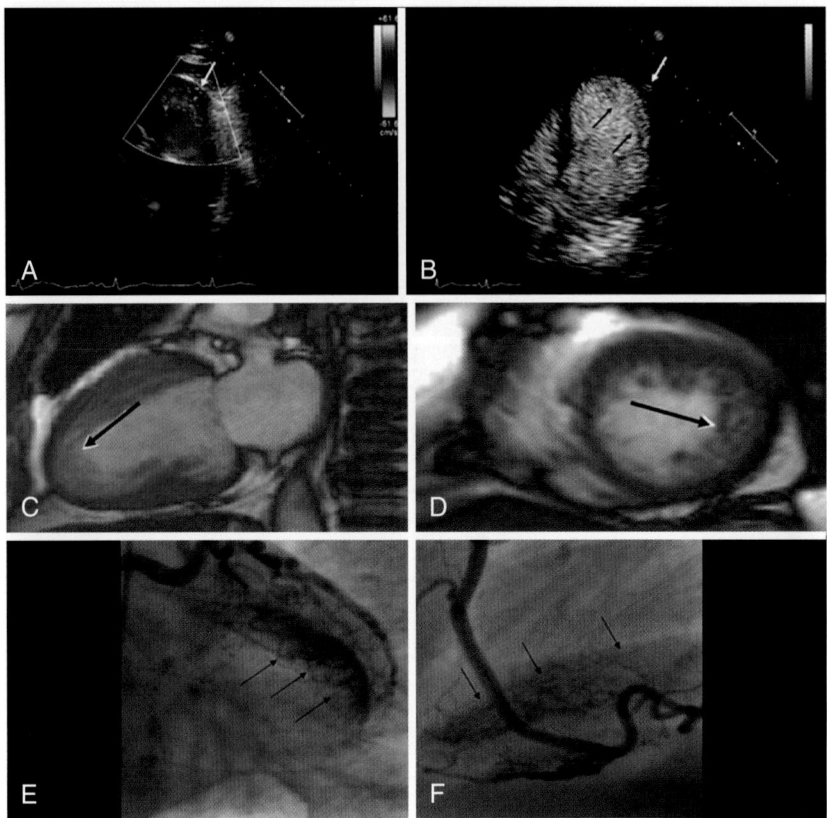

Figure 10-18. A 67-year-old man presented to our department with progressing dyspnea and effort angina for the past 3 months. **A** and **B,** The transthoracic echocardiogram showed hypertrabeculation of the left ventricular lateroapical region with a maximal ratio of noncompacted-to-compacted myocardium of 2.3. **C** and **D**, On cardiovascular MRI, the ratio was 2.6, supporting the diagnosis of noncompaction cardiomyopathy. Both imaging modalities clearly depicted the endocardial border of the noncompacted myocardium (*arrows*) and the flow within it. **E** and **F**, Interestingly, on coronary angiography, left ventricular opacification occurred after left and right coronary injections disclosing multiple coronary artery to left ventricular fistulae. There was no epicardial coronary obstructive disease. Reviewing the color Doppler and contrast echocardiogram images, this coronary malformation could already have been suspected because an unusually evident diastolic flow within the compacted layer of the myocardium (*white arrows*) was clearly shown. To our knowledge, this is the first report describing the association of noncompaction cardiomyopathy and multiple coronary–left ventricular fistulae in the same patient. We think that this case could demonstrate an arrest in embryogenic development somewhere between the regression of the myocardial sinusoids and the compaction of the myocardium and may be a continuum of only one disease. (Reprinted with permission from Dias V, Cabral S, Vieira M, et al. Noncompaction cardiomyopathy and multiple coronary arterioventricular fistulae: 1 or 2 distinct disease entities? *J Am Coll Cardiol.* 2011;57(25):e377.)

Surgical Intervention

Surgical fistula closure can be successful if CAVF is well defined and clear surgical access is believed to be technically achievable. Recurrence may be a problem if anatomic definition is suboptimal, and surgery may be difficult to perform owing to poorly visualized, typically distal fistulous connections. Surgical closure of audible CAVF with appropriate anatomy is recommended in all large CAVFs and in small to moderate CAVFs in the presence of symptoms of myocardial ischemia, threatening arrhythmia, unexplained ventricular dysfunction, or left atrial hypertension.

Catheterization-Based Intervention

Numerous reports of transcatheter closure with coils or detachable devices describe near or complete CAVF occlusion in attempted closure procedures. Criteria for transcatheter closure of CAVF are similar to those used for surgical closure of CAVF. Transcatheter closure of CAVF should be performed only in centers with particular expertise in such intervention.

Preintervention Evaluation after Surgical or Catheterization-Based Repair

Patients with CAVF, even after repair, may still have large, patulous epicardial conduits. Intermediate- and longer-term follow-up of these thin-walled, ectatic coronary arteries after either surgical or transcatheter repair appears mandated.

Alternative Testing to Detect Coronary Fistulae, Arteriovenous Malformations, and Right Atrial Tunnels

❒ **Echocardiography**

- Transthoracic echocardiography (TTE) is unlikely to depict a coronary artery fistula from beginning to end. The supplying ("feeder") coronary artery is likely dilated in its proximal portion and often is visible, especially in

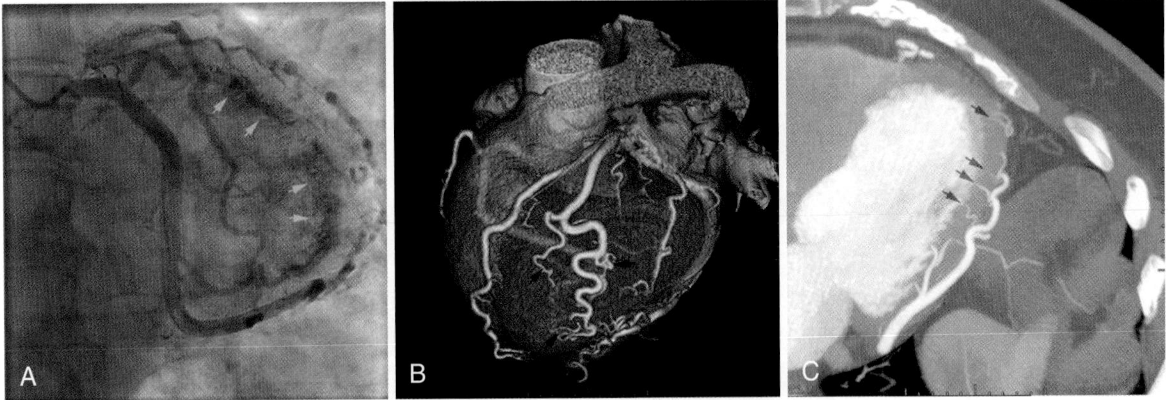

Figure 10-19. **A,** Invasive coronary angiogram of the left coronary artery. *White arrows* point to the semicircular blush of contrast in the subendocardium/left ventricular cavity. **B,** Three-dimensional volume-rendered CT images with semitransparent cardiac chambers. Black arrows point to distal tortuous branches of the large first diagonal branch of the left anterior descending coronary artery. **C,** Double oblique 15-mm maximum intensity projection. The image plane is parallel to the distal circumflex coronary artery and perpendicular to the lateral/inferolateral left ventricular myocardium. *Black arrows* point to some of the coronary artery fistulae. (Reprinted with permission from Mitchell GR, Morgan-Hughes G, Roobottom C. Coronary arterial microfistulae: a CT coronary angiography perspective. *J Cardiovasc Comput Tomogr.* 2010;4(4):279-280.)

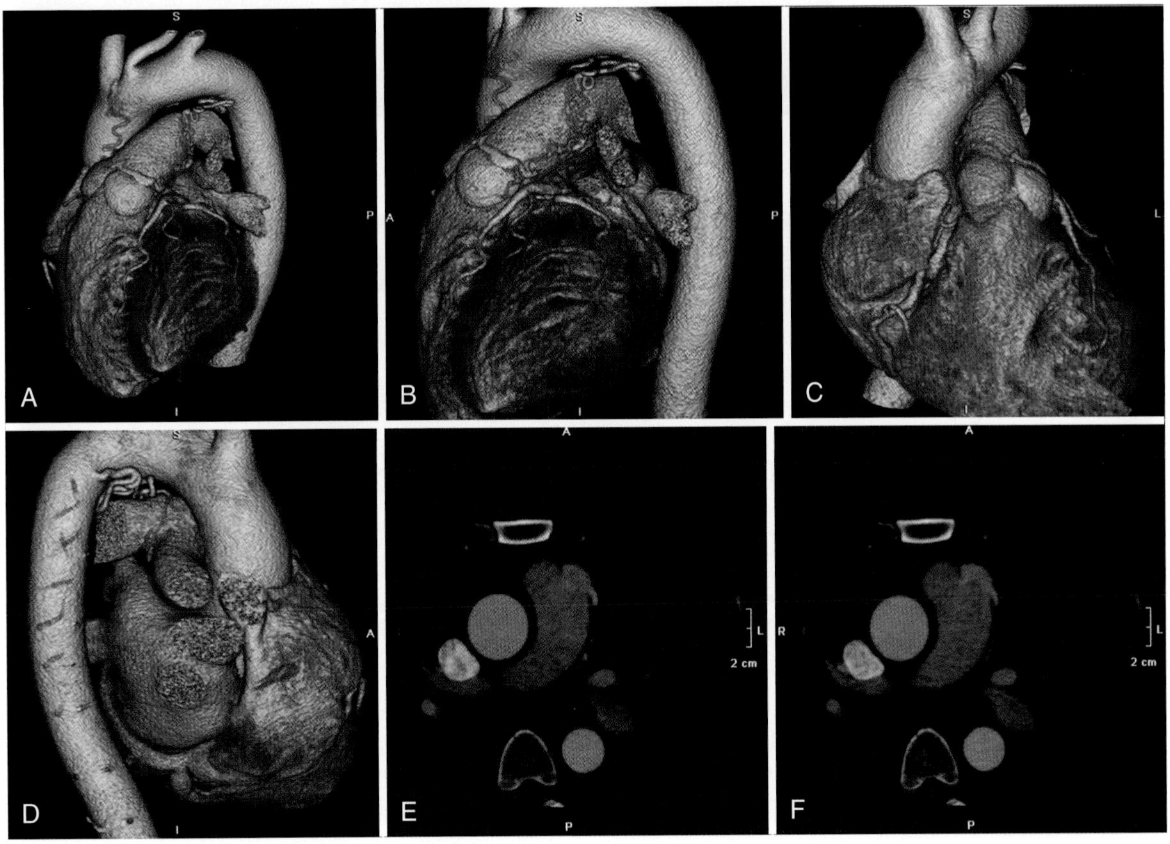

Figure 10-20. Composite image with multiple volume-rendered and axial CT angiographic images demonstrating a left anterior descending artery to main pulmonary artery fistula. This fistula enters the main pulmonary artery just above the level of the pulmonic valve. Multiple small web-like aortopulmonary communications are also seen extending from the undersurface of the aortic arch to the main pulmonary artery. These fistulous connections act as multiple small left-to-right shunts. See **Video 10-13.**

children, who are more easily imaged by TEE, and by TEE in adults. The influx of flow into the recipient chamber or vessel may be discerned by echocardiography, although this is variable.

- TTE is only mildly more likely to define aspects of coronary artery fistulae.[35,43] It may be better at depicting the recipient chamber if it is posterior, but is not as comprehensive as cardiac magnetic resonance (CMR) imaging or CT in its direct visualization of the fistula or the drainage from it.
- Overall, the strength of echocardiography is in identifying the abnormal flow returning into a chamber by use of color Doppler flow mapping. The weaknesses of echocardiographic

Figure 10-21. **A,** A 2-month-old infant with heart failure. Color flow mapping in short-axis view demonstrating aorta–right atrial tunnel (ARAT). **C,** Multislice CT angiographic reconstruction shows ARAT in the left aortic sinus, the tunnel's retroaortic course, and the tunnel's termination (*arrow*). **D,** Operative photograph demonstrates ARAT originating from the aorta and its termination in the right atrium below the SVC:RA junction. AO, aorta; RA, right atrium; RV, right ventricle; SVC, superior vena cava. (Reprinted with permission from Matter M, Elgamal MA, Abdel Rahman A, Almarsafawy H. Aortico-right atrial tunnel in an infant. *Pediatr Cardiol.* 2011;32(6):849-850.)

TABLE 10-1 ACCF 2010 Appropriateness Criteria for the Use of Cardiac Computed Tomography to Evaluate Coronary Fistulae

	APPROPRIATENESS RATING	INDICATION	MEDIAN SCORE
Evaluation of adult congenital heart disease	Appropriate	Assessment of anomalies of coronary arterial and other thoracic arteriovenous vessels	9
	Uncertain	None listed	
	Inappropriate	None listed	

Data from Taylor AJ, Cerqueira M, Hodgson JM, et al. ACCF/SCCT/ACR/AHA/ASE/ASNC/NASCI/SCAI/SCMR 2010 appropriate use criteria for cardiac computed tomography. A report of the American College of Cardiology Foundation Appropriate Use Criteria Task Force, the Society of Cardiovascular Computed Tomography, the American College of Radiology, the American Heart Association, the American Society of Echocardiography, the American Society of Nuclear Cardiology, the North American Society for Cardiovascular Imaging, the Society for Cardiovascular Angiography and Interventions, and the Society for Cardiovascular Magnetic Resonance. *J Am Coll Cardiol.* 2010;56(22):1864-1894.

planar imaging are (1) the two-dimensional depiction of the fistula, which is very much a three-dimensional structure and (2) the two-dimensional depiction of the surrounding structures.

- **Coronary angiography** (catheter-based) was the traditional diagnostic test, although whether or not it is the current gold-standard modality is unclear. Realistically, catheter angiography does generate some equivocal, ambiguous or incorrect interpretations.
- **MRI** was the original advanced imaging modality to assess proximal coronary anatomy and diameter, and has shown good agreement with conventional angiography,[53,54] although imperfect sensitivity (88%).[55] CCT and MRI appear roughly equivalent. Current use of MRI would be best limited to assessment of anomalies or suspected anomalies in patients with renal insufficiency or other contraindication to iodinated contrast material. Using steady-state free precession and magnetic resonance angiography pulse sequences, CMR is able to depict a large number of coronary fistulae, especially the large ones. Phase-contrast sequences image the flow direction/variation within the fistula and the site(s) of return of the fistula. The ability to determine by phase contrast technique the volumetric quantification of pulmonary artery and aortic flow enables accurate determination of the pulmonary to aortic flow ratio (Qp:Qs).

References

1. Angelini P. Normal and anomalous coronary arteries: definitions and classification. *Am Heart J.* 1989;117(2):418-434.
2. Abdelmoneim SS, Mookadam F, Moustafa SE, Holmes DR. Coronary artery fistula with anomalous coronary artery origin: a case report. *J Am Soc Echocardiogr.* 2007;20(3):e331-e334.
3. Yamanaka O, Hobbs RE. Coronary artery anomalies in 126,595 patients undergoing coronary arteriography. *Cathet.Cardiovasc. Diagn.* 1990;21(1):28-40.
4. Jung HS, Lee TK, Bae W, Yun CS, Park CH, Jang JB. Communicating bilateral coronary artery to pulmonary artery fistula with aneurysms. *Int J Cardiol.* 2009;150(3):e107-e109.
5. Pagni S, Austin EH, Abraham JS. Right coronary artery to superior vena cava fistula presenting with "steal" phenomenon. *Interact Cardiovasc Thorac Surg.* 2004;3(4):573-574.
6. Cevik C, Nugent K, Topkara VK, Otahbachi M, Jenkins LA. Left circumflex coronary artery to hepatic vein fistula: a case report and brief review of coronary vasculogenesis. *Cardiovasc Revasc Med.* 2009;10(3):179-182.
7. Kang WC, Moon 2nd C, Ahn TH, Shin EK. Identifying the course of a coronary-bronchial artery fistula using contrast-enhanced multi-detector row computed tomography. *Int J Cardiol.* 2008; 130(3):125-128.
8. Ozaki N, Wakita N, Inoue K, Yamada A. Surgical repair of coronary artery to pulmonary artery fistula with aneurysms. *Eur J Cardiothorac Surg.* 2009;35(6):1089-1090.
9. Papazoglou PD, Mitsibounas D, Nanas JN. Left anterior descending coronary artery-left ventricular fistula presenting as unstable angina and syncope. *Int J Cardiol.* 2004;96(1):121-122.
10. Dursun A, Demirbag R, Yildiz A, Sezen Y, Altiparmak IH, Yilmaz R. Diagnosis of the left circumflex coronary artery fistula drainage into the left ventricle by echocardiographic color Doppler flow imaging. *Int J Cardiol.* 2009;134(3):85-86.
11. Said SA, van der Werf T. Dutch survey of congenital coronary artery fistulas in adults: coronary artery-left ventricular multiple micro-fistulas multi-center observational survey in the Netherlands. *Int J Cardiol.* 2006;110(1):33-39.
12. Yeter E, Ozdemir L, Durmaz T, Akcay M. Multiple coronary artery-left ventricular fistulae: a pattern of anomalous coronary microvascularization. *Eur J Cardiothorac Surg.* 2007;32(4):662.
13. Murphy BP, Gilbert T. Case report: coronary steal secondary to a left main coronary artery-pulmonary artery fistula only manifest after coronary artery bypass surgery. *Int J Cardiol.* 2009;137(3): 47-48.
14. Hackett D, Hallidie-Smith KA. Spontaneous closure of coronary artery fistula. *Br Heart J.* 1984;52(4):477-479.
15. Deibler AR, Kuzo RS, Vohringer M, et al. Imaging of congenital coronary anomalies with multislice computed tomography. *Mayo Clin Proc.* 2004;79(8):1017-1023.
16. Bijulal S, Namboodiri N, Nair K, Ajitkumar VK. Native vessel angioplasty as treatment strategy for left internal mammary artery to pulmonary vasculature fistula producing coronary steal phenomenon. *Int J Cardiol.* 2009;133(1):e25-e27.
17. Musleh G, Jalal A, Deiraniya AK. Post-coronary artery bypass grafting left internal mammary artery to pulmonary artery fistula: a 6 year follow-up following successful surgical division. *Eur J Cardiothorac Surg.* 2001;20(6):1258-1260.
18. Scholz KH, Wiegand V, Rosemeyer P, Chemnitius JM, Kreuzer H. Aorto-coronary artery to coronary vein fistula with the potential of coronary steal as complication of saphenous vein jump bypass graft. *Eur J Cardiothorac Surg.* 1993;7(8):441-442.
19. Chiu SN, Wu MH, Lin MT, Wu ET, Wang JK, Lue HC. Acquired coronary artery fistula after open heart surgery for congenital heart disease. *Int J Cardiol.* 2005;103(2):187-192.
20. Garber PJ, Hussain F, Koenig JK, Maycher B, Jassal DS. Multimodality imaging of a coronary artery fistula after septal myomectomy in hypertrophic cardiomyopathy. *J Am Coll Cardiol.* 2001; 57(9):e95.
21. Wada T, Ohara T, Nakatani S, Sumita Y, Kobayashi J, Kitakaze M. A case of coronary artery fistula between a coronary artery and the left atrium following MAZE procedure. *J Am Soc Echocardiogr.* 2009;22(3):e323-e326.
22. McGoldrick JP, Wells FC. Type 1 aortic dissection with right coronary artery occlusion and fistula to right atrium and right ventricle. *Eur J Cardiothorac Surg.* 1990;4(9):514-516.
23. Hancock Friesen C, Howlett JG, Ross DB. Traumatic coronary artery fistula management. *Ann Thorac Surg.* 2000;69(6):1973-1982.
24. Ercan E, Tengiz I, Yakut N, Gurbuz A, Bozdemir H, Bozdemir G. Takayasu's arteritis with multiple fistulas from three coronary arteries to lung paranchima. *Int J Cardiol.* 2003;88(2-3):319-320.
25. Rahimi JA, Salehian O. A hungry thrombus. *J Am Coll Cardiol.* 2012;59(15):e29.
26. Fujimoto N, Onishi K, Tanabe M, et al. Two cases of giant aneurysm in coronary-pulmonary artery fistula associated with atherosclerotic change. *Int J Cardiol.* 2004;97(3):577-578.
27. Aydogan U, Onursal E, Cantez T, Barlas C, Tanman B, Gurgan L. Giant congenital coronary artery fistula to left superior vena cava and right atrium with compression of left pulmonary vein simulating cor triatriatum–diagnostic value of magnetic resonance imaging. *Eur J Cardiothorac Surg.* 1994;8(2):97-99.
28. Ozeki S, Utsunomiya T, Kishi T, et al. Coronary arteriovenous fistula presenting as chronic pericardial effusion. *Circ J.* 2002;66(8): 779-782.
29. Gamma R, Seiler J, Moschovitis G, et al. Giant coronary artery fistula complicated by cardiac tamponade. *Int J Cardiol.* 2006;107(3): 413-414.
30. Bauer HH, Allmendinger PD, Flaherty J, Owlia D, Rossi MA, Chen C. Congenital coronary arteriovenous fistula: spontaneous rupture and cardiac tamponade. *Ann Thorac Surg.* 1996;62(5):1521-1523.
31. Mutlu H, Serdar Kucukoglu M, Ozhan H, Kansyz E, Ozturk S, Uner S. A case of coronary artery fistula draining into the pericardium causing hematoma. *Cardiovasc Surg.* 2001;9(2):201-203.
32. Lee KM, Pichard AD, Lindsay Jr J. Acquired coronary artery-left ventricular pseudoaneurysm fistula after myocardial infarction. *Am J Cardiol.* 1989;64(12):824-825.
33. Puvaneswary M, Warner G, Pressley L, Hawker R. Coronary artery fistula in a patient with pulmonary atresia and tricuspid atresia clinical and MRI findings. *Heart Lung Circ.* 2004;13(3):317-321.
34. Lemke P, Urbanyi B, Wehr G, Hellberg K. Anomalous coronary artery fistula with simultaneous drainage to the left atrium and the coronary sinus. *Eur J Cardiothorac Surg.* 1997;11(4):793-795.
35. Vitarelli A, De Curtis G, Conde Y, et al. Assessment of congenital coronary artery fistulas by transesophageal color Doppler echocardiography. *Am J Med.* 2002;113(2):127-133.
36. Okmen AS. Bilateral coronary artery fistulas terminating at the same location case report. *Int J Cardiol.* 2007;116:253-254.
37. Jha NK, AlHabshan F, AlMutairi M, Godman M, Najm HK. Coronary artery fistula with coronary sinus obstruction and retrograde drainage. *Heart Lung Circ.* 2008;17:248-151.
38. Hatakeyama Y, Doi T, Shirasawa K, et al. Four coronary to pulmonary artery fistulas originating from the left main trunk and each of three coronary arteries (LAD, LCX and RCA) detected by the combination of coronary angiography and multislice computed tomography. *Int J Cardiol.* 2007;121(2):227-228.
39. Neema PK, Varma PK, Sinha PK, et al. Case 4–2006: coexistent hypertrophic obstructive cardiomyopathy, mitral stenosis, and coronary artery fistula. *J Cardiothorac Vasc Anesth.* 2006;20(4): 594-605.
40. Gowda RM, Vasavada BC, Khan IA. Coronary artery fistulas: clinical and therapeutic considerations. *Int J Cardiol.* 2006;107(1):7-10.
41. Hoffer E, Materne P, Henroteaux D, Markov M, Boland J. Successful percutaneous closure of multiple coronary artery fistulas with coils embolization in two adults. *Int J Cardiol.* 2007;122(3):e25-e28.
42. Tirilomis T, Aleksic I, Busch T, Zenker D, Ruschewski W, Dalichau H. Congenital coronary artery fistulas in adults: surgical treatment and outcome. *Int J Cardiol.* 2005;98(1):57-59.
43. Ishikawa Y, Niimi Y, Morita S. An unusual transesophageal echocardiographic finding after surgical correction of a coronary artery fistula. *J Cardiothorac Vasc Anesth.* 2005;19(5):693-694.
44. Guo DW, Cheng TO, Lin ML, Gu ZQ. Aneurysm of the sinus of Valsalva: a roentgenologic study of 105 Chinese patients. *Am Heart J.* 1987;114(5):1169-1177.
45. Sreedharan M, Baruah B, Dash PK. Aorta–right atrial tunnel—a novel therapeutic option. *Int J Cardiol.* 2006;107(3):410-412.
46. Sung YM, Merchant N. Imaging of congenital aorta-right atrial tunnel with electrocardiogram gated 64-multi-slice computed tomography. *Ann Thorac Surg.* 2011;92(2):743.
47. Matter M, Elgamal MA, Abdel Rahman A, Almarsafawy H. Aortico-right atrial tunnel in an infant. *Pediatr Cardiol.* 2011;32(6):849-850.
48. Turkay C, Golbasi I, Belgi A, Tepe S, Bayezid O. Aorta-right atrial tunnel. *J Thorac Cardiovasc Surg.* 2003;125(5):1058-1060.
49. Kalangos A, Beghetti M, Vala D, Chraibi S, Faidutti B. Aorticoright atrial tunnel. *Ann Thorac Surg.* 2000;69(2):635-637.
50. Taylor AJ, Cerqueira M, Hodgson JM, et al. ACCF/SCCT/ACR/AHA/ASE/ASNC/NASCI/SCAI/SCMR 2010 appropriate use criteria for cardiac computed tomography. A report of the American College of Cardiology Foundation Appropriate Use Criteria Task Force, the Society of Cardiovascular Computed Tomography, the American College of Radiology, the American Heart Association, the American Society of Echocardiography, the American Society of Nuclear Cardiology, the North American Society for Cardiovascular Imaging, the Society for Cardiovascular Angiography and Interventions, and the Society for Cardiovascular Magnetic Resonance. *J Am Coll Cardiol.* 2010;56(22):1864-1894.

51. Warnes CA, Williams RG, Bashore TM, et al. ACC/AHA 2008 guidelines for the management of adults with congenital heart disease: a report of the American College of Cardiology/American Heart Association Task Force on Practice Guidelines (Writing Committee to Develop Guidelines on the Management of Adults With Congenital Heart Disease). Developed in Collaboration With the American Society of Echocardiography, Heart Rhythm Society, International Society for Adult Congenital Heart Disease, Society for Cardiovascular Angiography and Interventions, and Society of Thoracic Surgeons. *J Am Coll Cardiol.* 2008;52(23):e1-e121.
52. Mavroudis C, Backer CL, Rocchini AP, Muster AJ, Gevitz M. Coronary artery fistulas in infants and children: a surgical review and discussion of coil embolization. *Ann Thorac Surg.* 1997;63(5): 1235-1242.
53. McConnell MV, Ganz P, Selwyn AP, Li W, Edelman RR, Manning WJ. Identification of anomalous coronary arteries and their anatomic course by magnetic resonance coronary angiography. *Circulation.* 1995;92(11):3158-3162.
54. Post JC, van Rossum AC, Bronzwaer JG, et al. Magnetic resonance angiography of anomalous coronary arteries. A new gold standard for delineating the proximal course? *Circulation.* 1995;92(11): 3163-3171.
55. Taylor AM, Thorne SA, Rubens MB, et al. Coronary artery imaging in grown up congenital heart disease: complementary role of magnetic resonance and x-ray coronary angiography. *Circulation.* 2000;101(14):1670-1678.
56. Burma O, Rahman A, Ilkay E. Coronary arteriovenous fistulas from both coronary arteries to pulmonary artery. *Eur J Cardiothorac Surg.* 2002;21(1):86.

Coronary Artery Aneurysms

Key Points

- CCT angiography is the test of choice to define coronary artery aneurysms.
- The common occurrence of mural thrombosis of larger coronary artery aneurysms renders cardiac CT particularly able to determine the full size of the coronary artery aneurysm, beyond the means of conventional coronary angiography and beyond that of CMR.

Coronary aneurysms have been identified in 0.5% to 4% of patients undergoing coronary angiograms.[1] The incidence among patients undergoing coronary CT angiography (CTA) has not been determined.

The most common definition of a coronary artery aneurysm is focal dilation of the artery, 1.5 times normal (adjacent reference segment or elsewhere maximal vessel) diameter, and limited to spherical or saccular dilation—a standard and borrowed convention of the definition of an aneurysm.[1] Although generally small (just millimeters in diameter), coronary artery aneurysms may be extremely large. Aneurysms measuring 12 *cm* have been found.[2,3]

Aneurysms are encountered most commonly in the right coronary artery but may be found in any coronary artery and may be multiple, especially in the setting of prior Kawasaki disease, where large aneurysms also are common.[4,5] The left main stem coronary artery appears to be the least common site for coronary aneurysms, although this site is heavily represented in the literature.[1,6-8]

Some reviews suggest male dominance of coronary aneurysms.[6]

Formation of coronary aneurysm after percutaneous coronary intervention is relatively common in patients with Kawasaki disease, and the incidence varies from 15% to 18%.[9]

ETIOLOGIES AND ASSOCIATIONS

- Half of all coronary artery aneurysms (50%) are associated with atherosclerotic coronary artery disease. Associated stenoses are common.[6,10,11]
- Coronary artery disease (CAD)–associated
  - Drug-eluting stents[9,12-14]
  - Cutting balloon[15]
  - Coronary ectasia
  - Extensive coronary calcification[16]
  - Saphenous bypass grafts[17]
- Vasculitis
  - Aortitis of all forms extending onto the proximal coronary arteries
  - Polyarteritis nodosa (PAN)
  - Kawasaki disease[1,2,14]
  - Hyperesoinophilic syndrome[18]
  - Other
- Vascular disease–or syndrome-associated
  - Fibromuscular dysplasia
  - Supravalvular aortic stenosis[19]
- Marfan syndrome[20]
- Infection (mycotic)[21]
- Coronary artery arteriovenous fistulae[22]
- Myocardial bridging[23]
- Idiopathic[24]

RISKS

The risk from coronary artery aneurysms appears to be due mainly to the development of mural thrombus within the aneurysm sac and subsequent embolization of thrombus down the ongoing coronary artery or branch vessels.[24] Because thromboembolism is the late outcome of large coronary aneurysms, the amount of embolized thrombus, and the ensuing coronary event, may be large.

- Acute coronary syndrome (ACS)[10]
- Myocardial infarction not associated with stenosis in the same vessel[25,26]
- Myocardial infarction and post-infarction tamponade[6]
- Rupture and tamponade[25,27]
- Myocardial infarction and right ventricular infarction/shock[25]
- Cardiac arrest[24,28]
- Sudden death[24,29]
- Breakdown of the wall of the aneurysm with:
  - Fistulization into an adjacent cavity
  - Pericardial tamponade

- ❒ Aneurysms also may compress adjacent structures:
  - Chambers[17,22,30,31]
  - Superior vena cava (SVC): SVC syndrome[32]
  - Pulmonary artery[33]
- ❒ Aortic insufficiency[3]
- ❒ Vasospasm elsewhere[6]
- ❒ Thrombosis of a bare-metal stent inserted into an unappreciated aneurysm with extensive mural thrombus, which may dissolve and result in stent dislodgement[34]

TREATMENT

- ❒ Prevention: Established for Kawasaki disease using intravenous gamma globulin and aspirin[35]
- ❒ Observation
- ❒ Active treatment
  - Anti-platelet and anticoagulation[36]
  - Percutaneous covered stent closure[8]
  - Percutaneous coil embolization (saphenous graft aneurysm)[17]
  - Surgical repair[15,21,37]
    - Ligation at the inflow and/or outflow and internal thoracic/mammary or saphenous bypass. Use of arterial conduits is anticipated to provide more lasting benefit to younger patients.[38]
    - Aneurysmectomy and end-to-end repair[33]
    - Resection with bypass[39]
    - Patch repair/reconstruction[40]

POTENTIAL CORONARY CTA FINDINGS OF CORONARY ARTERY ANEURYSMS

- ❒ Aneurysmal dilation
  - Solitary or multiple
  - Spherical or saccular
- ❒ Coronary ectasia
- ❒ Coronary stenoses
- ❒ Mural thrombus within the aneurysm
- ❒ Calcification of the aneurysm
- ❒ Fistulous drainage of the aneurysm
- ❒ Aneurysm located within a fistulous coronary anomaly
- ❒ Compression of adjacent chambers and structures
- ❒ Associated aneurysms of the aorta or other vessels

CCT IMAGES OF CORONARY ARTERY ANEURYSMS

Examples are shown in Figures 11-1 through 11-15 and **Videos 11-1 through 11-7.**

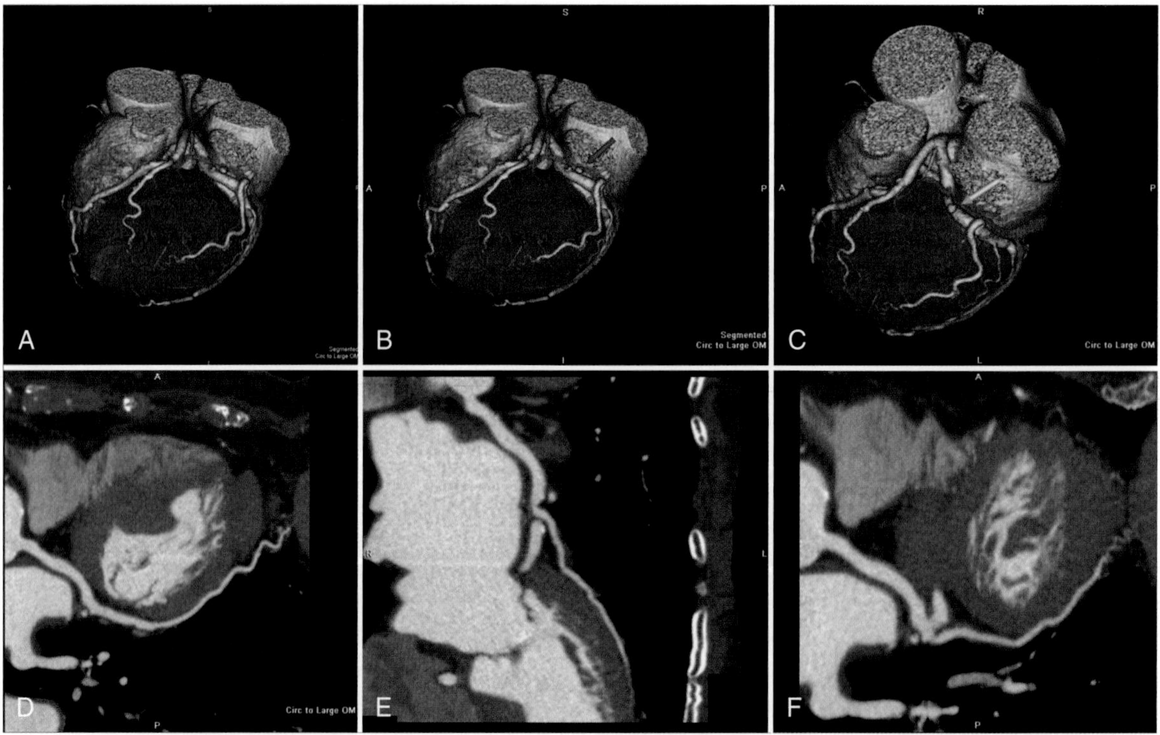

Figure 11-1. Multiple volume-rendered and curved reformatted cardiac CT images demonstrate a small focal aneurysm extending from the proximal circumflex artery in a patient with Kawasaki disease. There is multifocal ectasia of the proximal to mid-right coronary artery (RCA) and a mild (30%) stenosis of the mid-RCA.

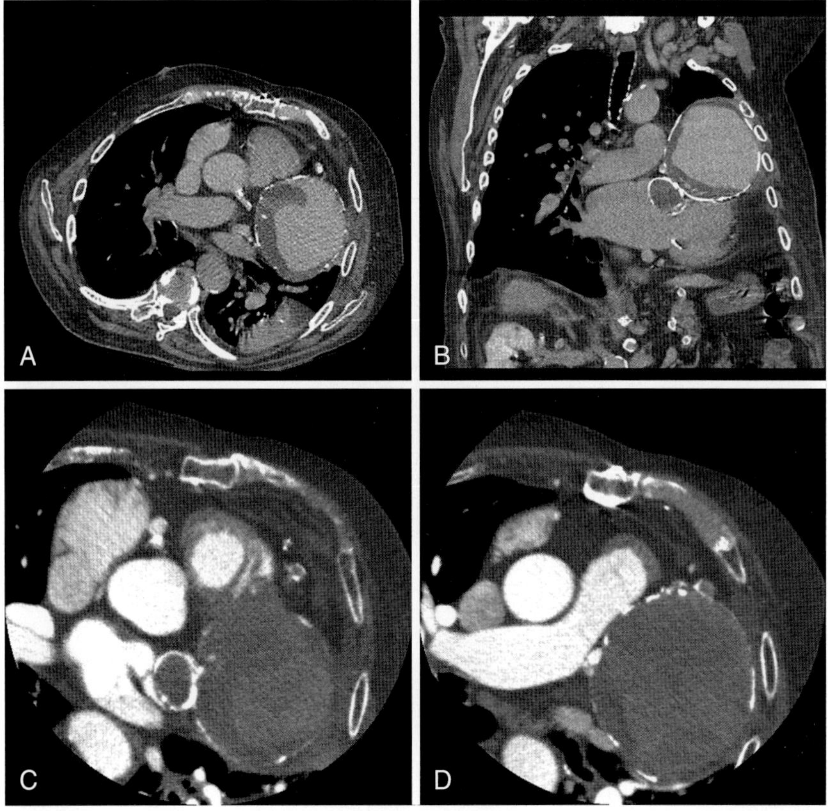

Figure 11-2. Chest CT (**A** and **B**) and cardiac CT (**C** and **D**). Two large, calcified, and extensively thrombus-containing coronary artery aneurysms are present, one arising off the left circumflex artery and the other off a diagonal branch of the left anterior descending artery.

CCT IMAGES OF KAWASAKI DISEASE–INCITED CORONARY ARTERY ANEURYSMS

Examples are shown in Figure 11-16 and **Video 11-8.**

CCT IMAGES OF SAPHENOUS VEIN GRAFT ANEURYSMS

Examples are shown in Figures 11-17 and 11-18.

CCT PROTOCOL POINTS

The standard CCT protocol is used.

IMAGING ALTERNATIVES

Cardiac MR is able to adequately image medium-sized (approximately 5 mm) and larger coronary artery aneurysms.

2011 AMERICAN COLLEGE OF CARDIOLOGY FOUNDATION APPROPRIATENESS CRITERIA FOR CCT

The American College of Cardiology Foundation (ACCF) has not specified approrpriateness criteria for CCT assessment of coronary aneurysms.

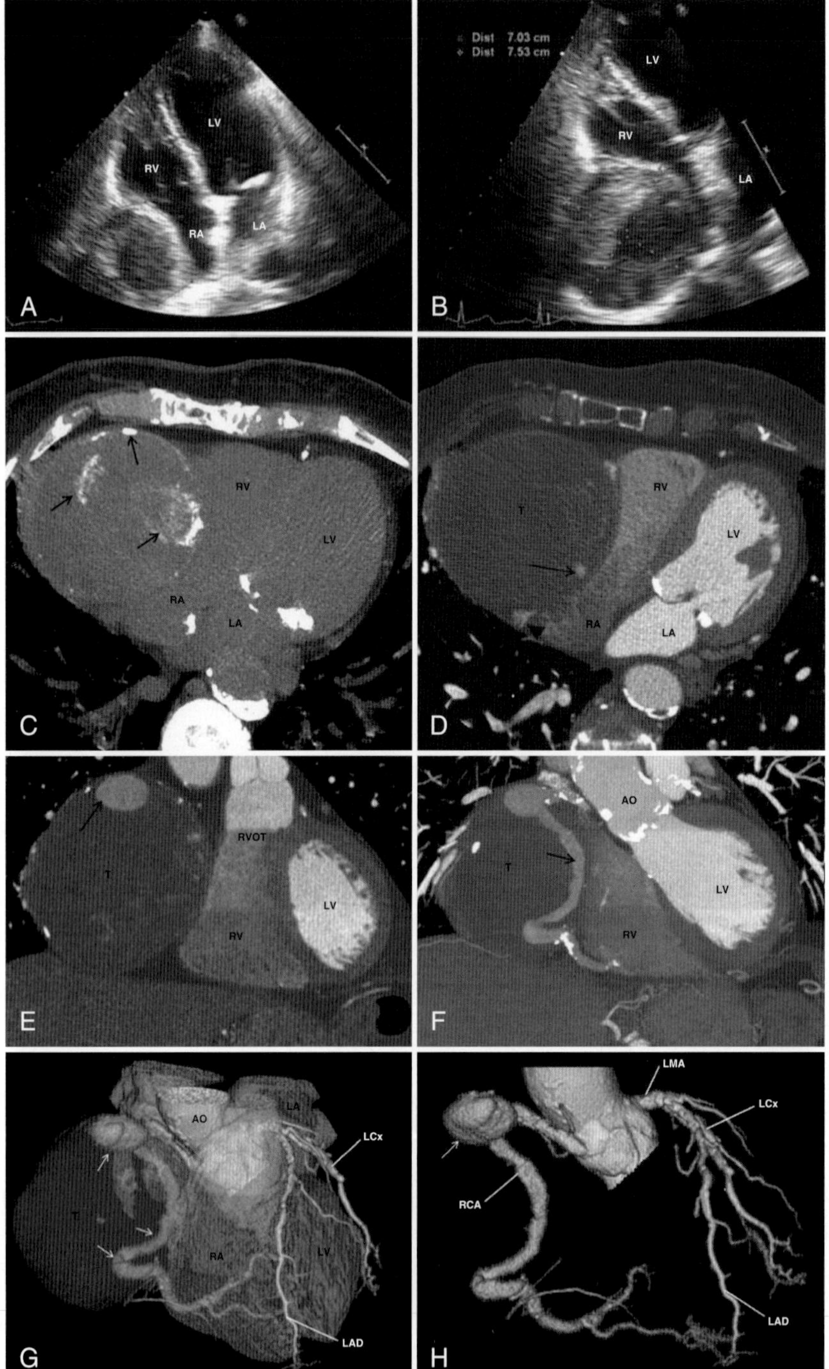

Figure 11-3. **A** and **B,** Two-dimensional echocardiography images show a large echogenic mass compressing the right atrium (RA) and tricuspid annulus. **C** and **D,** ECG-gated axial CT images. **C,** Before contrast injection, showing a large mass in the right atrioventricular groove; note peripheral and central calcifications (*arrows*). **D,** After contrast injection, a large mural thrombus with small eccentric residual lumen (*arrow*) is seen. Compression of the right atrium, right appendage (*arrowhead*), and right ventricle inlet are noted. Coronal multiplanar (**E**) and maximum intensity projection reconstructed images (**F**) show the maximal diameter of the giant right coronary artery aneurysm; the thrombus and lumen (*arrows*) can be appreciated. **G** and **H,** Three-dimensional volume-rendered reformats show the giant right coronary artery aneurysm in relation to the cardiac chambers and the angiographic view, demonstrating the residual lumen (*arrows*). Note that the actual size of the aneurysm is largely underestimated if evaluation is made only on the basis of the angiogram. AO, aorta; LA, left atrium; LAD, left anterior descending artery; LCx, left circumflex artery; LMA, left main coronary artery; LV, left ventricle; RCA, right coronary artery; RV, right ventricle; RVOT, right ventricle outflow tract; T, thrombus. (Reprinted with permission from Pasian SG, Tan KT, Pen V, et al. Giant right coronary artery aneurysm on 64-MDCT. *J Cardiovasc Med* (*Hagerstown*). 2010;11(7):544-546.)

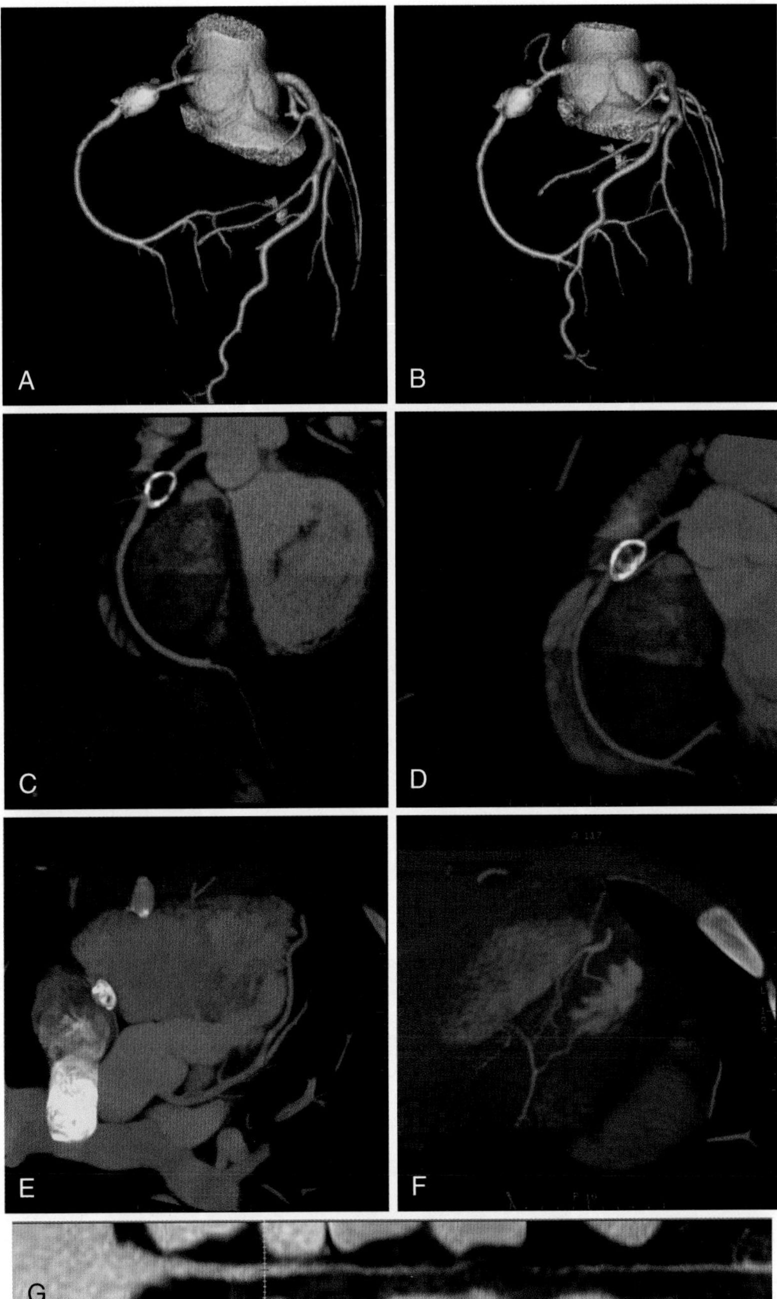

Figure 11-4. Composite images in a 21-year-old man with remote Kawasaki disease demonstrate a peripherally calcified and thrombosed proximal right coronary artery (RCA) aneurysm with immediate reconstitution of the RCA by sinoatrial node and conus branch collaterals. **See Video 11-8.**

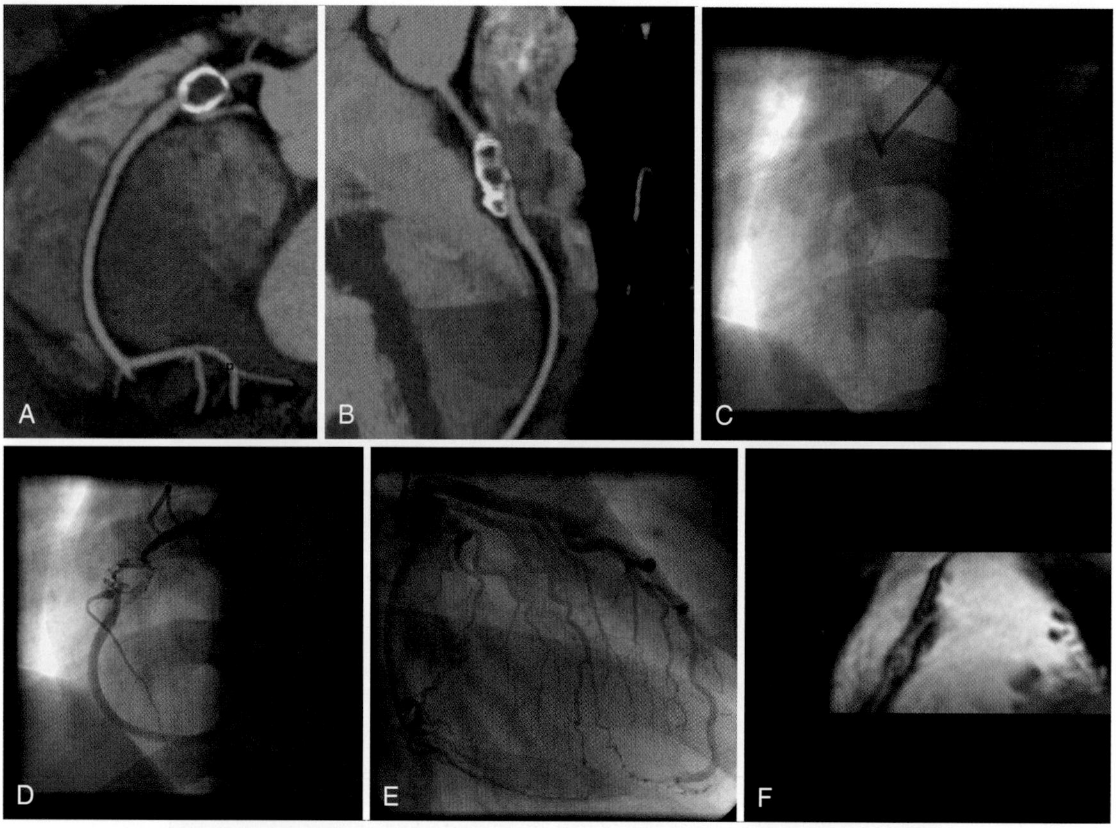

Figure 11-5. **A** and **B,** Cardiac CT images demonstrate a thrombosed and calcified aneurysm of the right coronary artery (RCA). **C** and **D**, Conventional angiography reveals the same, and better depicts the bridging collaterals. **E,** Angiography demonstrates filling of the RCA by left–to-right coronary collaterals as well. **F,** Coronary MR angiographic depiction of the thrombosed RCA aneurysm. **See Videos 11-1 and 11-2.**

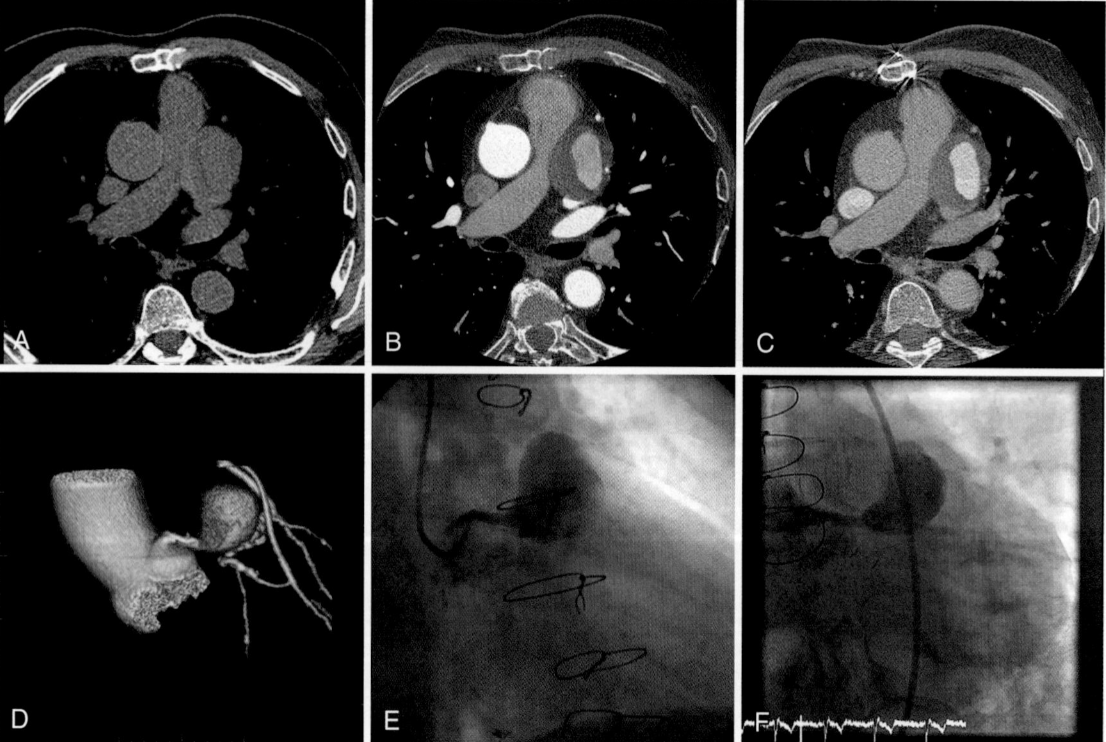

Figure 11-6. Cardiac CT (**A–C**) and conventional angiography (**E** and **F**). A large and partially thrombosed aneurysm arises from the left main stem coronary artery. The mural thrombus within the aneurysm, and thereby the true size of the aneurysm, is seen only on the axial cardiac CT image, not on the volume-rendered (**D**) or conventional angiography images. **See Videos 11-3 and 11-4.**

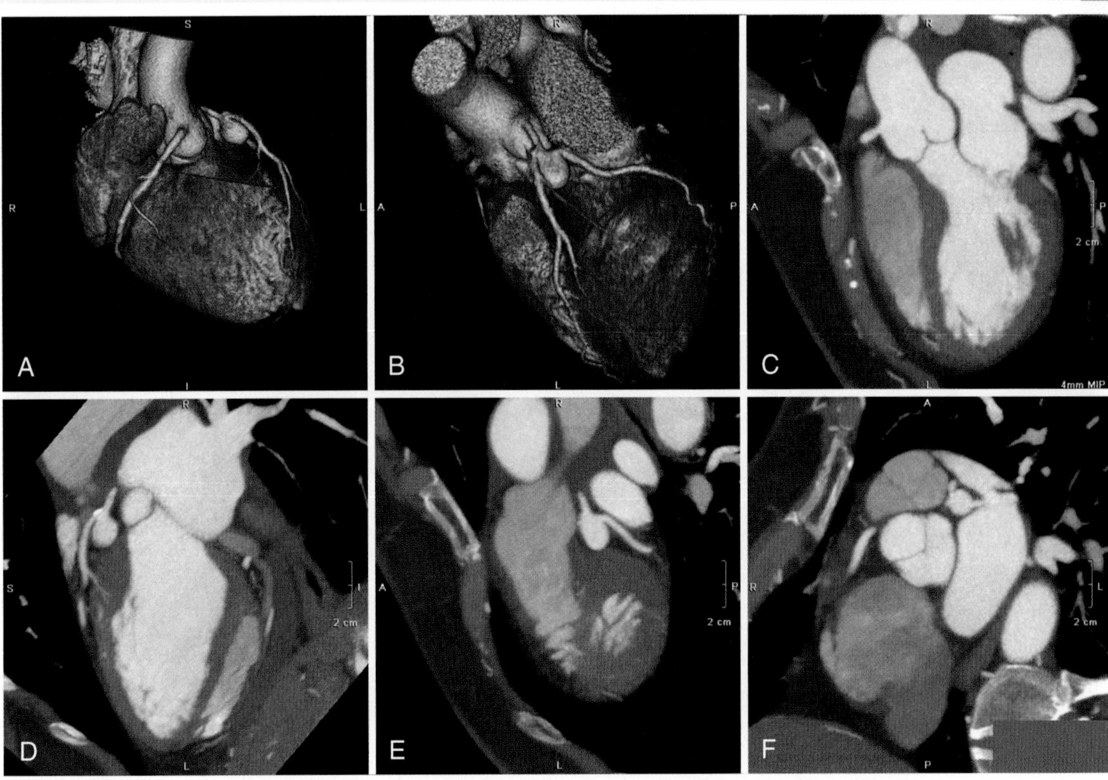

Figure 11-7. Multiple images from a cardiac CT study in a 52-year-old woman. The patient had no prior coronary intervention or surgery. A focal saccular aneurysm is seen arising from the distal left main coronary artery. The left anterior descending artery and circumflex artery arise off the saccular aneurysm. No evidence of thrombus or calcification was seen in the aneurysm. **See Video 11-5.**

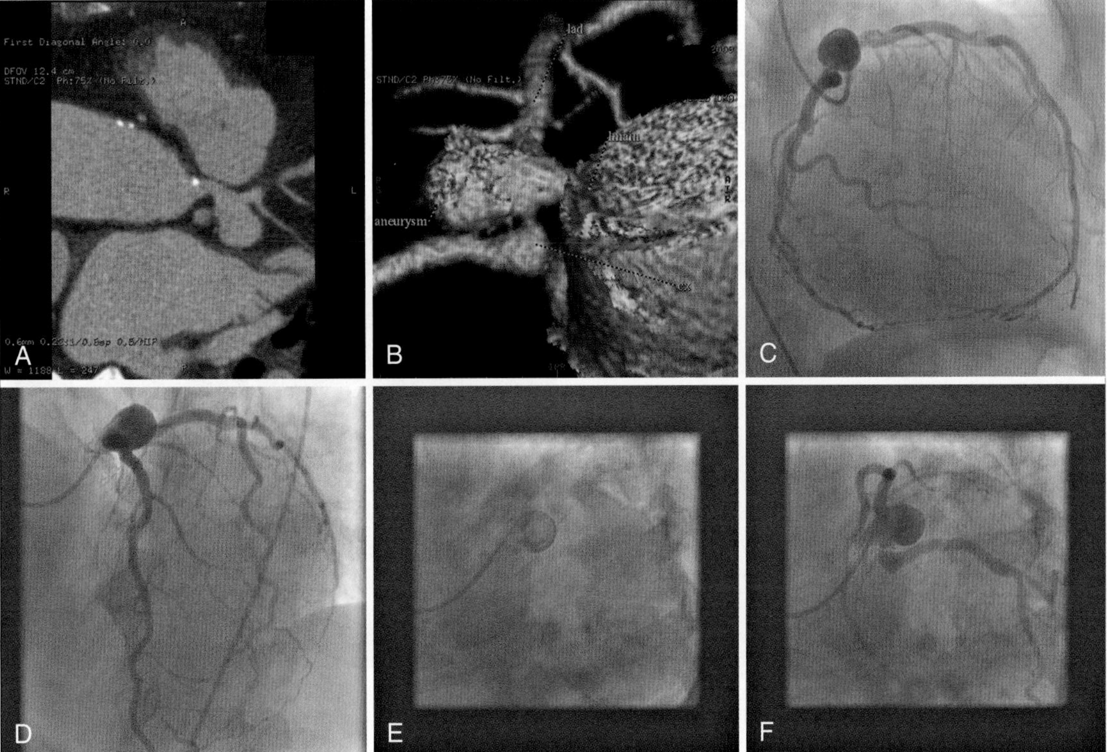

Figure 11-8. Composite curved reformatted and volume-rendered images in a 58-year-old woman with chest pain demonstrate a large aneurysm of the left main coronary artery, with an associated severe 70% stenosis at the origin of the circumflex artery. Multiple images from a conventional coronary angiogram demonstrate the aneurysm and the focal circumflex stenosis. Cine images from a left coronary catheterization show the large left main aneurysm and the tight focal circumflex stenosis. **See Video 11-6.**

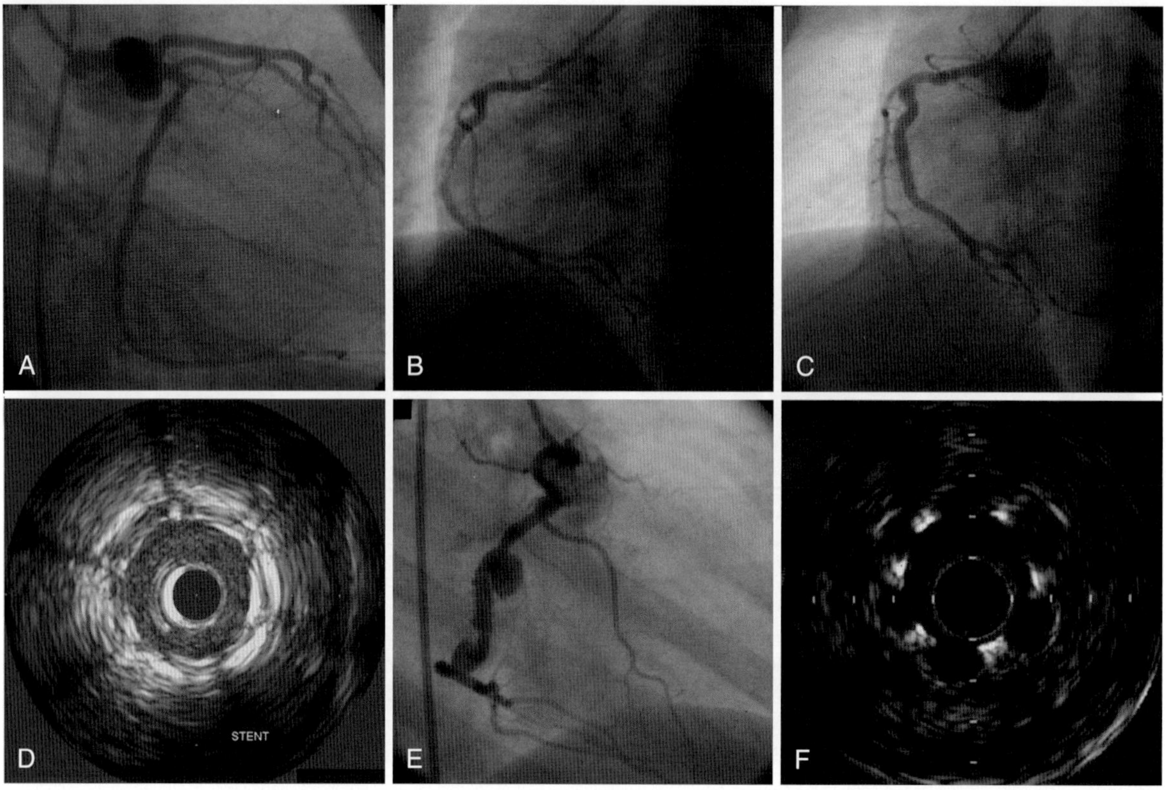

Figure 11-9. A 12-year-old girl with Kawasaki disease was admitted for percutaneous coronary intervention for her 90% mid-right coronary artery (RCA) stenosis (**B**). There was also a large coronary aneurysm (15.9 × 11.9 mm) of her left main coronary artery (**A**). The RCA stenosis was pre-dilated with a 3.0/15-mm Aqua T3 balloon (Cordis) at 6 atmospheres (atm), followed by deployment of a 3.0/18-mm Cypher stent at 16 atm and post-dilated with a 3.5/16-mm Extensor balloon at 16 atm (**C**). Intravascular ultrasound (IVUS) showed good stent apposition (**D**). The patient was prescribed clopidogrel for 3 months and aspirin for life. She remained asymptomatic, and a follow-up coronary angiogram was done 1 year later. Formation of two large eccentric and saccular neoaneurysms was found at the segments just proximal and distal to the stent; the sizes were 10.1 × 9.8 mm and 6.5 × 5.6 mm, respectively. Along the stented segment, smaller aneurysmal dilatations also were seen (**E**). IVUS confirmed the two large aneurysms with malapposition of the stent within the vessel (**F**). No neointimal hyperplasia within the stent was seen. (Reprinted with permission from Li SS, Cheng BC, Lee SH. Images in cardiovascular medicine. Giant coronary aneurysm formation after sirolimus-eluting stent implantation in Kawasaki disease. *Circulation.* 2005;112(8): e105-107, Figures 1 and 2.)

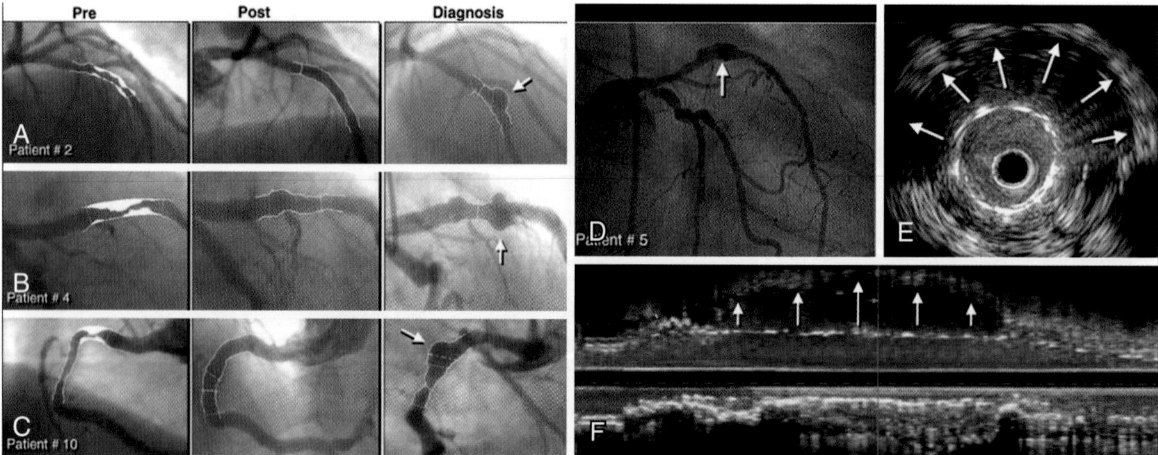

Figure 11-10. A–C, Angiographic images of three coronary aneurysms after drug-eluting stent implantation. *Left:* Before intervention (pre); *middle:* after drug-eluting stent implantation (post); *right:* at late follow-up, when coronary aneurysms (*white arrows*) were diagnosed. **D,** Angiographic image of a coronary aneurysm in the left anterior descending coronary artery (*arrow*). **E,** Intravascular ultrasound image shows a coronary aneurysm with severe incomplete apposition of the stent struts (*arrows*). **F,** Longitudinal reconstruction of the vessel disclosing the aneurysm and the full extent of malapposition (*arrows*). (Reprinted with permission from Alfonso F, Perez-Vizcayno MJ, Ruiz M, et al. Coronary aneurysms after drug-eluting stent implantation: clinical, angiographic, and intravascular ultrasound findings. *J Am Coll Cardiol.* 2009;53(22):2053-2060.)

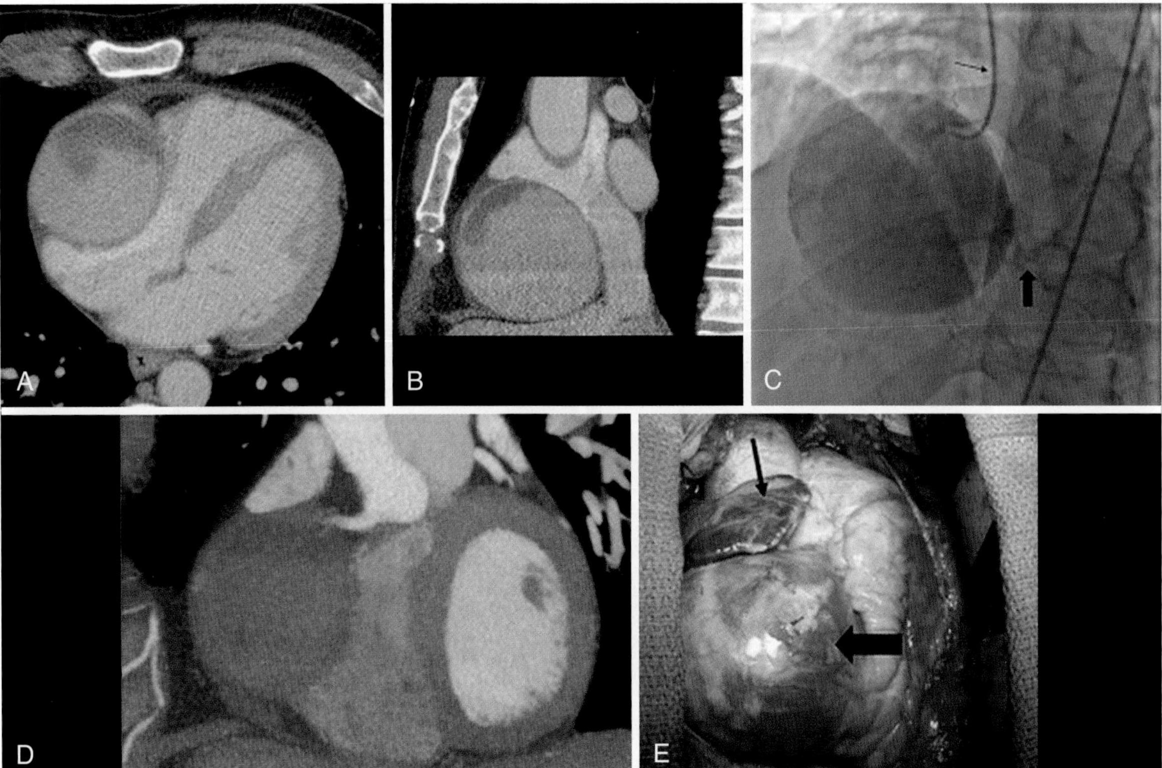

Figure 11-11. Delayed axial (**A**) and sagittal (**B**) images of cardiac CT scan performed 3 minutes after the initial contrast scan show a large area of decreased enhancement within the giant aneurysm, consistent with large thrombus burden. **C,** Selective catheterization of the right coronary artery in a 30-degree left anterior oblique (LAO) view. The image shows a 6-French catheter (*small black arrow*) engaging the ostium of the right coronary artery. There is a large (8 × 8 cm) mass filled with radiocontrast. Distal to this mass one can faintly appreciate the distal vessel (*large black arrow*) that was difficult to fill fully with contrast despite large-volume injections. **D,** Comparable multiplanar-reformatted image of the cardiac CT angiography in a 30-degree LAO projection. **E,** Intraoperative photograph of the subject before right coronary artery aneurysm resection and vein graft bypass. The aneurysm is obvious in this view (*large arrow*). Also appreciable is the right atrial appendage (*small arrow*). (Reprinted with permission from Gibbs B, Feuerstein IM, Tavaf H, Villines TC. Giant compressive coronary artery aneurysm delineated by cardiac CT. *J Cardiovasc Comput Tomogr.* 2009;3(5):348-350.)

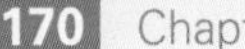

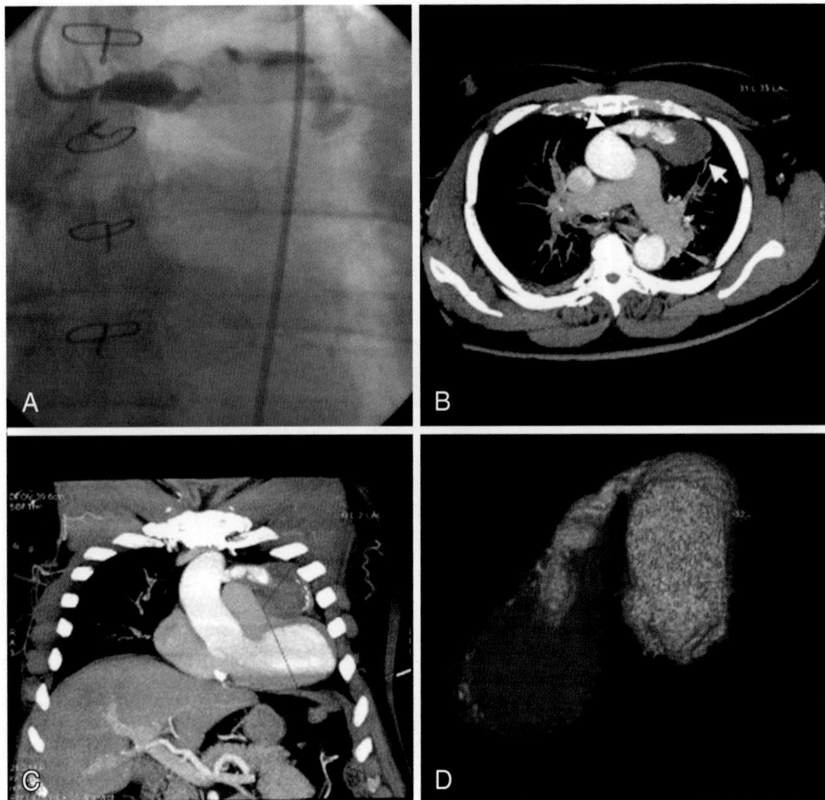

Figure 11-12. A 60-year-old man who had undergone saphenous vein grafting to the left anterior descending artery 23 years earlier complained of continuous chest pain for the past 48 hours. No ECG changes were observed, and laboratory tests showed normal troponin T and creatine kinase levels on admittance and at 8, 12, and 24 hours. Coronary angiography was performed and showed chronic total occlusion of the left anterior descending artery and a severely degenerated and occluded saphenous vein graft. Contrast-enhanced CT showed an extracardiac mass of 85 × 51 mm compressing the left atrium, corresponding to a giant aneurysmatic saphenous vein graft. The patient had severe obesity (160 cm, 100 kg, body mass index 39 kg/m^2) and was not considered a good surgical candidate. One week later, the patient was scheduled for percutaneous closure of a severely degenerated saphenous vein graft. One embolization coil was deployed through a right femoral artery access, allowing complete exclusion of the aneurysmatic graft. The patient did well and was discharged 24 hours later. (Reprinted with permission from Garcia-Lara J, Pinar-Bermudez E, Hurtado JA, Valdez-Chavarri M. Giant true saphenous vein graft aneurysm. *J Am Coll Cardiol.* 2009;54(20):1899.)

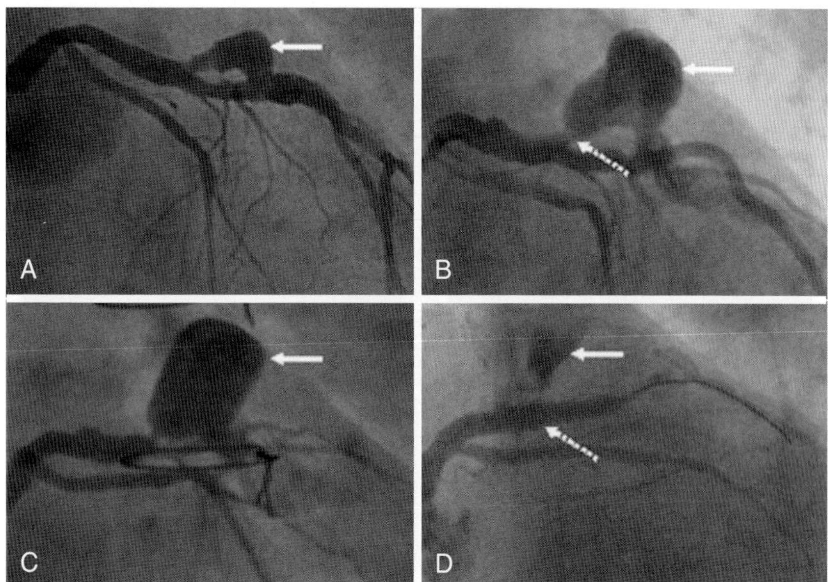

Figure 11-13. This case illustrates dramatic progressive dilatation of a left anterior descending artery (LAD) aneurysm, treated with a covered stent. A 63-year-old man with a background history remarkable for hypertension and previous smoking presented 18 months prior to the current presentation for elective coronary angiography for chest pain (**A**). This revealed an ectatic proximal LAD (*arrow*) with no significant flow-limiting lesions. Twelve months later, angina developed, and repeat angiography demonstrated a moderate to severe stenosis of the proximal LAD (*dotted arrow*) followed by significant aneurysmal dilation (*arrow*) of the LAD. There was moderate ostial circumflex disease (**B**). The patient was referred for coronary artery bypass graft surgery and received a left internal mammary artery graft to the LAD and a vein graft to the obtuse marginal circumflex artery. Six months later, the patient presented with further angina, and angiography (**C**) revealed further dilation (15 × 9 mm) of the LAD aneurysm (*arrow*) and occlusion of the left internal mammary graft. Given the rapidly progressive nature of the aneurysm, a single covered stent (**D**, *dotted arrow*) was placed over the mouth of the aneurysm, to obstruct blood flow into the sac and potentially reduce the risk of catastrophic rupture. (Reprinted with permission from Bhindi R, Testa L, Ormerod OJ, Banning AP. Rapidly evolving giant coronary aneurysm. *J Am Coll Cardiol.* 2009;53(4):371.)

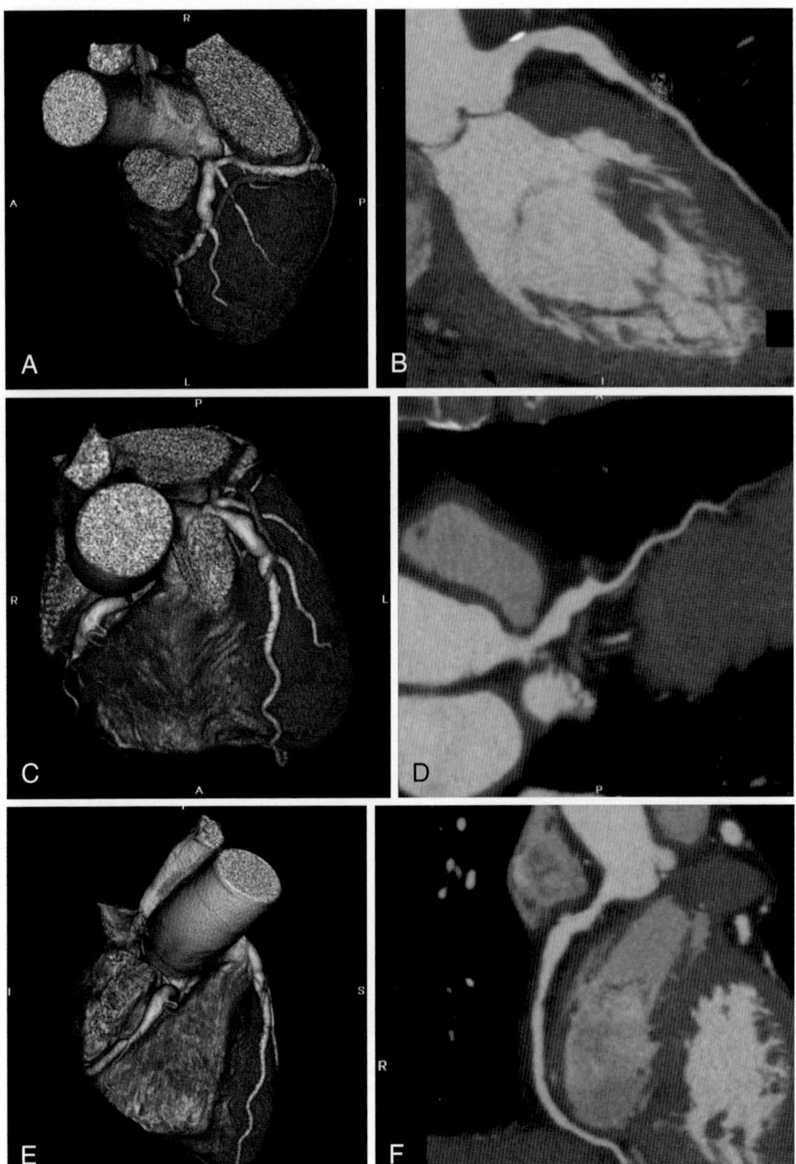

Figure 11-14. Multiple images from a cardiac CT study of a 34-year-old man with a prior history of Kawasaki disease. **A** and **B,** Fusiform ectasia of the left main coronary artery extending into the proximal circumflex artery. **C** and **D,** Fusiform ectasia of the left main artery extending into the proximal left anterior descending artery. **E** and **F,** Fusiform ectasia of the proximal RCA. **See Video 11-7.**

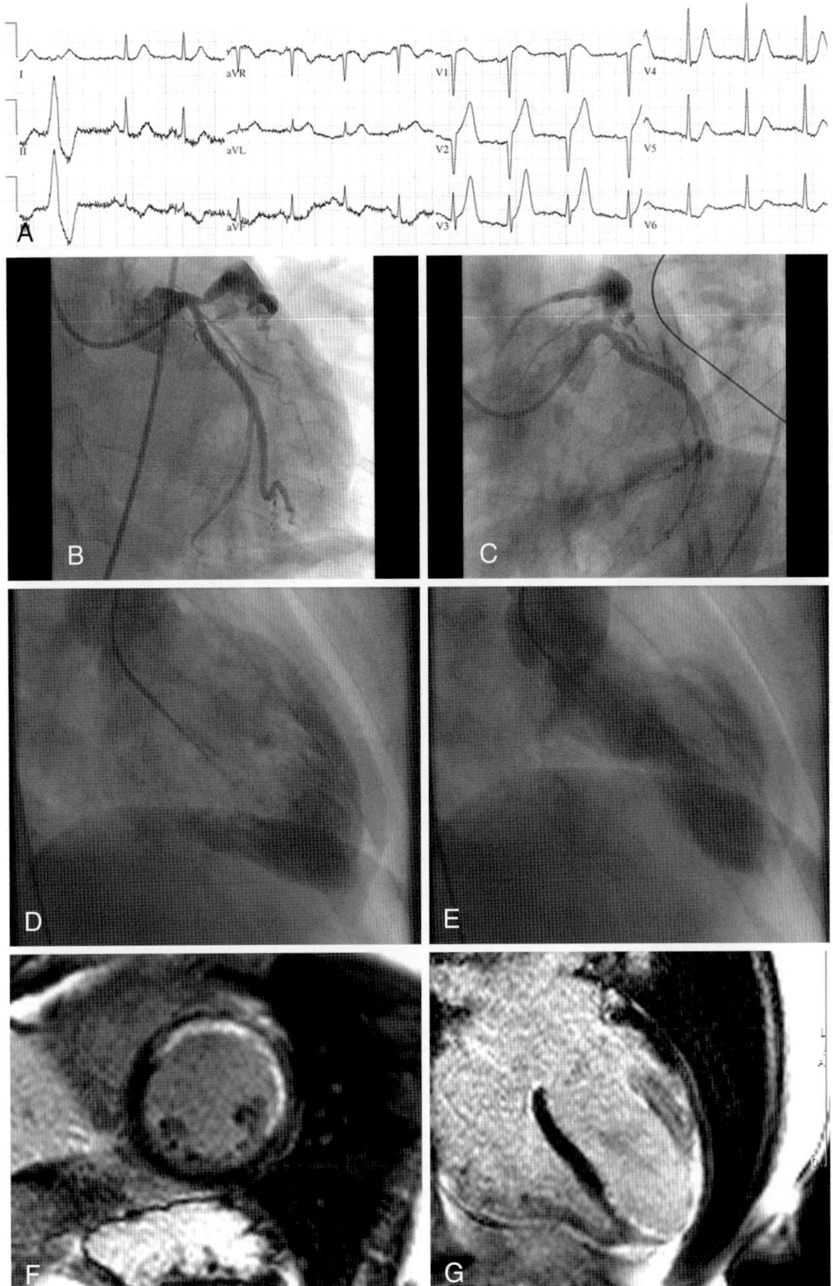

Figure 11-15. A 50-year-old man with an anterior ST-elevation myocardial infarction (STEMI) presentation. **A,** ECG shows anteroseptal ST elevation and Q-waves. **B** and **C,** Coronary angiography reveals a complex aneurysm of the left anterior descending artery (LAD), with an associated extensive anteroapical akinetic segment as seen by contrast ventriculography. **D** and **E,** CMR steady-state free precession sequences reveal an aneurysm of the left anterior descending coronary artery, which is apparent, but not readily appreciated in detail (course, lumen, intraluminal thrombus). **F** and **G,** CMR double inversion recovery images reveal transmural (>50%) late enhancement within the LAD distribution.

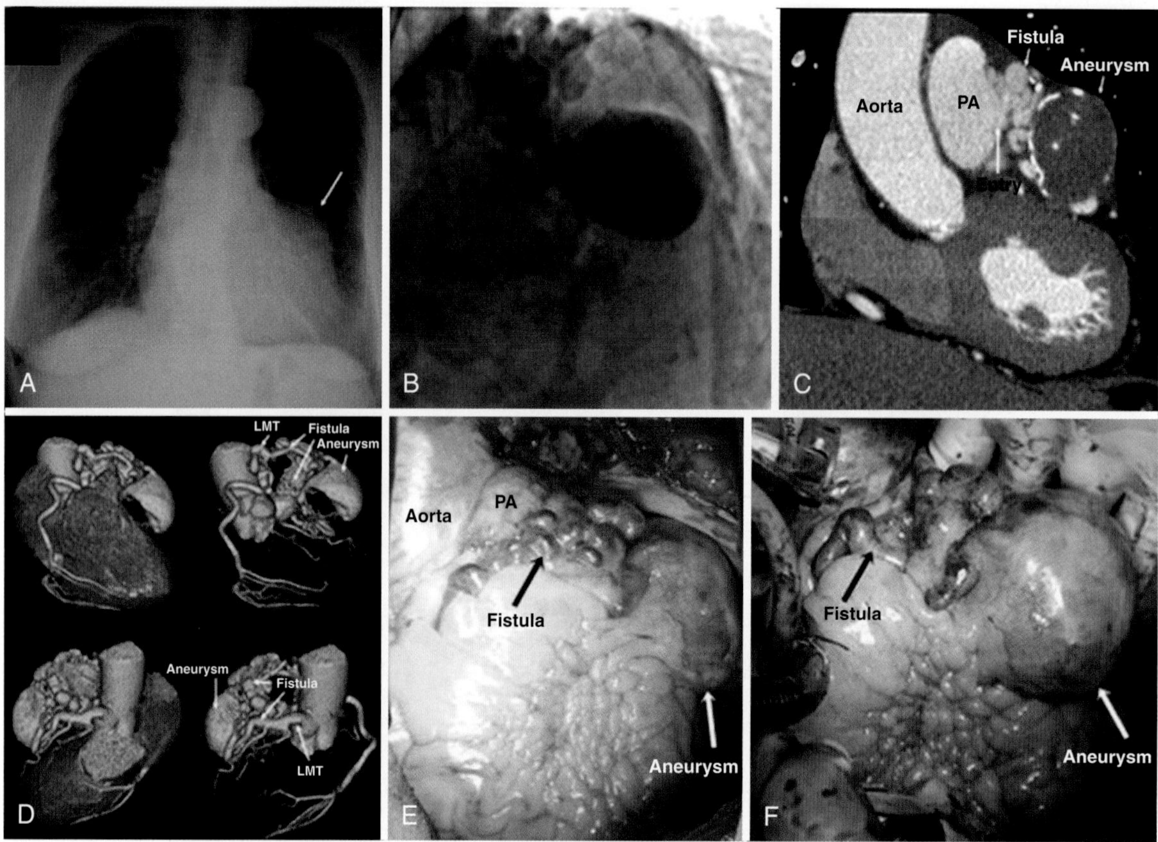

Figure 11-16. A 69-year-old woman with dyspnea. **A,** The chest radiograph was notable for a mass shadow. A transthoracic echocardiogram revealed a mosaic pattern in the pulmonary artery (PA). **B,** Multislice CT angiography and coronary angiography showed the giant aneurysm in the coronary artery fistula arising from the left main coronary trunk (LMT) and entering in the PA. The aneurysm measured 55 × 45 mm with calcification and thrombus formation (**C** and **D**). Cardiac catheterization revealed an oximetry step-up of 9% at the main PA, and a left-to-right shunt of 1.84:1 (Qp:Qs) was found. Aneurysmorrhaphy and closure of the fistula outlet from the PA were performed (**E** and **F**), and the symptoms disappeared, probably due to resolution of a coronary steal phenomenon. (Reprinted with permission from Maeda S, Nishizaki M, Hashiyama N, Mo M. Giant aneurysm in coronary artery fistula. *J Am Coll Cardiol.* 2009;54(24):e119.)

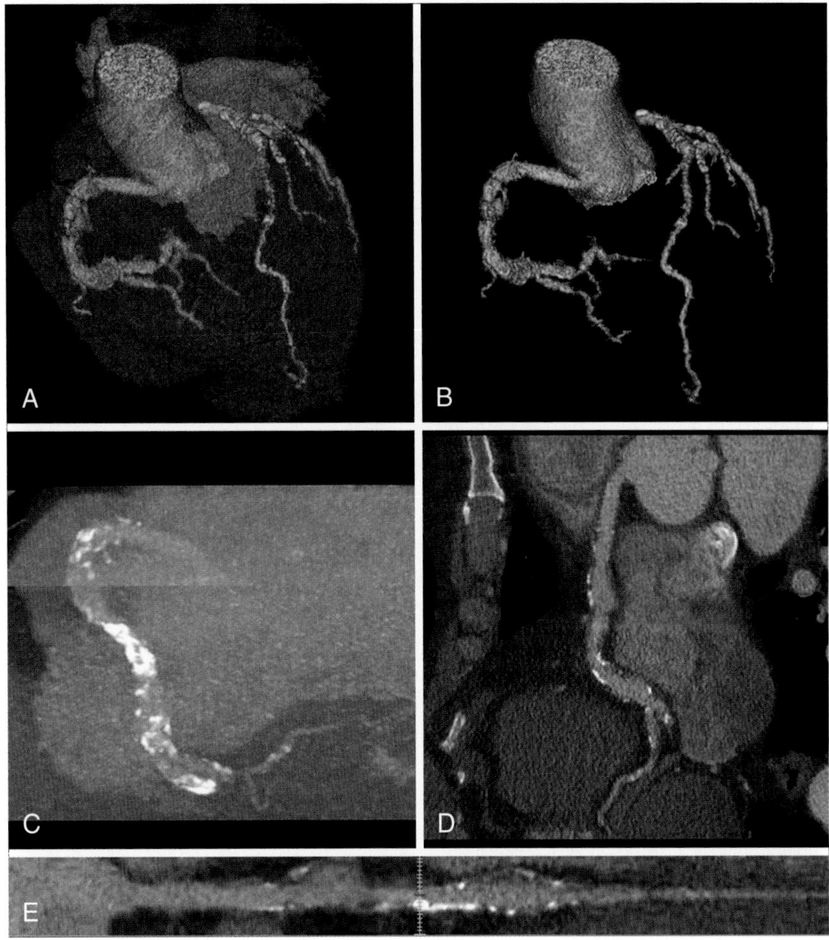

Figure 11-17. Multiple images from a cardiac CT study in a 52-year-old man with suspected coronary artery disease. These images demonstrate atherosclerotic ectasia of the right coronary artery (RCA). There are two focal areas of aneurysmal enlargement of the RCA. The more proximal aneurysm measures 14 mm, within the mid-RCA, and the second, seen in the distal RCA, measures 11 mm. Neither of these aneurysms demonstrates an associated stenosis. Extensive diffuse coronary artery calcification throughout the coronary artery tree (calcium score of 3572) suggests that the likely cause of these aneurysms was atherosclerotic disease.

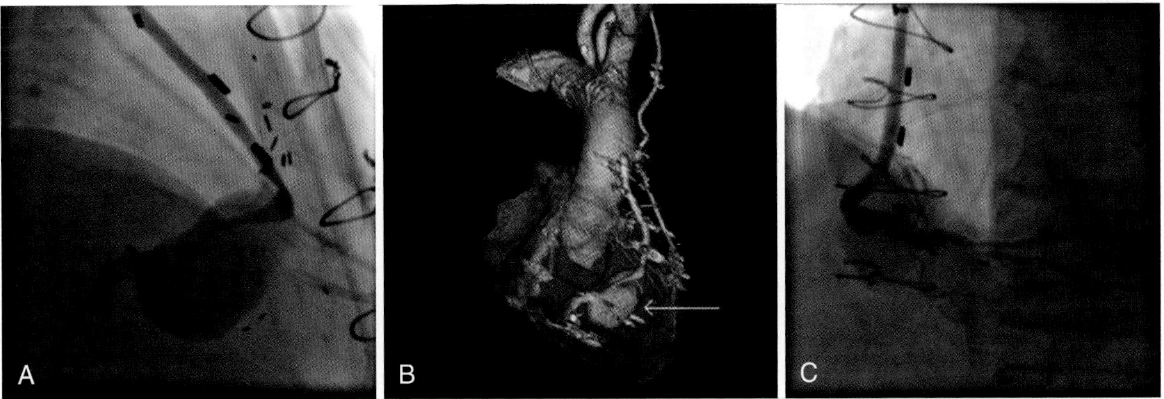

Figure 11-18. **A,** Coronary angiography demonstrates an aneurysm of a saphenous vein bypass graft. **B,** Volume-rendered cardiac CT image depicts the same saphenous vein graft aneurysm. **C,** Angiography post–covered stent exclusion of the vein graft aneurysm.

References

1. Gziut AI, Gil RJ. Coronary aneurysms. *Pol Arch Med Wewn.* 2008;118(12):741-746.
2. Canino-Rodriguez A, Cox RA. Giant coronary aneurysms in a young adult patient with Kawasaki disease. *P R Health Sci J.* 2008;27(4):382-386.
3. Hirooka K, Watanabe T, Ohnuki M. Giant coronary artery aneurysm complicated with aortic regurgitation. *Ann Thorac Surg.* 2009;87(3):935-936.
4. Khositseth A, Siripornpitak S, Pornkul R, Wanitkun S. Case report: Giant coronary aneurysm caused by Kawasaki disease: follow-up with echocardiography and multidetector CT angiography. *Br J Radiol.* 2008;81(964):e106-e109.
5. Peng Y, Zeng J, Du Z, Sun G, Guo H. Usefulness of 64-slice MDCT for follow-up of young children with coronary artery aneurysm due to Kawasaki disease: initial experience. *Eur J Radiol.* 2009;69(3):500-509.
6. Syed M, Lesch M. Coronary artery aneurysm: a review. *Prog Cardiovasc Dis.* 1997;40(1):77-84.
7. Abbate A, Patti G, Dambrosio A, Di Sciascio G. Left main coronary artery aneurysm: a case report and review of the literature. *Ital Heart J.* 2001;2(9):711-714.
8. Hayat SA, Ghani S, More RS. Treatment of ruptured coronary aneurysm with a novel covered stent. *Catheter Cardiovasc Interv.* 2009;74(2):367-370.
9. Stabile E, Escolar E, Weigold G, et al. Marked malapposition and aneurysm formation after sirolimus-eluting coronary stent implantation. *Circulation.* 2004;110(5):e47-e48.
10. Cohen R, Salengro E, Vignaux O, Bical O, Spaulding C. [Large coronary aneurysm diagnosed during an acute coronary syndrome. A case report and review of the literature]. *Arch Mal Coeur Vaiss.* 2006;99(3):247-250.
11. Pineda GE, Khanal S, Mandawat M, Wilkin J. Large atherosclerotic left main coronary aneurysm—a case report and review of the literature. *Angiology.* 2001;52(7):501-504.
12. Levisay JP, Roth RM, Schatz RA. Coronary artery aneurysm formation after drug-eluting stent implantation. *Cardiovasc Revasc Med.* 2008;9(4):284-287.
13. Alfonso F, Perez-Vizcayno MJ, Ruiz M, et al. Coronary aneurysms after drug-eluting stent implantation: clinical, angiographic, and intravascular ultrasound findings. *J Am Coll Cardiol.* 2009;53(22): 2053-2060.
14. Li SS, Cheng BC, Lee SH. Images in cardiovascular medicine. Giant coronary aneurysm formation after sirolimus-eluting stent implantation in Kawasaki disease. *Circulation.* 2005;112(8):e105-e107.
15. Bertrand OF, Mongrain R, Soualmi L, et al. Development of coronary aneurysm after cutting balloon angioplasty: assessment by intracoronary ultrasound. *Cathet Cardiovasc Diagn.* 1998;44(4): 449-452.
16. Okmen E, Sanli A, Kasikcioglu H, Uyarel H, Cam N. Left main coronary artery aneurysm associated with extensive coronary arterial calcification: case report and review. *Int J Cardiovasc Imaging.* 2004;20(3):231-235.
17. Garcia-Lara J, Pinar-Bermudez E, Hurtado JA, Valdez-Chavarri M. Giant true saphenous vein graft aneurysm. *J Am Coll Cardiol.* 2009;54(20):1899.
18. Puri R, Dundon BK, Leong DP, Khurana S, Worthley MI. Hypereosinophilic syndrome associated with multiple coronary aneurysms. *Int J Cardiol.* 2009;133(1):e43-e45.
19. Yilmaz AT, Arslan M, Ozal E, Byngol H, Tatar H, Ozturk OY. Coronary artery aneurysm associated with adult supravalvular aortic stenosis. *Ann Thorac Surg.* 1996;62(4):1205-1207.
20. Takeda K, Matsumiya G, Nishimura M, Matsue H, Tomita Y, Sawa Y. Giant circumflex coronary artery aneurysm associated with cystic medial necrosis in a non-Marfan patient. *Ann Thorac Surg.* 2007;83(2):668-670.
21. Takahashi Y, Sasaki Y, Shibata T, Bito Y, Suehiro S. Successful surgical treatment of a mycotic right coronary artery aneurysm complicated by a fistula to the right atrium. *Jpn J Thorac Cardiovasc Surg.* 2005;53(12):661-664.
22. Fujimoto N, Onishi K, Tanabe M, et al. Two cases of giant aneurysm in coronary-pulmonary artery fistula associated with atherosclerotic change. *Int J Cardiol.* 2004;97(3):577-578.
23. Meraj PM, Makaryus AN, Boxt LM. An unusual combination of myocardial bridging and coronary artery aneurysm identified on 64-detector coronary angiography. *Int J Cardiovasc Imaging.* 2007;23(5):649-653.
24. Villines TC, Avedissian LS, Elgin EE. Diffuse nonatherosclerotic coronary aneurysms: an unusual cause of sudden death in a young male and a literature review. *Cardiol Rev.* 2005;13(6):309-311.
25. Koike R, Oku T, Satoh H, et al. Right ventricular myocardial infarction and late cardiac tamponade due to right coronary artery aneurysm—a case report. *Jpn J Surg.* 1990;20(4):463-467.
26. Bouchiat C, Dussarat GV, Talard P. [Myocardial infarction and coronary artery aneurysm]. *Ann Cardiol Angeiol (Paris).* 1992;41(3): 145-149.
27. Ueyama K, Tomita S, Takehara A, Kamiya H, Mukai K, Kubota S. [A case of surgical treatment for cardiac tamponade caused by a ruptured coronary aneurysm accompanied by a coronary artery-pulmonary artery fistula]. *Kyobu Geka.* 2001;54(1):70-75.
28. Velasco M, Zamorano JL, Almeria C, Ferreiros J, Alfonso F, Sanchez-Harguindey L. [Multiple coronary aneurysms in a young man. A diagnostic approach via different technics]. *Rev Esp Cardiol.* 1999;52(1):55-58.
29. Virmani R, Burke AP, Farb A, Kark JA. Causes of sudden death in young and middle-aged competitive athletes. *Cardiol.Clin.* 1997; 15(3):439-466.
30. Gibbs B, Feuerstein IM, Tavaf H, Villines TC. Giant compressive coronary artery aneurysm delineated by cardiac CT. *J Cardiovasc Comput Tomogr.* 2009;3(5):348-350.
31. Kanamaru H, Sato Y, Inoue F, et al. Detection of coronary artery aneurysms, stenoses and occlusions by means of multislice spiral computed tomography in adolescents and young adults with Kawasaki disease. *J Am Coll Cardiol.* 2004;43(5): A330, Supplement.
32. Kumar G, Karon BL, Edwards WD, Puga FJ, Klarich KW. Giant coronary artery aneurysm causing superior vena cava syndrome and congestive heart failure. *Am J Cardiol.* 2006;98(7): 986-988.
33. Matsubayashi K, Asai T, Nishimura O, et al. Giant coronary artery aneurysm in the left main coronary artery: a novel surgical procedure. *Ann Thorac Surg.* 2008;85(6):2130-2132.
34. Sugimoto K, Kobayashi Y, Miyahara H, Kuroda N, Funabashi N, Komuro I. Early stent thrombosis because of stent dislodgement in a coronary artery aneurysm. *Circ J.* 2009;73(9):1759-1761.
35. Durongpisitkul K, Gururaj VJ, Park JM, Martin CF. The prevention of coronary artery aneurysm in Kawasaki disease: a meta-analysis on the efficacy of aspirin and immunoglobulin treatment. *Pediatrics.* 1995;96(6):1057-1061.
36. Suda K, Kudo Y, Sugawara Y, Ishii M, Matsuishi T. [Prevention of thrombosis of coronary aneurysms in patients with a history of Kawasaki disease]. *Nippon Rinsho.* 2008;66(2):355-359.
37. Mawatari T, Koshino T, Morishita K, Komatsu K, Abe T. Successful surgical treatment of giant coronary artery aneurysm with fistula. *Ann Thorac Surg.* 2000;70(4):1394-1397.
38. Iwamura T, Kikuchi K, Tambara K, et al. [Off-pump coronary artery bypass grafting for angina pectoris with coronary artery aneurysm due to Kawasaki disease: report of a case]. *Kyobu Geka.* 2009;62(6):500-503.
39. Ozler A, Tarhan IA, Kehlibar T, et al. Resection of a right coronary artery aneurysm with fistula to the coronary sinus. *Ann Thorac Surg.* 2008;85(2):649-651.
40. Patila T, Virolainen J, Sipponen J, Heikkila L. Resection and patch repair of a large saccular coronary artery aneurysm at the left main bifurcation. *Ann Thorac Surg.* 2009;87(1):297-299.

12 Coronary Artery Dissections

Key Points

- The conventional test of choice to identify coronary artery dissections is standard coronary angiography.
- Cardiac CT angiography shows some early ability to depict coronary artery dissection; validation is limited.

Although coronary artery dissections are rare overall (0.1–0.3% incidence in angiographic series),[1,2] when they do occur it is usually within the settings of the pregnant or peripartum state, blunt chest trauma, iatrogenesis, or severe exertion or stress, or associated with one of several medical conditions (see Etiologies and Associations).

Coronary artery dissections may be single[3] or multiple[4,5] and may involve all three coronary arteries[6,7] and the left main stem coronary artery.[8-11]

Repeated angiography may reveal regression or healing,[12-14] although progression has been described,[15] as has recurrence, and conventional catheter-based angiography may initiate coronary artery dissection.[16]

Some coronary artery dissections, usually iatrogenic ones, may propagate retrograde back into the aortic root.[17] Most spontaneous coronary artery dissections remain within the coronary tree.

ETIOLOGIES AND ASSOCIATIONS

- Hormone-associated[18]
  - Oral contraception–related[19]
  - Pregnancy-associated[9]
    - Mid-term[20]
    - Third trimester[15]
    - Twin pregnancy[21]
  - Peri-/postpartum–associated[22]
  - Post-abortion[23]
  - Menstruation-associated[24-26]
  - Postmenopausal[5,27,28]
- Nonhormone-associated
  - Iatrogenic
    - Coronary angiography[29]
    - Percutaneous coronary intervention
      - Plain old balloon angioplasty (POBA)
      - Coronary artery stenting (bare metal; drug-eluting)
      - Cutting balloon[30]
      - Intracoronary radiation[31]
      - Intravascular ultrasound (IVUS)
    - Cryoablation for atrial fibrillation[32]
    - Coronary artery bypass grafting
  - Drug abuse–associated
    - Cocaine abuse[31,33,34]
    - Ergotamine abuse[35]
  - Drug-associated
    - Fenfluramine[25]
    - 5-FU[36]
  - Hypertension-associated
    - Retching-associated[37]
    - Weight-lifting–associated[38]
  - Acute aortic dissection (type A)[39]
  - Acute aortic dissection, despite repair of the dissected aorta[40]
  - Supravalvular aortic stenosis[41]
  - Disease-associated
    - Active inflammatory bowel disease[42]
    - Systemic lupus erythematosus[43]
    - Polycystic kidney disease[44,45]
    - Renal transplantation–associated[46]
    - Anti-phospholipid antibody[14,47,48]
    - Alpha-1 antitrypsin–associated[49]
    - Pulmonary embolism[2]
  - Vascular disease–associated
    - Eosinophilic monoarteritis[3]
    - Fibromuscular dysplasia[29,50]
    - Coronary ectasia[4]
  - Inheritable connective tissue disorder
    - Marfan syndrome
    - Cystic medial necrosis[8]
  - Exertion
    - Skiing at altitude[10]
    - Wrestling[51]
    - Exercise/athleticism/strenuous workouts[52-56]

- Neurofibromatosis (type 1—vasculopathy-associated)[57]
- Stress-associated
  - Sleep deprivation (72 hours)[58]
  - Depression[59]
  - Emotional stress[60]
- Sexual intercourse[61]
- Blunt chest trauma[62-68]

CLINICAL PRESENTATIONS OF SPONTANEOUS DISSECTIONS

- ❒ Chest pain
- ❒ Stable angina[6,69] (likely due to organization/evolution of dissection into a coronary artery stenosis or occlusion)
- ❒ Acute coronary syndrome[70]
- ❒ Myocardial infarction (MI)[15,44,52,53]
  - ST-elevation myocardial infarction (STEMI)
  - Non-STEMI
- ❒ Transient ST elevation[71]
- ❒ Sudden death[3,72,73]
- ❒ Atrial fibrillation and tamponade due to rupture of the dissected artery[74]
- ❒ Tamponade due to rupture of the dissected artery[75]
- ❒ Aortic dissection–like[76]
- ❒ Stroke (due to coronary dissection resulting in MI)[77]

Ischemic presentations dominate. It has been suggested that inadvertent use of thrombolytics for STEMI due to spontaneous coronary dissection may predispose the coronary dissection to extension.[78] Arrhythmic presentations and sudden death are relatively common for this diagnosis. Rupture of the artery with tamponade has been described, as have other indirect complications or presentations. Multivascular occurrences (e.g., stroke, renovascular disease) should prompt consideration of vasculitides, including the inheritable variants and fibromuscular dysplasia.

TREATMENT

- ❒ Observation and medical treatment, without or with repeat imaging[12,13,79,80]
- ❒ Stenting[15,80-82]
- ❒ Surgical bypass or repair[5]

DIAGNOSTIC TESTING FOR CORONARY DISSECTIONS

Conventional angiography has been and remains the standard diagnostic test to diagnose coronary artery dissections, although, unfortunately, it may also *cause* coronary dissection. IVUS, performed at the time of angiography, is able to visualize a subset of coronary dissection cases that are ambiguously represented on angiography.[37] Transesophageal echocardiography (TEE) has detected spontaneous coronary dissection, but would be expected to have very limited ability to interrogate the coronary tree.[83] TEE would be able to image dissection of the aorta extending into a coronary artery, or coronary dissection extending into the aortic root.

Coronary CT angiography (CTA) has been used to image coronary artery dissections (see Figures 12-1 through 12-10).[9,53,63,64,84-92]

POTENTIAL CORONARY CTA FINDINGS IN CORONARY DISSECTION CASES

- ❒ Intimal flap
- ❒ True and false lumens
- ❒ Pseudoaneurysm formation of the artery[9,91]
- ❒ Signs of myocardial infarction
- ❒ Complications of myocardial infarction
- ❒ Aneurysm[93]
- ❒ Mural thrombi[86]

CORONARY CTA PROTOCOL SPECIFICS

Standard coronary CTA protocols may suffice for imaging of coronary dissection, although additional effort, such as multiple phase reconstructions, may be needed to depict more distal or branch vessel lesions, because proximal coronary anatomy is more amenable to the depiction of coronary dissection by current cardiac CT technology.

CARDIAC CT PROTOCOL POINTS

The standard cardiac CT protocol is utilized.

AMERICAN COLLEGE OF CARDIOLOGY FOUNDATION 2011 APPROPRIATENESS CRITERIA

No appropriateness criteria have been specified by the American College of Cardiology Foundation (ACCF) for suspected or proven coronary artery dissections.

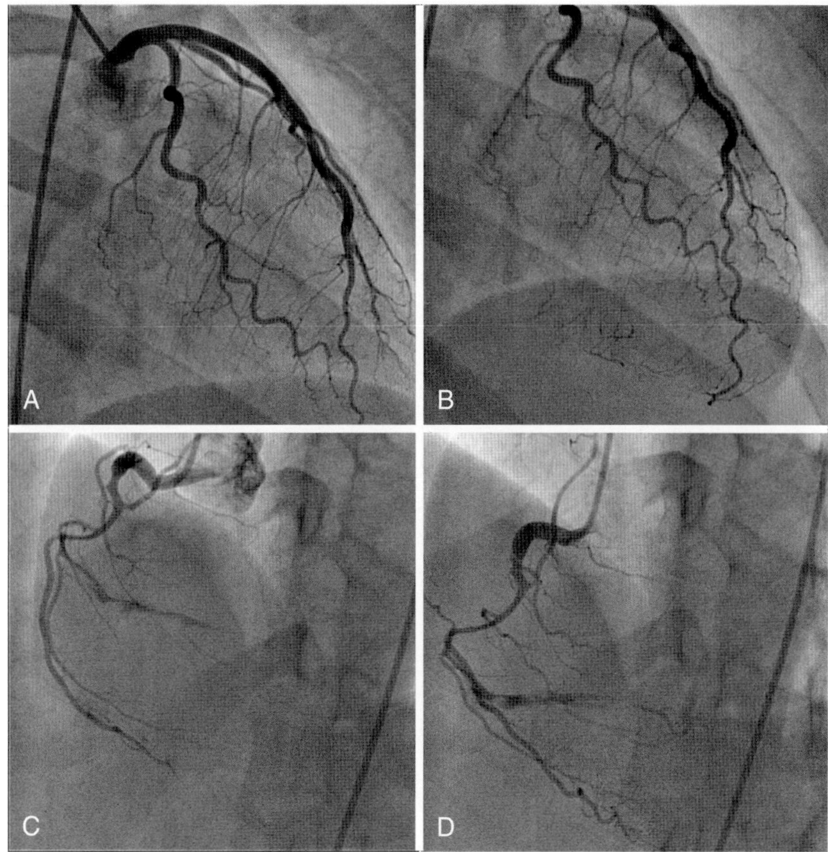

Figure 12-1. A 44-year-old woman presents with an acute coronary syndrome (ACS). Conventional coronary angiography demonstrates a normal left main and left anterior descending (LAD) coronary arteries (**A**), but with faint collateralization to the posterior descending coronary artery (PDA), primarily via septal perforators (**B**). **C** and **D,** Poor opacification of the right coronary artery (RCA) with an RCA dissection involving the proximal to mid-RCA. See Figure 12-2.

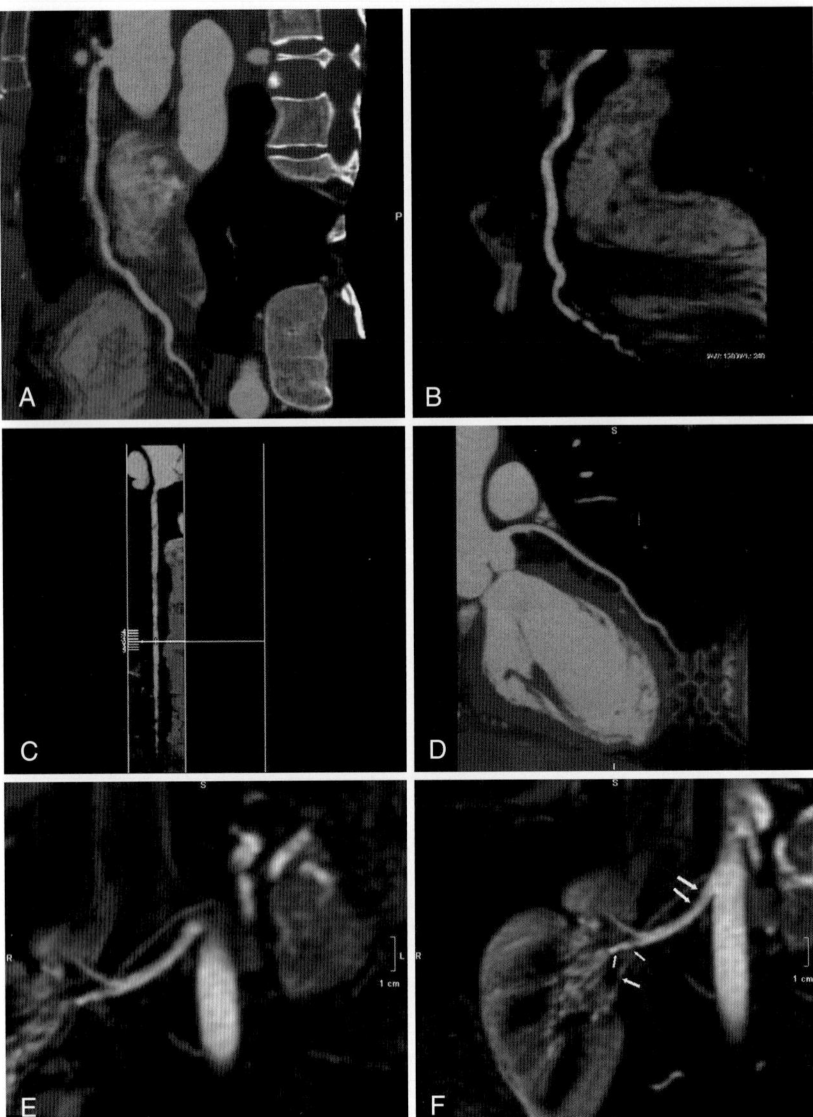

Figure 12-2. Same case as Figure 12-1. **A–D,** Multiple curved reformations from a cardiac CT confirm a normal left anterior descending artery and right coronary artery dissection with contrast in both lumens well demonstrated. Additionally, multifocal "beaded" stenoses in the posterior descending coronary artery are seen. These are not associated with any soft or calcified plaque and are suspicious for coronary artery involvement with fibromuscular dysplasia, and its basis or cause of the coronary dissection. **E–F,** Maximum intensity projection images from renal gadolinium-enhanced magnetic resonance angiography demonstrate mild beaded irregularity of the right renal artery consistent with fibromuscular dysplasia.

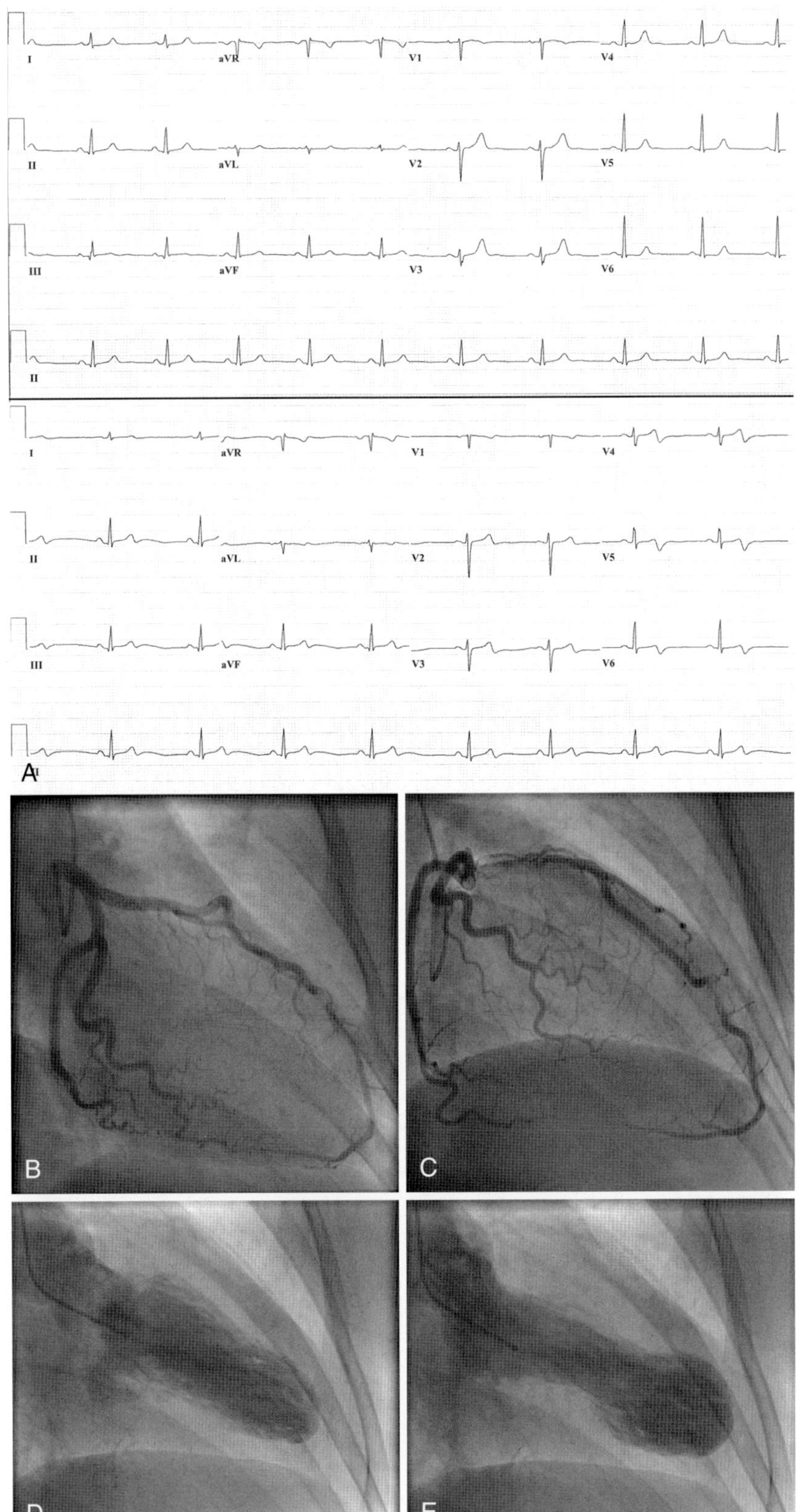

Figure 12-3. A 32-year-old woman 4 weeks postpartum presents with chest pain, toponin elevation, and an abnormal ECG. Apical akinesis was identified on echocardiography. The first and second ECGs on the first and second days in the hospital reveal evolution from extensive mild repolarization abnormalities to obviously biphasic T waves. Conventional angiographic images demonstrate a small localized mid- to distal left anterior descending artery dissection with akinesis of the left ventricular apex.

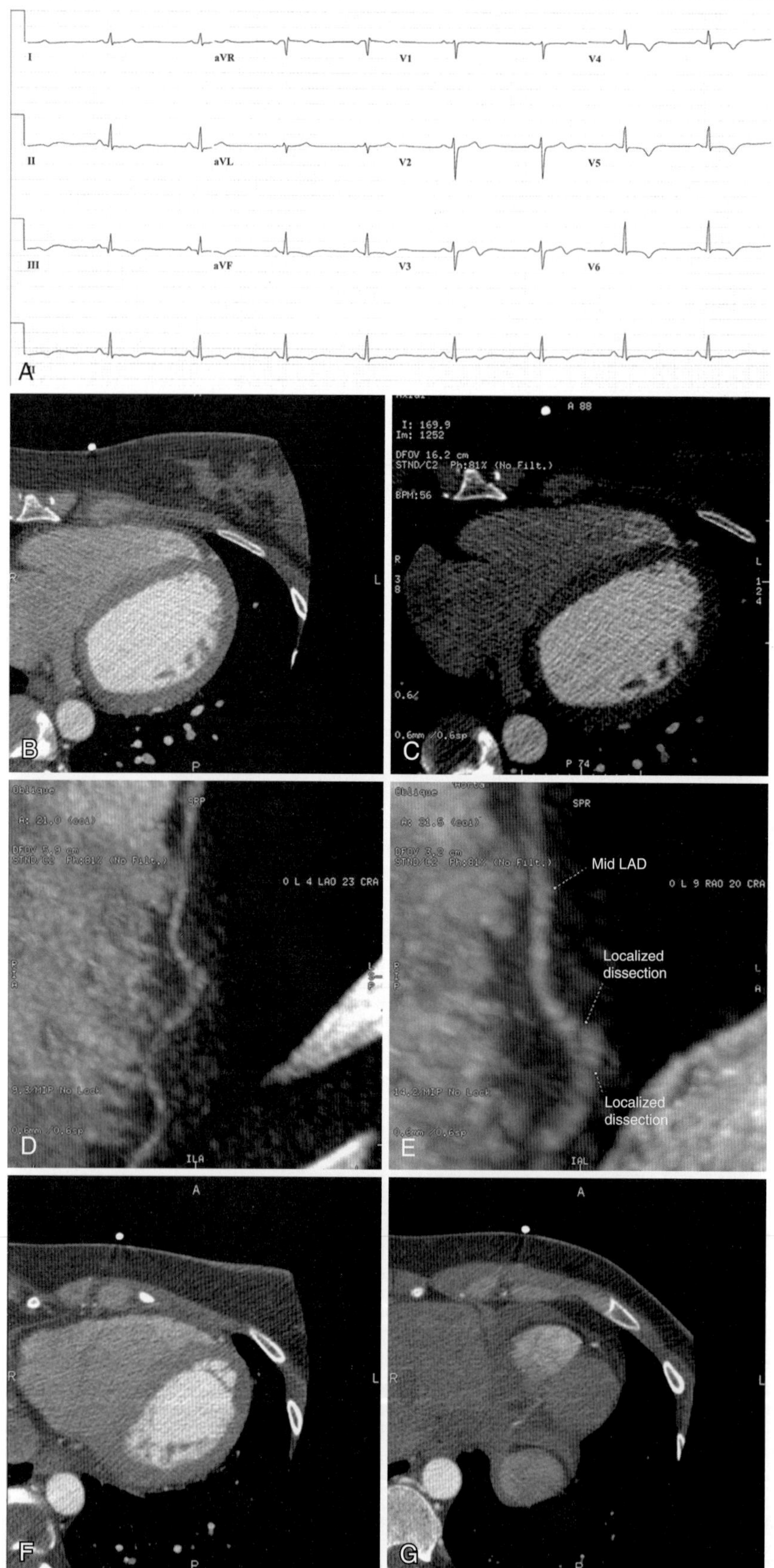

Figure 12-4. A 39-year-old woman with a bicuspid aortic valve, chest pain, and left main coronary artery dissection seen at conventional coronary angiography. Follow-up cardiac CT demonstrates a localized left main coronary artery dissection with a small associated false aneurysm. The false aneurysm has a small amount of thrombus within it. The patient went on to coronary artery bypass grafting (CABG). LAD, left anterior descending artery. See Figure 12-5.

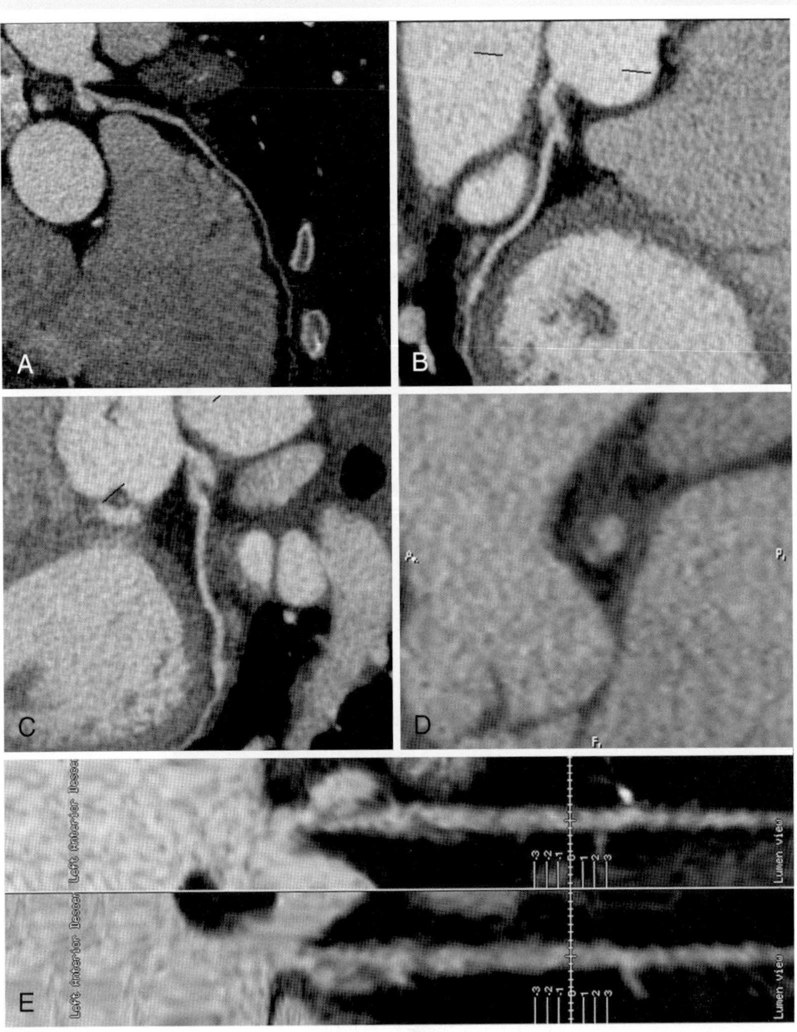

Figure 12-5. Same case as Figure 12-4. Ongoing intermittent chest pain associated with evolving ECG repolarization changes and rising troponin levels led to CT angiography evaluation 2 days later to rule out proximal extension of the dissection, or dissection of another vessel. Axial source images windowed differently demonstrate two contrast-filled lumina within the mid distal left anterior descending artery. Curved reformats demonstrate the focal dissection with no evidence of proximal or distal extension. Note how the dissection is "sandwiched" between two regions of superficial myocardial bridging.

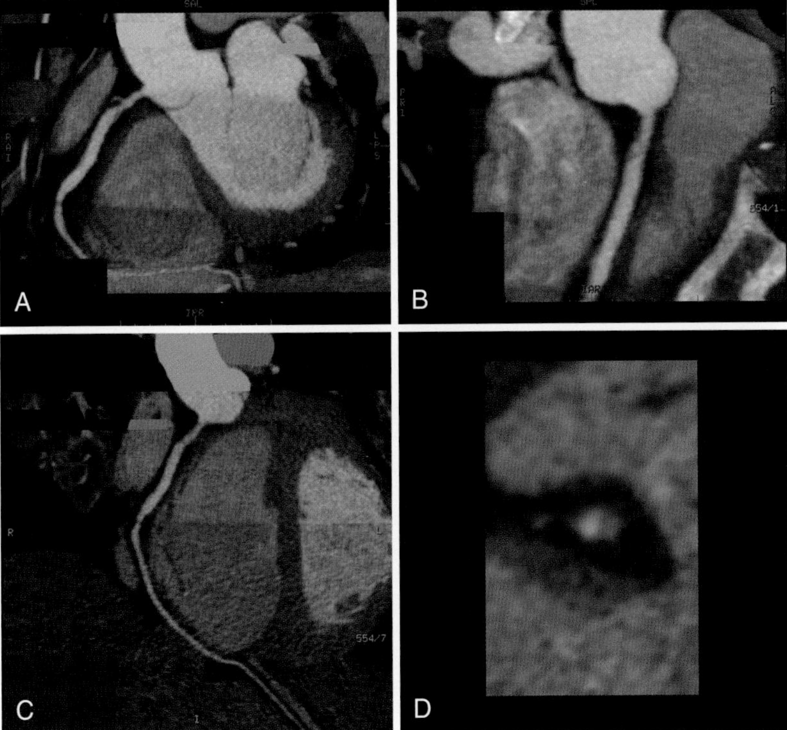

Figure 12-6. A 5-mm dissection is present in the proximal right coronary artery, seen on these curved multiplanar images and an intravascular ultrasound image.

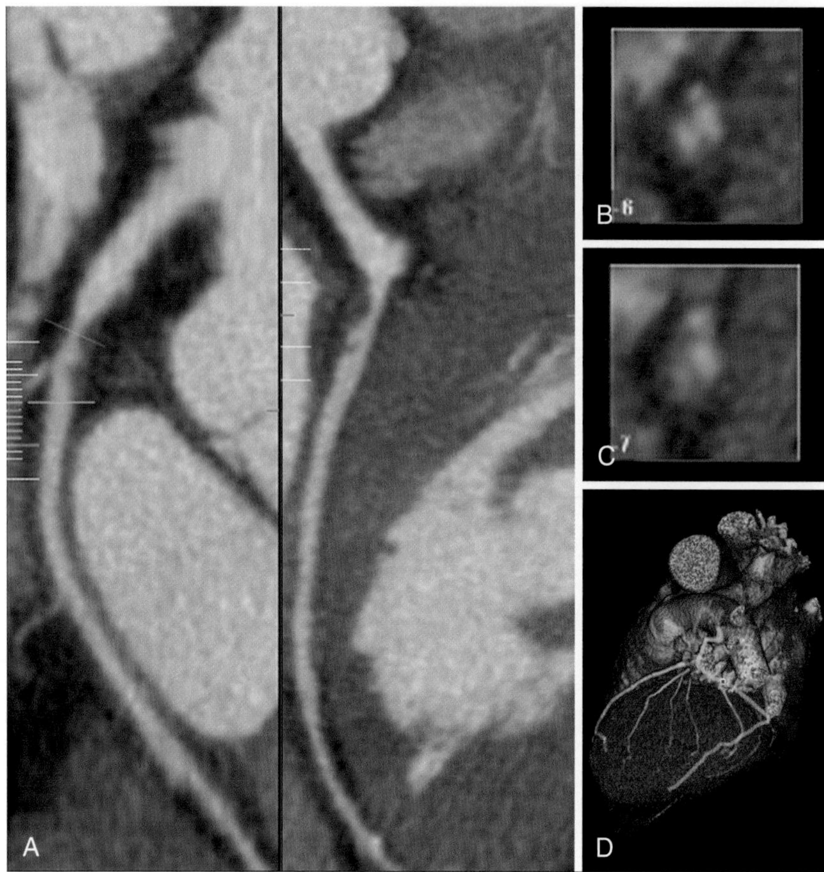

Figure 12-7. Curved multiplanar images (**A**) and "intravascular ultrasound" views (**B** and **C**) of a complex ulcerated and dissected proximal left circumflex artery lesion. **D,** Volume-rendered view.

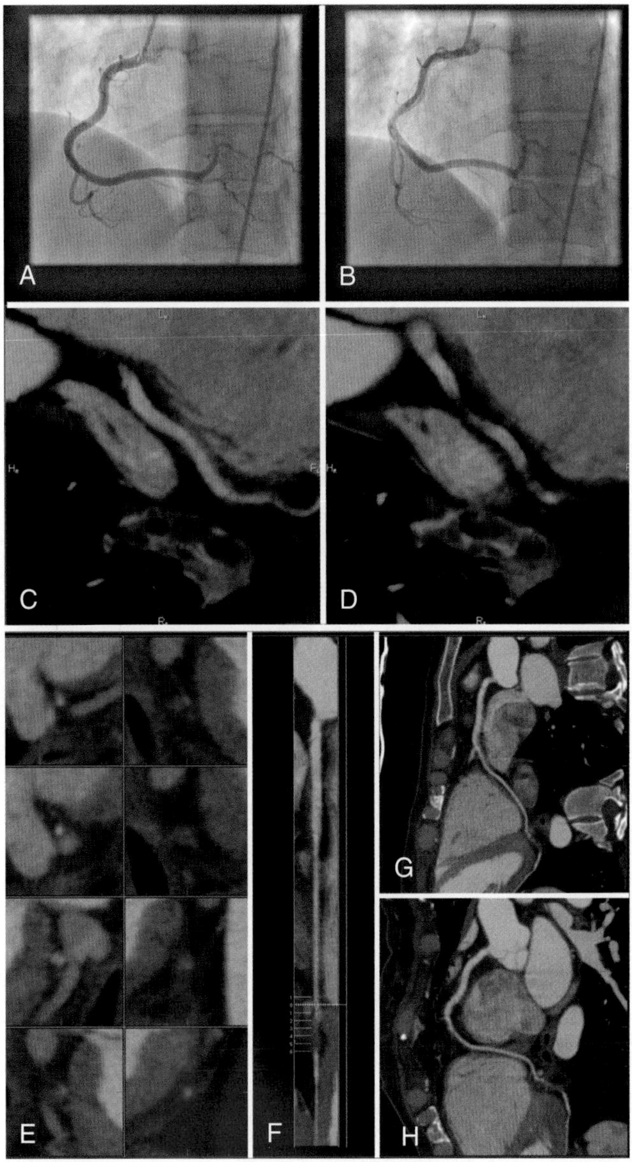

Figure 12-8. Conventional angiography and CT coronary angiography of a postpartum patient with a catheter-induced dissection of the right coronary artery.

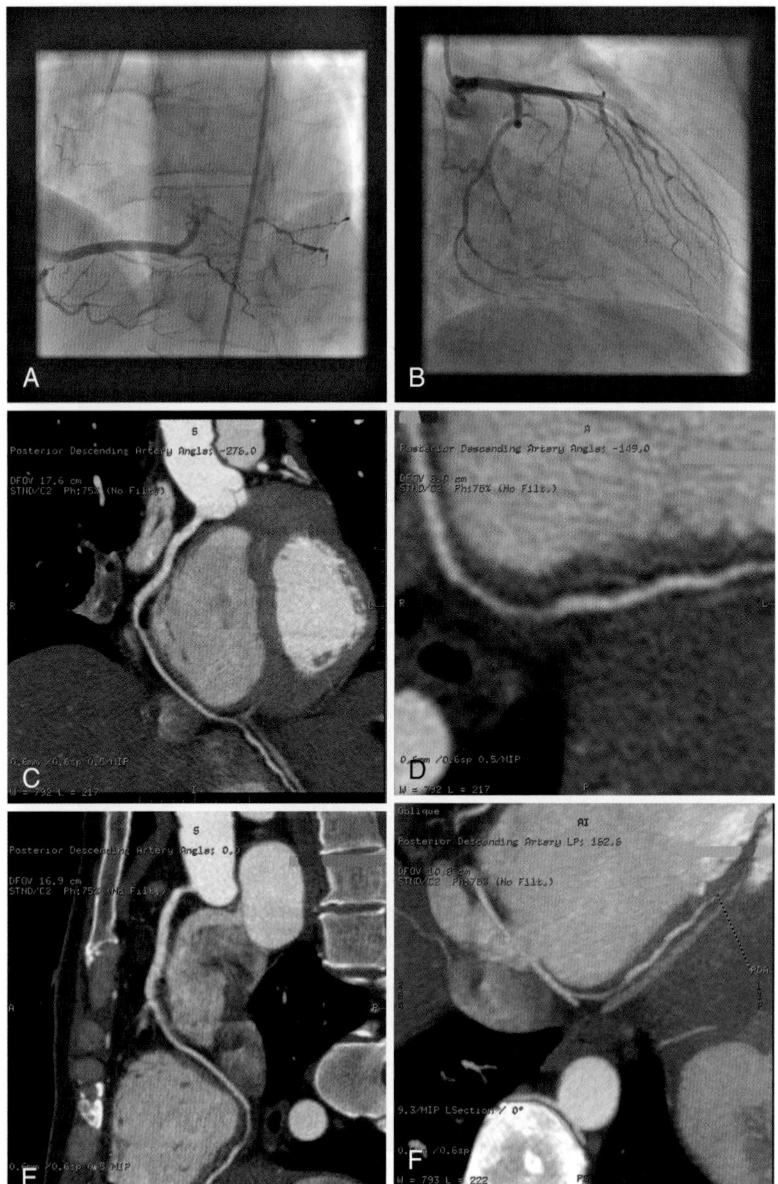

Figure 12-9. Conventional angiography and CT coronary angiography of a postpartum patient with spontaneous dissections of the posterolateral coronary artery branches.

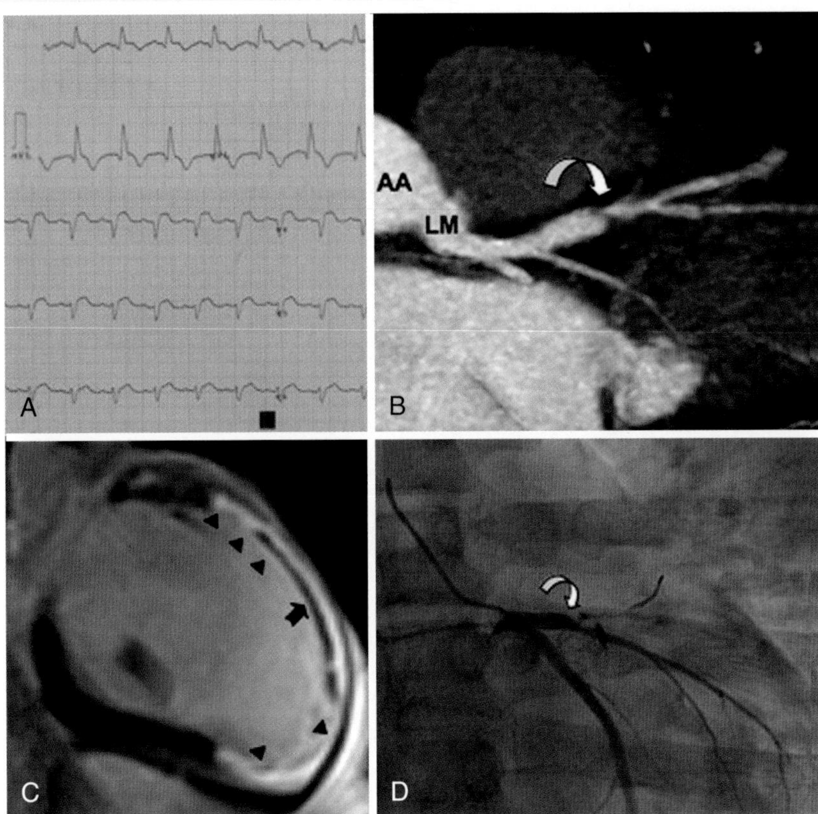

Figure 12-10. A 16-year-old boy involved in a car accident sustained a blunt chest trauma. He was admitted to the emergency department because of severe chest pain associated with remarkable elevation of the ST-segment in the anterior leads (**A**). A chest CT scan excluded pericardial, aortic, and major vessel disease while showing bilateral lung contusions. **B,** ECG-gated coronary CT angiography detected a dissection of the proximal left anterior descending artery (*curved arrow*), with distal opacification of the vessel. **C,** Late gadolinium enhancement cardiac MRI demonstrated an extensive acute transmural infarction of the anterior and apical wall of the left ventricle (*arrowheads*), with concomitant extensive microvascular damage (*black arrow*). Cine imaging showed regional akinesia of the anteroseptal left ventricular wall. **D,** Coronary angiography confirmed a focal dissection of the proximal left anterior descending artery (*curved arrow*). AA, ascending aorta; LM, left main coronary artery. (Reprinted with permission from Carbone I, Francone M, Galea N, et al. Images in cardiology. Computed-tomography and magnetic resonance imaging assessment of traumatic left anterior descending coronary dissection causing acute myocardial infarction. *J Am Coll Cardiol.* 2011;57(2):e3.)

References

1. Bulum J, Strozzi M, Smalcelj A. Spontaneous and catheter-induced secondary coronary artery dissection: a single-centre experience. *Acta Cardiol.* 2008;63(2):203-206.
2. Gul I, Basar E, Cetinkaya Y, Kasapkara A, Kalay N, Ozdogru I. Spontaneous coronary artery dissection and pulmonary thromboembolism: a case report. *Int J Cardiol.* 2007;118(1):e21-e23.
3. Stoukas V, Dragovic LJ. Sudden deaths from eosinophilic coronary monoarteritis: a subset of spontaneous coronary artery dissection. *Am J Forensic Med Pathol.* 2009;30(3):268-269.
4. Goz M, Soylemez N, Demirbag R. Images in cardio-thoracic surgery: multiple spontaneous coronary artery dissection presenting in association with coronary ectasia. *Eur J Cardiothorac Surg.* 2009;35(5):907.
5. Konstantinov IE, Saxena P, Shehatha J. Spontaneous multivessel coronary artery dissection: surgical management in a postmenopausal woman. *Tex Heart Inst J.* 2009;36(4):360-361.
6. Harikrishnan S, Ajithkumar VK, Tharakan JM. Spontaneous coronary artery dissection of all major coronary arteries. *Can J Cardiol.* 2007;23(4):313-314.
7. Ooi A, Lavrsen M, Monro J, Langley SM. Successful emergency surgery on triple-vessel spontaneous coronary artery dissection. *Eur J Cardiothorac Surg.* 2004;26(2):447-449.
8. Hirose H, Matsunaga I, Anjun W, Strong MD. Spontaneous left main coronary artery dissection, possibly due to cystic medial necrosis found in the internal mammary arteries. *Interact Cardiovasc Thorac Surg.* 2009;9(4):725-727.
9. Rahman S, Abdul-Waheed M, Helmy T, et al. Spontaneous left main coronary artery dissection complicated by pseudoaneurysm formation in pregnancy: role of CT coronary angiography. *J Cardiothorac Surg.* 2009;4:15.
10. Dworakowski R, Desai J, MacCarthy P. Spontaneous left main coronary artery dissection while skiing at altitude. *Eur Heart J.* 2009;30(7):868.
11. Unal M, Korkut AK, Kosem M, Ertunc V, Ozcan M, Caglar N. Surgical management of spontaneous coronary artery dissection. *Tex Heart Inst J.* 2008;35(4):402-405.
12. Kalra N, Greenblatt J, Ahmed S. Postpartum spontaneous coronary artery dissection (SCAD) managed conservatively. *Int J Cardiol.* 2008;129(2):e53-e55.
13. Erdim R, Gormez S, Aytekin V. Spontaneous healing of spontaneous coronary artery dissection: a case report. *J Invasive Cardiol.* 2008;20(8): E237-E238.
14. Reed RK, Malaiapan Y, Meredith IT. Spontaneous coronary artery dissection in a female with antiphospholipid syndrome. *Heart Lung Circ.* 2007;16(2):120-122.
15. Azzarelli S, Fiscella D, Amico F, Giacoppo M, Argentino V, Fiscella A. Multivessel spontaneous coronary artery dissection in a postpartum woman treated with multiple drug-eluting stents. *J Cardiovasc Med (Hagerstown).* 2009;10(4):340-343.
16. Eddinger J, Dietz WA. Recurrent spontaneous coronary artery dissection. *Catheter Cardiovasc Interv.* 2005;66(4):566-569.
17. Park IW, Min PK, Cho DK, Byun KH. Successful endovascular treatment of iatrogenic coronary artery dissection extending into the entire ascending aorta. *Can J Cardiol.* 2008;24(11):857-859.
18. Cano O, Almenar L, Chirivella M, Martinez L. Idiopathic spontaneous coronary artery dissection. Clinical and pathological correlate. *Int J Cardiol.* 2009;133(1):e18-e19.
19. Muretto P. Images in pathology. Spontaneous coronary artery dissection as cause of sudden cardiac death in a young woman with oral contraceptive use. *Int J Surg Pathol.* 2006;14(4):331.
20. Tang AT, Cusimano RJ. Spontaneous coronary artery dissection complicating midterm pregnancy. *Ann Thorac Surg.* 2004;78(2): e35.
21. Phillips LM, Makaryus AN, Beldner S, Spatz A, Smith-Levitin M, Marchant D. Coronary artery dissection during pregnancy treated with medical therapy. *Cardiol Rev.* 2006;14(3):155-157.
22. Hammond AS, Bailey PL. Acute spontaneous coronary artery dissection in the peripartum period. *J Cardiothorac Vasc Anesth.* 2006;20(6):837-841.
23. Iltumur K, Karahan Z, Ozmen S, Danis R, Toprak N. Spontaneous coronary artery dissection during hemodialysis in the post-abortion period. *Int J Cardiol.* 2008;127(2):e45-e47.
24. Skelding KA, Hubbard CR. Spontaneous coronary artery dissection related to menstruation. *J Invasive Cardiol.* 2007;19(6):E174-E177.

25. Goli AK, Koduri M, Haddadin T, Henry PD. Spontaneous coronary artery dissection in a woman on fenfluramine. *Rev Cardiovasc Med.* 2007;8(1):41-44.
26. Slight R, Behranwala AA, Nzewi O, Sivaprakasam R, Brackenbury E, Mankad P. Spontaneous coronary artery dissection: a report of two cases occurring during menstruation. *N Z Med J.* 2003;116(1181):U585.
27. Leone F, Macchiusi A, Ricci R, Cerquetani E, Reynaud M. Acute myocardial infarction from spontaneous coronary artery dissection: a case report and review of the literature. *Cardiol Rev.* 2004;12(1):3-9.
28. Salmo E, Callaghan J. Spontaneous coronary artery dissection in a healthy postmenopausal woman. *Med Sci Law.* 2002;42(2):126-128.
29. de Jong J, Piek J, van der Wal A. Multifocal arterial fibromuscular dysplasia causing coronary artery dissection following coronary angiography. *EuroIntervention.* 2009;5(1):166.
30. Niccoli G, Orr WP, Banning AP. Extensive right coronary artery dissection following cutting balloon treatment of in-stent restenosis. *J Invasive Cardiol.* 2002;14(4):209-211.
31. Kay IP, Sabate M, Van Langenhove G, et al. Outcome from balloon induced coronary artery dissection after intracoronary beta radiation. *Heart.* 2000;83(3):332-337.
32. Doguet F, Le Guillou V, Litzler PY, et al. Coronary artery dissection after surgical cryoablation procedure. *Ann Thorac Surg.* 2009;87(6):1946-1948.
33. Steinhauer JR, Caulfield JB. Spontaneous coronary artery dissection associated with cocaine use: a case report and brief review. *Cardiovasc Pathol.* 2001;10(3):141-145.
34. Eskander KE, Brass NS, Gelfand ET. Cocaine abuse and coronary artery dissection. *Ann Thorac Surg.* 2001;71(1):340-341.
35. Garcia Garcia C, Casanovas N, Recasens L, Miranda F, Bruguera J. Spontaneous coronary artery dissection in ergotamine abuse. *Int J Cardiol.* 2007;118(3):410-411.
36. Abbott JD, Curtis JP, Murad K, et al. Spontaneous coronary artery dissection in a woman receiving 5-fluorouracil—a case report. *Angiology.* 2003;54(6):721-724.
37. Velusamy M, Fisherkeller M, Keenan ME, Kiernan FJ, Fram DB. Spontaneous coronary artery dissection in a young woman precipitated by retching. *J Invasive Cardiol.* 2002;14(4):198-201.
38. Aghasadeghi K, Aslani A. Spontaneous coronary artery dissection in a professional body builder. *Int J Cardiol.* 2008;130(3):e119-e120.
39. Jo SH, Kang HJ, Koo BK. Coronary artery dissection associated with ascending aortic dissection. *Can J Cardiol.* 2008;24(8):643.
40. Funatsu T, Fukuda H, Takeuchi M, Masai M, Kawano S, Abe K. Progression of left coronary artery dissection during and after aortic replacement in acute type A aortic dissection: a case report. *Ann Thorac Cardiovasc Surg.* 2007;13(3):209-212.
41. van Son JA, Edwards WD, Danielson GK. Pathology of coronary arteries, myocardium, and great arteries in supravalvular aortic stenosis. Report of five cases with implications for surgical treatment. *J Thorac Cardiovasc Surg.* 1994;108(1):21-28.
42. Srinivas M, Basumani P, Muthusamy R, Wheeldon N. Active inflammatory bowel disease and coronary artery dissection. *Postgrad Med J.* 2005;81(951):68-70.
43. Kothari D, Ruygrok P, Gentles T, Occleshaw C. Spontaneous coronary artery dissection in an adolescent man with systemic lupus erythematosus. *Intern Med J.* 2007;37(5):342-343.
44. Basile C, Lucarelli K, Langialonga T. Spontaneous coronary artery dissection: one more extrarenal manifestation of autosomal dominant polycystic kidney disease? *J Nephrol.* 2009;22(3):414-416.
45. Itty CT, Farshid A, Talaulikar G. Spontaneous coronary artery dissection in a woman with polycystic kidney disease. *Am J Kidney Dis.* 2009;53(3):518-521.
46. Tsimikas S, Giordano FJ, Tarazi RY, Beyer RW. Spontaneous coronary artery dissection in patients with renal transplantation. *J Invasive Cardiol.* 1999;11(5):316-321.
47. Kiernan TJ, Rochford M. Postpartum spontaneous coronary artery dissection: an important clinical link with anticardiolipin antibody. *Int J Cardiol.* 2007;114(2):E75-E76.
48. Krishnamurthy M, Desai R, Patel H. Spontaneous coronary artery dissection in the postpartum period: association with antiphospholipid antibody. *Heart.* 2004;90(9):e53.
49. Martin Davila F, Delgado Portela M, Garcia Rojo M, et al. Coronary artery dissection in alpha-1-antitrypsin deficiency. *Histopathology.* 1999;34(4):376-378.
50. Brodsky SV, Ramaswamy G, Chander P, Braun A. Ruptured cerebral aneurysm and acute coronary artery dissection in the setting of multivascular fibromuscular dysplasia: a case report. *Angiology.* 2007;58(6):764-767.
51. Tacoy G, Sahinarslan A, Timurkaynak T. Spontaneous multivessel coronary artery dissection in a wrestler. *Anadolu Kardiyol Derg.* 2007;7(2):193-195.
52. Kurum T, Aktoz M. Spontaneous coronary artery dissection after heavy lifting in a 25-year-old man with coronary risk factors. *J Cardiovasc Med (Hagerstown).* 2006;7(1):68-70.
53. Cardenas GA, Grines CL, Sheldon M, Goldstein JA. Spontaneous coronary artery dissection. *South Med J.* 2008;101(4):442-446.
54. Kalaga RV, Malik A, Thompson PD. Exercise-related spontaneous coronary artery dissection: case report and literature review. *Med Sci Sports Exerc.* 2007;39(8):1218-1220.
55. Umman S, Olcay A, Sezer M, Erdogan D. Exercise-induced coronary artery dissection treated with an anticoagulant and antiaggregants. *Anadolu Kardiyol Derg.* 2006;6(4):385-386.
56. Ellis CJ, Haywood GA, Monro JL. Spontaneous coronary artery dissection in a young woman resulting from an intense gymnasium "work-out.". *Int J Cardiol.* 1994;47(2):193-194.
57. Giugliano GR, Sethi PS. Spontaneous left anterior descending coronary artery dissection in a patient with neurofibromatosis. *J Invasive Cardiol.* 2009;21(6):e103-e105.
58. Suh SY, Kim JW, Choi CU, et al. Complete angiographic resolution of spontaneous coronary artery dissection associated with sleep deprivation. *Int J Cardiol.* 2007;119(2):e38-e39.
59. Ho YD, Koizumi T, Lee DP. Spontaneous coronary artery dissection in a woman with depression without coronary atherosclerotic risk factors. *J Invasive Cardiol.* 2007;19(6):E166-E168.
60. Anisman SD, Joelson JM. Left main coronary artery dissection associated with emotional stress. *Dis Mon.* 2006;52(6):227-253.
61. Schifferdecker B, Pacifico L, Ramsaran EK, Folland ED, Spodick DH, Weiner BH. Spontaneous coronary artery dissection associated with sexual intercourse. *Am J Cardiol.* 2004;93(10):1323-1324.
62. Li CH, Chiu TF, Chen JC. Extensive anterolateral myocardial infarction caused by left main coronary artery dissection after blunt chest trauma: a case report. *Am J Emerg Med.* 2007;25(7):858 e853-e855.
63. Sato Y, Matsumoto N, Komatsu S, et al. Coronary artery dissection after blunt chest trauma: depiction at multidetector-row computed tomography. *Int J Cardiol.* 2007;118(1):108-110.
64. Smayra T, Noun R, Tohme-Noun C. Left anterior descending coronary artery dissection after blunt chest trauma: assessment by multi-detector row computed tomography. *J Thorac Cardiovasc Surg.* 2007;133(3):811-812.
65. Ryu JK, Kim KS, Lee JB, Choi JY, Chang SG, Ko S. Coronary artery stenting in a patient with angina pectoris caused by coronary artery dissection after blunt chest trauma. *Int J Cardiol.* 2007;114(3):e89-e90.
66. Hobelmann A, Pham JC, Hsu EB. Case of the month: Right coronary artery dissection following sports-related blunt trauma. *Emerg Med J.* 2006;23(7):580-581.
67. Patila T, Virolainen J, Sipponen J, Heikkila L. Resection and patch repair of a large saccular coronary artery aneurysm at the left main bifurcation. *Ann Thorac Surg.* 2009;87(1):297-299.
68. Carbone I, Francone M, Galea N, Benedetti G, Frustaci A. Images in cardiology. Computed-tomography and magnetic resonance imaging assessment of traumatic left anterior descending coronary artery dissection causing acute myocardial infarction. *J Am Coll Cardiol.* 2011;57(2):e3.
69. Chang SM, Huh A, Bianco JA, Wann LS. Spontaneous coronary dissection on multiple detector computed tomography (MDCT). *J Cardiovasc Comput Tomog.* 2007;1:60-61.
70. Monte I, Grasso S, Scandura S, Mangiafico S, Tamburino C. Spontaneous coronary artery dissection: a report of two atypical cases. *Heart Vessels.* 2009;24(5):380-384.
71. Tsiamis E, Toutouzas K, Stefanadis C. Spontaneous coronary artery dissection in a pre-menopausal woman presenting with transient ST segment elevation. *Heart.* 2003;89(11):1326.
72. Bicer M, Saba D, Ozdemir B, Ercan A. Idiopathic spontaneous coronary artery dissection: a case report. *Thorac Cardiovasc Surg.* 2008;56(8):486-488.
73. Bergen E, Huffer L, Peele M. Survival after spontaneous coronary artery dissection presenting with ventricular fibrillation arrest. *J Invasive Cardiol.* 2005;17(10):E4-E6.
74. Hayes CR, Lewis D. Spontaneous coronary artery dissection of the left circumflex artery causing cardiac tamponade and presenting with atrial fibrillation: a case report and review of the literature. *Angiology.* 2007;58(5):630-635.
75. Badmanaban B, McCarty D, Mole DJ, McKeown PP, Sarsam MA. Spontaneous coronary artery dissection presenting as cardiac tamponade. *Ann Thorac Surg.* 2002;73(4):1324-1326.
76. Kim SH, Kim MK, Kim EJ, Park WJ, Choi YJ, Rhim CY. Spontaneous coronary artery dissection mimicking acute aortic dissection. *Angiology.* 2008;59(3):382-384.
77. Jaigobin C, Silver FL. Stroke secondary to post-partum coronary artery dissection. *Can J Neurol Sci.* 2003;30(2):168-170.

78. Zupan I, Noc M, Trinkaus D, Popovic M. Double vessel extension of spontaneous left main coronary artery dissection in young women treated with thrombolytics. *Catheter Cardiovasc Interv.* 2001;52(2):226-230.
79. Satoda M, Takagi K, Uesugi M, et al. Acute myocardial infarction caused by spontaneous postpartum coronary artery dissection. *Nat Clin Pract Cardiovasc Med.* 2007;4(12):688-692.
80. Sarmento-Leite R, Machado PR, Garcia SL. Spontaneous coronary artery dissection: stent it or wait for healing? *Heart.* 2003;89(2):164.
81. Chue CD, Routledge HC, Townend JN. Spontaneous coronary artery dissection and the role for percutaneous coronary intervention: to treat or not to treat? *J Invasive Cardiol.* 2009;21(3): E44-E47.
82. Vale PR, Baron DW. Coronary artery stenting for spontaneous coronary artery dissection: a case report and review of the literature. *Cathet Cardiovasc Diagn.* 1998;45(3):280-286.
83. Lerakis S, Manoukian S, Martin RP. Transesophageal echo detection of postpartum coronary artery dissection. *J Am Soc Echocardiogr.* 2001;14(11):1132-1133.
84. Chang SM, Fuh A, Bianco JA, Wann LS. Spontaneous coronary artery dissection on multiple detector computed tomography (MDCT). *J Cardiovasc Comput Tomogr.* 2007;1(1):60-61.
85. Nambi P, Sengupta R, Cheong BY. Previous left main coronary artery dissection: detected upon multislice computed tomography. *Tex Heart Inst J.* 2008;35(3):365-366.
86. Park SM, Koh KK, Kim JH, Yoon KH, Chung WJ, Kang WC. Myocardial infarction with huge mural thrombus due to spontaneous coronary artery dissection detected by 64-multidetector computed tomography. *Int J Cardiol.* 2008;127(2):e73-e75.
87. Lubarsky L, Jelnin V, Roubin GS, Hecht HS. Spontaneous right coronary artery dissection: evaluation by 64-slice multidetector computed tomographic angiography. *J Invasive Cardiol.* 2007;19(6): 280-281.
88. Kantarci M, Ogul H, Bayraktutan U, Gundogdu F, Bayram E. Spontaneous coronary artery dissection: noninvasive diagnosis with multidetector CT angiography. *J Vasc Interv Radiol.* 2007;18(5): 687-688.
89. Dwyer N, Galligan L, Harle R. Spontaneous coronary artery dissection and associated CT coronary angiographic findings: a case report and review. *Heart Lung Circ.* 2007;16(2):127-130.
90. Komatsu S, Omori Y, Hirayama A, et al. Coronary artery dissection following angioplasty detected by multi-detector row computed tomography: evaluation using the Plaque Map system. *Int J Cardiol.* 2007;115(3):404-405.
91. Chabrot P, Motreff P, Boyer L. Postpartum spontaneous coronary artery dissection: a case of pseudoaneurysm evolution detected on MDCT. *AJR Am J Roentgenol.* 2006;187(6):W660.
92. Manghat NE, Morgan-Hughes GJ, Roobottom CA. Spontaneous coronary artery dissection: appearance and follow-up on multidetector row CT coronary angiography. *Clin Radiol.* 2005;60(10): 1120-1125.
93. Takaseya T, Nishimi M, Kawara T, et al. Spontaneous coronary artery dissection causing myocardial infarction and left ventricular aneurysm. *Circ J.* 2002;66(10):972-973.

13 Coronary Ostial and Left Main Stem Lesions, Spasm, and Thrombus

Key Points

- Cardiac CT is best suited to imaging the larger-caliber coronary segments, such as proximal coronary arteries, ostial lesions, and the left main stem coronary artery.
- The ambiguities in a subset of coronary ostial lesions as assessed by conventional angiography may potentially be resolvable by CCT.
- Aortic diseases associated with ostial coronary involvement are well assessed by CCT.
- Ostial compression by extrinsic structures also is potentially well evaluated by CCT.

Lesions of the coronary artery ostia and of the left main stem coronary artery are of higher clinical and angiographic risk.[1]

Left main coronary ostial lesions are notable for being found more commonly among middle-aged women with fewer conventional coronary artery risk factors and for lower long-term patency of internal thoracic grafts.[2]

Although conventional angiography is the gold standard for assessment of ostial and left main stem lesions, numerous aspects of conventional angiography for the assessment of these lesions may be challenging when trying to obtain definitive imaging characterization, especially to assess membrane-like lesions, complex courses, eccentric luminal geometry (slit-like orifices), and extremely proximal or ostial lesions. Intravascular ultrasound (IVUS), coronary CT angiography (CTA), and coronary MR angiography (MRA) have all been used in attempts to resolve ambiguous cases.[3]

The left main stem coronary artery, when investigated by cardiac CT studies of 70 consecutive cases, was seen to be elliptical at its ostium in 94%, at its mid-portion in 73%, and at its distal portion in 77% of cases. The most common morphology is biconcave, followed by tapering, combined morphology, and, least commonly, funnel-shaped. In 72% of cases, the ostium of the left main stem arises from the middle one third of the aortic sinus, in 22% it arises from the posterior third of the sinus, and in 4% it arises from the anterior third. In men, significant correlation is found between left main stem cross-sectional area and body weight, height, and body surface, whereas there is no such correlation in women. Left main stem ostial angulation is a normal finding/variant associated with posterior position of the ostium.[4]

CCT is best suited to imaging the larger-caliber coronary segments—hence its suitability to assess the left main stem in particular, as has been advocated by some.[5] In general, for the assessment of minimal lesional diameter (r = 0.77, $P < .01$), minimal lumen area (r = 0.93, $P < .01$), lumen area stenosis (r= 0.83, $P< .01$) and plaque burden (r = 0.94, $P < .01$), CCT findings correlate well with those of IVUS.[3]

Among asymptomatic patients, an IVUS minimal luminal diameter and minimal luminal area of 2.8 mm and 5.9 mm^2, respectively, strongly predict the physiologic significance of a left main stem coronary lesion; a fractional flow reserve of 0.75 is strongly associated with survival and event-free survival.[6]

The prevalence of significant stenotic disease of the left main stem is influenced principally by the nature of the referral population, but has been suggested to be 2% by one series of 1000 consecutive cases.[7,8] The dichotomization of left main stem disease into significant versus nonsignificant based on 50% stenosis has been queried by some.[8]

The use of cardiac CTA to image the left main stem coronary artery post-stenting has shown some validation.[9] However, numerous considerations still need resolution[10]:

- Complex (distal) left main stem coronary artery stenting of LMCA bifurcation lesions that achieve overlapping or adjacent ("crush") stents would be expected to yield greater artifacts and more potential for error, and have not been well described in the literature.

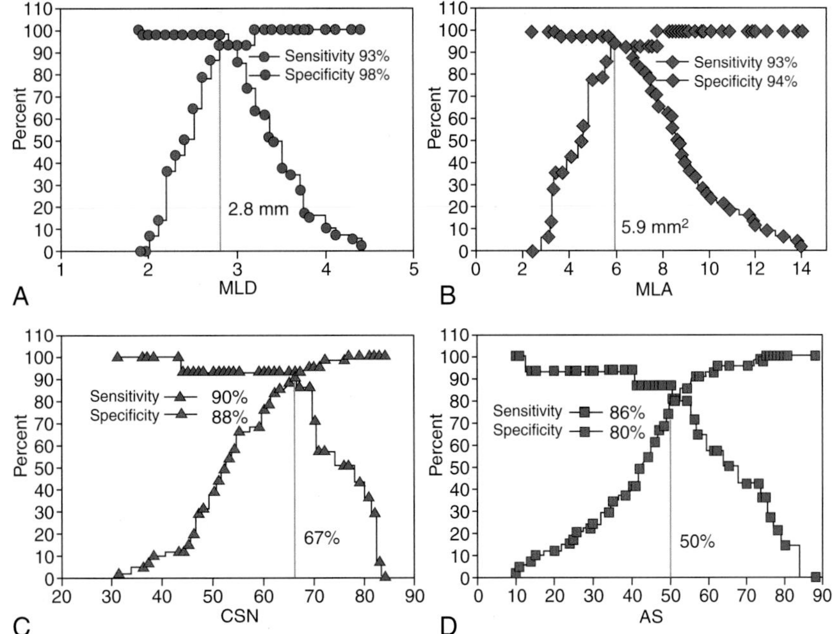

Figure 13-1. An intravascular ultrasound (IVUS) minimum luminal diameter (MLD) of 2.8 mm and a minimum luminal area (MLA) of 5.9 mm^2 strongly predict the physiologic significance of left main coronary artery stenosis. Sensitivity and specificity curves of the ischemic cut-point of fractional flow or reserve (FFR) and IVUS parameters are shown. **A,** Best agreement with the FFR cut-point of 0.75 was found when MLD by IVUS was 2.8 mm (sensitivity, 93%; specificity, 98%). **B,** Best agreement with the FFR cut-point of 0.75 was found when MLA by IVUS was 5.9 mm^2 (sensitivity, 93%; specificity, 94%). **C,** Best agreement with FFR was found when cross-sectional narrowing (CSN)—calculated as plaque plus media cross-sectional area (CSA) divided by the external elastic membrane CSA—was 67% (sensitivity, 90%; specificity, 88%). **D,** Best agreement with FFR was found when area stenosis (AS; calculated as the reference-lumen CSA-lesion MLA × 100/reference-lumen CSA) by IVUS was 50% (sensitivity, 86%; specificity 80%). (Reprinted with permission from Jasti V, Ivan E, Yalamanchili V, et al. Correlations between fractional flow reserve and intravascular ultrasound in patients with an ambiguous left main coronary artery stenosis. *Circulation.* 2004;110(18):2831-2836.)

- Prominent calcium within left main stem lesions presents another difficulty for the assessment of LMCA lesions, as with all coronary lesions.
- A 1-mm error in ascertaining restenosis of the LMCA would incur, on average, quite a significant (~20%) error of restenosis severity.

The relationship between LMCA IVUS determinations of stenosis severity with fractional flow reserve determinations of severity is presented in Figure 13-1.

ETIOLOGY OF CORONARY ARTERY OSTIAL LESIONS

- Congenital
  - Isolated atresia of the coronary ostia[11-13]
  - Associated with supravalvular aortic stenosis[14-16]
- Aorto-arteritis[17]
- Takayasu arteritis[18,19]
- Relapsing polychondritis[20]
- Syphilis[21-24]
- Post-radiation[1,25-28]
- Post–aortic valve replacement (AVR)[29]
- Post-AVR/intracoronary cardioplegia perfusion[30,31]
- Post–freestyle stentless bioprosthesis[32]
- Trauma
- Stenting/restenosis
- Spasm[33]

ETIOLOGY OF LEFT MAIN STEM LESIONS

- Intrinsic lesions
  - Congenital
    - Atresia[11-13,34]
    - Anomalous right-sided origin[35]
    - Anomalous origin from the pulmonary artery (ALCAPA)[36]
    - Anomalous fistula of the LMCA to the pulmonary artery[37]
    - Kinking
  - Atherosclerotic[38,39]
  - Thrombotic
  - Stenting
  - Restenotic
    - Restenosis[40]
    - In-stent restenosis[9,10]
  - Post-surgical
    - Post-AVR[29]
    - Post-AVR/coronary perfusion[30,31]
    - Post–aortic root reconstruction

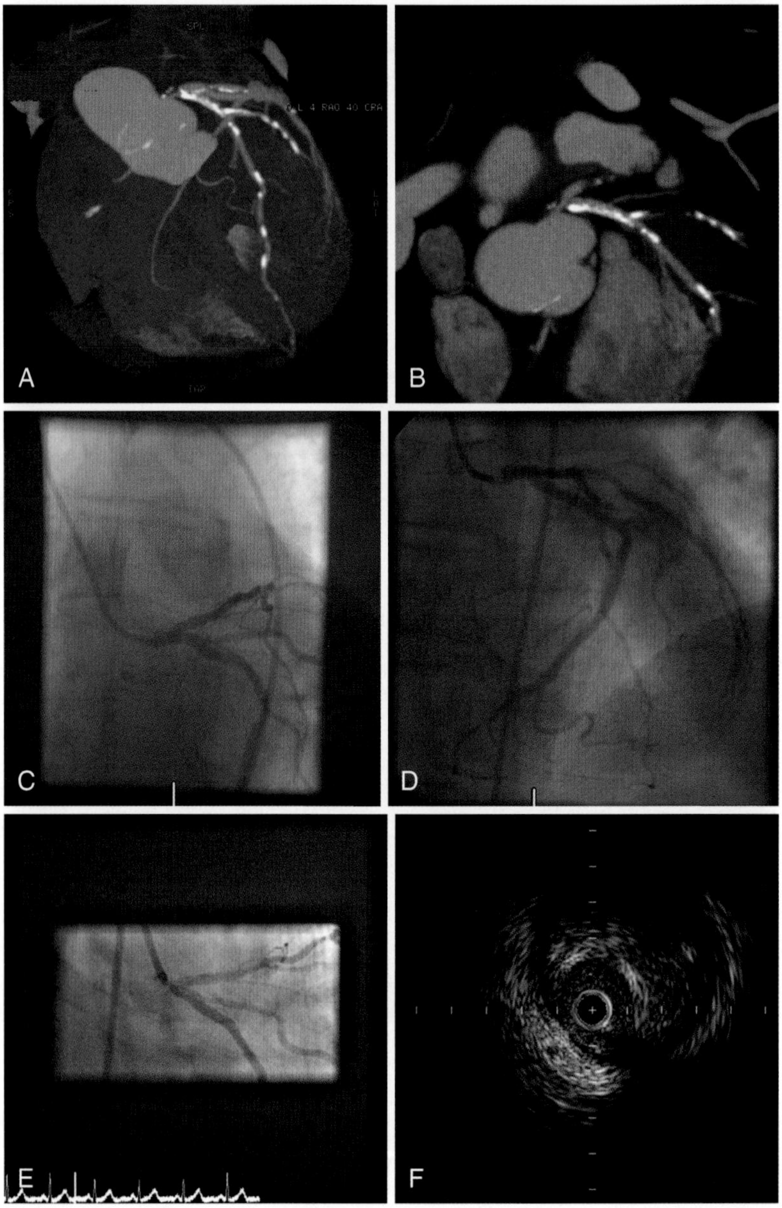

Figure 13-2. A 63-year-old man with symptoms of typical stable angina, CCS Class III, and a negative myocardial perfusion scan. **A** and **B,** CT coronary angiography demonstrating a mixed calcified/noncalcified plaque of significant stenosis at the ostium of the left main stem coronary artery. On the basis of these findings the patient was referred for coronary angiography. **C** and **D,** First angiogram, different views. The study was reported as "normal." **E** and **F,** Second angiogram 2 weeks later, with intravascular ultrasound (IVUS). The IVUS image at the ostial left main stem reveals a significant (70–80%) stenosis from a large volume of plaque. Note the lucent internal elastic lamina layer that references the actual vessel wall. More careful angiography demonstrates the same finding, which was poorly represented on the initial angiogram, as the catheter tip was distal to the lesion and the back-blow never clearly outlined the stenosis.

    - Surgical gelatin-resorcin-formalin glue[41,42]
    - End-to-end anastomosis of the LMCA onto a Freestyle (Medtronic) or Toronto SPV (St. Jude Medical) aortic valve/root[32]
    - Post–aortic valve and root repair[43]
    - Post–Bentall repair aneurysms, stenosis, and dehiscence[41,44]
  - Dissection
    - Aortic dissection
    - Spontaneous coronary dissection[5,45]
  - Post-syphilitic[21-24]
  - Post-radiation[25-28]
  - Aortitis: Takayasu arteritis[18,19]
  - Spasm[33]
- ❒ Extrinsic lesions
  - Pulmonary artery compression of the LMCA
    - Pulmonary hypertension[46-50]
    - Eisenmenger syndrome[51]
    - Pulmonary artery dilation[46]
    - Main pulmonary artery aneurysm[52]
  - Right pulmonary artery stenting[53]
  - Post-pericardiotomy syndrome[54]

CORONARY CTA

Coronary CTA has documented:

- ❒ Left main stem patency, stenosis, restenosis, and ostial stent-related problems of the left main stem coronary artery (Figs. 13-2 and 13-3)
- ❒ In-stent restenosis of the left main stem coronary artery (Figs. 13-4 through 13-6)

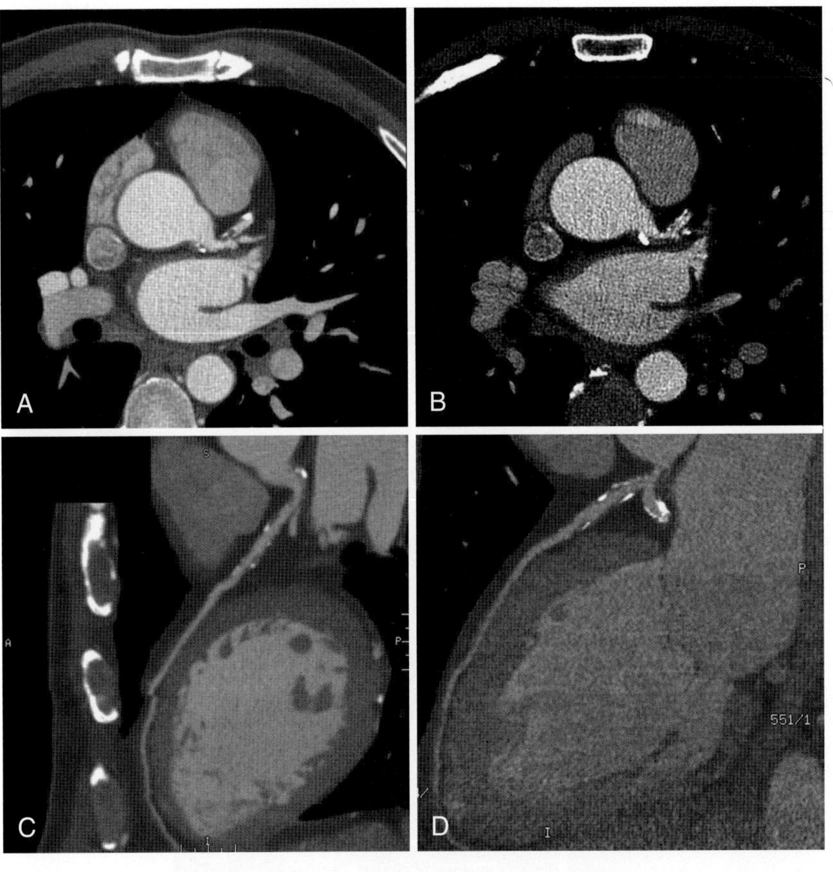

Figure 13-3. A 52-year-old man with a known history of coronary artery disease. The patient had previously undergone stenting of the proximal right coronary artery (RCA) and proximal circumflex arteries. At the time of the circumflex artery stenting, an iatrogenic dissection of the left main coronary artery occurred. The patient was treated conservatively for this. A follow-up cardiac CT study 1 year later (**A** and **C**) demonstrated a small amount of mixed plaque at the origin of the left main coronary artery, causing a mild 30% stenosis. There was no evidence of a residual dissection. A second follow-up study at 36 months (**B** and **D**) demonstrates interval worsening of left main coronary artery disease, with more extensive soft and calcified plaque, and the development of a significant 50% to 60% left main stenosis.

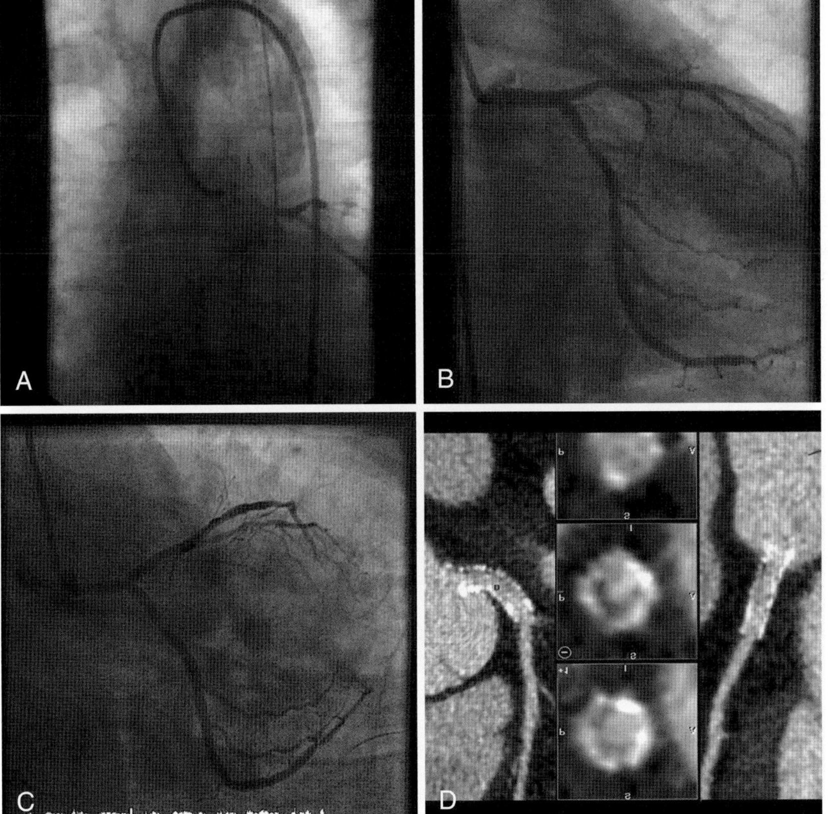

Figure 13-4. A 63-year-old man presented with an acute coronary syndrome. An initial angiogram (**A**) demonstrated thrombosis of the left main coronary artery, which led to immediate percutaneous intervention of the left main coronary artery (**B**). The patient presented with recurrent angina 4 months later. **C,** A repeat conventional angiogram showed mild in-stent restenosis involving the inferior potion of the left main stent. **D,** A subsequent cardiac CT study in follow-up confirms the mild in-stent restenosis of the left main coronary artery as subtle low attenuation along the inferior aspect of the stent, but no further progression.

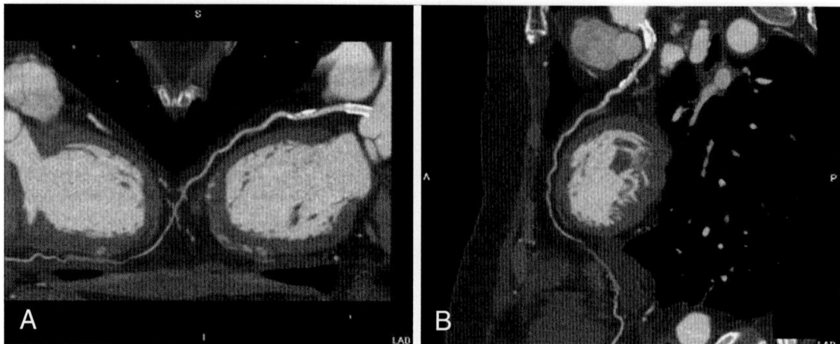

Figure 13-5. Multiplanar reformations of a patient with a stented left main stem coronary artery. The proximal aspect of the stent sits 3 to 4 mm back in the aortic root. There is mild to moderate mixed disease of the proximal left anterior descending artery.

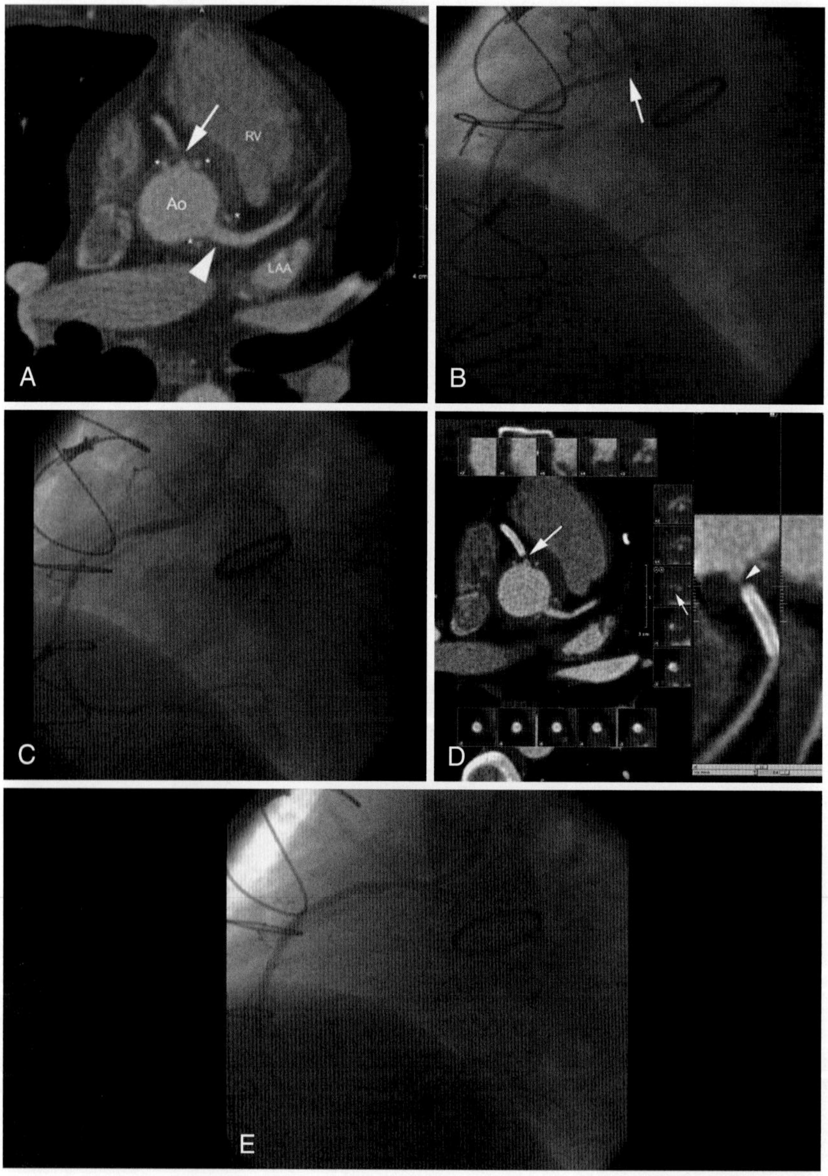

Figure 13-6. A 51-year-old man 1 year following a Bentall procedure with coronary button implantation using reinforcement with BioGlue (CryoLife), was experiencing atypical chest pains. **A,** CT axial oblique image showing ostial right coronary artery (RCA) stenosis after a Bentall procedure (*arrow*). The left main artery (*arrowhead*) also is seen. **B,** Right coronary angiogram in the left anterior oblique view shows ostial RCA stenosis (*arrow*). **C,** Right coronary angiogram after stenting of the RCA stenosis. **D,** RCA ostial stenosis was shown proximal to the previously deployed stent on CT axial oblique and cross-sectional images (*arrows*) and curved multiplanar reformatted images (*arrowhead*). **E,** Right coronary angiogram in left anterior oblique view shows ostial stenosis proximal to stent and mild in-stent restenosis. Ao, aorta; LAA, left atrial appendage; RV, right ventricle; *, coronary button markers. (Reprinted with permission from Shenoda M, Barack BM, Toggart E, Chang DS. Use of coronary computed tomography angiography to detect coronary ostial stenosis after Bentall procedure. *J Cardiovasc Comput Tomogr.* 2009;3(5):340-343).

- Catheter-induced spasm of the left main stem coronary artery (Figs. 13-7 through 13-9)
- Left main stem ostial stenosis due to Takayasu arteritis[18] (Figs. 13-10 through 13-12)
- Left main stem ostial stenosis due to relapsing polychondritis (Figs. 13-13 and 13-14)
- Left main stem ostial stenosis due to syphilis (Fig. 13-15)
- Left main stem dissection[45]
- Left main stem, intra- and extracoronary aortic thrombus[55,56] (Fig.13-16)
- Post–coronary reimplantation (Bentall procedure), dilation, stenosis, and dehiscences (Fig. 13-17)
- Ostial stenosis due to radiation or post-surgery (Figs. 13-18 and 13-19)
- Sterile and mycotic false aneurysms of the left main stem coronary artery (Fig. 13-20)
- Extrinsic compression by masses of the left main stem/ left coronary artery
- Kinking / eccentric ostia (Figs. 13-21 through 13-24)
- Abnormally high coronary ostia (Fig. 13-25)
- Abnormally shaped coronary ostia due to encroachment by an AVR valve ring (Fig. 13-26)
- Extrinsic compression of the left main stem associated with primary pulmonary hypertension and prominent dilation of the main pulmonary artery (Fig. 13-27)

Text continued on page 208

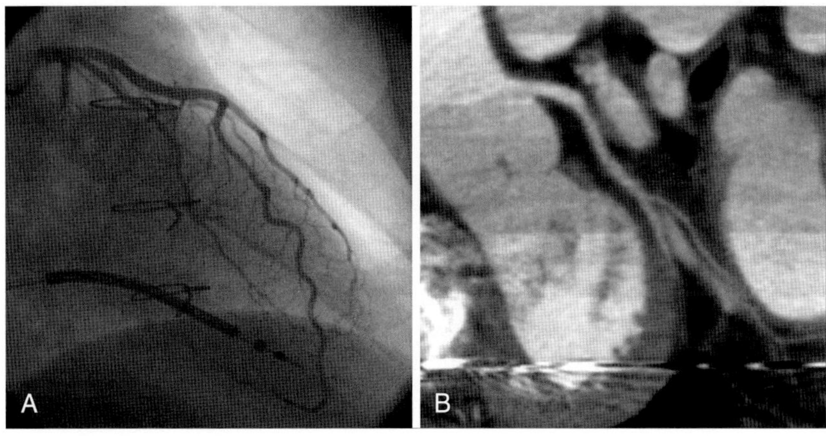

Figure 13-7. A 65-year-old man with a prior ventricular fibrillation cardiac arrest and an implantable cardioverter defibrillator. Coronary angiography reveals occlusion of the proximal left circumflex; CT angiography demonstrates patency and no plaques within the left circumflex, establishing a strong case that the occlusion at the time of angiography was due to spasm.

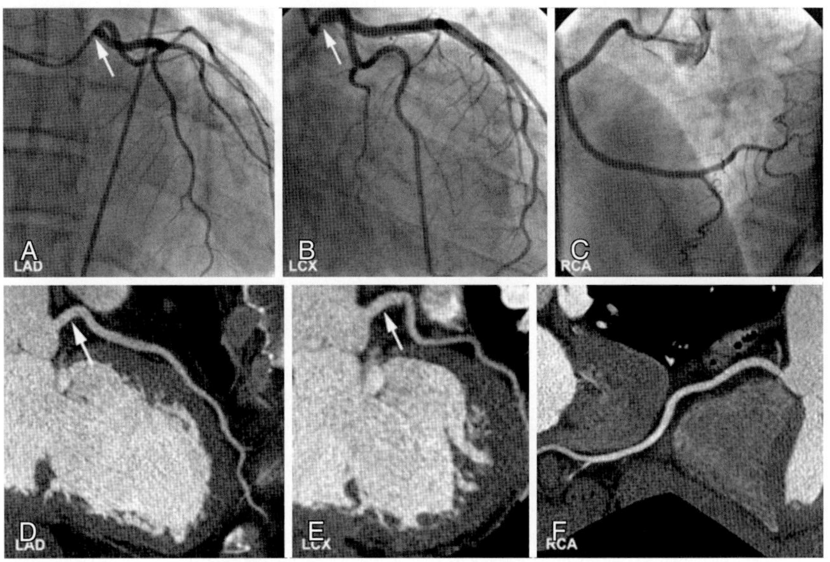

Figure 13-8. **A–C,** Conventional coronary angiography showing left anterior descending (LAD) artery, left circumflex (LCX) artery, and right coronary artery (RCA) with isolated high-grade ostial stenosis of the left main coronary artery (*arrow*). **D–F,** Curved multiplanar reconstructions of LAD, LCX, and RCA in CT angiography showing a completely normal left main coronary artery (*arrow*), thereby proving catheter-induced spasm as the underlying reason for the false-positive lumen narrowing in invasive catheterization. (Reprinted with permission from Pflederer T, Marwan M, Ropers D, et al. CT angiography unmasking catheter-induced spasm as a reason for left main coronary artery stenosis. *J Cardiovasc Comput Tomogr.* 2008;2(6):406-407.)

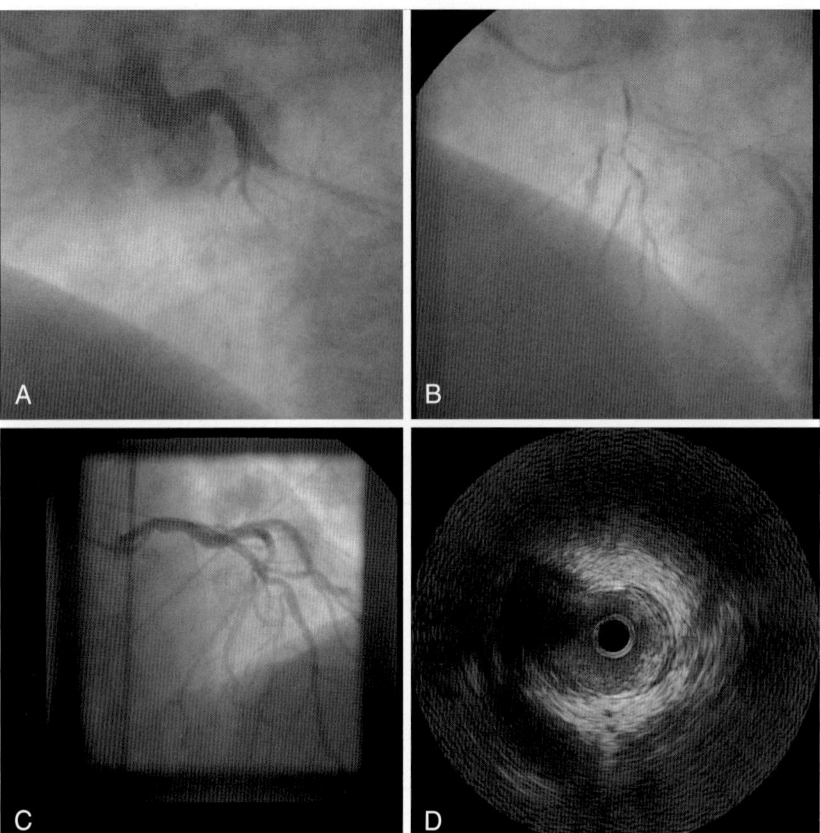

Figure 13-9. An angiographic case of left coronary artery spasm. **A,** On the first injection, the caliper of the left main stem is seen. Within a few seconds, the left main stem artery has occluded and the entire left coronary tree is also in severe spasm. Ventricular fibrillation ensued. **C,** After defibrillations, and intracoronary nitroglycerin, the examination was resumed. **D,** An eccentric lesion at the ostium to the left coronary artery is evident on the angiogram and on the intravascular ultrasound image.

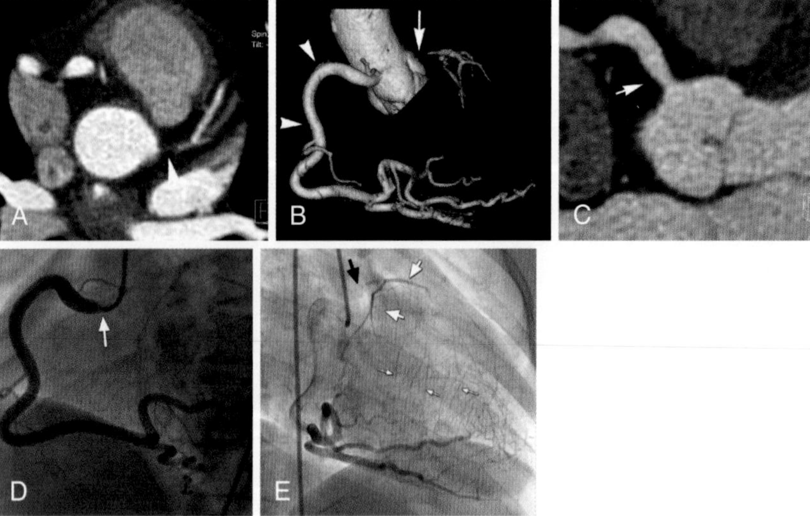

Figure 13-10. Occlusion of the left main coronary artery in Takaysu arteritis. Coronary CT and invasive angiography of a patient with Takayasu arteritis (Numano type IIb) with an ostial occlusion of the left main coronary artery and right coronary artery dilation as a compensatory mechanism. **A,** Coronary CT angiographic axial image at the origin of the left main coronary trunk shows lack of opacification of the vessel (*arrow*), associated with negative remodeling. The vessel reconstitutes distally. **B,** Conversely, the right coronary artery (*arrowheads*) is diffusely dilated as a compensatory mechanism, as demonstrated in this volume-rendered image, but its origin also shows mild tapering, as seen in the multiplanar reformat (**C**; *arrow*). Note the absence of contrast material within the lumen of the left main coronary trunk (**B**; *arrow*). **D** and **E,** Conventional coronary angiography confirms the right coronary ectasia and its tapering at the origin (**D**; *arrow*) and the occlusion of the left main trunk (**E**; *black arrow*). Multiple collaterals (*small white arrows*) to the left coronary circulation coming from the right coronary artery and reconstituting the mid-distal left anterior descending and left circumflex coronary arteries (*large white arrows*) also are seen. Most significant coronary lesions in patients with Takayasu arteritis are ostial and noncalcified, as they were in this case. (Reprinted with permission from Soto ME, Meléndez-Ramírez G, Kimura-Hayama E, et al. Coronary CT angiography in Takayasu arteritis. *J Am Coll Cardiol.* 2011;4(9):958-966).

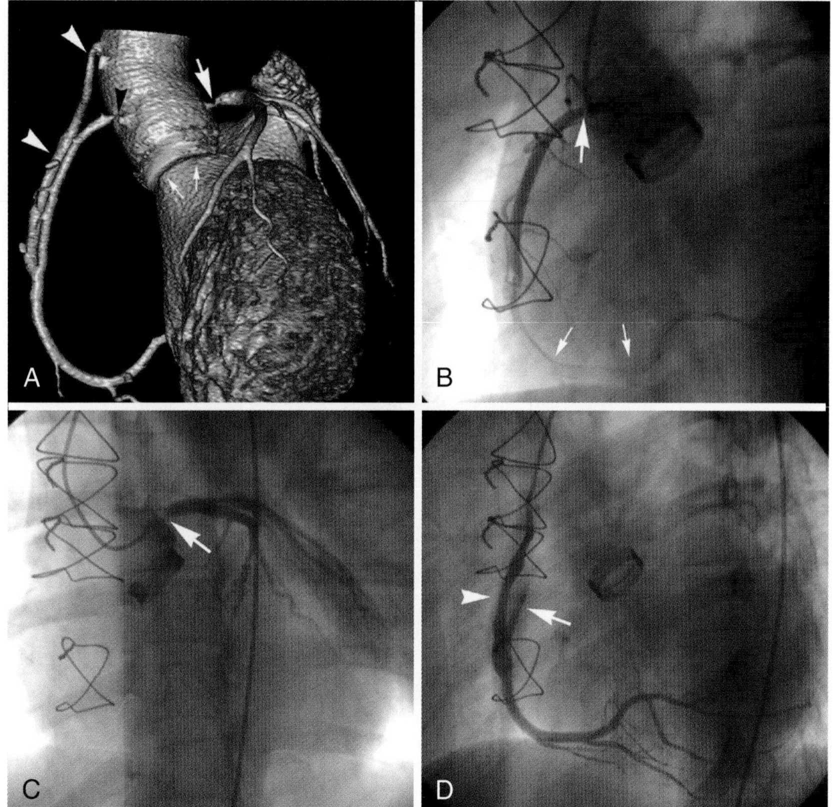

Figure 13-11. Significant proximal coronary artery lesions in Takaysu arteritis (TA). Coronary CT and conventional angiography of a patient with TA (Numano type V) and significant noncalcified lesions in the proximal right and left coronary arteries. This 31-year-old woman with TA had a history of surgical revascularization (vein graft to right coronary artery) and aortic valve replacement 3 years previously. **A,** CT volume-rendered image clearly demonstrates two areas of focal stenosis in the proximal right (*black arrowhead*) and left (*large white arrow*) coronary arteries, a patent vein graft to the mid-right coronary artery (*white arrowheads*), and the metallic aortic valve ring (*small arrows*). **B–D,** Conventional coronary angiography confirms both semiocclusive stenoses at the origins of the right and left coronary arteries (*arrows* in **B** and **C**). Also notice the slow filling of the distal right coronary artery (**B**; *small arrows*) due to the decreased flow velocity. More than 90% of coronary lesions in TA are ostial or proximal, in accordance with the theory of a direct extension of aortic disease. (Reprinted with permission from Soto ME, Meléndez-Ramírez G, Kimura-Hayama E, et al. Coronary CT angiography in Takayasu arteritis. *J Am Coll Cardiol.* 2011;4(9):958-966).

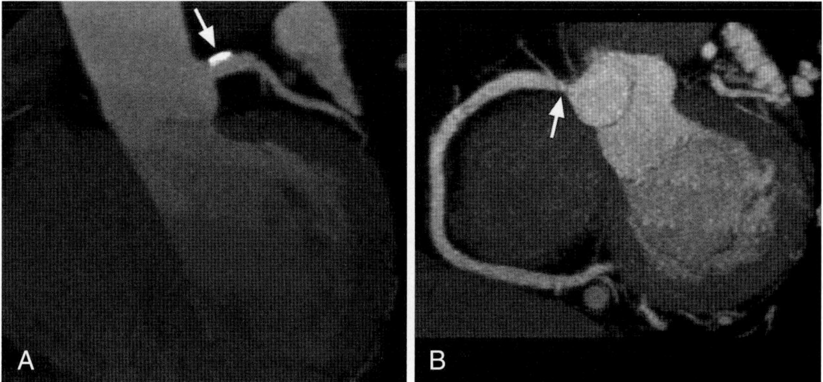

Figure 13-12. Nonstenotic coronary lesions in Takayasu arteritis. **A,** Multiplanar reconstructed image obtained by coronary CT angiography shows a completely calcified plaque at the origin of the left main coronary artery, without significant stenosis (*arrow*), in a 58-year-old patient. **B,** Multiplanar reconstructed coronary CT angiographic image shows noncalcified plaque, without significant stenosis, at the ostium of the right coronary artery (*arrow*) in a 26-year-old patient. (Reprinted with permission from Soto ME, Meléndez-Ramírez G, Kimura-Hayama E, et al. Coronary CT angiography in Takayasu arteritis. *J Am Coll Cardiol.* 2011;4(9):958-966).

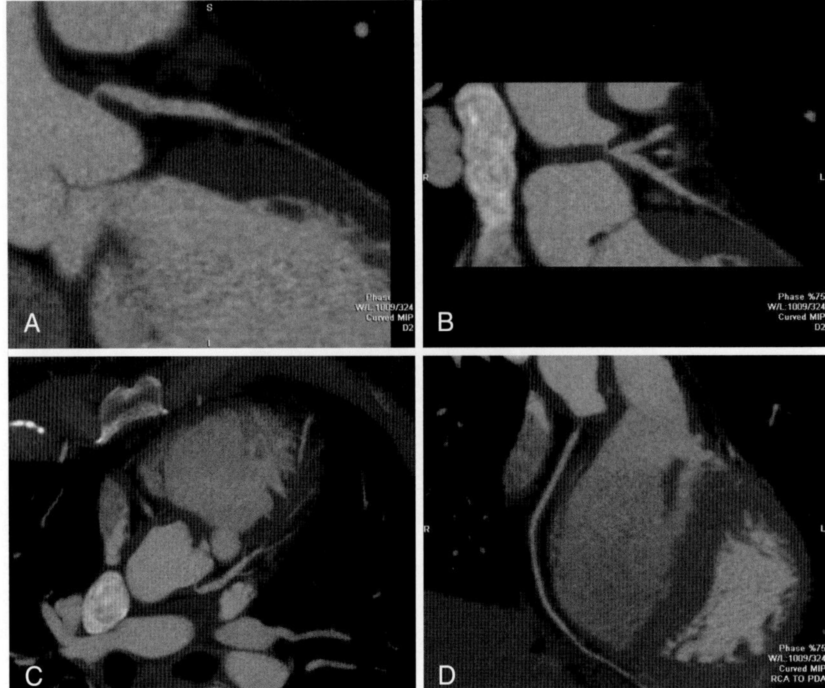

Figure 13-13. Composite CT images from a cardiac CT study in a patient with relapsing polychondritis. A moderate amount of soft tissue thickening is seen involving the aortic root. This had resulted in severe ostial stenosis to both the left main and the right coronary arteries.

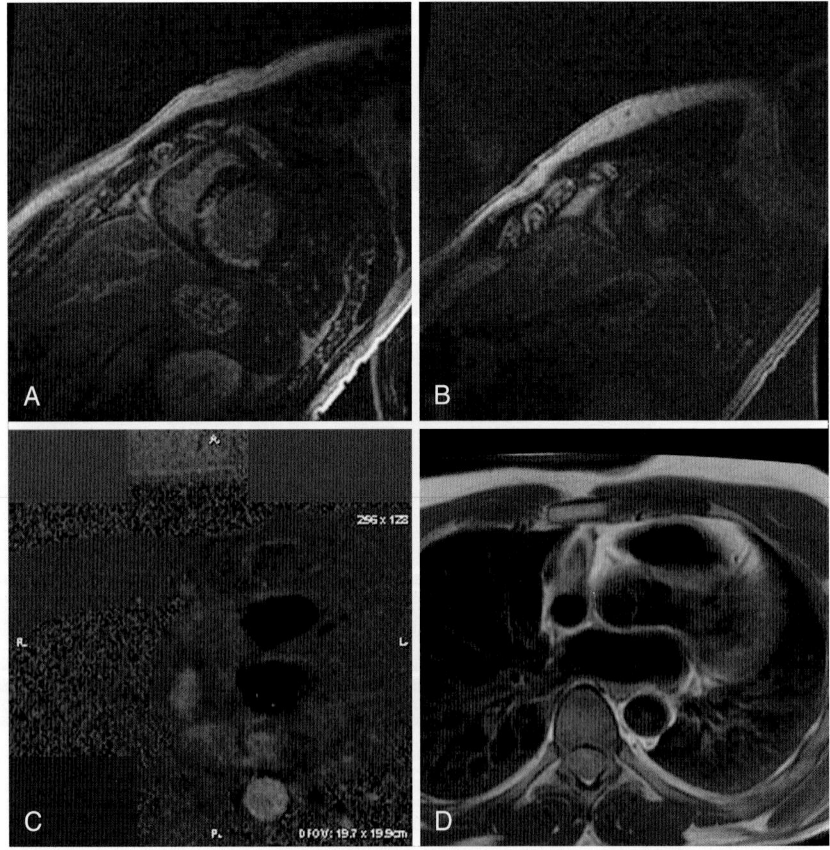

Figure 13-14. Composite MRI study of the same patient as in Figure 13-15 demonstrates a poorly defined proximal right coronary artery (RCA) on the double inversion recovery image in the right lower quadrant, with no identifiable flow in the RCA on phase contrast imaging (of lower left quadrant). Delayed enhanced images demonstrate a near full-thickness basal septal and inferior wall infarct. This is likely a consequence of the patient's underlying severe ostial RCA disease. There is no evidence of an infarct in the left anterior descending and circumflex artery territories.

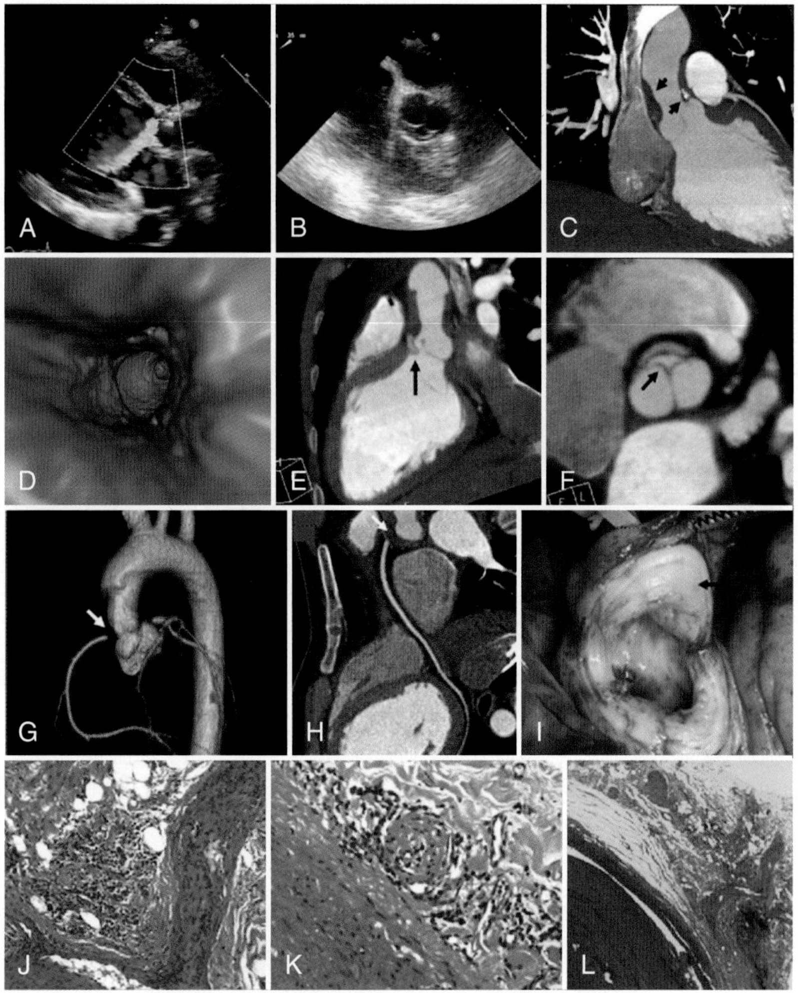

Figure 13-15. A 34-year-old man was referred to our hospital with dyspnea, palpitations, and a diastolic murmur. **A** and **B,** Transthoracic and transesophageal echocardiography showed severe aortic regurgitation and suggested wall thickening of the ascending aorta. **C,** Cardiac CT confirmed circumferential aortic wall thickening (8 mm), partly calcified and resulting in aorta lumen narrowing (16 mm). **D,** Virtual navigation in the proximal aorta. The right cusp of the aortic valve was stuck by its tip to the wall (**E**), causing a large closing defect in diastole (**F**). Extension to the right coronary ostium caused occlusive stenosis, which was demonstrated on three-dimensional volume rendering (**G**) and curvilinear (**H,** *arrow*) analyses. Syphilitic serologies *Treponema pallidum* hemagglutination assay (TPHA) and Venereal Disease Research Laboratories (VDRL) were highly positive, and after 3 weeks of penicillin treatment, surgical replacement of the ascending aorta and aortic valve with bypass graft to the right coronary artery was performed. Operative findings (**I,** *arrow*) and pathology findings (**J–L**) were consistent with aortic wall thickening by syphilitic inflammatory gummas. (Reprinted with permission from Bouvier E, Tabet J-Y, Malergue MC, et al. Syphilitic aortic regurgitation and ostial coronary occlusion. *J Am Coll Cardiol.* 2011;57(24):e375.)

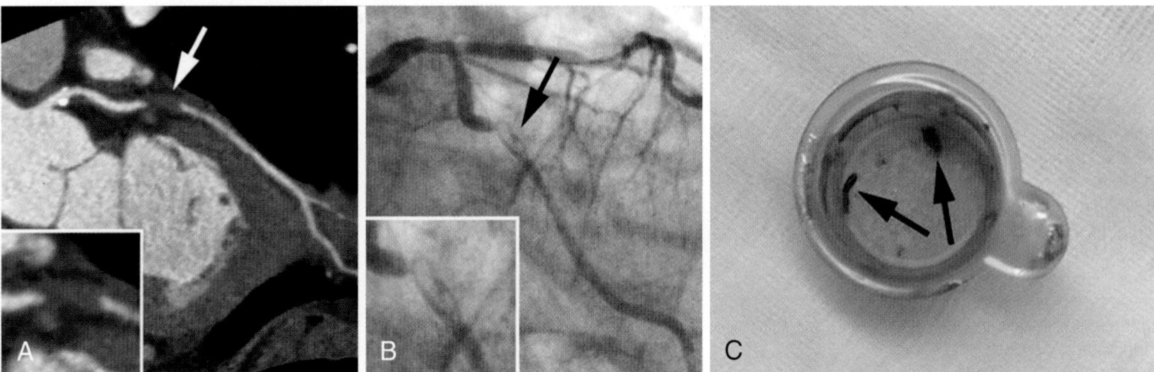

Figure 13-16. **A,** Coronary CT angiography. Curved multiplanar reconstruction images of the left main and left circumflex coronary arteries. An interruption of the contrast-enhanced lumen is appreciated (*arrow* and *inset*). The lesion has a relatively low CT attenuation (55 Hounsfield units) and shows pronounced "positive remodeling" as a consequence of intracoronary thrombosis, most likely because of plaque rupture. **B,** Corresponding invasive coronary angiogram confirms the presence of a thrombus in the lesion (*arrow* and *inset*). **C,** By using a vacuum extraction device, fragments of red thrombus could be retrieved from the left circumflex coronary artery (*arrows*). (Reprinted with permission from Achenbach S, Marwan M. Intracoronary thrombus. *J Cardiovasc Comput Tomogr.* 2009;3(5):344-345.)

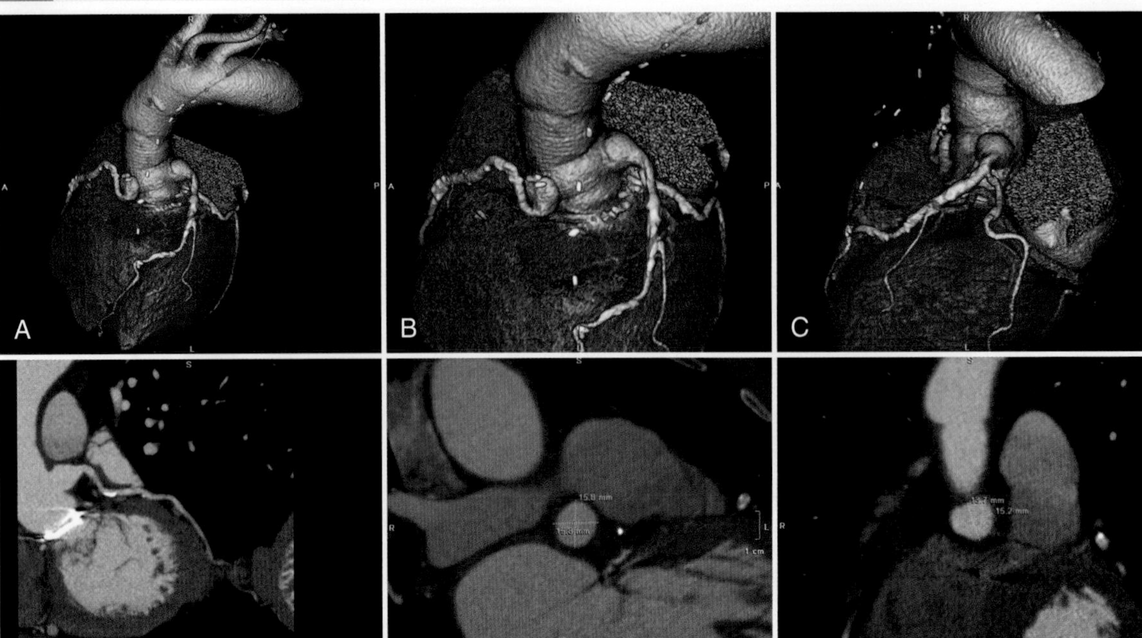

Figure 13-17. A 67-year-old man with aortic valve stenosis and descending aortic aneurysm. Preoperative coronary angiography demonstrated a 50% stenosis in the proximal left anterior descending artery (LAD). The patient underwent a Bentall procedure with a left internal mammary artery to LAD graft, and buttonhole reimplantation of both coronary artery ostia. Follow-up echocardiography was suspicious for coronary buttonhole aneurysms. Composite images from a cardiac CT study demonstrate moderate-sized buttonhole aneurysms at the implantation sites of both the left main and right coronary arteries. Both aneurysms measured approximately 1.5 cm. No complication is seen at the anastomotic site of the descending aortic graft. There has been interval occlusion of the left internal mammary artery graft.

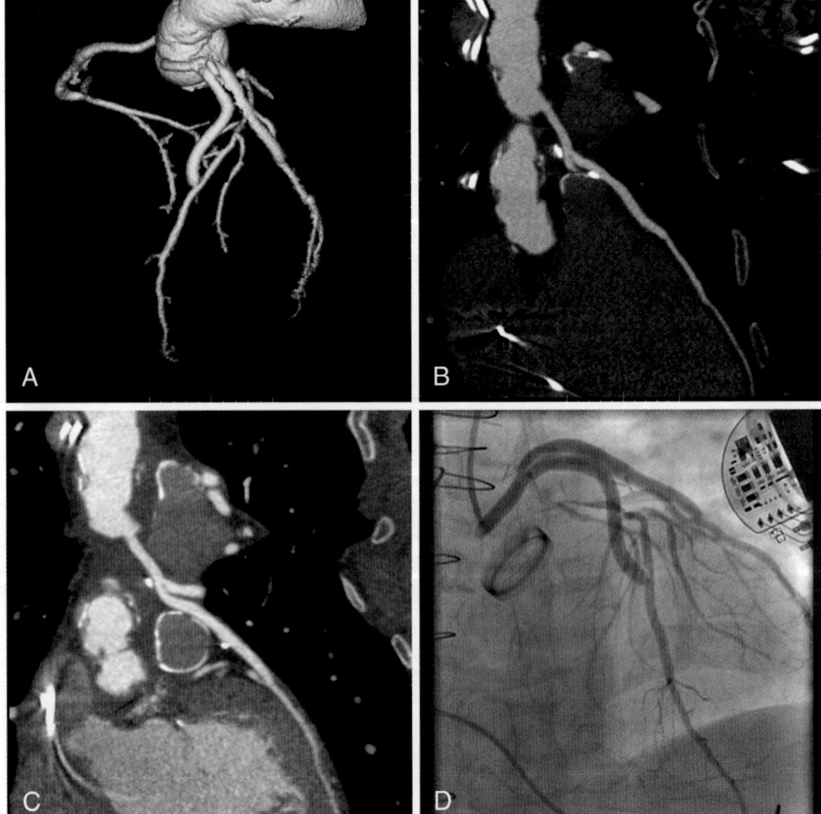

Figure 13-18. A 42-year-old man with a prior history of aortic valve and aortic root replacement secondary to severe aortic stenosis from extensive mediastinal irradiation due to Hodgkin disease. Coronary artery bypass grafting was performed at the time of the patient's aortic surgery. Four years after surgery the patient presents with chest pain. The volume-rendered and curved reformatted images demonstrate a patent saphenous vein bypass graft extending to the left anterior descending artery. A jump graft from the saphenous vein graft to an obtuse marginal branch also is noted with no evidence of a complication. A conventional angiogram confirms these findings.

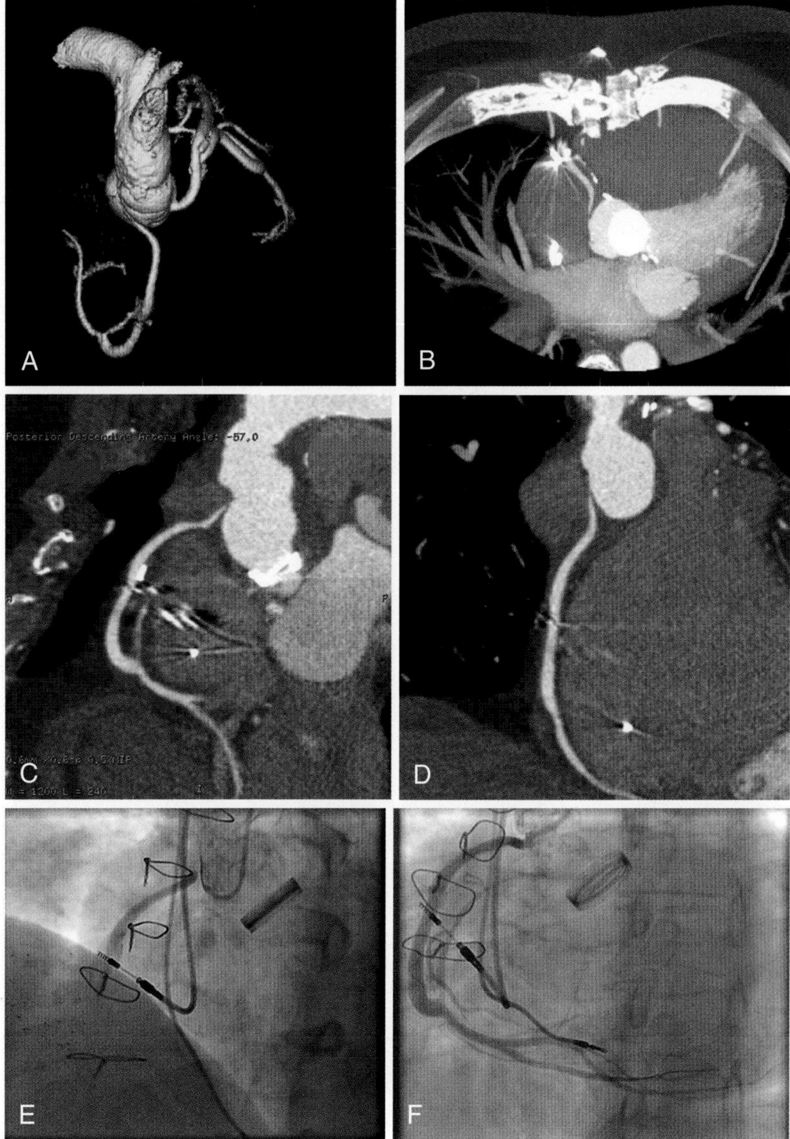

Figure 13-19. A 42-year-old man with a prior history of aortic valve and aortic root replacement secondary to severe aortic stenosis from extensive mediastinal irradiation due to Hodgkin disease. Coronary artery bypass grafting was performed at the time of the patient's aortic surgery. The patient now presents with chest pain. Multiple cardiac CT images (**A–D**) demonstrate a severe ostial right coronary artery (RCA) graft stenosis/near occlusion. The patient went on to have conventional coronary angiography. Image **E** demonstrates difficulty cannulating the ostium and poor filling of the RCA. The patient subsequently underwent angioplasty and stenting of the RCA ostium (**F**).

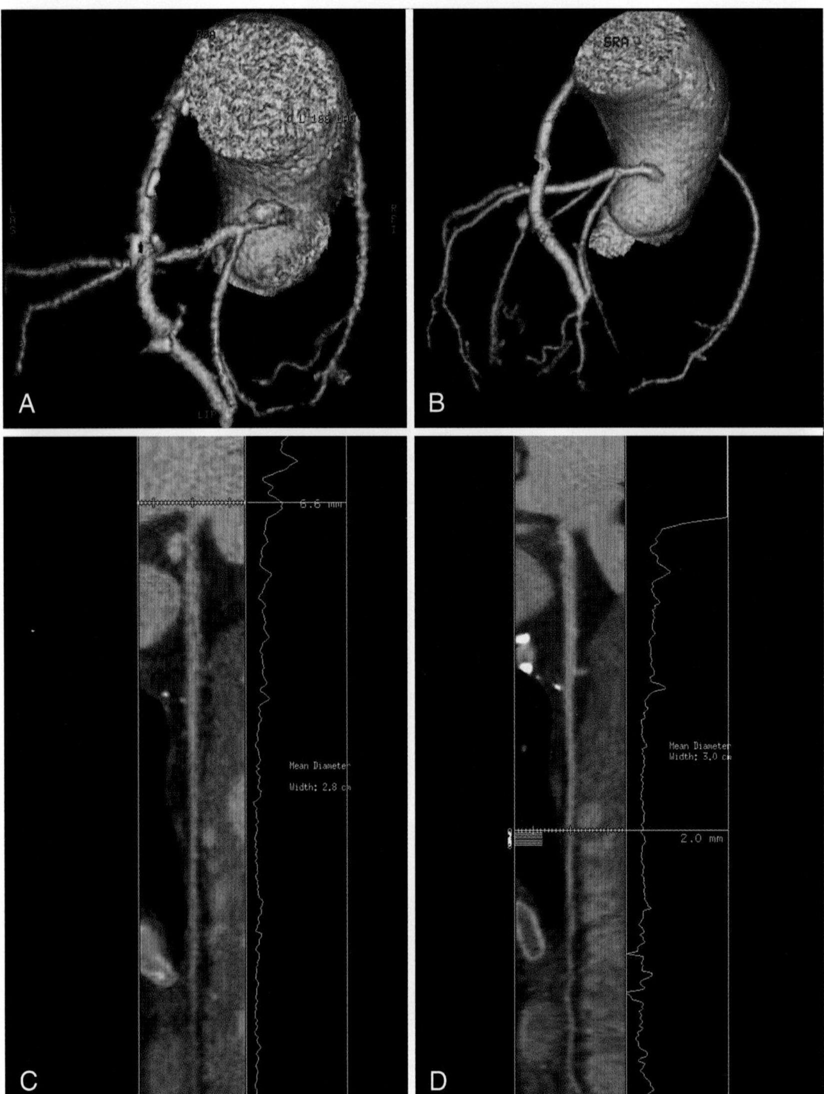

Figure 13-20. Left and right images 1 year apart. **A** and **C,** A pea-sized false aneurysm off the left main stem coronary artery, the result of a prior catheter-induced coronary dissection, is seen. The patient had undergone coronary bypass because of the lesion. **B** and **D,** One year later, the false aneurysm has healed, apparently entirely.

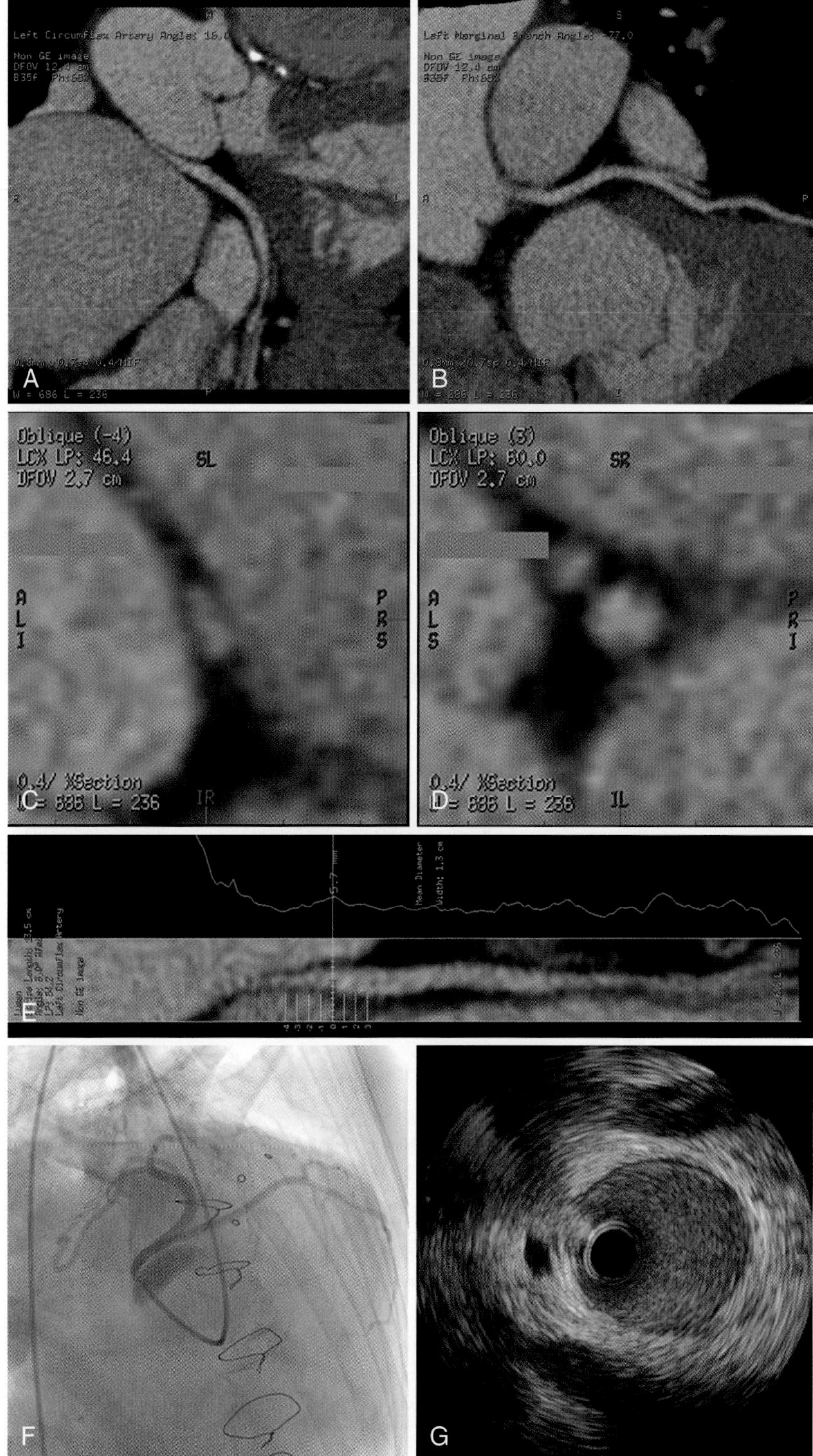

Figure 13-21. A 31-year-old woman with a history of repaired tetralogy of Fallot and a single (right) pulmonary artery presented with exertional chest pain and dyspnea. A stress myocardial perfusion study showed a perfusion abnormality in the left coronary circulation. Composite cardiac CT images demonstrate an eccentric slit-like stenosis of the proximal left main coronary artery as it is "trapped" between a markedly enlarged right pulmonary artery and the left sinus of Valsalva. A corresponding cardiac catheterization and intravascular ultrasound study did not confirm the findings seen on the CT study. Eventually, as symptoms worsened, the patient underwent surgical revascularization of the left coronary artery, with symptomatic relief.

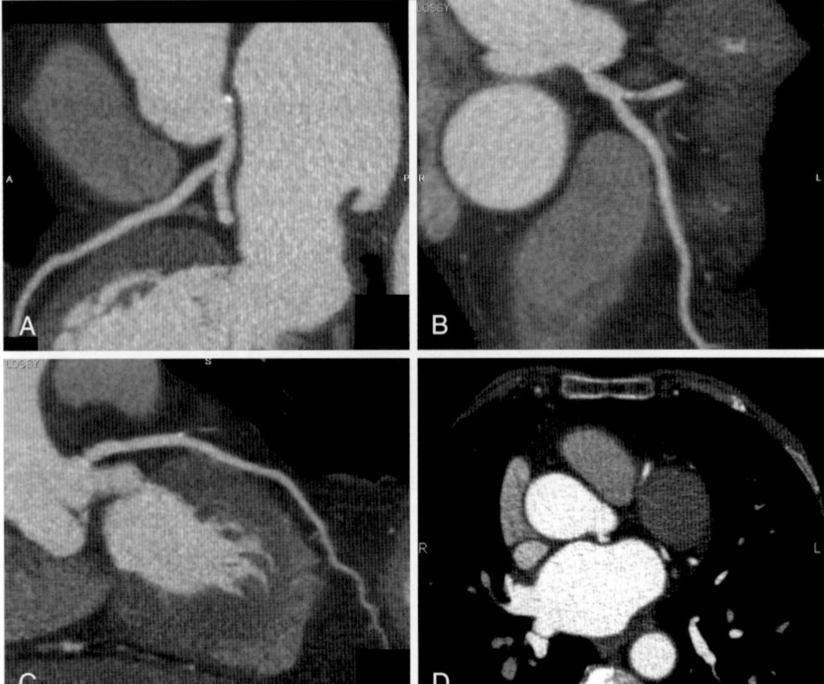

Figure 13-22. Multiple perpendicular cross-sectional images through the left main stem coronary artery demonstrate focal calcification above the left main stem origin and a band-like narrowing of the left main stem ostium, resulting in approximately 50% narrowing of the lumen. The lack of any soft or calcified plaque involving the ostial left main stem suggests that the narrowing is anatomic rather than atherosclerosis-related.

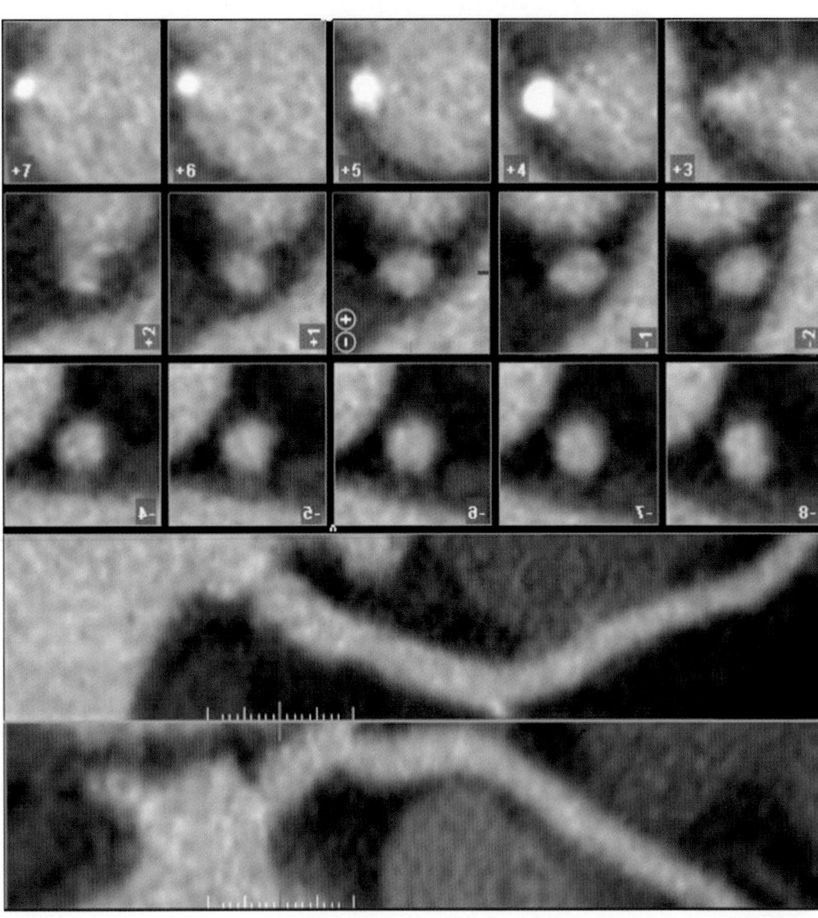

Figure 13-23. "IVUS" cross-sectional and curved multiplanar images demonstrate a focal kinking/band-like narrowing of the left main stem coronary ostium.

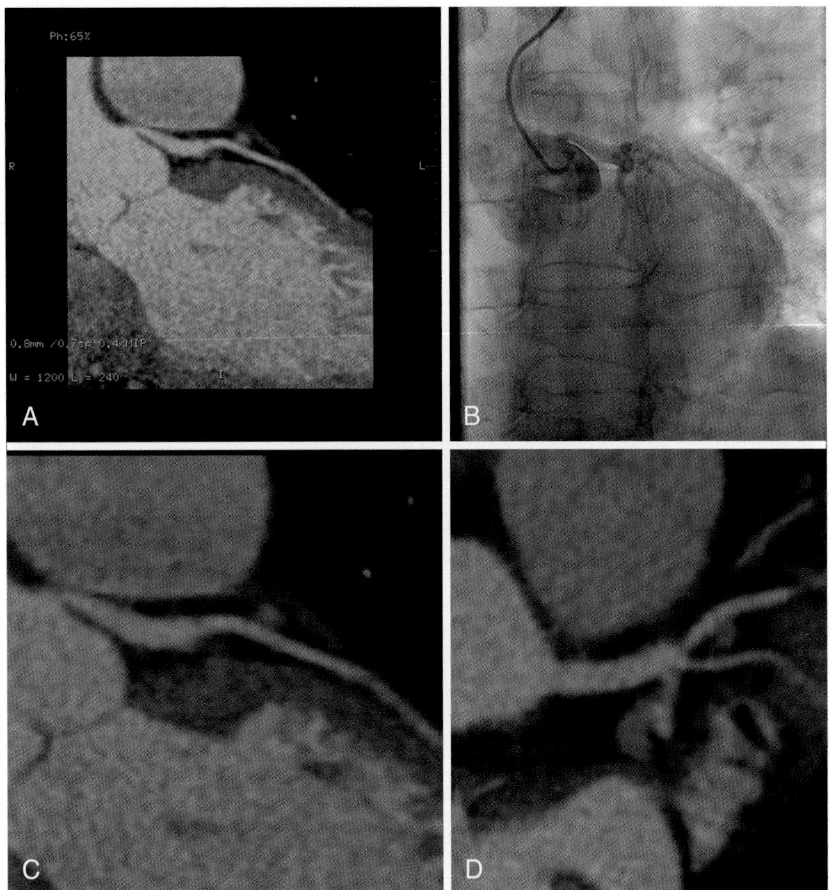

Figure 13-24. A 51-year-old man with a history of sclerosing cholangitis and portal hypertension presented with atypical chest pain and a left anterior descending artery (LAD) territory perfusion abnormality on a myocardial perfusion study. Multiple curved reformatted cardiac CT images demonstrate a high origin of the left main coronary artery from the left sinus of Valsalva. **A,** Note the marked enlargement of the right pulmonary artery, which compresses the left main coronary artery and causes a moderate to severe eccentric left main stenosis of 50% to 60%. This was confirmed on conventional angiography (**B**). Note the lack of any coronary artery plaque in this stenosis caused by the juxtaposition of the left main coronary artery and right pulmonary artery.

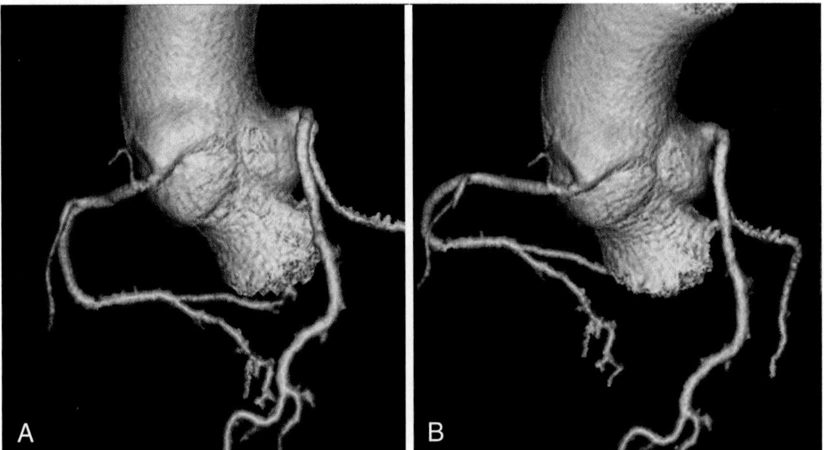

Figure 13-25. A 28-year-old woman with a known history of Marfan syndrome. A dedicated CT angiogram of the thorax was performed to evaluate the patient's aortic root and ascending aorta. No evidence was found of enlargement of the sinuses of Valsalva, or an ascending aortic aneurysm. Note is made of unusual origins of the coronary arteries bilaterally. They do not arise from the mid-sinuses of Valsalva proper, but from the superior portions of the sinuses in the region of the sinotubular junction. Both the right and left coronary artery ostia have focal patulous areas of dilatation associated with them. The diagnosis was an unusual variant of coronary artery ostia anatomy.

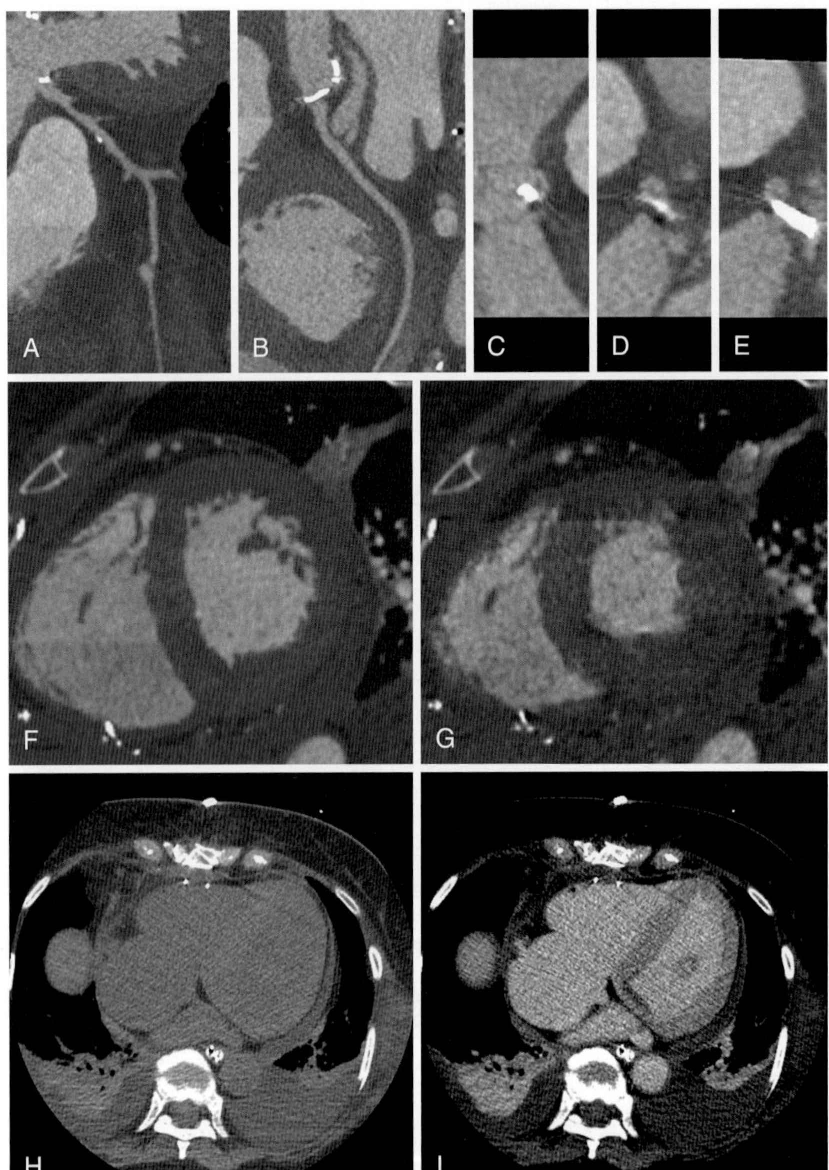

Figure 13-26. Multiple cardiac CT images and the patient post by prosthetic aortic valve replacement (AVR). After undergoing AVR, the patient had difficulty coming off the bypass pump. An intraoperative echocardiogram demonstrated akinesis of the anterior wall. A left internal mammary artery (LIMA) graft was placed, and the patient's left ventricle (LV) function subsequently improved. A postoperative cardiac CT study was obtained. **A,** The origin of the left main coronary artery extending into the LAD. The tip of the valve ring can be seen extending, also into the left main coronary artery. **B,** The valve ring overriding the os of the left main coronary artery. **C–E,** Cross-sectional images demonstrate a similar finding, with almost 50% of the left main ostium being impinged upon by the valve ring. **F** and **G** demonstrate thickening, but hypokinesis to dyskinesis of the inferoseptum. **H,** A precontrast image demonstrates a homogeneous attenuation of the left ventricle. **I,** A delayed image from the study demonstrates a well-defined subendocardial hypodensity involving the basal inferior and inferolateral walls. This likely reflects a myocardial infarction. The diagnosis was obstruction of the left main ostium by a low-positioned aortic valve ring, and subsequent myocardial infarction.

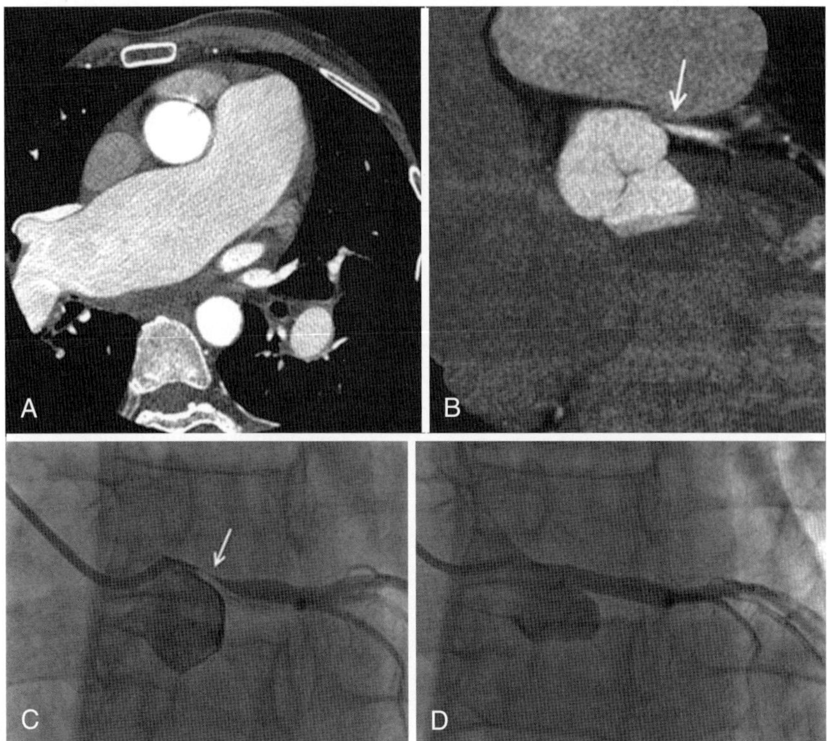

Figure 13-27. A 61-year-old man with known primary pulmonary arterial hypertension had typical angina when lying on his back. Strangely, in the left lateral decubitus position, the pain disappeared completely. Coronary 64-slice multidetector CT showed (**A**) major dilation of the pulmonary artery trunk inducing (**B**) left main artery compression (*arrow*), which was confirmed by (**C**) coronary angiography. **D,** Angioplasty was performed, resulting in complete relief of the pain. Such compression of the left main artery by an enlarged pulmonary artery is not a recent finding, but seldom has been described. The position-related character of the angina, which disappeared when the patient turned on his left side, can be explained by a change in the anatomic relationship between the aneurysmal pulmonary artery and the left main artery. The prevalence of left main artery stenosis may be underestimated and partially may explain the chest pain often associated with pulmonary arterial hypertension. (Reprinted with permission from Doyen D, Moceri P, Moschietto S, et al. Left main coronary artery compression associated with primary pulmonary hypertension. *J Am Coll Cardiol*. 2012;60(6):559.)

TABLE 13-1 ACCF 2010 Appropriateness Criteria for the Evaluation of Coronary Ostial and Left Main Stem Coronary Arteries

	APPROPRIATENESS RATING	INDICATION	MEDIAN SCORE
Evaluation of intra- and extracardiac structures	Appropriate	Prior left main coronary stent Stent diameter ≥ 3 mm	7
	Uncertain	Stent diameter ≥ 3 mm Time since PCI ≥ 2 yr	4
	Inappropriate	Stent diameter < 3 mm Time since PCI < 2 yr	2
		Stent diameter < 3 mm Time since PCI ≥ 2 yr	2
		Stent diameter ≥ 3 mm Time since PCI < 2 yr	2

Data from Taylor AJ, Cerqueira M, Hodgson JM, et al. ACCF/SCCT/ACR/AHA/ASE/ASNC/NASCI/SCAI/SCMR 2010 appropriate use criteria for cardiac computed tomography. A report of the American College of Cardiology Foundation Appropriate Use Criteria Task Force, the Society of Cardiovascular Computed Tomography, the American College of Radiology, the American Heart Association, the American Society of Echocardiography, the American Society of Nuclear Cardiology, the North American Society for Cardiovascular Imaging, the Society for Cardiovascular Angiography and Interventions, and the Society for Cardiovascular Magnetic Resonance. *J Am Coll Cardiol.* 2010;56(22):1864-1894.

TREATMENT OF CORONARY OSTIAL LESIONS

- Medical
- Interventional
  - Stenting following adjunctive atherectomy[57]
  - Stenting[58]
- Surgical
  - Bypass grafting[21]
  - Saphenous vein patch angioplasty[59]
  - Rhombic-shaped pulmonary autograft patch angioplasty[60]

CCT PROTOCOL POINTS

- The standard CCT protocol is utilized.
- See Table 13-1.

References

1. Bensaid J, Benabbou M, Goburdhun C, Medard C, Guillon A, el Kenz A. [Ostial stenosis of the common trunk of the left coronary artery 20 years after mediastinal irradiation]. *Ann Cardiol Angeiol (Paris).* 1998;47(10):732-734.
2. Arima M, Kanoh T, Okazaki S, Iwama Y, Matsuda S, Nakazato Y. Long-term clinical and angiographic follow-up in patients with isolated ostial stenosis of the left coronary artery. *Circ J.* 2009; 73(7):1271-1277.
3. Dragu R, Kerner A, Gruberg L, et al. Angiographically uncertain left main coronary artery narrowings: correlation with multidetector computed tomography and intravascular ultrasound. *Int J Cardiovasc Imaging.* 2008;24(5):557-563.
4. Zeina AR, Rosenschein U, Barmeir E. Dimensions and anatomic variations of left main coronary artery in normal population: multidetector computed tomography assessment. *Coron Artery Dis.* 2007;18(6):477-482.
5. Ando G, Saporito F, Cerrito M, et al. Imaging of left main coronary artery dissection with multislice computed tomography. *Int J Cardiol.* 2007;115(3):e111-e113.
6. Jasti V, Ivan E, Yalamanchili V, Wongpraparut N, Leesar MA. Correlations between fractional flow reserve and intravascular ultrasound in patients with an ambiguous left main coronary artery stenosis. *Circulation.* 2004;110(18):2831-2836.
7. Gemici G, Guneysu T, Eroglu E, et al. Prevalence of left main coronary artery disease among patients referred to multislice computed tomography coronary examinations. *Int J Cardiovasc Imaging.* 2009;25(4):433-438.
8. van der Wall EE, Schuijf JD, Jukema JW, Bax JJ, Schalij MJ. Non-significant left main disease; truly non-significant? *Int J Cardiovasc Imaging.* 2009;25(4):439-442.
9. van Mieghem CA, Cademartiri F, Mollet NR, et al. Multislice spiral computed tomography for the evaluation of stent patency after left main coronary artery stenting: a comparison with conventional coronary angiography and intravascular ultrasound. *Circulation.* 2006;114(7):645-653.
10. Kimmelstiel C. Multislice computed tomography after left main drug-eluting stenting: are we putting the cart before the horse? *Circulation.* 2006;114(7):616-619.
11. Knobel B, Rosman P, Kriwisky M, Tamari I. Sudden death and cerebral anoxia in a young woman with congenital ostial stenosis of the left main coronary artery. *Catheter Cardiovasc Interv.* 1999;48(1):67-70.
12. Levisman J, Budoff M, Karlsberg R. Congenital atresia of the left main coronary artery: cardiac CT. *Catheter Cardiovasc Interv.* 2009;74(3):465-467.
13. Nicol ED, Lyne J, Rubens MB, Padley SP. Yen Ho S. Left main coronary atresia: a more commonly identified condition after the advent of 64-slice CT coronary angiography? *J Nucl Cardiol.* 2007; 14(5):715-718.
14. Goel P, Madhu Sankar N, Rajan S, Cherian KM. Coarctation of the aorta, aortic valvar stenosis, and supravalvar aortic stenosis with left coronary artery ostial stenosis: management using a staged hybrid approach. *Pediatr Cardiol.* 2001;22(1):83-84.
15. Roberts WC. The status of the coronary arteries in fatal ischemic heart disease. *Cardiovasc Clin.* 1975;7(2):1-24.
16. Yilmaz AT, Arslan M, Ozal E, Byngol H, Tatar H, Ozturk OY. Coronary artery aneurysm associated with adult supravalvular aortic stenosis. *Ann Thorac Surg.* 1996;62(4):1205-1207.
17. Lanjewar C, Kerkar P, Vaideeswar P, Pandit S. Isolated bilateral coronary ostial stenosis—an uncommon presentation of aortoarteritis. *Int J Cardiol.* 2007;114(3):e126-e128.
18. Cavalli G, Luzza F, Carerj S, Fiumara F, Oreto G. Ostial stenosis of the left coronary artery in Takayasu's arteritis detected by multislice computed tomography. *Int J Clin Pract.* 2008;62(1):162.
19. Bottio T, Cardaioli P, Ossi E, Casarotto D, Thiene G, Basso C. Left main trunk ostial stenosis and aortic incompetence in Takayasu's arteritis. *Cardiovasc Pathol.* 2002;11(5):291-295.
20. Stein JD, Lee P, Kuriya B, et al. Critical coronary artery stenosis and aortitis in a patient with relapsing polychondritis. *J Rheumatol.* 2008;35(9):1898-1900.
21. Tanaka K, Takeda M, Nagayama K. Composite Y-graft for syphilitic ostial stenosis in left main coronary artery. *Asian Cardiovasc Thorac Ann.* 2007;15(2):159-161.
22. Kennedy JL, Barnard JJ, Prahlow JA. Syphilitic coronary artery ostial stenosis resulting in acute myocardial infarction and death. *Cardiology.* 2006;105(1):25-29.
23. Hirata K, Ikenaga S, Ikeda Y, et al. [Left coronary ostial stenosis caused by syphilitic aortitis]. *Kyobu Geka.* 2005;58(6):481-485.
24. Aizawa H, Hasegawa A, Arai M, et al. Bilateral coronary ostial stenosis and aortic regurgitation due to syphilitic aortitis. *Intern Med.* 1998;37(1):56-59.
25. Fuzellier JF, Mauran P, Metz D. Radiation-induced bilateral coronary ostial stenosis in a 17-year-old patient. *J Card Surg.* 2006;21(6): 600-602.
26. Sachithanandan A, Ahmed A, O'Kane H. Bilateral isolated coronary ostial stenosis following mediastinal irradiation. *Asian Cardiovasc Thorac Ann.* 2004;12(1):78-80.
27. Notaristefano S, Giombolini C, Santucci S, et al. Radiation-induced ostial stenosis of the coronary artery as a cause of acute coronary syndromes: a novel mechanism of thrombus formation? *Ital Heart J.* 2003;4(5):341-344.
28. Aronow H, Kim M, Rubenfire M. Silent ischemic cardiomyopathy and left coronary ostial stenosis secondary to radiation therapy. *Clin Cardiol.* 1996;19(3):260-262.
29. Pillai JB, Pillay TM, Ahmad J. Coronary ostial stenosis after aortic valve replacement, revisited. *Ann Thorac Surg.* 2004;78(6): 2169-2171.
30. Bjork V, Henze A, Szamosi A. Coronary ostial stenosis: a complication of aortic valve replacement of coronary perfusion. *Scand J Thorac Cardiovasc Surg.* 1976;10(1):1-6.
31. Pennington DG, Dincer B, Bashiti H, et al. Coronary artery stenosis following aortic valve replacement and intermittent intracoronary cardioplegia. *Ann Thorac Surg.* 1982;33(6):576-584.
32. Tsukiji M, Akasaka T, Wada N, et al. [Bilateral coronary ostial stenosis after aortic valve replacement with freestyle stentless bioprosthesis: a case report]. *J Cardiol.* 2004;44(5):207-213.
33. Arima M, Kanoh T, Kawano Y, et al. Isolated coronary ostial stenosis associated with coronary vasospasm. *Jpn Circ J.* 2000;64(12): 985-987.
34. Saito T, Motohashi M, Matsushima S, et al. Left main coronary artery atresia diagnosed by multidetector computed tomography. *Int J Cardiol.* 2009;135(1):e27-e29.
35. Ropers D, Ping DC, Achenbach S. Right-sided origin of the left main coronary artery: typical variants and their visualization by cardiac computerized tomography. *JACC Cardiovasc Imaging.* 2008; 1(5):679-681.
36. Coche E, Muller P, Gerber B. Anomalous origin of the left main coronary artery from the main pulmonary artery (ALCAPA) illustrated before and after surgical correction on ECG-gated 40-slice computed tomography. *Heart.* 2006;92(9):1193.
37. Funabashi N, Komuro I. Aberrant fistula arteries from the left main branch and right coronary artery to the left pulmonary arterial sinus demonstrated by multislice computed tomography. *Int J Cardiol.* 2006;106(3):428-430.
38. Cademartiri F, La Grutta L, Malago R, et al. Assessment of left main coronary artery atherosclerotic burden using 64-slice CT coronary angiography: correlation between dimensions and presence of plaques. *Radiol Med.* 2009;114(3):358-369.
39. Rodriguez-Granillo GA, Rosales MA, Degrossi E, Durbano I, Rodriguez AE. Multislice CT coronary angiography for the detection of burden, morphology and distribution of atherosclerotic plaques in the left main bifurcation. *Int J Cardiovasc Imaging.* 2007;23(3):389-392.
40. Kalangos A. Left coronary ostial stenosis caused by focal intimal fibrosis. *Ann Intern Med.* 1999;131(9):717.

41. Shenoda M, Barack BM, Toggart E, Chang DS. Use of coronary computed tomography angiography to detect coronary ostial stenosis after Bentall procedure. *J Cardiovasc Comput Tomogr.* 2009; 3(5):340-343.
42. Kiyama H, Ohshima N, Sakurada M, Kagawa N, Imazeki T, Yamada T. [A case of progressive right coronary ostial stenosis after Carrel patch method using gelatin-resorcin-formalin glue]. *Kyobu Geka.* 1998;51(2):102-105.
43. Han SW, Kim HJ, Kim S, Ryu KH. Coronary ostial stenosis after aortic valvuloplasty (comprehensive aortic root and valve repair). *Eur J Cardiothorac Surg.* 2009;35(6):1099-1101.
44. Trivi M, Albertal J, Vaccarino G, Albertal M, Navia D. Ostial stenosis after Bentall technique using glue: percutaneous stenting may be ineffective. *Interact Cardiovasc Thorac Surg.* 2007;6(4):511-513.
45. Nambi P, Sengupta R, Cheong BY. Previous left main coronary artery dissection: detected upon multislice computed tomography. *Tex Heart Inst J.* 2008;35(3):365-366.
46. Pina Y, Exaire JE, Sandoval J. Left main coronary artery extrinsic compression syndrome: a combined intravascular ultrasound and pressure wire. *J Invasive Cardiol.* 2006;18(3):E102-E104.
47. Patrat JF, Jondeau G, Dubourg O, et al. Left main coronary artery compression during primary pulmonary hypertension. *Chest.* 1997;112(3):842-843.
48. Safi M, Eslami V, Shabestari AA, et al. Extrinsic compression of left main coronary artery by the pulmonary trunk secondary to pulmonary hypertension documented using 64-slice multidetector computed tomography coronary angiography. *Clin Cardiol.* 2009;32(8): 426-428.
49. Dodd JD, Maree A, Palacios I, et al. Images in cardiovascular medicine. Left main coronary artery compression syndrome: evaluation with 64-slice cardiac multidetector computed tomography. *Circulation.* 2007;115(1):e7-e8.
50. Doyen D, Moceri P, Moschietto S, Cerboni P, Ferrari E. Left main coronary artery compression associated with primary pulmonary hypertension. *J Am Coll Cardiol.* 2012;60(6):559.
51. Dubois CL, Dymarkowski S, Van Cleemput J. Compression of the left main coronary artery by the pulmonary artery in a patient with the Eisenmenger syndrome. *Eur Heart J.* 2007; 28(16):1945.
52. Decuypere V, Delcroix M, Budts W. Left main coronary artery and right pulmonary vein compression by a large pulmonary artery aneurysm. *Heart.* 2004;90(4):e21.
53. Hamzeh RK, El-Said HG, Moore JW. Left main coronary artery compression from right pulmonary artery stenting. *Catheter Cardiovasc Interv.* 2009;73(2):197-202.
54. De Scheerder I, De Buyzere M, Clement D. Association between post-pericardiotomy syndrome and coronary occlusion after aortic valve replacement. *Br Heart J.* 1985;54(4):445-447.
55. Von Dem Bussche N, Isaacs DL, Goodman ET, Hassankhani A, Mahmud E. Imaging of intracoronary thrombus by multidetector helical computed tomography angiography. *Circulation.* 2004; 109(3):432.
56. Achenbach S, Marwan M. Intracoronary thrombus. *J Cardiovasc Comput Tomogr.* 2009;3(5):344-345.
57. Bramucci E, Repetto A, Ferrario M, et al. Effectiveness of adjunctive stent implantation following directional coronary atherectomy for treatment of left anterior descending ostial stenosis. *Am J Cardiol.* 2002;90(10):1074-1078.
58. Chen M, Hong T, Huo Y. Stenting for left main stenosis in a child with anomalous origin of left coronary artery: case report. *Chin Med J (Engl).* 2005;118(1):80-82.
59. Botsios S, Maatz W, Sprengel U, Heuer H, Walterbusch G. Patch angioplasty for isolated ostial stenosis of the left main coronary artery. *J Card Surg.* 2008;23(6):743-746.
60. Miura T, Yamazaki K, Kihara S, et al. Extensive patch angioplasty of the left main ostial stenosis using a rhombic-shaped pulmonary autograft. *Ann Thorac Cardiovasc Surg.* 2008;14(4):263-266.
61. Taylor AJ, Cerqueira M, Hodgson JM, et al. ACCF/SCCT/ACR/AHA/ASE/ASNC/NASCI/SCAI/SCMR 2010 appropriate use criteria for cardiac computed tomography. A report of the American College of Cardiology Foundation Appropriate Use Criteria Task Force, the Society of Cardiovascular Computed Tomography, the American College of Radiology, the American Heart Association, the American Society of Echocardiography, the American Society of Nuclear Cardiology, the North American Society for Cardiovascular Imaging, the Society for Cardiovascular Angiography and Interventions, and the Society for Cardiovascular Magnetic Resonance. *J Am Coll Cardiol.* 2010;56(22):1864-1894.

14 Determination of Coronary Calcium

Key Points

- Initially, CT assessment of coronary artery disease was done via assessment of the burden of coronary artery calcium as a surrogate of coronary atherosclerotic plaque severity assessment.
- The coronary artery calcium burden is associated, on average, with the severity of CAD plaque stenosis, but with a problematically wide standard error.
- Calcium scoring improves classification of patients deemed to be at intermediate risk by conventional risk factor assessment.
- Outcome improvement or cost-effectiveness benefits have not yet been established. Weintraub[52] states that "the question is not whether coronary calcium scoring adds additional information but whether it is enough to justify its use—and in which patient groups."
- Calcium scoring can be accomplished by several scoring methods:
  - The Agatston score should probably not be abandoned entirely, as it has the greatest amount of literature behind it.
  - Calcium mass offers the greatest reproducibility, and its value is easily interchanged with that of the Agatston score.

In many laboratories, calcium scoring is performed before coronary CT angiography (CTA) is (contingently) performed. If the score (for example, the Agatston score) is above a certain amount (for example, >600) the coronary CTA is not performed, because the CTA image quality is not likely to be adequate in the presence of extensive calcification. Thus, calcium scoring as an initial scan may obviate the radiation exposure of CTA.

According to the 1996 ACC/AHA Consensus Statement, "coronary calcification is part of the development of atherosclerosis; it occurs exclusively in atherosclerotic arteries and is absent in the normal vessel wall."[1] Calcium is a component of some, but not all, coronary atherosclerotic plaques. Calcium accounts for, on average, approximately 20% of the plaque volume, but there is wide variation in the amount of calcium within plaques, and a large plaque or severe stenosis may exist without calcification.[2]

In general (but not always), coronary calcium correlates with plaque volume.[3] CT determinations of coronary calcium compared with those obtained by intravascular ultrasound (IVUS) are excellent.[4,5]

CT scanning is exquisitely sensitive to the presence of calcification and is easily the best test to detect calcification. The ability of CT to image, and then to quantify, coronary calcium with a calcium "score" launched an entire field of investigation.

Other cardiac structures within the heart and potentially near the coronary arteries, such as the aortic root, valve annuli, valves, pericardium, and myocardium, may calcify, as may other vessels.

CALCIUM ASSESSMENT BY CARDIOVASCULAR CT IS POSSIBLE BY DIFFERENT METHODS

Cardiovascular CT may be used to assess calcium by any of the following methods:

- Agatston score
- Volume score
- Calcium mass score

Agatston Score

The Agatston score, the original means by which coronary calcification was quantified, was derived from the use of electron beam CT (EBCT) scanning. Calcium scoring by EBCT and cardiac CT, though, are not wholly equivalent.

Most of the literature on coronary calcification was derived using Agatston scoring on now-obsolete EBCT equipment. The determination of coronary calcification by other scores has less presence in the literature.

The Agatston score was derived from two-dimensional axial scans with 3-mm slice thickness, with calcium weighted according to its density as determined by HU (higher weight for greater HUs).[6]

The first problem encountered with calcium scoring by the Agatston EBCT method was reproducibility: its accuracy was ±14% to ±51%[7]

TABLE 14-1 Variation of Agatston Score and Mass Score by EBCT and CCT

	EBCT	CCT PROSPECTIVE	CCT RETROSPECTIVE	CCT RETROSPECTIVE	CCT RETROSPECTIVE
Width	3 mm	4 x 2.5 mm	4 x 2.5 mm	4 x 2.5 mm	4 x 1.0 mm
Agatston Score					
Mean	35.5	20.8	21.6	24.1	28.8
σ	3.3	5.8	6.1	4.8	1.6
CV(%)	9.3	27.9	28.3	19.8	5.9
HA Mass					
Mean	6.3	3.9	4.2	4.8	4.9
σ	0.3	0.9	1.0	0.8	0.2
CV(%)	5.3	22.2	23.9	16.1	4.1

CCT, cardiac CT; CV(%), mean coefficient of variance = σ/mean[10]; EBCT, electron beam CT; HA, hydroxyapatite.

(±40% average). Reproducibility even by now-obsolete four-slice CCT appeared superior: ±20%,[8] and by 16-slice CCT reproducibility was even greater: ±13%.[9] The better reproducibility of Agatston score by CCT may be the result of better spatial resolution.[10]

The Agatston score is vulnerable to the partial volume effect. Phantom studies suggest that body size and level of scanning influence attenuation and calcium score.[11] As the intra- and interobserver variability of coronary artery calcium scores by EBCT technology are low, ECG gating should be used to reduce the variability.[12]

Agatston calcium scoring is influenced by the different equipment used for the scan.

In general, the literature suggests that coronary calcium scores lower than 400 by CCT and EBCT are similar[11] but that older-generation CCT may not yield the same correlation[13] as do more contemporary CCT scanners.[11]

Problems with the Agatston score include:

- ❒ Susceptibility to partial volume effects
- ❒ Submitral annular calcium sampling
- ❒ Effects of slice thickness
- ❒ Effects of cardiac motion
- ❒ Very long breath-holds needed in EBCT systems
- ❒ Variability depending on the type and make of equipment used

Use of average density improves reproducibility.[14]

Calcium Volume

The calcium volume score is the product of the number of voxels exceeding threshold multiplied by the volume of a voxel. It is theoretically independent of slice thickness—an improvement over the Agatston score. Calcium volume appears more reproducible than Agatston score: ±14%.[8] However, calcium volume does not have as much literature to back it up.

Calcium ("Hydroxyapatite" or "Mineral") Mass

Use of calcium or hydroxyapatite (HA) mass as a measure of the total amount of calcification offers improvements over the Agatston score but does not have as much literature to support it. It has become a preferred means of describing coronary calcium because it:

- ❒ Automatically adjusts/corrects for partial volume effects
- ❒ Is less affected by scan parameters
- ❒ Has the best reproducibility: ±9%[8]
- ❒ Correlates well with Agatston score: $r^2 = 0.97$, $y - 0.1922x$ (Table 14-1)[10]

Mass score is 0.2 times the Agatston score.

Protocol of Coronary Artery Identification, Marking, and Calcium Scoring

Calcium Scoring Protocol

- ❒ Scanning
  - Breath-hold
  - 3-mm slices
  - 55 mA, 120 kV
- ❒ Software analysis
  - Establish the cutoff for determining (coronary) calcium; usually 130 HU
  - Select the score (e.g., Agatston, volume, or mass)
  - Review on axial images: scroll from the top down
  - Use the available software to:
    - "Highlight" the coronary arteries (software algorithms)
    - Select each coronary artery one after the other
    - Mark the calcification that is to be included in the scoring
    - Calculate the score specific to each artery, and the total score.
    - See Figures 14-1 through 14-6.

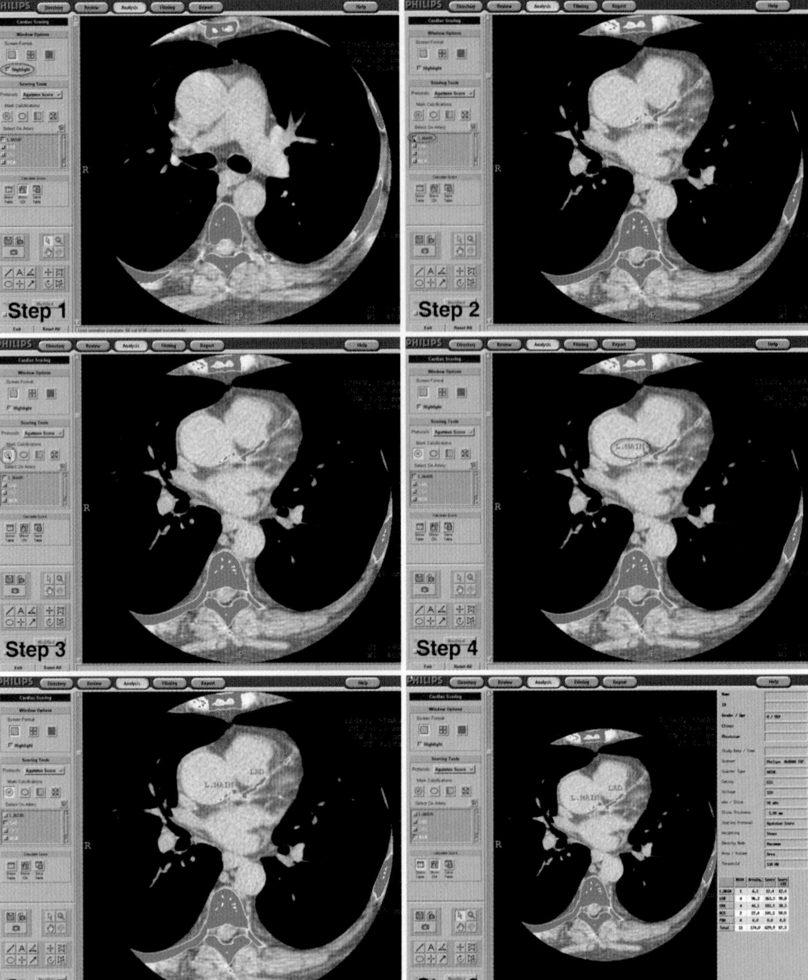

Figure 14-1. *Step 1:* Select: "Highlight" from the menu. Scrolling up and down through the heart, the coronary arteries, if calcified >130 HU, will become color-encoded. Here, above the coronary arteries, none appear color-encoded. *Step 2:* Select an artery from the menu. Here the left main coronary artery is selected from the menu. The imaging algorithms have identified calcium (using the 130 HU cutoff) in the aortic wall, the left main coronary artery (LMCA), and the left anterior descending artery (LAD). *Step 3:* Mark the calcification relevant to the selected artery, using the "mark calcification" cursor. *Step 4:* The artery and the calcification specific to it are identified by the process of highlighting, artery identification, and calcium marking. *Step 5:* Repeat selection of artery and marking with cursor, artery by artery (LMCA, LAD, left circumflex, right coronary). *Step 6:* Calcium scoring quantification.

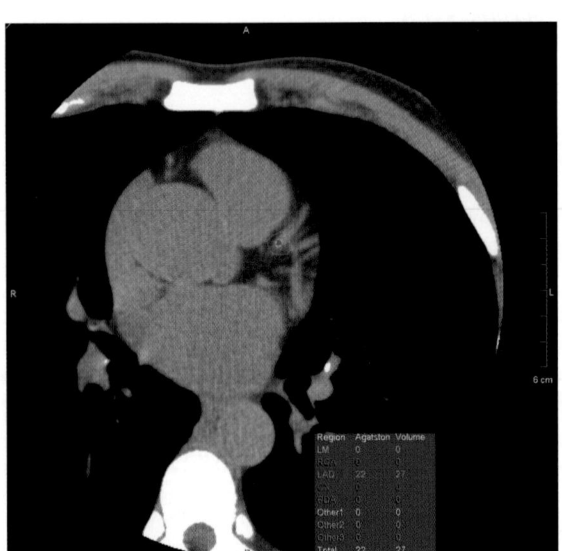

Figure 14-2. Automated coronary calcium Agatston scoring and calcium volume determinations. Note the red pixellation on the proximal LAD denoting calcium detection.

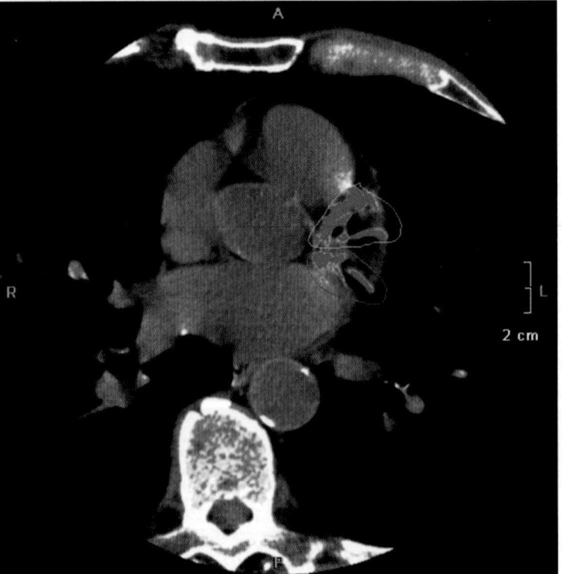

Figure 14-3. Manual separation of left anterior descending (traced green line) and left circumflex (traced blue line) automated coronary calcium detection (red pixels).

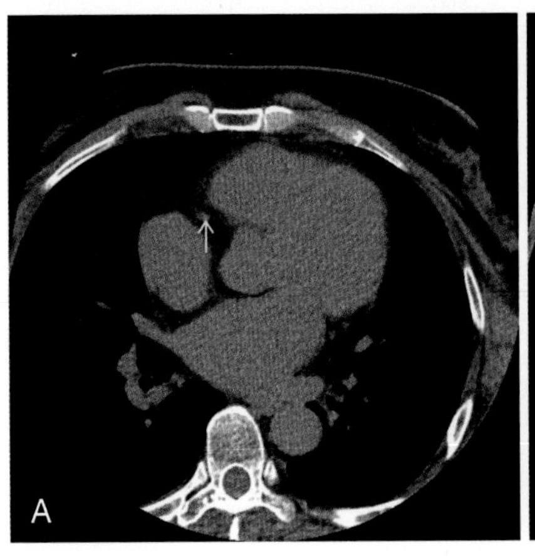

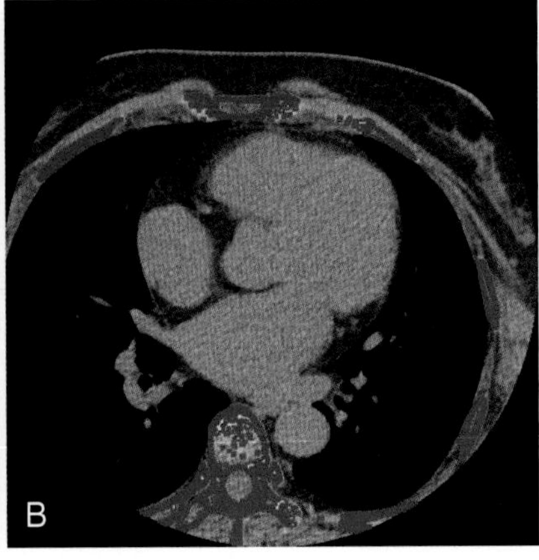

Figure 14-4. Coronary calcification despite a "zero" Agatston score. **A,** Note the visually apparent focus of calcification in the proximal right coronary artery (RCA; *yellow arrow*). **B,** With the Agatston filter on, which selects voxels with an attenuation > 130 HU, the ribs and spine have been automatically depicted (*red pixelated regions*). Despite the visually apparent calcification within the proximal RCA, the filter has missed the RCA calcification, as the mean voxel attenuation within the RCA is <130 HU due to partial volume averaging of the calcium with lower attenuation material.

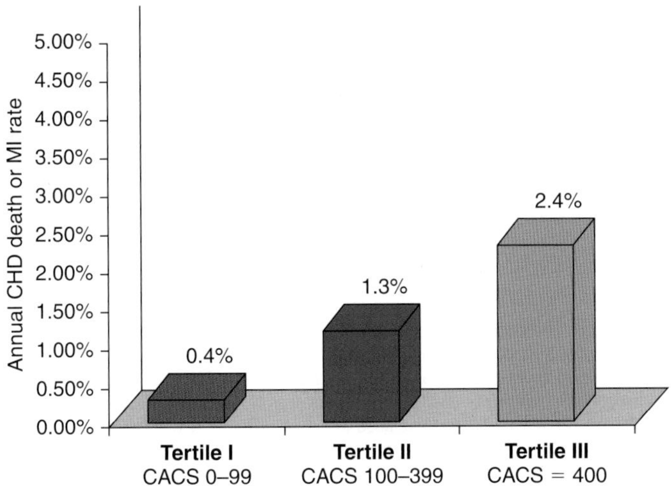

Figure 14-5. Estimated annual risk of coronary heart disease (CHD) death or myocardial infarction (MI) rate. Rate shown is by tertile of the Agatston score in patients at intermediate risk for a CHD event, using definitions of an intermediate Framingham Risk Score (FRS). Intermediate FRS has been variably defined as 10% to 20% risk or more than one cardiac risk factor. (From *Circulation.* 2007;115:402-426; originally published online January 12, 2007; doi: 10.1161/CIRCULATIONAHA..107.181425.)

Coronary Calcium and Electron Beam CT Studies

Adjusting for other risk factors, calcium scoring is a modest predictor of coronary events.[15] CT coronary angiography trumps calcium scoring because it provides independent and incremental value in the prediction of all-cause mortality and a diagnosis.[16]

By convention, a risk of more than 2% per year constitutes "high risk"[17] and legitimizes the use of "aggressive interventions."[18]

Improved Stratification of Intermediate-Risk Patients. The main advantage of calcium scoring is that it provides improved risk assessment of intermediate-risk patients by conventional risk assessment schemes—for example, to "upgrade" them to high risk, and have them benefit from aggressive interventions. The ability of calcium scoring to add incremental information on coronary risk beyond conventional risk factor assessment has been demonstrated.[19-24]

In general, there is no strong correlation between coronary calcium and conventional risk factor assessment, suggesting that these two strategies assess by different and what potentially may be complementary means. As predicted by correlation of coronary calcium score and Framingham Risk Score, as well as Adult Treatment Panel III (ATP III) from the National Cholesterol Education Program (NCEP) and PROspective CArdiovascular Münster Study (PROCAM), the 10-year risk events rate is low (0.19–0.28), with elevated coronary calcium scoring present in many patients with lower risk as predicted by traditional risk factors.[25]

Observational Data on Calcium Scoring, Usually by Electron Beam CT, and Coronary Disease

- Baseline plaque burden determines coronary artery calcium (CAC) progression.[26]
- Coronary calcification has both racial[27] and genetic[28] predisposition.

Observational Data on Calcium Scoring, Usually by Electron Beam CT, and Coronary Disease Outcomes

- Among patients younger than 60 years of age with a first infarct, CAC levels were greater than in aged-matched controls (529 ± 901 vs. 119 ± 213; $P < .001$). CAC scores above the 50th

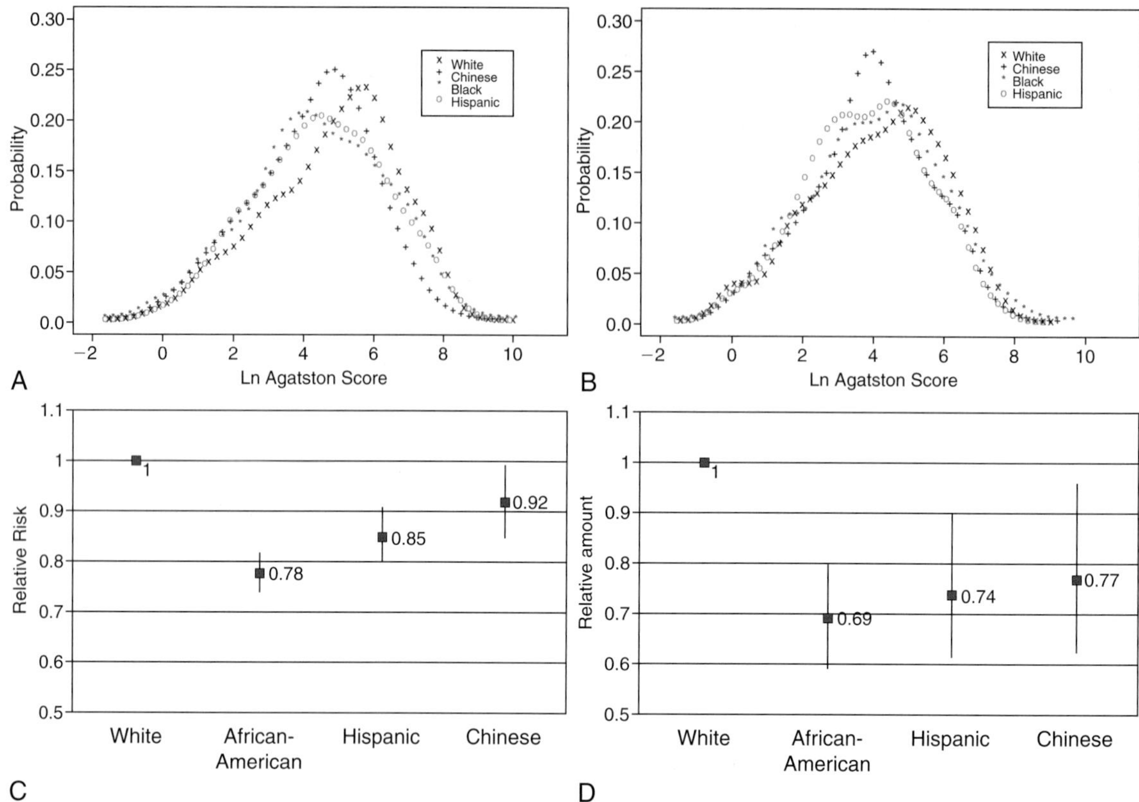

Figure 14-6. Results from the Multi-Ethnic Study of Atherosclerosis (MESA). **A,** Distribution of coronary calcification among those with detectable calcification by ethnicity, men. **B,** Distribution of coronary calcification among those with detectable calcification by ethnicity, women. **C,** Relative risk for presence of coronary calcification by ethnicity, compared with whites. 95% CIs shown. Adjusted for age, gender, education, body mass index (BMI), low-density lipoprotein (LDL) cholesterol, high-density lipoprotein (HDL) cholesterol, smoking, hypertension, diabetes, reported treatment for high cholesterol, and center. **D,** Relative coronary calcium amount, as measured by Agatston score, by ethnicity compared with whites, among those with detectable calcification. Relative amounts measured by Agatston scores. 95% CIs shown. Adjusted for age, gender, education, BMI, LDL cholesterol, triglycerides, smoking, hypertension, diabetes, reported treatment for high cholesterol, and center. (Reprinted with permission from Bild DE, Detrano R, Peterson D, et al. Ethnic differences in coronary calcification: the Multi-Ethnic Study of Atherosclerosis (MESA). *Circulation.* 2005;111(10):1313-1320.)

percentile were present in 87% of infarct patients and in 47% of controls, and above the 90th percentile in 61% of infarct patients and 6% of controls.[29]

- Progression of coronary calcium scoring is greater (RR: 17.2-fold) in patients who experienced myocardial infarction (MI) versus those who did not.[30,31]
- Annual change in coronary calcium scoring is greater in patients who experienced a coronary event.[17] Among asymptomatic middle-aged individuals, the CAC scores of individuals who experienced MI, revascularization, or death were significantly higher: 764 ± 935 vs. 135 ± 432 ($P < .0001$). A coronary calcium score of 160 was associated with odds ratios of 16 for nonfatal MI and 22 for death.[32] Yet the South Bay Heart Watch Study reported an odds ratio of 3.1 ($P < .07$) prediction of nonfatal MI and death, a level short of significance.[33]
- Association of CAC and risk prediction is present even among the elderly, as reported by the Rotterdam Coronary Calcification Study.[34,35]
- A high calcium score is three times more predictive of infarction/death than is a severe single-photon emission CT (SPECT) abnormality (25% vs. 7.5%; $P < .0001$).[36]
- An extremely high CAC (>1000) poses a high risk of MI or death (36% with 28 months), greater than risk predicted by historical control MPI data.[36]
- Screening patients presenting in the Emergency Department with chest pain by calcium scoring. If the calcium score is 0, the risk is low,[37] as long as the prevalence of disease is low.[38]
- Combined use of calcium scoring and measurement of plasma C–reactive protein assists in stratifying intermediate risk (nondiabetic) patients as each contributes independent risk prediction of cardiovascular events.[39]
- A wide range of calcium scores is observed in older adults.[40]
- A positive family history is associated with higher CAC scores.[41]
- Coronary vasodilator response correlates inversely with the presence and severity of CAC scores.[42]

- ❐ No major differences among racial or ethnic groups have been convincingly demonstrated in regard to the predictive value of CAC.[43]

In the Multi-Ethnic Study of Atherosclerosis (MESA)—which included 6722 patients: 38.6% white, 27.7% black, 21.9% Hispanic, and 11.9% Chinese—increasing calcium scores were shown across ethnicities to correlate with increasing coronary risk of major events (myocardial infarction or death from coronary heart disease).[43] No major differences were observed among racial and ethnic groups in the predictive value of calcium scoring.[43] Whether or not calcium predicted or contributed to risk,[44] whether or not renal dysfunction contributed to the observations,[45] and whether or not the study was underpowered with respect to its predetermined event rate[46] engendered discussion. Differences were detected in the presence and quantity of calcium that were not explained by conventional coronary risk factors. The amount of coronary calcification (Agatston score > 0) was greatest among whites[27] (see Figs. 14-5 and 14-6). The MESA website (http://www.mesa-nhlbi.org/CACReference.aspx) has on-line calculators of measured CAC as a percentile of age, gender, value according to race, and "arterial age."

Experimental Data on Calcium Scoring, Usually by EBCT, and Coronary Disease Outcomes

- ❐ Treatment with low-dose atorvastatin and vitamins C and E does not reduce CAC progression (St. Francis Heart Study).[47]
- ❐ Effect of lipid lowering on coronary calcium scoring as see on EBCT
  - Median annualized rate of coronary calcium scoring increase in untreated vs. statin-treated: 25% vs. 9%
  - The extent to which plaque volume decreased, stabilized, or increased related directly to treatment with statins[48]
  - Calcified plaques are more resistant to medical interventions,[49] because they contain less lipid.
- ❐ Progression rates[50]
  - Treated (all risk factors): 15 ± 8%
  - Untreated: 39 ± 12%/year

A relation of on-treatment cholesterol levels (under standard and intensive atorvastatin regimens) and CAC progression by EBCT was not demonstrated (over a 12-month period).[51]

Outcomes Data on Calcium Scoring, Usually by Electron Beam CT, and Coronary Disease Outcomes

- ❐ There are no outcomes data on calcium scoring versus coronary disease outcomes to date.[52]
- ❐ The most relevant outcomes data on calcium scoring is that intermediate-risk (10-year 10–120% risk) patients, by Framingham scoring, would have better survivals if they were to undergo CT and were reclassified.[19,53]

Cost-effectiveness Data on Calcium Scoring, Usually by Electron Beam CT, and Coronary Disease Outcomes. There are no cost-effectiveness data to date.[52]

Caveats, Concerns, and Controversy

However, a calcium score of 0 does not always predict no/low risk.[19,54]

- ❐ Core-64[54]
  - Of 72 patients with a calcium score of 0:
    - 56% had a stenosis >50%
    - a calcium score of 0 has limited negative predictive value for stenosis <50% (Fig. 14-7; Table 14-2)
- ❐ One study showed a marginal benefit in older patients.[55]
- ❐ Coronary calcium percentiles versus scores are more effective at predicting risk.[56]
- ❐ Concern over self-referral[57]
- ❐ Informing patients of their EBCT results to improve their motivation to change modifiable risk factors does not improve cardiovascular risk at 1 year.[58]
- ❐ There does not appear to be incremental value in predicting patient events by CAC to patients with negative myocardial perfusion tests.[59]
- ❐ Concern over heterogeneity in study composition in meta-analysis.[60]
- ❐ Guidelines published by the American College of Cardiology (ACC) with the American Heart Association (AHA) and by the American College of Cardiology Foundation (ACCF) with the AHA have been restrained in recommendations for calcium scoring.[34,61]
- ❐ Controversy and rebuttals.[62] ACC/AHA Expert Consensus.[61]
- ❐ The weight of evidence suggests that CAC scores are not reliable predictors of cardiac events.[63]
- ❐ ACC/AHA rebuttal of prognostic odds ratio for death or MI was 2.0 (CI: 0.5–8.2, $P > .20$)using a more rigorous analysis of the St. Francis data.[47]

CCT PROTOCOL POINTS

- ❐ Non-contrast enhanced scanning is utilized.
- ❐ For ACCF appropriateness criteria see Table 14-3.

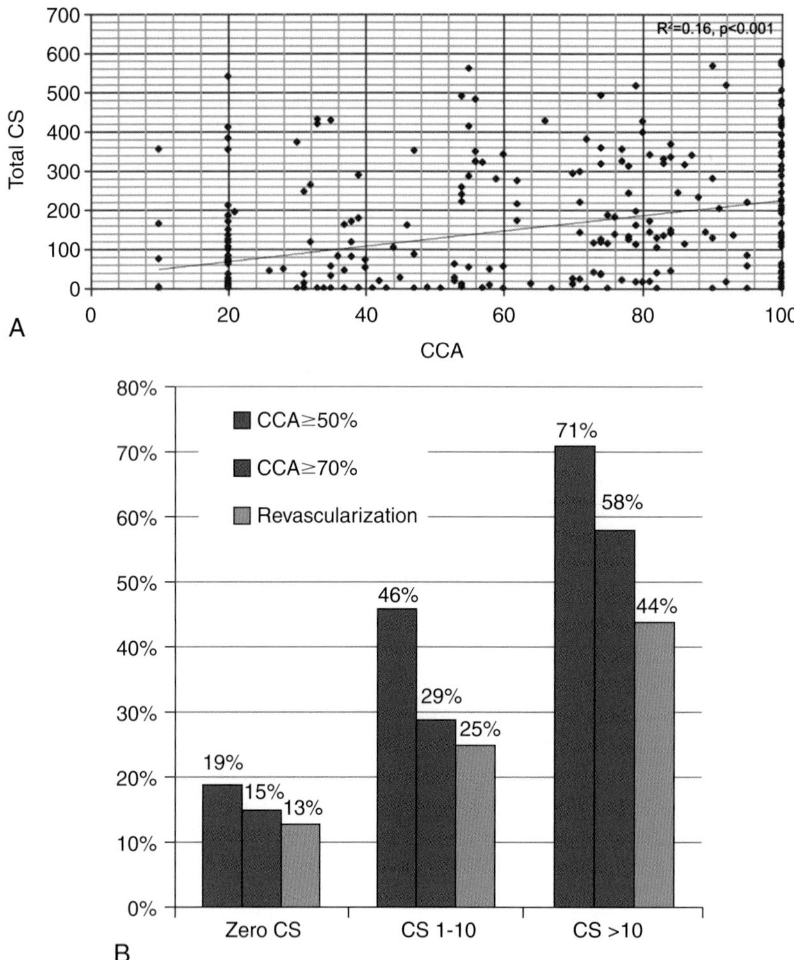

Figure 14-7. **A,** Individual values of calcium scoring and maximum coronary stenosis in subjects. Linear regression plot showing the poor correlation between the maximum degree of coronary stenosis by conventional coronary angiogram (CCA) and the calcium score (CS) in a patient. **B,** Prevalence of obstructive coronary artery disease (CAD) and need for clinically indicated revascularization among patients in different CS categories. As the calcium score increases, the prevalence of obstructive coronary artery disease and revascularization also increases ($P < .001$ for all trends). Note that the group of patients with a calcium score of 0 has a high prevalence of obstructive CAD and revascularization. The blue bars indicate CCA 50%; the red bars indicate CCA 70%; and the green bars indicate revascularization. (Reprinted with permission from Gottlieb I, Miller JM, Arbab-Zadeh A, et al. The absence of coronary calcification does not exclude obstructive coronary artery disease or the need for revascularization in patients referred for conventional coronary angiography. *J Am Coll Cardiol.* 2010;55:627-634.)

TABLE 14-2 A Calcium Score of 0 to Predict <50% Stenosis

SENSITIVITY (%)	SPECIFICITY (%)	NPV (%)	PPV (%)
45	91	68	81

Data from Gottlieb I, Miller JM, Arbab-Zadeh A, et al. The absence of coronary calcification does not exclude obstructive coronary artery disease or the need for revascularization in patients referred for conventional coronary angiography. *J Am Coll Cardiol.* 2010;55:627-634.

TABLE 14-3 ACCF 2010 Appropriateness Criteria for the Use of Cardiac Computed Tomography to Evaluate Coronary Calcium Score

INDICATION		APPROPRIATE USE SCORE (1–9)
Detection of CAD/Risk Assessment in Asymptomatic Individuals Without Known CAD—Noncontrast CT for CCS	Family history of premature CHD Low global CHD risk estimate	Appropriate (7)
	Asymptomatic No known CAD Intermediate global CHD risk estimate	Appropriate (7)
Detection of CAD/Risk Assessment in Asymptomatic Individuals Without Known CAD—Noncontrast CT for CCS	Asymptomatic No known CAD High global CHD risk estimate	Uncertain (4)

	GLOBAL CHD RISK ESTIMATE	LOW	INTERMEDIATE	HIGH
Noncontrast CT for CCS	Family history of premature CHD	Appropriate (7)		
	Asymptomatic No known CAD	Inappropriate (2)	Appropriate (7)	Uncertain (4)

CAD, Coronary artery disease; CCS, coronary calcium score; CHD, coronary heart disease.

Reprinted with permission from Taylor AJ, Cerqueira M, Hodgson JM, et al. ACCF/SCCT/ACR/AHA/ASE/ASNC/NASCI/SCAI/SCMR 2010 appropriate use criteria for cardiac computed tomography. A report of the American College of Cardiology Foundation Appropriate Use Criteria Task Force, the Society of Cardiovascular Computed Tomography, the American College of Radiology, the American Heart Association, the American Society of Echocardiography, the American Society of Nuclear Cardiology, the North American Society for Cardiovascular Imaging, the Society for Cardiovascular Angiography and Interventions, and the Society for Cardiovascular Magnetic Resonance. *J Am Coll Cardiol.* 2010;56(22):1864-1894.

References

1. O'Rourke RA, Brundage BH, Froelicher VF, et al. American College of Cardiology/American Heart Association Expert Consensus Document on electron-beam computed tomography for the diagnosis and prognosis of coronary artery disease. *J Am Coll Cardiol.* 2000;36(1):326-340.
2. Rumberger JA, Simons DB, Fitzpatrick LA, Sheedy PF, Schwartz RS. Coronary artery calcium area by electron-beam computed tomography and coronary atherosclerotic plaque area. A histopathologic correlative study. *Circulation.* 1995;92(8):2157-2162.
3. Achenbach S, Ropers D, Hoffmann U, et al. Assessment of coronary remodeling in stenotic and nonstenotic coronary atherosclerotic lesions by multidetector spiral computed tomography. *J Am Coll Cardiol.* 2004;43(5):842-847.
4. Schmermund A, Baumgart D, Adamzik M, et al. Comparison of electron-beam computed tomography and intracoronary ultrasound in detecting calcified and noncalcified plaques in patients with acute coronary syndromes and no or minimal to moderate angiographic coronary artery disease. *Am J Cardiol.* 1998;81(2):141-146.
5. Ehara S, Kobayashi Y, Yoshiyama M, et al. Spotty calcification typifies the culprit plaque in patients with acute myocardial infarction: an intravascular ultrasound study. *Circulation.* 2004;110(22):3424-3429.
6. Agatston AS, Janowitz WR, Hildner FJ, Zusmer NR, Viamonte Jr M, Detrano R. Quantification of coronary artery calcium using ultrafast computed tomography. *J Am Coll Cardiol.* 1990;15(4):827-832.
7. Wang S, Detrano RC, Secci A, et al. Detection of coronary calcification with electron-beam computed tomography: evaluation of interexamination reproducibility and comparison of three image-acquisition protocols. *Am Heart J.* 1996;132(3):550-558.
8. Hong C, Bae KT, Pilgram TK. Coronary artery calcium: accuracy and reproducibility of measurements with multi-detector row CT–assessment of effects of different thresholds and quantification methods. *Radiol.* 2003;227(3):795-801.
9. Horiguchi J, Yamamoto H, Akiyama Y, et al. Variability of repeated coronary artery calcium measurements by 16-MDCT with retrospective reconstruction. *AJR Am J Roentgenol.* 2005;184(6):1917-1923.
10. Ulzheimer S, Kalender WA. Assessment of calcium scoring performance in cardiac computed tomography. *Eur Radiol.* 2003;13(3):484-497.
11. Stanford W, Thompson BH, Burns TL, Heery SD, Burr MC. Coronary artery calcium quantification at multi-detector row helical CT versus electron-beam CT. *Radiol.* 2004;230(2):397-402.
12. Lu B, Zhuang N, Mao SS, et al. EKG-triggered CT data acquisition to reduce variability in coronary arterial calcium score. *Radiol.* 2002;224(3):838-844.
13. Goldin JG, Yoon HC, Greaser III LE, et al. Spiral versus electron-beam CT for coronary artery calcium scoring. *Radiol.* 2001;221(1):213-221.
14. Shemesh J, Apter S, Stolero D, Itzchak Y, Motro M. Annual progression of coronary artery calcium by spiral computed tomography in hypertensive patients without myocardial ischemia but with prominent atherosclerotic risk factors, in patients with previous angina pectoris or healed acute myocardial infarction, and in patients with coronary events during follow-up. *Am J Cardiol.* 2001;87(12):1395-1397.
15. Wong ND, Hsu JC, Detrano RC, Diamond G, Eisenberg H, Gardin JM. Coronary artery calcium evaluation by electron beam computed tomography and its relation to new cardiovascular events. *Am J Cardiol.* 2000;86(5):495-498.
16. Ostrom MP, Gopal A, Ahmadi N, et al. Mortality incidence and the severity of coronary atherosclerosis assessed by computed tomography angiography. *J Am Coll Cardiol.* 2008;52(16):1335-1343.
17. Greenland P, Smith Jr SC, Grundy SM. Improving coronary heart disease risk assessment in asymptomatic people: role of traditional risk factors and noninvasive cardiovascular tests. *Circulation.* 2001;104(15):1863-1867.
18. Smith Jr SC, Greenland P, Grundy SM. AHA Conference Proceedings. Prevention conference V: Beyond secondary prevention: identifying the high-risk patient for primary prevention: executive summary. American Heart Association. *Circulation.* 2000;101(1):111-116.
19. Greenland P, LaBree L, Azen SP, Doherty TM, Detrano RC. Coronary artery calcium score combined with Framingham score for risk prediction in asymptomatic individuals. *JAMA.* 2004;291(2):210-215.
20. Arad Y, Goodman KJ, Roth M, Newstein D, Guerci AD. Coronary calcification, coronary disease risk factors, C-reactive protein, and atherosclerotic cardiovascular disease events: the St. Francis Heart Study. *J Am Coll Cardiol.* 2005;46(1):158-165.
21. Kondos GT, Hoff JA, Sevrukov A, et al. Electron-beam tomography coronary artery calcium and cardiac events: a 37-month follow-up of 5635 initially asymptomatic low- to intermediate-risk adults. *Circulation.* 2003;107(20):2571-2576.
22. Shaw LJ, Raggi P, Schisterman E, Berman DS, Callister TQ. Prognostic value of cardiac risk factors and coronary artery calcium screening for all-cause mortality. *Radiol.* 2003;228(3):826-833.
23. Raggi P, Cooil B, Callister TQ. Use of electron beam tomography data to develop models for prediction of hard coronary events. *Am Heart J.* 2001;141(3):375-382.

24. Budoff MJ, Diamond GA, Raggi P, et al. Continuous probabilistic prediction of angiographically significant coronary artery disease using electron beam tomography. *Circulation.* 2002;105(15):1791-1796.
25. Achenbach S, Nomayo A, Couturier G, et al. Relation between coronary calcium and 10-year risk scores in primary prevention patients. *Am J Cardiol.* 2003;92(12):1471-1475.
26. Schmermund A, Baumgart D, Mohlenkamp S, et al. Natural history and topographic pattern of progression of coronary calcification in symptomatic patients: an electron-beam CT study. *Arterioscler Thromb Vasc Biol.* 2001;21(3):421-426.
27. Bild DE, Detrano R, Peterson D, et al. Ethnic differences in coronary calcification: the Multi-Ethnic Study of Atherosclerosis (MESA). *Circulation.* 2005;111(10):1313-1320.
28. Wagenknecht LE, Bowden DW, Carr JJ, Langefeld CD, Freedman BI, Rich SS. Familial aggregation of coronary artery calcium in families with type 2 diabetes. *Diabetes.* 2001;50(4):861-866.
29. Pohle K, Ropers D, Maffert R, et al. Coronary calcifications in young patients with first, unheralded myocardial infarction: a risk factor matched analysis by electron beam tomography. *Heart.* 2003;89(6):625-628.
30. Raggi P, Callister TQ, Shaw LJ. Progression of coronary artery calcium and risk of first myocardial infarction in patients receiving cholesterol-lowering therapy. *Arterioscler Thromb Vasc Biol.* 2004;24(7):1272-1277.
31. Raggi P, Cooil B, Shaw LJ, et al. Progression of coronary calcium on serial electron beam tomographic scanning is greater in patients with future myocardial infarction. *Am J Cardiol.* 2003;92(7):827-829.
32. Arad Y, Spadaro LA, Goodman K, Newstein D, Guerci AD. Prediction of coronary events with electron beam computed tomography. *J Am Coll Cardiol.* 2000;36(4):1253-1260.
33. Wexler L, Brundage B, Crouse J, et al. Coronary artery calcification: pathophysiology, epidemiology, imaging methods, and clinical implications. A statement for health professionals from the American Heart Association. Writing Group. *Circulation.* 1996;94(5):1175-1192.
34. Vliegenthart R, Oudkerk M, Song B, van der Kuip DA, Hofman A, Witteman JC. Coronary calcification detected by electron-beam computed tomography and myocardial infarction. The Rotterdam Coronary Calcification Study. *Eur Heart J.* 2002;23(20):1596-1603.
35. Vliegenthart R, Oudkerk M, Hofman A, et al. Coronary calcification improves cardiovascular risk prediction in the elderly. *Circulation.* 2005;112(4):572-577.
36. Wayhs R, Zelinger A, Raggi P. High coronary artery calcium scores pose an extremely elevated risk for hard events. *J Am Coll Cardiol.* 2002;39(2):225-230.
37. Georgiou D, Budoff MJ, Kaufer E, Kennedy JM, Lu B, Brundage BH. Screening patients with chest pain in the emergency department using electron beam tomography: a follow-up study. *J Am Coll Cardiol.* 2001;38(1):105-110.
38. Raggi P, Callister TQ, Cooil B, Russo DJ, Lippolis NJ, Patterson RE. Evaluation of chest pain in patients with low to intermediate pretest probability of coronary artery disease by electron beam computed tomography. *Am J Cardiol.* 2000;85(3):283-288.
39. Park R, Detrano R, Xiang M, et al. Combined use of computed tomography coronary calcium scores and C-reactive protein levels in predicting cardiovascular events in nondiabetic individuals. *Circulation.* 2002;106(16):2073-2077.
40. Newman AB, Naydeck BL, Sutton-Tyrrell K, Feldman A, Edmundowicz D, Kuller LH. Coronary artery calcification in older adults to age 99: prevalence and risk factors. *Circulation.* 2001;104(22):2679-2684.
41. Nasir K, Budoff MJ, Wong ND, et al. Family history of premature coronary heart disease and coronary artery calcification: Multi-Ethnic Study of Atherosclerosis (MESA). *Circulation.* 2007;116(6):619-626.
42. Wang L, Jerosch-Herold M, Jacobs Jr DR, Shahar E, Detrano R, Folsom AR. Coronary artery calcification and myocardial perfusion in asymptomatic adults: the MESA (Multi-Ethnic Study of Atherosclerosis). *J Am Coll Cardiol.* 2006;48(5):1018-1026.
43. Detrano R, Guerci AD, Carr JJ, et al. Coronary calcium as a predictor of coronary events in four racial or ethnic groups. *N Engl J Med.* 2008;358(13):1336-1345.
44. Littmann L. Coronary calcium and events in four ethnic groups. *N Engl J Med.* 2008;359(2):202; author reply 204.
45. Burtey S, Dussol B, Brunet P. Coronary calcium and events in four ethnic groups. *N Engl J Med.* 2008;359(2):202-203; author reply 204.
46. Goyal SK, Punnam SR. Coronary calcium and events in four ethnic groups. *N Engl J Med.* 2008;359(2):203; author reply 204.
47. Arad Y, Spadaro LA, Roth M, Newstein D, Guerci AD. Treatment of asymptomatic adults with elevated coronary calcium scores with atorvastatin, vitamin C, and vitamin E: the St. Francis Heart Study randomized clinical trial. *J Am Coll Cardiol.* 2005;46(1):166-172.
48. Callister TQ, Raggi P, Cooil B, Lippolis NJ, Russo DJ. Effect of HMG-CoA reductase inhibitors on coronary artery disease as assessed by electron-beam computed tomography. *N Engl J Med.* 1998;339(27):1972-1978.
49. Nicholls SJ, Tuzcu EM, Wolski K, et al. Coronary artery calcification and changes in atheroma burden in response to established medical therapies. *J Am Coll Cardiol.* 2007;49(2):263-270.
50. Budoff MJ, Lane KL, Bakhsheshi H, et al. Rates of progression of coronary calcium by electron beam tomography. *Am J Cardiol.* 2000;86(1):8-11.
51. Schmermund A, Achenbach S, Budde T, et al. Effect of intensive versus standard lipid-lowering treatment with atorvastatin on the progression of calcified coronary atherosclerosis over 12 months: a multicenter, randomized, double-blind trial. *Circulation.* 2006;113(3):427-437.
52. Weintraub WS. Coronary artery calcium and cardiac events: is electron-beam tomography ready for prime time? *Circulation.* 2003;107(20):2528-2530.
53. Hecht HS, Budoff MJ, Berman DS, Ehrlich J, Rumberger JA. Coronary artery calcium scanning: clinical paradigms for cardiac risk assessment and treatment. *Am Heart J.* 2006;151(6):1139-1146.
54. Gottlieb I, Miller JM, Arbab-Zadeh A, et al. The absence of coronary calcification does not exclude obstructive coronary artery disease or the need for revascularization in patients referred for conventional coronary angiography. *J Am Coll Cardiol.* 2010;55:627-634.
55. Detrano RC, Wong ND, Doherty TM, et al. Coronary calcium does not accurately predict near-term future coronary events in high-risk adults. *Circulation.* 1999;99(20):2633-2638.
56. Raggi P, Callister TQ, Cooil B, et al. Identification of patients at increased risk of first unheralded acute myocardial infarction by electron-beam computed tomography. *Circulation.* 2000;101(8):850-855.
57. Taylor AJ, O'Malley PG. Self-Referral of Patients for Electron-Beam Computed Tomography to Screen for Coronary Artery Disease. *N Engl J Med.* 1998;339(27):2018-2020.
58. O'Malley PG, Feuerstein IM, Taylor AJ. Impact of electron beam tomography, with or without case management, on motivation, behavioral change, and cardiovascular risk profile: a randomized controlled trial. *JAMA.* 2003;289(17):2215-2223.
59. Rozanski A, Gransar H, Wong ND, et al. Clinical outcomes after both coronary calcium scanning and exercise myocardial perfusion scintigraphy. *J Am Coll Cardiol.* 2007;49(12):1352-1361.
60. O'Malley PG, Taylor AJ, Jackson JL, Doherty TM, Detrano RC. Prognostic value of coronary electron-beam computed tomography for coronary heart disease events in asymptomatic populations. *Am J Cardiol.* 2000;85(8):945-948.
61. O'Rourke RA, Brundage BH, Froelicher VF, et al. American College of Cardiology/American Heart Association Expert Consensus document on electron-beam computed tomography for the diagnosis and prognosis of coronary artery disease. *Circulation.* 2000;102(1):126-140.
62. Guerci AD, Arad Y. Electron beam computed tomography for the diagnosis and prognosis of coronary artery disease. *Circulation.* 2001;103(16):E87.
63. Redberg RF. Coronary artery calcium: should we rely on this surrogate marker? *Circulation.* 2006;113(3):336-337.

Pericardial Diseases

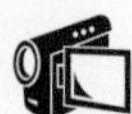

Key Points

- CCT is a superb test for assessing the structural aspects of pericardial diseases, including thickening, calcification, effusion, cysts, absence, masses, and malignancy.
- CCT is a poor test for identifying the functional aspects of pericardial diseases.
- CCT is best able to image the normal pericardium over the right ventricular free wall, where it is most likely to be offset by under- and overlying fat layers.
- Pericardial thickening can be seen by CCT, but this is not synonymous with constriction, because
  - Thickened pericardium may not constrict the heart.
  - About 20% of cases of constriction do not appear to have thickened pericardium.
  - Older definitions of pericardial thickening by CCT (and MRI) were not realistic and were actually misleading. Normal pericardial thickness is 1 mm. Current CCT imaging is able to depict pericardium nearly as it exists.

Pericardial diseases are numerous and diverse, and imaging has a central role in their evaluation. Currently, echocardiography is the principal test for pericardial disease assessment, because two-dimensional imaging and Doppler assessment are highly feasible by echocardiography, the test is portable, and it can be used to guide drainage procedures. However, several forms of pericardial disease—notably pericarditis and constrictive pericarditis, as well as cysts and congenital absence of the pericardium—remain elusive to delineation by echocardiography. With regard to pericardial diseases in general, the drawbacks of echocardiography include limited field of view and poor tissue plane recognition.

Pericardial diseases are usually investigated with combined physiologic and anatomic approaches. Cardiac catheterization offers only assessment of physiology (as well as depiction of calcium), whereas echocardiography and cardiac MR (CMR) offer assessment of physiology and anatomy, and CT offers depiction of anatomy and very limited surrogate markers for physiology. The choice of which test or combination of tests to use is determined by the disorder and its findings.

NORMAL PERICARDIUM

The normal pericardium consists of:

- A thin (<1 mm) fibrous layer (the parietal pericardium) that limits displacement of the heart within the chest, provides a barrier to disease (infection, inflammation and malignancy), and also limits distention of the heart chambers
- 15 to 50 mL of pericardial fluid that serves as a lubricant
- An extremely thin layer (cell monolayer—the "visceral pericardium") on the epicardial surface of the heart itself and on the inside of the parietal pericardial layer

There is potentially a space between the layers of the pericardium that may accumulate fluid if forces that favor fluid formation exceed those that favor removal.

The anatomic extent of the pericardium is complex: the pericardium and its space extend up along all of the vessels that connect to the heart:

- Up the ascending aorta to the innominate artery
- Up the pulmonary artery to or past the bifurcation
- Up the superior vena cava a few centimeters
- Down the inferior vena cava (IVC) a few centimeters
- Back along the pulmonary veins for a few centimeters

Thus, pericardial fluid can accumulate in numerous recesses well away from the heart chambers. Lack of knowledge of pericardial anatomy can lead to confusion regarding the cause of this fluid when it is present.

In addition, the covering of the heart proper by the pericardium is complex: a small part of the posterior aspect of the left atrium is *extra*pericardial (i.e., not within the pericardial space).

True normal pericardial thickness is less than 1 mm. The medical literature previously stated that "normal" pericardial thickness by MRI and by CT is

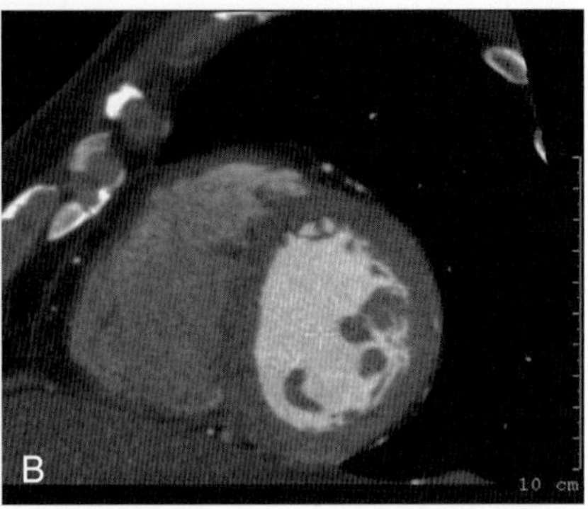

Figure 15-1. **A,** Contrast-enhanced axial view of the lower heart. The pericardium is seen as a thin (<1 mm) high-attenuation line starting around the right atrioventricular groove, and extending around the right ventricular free wall to the left ventricular (LV) apex. On this and many hearts, the normal pericardium is only well seen over the RV free wall, and tends to be poorly seen over the LV free wall, where there is less fat. **B,** Contrast-enhanced sagittal view of the heart. Again, the pericardium is seen over the right ventricle, between layers of low-attenuation fat. Some faint detection of the pericardium over the anterior interventricular groove is seen, because the groove contains fat.

less than 4 mm,[1] in contradistinction to what is seen in the operating room every day: normal pericardium has the thickness of paper. The older CT literature struggled with imaging that inevitably included translational artifact due to inadequate temporal resolution; therefore, the motion of the pericardium during acquisition rendered its image thicker than it truly was. Current cardiac CT (CCT) has much better spatial and temporal resolution and is capable of depicting the pericardium at close to its true thickness. By current ECG-gated CCT, normal pericardial thickness is about 1 mm.

Over some surfaces of the heart, usually the right heart, the parietal pericardium is sandwiched between layers of underlying epicardial fat and overlying pericardial fat, and when it is, the parietal pericardium can be distinguished from the myocardium and adjacent lung by its higher attenuation coefficient. In the absence of either the over- or the underlying fat layer, the thickness of the parietal pericardium cannot be established. In the absence of both underlying epicardial and overlying pericardial fat, the parietal pericardium cannot be identified as present or absent.

Pericardium over the left ventricular (LV) free wall may not be evident on CT, because there is little fat to make the pericardium stand out. Potential thickening is therefore usually assessed over the right ventricular (RV) free wall.

For CCT images of normal pericardium, see Figures 15-1 and 15-2.

PERICARDIAL CALCIFICATION

CCT is the preeminent test for detecting cardiac calcification, including pericardial calcification. Pericardial calcification is not synonymous with pericardial constriction. For CCT images of pericardial calcification, see Figures 15-3 through 15-7.

PERICARDIAL THICKENING

CCT is the best test for detecting pericardial thickening. It is important to recall that pericardial thickening is not present in 20% of constriction cases and that it may be present in the absence of constrictive physiology. Pericardial calcification is not synonymous with pericardial constriction. For CCT images of pericardial calcification, see Figure 15-8.

PERICARDITIS

Pericarditis is defined as inflammation of either or both of the pericardial layers. It usually occurs with little or no increase in the amount of pericardial fluid and only mild pericardial thickening; hence, imaging modalities have little to contribute directly toward the diagnosis of the average case of pericarditis. MRI is superior to CCT in distinguishing pericardial fluid from pericardial thickening. However, due to its increased spatial resolution, CCT may, in fact, be superior in identifying subtle pericardial nodularity. Subtle "stranding" of the epicardial fat also may be seen as a marker of peri- or epicardial inflammatory change and is better appreciated on CCT than on CMR.

For CCT images of pericarditis, see Figure 15-9 and **Videos 15-1 and 15-2.**

Pericardial Effusions

Echocardiography, CCT, and MRI are all capable of depicting pericardial effusions, and, importantly, of distinguishing them from pleural effusions, which have no risk of tamponade. Echocardiography and MRI are superior to CCT in distinguishing pericardial fluid from pericardial thickening. CCT also is less able to characterize pericardial fluid by appearance than are echocardiography and MRI. Fine specular echoes seen on either transthoracic or transesophageal echocardiography are strongly suggestive of blood, and wobbly, fine specular echoes

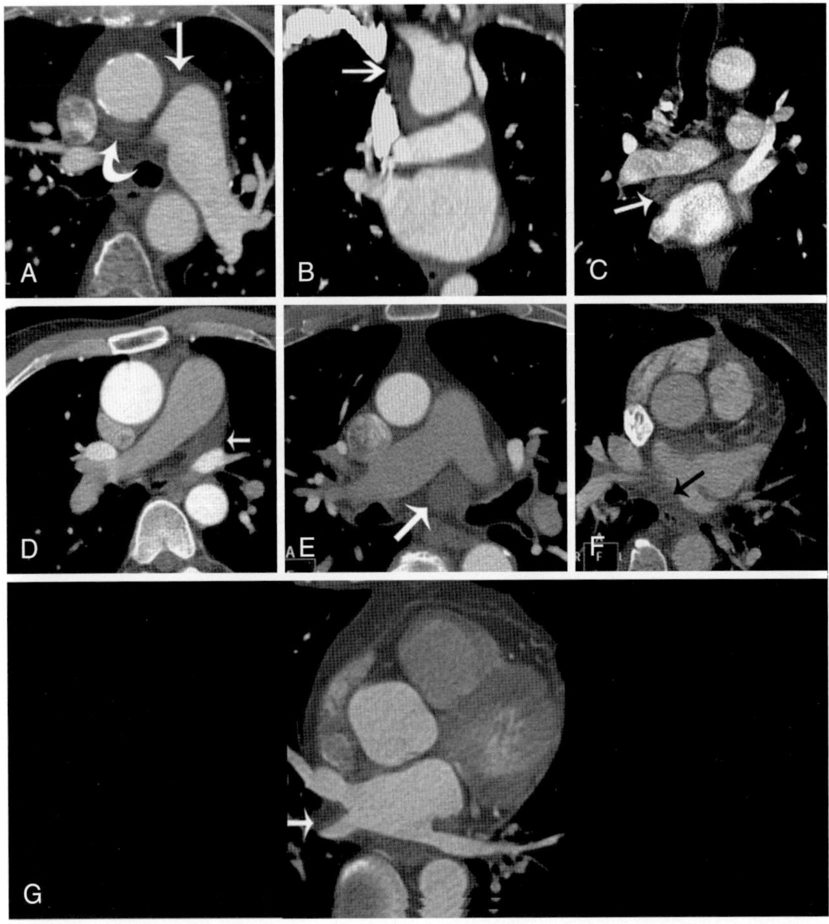

Figure 15-2. CT scan appearances of the various normal pericardial sinuses and recesses. **A,** Axial image shows anterior (*arrow*) and posterior (*curved arrow*) superior aortic recesses. **B,** Coronal image shows lateral superior aortic recess (*arrow*). **C,** Coronal image shows a right pulmonary artery recess (*arrow*) posterior to the right pulmonary artery. **D,** Axial image shows the left pulmonary artery recess (*arrow*) below the left pulmonary artery. **E,** Axial image shows the oblique sinus (*arrow*). **F,** Axial image shows posterior pericardial recess (*arrow*), which continues inferiorly with the oblique sinus. **G,** Axial image shows the right pulmonic vein recess (*arrow*), anterior to the right inferior pulmonary vein. (Reprinted with permission from Rajiah P, Kanne JP. Computed tomography of the pericardium and pericardial disease. *J Cardiovasc Comput Tomogr.* 2010;4(1):3-18.)

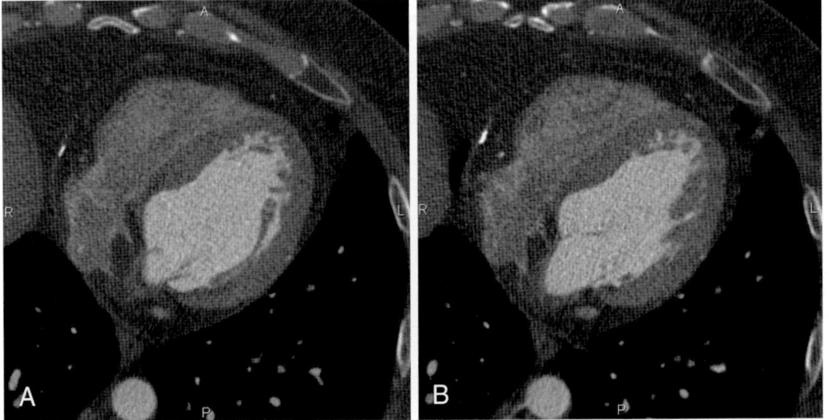

Figure 15-3. Composite images from a cardiac CT examination for coronary disease evaluation demonstrate a mild amount of pericardial calcification anterior to the right atrium. The cardiac chambers appear normal on this prospectively acquired study. No effusion is present. In isolation, pericardial calcification does not denote the presence of constrictive physiology.

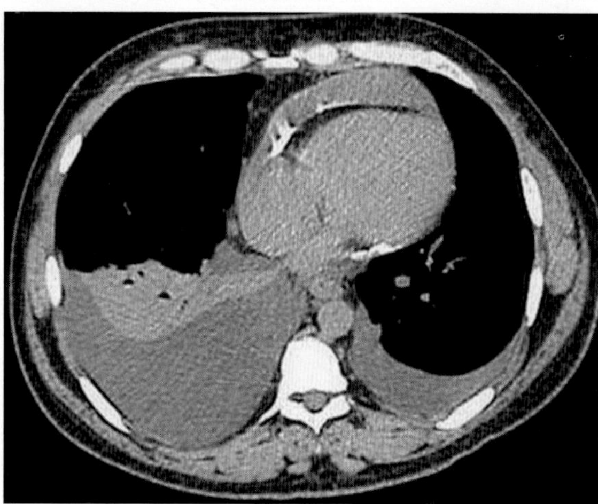

Figure 15-4. Non–contrast-enhanced axial view. There are regions of calcification on the pericardium at the right and left atrioventricular grooves, and over the right ventricular free wall. There is also an anterior pericardial effusion, and bilateral pleural effusions. The diagnosis was effuso-constrictive pericarditis.

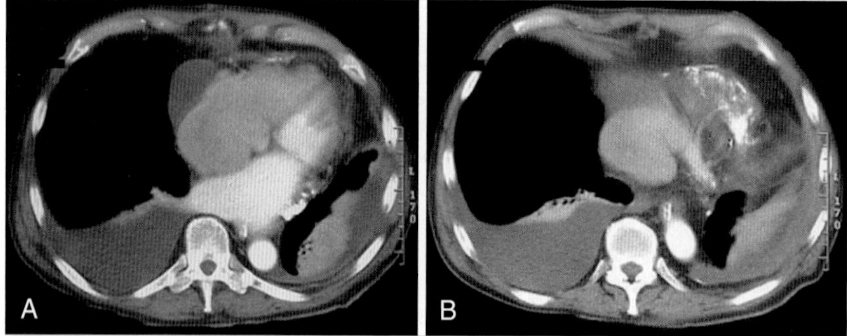

Figure 15-5. Contrast-enhanced axial views at two different levels. **A,** There are regions of calcification over the right ventricular free wall and lateral to the left atrium. There is a small effusion to the right side of the right atrium. **B,** This view cuts under the diaphragmatic surface of the right ventricle; more extensive patchy calcification is seen. The diagnosis was effuso-constrictive pericarditis.

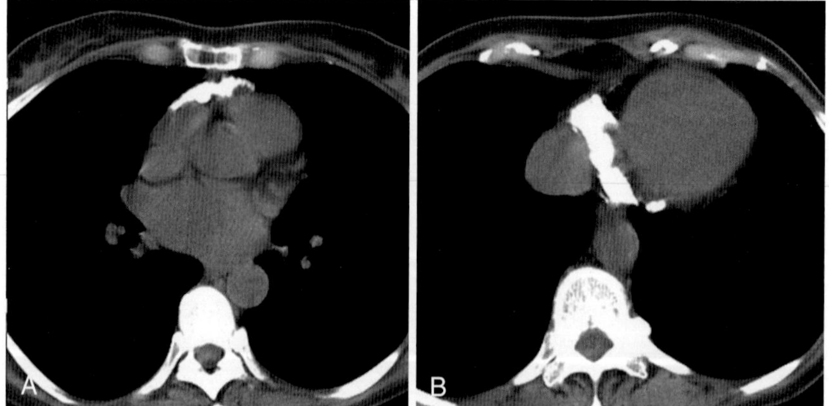

Figure 15-6. Non–contrast-enhanced axial views of two different cases. **A,** At the right ventricular outflow tract level, there is a thick plate of contiguous calcium over the anterior pericardium and no thickening or calcification elsewhere. There was no associated constrictive physiology despite attempts to prove it. **B,** A thick plate of contiguous calcium is seen along the atrioventricular groove, and no thickening or calcification elsewhere. There was no associated constrictive physiology despite attempts to prove it. The diagnosis was localized calcific pericardium without constrictive physiology.

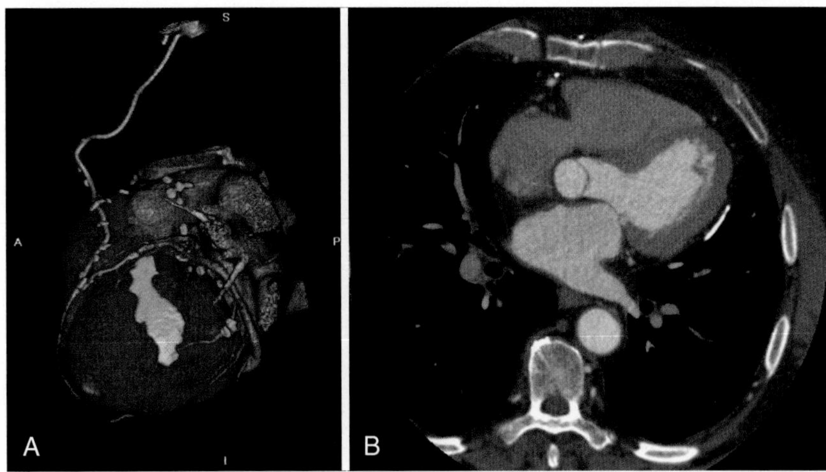

Figure 15-7. A 68-year-old man experienced chest pain 2 years post–triple bypass surgery: left internal mammary artery (LIMA) to left anterior descending artery (LAD), saphenous vein graft (SVG) to right coronary artery (RCA), and saphenous vein graft (SVG) to the second obtuse marginal branch (OM2). Composite images from a cardiac CT study demonstrate a platelike area of pericardial calcification overlying the lateral wall of the left ventricle. **A,** The volume-rendered image demonstrates a patent LIMA to LAD graft, and the calcium is seen "en-face." **B,** The axial source image demonstrates a patent SVG graft in the right atrioventricular groove, a patent left circumflex graft in the left atrioventricular groove, and the plate of calcium in cross-section. In isolation, pericardial calcification does not denote constrictive (compressive) physiology.

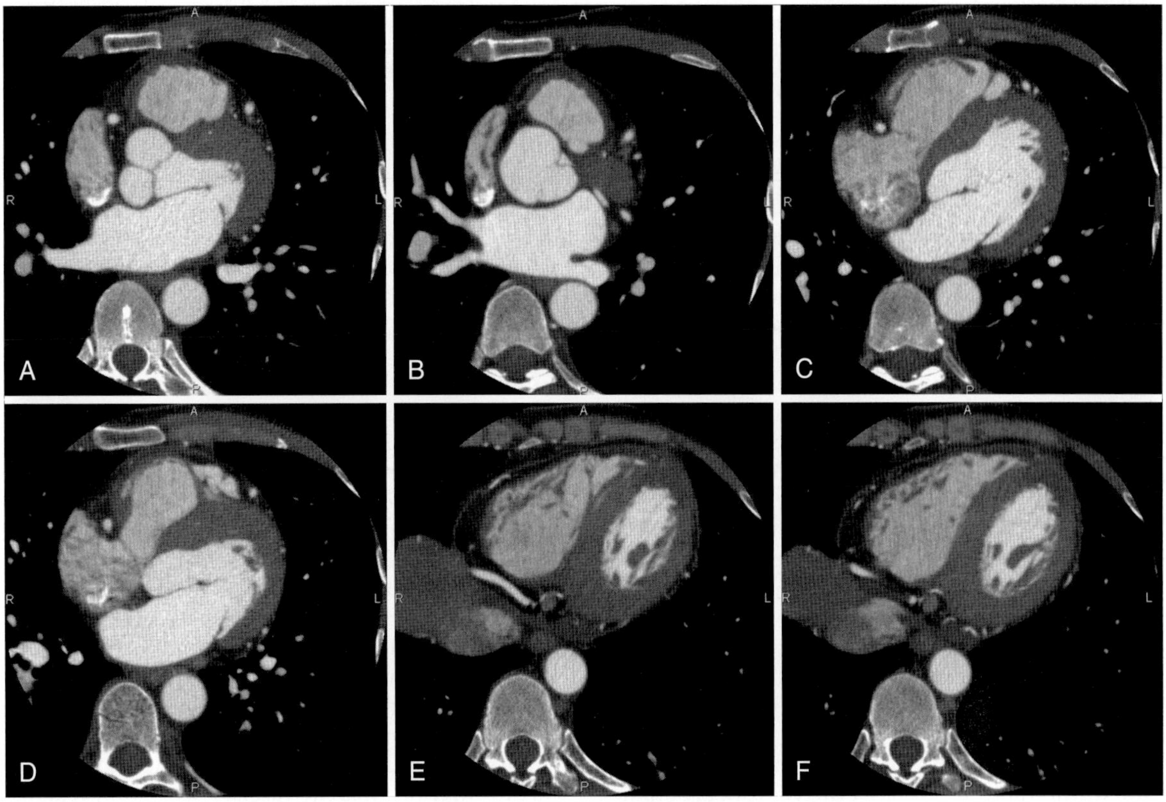

Figure 15-8. Mild pericardial thickening.

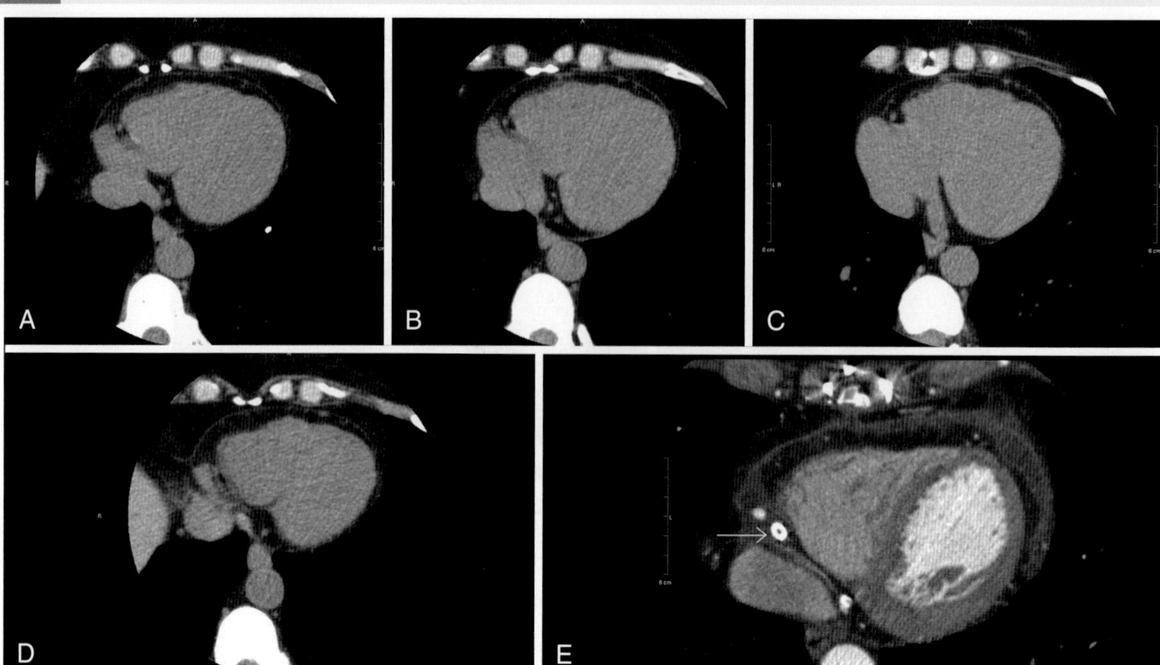

Figure 15-9. A patient with acute chest pain and nonspecific ST segment elevation. **A–D,** Composite images from the calcium score component of a cardiac CT. No coronary artery calcification was detected. There are focal areas of nodular thickening involving the pericardium. Additionally, the pericardium is seen virtually in toto around the heart. Incidental note is made of a calcified left lower lobe granuloma. **E,** A single image from a cardiac CT study in a patient with purulent pericarditis post–coronary artery bypass grafting. A pericardial drain (*arrow*) is seen in place. Note is made of a moderate pericardial effusion, with split pericardial sign and enhancement of the parietal and visceral pericardium. There is subtle stranding of the epicardial and parietal pericardial fat, suggesting inflammatory change. **See Videos 15-1 and 15-2.**

are suggestive of blood clot. Low T1-weighted signal intensity on MRI is consistent with transudative effusions, and medium or high T1-weighted signal intensity on MRI is consistent with exudative and hemorrhagic effusions. Simple pericardial fluid, as in simple pleural effusions, has a uniform, low attenuation value, usually less than 20 HU. Pericardial effusions with attenuation values greater than 20 HU should be considered complicated until proven otherwise. Use of a threshold as low as 10 HU is not clinically accurate.[2] Hemorrhagic pericardial effusions often demonstrate heterogeneous mixed attenuation, with regions measuring more than 50 HU. Often a complicated pericardial effusion provides the corollary of the "split pleura" sign where a complex pericardial effusion demonstrates enhancement of the parietal and visceral pleura.

For CCT images of pericardial effusions, see Figure 15-10.

Pericardial Tamponade

Due to the rapid motions of the right heart chamber free wall collapse in pericardial tamponade, their appearance is depicted poorly without ECG gating. Even with ECG gating, brief right atrial systolic collapse or right ventricular diastolic collapse may not be depicted adequately due to representation of the cardiac cycle by an inadequate number of phases. Even if CCT is the least capable imaging modality to assess the physiologic consequences of pericardial tamponade, the presence of a moderate sized effusion, visible right heart chamber collapse, and evidence of elevated central venous pressure make a fair case for consideration of tamponade,

CONSTRICTIVE PERICARDITIS

CCT findings are useful for the recognition of constrictive pericarditis.

Thickened pericardium is a usual finding. Notably, however, pericardial thickening may occur from past disease or surgery and not result in the physiologic disturbances of constriction; therefore, pericardial thickening is not specific for constriction. The distribution of thickening often is variable. Pericardium of normal thickness does not exclude constrictive pericarditis—about 20% of cases have normal pericardial thickness, but inadequately compliant pericardium. Constrictive pericarditis may be an acute disease process with active inflammation (which reduces pericardial compliance) or active infection (e.g., tuberculosis) or a chronic disease process due to prior inflammation or infection. In the former cases, there would be no calcification, whereas in the latter there may be.

The etiology of constrictive pericarditis depends on the nature of the population. Common causes include prior open heart surgery, prior pericarditis

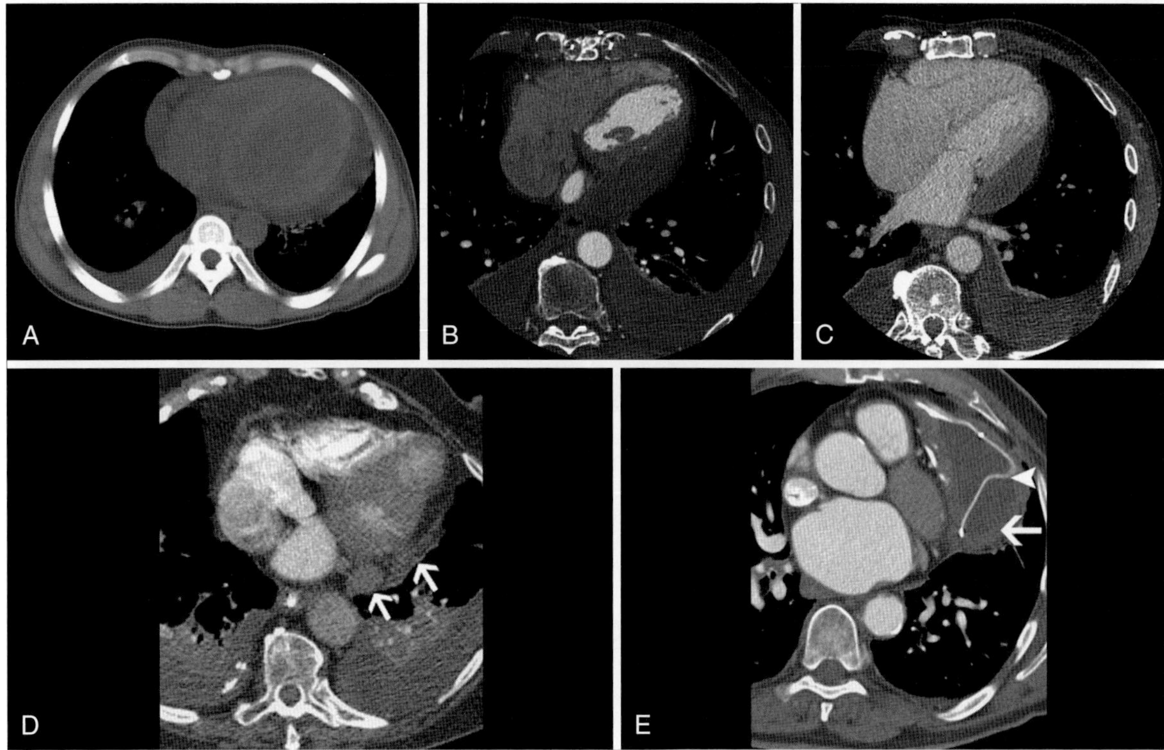

Figure 15-10. **A,** Noncontrast axial image shows a moderate-sized pericardial effusion, and a small right pleural effusion. The greater attenuation of the myocardium than the blood pool is consistent with anemia, which was present due to renal failure. **B,** Contrast-enhanced axial cardiac CT images. First-pass scanning reveals a localized ("loculated") pericardial effusion, which indents the left heart chambers, consistent with localized cardiac compression. **C,** Delayed scan. Note the late enhancement of the parietal pericardium over the localized pericardial effusion. **D** and **E,** Loculated pericardial fluid collections. **D,** CT image of a 72-year-old woman shows two small loculations of pericardial fluid (*arrows*) posterior to the left ventricle. **E,** CT image of a 54-year-old man shows a large seroma (*arrow*) surrounding an epicardial pacemaker lead (*arrowhead*). (Reprinted with permission from Rajiah P, Kanne JP. Computed tomography of the pericardium and pericardial disease. *J Cardiovasc Comput Tomogr.* 2010;4(1):3-18.)

of any etiology, and tuberculosis. Approximately one third of cases are idiopathic.

Careful attention to the distribution of the thickening provides a "roadmap" for the surgeon to follow to free up the constrictive chamber. Calcification of the pericardium in anyone considered to have constrictive pericarditis is important and is best mapped with initial noncontrast views. Because MRI is relatively insensitive to calcification, CCT is the preferred advanced imaging modality for patients who can tolerate iodinated contrast; conversely, if contrast tolerance is an issue, MRI is the preferred test.

CT Findings of Pericardial Constriction

- Pericardial thickening in most cases.
- Regional or focal distortion of the ventricles. Compression by overlying compressive pericardium of the RV is more common than of the LV, due to its thinner wall.
- Tubular-shaped ventricles
- Dilated atria
- Ascites
- Pleural effusions
- Dilated IVC, dilated hepatic veins
- Hepatic venous congestion
- Reflux of contrast dye into the IVC consistent with elevated right atrial pressure

The complex motions of the septum in constrictive pericarditis (early and late diastolic septal dips, inspiratory septal shift) are not as well shown by cardiac CT as they are by CMR or echocardiography. This is due primarily to the poorer temporal resolution of CT relative to echocardiography and CMR. The temporal resolution of echocardiography is in the range of 20 msec. Steady-state cine gradient echo imaging in MR has an approximate temporal resolution of 30 to 50 msec. Current typical 64-slice cardiac CT scanners have gantry rotation times of about 350 msec. With partial reconstruction of the image, effective temporal resolution for retrospective cardiac CT is in the range of 150 to 200 msec. Newer scanners with faster gantry rotation times and dual source configurations have improved temporal resolution so that it now approaches that of CMR at 50 to 100 msec.

Some cases of pericardial constriction involve compression by both pericardial fluid and one or both layers of the pericardium (i.e., effuse-constrictive pericarditis).

For CCT images of pericardial constriction, see Figures 15-11 to 15-17 and **Videos 15-3 through 15-5.**

Text continued on page 230

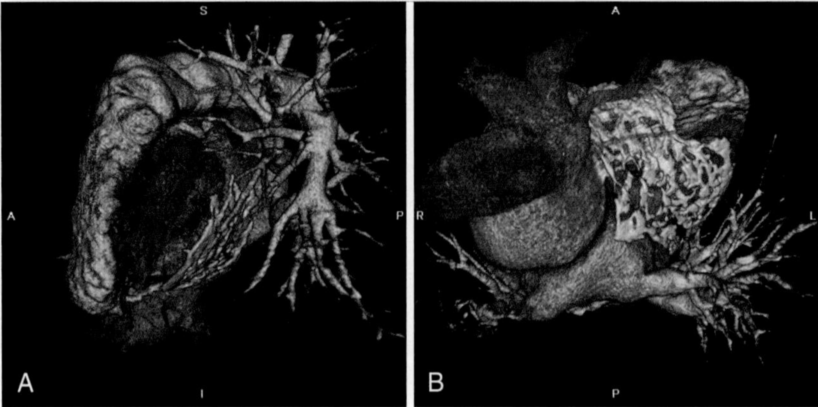

Figure 15-11. Two volume-rendered images from a cardiac CT examination demonstrate small-volume right and left ventricles, with a lace-like area of pericardial calcification extending along the inferior and left lateral atrioventricular (AV) groove. There is marked enlargement of the inferior vena cava (IVC) and intrahepatic veins. The diagnosis was calcific constrictive pericarditis.

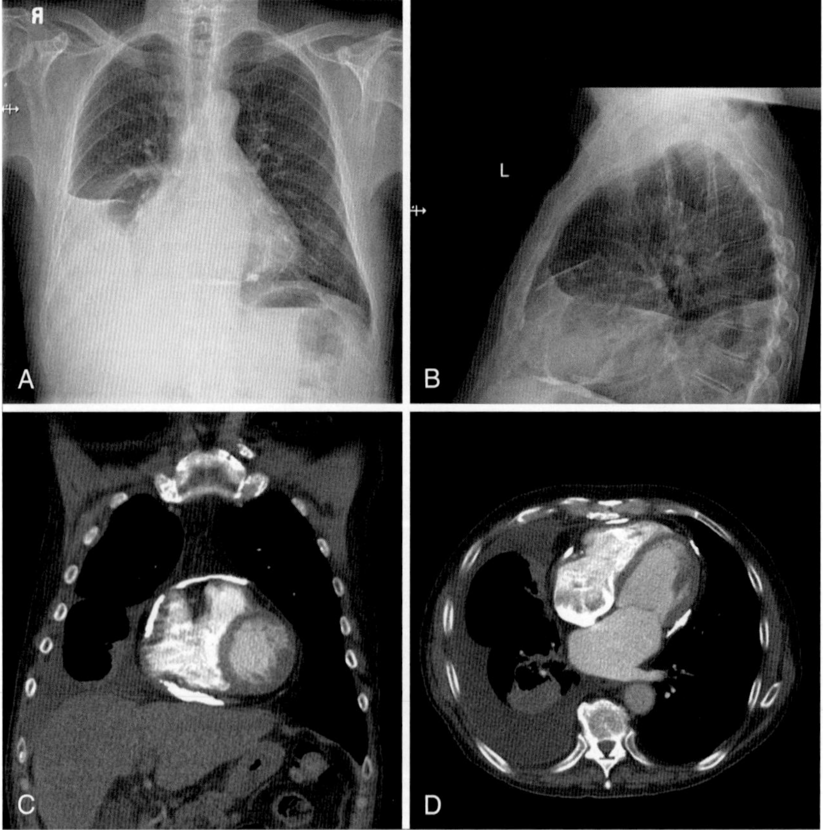

Figure 15-12. Posteroanterior (**A**) and lateral (**B**) chest radiographs of a patient with shortness of breath. There is a large right pleural effusion, and atelectatic change is seen in the right lower lung. Extensive curvilinear calcification is seen projecting over the cardiac silhouette, consistent with pericardial calcification. The patient proceeded to a chest CT study (**C** and **D**), which confirmed multiple foci of pericardial calcification. There is no evidence of a pericardial effusion. There is at least moderate biatrial dilatation and a small somewhat spade-shaped–appearing right ventricle. These findings are suggestive of constrictive pericarditis. A moderate to large right pleural effusion is seen. Atelectatic change in the right lower lobe has a somewhat rounded configuration, with vessels coursing to it, indicative of rounded atelectasis. The presence of round atelectasis suggests that the underlying pleural effusion is likely chronic or preexistent.

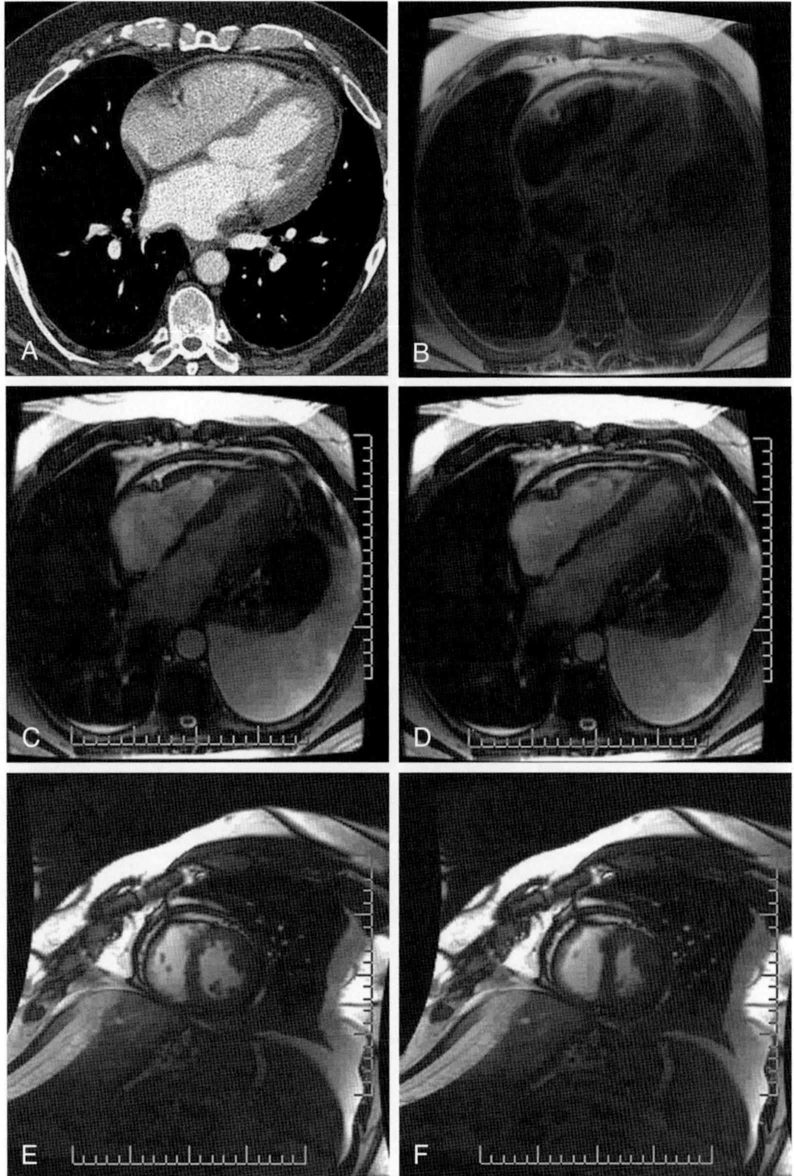

Figure 15-13. Comparative images from a case of proven constrictive pericarditis. **A,** Contrast-enhanced CT four-chamber view. There is fat both beneath and above the parietal pericardium over the right ventricle, revealing thickening of the pericardium. There are no other findings on the CT scan supportive of constriction. Along the posterior wall of the left ventricle there is a lower-attenuation thickening that may be an effusion. **B,** T1-weighted black blood image corresponding to the CT scan image. The "fat sandwich" nicely delineates the thickened parietal pericardium. In the interval of time since the CT scan, a pleural effusion has developed. **C** and **D,** Steady-state free precession (SSFP) cine sequence—systole (**C**) and diastole (**D**)—depicting the right-to-left septal displacement (diastolic septal dip) of ventricular interdependence. **E** and **F,** Short-axis views of the right-to-left septal displacement (diastolic septal dip) of ventricular interdependence (systole, **E,** and diastole, **F**).

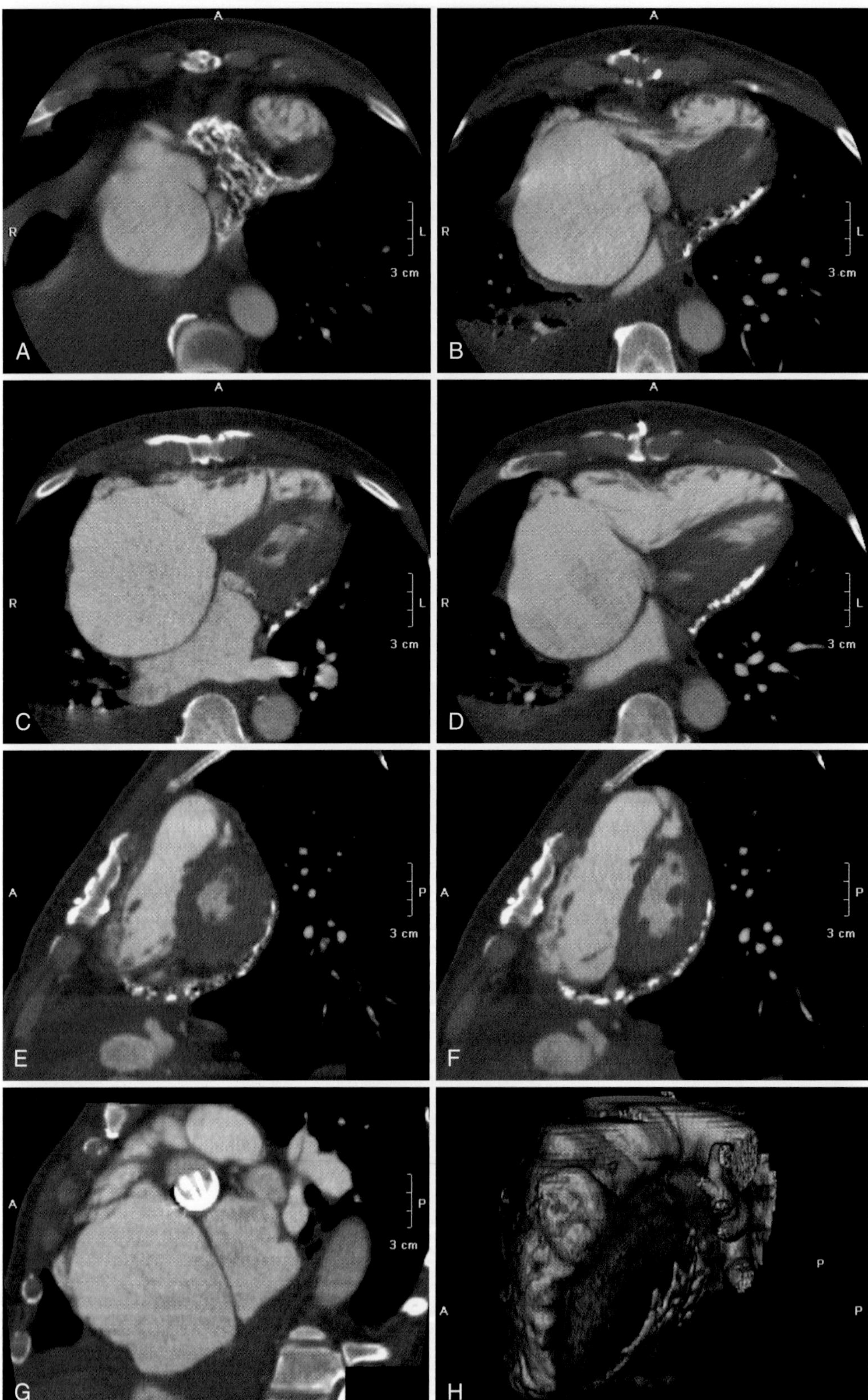

Figure 15-14. Multiple axial and reformatted images from a cardiac CT study in a patient suspected of constrictive pericarditis post–aortic valve replacement. Small-volume ventricles are noted bilaterally with flattening of the intraventricular septum. Marked enlargement of the left atrium and intrahepatic veins. There is extensive calcification in the inferior atrioventricular groove extending along the lateral margin of the left ventricle. Large right pleural effusion and small left pleural effusion are present. Calcific constrictive pericarditis. **See Videos 15-3 through 15-5.**

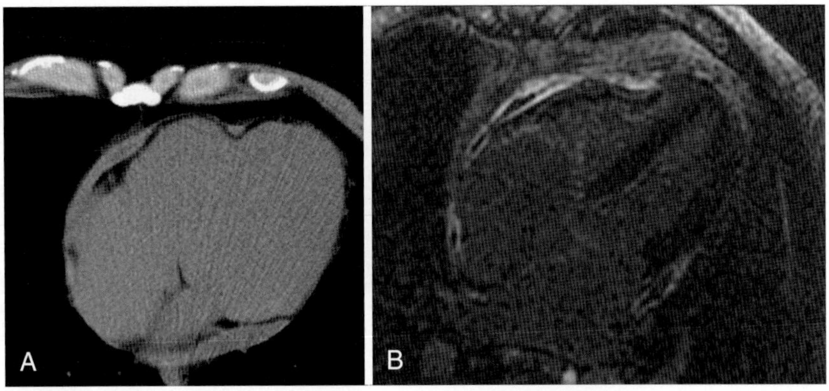

A B

Figure 15-15. A 49-year-old man with a long history of rheumatoid arthritis with shortness of breath. Echocardiography demonstrated nondilated, but hypokinetic, right and left ventricles. Because of a prior severe allergic reaction to iodinated contrast, a gated noncontrast CT was performed. No coronary calcium is present, but moderate thickening of the pericardium is noted. A cardiac MRI confirms the thickened, enhancing pericardium, as well as some deformity of the right ventricular free wall, and functional evaluation consistent with constrictive pericarditis.

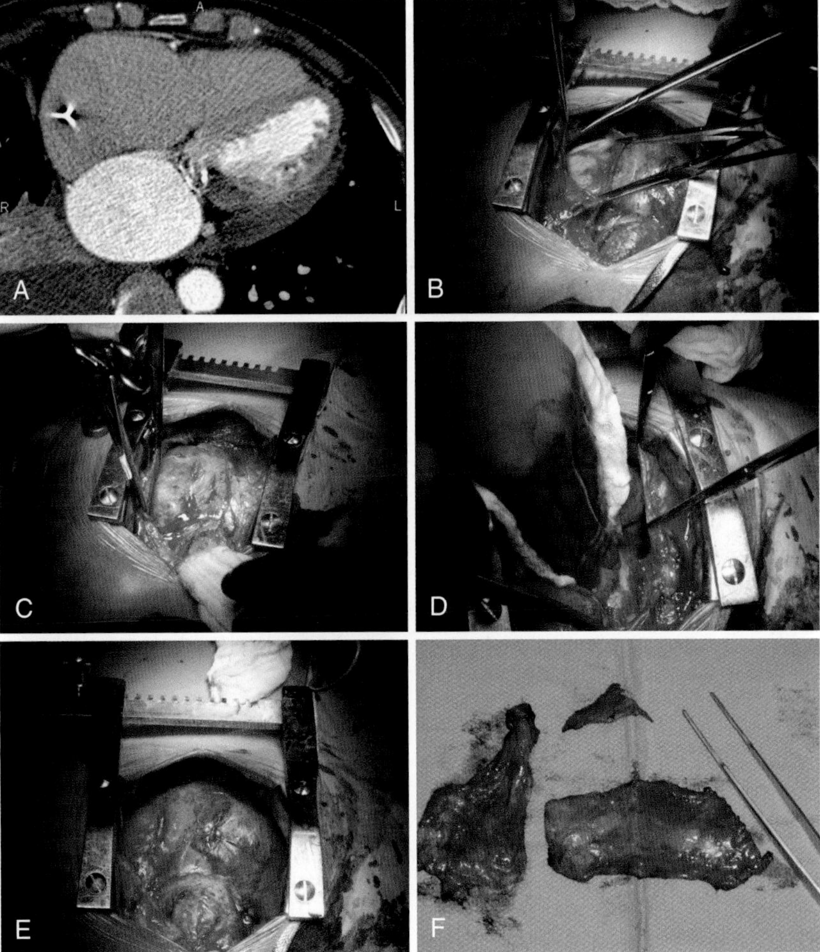

Figure 15-16. A case of surgically proven constrictive pericarditis with near-normal pericardial thickness was seen on preoperative ECG-gated CT scanning (**A**) and only mildly thickened pericardial thickness was seen at surgery. The constriction was due to prior open heart surgery (mechanical mitral valve replacement 17 years previously for mixed rheumatic mitral valve disease). Due to the chronic atrial fibrillation, the right atrium is so thin that it is nearly transparent. Note the dark venous blood in the right atrium in **E**.

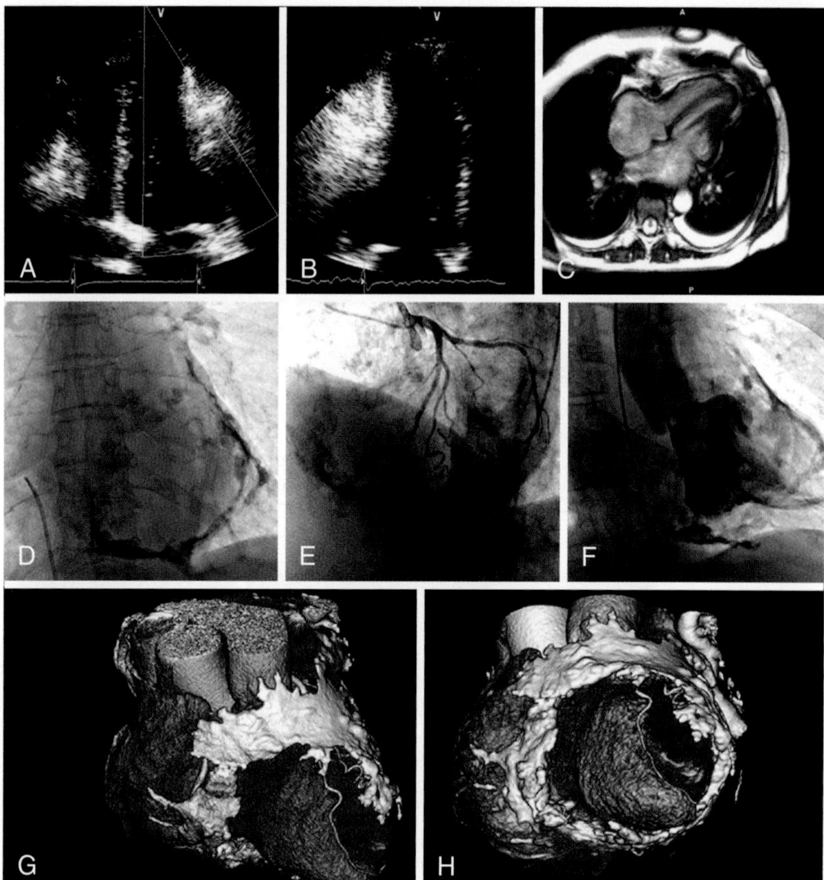

Figure 15-17. A 70-year-old woman presented with worsening dyspnea on minimal exertion and an echocardiogram notable for possible basal aneurysm (**A** and **B**). A chest radiograph showed diffuse pericardial calcification, and a cardiac MRI scan showed biatrial enlargement and a thickened pericardium compressing the mid- to apical left ventricle (**C**). Fluoroscopy revealed a band of pericardial calcification (**D–F**), and simultaneous right and left heart catheterization demonstrated equalization of pressures, respirophasic discordance of the ventricular pressure tracings, and a square root sign with a steep right atrial "y" descent suggesting constrictive physiology. Ventriculography showed compression of the mid- to apical left ventricle, giving an unusual appearance that could be misinterpreted as a basal aneurysm (**F**). Cardiac CT angiography revealed severe pericardial calcification in a belt-like pattern around the mid-ventricle (**G, H**). Unfortunately, the patient died perioperatively. She had no history of tuberculosis or mediastinal radiation. (Reprinted with permission from Blaha MJ, Panjrath G, Chacko M, Schulman SP. Localized calcific constrictive pericarditis masquerading as a basal aneurysm. *J Am Coll Cardiol.* 2011;57(18):e65.)

Pericardial Cysts

Pericardial cysts are well-marginated, thin-walled structures containing water-like fluid that are four times more likely to be located at the right than the left costophrenic angle. They may be located anywhere on either side of the midline, including the mediastinum. Some cysts are lobulated. Both CCT and MRI are able to depict the thin-walled capsule of the cyst. Hyperdense cysts often contain proteinaceous material and can be difficult to diagnose on a single contrast-enhanced CT scan. A pre-constrast study followed by a post-contrast study can confirm whether the cyst enhances. A proteinaceous cyst may demonstrate increased pre-contrast attenuation (>30 HU), but should not demonstrate any significant enhancement post-contrast. MRI is better able to characterize the fluid as water-like, and may be better able to evaluate any complication of the cyst such as hemorrhage or infection. Echocardiography is not well suited to imaging most cysts, as lung may be interposed between the cyst and the chest wall.

For CCT images of pericardial cysts, see Figures 15-18 through 15-21.

CONGENITAL ABSENCE OF THE PERICARDIUM

Congenital absence of the pericardium is a rare disorder that may encompass complete absence or, more commonly, partial absence of the pericardium. Pericardial defects occur as a result of maldevelopment of the pleuropericardial membrane, most commonly on the left. The most widely accepted theory for the etiology of these defects is persistence of the pleuropericardial channel due to premature atrophy of the left common cardinal vein (duct of Cuvier). The size of the defect is determined by the timing of the premature atrophic event.[3] It also has been proposed that some defects may arise secondary to a traction-induced tear in the pleuropericardial membrane during embryogenesis rather than failure of the foramen to close.[4]

Complete absence of the pericardium leads to abnormal leftward and posterior positioning of the heart in the chest and, therefore, abnormal vectors on surface ECG recording and abnormal appearance on imaging such as chest radiographs, but often it is clinically occult.

Figure 15-18. **A,** Contrast-enhanced axial view of the lower heart. There is a thin-walled structure immediately adjacent to the heart at the right costodiaphragmatic junction (note the dome of the right diaphragm) that does not enhance. There is an intimal flap in the descending aorta. Right-sided pericardial cyst (and acute aortic dissection). **B,** Contrast-enhanced axial view of the lower heart. There is a thin-walled structure immediately adjacent to the heart at the left costodiaphragmatic junction. Right-sided pericardial cyst. **C,** Contrast-enhanced axial view of the upper chest. There is a thin-walled structure immediately to the right and anterior to the innominate vein. A pericardial (anterior mediastinal) cyst.

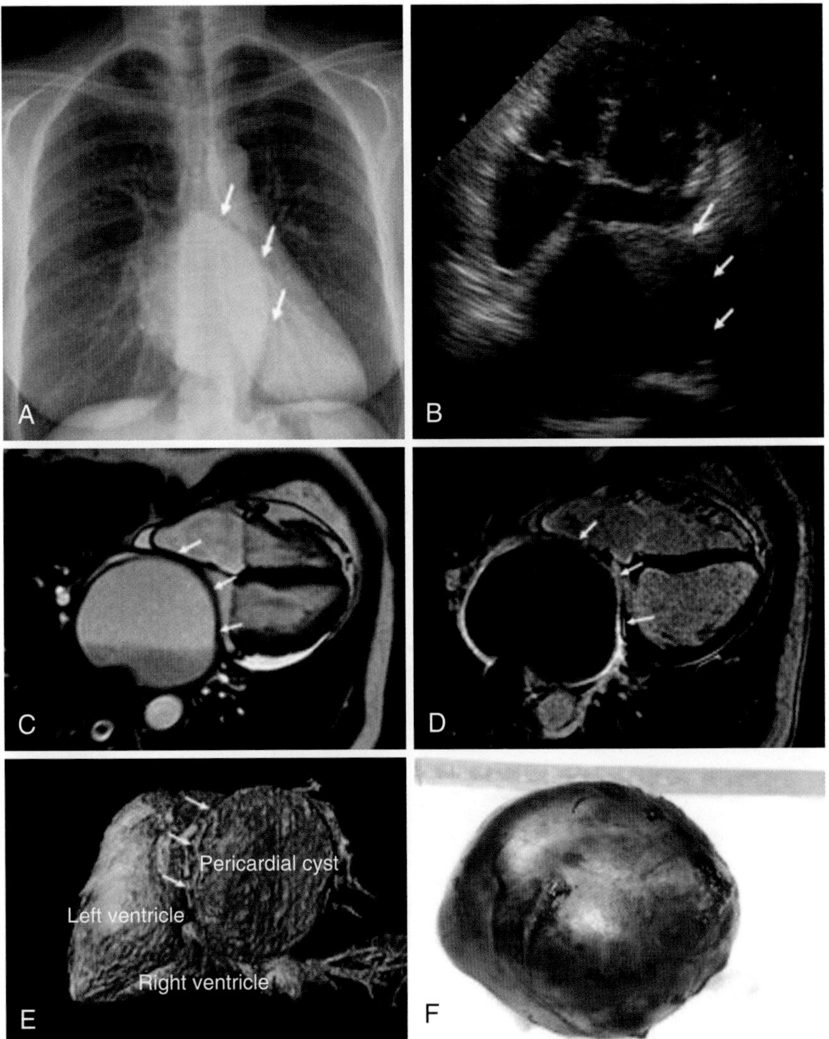

Figure 15-19. A 59-year-old woman presented with atrial flutter and presyncope. A chest roentgenogram and an echocardiogram showed a large intrathoracic mass (**A** and **B**, *arrows*). Cardiac MRI with steady-state free precession sequences, T2-weighted images, and inversion recovery images, as well as three-dimensional whole-heart acquisition, were performed for further characterization of the lesion. The diagnosis of a pericardial cyst (*arrows* in cardiac MRI [**C**] and cardiac CT [**D**]) was made and was confirmed at surgery as well as histologically. Postoperatively, the patient was in sinus rhythm again. Pericardial cysts are rare, benign intrathoracic lesions with a prevalence of 1 in 100,000. For asymptomatic patients, conservative management with short follow-up periods is recommended. However, for symptomatic patients or for patients suffering from complications, surgery should be considered. (Reprinted with permission from Neizel M, Krüger S, Spillner J, et al. A giant pericardial cyst as unusual cause for atrial flutter. *J Am Coll Cardiol.* 2010;55(11):1160.)

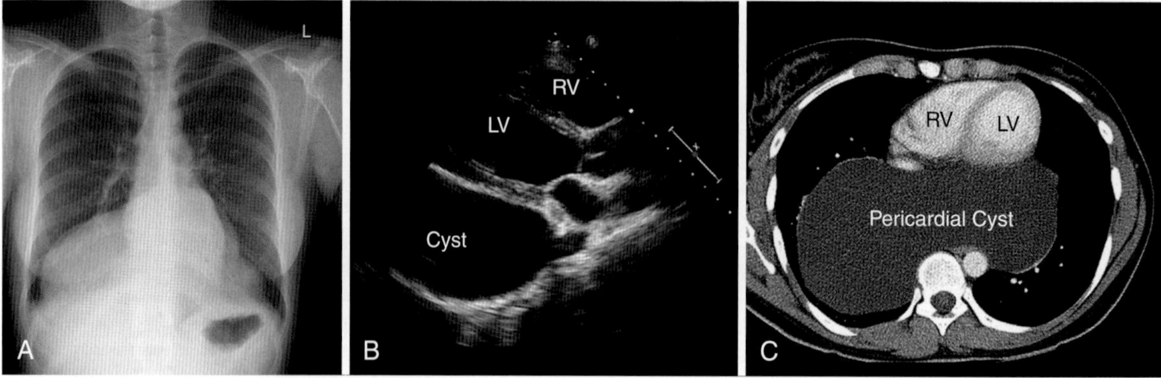

Figure 15-20. A 22-year-old woman presented with syncope. The results of physical examination and electrocardiography were unremarkable. **A,** A chest radiograph revealed a markedly increased cardiac silhouette. **B,** Two-dimensional transthoracic echocardiography showed normal-sized cardiac chambers and a large echo-free space behind the heart. **C,** Contrast-enhanced CT examination revealed a large fluid attenuation mass within the posterior mediastinum measuring 21.5 × 11.4 × 14.2 cm consistent with pericardial cyst. Needle aspiration revealed clear fluid and no malignant or inflammatory cells. LV, left ventricle; RV, right ventricle. (Reprinted with permission from Thanneer L, Saric M, Perk G, et al. A giant pericardial cyst. *J Am Coll Cardiol.* 2011; 57(17):1784.)

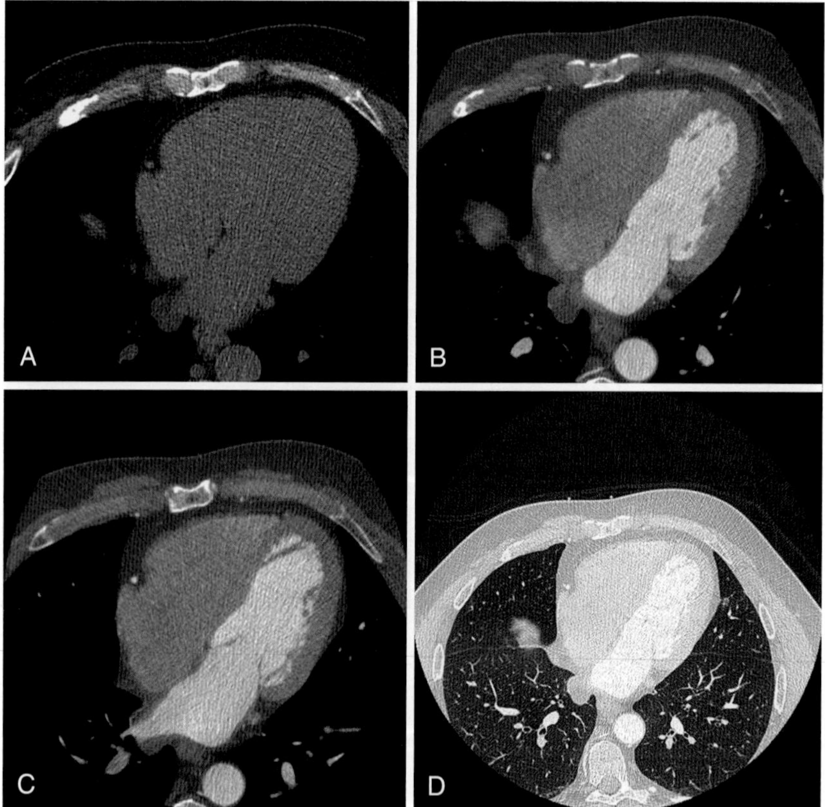

Figure 15-21. A 43-year-old man with chest pain. **A,** Noncontrast calcium score image demonstrates a focal region of low attenuation adjacent to the right aspect of the left atrium. This has a Hounsfield unit measurement of 11. **B,** CT angiography image demonstrates no enhancement within this rounded low-attenuation region. **C,** CT image obtained slightly more inferiorly demonstrates the right lower lobe pulmonary vein coursing through the lobulated area of low attenuation. **D,** Lung windows demonstrate the aforementioned nodule appearing as a lung nodule. The diagnosis was normal pericardial recess around the left inferior pulmonary vein mimicking a lung nodule, which may also be misdiagnosed as a pericardial cyst or foregut duplication cyst.

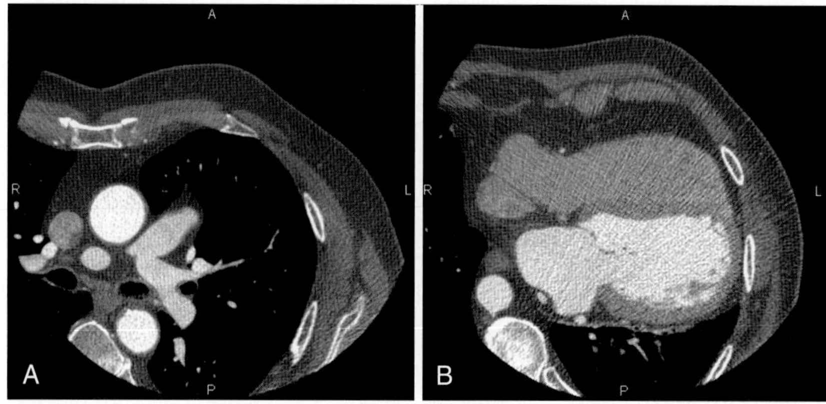

Figure 15-22. Two images from a gated cardiac CT study demonstrate shift of the mediastinum into the left hemithorax, and extension of a "tongue of lung" interposed between the aorta and main pulmonary artery. These findings are characteristic of left pericardial absence. Of note, portions of the right sided pericardium are visible.

In partial absence of the pericardium, it usually is the left-sided pericardium that is affected. Such a partial absence is a rare cause of chest pain and, very rarely, of death, should the left atrial appendage herniate out of the pericardial defect and become incarcerated. The left atrial appendage may appear as large as the pulmonary artery. An aneurysm of the left atrial appendage is as rare as, and has similar appearance to, partial absence of the pericardium on the chest radiograph.

The surface of the heart, where there is absence of the pericardium, may exhibit a slightly lumpy character, due to the topographic variation of the epicardial surface of the heart caused by fat and vessels.

CT imaging often demonstrates the heart as being significantly displaced into the left hemithorax. Occasionally, as the heart is displaced to the left, its axis can rotate to the right. A pathognomonic sign for left pericardial absence is the presence of interposed lung between the ascending aorta and the main pulmonary artery under the LV and between it and the diaphragm. In the normal situation, pericardium resides over this region and does not allow the adjacent lung to extend into this space.[5,6]

Both CCT and MRI may fail to visualize pericardium over the left heart even in normal cases, especially if there is a paucity of peri- or epicardial fat; hence, the appearance of absence of pericardium over the left heart (atrial or ventricular levels) does not establish the diagnosis.

Patients with congenital pericardial absence also may have other associated congenital defects, including tetralogy of Fallot, atrial septal defects, patent ductus arteriosus, congenital mitral stenosis, partial anomalous pulmonary venous return, and pulmonary sequestration.[3]

For CCT images of congenital absence of the pericardium (and traumatic pericardial defects), see Figures 15-22 and 15-23.

INTRAPERICARDIAL FAT QUANTIFICATION

Intrapericardial fat is purported to be a risk factor for cardiovascular disease.[7] Semi-automated CCT volumetric quantification of intrapericardial fat is highly reproducible.[8]

NEOPLASTIC PERICARDIAL DISEASE

Metastatic pericardial disease occurs far more commonly than do primary pericardial tumors. Autopsy series in patients with a known antecedent primary malignancy identify the presence of pericardial metastases in 10% to 12% of cases.[9,10] The pericardium may be seeded by direct invasion from bronchogenic carcinoma or a mediastinal malignancy. More distant seeding occurs via the bloodstream or lymphatics. The most common primary sources for pericardial metastases are lung and breast cancers, followed by lymphoma and melanoma.[10] Direct invasion may be associated with a pericardial effusion. The pericardium demonstrates irregular thickening or an associated mass or masses. If pre-contrast imaging has been performed, the pericardial thickening or mass can demonstrate enhancement after contrast administration, helping to distinguish it from bland pericardial clot. Distant metastases can give a multinodular appearance to the pericardium.

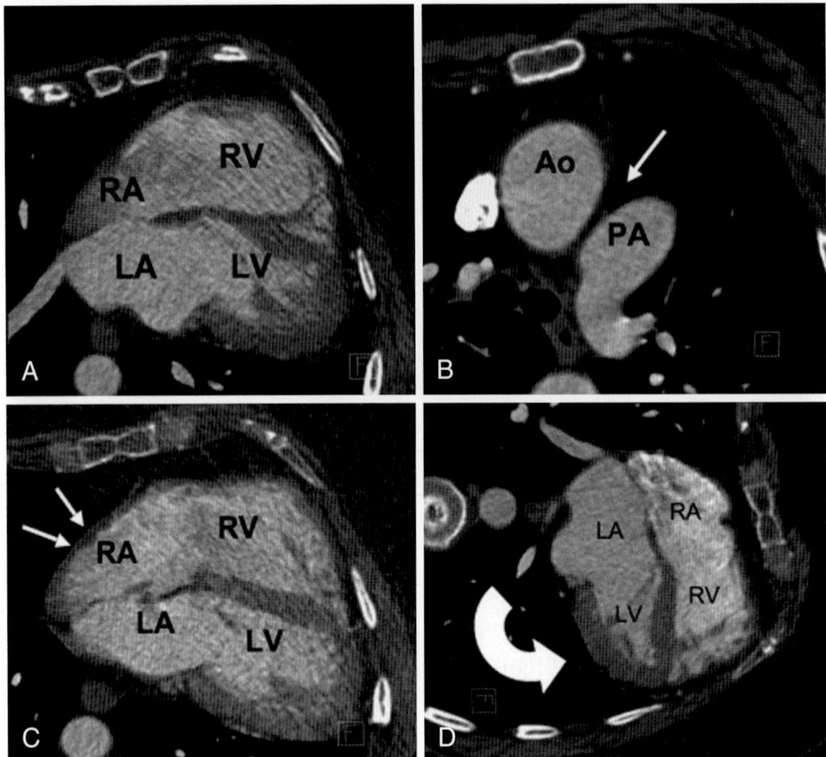

Figure 15-23. **A,** Axial supine image at the level of the right inferior pulmonary vein shows dilation of the right heart chambers and extreme levoposition. The cardiac apex is excessively mobile on cine images. **B,** Axial supine image at the level of the aortopulmonary window shows interposition of lung tissue between the aorta (Ao) and main pulmonary artery (PA; *arrow*), which is pathognomonic of absent pericardium in this region. **C,** Axial supine image at the level of the right atrium (RA) shows a short slip of pericardium overlying the right atrium (*arrows*). **D,** Axial left lateral decubitus image at the level of the right inferior pulmonary vein shows rightward shift of the cardiac apex (*curved arrow*). LA, left atrium; LV, left ventricle; RV, right ventricle. (Reprinted with permission from Hoey ET, Yap KS, Darby MJ, et al. Complete left pericardial defect: evaluation with supine and decubitus dual source CT. *J Cardiovasc Comput Tomogr.* 2009;3(6):417-419.)

Primary pericardial tumors are rare. The pericardium is lined by mesothelial cells, and primary mesotheliomas have been reported.[11] Other possible primary malignancies include lymphoma and lipoma or liposarcoma. In the absence of a known primary malignancy, biopsy and histologic evaluation often is necessary to obtain a definitive diagnosis.

Tumor encasement of the heart may produce compressive or constrictive physiology. Any case of pericardial constriction presenting with markedly thickened pericardium and no known primary tumor should beg consideration of pericardial mesothelioma within the differential diagnosis (Fig. 15-24).

OTHER INTRAPERICARDIAL MASSES

Hematomas and organized pericardial hematomas, which may calcify, are sometimes encountered, especially in patients who previously underwent open heart surgery (Fig. 15-25).

PNEUMOPERICARDIUM

Pneumopericardium may result from percutaneous or surgical procedures, fistulization from the esophagus or bowel into the pericardium, or gas-forming infection. Pneumopericardium is readily detected by CCT. For CCT images of pneumopericardium, see Figure 15-26.

INTRAPERICARDIAL BOWEL HERNIATION

With abdominal blunt trauma, bowel may herniate through a diaphragmatic defect into the pericardial space. Although there is visibly air within the pericardial space, the findings differ from those of pneumopericardium per se, because the bowel wall also is evident. See Figure 15-26.

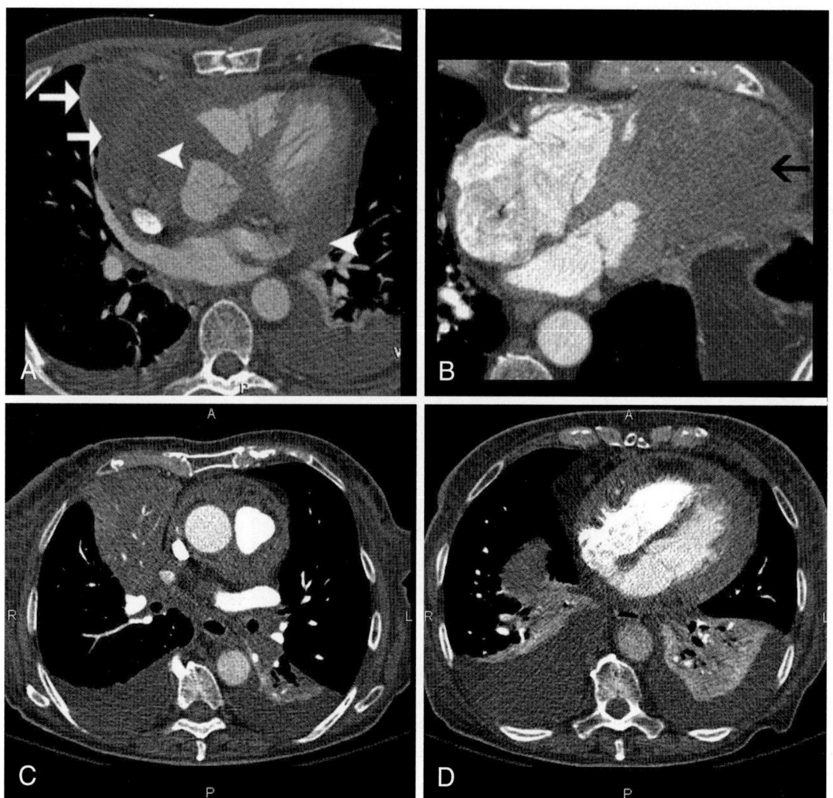

Figure 15-24. **A,** Mesothelioma. Axial CT image of a 56-year-old man shows a heterogeneously enhancing mass in the pericardium (*arrows*), predominantly in the right and anterior aspects, with associated high-attenuation effusion (*arrowheads*) that was confirmed on pathology to be malignant mesothelioma. Bilateral pleural effusions are present. **B,** Synovial cell sarcoma. Axial CT image shows a large, heterogeneously enhancing mass (*arrow*) in the pericardium, predominantly near the apex of the left ventricle, which on biopsy was proven to be a synovial cell sarcoma. **C** and **D,** Two images from a cardiac CT study demonstrate marked circumferential pericardial thickening and irregularity and infiltration of the pericardial and epicardial fat. Thickening extending along the central airways is also noted. There is atelectasis of the right middle lobe, right lower lobe, and left lower lobe in conjunction with moderate bilateral pleural effusions in a patient with known underlying bronchogenic carcinoma. This appearance is typical for pericardial metastatic infiltration. (Reprinted with permission from Rajiah P, Kanne JP. Computed tomography of the pericardium and pericardial disease. *J Cardiovasc Comput Tomogr.* 2010;4(1):3-18.)

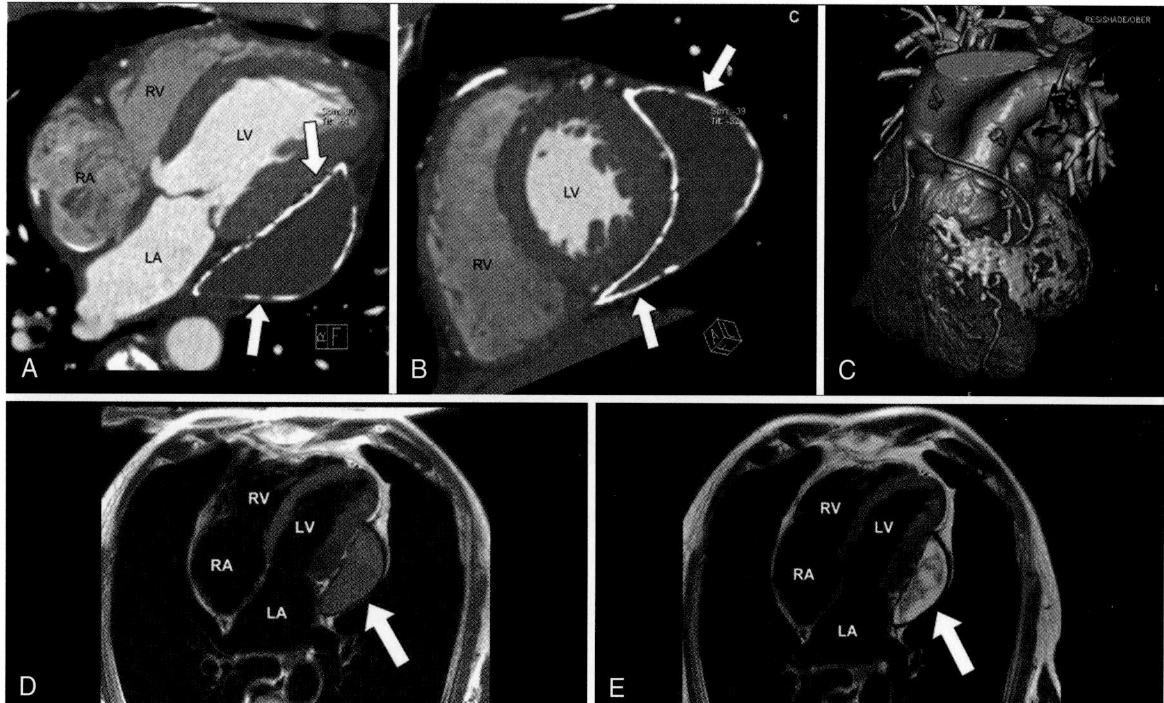

Figure 15-25. Organized hematoma within the pericardial space. Contrast-enhanced 64-slice multidetector CT showing intrapericardial mass (**A,** *arrow*) with calcified borders. **A,** Four-chamber view, long axis. **B,** Two-chamber view, short axis (intrapericardial mass, *arrow*). **C,** Three-dimensional reconstructions. **A** through **C** demonstrate the intrapericardial calcified mass adjacent to the left ventricle. MRI T1-weighted spin-echo image, 4-chamber view showing a circumscribed intrapericardial structure of the left myocardium (**D,** *arrow*), corresponding to an organized and calcified hematoma after aortocoronary bypass surgery. At the lateral wall of the left ventricle a structure appearing similar in signal intensity to the myocardium is shown. **E,** T2-weighted short T1 inversion recovery image, four-chamber view, showing a high signal intensity of the mass. LA, left atrium; LV, left ventricle; RA, right atrium; RV, right ventricle. (Reprinted with permission from Wechsel M, Ropers D, Ropers U, et al. Organized intrapericardial hematoma after coronary artery bypass surgery. *J Cardiovasc Comput Tomogr.* 2008;2(5):328-331.)

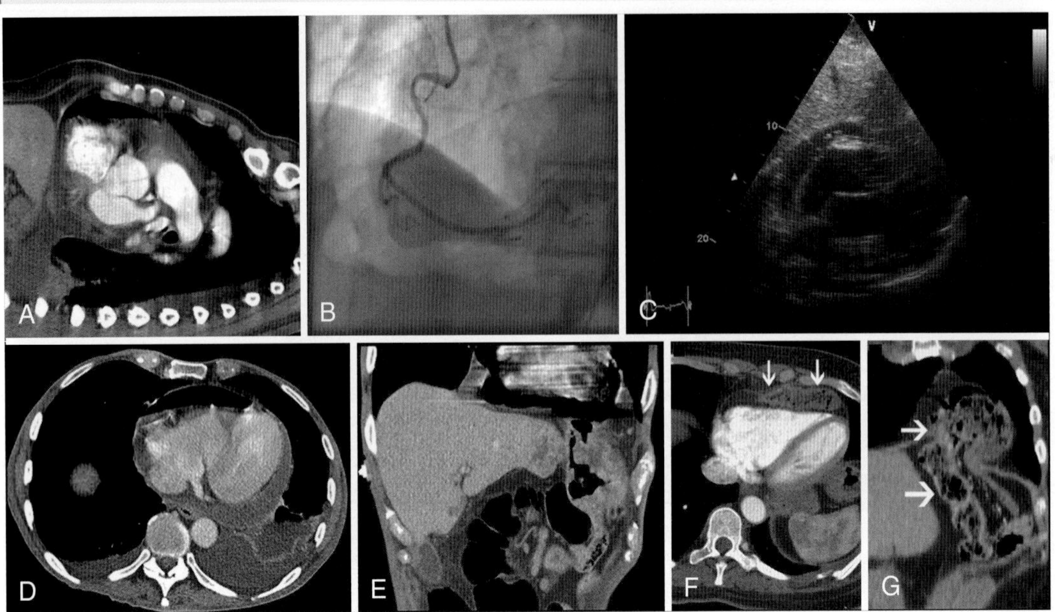

Figure 15-26. **A,** Noncontrast sagittal image. There is a moderate-sized pericardial effusion, anterior pneumopericardium (from a pericardial "tap"), and a left pleural effusion. **B–E** (different case), A 70-year-old man presented with chest pain and inferolateral ST segment elevation on electrocardiogram via primary percutaneous coronary intervention service. He had gastric cancer, palliated with radiotherapy. A coronary angiogram showed unobstructed arteries and a radiolucent pericardial space with a craggy surface (**B**). Echocardiography was hindered by trapped pericardial air. Subcostal views showed a pericardial effusion containing air bubbles, no tamponade, and thickening around the right atrium consistent with malignant infiltration (**C**). A contrast-enhanced CT scan showed hydropneumopericardium (**D**), produced by a fistulous tract between the gastric fundus and the pericardial space (**E**). The opening of this fistula likely caused the acute onset of chest pain. Radiation therapy in the oncologic patient is a predisposing factor for such fistula formation. The patient was treated palliatively and died the next day. This case highlights the value of CT in the investigation of pericardial disease. **F** and **G** (different case), Traumatic defect in the pericardium. Axial (**F**) and coronal (**G**) CT images of a 31-year-old man with traumatic diaphragmatic injury show a pericardial defect, resulting in herniation of the transverse colon (*arrows*) into the pericardial cavity. (**A–E** reprinted with permission from Prasad R, Little M, David S, O'Sullivan M. Acute pneumopericardium. *J Am Coll Cardiol.* 2011;57(12):1399; **F** and **G** reprinted with permission from Rjiah P, Kanne JP. Computed tomography of the pericardium and pericardial disease. *J Cardiovasc Comput Tomogr.* 2010;4(1):3-18.)

CCT PROTOCOL POINTS

- The standard CCT protocol is utilized (Table 15-1).
- If there is suspicion of a pericardial or cardiac mass, obtaining a pre-contrast study should be considered to evaluate for enhancement in a mass/cyst or complex pericardial effusion.
- A delayed study (30–60 seconds) post–contrast administration also should be considered, to demonstrate late enhancement as a sign of inflammation or infection.
- Right and left ventricular function and septal motion can be assessed with a helical CTA acquisition if clinically indicated. (MRI is contraindicated, and echocardiography is suboptimal.)

TABLE 15-1 ACCF 2010 Appropriateness Criteria for the Use of Cardiac Computed Tomography to Evaluate Pericardial Diseases

	APPROPRIATENESS RATING	INDICATION	MEDIAN SCORE
Evaluation of intra- and extracardiac structures	Appropriate	Evaluation of pericardial anatomy	8
		Evaluation of cardiac mass (suspected tumor or thrombus)	8
		Inadequate images from other noninvasive methods	
	Uncertain	None listed	
	Inappropriate	Initial evaluation of cardiac mass (suspected tumor or thrombus)	3

Data from Taylor AJ, Cerqueira M, Hodgson JM, et al. ACCF/SCCT/ACR/AHA/ASE/ASNC/NASCI/SCAI/SCMR 2010 appropriate use criteria for cardiac computed tomography. A report of the American College of Cardiology Foundation Appropriate Use Criteria Task Force, the Society of Cardiovascular Computed Tomography, the American College of Radiology, the American Heart Association, the American Society of Echocardiography, the American Society of Nuclear Cardiology, the North American Society for Cardiovascular Imaging, the Society for Cardiovascular Angiography and Interventions, and the Society for Cardiovascular Magnetic Resonance. *J Am Coll Cardiol.* 2010;56(22):1864-1894.

References

1. Masui T, Finck S, Higgins CB. Constrictive pericarditis and restrictive cardiomyopathy: evaluation with MR imaging. *Radiol.* 1992; 182(2):369-373.
2. Abramowitz Y, Simanovsky N, Goldstein MS, Hiller N. Pleural effusion: characterization with CT attenuation values and CT appearance. *AJR Am J Roentgenol.* 2009;192(3):618-623.
3. Southworth H, Stevenson CS. Congenital defects of the pericardium. *Arch Int Med.* 1938;61:223-240.
4. Kaneko Y, Okabe H, Nagata N. Complete left pericardial defect with dual passage of the phrenic nerve: a challenge to the widely accepted embryogenic theory. *Pediatr Cardiol.* 1998;19(5): 414-417.
5. Gatzoulis MA, Munk MD, Merchant N, Van Arsdell GS, McCrindle BW, Webb GD. Isolated congenital absence of the pericardium: clinical presentation, diagnosis, and management. *Ann Thorac Surg.* 2000;69(4):1209-1215.
6. Hoey ET, Yap KS, Darby MJ, Mankad K, Puppala S, Sivananthan MU. Complete left pericardial defect: evaluation with supine and decubitus dual source CT. *J Cardiovasc Comput Tomogr.* 2009;3(6):417-419.
7. Taguchi R, Takasu J, Itani Y, et al. Pericardial fat accumulation in men as a risk factor for coronary artery disease. *Atherosclerosis.* 2001;157(1):203-209.
8. Nichols JH, Samy B, Nasir K, et al. Volumetric measurement of pericardial adipose tissue from contrast-enhanced coronary computed tomography angiography: a reproducibility study. *J Cardiovasc Comput Tomogr.* 2008;2(5):288-295.
9. Abraham KP, Reddy V, Gattuso P. Neoplasms metastatic to the heart: review of 3314 consecutive autopsies. *Am J Cardiovasc Pathol.* 1990;3(3):195-198.
10. Klatt EC, Heitz DR. Cardiac metastases. *Cancer.* 1990;65(6): 1456-1459.
11. Oreopoulos G, Mickleborough L, Daniel L, De Sa M, Merchant N, Butany J. Primary pericardial mesothelioma presenting as constrictive pericarditis. *Can J Cardiol.* 1999;15(12):1367-1372.

16 Assessment of Native Cardiac Valves

Key Points

- Cardiac CT is able to image aortic valve morphology and to depict aortic valve area by planimetry.
- CCT is able to depict the stenotic orifice of mitral stenosis and to determine by planimetry the severity of mitral stenosis, but the coexistence of atrial fibrillation with mitral valve disease is an impediment to doing so.
- The CCT description of regurgitant lesions and their severity is in a preliminary phase.
- CCT may contribute indirectly to the assessment of native valve regurgitant disease by quantifying ventricular volumes and ejection fraction.
- CCT determination of aortic root and ascending aortic detail may assist in defining the nature of aortic insufficiency and therefore in surgical planning.
- CCT is able to exclude, with high negative predictive value, the presence of coexistent coronary artery disease, with the caveat that atrial fibrillation complicating mitral valve disease is a potential impediment to image quality.

At the present time only preliminary data exist on the evaluation of cardiac valves by cardiac CT (CCT), although contemporary CCT, if cardiac gated, can yield excellent images of native valves. Valve disease, however, is subject to many of the factors that present significant technical limitations or usual exclusions to CCT. Atrial fibrillation, which often coexists with mitral value disease, is an example of such a factor.

One critical deficiency of CCT in the assessment of valves is its inability to assess the hemodynamic function or dysfunction of the valve or prosthesis, because CCT lacks physiologic assessment capability (such as flow velocity, volume, or pressure recording). The role of CCT may be to ascertain and quantify stenotic orifice areas. Quantification of (most, particularly mitral) regurgitant orifices is, for the foreseeable future, beyond the technical means of CCT technology, although structurally simpler regurgitant orifices, such as perforations of the aortic valve, appear to be displayed well by optimized thin oblique multiplanar reformatted images and thin-slab volumetric reconstructions using the blood pool inversion method.[1,2]

Cine CT is the best means for assessing cardiac valves, and contrast enhancement improves image quality and diagnostic confidence[3] and also improves measurement of aortic valve annulus diameter.[3] The aortic and pulmonary valves, which exhibit one opening/closing motion per cardiac cycle and are smaller and simpler structures than the mitral and tricuspid valves, generally are well visualized. The mitral and tricuspid valves generally are visualized less completely and convincingly, as they exhibit two opening and closing motions per cardiac cycle, and they are much larger and more complex structures.

Valve-associated structures that have very high-speed or erratic motion, especially when they are small (such as flail leaflets and flail chordae, and many vegetations), cannot be seen as readily by CCT due to temporal resolution limitations. Calcification is a common confounder of valve lesion assessment and is almost invariably present in degenerative valve lesions such as aortic valve stenosis and older rheumatic valve lesions. Extensive submitral calcification (mitral annular calcification) or nearby mechanical (metallic) valve prostheses as well as pacemaker leads and implantable cardioverter defibrillators (ICDs) may all result in problematic artifacts to cardiac CT imaging. Atrial fibrillation is an unwelcome and frequently occurring complication of mitral valve disease.

AORTIC VALVE

Aortic valve morphology appears to be well evaluated by CCT. Leaflet thickness, leaflet number, leaflet suspension, and calcification, as well as annular and aortic root architecture, can be determined.

Congenital Morphology

Bicuspid aortic valve morphology is readily apparent. In the cine mode, the leaflets of a normal trileaflet valve open symmetrically to a triangular orifice. A functionally bicuspid valve with a raphe will appear similar to a trileaflet valve in diastole, but in systole will open to an elliptical orifice. A normal aortic valve is 1 to 2 mm thick and is not calcified. Thin (<1 mm) slices are useful for aortic valve morphologic determinations. It is imperative to assess the valve in systole to distinguish a third commissure (normal) from a raphe (functionally bicuspid valve).

Congenitally quadricuspid aortic valves also are readily recognized by CCT, as is the commonly associated central regurgitant orifice.[4,5]

For images of aortic valve morphology, see Figures 16-1 to 16-4 and **Videos 16-1 through 16-4.**

Aortic Stenosis

A stenotic aortic valve is apparent by cine CT because of its doming motion (if bicuspid), calcification, thickening, and reduced systolic orifice. The uncommon occurrence of atrial fibrillation in aortic stenosis (AS) reduces one challenge of the CCT assessment of AS.

Calcium Scoring of the Aortic Valve and Aortic Stenosis

Calcification is arbitrarily and variably defined, usually as greater than 130 HU.[6,7] Severe calcification (score > 3700) is consistent with stenosis,[8] but does not quantitate it or assess for the degree of concurrent aortic insufficiency. Studies suggest that the extent of valve calcification has overall reproducibility within 8%,[3] correlates with extent of valve dysfunction (both gradient; $r^2 = 0.77$ and area $r^2 = 0.73$),[7] has some prognostic value,[1] and is equally well assessed radiologically on noncontrast and contrast images.[1] However, calcium score is clinically not a surrogate for other traditional hemodynamic parameters of aortic stenosis and also may not be specific for

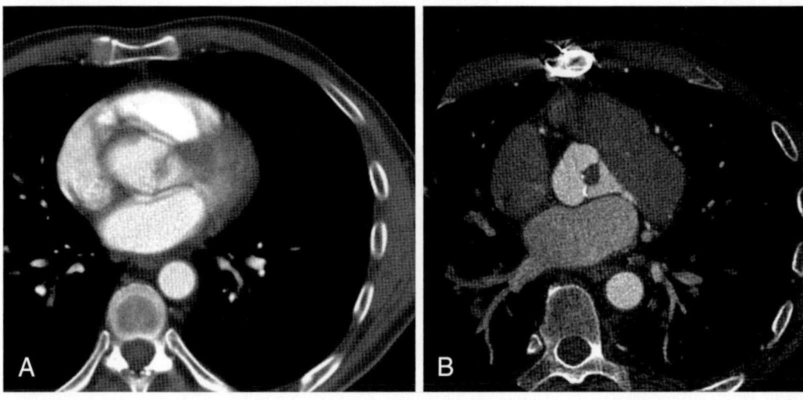

Figure 16-1. Two CT images in a 42-year-old man with a history of a descending aortic aneurysm (not shown). These images demonstrate the value of an ECG-gated acquisition (**B**) for evaluation of the aortic root. A moderate-sized focal area of thickening involving the aortic valve leaflets and mild aortic valve calcification are much better appreciated on the gated study on the right.

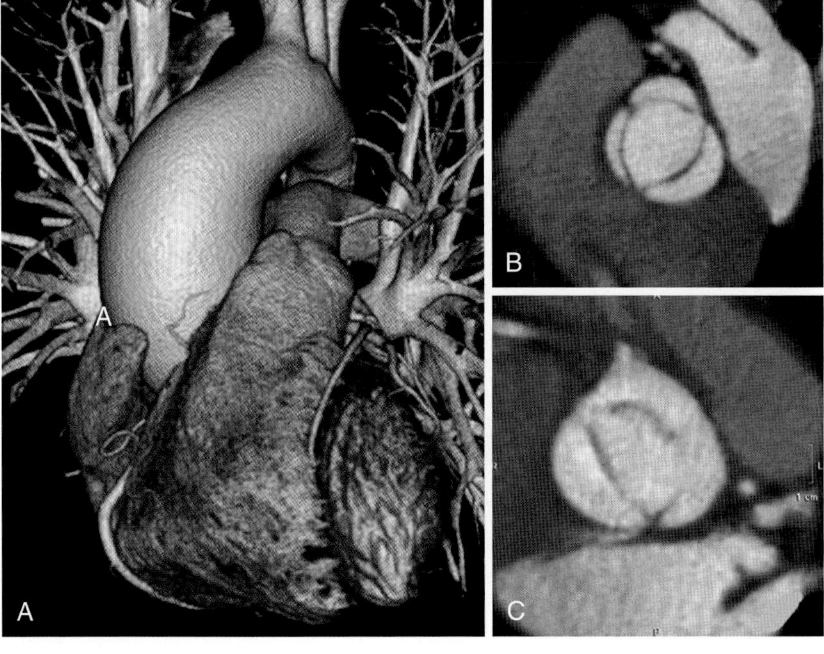

Figure 16-2. Composite images from a CCT examination in a patient with a functionally bicuspid aortic valve and an associated bicuspid aortopathy. The aneurysm of the ascending aorta is apparent on the 3D volume-rendered image (**A**). The bicuspid value is apparent by its elliptical shape in systole (**B, C**). CT angiography demonstrated normal coronary arteries.

aortic stenosis, as a calcific valve may also only be insufficient or may have little hemodynamic impairment. The real relevance of calcium for CCT is that when present in great excess in senile calcific degenerative AS, it impairs the planimetry of the orifice.

Aortic Valve Orifice Planimetry

Small single-center series using 16-CT have established that it is feasible to use planimetry to determine the stenotic aortic valve area, with good correlation (r = 0.89; P < .001) with transthoracic echocardiographic (TTE) estimates of aortic valve area.[9] Planimetry of a valve always assumes that the orifice is planar and is subject to many of the vicissitudes of planimetry seen with transesophageal echocardiography (TEE) and in addition, to the partial volume averaging effects of valve calcium. As indicated, aortic valve calcification is a common and nearly inevitable concurrence in aortic stenosis. However, CCT planimetry of the aortic valve is robust when compared to TEE, because volumetric acquisition of the valve moving in four-dimensional imaging allows for greater assurance that the valve is imaged at the truly most stenotic plane.

Another single-center series of 48 patients (40-slice CCT), mean age 62 ± 13 years, with and without AS, undergoing TTE, TEE, CCT, and cardiac MR (CMR) yielded high correlations by CCT with CMR (Tables 16-1 and 16-2).[10]

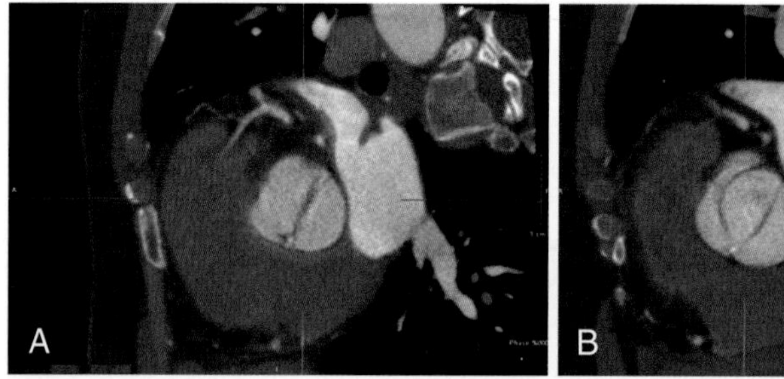

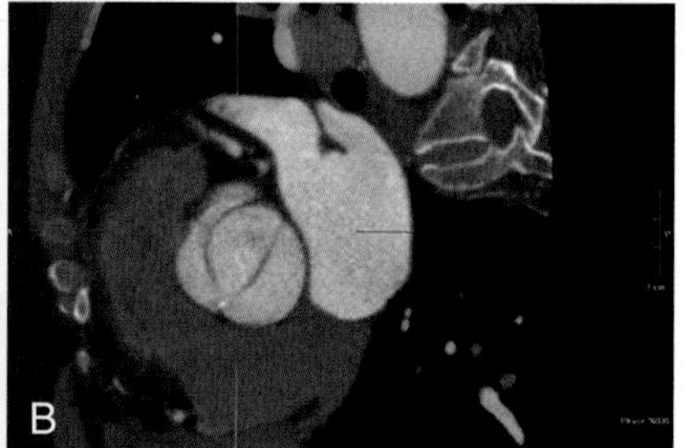

Figure 16-3. Two double-oblique images from a cardiac CT study demonstrating a functionally bicuspid aortic valve with a small fused raphe (**A**, diastole; **B**, systole). Small amounts of aortic valve calcification are noted. A wide "fish-mouth" appearance to the aortic valve is noted with no evidence of a reduction in the aortic valve area. **See Videos 16-1 through 16-3.**

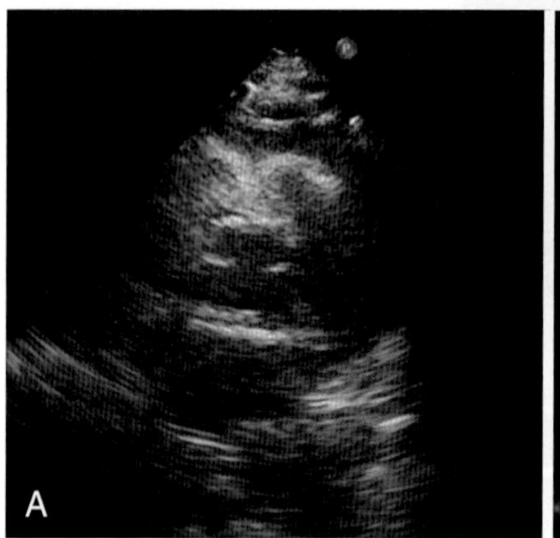

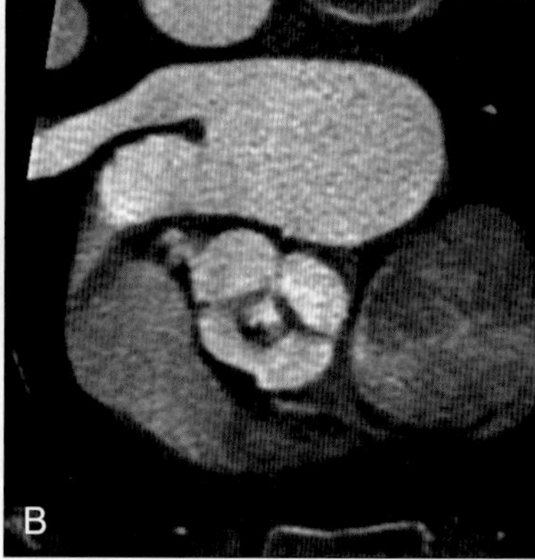

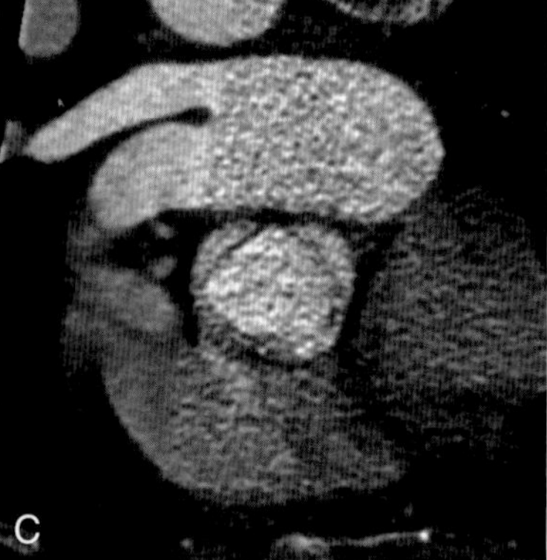

Figure 16-4. A quadricuspid aortic valve, poorly seen on transthoracic echocardiography, but adequately imaged by CCT in diastole (**B**) and in systole (**C**). **See Video 16-4.**

TABLE 16-1 Cardiac CT versus Cardiac MR for the Depiction of Aortic Valve Area

SENSITIVITY (%)	SPECIFICITY (%)	ACCURACY (%)	NPV (%)	PPV (%)
100	100	100	97	96

Data from Pouleur AC, le Polain de Waroux JB, Pasquet A, Vanoverschelde JL, Gerber BL. Aortic valve area assessment: multidetector CT compared with cine MR imaging and transthoracic and transesophageal echocardiography. *Radiology.* 2007;244(3):745-754.

TABLE 16-2 CCT versus CMR, TTE, and TEE for the Depiction of Aortic Valve Area

	CMR	TTE	TEE
CCT AVA versus	r = 0.98, P < .01	r = 0.96, P < .01	r = 0.98, P < .01

AVA, aortic valve area; CCT, cardiac CT; CMR, cardiac MR; TEE, transesophageal echocardiography; TTE, transthoracic echocardiography. Data from Pouleur AC, le Polain de Waroux JB, Pasquet A, Vanoverschelde JL, Gerber BL. Aortic valve area assessment: multidetector CT compared with cine MR imaging and transthoracic and transesophageal echocardiography. *Radiology.* 2007;244(3):745-754.

For Bland-Altman plots of linear regression and limits of agreement between CCT-derived and echocardiography- or CMR-derived estimates of aortic valve area, see Figure 16-5.

Another single-center small series using 64-CT showed good correlation with TEE.[9]

The overall correlation of CCT and TEE measurements of aortic valve area (AVA) as determined by a meta-analysis is 0.99, $P < .001$.[11]

Delineation of Left Ventricular Outflow Tract Anatomy

The delineation of subaortic geometry by CCT is highly feasible, describing the elliptical orifice shape[12] and lesions such as muscular subaortic stenosis,[13] although less has been established about the ability of CCT to assess subaortic membranes.

CCT determination by planimetry of the AVA tends to overestimate AVA when compared with TTE (Fig. 16-6).[14] The recognition that the left ventricular outflow tract (LVOT) has an elliptical rather than round cross-section likely underlies the reason for the difference between CCT and TTE measurements of AVA, because CCT determines true LVOT area, whereas TTE determination of the LVOT "diameter" from the parasternal long-axis view yields the lesser diameter (dimension).

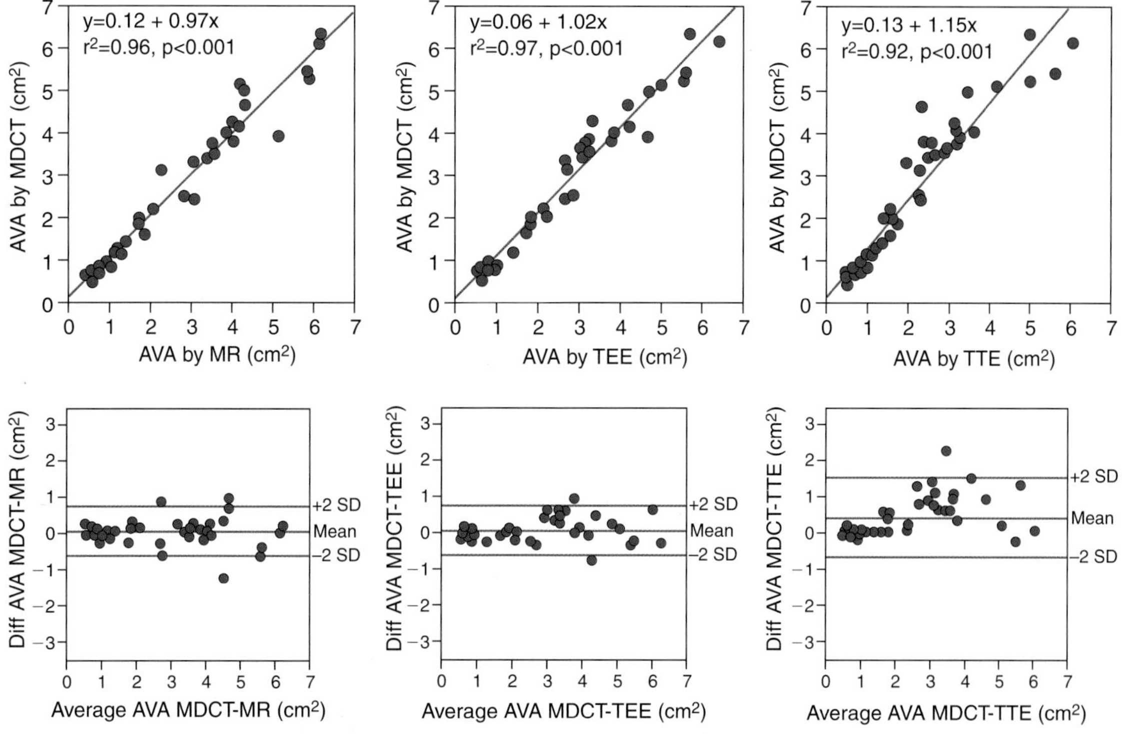

Figure 16-5. Bland-Altman plots of linear regression and limits of agreement between aortic valve area (AVA) estimates derived with multidetector CT (MDCT) and those derived with MR imaging, transesophageal echocardiography (TEE), and transthoracic echocardiography (TTE). AVA derived with multidetector CT planimetry correlated well with AVA derived with MR planimetry, TEE planimetry, and continuity equation TTE. Plots show no significant difference (bias) in AVA derived by using multidetector CT planimetry versus that derived by using MR planimetry and TEE planimetry but significantly overestimated planimetric values compared with continuity equation TTE values. Diff, difference. (Reprinted with permission from Pouleur AC, le Polain de Waroux JB, Pasquet A, et al. Aortic valve area assessment: multidetector CT compared with cine MR imaging and transthoracic and transesophageal echocardiography. *Radiology.* 2007;244(3):745-754.)

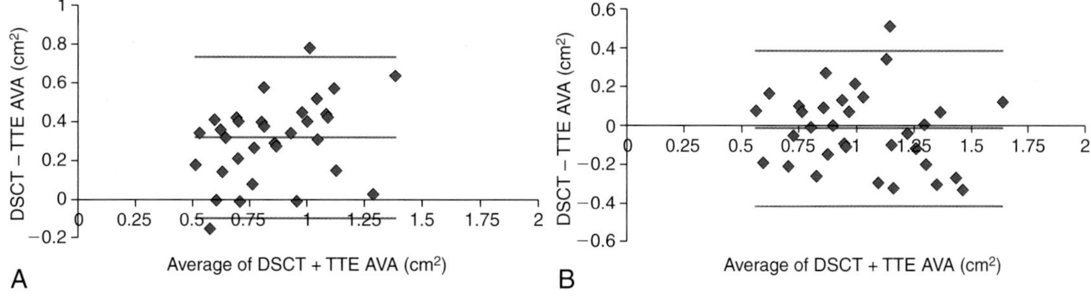

Figure 16-6. Bland-Altman analysis of aortic valve orifice area (AVA) determination by dual-source CT (DSCT; planimetry) and transthoracic echocardiography (TTE; continuity equation) in 35 patients with aortic valve stenosis. **A,** Between the two techniques, there is a systematic bias with overestimation of the orifice area by CT compared with TTE (mean absolute difference: 0.32 ± 0.19 cm^2). **B,** The bias is reduced significantly when flow velocities measured by TTE and the exact left ventricular outflow tract area as determined by CT are entered into the continuity equation (0.16 ± 0.12 cm^2). (Reprinted with permission from Pflederer T, Achenbach S. Aortic valve stenosis: CT contributions to diagnosis and therapy. *J Cardiovasc Comput Tomogr.* 2010;4(6):355-364.)

For images of stenotic aortic valves imaged by CCT, aortic valve areas measured by CCT, and calcium volume correlation with aortic stenosis severity, see Figures 16-7 through 16-10 and **Video 16-5.**

Subvalvular Stenosis

CCT is able to image subvalvular membranes and muscular subaortic obstruction (Figs. 16-11 through 16-13).

Supravalvular Stenosis

CCT is able to image supravalvular aortic membranes and muscular subaortic obstruction (Fig. 16-14).

Planning of Percutaneous Aortic Valve Replacement

See Chapter 17 for more information on planning percutaneous aortic valve replacement.

Aortic Insufficiency

The role of CCT in the assessment of aortic insufficiency has been only preliminarily demonstrated.

Etiology of Aortic Insufficiency

The aortic root and the valve-related mechanism or etiology of aortic insufficiency can be well imaged by CCT.

Severity of Aortic Insufficiency

In limited studies (single-center, small numbers, limited range of pathology), determination of the regurgitant orifice and categorization thereby of severity have yielded fair[15,16] and good[17,18] correlations with CTA estimates of regurgitant orifice size and severity.

Other Aortic Valve Lesions

The clinical contribution of CCT toward other aortic valve/root pathologies has not been

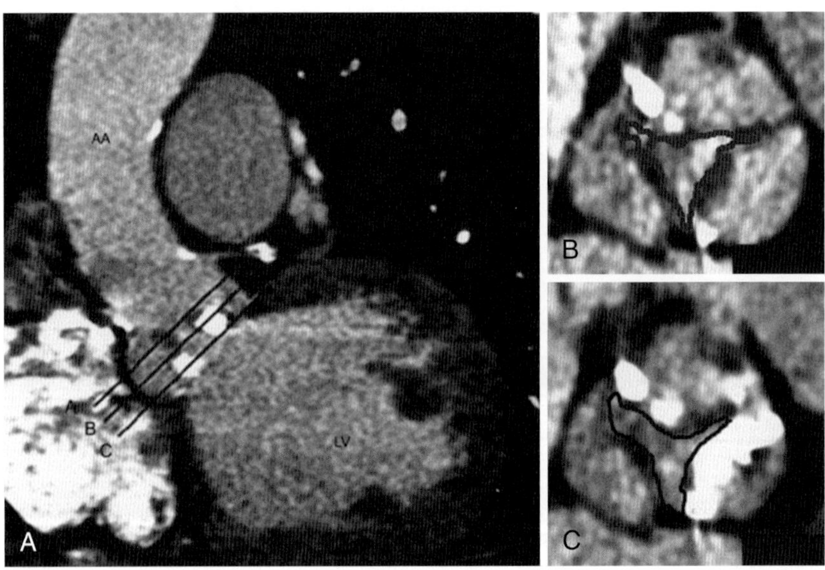

Figure 16-7. Quantification of aortic valve area (AVA) ("planimetry"). The AVA was reconstructed at three cross-sectional transverse levels (A to C). The smallest AVA value was taken for effective AVA. AA, ascending aorta; LV, left ventricle. (Reprinted with permission from Feuchtner GM, Dichtl W, Friedrich GJ, et al: Multislice computed tomography for detection of patients with aortic valve stenosis and quantification of severity. *J Am Coll Cardiol* 2006;47(7):1410-1417.)

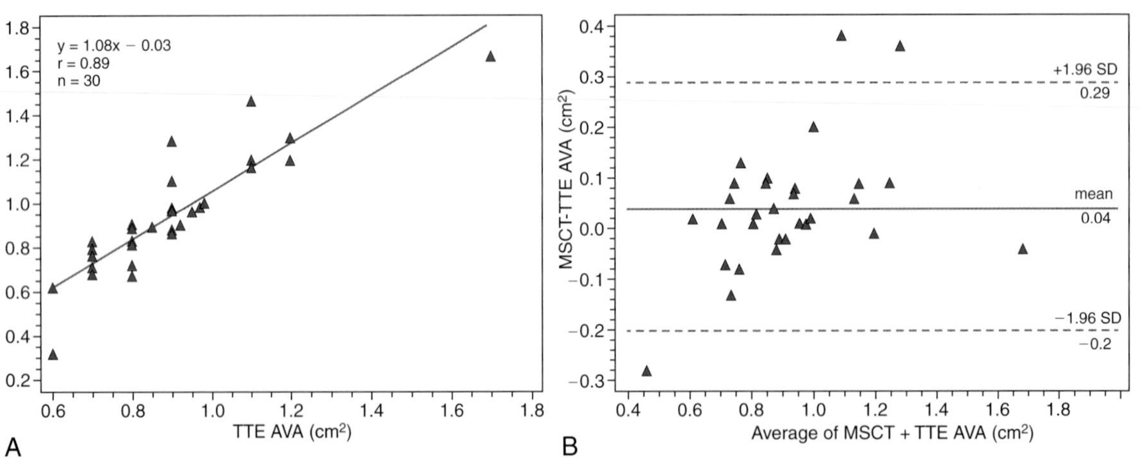

Figure 16-8. A, Linear regression analysis illustrates a good correlation of aortic valve area (AVA) derived by multislice CT (MSCT) ($r = 0.89$; $P < .001$) compared with transthoracic echocardiography (TTE). **B,** Bland-Altman plot demonstrates a good intermodality agreement between MSCT and TTE with a slight overestimation of AVA by MSCT (+0.04 cm^2). (Reprinted with permission from Feuchtner GM, Dichtl W, Friedrich GJ, et al. Multislice computed tomography for detection of patients with aortic valve stenosis and quantification of severity. *J Am Coll Cardiol.* 2006;47(7):1410-1417.)

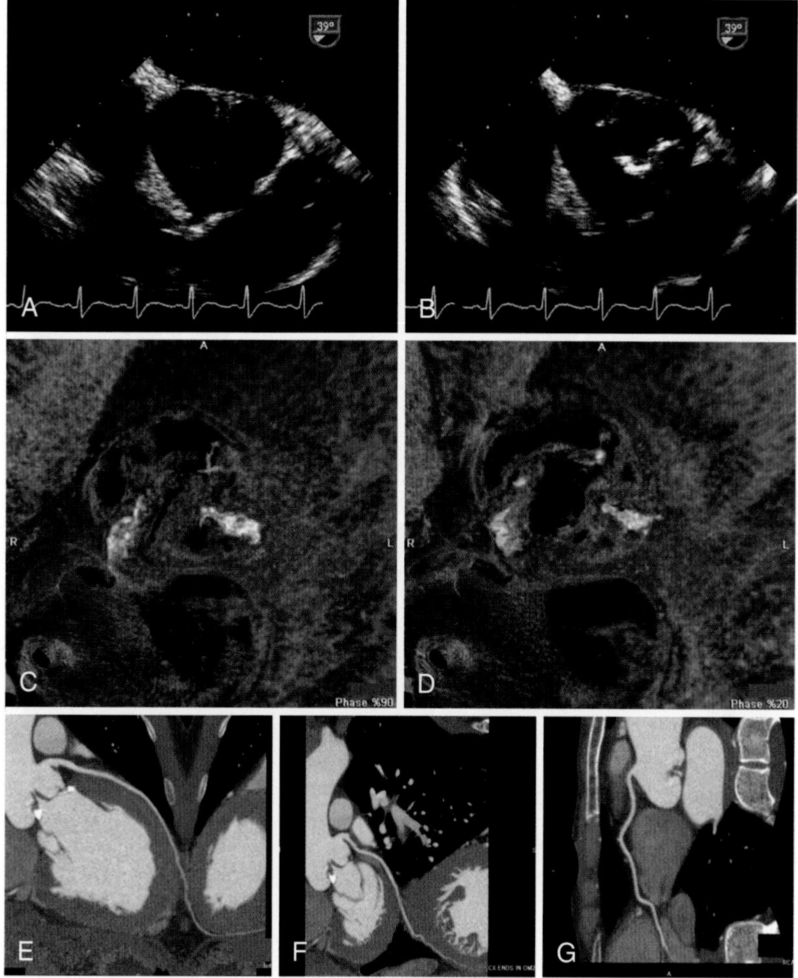

Figure 16-9. A 42-year-old man with symptomatic aortic stenosis was referred for CT coronary angiography. The aortic valve appearance was obtained in diastole and systole by retrospectively gated CTA, which yielded depictions of the valve and its systolic orifice similar to those obtained by transesophageal echocardiography. The valve leaflets are thickened and eccentrically calcified, and there is a calcified "raphe" (a fused or nondivided commissure) at 4 o'clock. CTA did not demonstrate coronary artery disease.

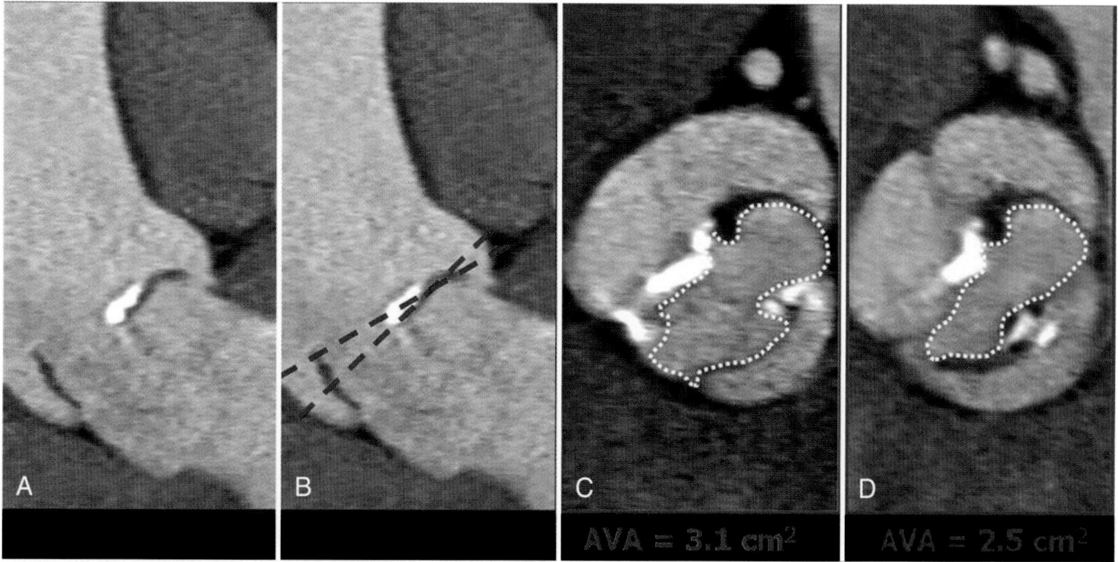

Figure 16-10. An aortic valve with dysmorphic anatomy. The valvular orifice plane deviates from the plane of the aortic annulus (**A** and **B**). Measuring the orifice area in a plane parallel to the annulus (*red line*) would lead to overestimation of the orifice (**C**). For correct planimetry, a multiplanar reconstruction must be performed exactly in the plane described by the borders of the aortic cusps (*blue line*, **D**). AVA, aortic valve orifice area. (Reprinted with permission from Pflederer T, Achenbach S. Aortic valve stenosis: CT contributions to diagnosis and therapy. *J Cardiovasc Comput Tomogr.* 2010;4(6):355-364.)

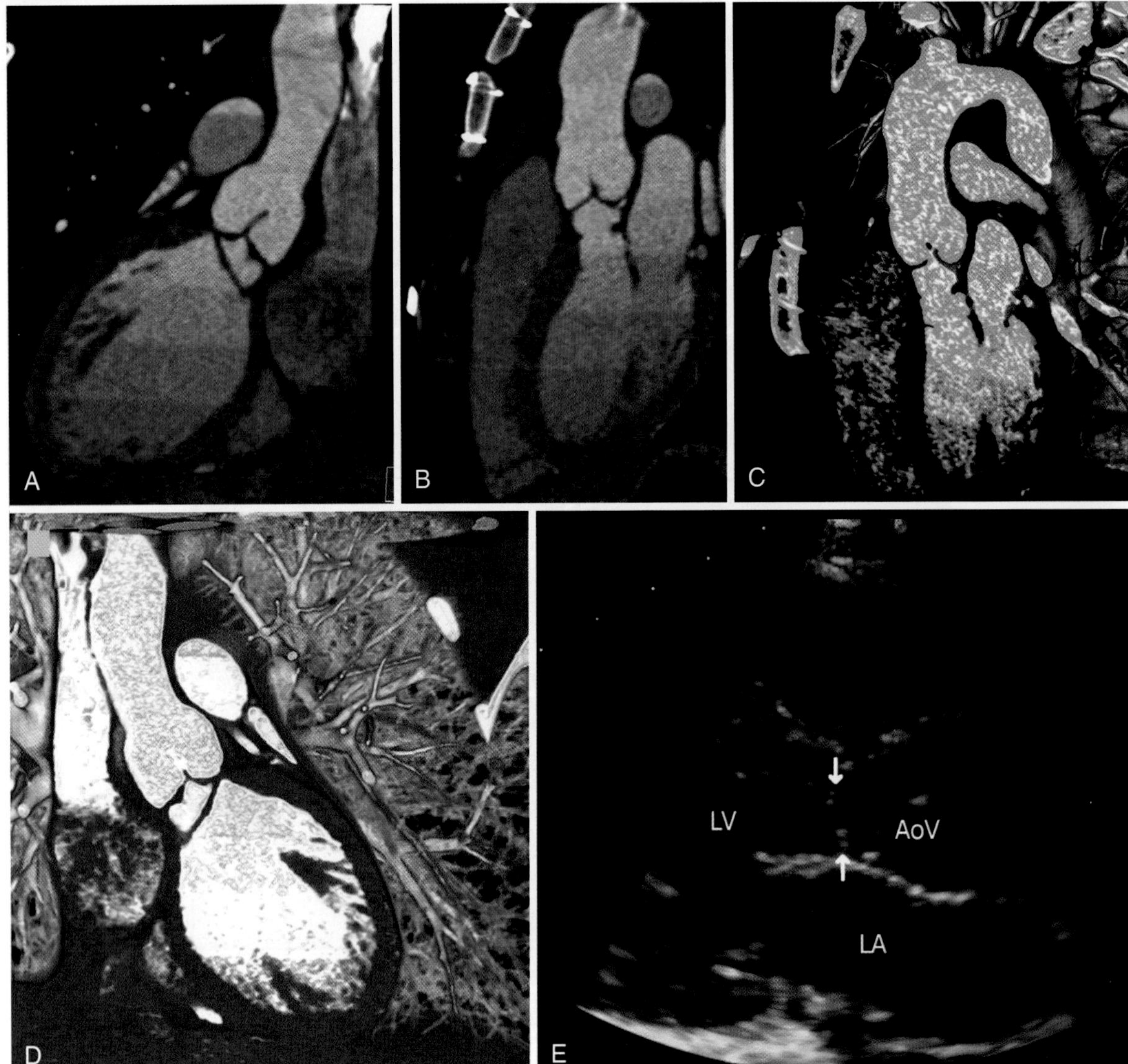

Figure 16-11. Maximum-intensity projection images (**A** and **B**) and volume-rendered images (**C** and **D**) show the recurrent subaortic membrane that caused obstruction of the left ventricular outflow tract and thickening of the aortic valve leaflets. Echocardiographic image (**E**), acquired in a zoomed-up parasternal long axis view, shows a discrete subaortic membrane (*between arrows*). The membrane is circumferential, with an attachment to the anterior leaflet of the mitral valve (*lower arrow*). AoV, aortic valve; LA, left atrium; LV, left ventricle. (Reprinted with permission from Takx R, Schoepf UJ, Friedman B, et al: Recurrent subaortic membrane causing subvalvular aortic stenosis 13 years after primary surgical resection. *J Cardiovasc Comput Tomogr.* 2011;5(2):127-128.)

established, but CCT should be able to contribute to the imaging of such lesions as:

- Sinus of Valsalva aneurysm
- Sinus of Valsalva fistula
- Sinus of Valsalva thrombus
- Fibroelastomas that are ambiguous by TEE (see Chapter 18)

MITRAL VALVE

The mitral valve is a more complex and far larger structure than the aortic valve and often is referred to as an "apparatus" because of all of its various components:

- Anterior and posterior leaflets
- Chordae tendineae
- Annulus
- Anterolateral and posteromedial commissure
- Anterolateral and posteromedial papillary muscles
- Subtending myocardium

CCT is able to image mitral valve components, contingent on many of the usual demands on CCT such as heart rate and rhythm. Atrial fibrillation, and its higher than usual ventricular response, and cardiac cycle length variability and

Figure 16-12. Axial (**A**) and three-chamber (**B**) multiplanar reformatted images from preoperative cardiac CT demonstrate a discrete membrane within the left ventricular outflow tract (LVOT; *black arrows*). **C,** Intraoperative transesophageal echocardiography (TEE) during systole demonstrates a high-velocity turbulent jet emanating from a discrete focal narrowing of the LVOT (*white arrow*). **D,** Three-dimensional volume-rendered thick slab image using blood pool inversion (BPI) technique at the level of the LVOT oriented in the same perspective as the TEE image in **C**. Note the discrete membranous narrowing (*white arrows*) within the LVOT approximately 1 cm below the aortic valve. This membrane extended posteriorly from the basal anteroseptal wall across the membranous interventricular septum to the mitral–aortic intervalvular fibrosa (*). Ao, aorta; LA, left atrium. (Reprinted with permission from Entrikin DW, Kon N, Carr JJ. Discrete membranous subaortic stenosis demonstrated by cardiac CT. *Society of Cardiovascular Computed Tomography Case of the Month*, April 2010. http://archive.constantcontact.com/fs027/1101901294184/archive/1103233525137.html.)

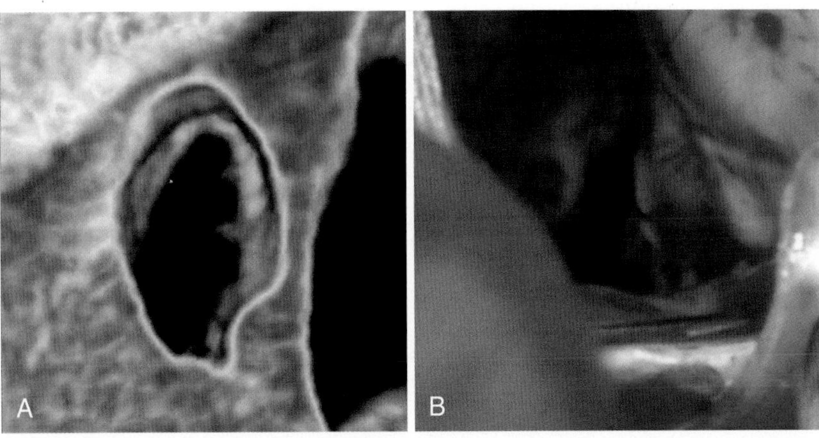

Figure 16-13. **A,** Blood pool inversion image from an aortotomy perspective looking below the aortic valve into the left ventricular outflow tract demonstrates an incomplete subvalvular membrane from 9 o'clock to 5 o'clock. **B,** Corresponding intraoperative photo. (Reprinted with permission from Entrikin DW, Kon N, Carr JJ. Discrete membranous subaortic stenosis demonstrated by cardiac CT. *Society of Cardiovascular Computed Tomography Case of the Month*, April 2010. http://archive.constantcontact.com/fs027/1101901294184/archive/1103233525137.html.)

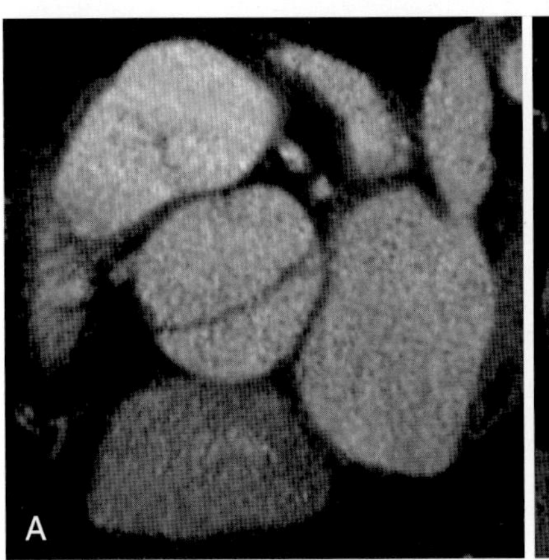

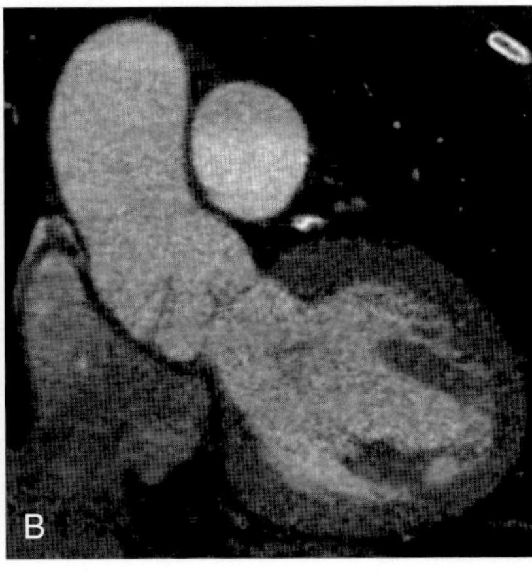

Figure 16-14. Cardiac CT in a patient with prior echocardiography demonstrating linear filamentous structure in the supravalvular aorta. A very fine linear membrane is seen within the supravalvular aorta. There is no associated calcification, no evidence of extension of this process, and no surrounding intramural hematoma. This remained unchanged over multiple subsequent follow-up studies and was thought to represent a nonobstructing supravalvular membrane.

excessive heart rate increment during scanning are particularly common in mitral valve disease.

The contribution of CCT to the imaging of mitral disease has not yet been entirely defined. TTE and TEE, on the other hand, leave few questions unanswered, other than the etiology of mitral regurgitation in about 20% of cases. Still, CCT visualization of the mitral valve and its lesions, such as clefts and associated lesions, is impressive.[19]

For CCT images of mitral valve morphology, see Figure 16-15.

Congenital Mitral Valve Anomalies

For CCT images of a congenital mitral arcade, see Figure 16-16; for images of a cleft mitral valve, see Figure 16-17.

Mitral Stenosis

As with the aortic valve, CCT is better suited to assessing stenosis than insufficiency. Volumetric acquisition lends itself to identification of the true level of stenosis (valve leaflet or subvalvular).

A small single-center series using 16-CT, after the exclusion of patients who had atrial fibrillation, calcified valves, nonfeasible planimetry, or renal dysfunction, or who were pregnant, demonstrated good correlation with TTE determinations of mitral valve area (r = 0.88; $P < .0001$).[20]

Any associated degree of mitral insufficiency is outside the scope of what CCT can currently assess.

For CCT images of stenotic mitral valves and plots of CCT compared with echo regression and limits of agreement plots, see Figures 16-18 and 16-19.

Mitral Insufficiency

The complexity of the mitral valve and its motion present a higher challenge to CCT, and no role has yet been proposed or established for CCT evaluation of mitral insufficiency.

Submitral Calcification

The extent of submitral or mitral annular calcification is readily depicted by CCT.[21] For CCT images of submitral calcification, see Figures 16-20 and 16-21.

TRICUSPID VALVE DISEASE

Tricuspid Insufficiency

Reflux of contrast into the inferior vena cava (IVC) following upper extremity injection is an older sign of tricuspid regurgitation (TR), as it can seldom be explained otherwise (sensitivity 90% and specificity 100%). The extent of reflux as seen by CT approximates the severity of TR as assessed by echocardiography (r = 0.56) and its

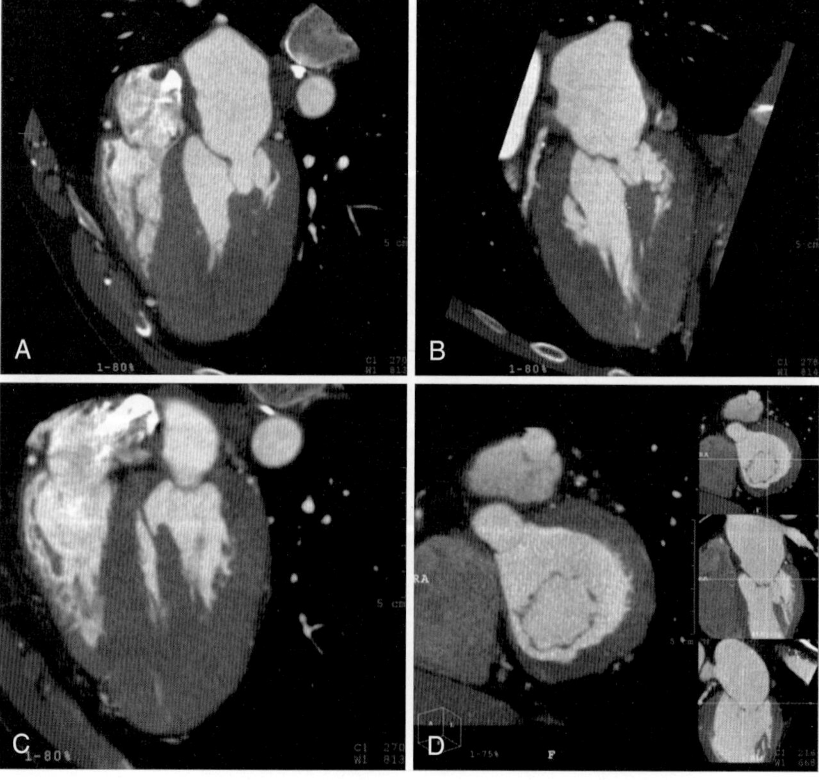

Figure 16-15. A, Contrast-enhanced maximum intensity projection (MIP) image of the mitral apparatus in diastole. The anterior and posterior leaflets, the chordae to each leaflet, and the posteromedial papillary muscle are well seen. **B,** Contrast-enhanced MIP image of the mitral apparatus in diastole. The anterior and posterior leaflets, the chordae to each leaflet, and the posteromedial papillary muscle and its attachments are well seen. **C,** Contrast-enhanced MIP image of the mitral apparatus in diastole. The details of the posteromedial papillary muscle architecture, including, in this image, an accessory chordae attaching to the basal septum, are well seen. **D,** Contrast-enhanced MIP image of the mitral orifice in diastole. The full opening of the anterior and posterior leaflets and their normal thickness are well seen.

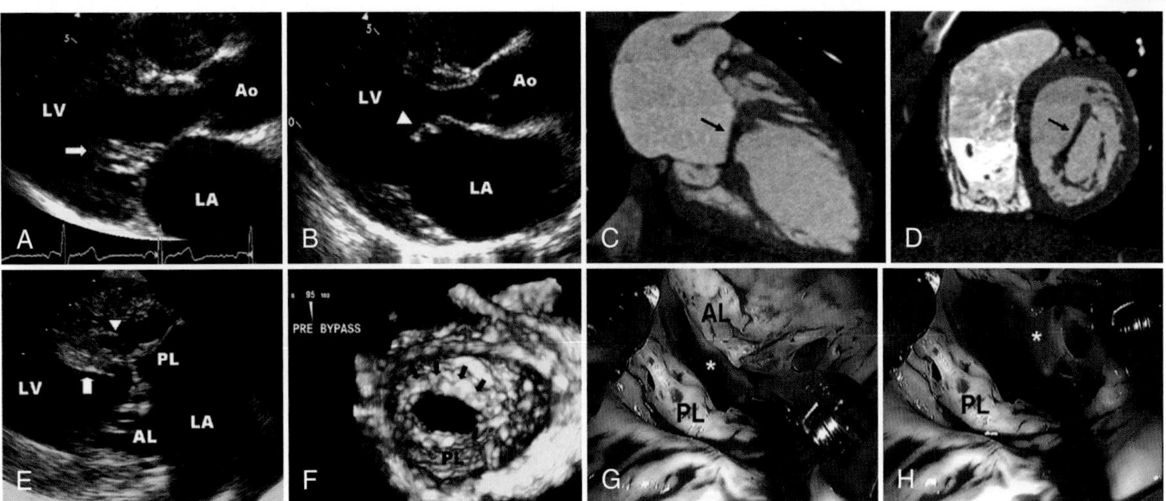

Figure 16-16. A 25-year-old woman who had experienced heart failure in infancy presented with progressive exertional dyspnea. Transthoracic echocardiography revealed severe mitral regurgitation and thickening of the mitral valve and subvalvular apparatus (**A**, *arrow*), with apparent "hockey-stick" diastolic deformity of the anterior mitral leaflet (AL) (**B**, *arrowhead*) suggestive of rheumatic involvement. The patient was referred for surgery. ECG-gated cardiac CT performed for preoperative coronary artery evaluation unexpectedly demonstrated elongated papillary muscles connected along the free edge of the AL by a bridge of abnormal tissue (**C** and **D**, *arrows*), with restricted AL mobility. Intraoperative transesophageal echocardiography showed similar findings with elongated papillary muscle in direct continuity with the AL (**E**, *arrow*) and thick, shortened chordae between the papillary muscle and the posterior leaflet (PL) (**E**, *arrowhead*) with formation of an anterior fibrous arcade on three-dimensional left ventricular (LV) perspective reconstruction (**F**, *arrows*). Robot-assisted minimally invasive surgery confirmed anomalous mitral arcade with direct continuity of both anterolateral (*, **G**) and posteromedial (*, **H**) papillary muscles with the AL. The native valve was replaced with a mechanical prosthesis, and the patient recovered uneventfully. Ao, aorta; LA, left atrium. (Reprinted with permission from Morris MF, Williamson E, Topilsky Y, et al. Multi-imaging assessment of the congenital mitral arcade. *J Am Coll Cardiol.* 2011;57(18):1854.)

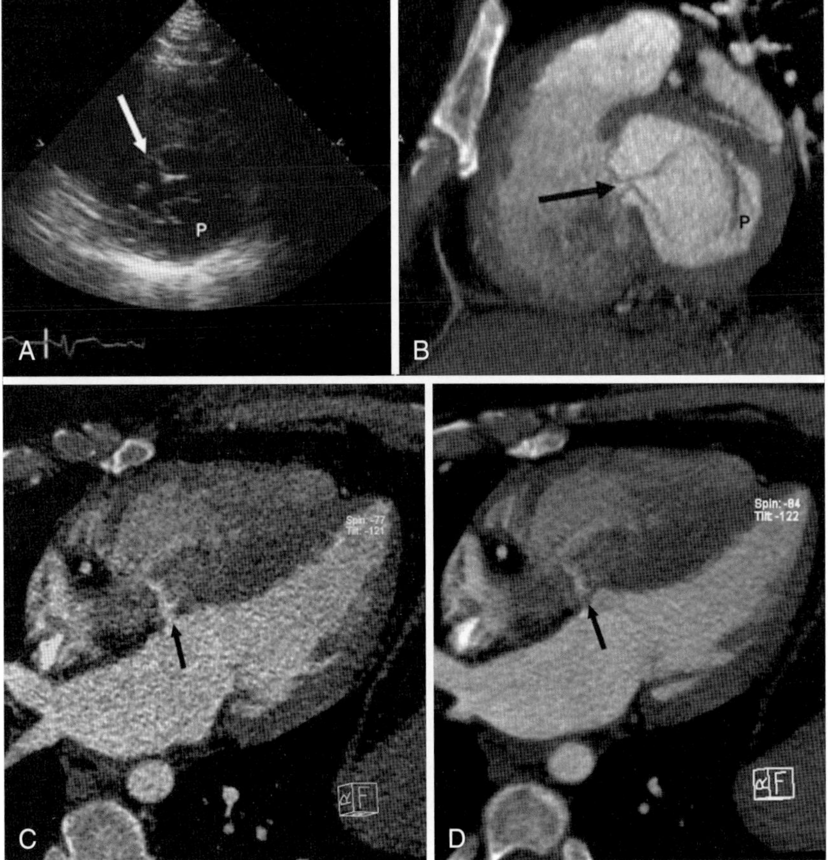

Figure 16-17. Short-axis echocardiographic (**A**) and CT (**B**) images of the cleft mitral valve. **A,** Two-dimensional left ventricular short-axis echocardiographic image at the level of the mitral valve shows a cleft within the anterior mitral valve leaflet extending into the mitral annulus (*arrow*). P, posterior leaflet. **B,** Early diastolic short-axis multiplanar reformation in the mitral valve plane shows the cleft within the anterior mitral valve leaflet *(arrow)*, which extends into the mitral annulus. **C** and **D,** Multiplanar reformation of end-diastolic multidetector CT data sets in four-chamber views show a contrast jet passing from the left atrium into the right heart (*arrows*). Note: poor contrast-to-noise ratio is the result of the patient's obesity. (Reprinted with permission from Durst R, Avelar E, Sollis J, King ME, Abbara S. Cleft mitral valve appearance on cardiac computed tomography. *J Cardiovasc Comput Tomogr.* 2008;2(5):341-342.)

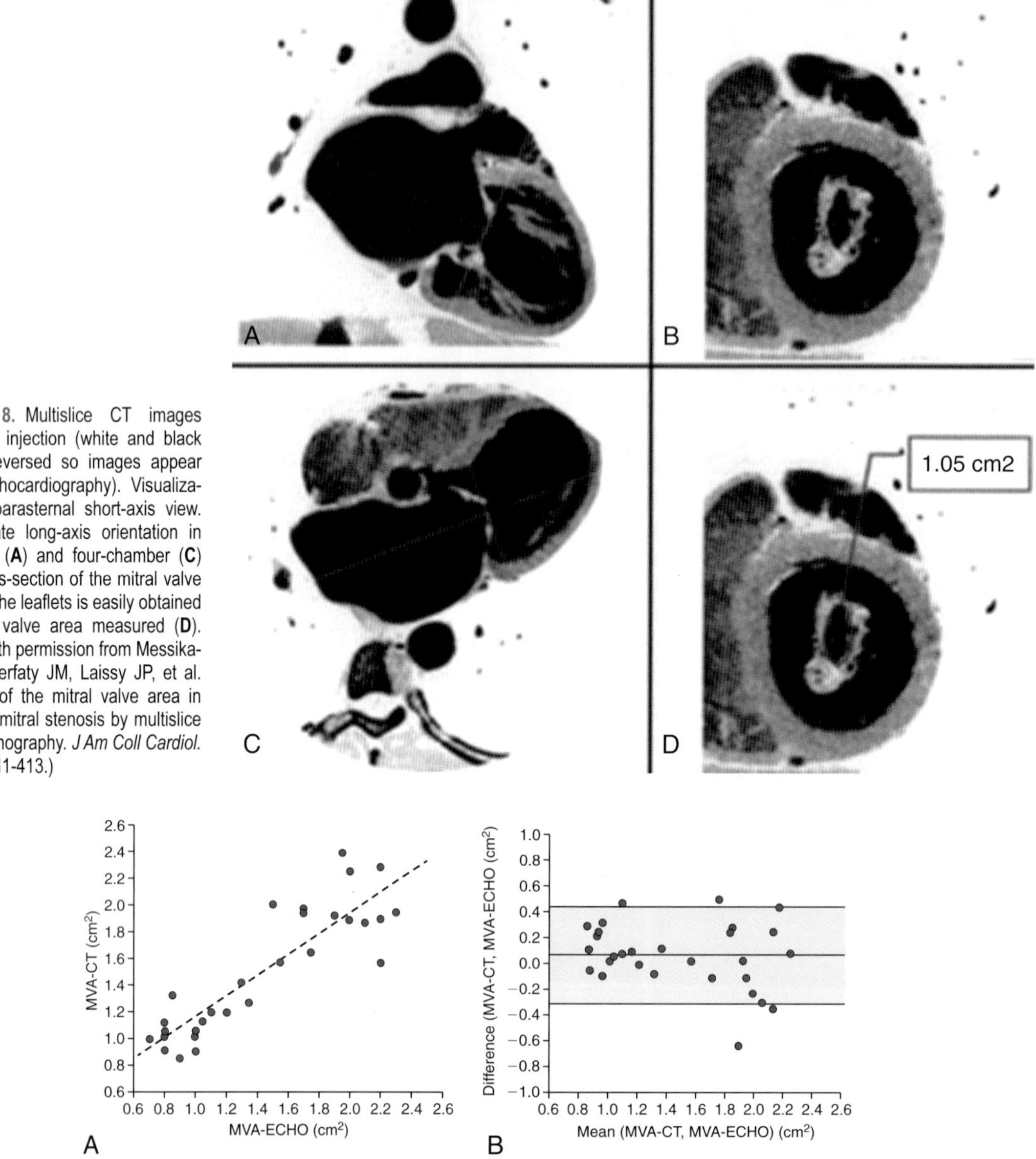

Figure 16-18. Multislice CT images with contrast injection (white and black colors are reversed so images appear similar to echocardiography). Visualization of the parasternal short-axis view. After adequate long-axis orientation in two-chamber (**A**) and four-chamber (**C**) views, a cross-section of the mitral valve at the tips of the leaflets is easily obtained (**B**) and the valve area measured (**D**). (Reprinted with permission from Messika-Zeitoun D, Serfaty JM, Laissy JP, et al. Assessment of the mitral valve area in patients with mitral stenosis by multislice computed tomography. *J Am Coll Cardiol.* 2006;48(2):411-413.)

Figure 16-19. **A,** Correlation between mitral valve area assessed by CTA (MVA-CT) and by two-dimensional echocardiography (MVA-ECHO) (r = 0.88, P < .001). **B,** Quality control plots using Bland-Altman analysis for the two methods. The *yellow circles* represent patients with calcified mitral valves, and the *blue circles* stand for those with noncalcified mitral valves. (Reprinted with permission from Messika-Zeitoun D, Serfaty JM, Laissy JP, et al: Assessment of the mitral valve area in patients with mitral stenosis by multislice computed tomography. *J Am Coll Cardiol.* 2006;48(2):411-413.)

driving pressure (pulmonary artery systolic pressure; r = 0.69).[22] However, the extent of reflux of dye into the IVC also correlates with the degree of right ventricular systolic hypertension.[23] The use of power injectors at higher rates increases the observation of dye reflux into the IVC.

CCT is able to determine the right and left ventricular end-systolic and end-diastolic volumes. If one makes the assumption that there is no PI, no MR, and no AI, then the stroke volume difference between the two ventricles, if greater for the right ventricle, represents the tricuspid regurgitant volume.

CARDIAC CT BEFORE VALVE SURGERY

Preliminary series have investigated the utility of CCT in the pre–valve replacement scenario, using the test for its negative predictive value. Predictably, studies have focused on aortic valve disease, which usually is not complicated by atrial fibrillation. Using 16-CCT[24-26] and 64-CT,[27] both the negative predictive value of low calcium scores and the absence of significant CTA-detected coronary artery disease have been investigated, with the evolution clearly moving toward CTA and away from the use of calcium scoring alone. Larger

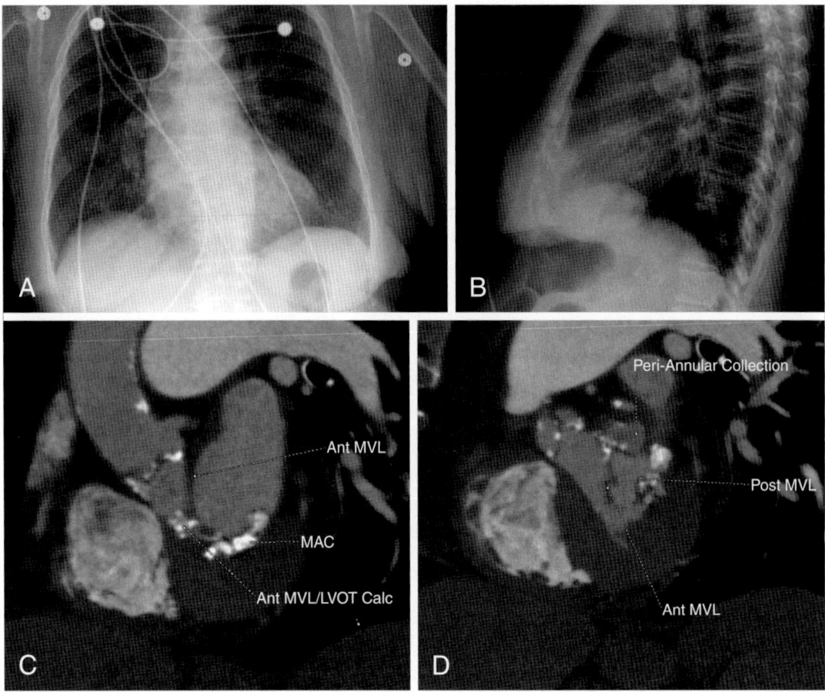

Figure 16-20. The frontal (**A**) and especially the lateral (**B**) chest radiograph reveal mitral annular calcification (MAC). **C** and **D,** The contrast-enhanced CT maximum intensity projection images reveal calcification of the aorta, the aortic valve, and complex heterogeneous calcification of the mitral annulus. Ant, anterior; Calc, calcification; LVOT, left ventricular outflow tract; MVL, mitral valve leaflet; Post, posterior.

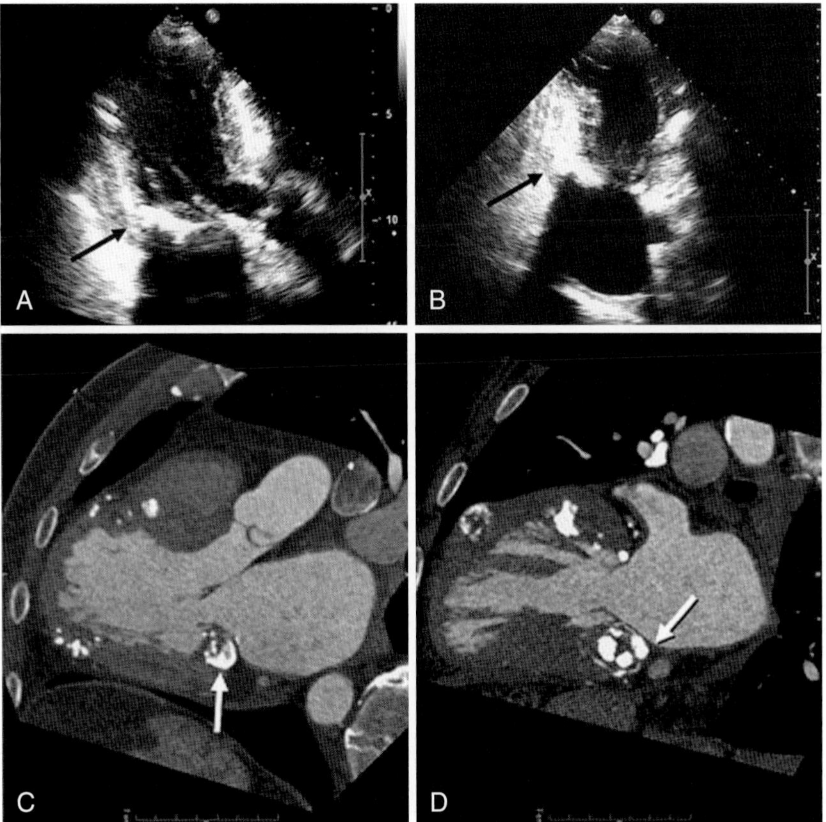

Figure 16-21. Transthoracic echocardiogram showing a posterior hyperechoic lesion with central lucency and ECG-gated cardiac CT with multiple foci of heterogeneous calcification. Arrows indicate heterogeneous submitral calcification. (Reprinted with permission from Salisbury AC, Shapiro BP, Martinez MW: Extensive myocardial and mitral annular calcification leading to mitral regurgitation and restrictive cardiomyopathy: an unusual case of caseous calcification of the mitral annulus. *J Cardiovasc Comput Tomogr.* 2009;3(5):351-353.)

TABLE16-3 ACCF 2010 Appropriateness Criteria for the Use of Cardiac Computed Tomography to Evaluate Infective Endocarditis and Valve Tumors

	APPROPRIATENESS RATING	INDICATION	MEDIAN SCORE
Evaluation of intra- and extracardiac structures	Appropriate	Characterization of native cardiac valves Suspected clinically significant valvular dysfunction Inadequate images from other noninvasive methods	8
		Characterization of prosthetic cardiac valves Suspected clinically significant valvular dysfunction Inadequate images from other noninvasive methods	8
		Evaluation of cardiac mass (suspected tumor or thrombus) Inadequate images from other noninvasive methods	8
		Coronary evaluation before noncoronary cardiac surgery Intermediate pretest probability of coronary artery disease	7
	Uncertain	None listed	
	Inappropriate	Initial evaluation of cardiac mass (suspected tumor or thrombus)	3

Data from Taylor AJ, Cerqueira M, Hodgson JM, et al. ACCF/SCCT/ACR/AHA/ASE/ASNC/NASCI/SCAI/SCMR 2010 appropriate use criteria for cardiac computed tomography. A report of the American College of Cardiology Foundation Appropriate Use Criteria Task Force, the Society of Cardiovascular Computed Tomography, the American College of Radiology, the American Heart Association, the American Society of Echocardiography, the American Society of Nuclear Cardiology, the North American Society for Cardiovascular Imaging, the Society for Cardiovascular Angiography and Interventions, and the Society for Cardiovascular Magnetic Resonance. *J Am Coll Cardiol.* 2010;56(22):1864-1894.

series are needed to confirm that the negative predictive value remains excellent in a broader patient population.[26] The use of CCT for detection of aortic valve disease seems more readily achievable than that for mitral valve disease, with its far higher incidence of atrial fibrillation and its incumbent CCT imaging challenges.

CCT PROTOCOL POINTS

- Helical scanning to obtain both systolic and diastolic images is needed to determine aortic valve morphology and planimetered orifice area.
- See Table 16-3.

References

1. Entrikin DW, Ntim WO, Kon ND, Carr JJ. Endocarditis with perforation of a bicuspid aortic valve as shown by cardiac-gated multidetector computed tomography. *J Cardiovasc Comput Tomogr.* 2007;1(3):177-180.
2. Entrikin DW, Carr JJ. Blood pool inversion volume-rendering technique for visualization of the aortic valve. *J Cardiovasc Comput Tomogr.* 2008;2(6):366-371.
3. Willmann JK, Weishaupt D, Lachat M, et al. Electrocardiographically gated multi-detector row CT for assessment of valvular morphology and calcification in aortic stenosis. *Radiol.* 2002;225(1):120-128.
4. Bettencourt N, Sampaio F, Carvalho M, et al. Primary diagnosis of quadricuspid aortic valve with multislice computed tomography. *J Cardiovasc Comput Tomogr.* 2008;2(3):195-196.
5. Mousavi N, Tam JW, Kirkpatrick IDC, Maycher B, Jassal DS. Multimodality imaging of a quadricuspid aortic valve. *J Am Coll Cardiol.* 2008;52:A3-A6.
6. Messika-Zeitoun D, Aubry MC, Detaint D, et al. Evaluation and clinical implications of aortic valve calcification measured by electron-beam computed tomography. *Circulation.* 2004;110(3):356-362.
7. Morgan-Hughes GJ, Owens PE, Roobottom CA, Marshall AJ. Three dimensional volume quantification of aortic valve calcification using multislice computed tomography. *Heart.* 2003;89(10):1191-1194.
8. Cowell SJ, Newby DE, Burton J, et al. Aortic valve calcification on computed tomography predicts the severity of aortic stenosis. *Clin. Radiol.* 2003;58(9):712-716.
9. Feuchtner GM, Dichtl W, Friedrich GJ, et al. Multislice computed tomography for detection of patients with aortic valve stenosis and quantification of severity. *J Am Coll Cardiol.* 2006;47(7):1410-1417.
10. Pouleur AC, le Polain de Waroux JB, Pasquet A, Vanoverschelde JL, Gerber BL. Aortic valve area assessment: multidetector CT compared with cine MR imaging and transthoracic and transesophageal echocardiography. *Radiology.* 2007;244(3):745-754.
11. Shah RG, Novaro GM, Blandon RJ, Whiteman MS, Asher CR, Kirsch J. Aortic valve area: meta-analysis of diagnostic performance of multi-detector computed tomography for aortic valve area measurements as compared to transthoracic echocardiography. *Int J Cardiovasc Imaging.* 2009;25(6):601-609.
12. Doddamani S, Grushko MJ, Makaryus AN, et al. Demonstration of left ventricular outflow tract eccentricity by 64-slice multi-detector CT. *Int J Cardiovasc Imaging.* 2009;25(2):175-181.
13. Stolzmann P, Scheffel H, Bettex D, et al. Subvalvular aortic stenosis: comprehensive cardiac evaluation with dual-source computed tomography. *J Thorac Cardiovasc Surg.* 2007:240-241.
14. Pflederer T, Achenbach S. Aortic valve stenosis: CT contributions to diagnosis and therapy. *J Cardiovasc Comput Tomogr.* 2010;4(6):355-364.
15. Jassal DS, Shapiro MD, Neilan TG, et al. 64-slice multidetector computed tomography (MDCT) for detection of aortic regurgitation and quantification of severity. *Invest Radiol.* 2007;42(7):507-512.
16. Feuchtner GM, Dichtl W, Schachner T, et al. Diagnostic performance of MDCT for detecting aortic valve regurgitation. *AJR Am J Roentgenol.* 2006;186(6):1676-1681.
17. Feuchtner GM, Dichtl W, Muller S, et al. 64-MDCT for diagnosis of aortic regurgitation in patients referred to CT coronary angiography. *AJR Am J Roentgenol.* 2008;191(1):W1-7.

18. Alkadhi H, Desbiolles L, Husmann L, et al. Aortic regurgitation: assessment with 64-section CT. *Radiology*. 2007;245(1):111-121.
19. Durst R, Avelar E, Sollis J, King ME, Abbara S. Cleft mitral valve appearance on cardiac computed tomography. *J Cardiovasc Comput Tomogr*. 2008;2(5):341-342.
20. Messika-Zeitoun D, Serfaty JM, Laissy JP, et al. Assessment of the mitral valve area in patients with mitral stenosis by multislice computed tomography. *J Am Coll Cardiol*. 2006;48(2):411-413.
21. Salisbury AC, Shapiro BP, Martinez MW. Extensive myocardial and mitral annular calcification leading to mitral regurgitation and restrictive cardiomyopathy: an unusual case of caseous calcification of the mitral annulus. *J Cardiovasc Comput Tomogr*. 2009; 3(5):351-353.
22. Groves AM, Win T, Charman SC, Wisbey C, Pepke-Zaba J, Coulden RA. Semi-quantitative assessment of tricuspid regurgitation on contrast-enhanced multidetector CT. *Clin Radiol*. 2004;59(8): 715-719.
23. Dusaj RS, Michelis KC, Terek M, et al. Estimation of right atrial and ventricular hemodynamics by CT coronary angiography. *J Cardiovasc Comput Tomogr*. 2011;5(1):44-49.
24. Reant P, Brunot S, Lafitte S, et al. Predictive value of noninvasive coronary angiography with multidetector computed tomography to detect significant coronary stenosis before valve surgery. *Am J Cardiol*. 2006;97(10):1506-1510.
25. Manghat NE, Morgan-Hughes GJ, Broadley AJ, et al. 16-detector row computed tomographic coronary angiography in patients undergoing evaluation for aortic valve replacement: comparison with catheter angiography. *Clin Radiol*. 2006;61(9):749-757.
26. Gilard M, Cornily JC, Pennec PY, et al. Accuracy of multislice computed tomography in the preoperative assessment of coronary disease in patients with aortic valve stenosis. *J Am Coll Cardiol*. 2006;47(10):2020-2024.
27. Meijboom WB, Mollet NR, van Mieghem CA, et al. Pre-operative computed tomography coronary angiography to detect significant coronary artery disease in patients referred for cardiac valve surgery. *J Am Coll Cardiol*. 2006;48(8):1658-1665.

17 Assessment of Prosthetic Heart Valves

Key Points

- Cardiac CT is able to image both biologic and mechanical cardiac valve prostheses.
- Helical CCT scanning enables recognition of normal or impaired occluder motion.
- Thrombus or pannus on mechanical valves can be depicted by CCT scanning.
- Atrial fibrillation is more common in patients with mitral prostheses, making CCT scanning less useful in such cases.
- Hemodynamic limits of patients with prosthetic valve dysfunction will preclude many from undergoing CCT scanning.

Currently, only preliminary data are available on the evaluation of prosthetic cardiac valves by CCT, although contemporary CCT, if cardiac gated, can yield excellent images of many prosthetic valves. Prosthetic valve disease, though, is prone to many of the factors that pose significant technical limitations or usual exclusions to cardiac CT, such as a high incidence of atrial fibrillation associated with prostheses in the mitral valve position, in particular.

Retrospectively gated helical imaging is the best means to assess prosthetic, especially mechanical, valves, and contrast enhancement improves image quality and diagnostic confidence.[1]

PROSTHETIC VALVES

Transthoracic echocardiography (TTE) and especially transesophageal echocardiography (TEE) have been the mainstays of bioprosthetic and mechanical prosthetic valve assessment, by virtue of the combination of two-dimensional imaging and spectral and color Doppler modalities. However the limitations of echocardiography are real, and these limitations are regularly encountered in busy laboratories and hospitals:

- Inability to resolve transvalvular versus paravalvular insufficiency
- Inability to image thrombus or pannus within the valve ring of a mechanical aortic valve prosthesis
- Inability to distinguish thrombus from pannus
- Inability to image an abscess on the far side of an aortic valve replacement (AVR) ring because shadowing or reverberation from the ring is projected onto the far root
- Inability to image an AVR well because of a mechanical mitral valve replacement (MVR) projecting reverberation artifact and shadowing onto the AVR
- Inability to adequately image the occluders of an AVR to determine their excursion
- Inability to distinguish postoperative inflammatory changes and hematomas from early infection-related changes
- Inability to assess the pulmonic valve by TEE due to near-field shadowing and reverberations from an AVR

Among a series of 170 patients with 208 mechanical prostheses who underwent surgery, echocardiographic diagnostic errors were encountered in 7% of MVRs and 15% of AVRs. The most common mistakes were the following[2]:

- Lack of surgical confirmation of paravalvular insufficiency: 36% of errors
- Failure to identify pannnus overgrowth: 4% of errors
- Failure to identify thrombus/pannus overgrowth: 4% of errors
- Failure to identify vegetations: 4% of errors
- Failure to identify ball variance: 4% of errors
- Erroneous diagnoses: 28% of errors
- AVR misclassification of aortic insufficiency (AI) as transvalvular: 28% of errors
- AVR misclassification of AI as paravalvular: 8% of errors

Although the primary means of assessing valve prostheses remains echocardiographic, there appears to be a complementary role for CCT, because most prosthetic valves are well imaged by CCT,[3] which is not necessarily the case with TTE and TEE. Some very old models of mechanical prostheses contain a large amount of ferrous metal

TABLE 17-1 The Opening, Closing, and Range of Occluder Motion for Different Tilting Disc Models of Mechanical Valve Replacements

MODEL	OPENING ANGLE (°)	CLOSING ANGLE (°)	EXCURSION (°)
Bileaflet Hemidisc Occluder			
Carbomedics (Sorin Group, Milan, Italy)	78	35	43
St. Jude Medical (St. Paul, MN)	85	35	50
Single Tilting Disc Occluder			
Bjork-Shiley (Irvine, CA)	60	0	60
Medtronic-Hall (Minneapolis, MN)	60	0	60
Omniscience (Medical CV, Ivea Grove Heights, MN)	60	0	60

that generates prohibitive artifact. Most contemporary bileaflet occluder "mechanical" valves are so well seen that it is necessary to have a high degree of familiarity with the structure and motion of different models to understand the imaging findings.

Assessing the opening angle of the occluder elements of a mechanical prosthesis is one of the traditional means of establishing the normality of mechanical prosthesis function, or, alternatively, obstruction by thrombus, pannus, or both; vegetations; tissue; or primary mechanical failure.[4-6] Fluoroscopy or cineradiology can measure the opening angle accurately (difference between real and measured opening angles: -0.7 ± 1.8 degrees) and with high reproducibility (to within -0.1 ± 0.8 degrees).[5] Pressure gradient recording or Doppler calculations of gradients by TTE or TEE[7] are complementary to two-dimensional imaging findings by CT.

The opening and closing angles of mechanical prosthesis occluder motion can be accurately assessed or measured using CCT.[3]

Obstructing pannus or thrombus also can be identified using CCT.[3,7,8]

The opening, closing, and range of occluder motion vary for different tilting disc models of mechanical valve replacements (Table 17-1).

Current bileaflet occluder mechanical valves (e.g., those manufactured by St. Jude Medical, Inc., St. Paul, MN, or Carbomedics) generate little artifact, and the sewing ring and occluders are clearly imaged with non–contrast-enhanced imaging. Single tilting disc valves also can be well imaged.[9] The motion of the occluders can thus be assessed for obstruction due to thrombus or pannus on cine imaging. The opening angle is established with reference to the plane of the base of the sewing ring.[9] Cardiac CT is able to accurately determine the opening angle.

Identification of thrombus or pannus requires contrast enhancement of the blood pool.

Assessment of occluder motion of bileaflet mechanical valves in the aortic position is difficult by TEE because the valve ring is oriented away from the probe, and fluoroscopy is variably able to convincingly depict occluder motion; hence, CCT may provide a novel contribution.

The wire struts of bioprostheses (e.g., Edwards Lifesciences, Irvine, CA) are easily seen, and the leaflets also may be seen. The heavy metal struts (stents) of some models may generate artifacts.

Complications of valve replacement surgery such as pseudoaneurysms of the left ventricular outflow tract and ascending aorta are well depicted by CCT.[10]

For images of normal bileaflet occluder prosthetic mechanical heart valves, see Figures 17-1 through 17-4; **Video 17-1.**

For images of single tilting disc prosthetic mechanical heart valves, see Figures 17-5 and 17-6; **Videos 17-2** and **17-3.**

For images of obstructed bileaflet occluder prosthetic mechanical heart valves, see Figures 17-7 through 17-9; **Videos 17-4** through **17-7.**

For images of false aneurysms or pseudoaneurysms associated with prosthetic mechanical heart valves, see Figures 17-10 through 17-13; **Videos 17-8** through **17-16.**

For images of a rocking mechanical heart valve, see Figure 17-14.

CARDIAC CT BEFORE PERCUTANEOUS AORTIC VALVE REPLACEMENT

In the planning of transcatheter AVR, many aspects of the aortic valve and root morphology, not just the size of the annulus, must be well understood. TEE is the current choice for planning insofar as understanding cardiac details, and it affords good clinical results.[11] CT is increasingly used as well for cardiac planning, and is critical in planning and establishing the feasibility of peripheral vascular access. The scan includes a field of view from the aortic arch to the common femoral artery. As transcatheter aortic valve implantation (TAVI) is growing in popularity,

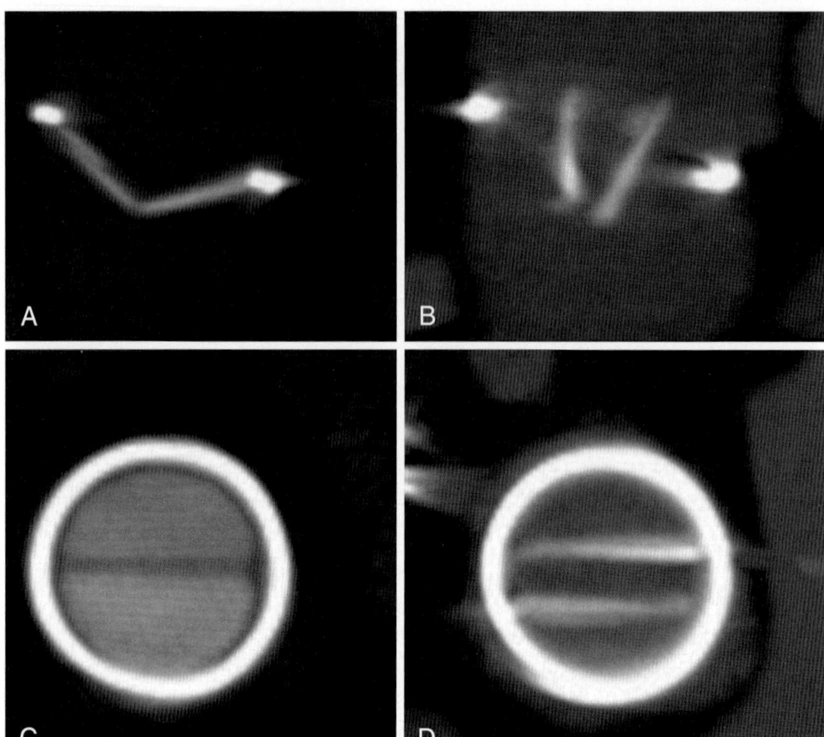

Figure 17-1. Aortic valve replacement (Carbomedics) in the closed (**A** and **C**) and open (**B** and **D**) positions. Normally, as in this example, the closed position of each occluder is 35 degrees, and the open is 78 degrees. The sewing ring is clearly seen, as are the two occluders.

so is understanding of the optimal use of TEE and CCT in planning of the procedure.

Detailed understanding of the patient's anatomy is essential to predict the final size of the prosthetic valve, the displacement of the native calcified leaflets, and the sealing around the prosthesis.[12-17] Undersizing of the prosthesis is a risk factor for paraprosthetic AI[18] and for dislodgement.

❐ Determination of aortic annular size:
- By TEE:
  - The long-axis three-chamber plane (120–140 degrees) is used to determine annulus diameter. TEE was the initial standard for planning, and affords good clinical results.[11]
- By CCT:
  - The long-axis three-chamber plane is used to make annular dimension measurements.
  - Contrast-enhanced measurements of the aortic valve annulus appear to be accurate and superior to non–contrast-enhanced images.[1,19]
  - Measurements of aortic annulus diameter using TTE, TEE, and CCT are close but not identical. CCT dimensions are very close to those of TEE but are significantly greater. Measurement differences have significant potential implications for the procedure.[11]
  - Double-oblique image reformation will depict the annulus in true cross-section, and reveal that there tends to be a major and a minor dimension of the left ventricular outflow tract rather than a single diameter.
- The optimal means by which to size a prosthesis is evolving. An important anatomic detail is that the aortic root is not actually round. The minor dimension is relatively anteroposterior, and is therefore the one depicted in a TEE outflow/three-chamber view. The major dimension typically is orthogonal to it. Therefore, it appears that TEE single-dimension measurements may lead to undersizing of the prosthesis and consequent risk of paraprosthesis aortic insufficiency. Analysis of receiver-operating characteristic models demonstrates that CT-derived cross-sectional parameters (maximal cross-sectional diameter minus prosthesis size (AUC 0.82 [0.69–0.94; $P < .001$]) and circumference-derived cross-sectional diameter minus prosthesis size (AUC 0.81 [0.70–0.94; $P < .001$]) have discriminating value for predicting post-TAVI paraprosthesis AI, whereas the traditional TEE-derived diameter measure is nondiscriminatory. Furthermore, prospective application of CT sizing appears to result in less paraprosthetic (greater than mild severity) AI (7.5% vs. 22%; $P = .045$).[20]
- Moderate or severe paraprosthetic AI is associated with annular undersizing.[18] Difference in TAVI prosthesis size and CCT annular size is predictive of paraprosthetic AI:
  - Diameter: area under the curve (AUC): 0.81 (0.68–0.88)

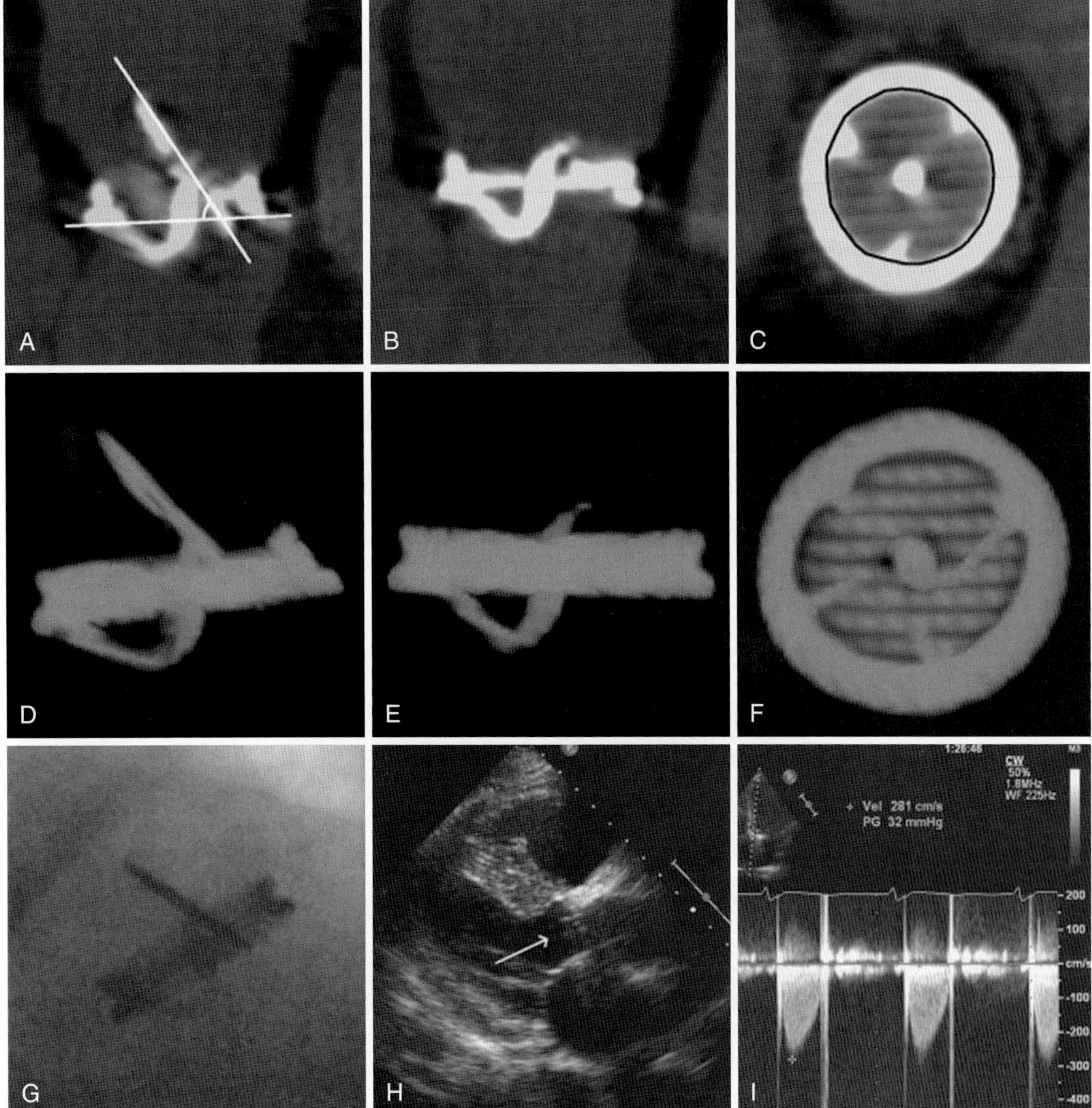

Figure 17-2. A single-disc aortic valve replacement with elevated gradient. The valve opens normally, with lines showing the baseline of the valve annulus and the open disc; the opening angle is measured with these two lines (**A**). The valve closes normally to the plane of the annulus on CT (**B**). The valve geometric orifice area was measured from the short axis view of the valve, as marked by the *black circle* (**C**). Thick maximum intensity projection images are useful for qualitative assessment of disc motion and confirmation of appropriate orientation for measurement of disc excursion. Representative images are shown during systole (**D**) and diastole (**E**); the valve can be viewed from multiple orientations (**F**). Disc opening (**G**) and closure is confirmed with cinefluoroscopy. On echocardiography, the valve cannot be well visualized (*arrow*) and assessment of disc function is not possible (**H**); with Doppler scanning, an elevated gradient is observed (**I**). On the basis of the normal disc excursion on CT and the elevated gradient and low effective orifice area index on echocardiography, this patient meets criteria for patient–prosthesis mismatch. In addition, after correction for pressure recovery, the effective orifice area of 1.3 cm^2 increases to 1.6 cm^2, suggesting pressure recovery may also be contributing to the gradient. (Reprinted with permission from LaBounty TM, Agarwal PP, Chughtai A, et al. Hemodynamic and functional assessment of mechanical aortic valves using combined echocardiography and multidetector computed tomography. *J Cardiovasc Comput Tomogr.* 2009;3(3):161-167.)

  - Area: AUC: 0.80, 95% CI: 0.65-0.90
  - Circumference: AUC: 0.76 (0.59-0.91)
- Eccentricity of the annulus does not appear to be associated with increased paraprosthetic AI using CCT assessment of annular size. With respect to mean diameter and to area, one third (35%) of cases may be undersized compared with CCT-derived mean diameter and area.[18]

❒ Three-dimensional morphology of the aortic root:
- If the sinuses have three-sinus morphology, all three diameters are measured, and if the architecture is symmetric, the largest is reported.[21]
- If the sinuses have asymmetric architecture, e.g., bicuspid, both the minor and major dimensions are measured and reported.[21]

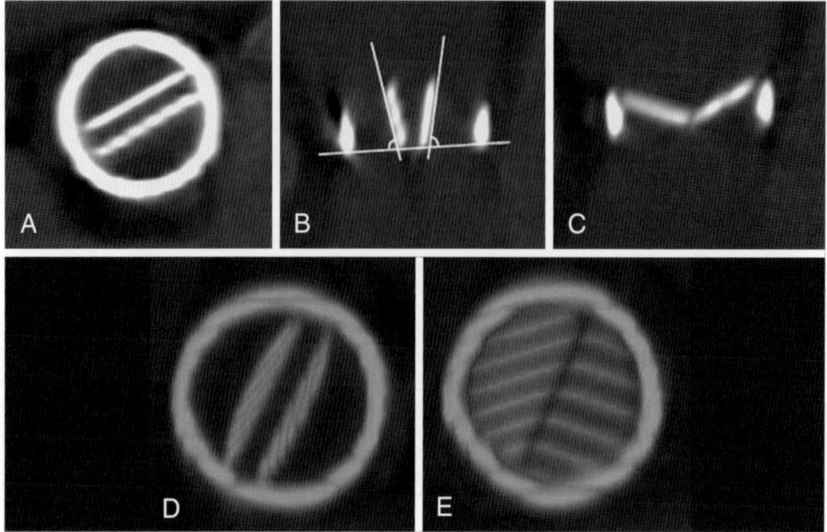

Figure 17-3. Example of a bileaflet aortic valve replacement with elevated gradient. The short axis of the valve (**A**) is used to measure the geometric orifice area. The valve discs open normally on CT (**B**); the opening angles are measured with the lines with the valve annulus as a baseline. The valve discs close normally on CT (**C**). Thick maximum intensity projection images permit qualitative confirmation of disc opening (**D**) and closing (**E**). On the basis of the normal valve function on CT and elevated gradient and low effective orifice area index on echocardiography, this patient meets the criteria for patient–prosthesis mismatch. (Reprinted with permission from LaBounty TM, Agarwal PP, Chughtai A, et al. Hemodynamic and functional assessment of mechanical aortic valves using combined echocardiography and multidetector computed tomography. *J Cardiovasc Comput Tomogr.* 2009;3(3):161-167.)

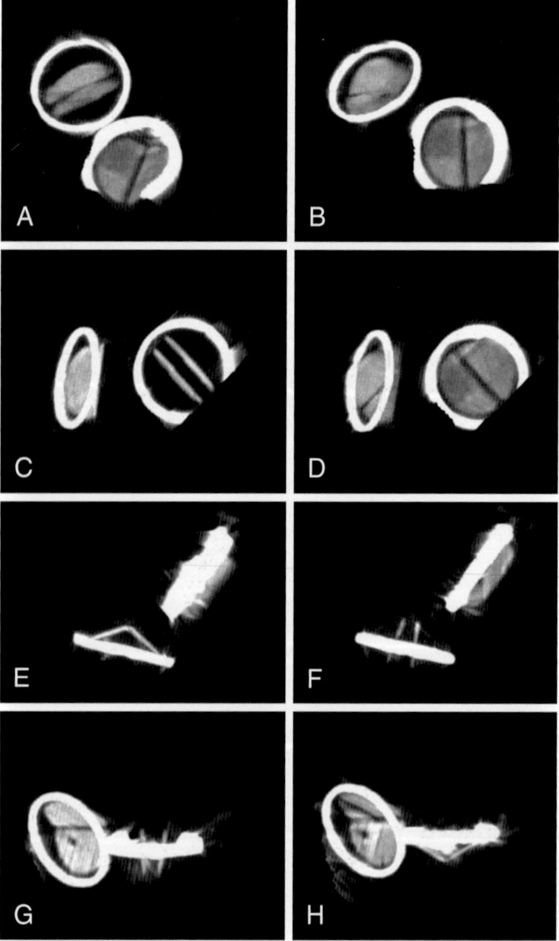

Figure 17-4. Multiple reconstructed images from a cardiac CT data set have been obtained demonstrating prosthetic aortic and mitral valve replacements with St. Jude valves (St. Jude Medical, St. Paul, MN). These images demonstrate normal movement of the prostheses at various angles. Extreme thresholding has been used to eliminate all soft tissues and cardiac chambers. **See Video 17-1.**

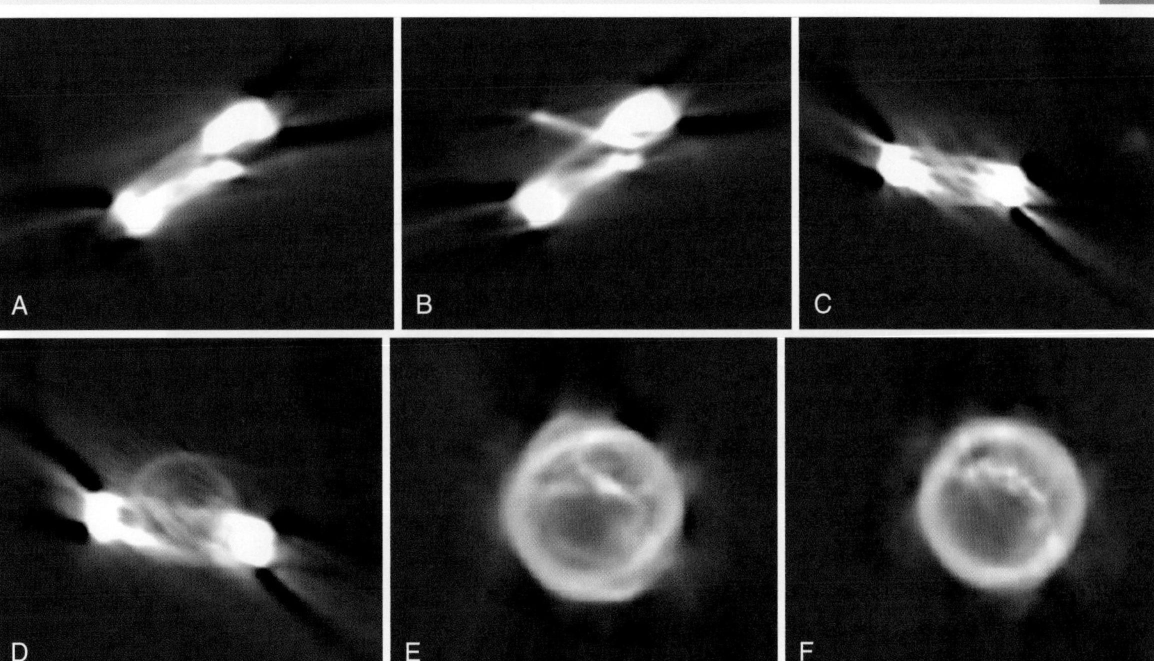

Figure 17-5. Multiple cardiac CT images through a Bjork-Shiley prosthetic aortic valve demonstrate a stuck aortic valve leaflet. Note: Window width level has been optimized to view the metallic components of the prosthetic aortic valve. See Figure 17-6 and **Videos 17-2 and 17-3.**

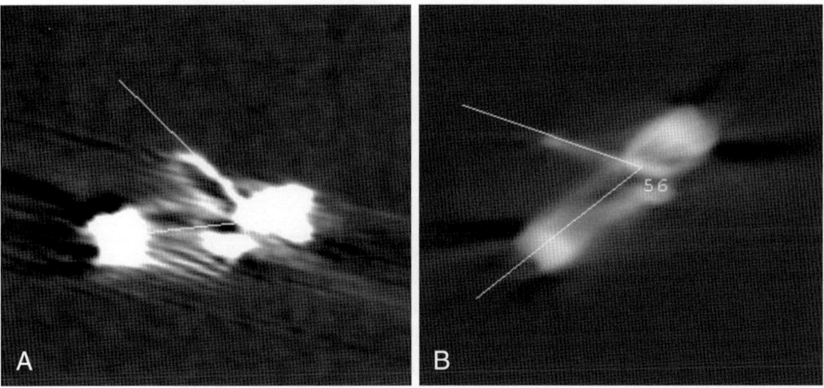

Figure 17-6. Because of the high-resolution data set acquired on the CT study, and the four-dimensional volumetric data set, double oblique reformations allow accurate evaluation of prosthetic valve function and accurate measurement of opening angles of the valve leaflets. See Figure 17-7 and **Videos 17-2 and 17-3.**

- Elliptical imaging-defined annulus (inferior virtual basal ring):
  - For implantation of Edwards Sapien valves (Edwards Lifesciences, Irvine, CA), aortic annuli must be 18 to 25 mm in diameter.[22]
  - For implantation of the CoreValve device, (Medtronic, Minneapolis, MN) aortic annuli must be between 20 and 27 mm in diameter.[22]
  - Larger aortic annular sizes constitute a contraindication to TAVI.[22]
- The origins of the coronary arteries from the sinuses of Valsalva
- The vertical height distance between the annulus and the coronary ostia in relation to the length of the valve leaflets
- The aortic valve leaflets
- The sinotubular junction geometry and dimension
- Peripheral vascular access anatomy. Severe tortuosity and stenoses, as well as small diameters (<6–9 mm, device-dependent) must be excluded if transfemoral access is to be employed.[21]

Post-procedure, procedural imperfections such as the extent and distribution of undersizing and incomplete apposition of CoreValve are well demonstrated by contrast-enhanced cardiac CT[19] as are complications such as left ventricular outflow tract pseudoaneurysms.[23]

The impact of the newest scanners on procedure planning has yet to be determined.

Text continued on page 264

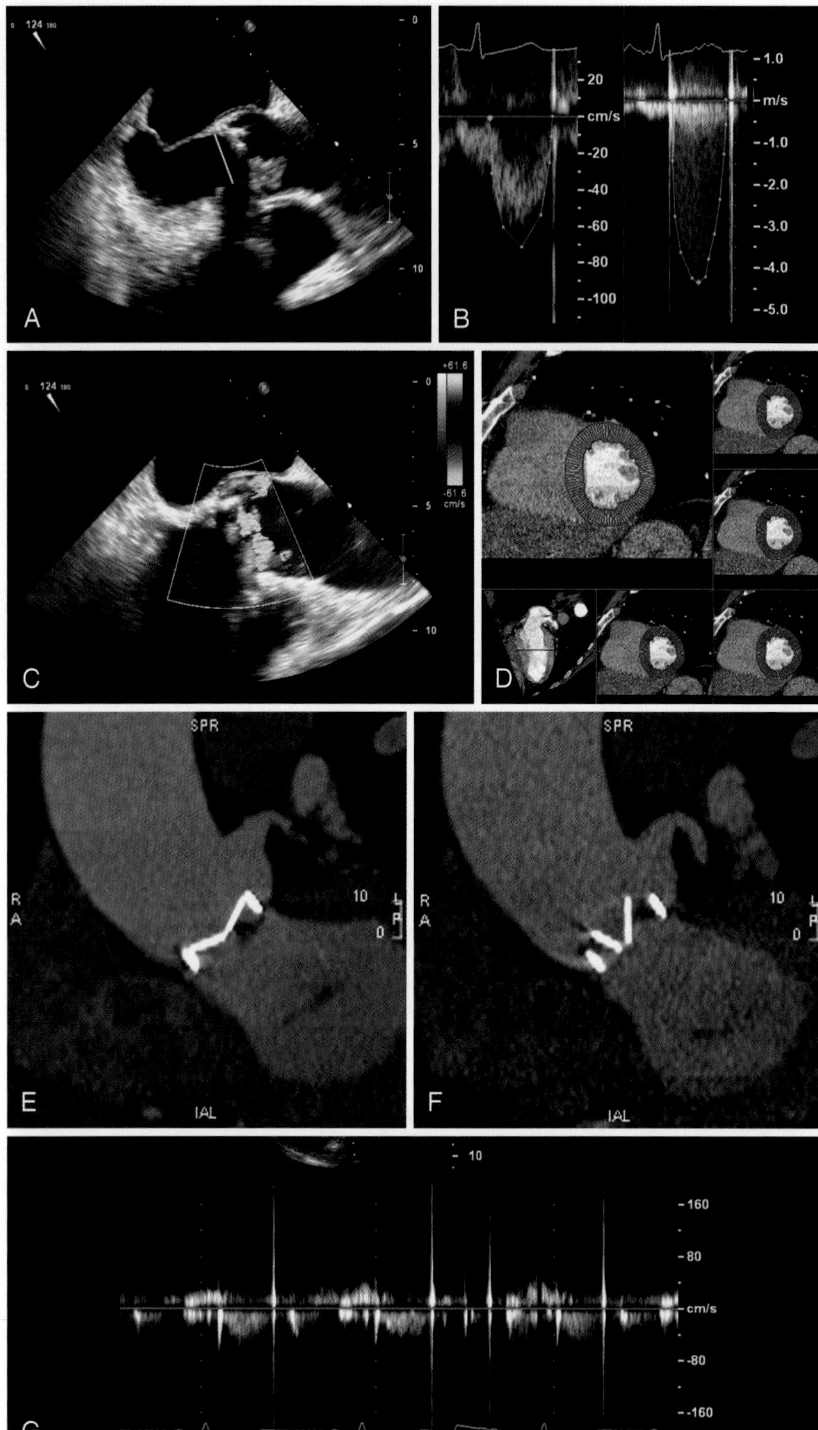

Figure 17-7. A 47-year-old man with prior mechanical aortic valve replacement (AVR) who had not been taking his warfarin for 5 years. Echocardiographic and CT images depicting obstruction of the bileaflet mechanical AVR. **A,** Transesophageal echocardiography (TEE) of the left ventricular outflow tract (LVOT) view yields the LVOT diameter (2.1 cm), and demonstrates a large (2 cm) thrombus on the AVR. **B,** Spectral profiles of the LVOT (V1) and transvalvular (V2) flow, which yield an effective orifice area of 0.6 cm^2 (0.785 × 2.1^2 × 0.74 /4.45 = 0.6 cm^2). **C,** Color Doppler flow mapping reveals highly eccentric flow across the AVR, consistent with obstruction of the hemidisc occluders. **D,** Cardiac CT images reveal concentric left ventricular hypertrophy consistent with aortic valve obstruction. Diastole (**E**), systole (**F**): The occluders close to normal angles, but open less than normal. **G,** Spectral recording of flow across the AVR yielding diminished or absent opening clicks, but present closing clicks, consistent with obstruction. See Figure 17-8 and **Video 17-4.**

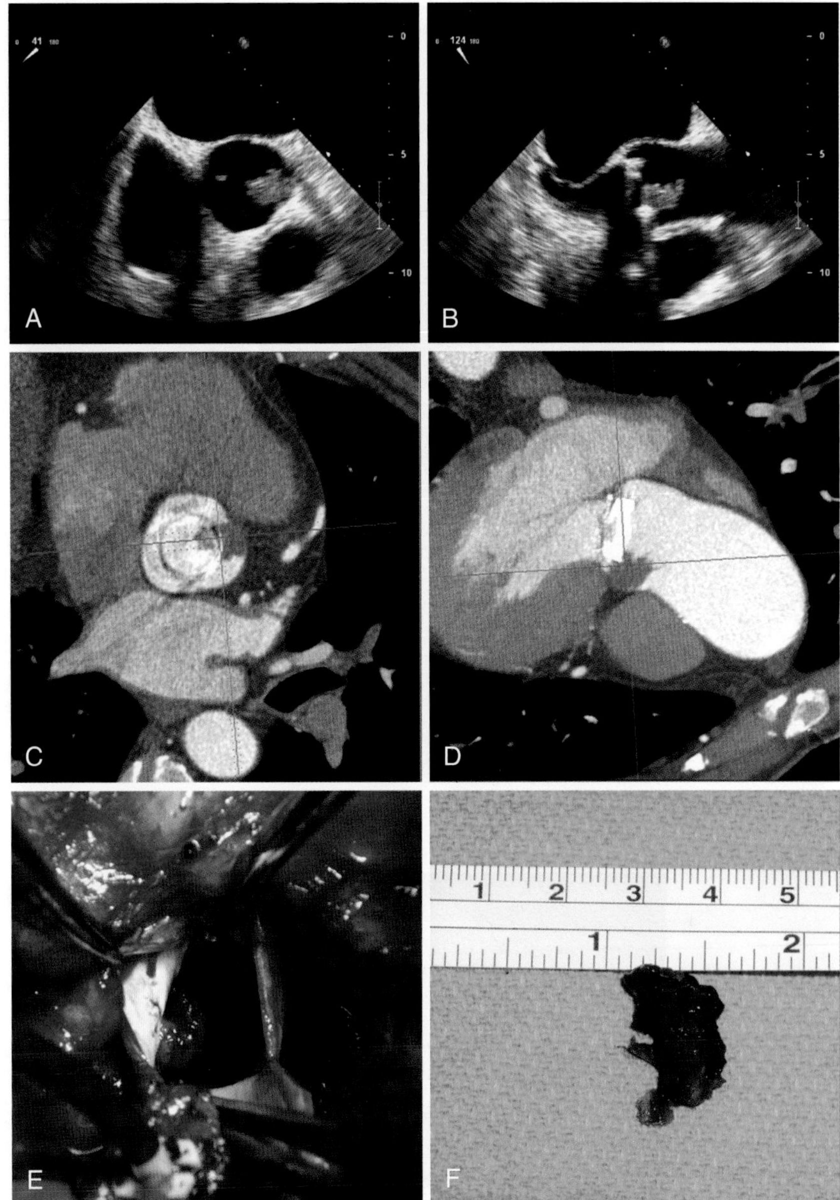

Figure 17-8. Same patient as Figure 17-7. **A** and **B,** Transesophageal echocardiographic views of a large thrombus on the ring of a bileaflet mechanical AVR. The thrombus is approximately 2 cm in size and sits into the valve orifice as well. **C** and **D**, Contrast-enhanced cardiac CT images of the thrombus. **E** and **F,** Surgical images of the same thrombus. **See Videos 17-5, 17-6, and 17-7.**

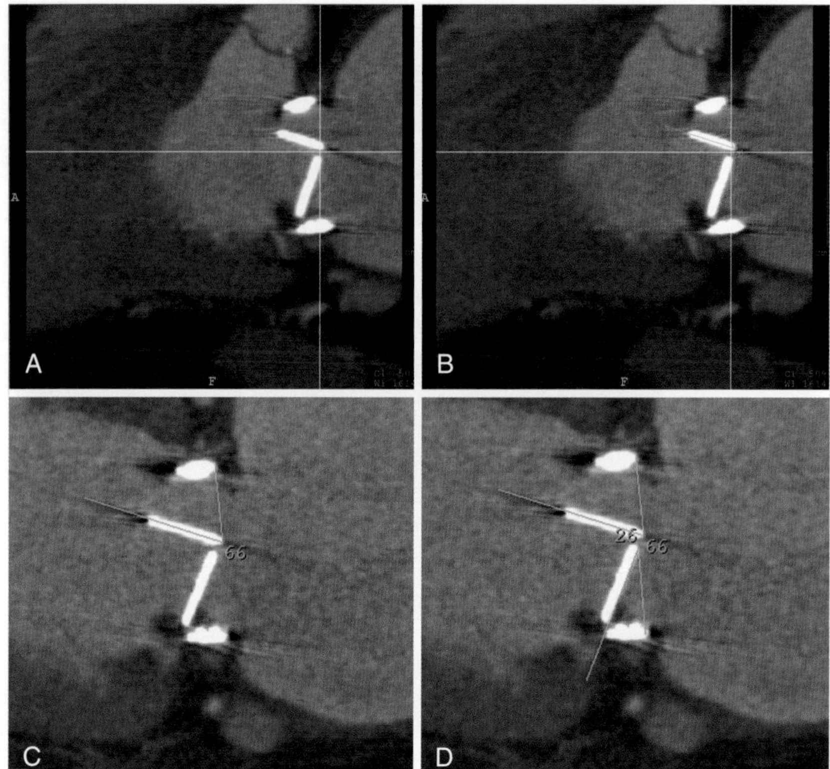

Figure 17-9. Multiple reconstructed images through the four-dimensional cardiac CT data set demonstrate angular evaluation of prosthetic valve motion. There is limited motion of the inferior leaflet, with an associated soft tissue pannus.

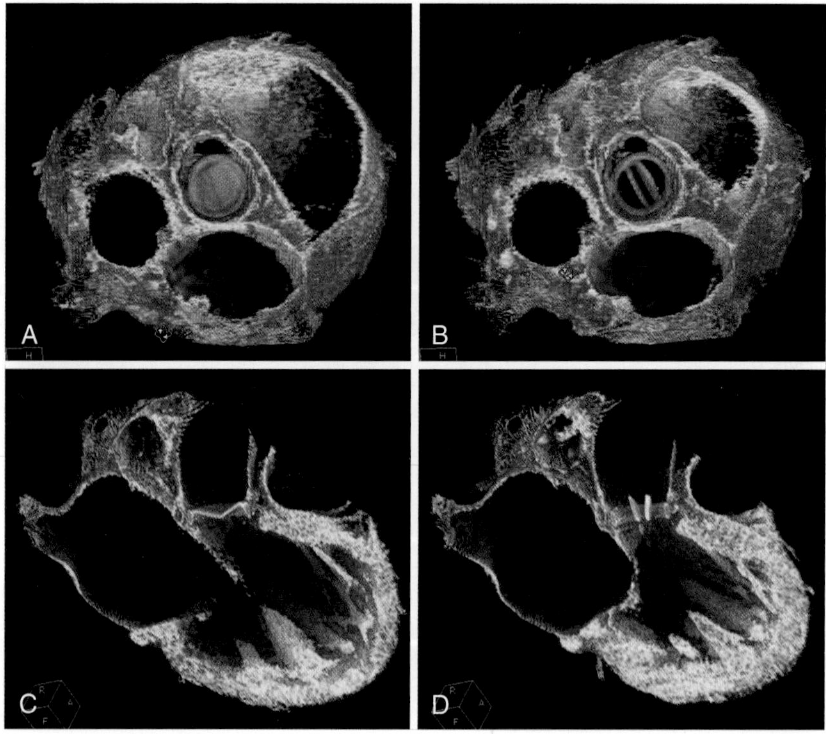

Figure 17-10. Composite image with volume-rendered data set of an aortic St. Jude's mitral valve (St. Jude's Medical, Inc., St. Paul, MN). While the intrinsic prosthesis function is normal (occluder motion is symmetric), note the moderate perivalvular leak, best seen on the axial reformations. (Reprinted with permission from Konen E, Goitein O, Feinberg MS, et al. The role of ECG-gated MDCT in the evaluation of aortic and mitral mechanical valves: initial experience. *AJR Am J Roentgenol.* 2008;191(1):26-31). **See Videos 17-8 and 17-9.**

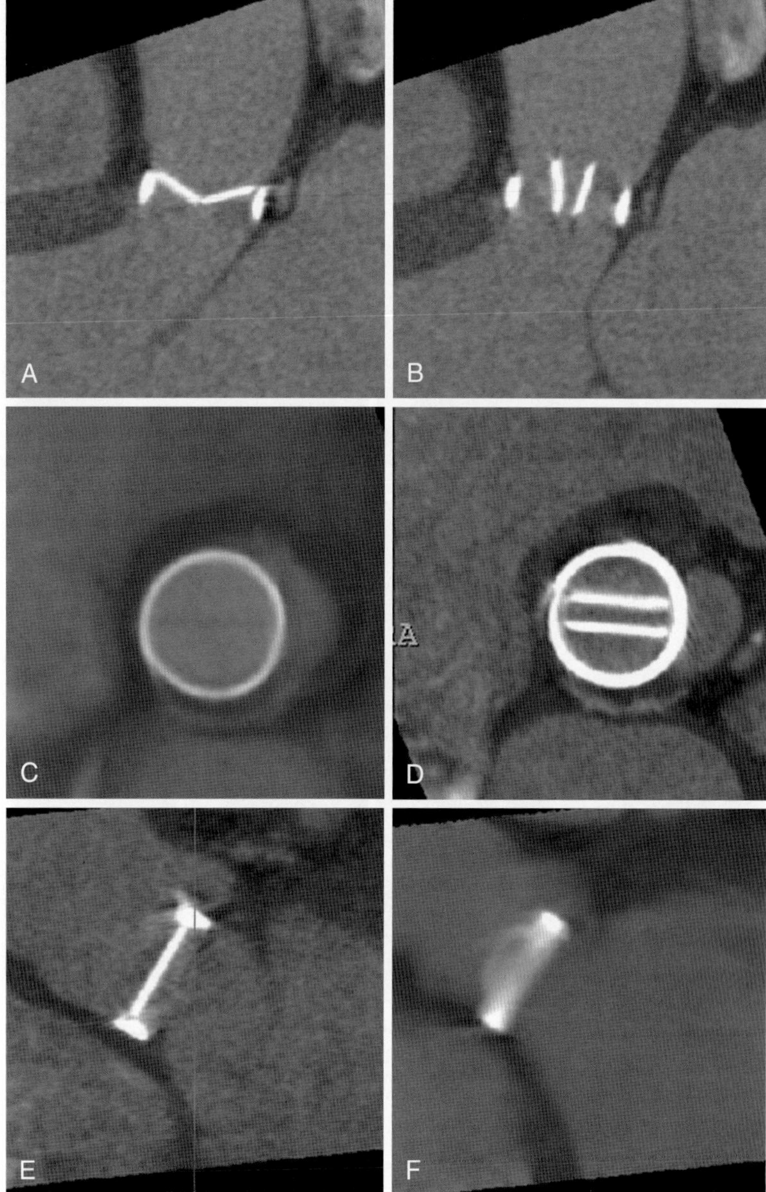

Figure 17-11. Multiple reconstructed data sets from cardiac CT study demonstrate normal valve motion of a St. Jude aortic valve (St. Jude Medical, St. Paul, MN), but with a moderate perivalvular collection/leak. (Reprinted with permission from Konen E, Goitein O, Feinberg MS, et al. The role of ECG-gated MDCT in the evaluation of aortic and mitral mechanical valves: initial experience. *AJR Am J Roentgenol.* 2008;191(1):26-31.) **See Videos 17-10 through 17-12.**

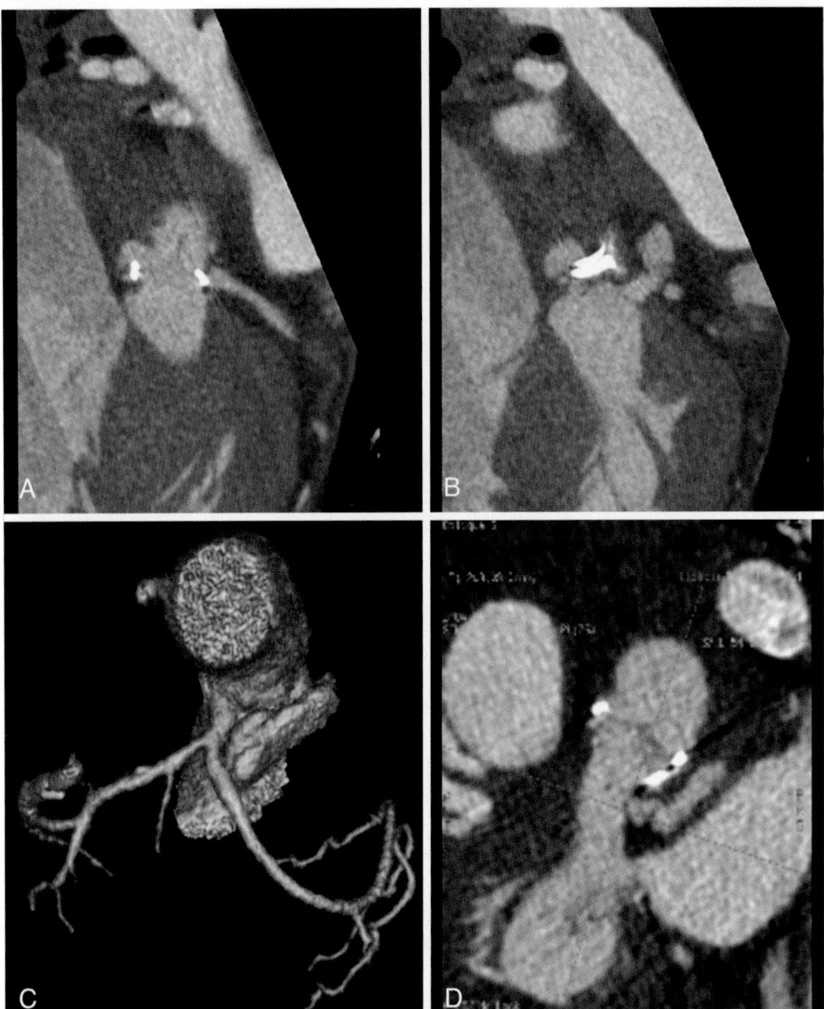

Figure 17-12. Multiplanar and 3D reformatted images of a patient 2 weeks following aortic valve bioprosthesis insertion. Arising in close proximity to the left main stem coronary artery, but not seen to be compressing it (although the acquisition is in diastole), there is a 3.5-cm tall false aneurysm with its neck arising from the inferior aspect of the sewing ring, and extending superiorly. **See Videos 17-13 and 17-14.**

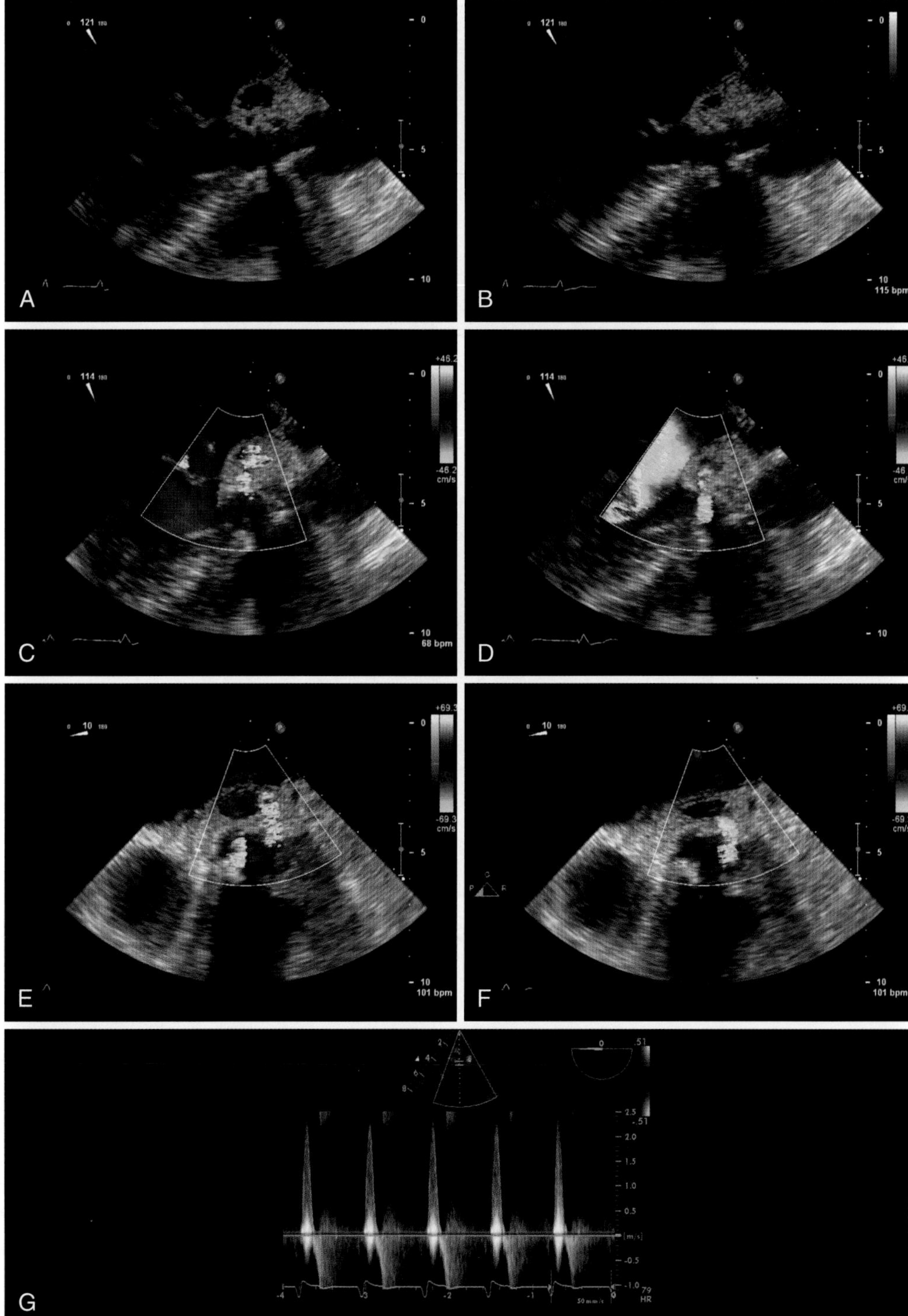

Figure 17-13. Transesophageal echocardiographic (TEE) images of the same patient as in Figure 17-14. **A**, **C**, **E**, systole; **B**, **D**, **F**, diastole. Note the systolic bulging of the false aneurysm off the posterior aortic root (**A**), the systolic flow into the false aneurysm via a neck at the inferior aspect of the sewing ring (**C**, **E**), and the diastolic decompression of the false aneurysm, with flow back out of it (**D**, **F**). The lower image is a spectral display of the reciprocating flow in the neck. **See Videos 17-15 and 17-16.**

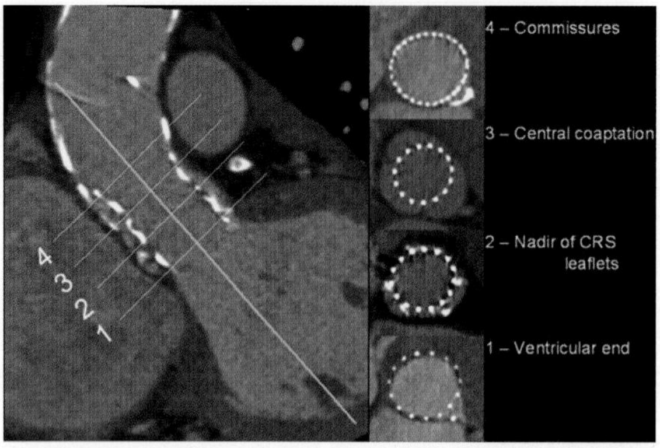

Figure 17-14. Levels of measurement of the CoreValve ReValving System (CRS) on multislice CT (MSCT). The appearance of the CRS is shown on MSCT (coronal cut plane) after implantation, with levels 1, 2, 3, and 4 where the dimensions were measured. (Reprinted with permission from Schultz CJ, Weustink A, Piazza N, et al. Geometry and degree of apposition of the CoreValve ReValving system with multislice computed tomography after implantation in patients with aortic stenosis. *J Am Coll Cardiol.* 2009;54(10):911-918)

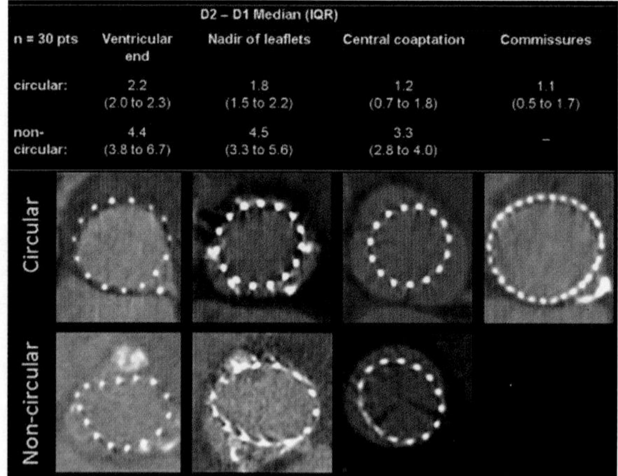

	D2 – D1 Median (IQR)			
n = 30 pts	Ventricular end	Nadir of leaflets	Central coaptation	Commissures
circular:	2.2 (2.0 to 2.3)	1.8 (1.5 to 2.2)	1.2 (0.7 to 1.8)	1.1 (0.5 to 1.7)
non-circular:	4.4 (3.8 to 6.7)	4.5 (3.3 to 5.6)	3.3 (2.8 to 4.0)	–

Figure 17-15. Axial shape and dimensions of the CRS (CoreValve ReValving System) at various levels. D1, smallest diameter; D2, largest diameter; IQR, interquartile range. (Reprinted with permission from Schultz CJ, Weustink A, Piazza N, et al. Geometry and degree of apposition of the CoreValve ReValving system with multislice computed tomography after implantation in patients with aortic stenosis. *J Am Coll Cardiol.* 2009;54(10):911-918)

For images of TAVI planning, see Figures 17-15 through 17-21.

POST–ROSS PROCEDURE

CCT is able to image some structural, but not functional, complications of the Ross procedure, such as calcification and false aneurysms (Figs. 17-22 and 17-23).

CCT PROTOCOL POINTS

- Post-processing: window optimization is important to depict soft tissue, such as thrombus or pannus, on prosthetic valves.
- Helical or retrospective scanning is needed to determine mechanical prosthetic valve occluder motion and opening and closing angles.
- See Table 17-2.

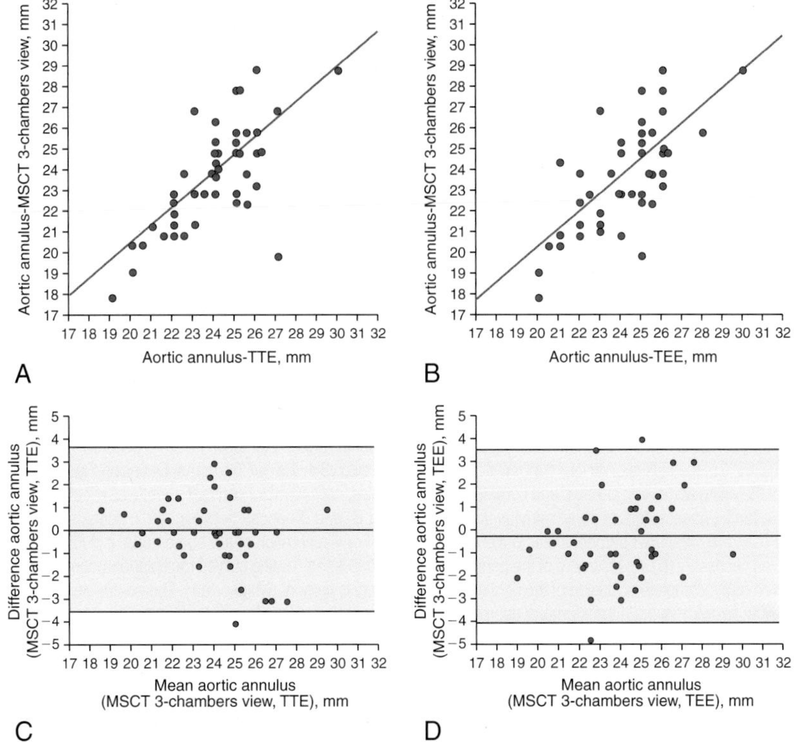

Figure 17-16. Correlations between echocardiographic and multislice CT (MSCT) measurements of the aortic annulus diameter. Correlations between the aortic annulus measured by MSCT using a three-chamber view and transthoracic echocardiography (TTE, **A**) and transesophageal echocardiography (TEE, **B**). The solid line indicates the regression line. Quality control plots using Bland-Altman analysis for the two methods, TTE (**C**) and TEE (**D**). The middle line represents the mean, the upper line represents +2 standard deviations, and the lower line represents –2 standard deviations. (Reprinted with permission from Messika-Zeitoun D, Serfaty JM, Brochet E, et al. Mutimodal assessment of the aortic annulus diameter: implications for transcatheter aortic valve implantation. *J Am Coll Cardiol.* 2010;55:186-194.)

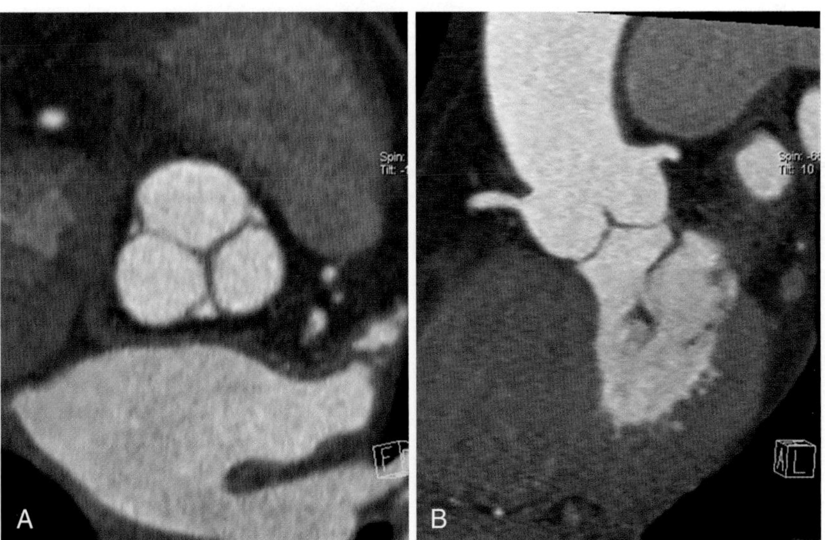

Figure 17-17. Contrast-enhanced CT provides high spatial resolution in all three dimensions and thus excellent visualization of the aortic valve (**A**) and aortic root (**B**). (Reprinted with permission from Pflederer T, Achenbach S. Aortic valve stenosis: CT contributions to diagnosis and therapy. *J Cardiovasc Comput Tomogr.* 2010;4(6):355-364.)

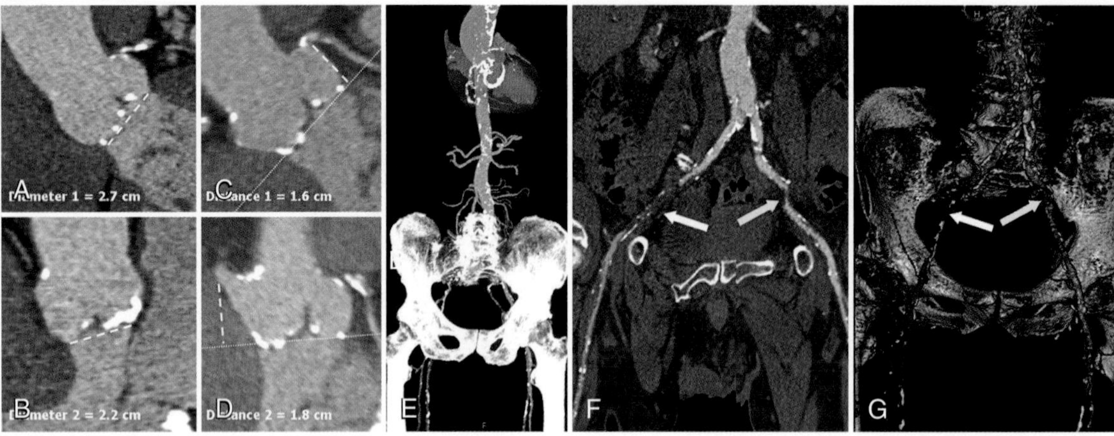

Figure 17-18. Example of a dual-source CT examination for planning a transcatheter aortic valve implantation (TAVI) procedure. High-pitch spiral data acquisition was used, prospectively triggered at 60% of the R-R interval (2 × 128 × 0.6 mm collimation, pitch 3.4, 100 kV, 320 mAs; Definition Flash, Siemens Healthcare, Forchheim, Germany). For assessment of the entire aorta, iliac arteries, and common femoral arteries, only 40 mL of contrast agent was injected (flow rate 4 mL/s). The estimated effective radiation dose was 4.3 mSv. Assessment of aortic annulus diameters (**A** and **B**) and distances between aortic annulus and coronary ostia (**C** and **D**) were made. Distances to coronary ostia are measured perpendicular to the annulus plane. For visualization of the entire aorta, including iliac and femoral arteries, a scan time of less than 2 seconds was necessary (**E**). Assessment of the peripheral arteries is illustrated using curved multiplanar reconstructions (**F**) and three-dimensional volume-rendered reconstruction (**G**). A complete occlusion of the right external iliac artery is present (*white arrow*). The contralateral side shows a high-grade stenosis of the external iliac artery (*yellow arrow*), making a transfemoral approach for TAVI impossible. Therefore, a transapical route was chosen in this patient. (Reprinted with permission from Pflederer T, Achenbach S. Aortic valve stenosis: CT contributions to diagnosis and therapy. *J Cardiovasc Comput Tomogr.* 2010;4(6):355-364.)

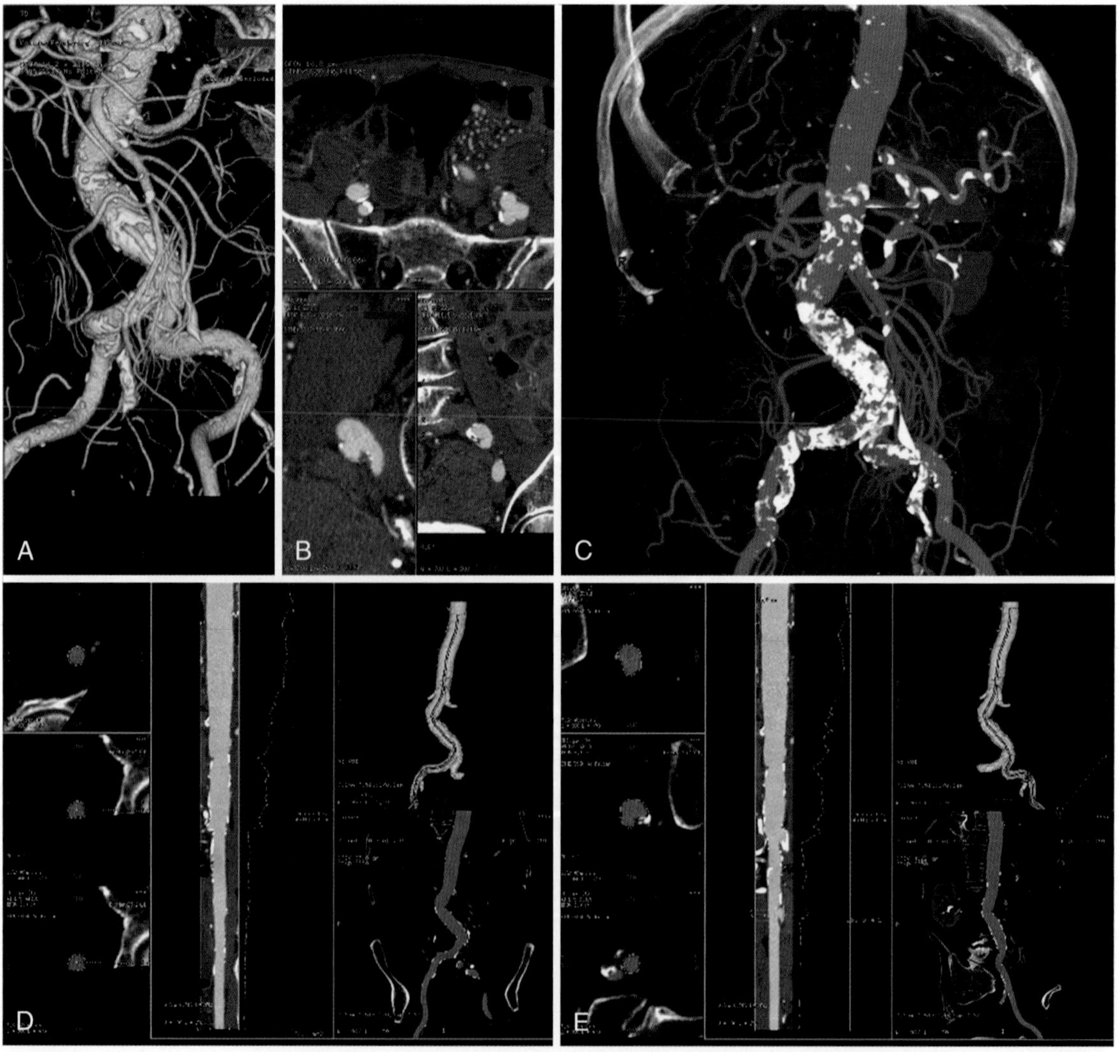

Figure 17-19. Peripheral access assessment for a prospective transcatheter aortic valve implantation case. Tortuosity and calcification of the distal aorta and iliofemoral vessels are seen. The right iliac artery is unremarkable, other than for its moderate tortuosity and calcification. The left iliac artery is notable for a small false aneurysm.

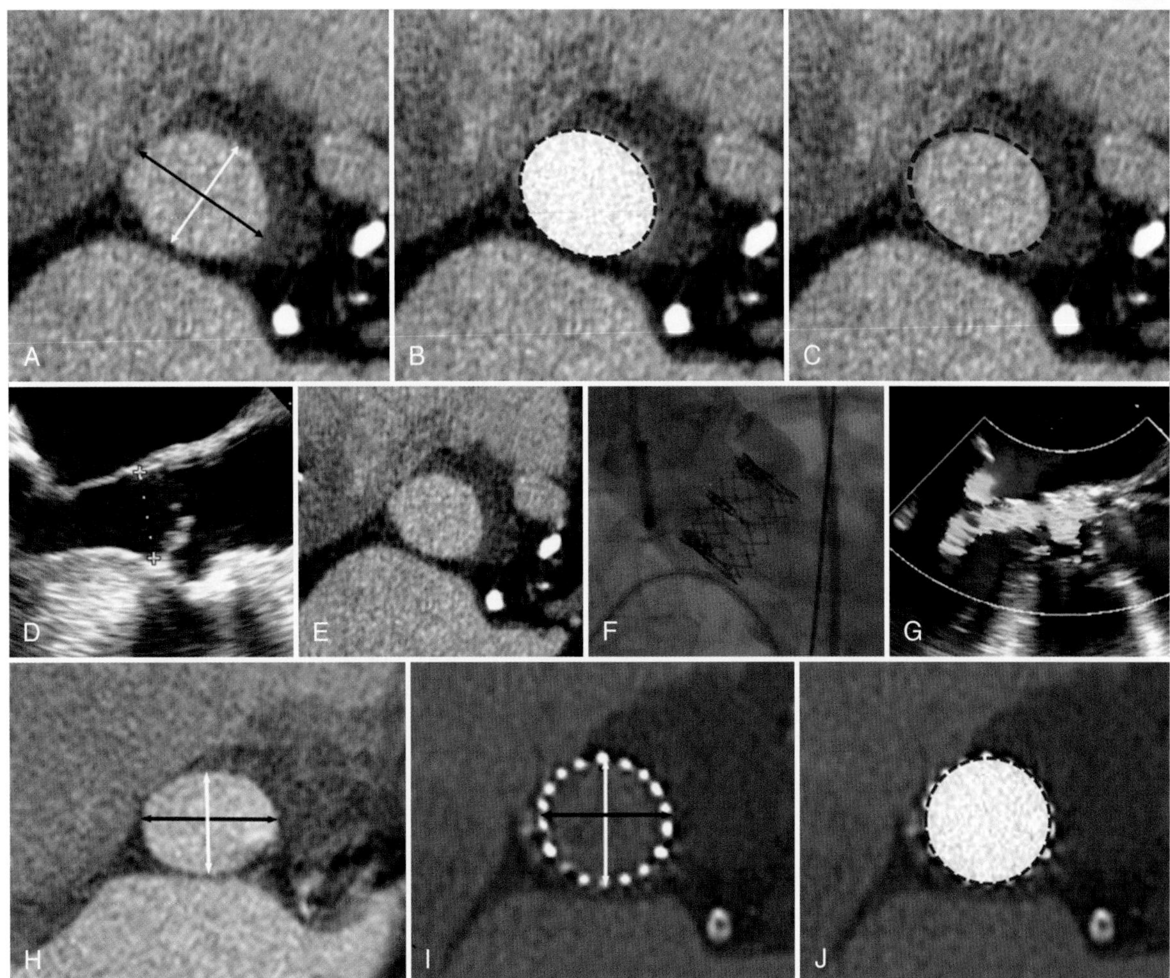

Figure 17-20. Three-dimensional multidetector CT (MDCT) aortic annular measurements. **A,** Short and long diameters provide a mean annulus diameter and annular eccentricity. **B,** Annular area. **C,** Annular circumference. Case example of transcatheter heart valve (THV) undersizing causing significant paravalvular aortic regurgitation (PAR). **D,** A 23-mm Sapien XT (Edwards Lifesciences, Irvine, CA) valve was selected based on a transesophageal (TEE) annular diameter of 22 mm. **E,** The MDCT mean annular diameter is 25 mm (22-28 mm) and the area is 4.90 cm^2. The THV is undersized by 2 mm relative to the mean diameter and by 15% relative to the annular area. **F,** The THV appears undersized on aortic root angiography. **G,** Moderate PAR on echocardiography. The effect of aortic annular eccentricity and THV oversizing on THV expansion and eccentricity as demonstrated by matched pre- and post transcatheter aortic valve replacement (TAVR) MDCT in an individual patient. **H,** At baseline, the aortic annulus is eccentric (29%) with a mean diameter of 20.5 mm (17.0 mm × 24.1 mm) and area of 3.45 cm^2. **I,** Following implantation of a 23-mm THV, MDCT shows a circular implant (23.2 mm × 23.5 mm, eccentricity 1.3%). **J,** Even though the THV is oversized relative to the annular area by 20%, the THV is fully expanded with an expansion ratio of 103.6% (THV area = 4.30 cm^2). (Reprinted with permission from Willson AB, Webb JG, Labounty TM, et al. 3-dimensional aortic annular assessment by multidetector computed tomography predicts moderate or severe paravalvular regurgitation after transcatheter aortic valve replacement: a multicenter retrospective analysis. *J Am Coll Cardiol.* 2012;59(14):1287-1294).

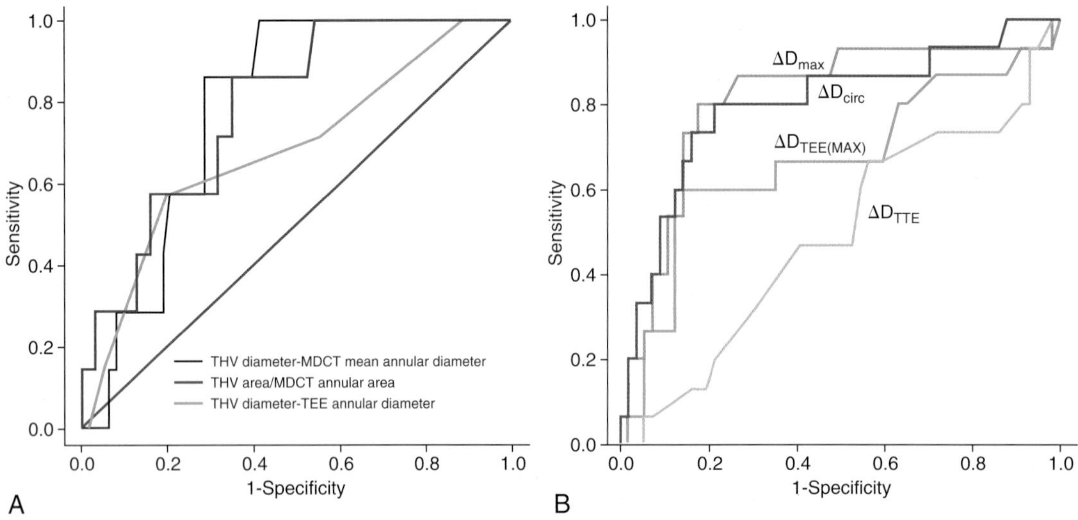

Figure 17-21. A, Area under the receiver-operating characteristic curves for prediction of paravalvular aortic regurgitation (PAR). Multidirectional CT (MDCT) mean diameter (0.81, 95% confidence interval [CI]: 0.68 to 0.88), MDCT area (0.80, 95% CI: 0.65 to 0.90), and transesophageal echocardiography (TEE) diameter (0.70, 95% CI: 0.51 to 0.88). **B,** Superimposed receiver operating characteristic curves evaluating predictive value of cross-sectional CT and standard echocardiographic measurements for post–transcatheter aortic valve replacement (TAVR) paravalvular regurgitation (>mild). The cross-sectional CT-derived parameters (D_{circ} and D_{max}) had a considerably greater discriminatory value (with larger areas under the curve) for significant paravalvular regurgitation (>mild) than two-dimensional echocardiography–derived measurements ($D_{TEE(MAX)}$ and D_{TTE}). MDCT, multidirectional CT; TEE, transesophageal echocardiography; THV, transcatheter heart valve; TTE, transthoracic echocardiography. (**A** reprinted with permission from Willson AB, Webb JG, Labounty TM, et al. 3-dimensional aortic annular assessment by multidetector computed tomography predicts moderate or severe paravalvular regurgitation after transcatheter aortic valve replacement: a multicenter retrospective analysis. *J Am Coll Cardiol.* 2012;59(14):1287-1294. **B** reprinted with permission from Jilaihawi H, Kashif M, Fontana G, et al. Cross-sectional computed tomographic assessment improves accuracy of aortic annular sizing for transcatheter aortic valve replacement and reduces the incidence of paravalvular aortic regurgitation. *J Am Coll Cardiol.* 2012;59(14):1275-1286.)

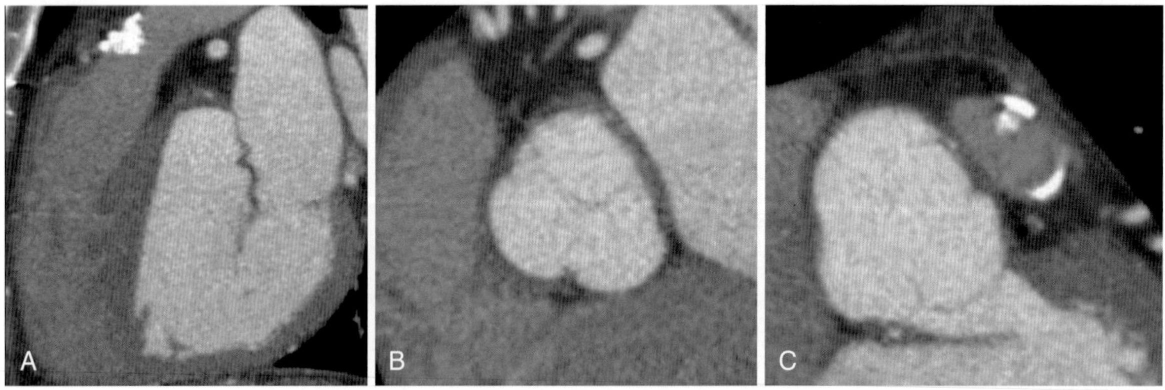

Figure 17-22. Multiple images from a cardiac CT study in a patient post–Ross procedure demonstrate a well-seated transposed pulmonic valve within the aorta. A small residual right ventricular outflow tract and main pulmonary artery segment are noted with high-attenuation material around the pulmonic valve plane. This could represent a postsurgical calcification, or postsurgical metallic suture or clip material.

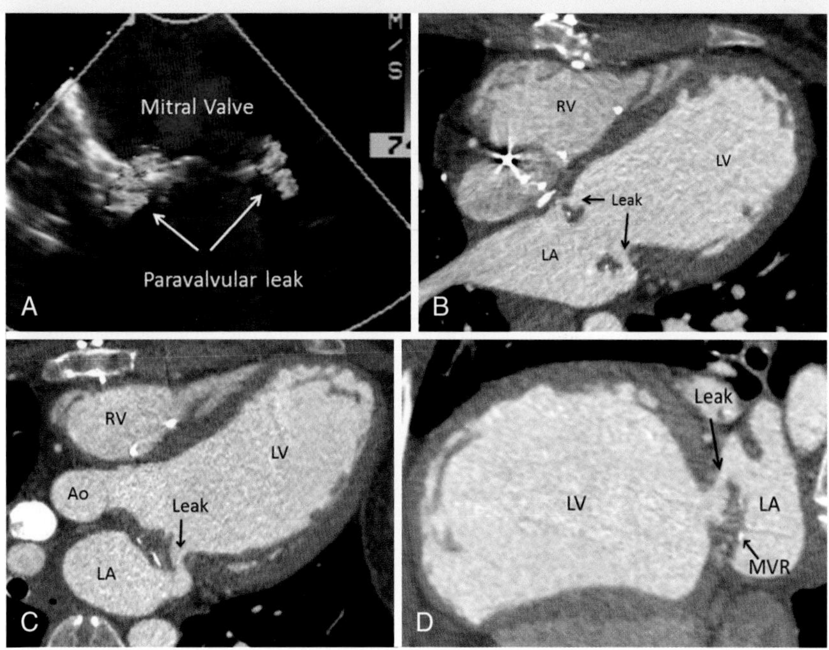

Figure 17-23. A 21-year-old woman had a complete atrioventricular canal repair and subsequent bioprosthetic mitral valve replacements (MVR) 5 and 14 years afterward. She had shortness of breath for the past 2 years while dancing, and transthoracic echocardiography showed a mitral diastolic gradient of 9 mm Hg with mild paravalvular mitral insufficiency. Left ventricular size and function were normal. **A,** Transesophageal echocardiography (TEE) showed a mild to moderate parvalvular leak. An exercise echocardiogram was performed to better understand the cause for dyspnea. At 4 minutes, her heart rate was 157, her right ventricular systolic pressure rose from a normal of 23 to more than 50, and the mean mitral gradient was greater than 30 mm Hg. Because of the uncertainty of the apparent physiology of mitral stenosis with normal-appearing leaflets, cardiac CT angiography (CTA) (4 mSv, 100 kV with function) was ordered to obtain ventricular volumes. Cardiac MRI (CMR) was not performed because a pacemaker was present. The left ventricular (LV) end-diastolic volume was enlarged (indexed for body surface area). The LV end-systolic volume index was also prominently increased, with a left ventricular ejection fraction (LVEF) of 53%. Comparing left and right ventricular volumes, the mitral regurgitant fraction was 50%. Prominent paravalvular leaks were seen (**B**) around the medial 2-mm, and lateral 4-mm, annulus (**C**). Oblique views (obtained by placing and rotating the crosshairs on the observed defects) demonstrate the irregular unobstructed path between the LV and left atrium (**D**). Large paravalvular leaks were confirmed during a repeat MVR. The patient had excellent postoperative symptom relief. Cardiac CT angiography (CTA) provides volumetric information for accurate ejection fractions and biventricular volumes. In this case, the enlarged left ventricle (corrected for the patient's size) and the difference between the left and right ventricular volumes was consistent with severe mitral regurgitation (MR). In addition, cardiac CTA allowed us to find the three paravalvular leaks (source of MR) and recognize that the TEE underestimated its severity. It is assumed that the elevated diastolic mitral gradient was created by increased diastolic flow from severe MR. Cardiac CTA was used here as a substitute in a patient with a CMR contraindication and had a unique advantage due to its superior spatial resolution and limited artifacts in the setting of a prosthetic valve. Ao, aorta. (Reprinted with permission from Lesser JR, Schwartz RS, Flygenring BJ, et al. Bioprosthetic mitral valve disease clarified by cardiac CT. *Society of Cardiovascular Tomography Case of the Month.* August 2012. http://archive.constantcontact.com/fs027/1101901294184/archive/ss1110790704413.html.)

TABLE 17-2 ACCF Appropriateness Criteria for the Use of Cardiac Computed Tomography to Evaluate Prosthetic Heart Valves

	APPROPRIATENESS RATING	INDICATION	MEDIAN SCORE
Evaluation of intracardiac and extracardiac structures	Appropriate	Characterization of prosthetic cardiac valves Suspected clinically significant valvular dysfunction Inadequate images from other noninvasive methods	8
		Evaluation of cardiac mass (suspected tumor or thrombus)	8
		Inadequate images from other noninvasive methods	8
		Coronary evaluation before noncoronary cardiac surgery Intermediate pretest probability of coronary artery disease	7
	Uncertain	None listed	
	Inappropriate	Initial evaluation of cardiac mass (suspected tumor or thrombus)	3

Data from Taylor AJ, Cerqueira M, Hodgson JM, et al. ACCF/SCCT/ACR/AHA/ASE/ASNC/NASCI/SCAI/SCMR 2010 appropriate use criteria for cardiac computed tomography. A report of the American College of Cardiology Foundation Appropriate Use Criteria Task Force, the Society of Cardiovascular Computed Tomography, the American College of Radiology, the American Heart Association, the American Society of Echocardiography, the American Society of Nuclear Cardiology, the North American Society for Cardiovascular Imaging, the Society for Cardiovascular Angiography and Interventions, and the Society for Cardiovascular Magnetic Resonance. *J Am Coll Cardiol.* 2010;56(22):1864-1894.

References

1. Willmann JK, Weishaupt D, Lachat M, et al. Electrocardiographically gated multi-detector row CT for assessment of valvular morphology and calcification in aortic stenosis. *Radiology.* 2002;225(1):120-128.
2. Faletra F, Constantin C, De Chiara F, et al. Incorrect echocardiographic diagnosis in patients with mechanical prosthetic valve dysfunction: correlation with surgical findings. *Am J Med.* 2000;108(7):531-537.
3. Konen E, Goitein O, Feinberg MS, et al. The role of ECG-gated MDCT in the evaluation of aortic and mitral mechanical valves: initial experience. *AJR Am J Roentgenol.* 2008;191(1):26-31.
4. Aoyagi S, Nishimi M, Kawano H, et al. Obstruction of St Jude Medical valves in the aortic position: significance of a combination of cineradiography and echocardiography. *J Thorac Cardiovasc Surg.* 2000;120(1):142-147.
5. Verdel G, Heethaar RM, Jambroes G, van der Werf T. Assessment of the opening angle of implanted Bjork-Shiley prosthetic valves. *Circulation.* 1983;68(2):355-359.
6. Montorsi P, Cavoretto D, Repossini A, Bartorelli AL, Guazzi MD. Valve design characteristics and cine-fluoroscopic appearance of five currently available bileaflet prosthetic heart valves. *Am J Card Imaging.* 1996;10(1):29-41.
7. Girard SE, Miller Jr FA, Orszulak TA, et al. Reoperation for prosthetic aortic valve obstruction in the era of echocardiography: trends in diagnostic testing and comparison with surgical findings. *J Am Coll Cardiol.* 2001;37(2):579-584.
8. Teshima H, Hayashida N, Fukunaga S, et al. Usefulness of a multidetector-row computed tomography scanner for detecting pannus formation. *Ann Thorac Surg.* 2004;77(2):523-526.
9. LaBounty TM, Agarwal PP, Chughtai A, Kazerooni EA, Wizauer E, Bach DS. Hemodynamic and functional assessment of mechanical aortic valves using combined echocardiography and multidetector computed tomography. *J Cardiovasc Comput Tomogr.* 2009;3(3):161-167.
10. Trivi M, Albertal J, Vaccarino G, Albertal M, Navia D. Ostial stenosis after Bentall technique using glue: percutaneous stenting may be ineffective. *Interact Cardiovasc Thorac Surg.* 2007;6(4):511-513.
11. Messika-Zeitoun D, Serfaty JM, Brochet E, et al. Mutimodal assessment of the aortic annulus diameter: implications for transcatheter aortic valve implantation. *J Am Coll Cardiol.* 2010;55(3):186-194.
12. Tuzcu EM, Kapadia SR, Schoenhagan P. Multimodality quantitative imaging of aortic root for transcatheter aortic valve implantation. *J Am Coll Cardiol.* 2010;55(3):195-197.
13. Schoenhagen P, Tuzcu EM, Kapadia SR, Desai MY, Svensson LG. Three-dimensional imaging of the aortic valve and aortic root with computed tomography: new standards in an era of transcatheter valve repair/implantation. *Eur Heart J.* 2009;30(17):2079-2086.
14. Tops LF, Van de Veire NR, Schuijf JD, et al. Noninvasive evaluation of coronary sinus anatomy and its relation to the mitral valve annulus: implications for percutaneous mitral annuloplasty. *Circulation.* 2007;115(11):1426-1432.
15. Kronzon I, Sugeng L, Perk G, et al. Real-time 3-dimensional transesophageal echocardiography in the evaluation of post-operative mitral annuloplasty ring and prosthetic valve dehiscence. *J Am Coll Cardiol.* 2009;53(17):1543-1547.
16. Akhtar M, Tuzcu EM, Kapadia SR, et al. Aortic root morphology in patients undergoing percutaneous aortic valve replacement: evidence of aortic root remodeling. *J Thorac Cardiovasc Surg.* 2009;137(4):950-956.
17. Wood DA, Tops LF, Mayo JR, et al. Role of multislice computed tomography in transcatheter aortic valve replacement. *Am J Cardiol.* 2009;103(9):1295-1301.
18. Willson AB, Webb JG, Labounty TM, et al. 3-dimensional aortic annular assessment by multidetector computed tomography predicts moderate or severe paravalvular regurgitation after transcatheter aortic valve replacement: a multicenter retrospective analysis. *J Am Coll Cardiol.* 2012;59(14):1287-1294.
19. Schultz CJ, Weustink A, Piazza N, et al. Geometry and degree of apposition of the CoreValve ReValving system with multislice computed tomography after implantation in patients with aortic stenosis. *J Am Coll Cardiol.* 2009;54(10):911-918.
20. Jilaihawi H, Kashif M, Fontana G, et al. Cross-sectional computed tomographic assessment improves accuracy of aortic annular sizing for transcatheter aortic valve replacement and reduces the incidence of paravalvular aortic regurgitation. *J Am Coll Cardiol.* 2012;59(14):1275-1286.
21. Schoenhagen P, Kapadia SR, Halliburton SS, Svensson LG, Tuzcu EM. Computed tomography evaluation for transcatheter aortic valve implantation (TAVI): imaging of the aortic root and iliac arteries. *J Cardiovasc Comput Tomogr.* 2011;5(5):293-300.
22. Pflederer T, Achenbach S. Aortic valve stenosis: CT contributions to diagnosis and therapy. *J Cardiovasc Comput Tomogr.* 2010;4(6):355-364.
23. Tsai IC, Hsieh SR, Chern MS, et al. Pseudoaneurysm in the left ventricular outflow tract after prosthetic aortic valve implantation: evaluation upon multidetector-row computed tomography. *Tex Heart Inst J.* 2009;36(5):428-432.

18 Assessment of Infective Endocarditis and Valvular Tumors

Key Points

- There have been few studies of the yield and contribution of CCT to the evaluation of infective endocarditis, but vegetations can be imaged, and several structural complications of endocarditis have been well described.
- The use of CCT to establish the absence of significant coronary artery disease in patients with complicated cases of aortic valve endocarditis who are to undergo surgery is appealing because it obviates the need for catheter-based coronary angiography.
- Fibroelastomas of the aortic valve also can be depicted by CCT.

INFECTIOUS ENDOCARDITIS

Although it is still early in the process of validating cardiac CT (CCT), this test may have a role to play in the assessment of aortic valve endocarditis—less to assess vegetations than to assess the aortic root for abscesses. The erratic oscillatory motion of many vegetations, and their irregular surfaces, render the lesions underrepresented, principally due to partial volume averaging effects.

Complications of endocarditis such as vegetations, abscesses, and fistulas[1] can be imaged by CCT (Table 18-1). Although cardiac MR (CMR) previously was better validated for the detection of root complications of endocarditis,[2] current CCT technology appears considerably more promising.[3] Root abscess lesions can be imaged by CCT[3,4] if they are not seen by transesophageal echocardiography (TEE), but metallic prosthetic valve material may impart image artifact in the vicinity of a ring abscess. CMR suffers from the same effect, probably to a greater degree.

Transthoracic echocardiography (TTE) and TEE remain the principal tests for assessing the presence of vegetations, abscesses, and fistulas. These tests do have limitations, however, especially in the presence of aortic valve prostheses, where the prosthesis is imaged edge-on and the sewing ring, in particular, may acoustically shadow the far side structures or cover them in reverberation artifact, thus obscuring relevant findings.[5-8] Minor degrees of perivalvular insufficiency, while commonly seen in endocarditis, are not specific for this condition.[9,10] It may be difficult to distinguish postoperative inflammatory changes and hematomas from infectious changes by TEE and probably by any modality.[11-13] When compared with surgical findings, incorrect echocardiographic diagnosis was found in 7% of mitral mechanical valve cases and in 15% of aortic valve mechanical prosthesis cases.[14]

The predictive value of CCT for the diagnosis of all anatomic echocardiographic findings of endocarditis has been published (Table 18-2).[10]

VEGETATIONS

Valvular vegetations can be imaged by CCT (Figs. 18-1 through 18-5; **Video 18-1**).

STRUCTURAL COMPLICATIONS OF ENDOCARDITIS

- Abscesses and fistulas can be imaged by CCT.
- For images of valvular endocarditic perforations, see Figures 18-6 through 18-8; **Videos 18-2 through 18-5.**
- For images of endocarditic abscesses, see Figures 18-9 through 18-12; **Videos 18-6 through 18-11.**
- For images of false aneurysms, see Figures 18-13 through 18-15.
- For images of a Gerbode defect (left ventricle to right atrium fistula), see Figures 18-16 through 18-21; **Videos 18-12 and 18-13.**

CORONARY ANGIOGRAPHY

The presence of aortic valve vegetations or an aortic root abscess may make conventional

TABLE 18-1 64-CT for the Detection of Valvular Lesions and Abscesses of Endocarditis*

	SENSITIVITY (%)	SPECIFICITY (%)	PPV (%)	NPV (%)	INTERMODALITY AGREEMENT
Valvular abnormalities	97	98	97	88	$\kappa = 0.84$
Vegetations	96				
Abscesses	100				
Perforations ≤ 2 mm	0				
Mobility of vegetations	96				
Correlation of size versus TEE					$r = 0.95$, $P < .001$
Per-valve basis for the detection of vegetations, abscesses/pseudoaneurysms	96	97	96	97	
TEE	100	100	100	100	

*$n = 37$ patients with suspected IE; TEE versus CCT, 29 cases proven to have definite IE
IE, infective endocarditis; NPV, negative predictive value; PPV, positive predictive value; TEE, transesophageal echocardiography.
Data from Feuchtner GM, Stolzmann P, Dichtl W, et al. Multislice computed tomography in infective endocarditis: comparison with transesophageal echocardiography and intraoperative findings. *J Am Coll Cardiol.* 2009;53(5):436-444.

TABLE 18-2 Positive Predictive Value of the Echocardiographic Findings of Prosthetic Value Endocarditis

	TRUE POSITIVES	FALSE POSITIVES	PPV (%)
Vegetations	17	1	94
Abscesses	19	1	96
Dehiscences	4	0	100
Pseudoaneurysms	3	0	100
Fistulas	2	0	100
Perivalvular leaks			
Mild regurgitation	1	1	6
Moderate to severe regurgitation	15	0	100
All echocardiographic findings	61	16	94

PPV, positive predictive value.
Data from Ronderos RE, Portis M, Stoermann W, Sarmiento C. Are all echocardiographic findings equally predictive for diagnosis in prosthetic endocarditis? *J Am Soc Echocardiogr.* 2004;17(6):664-669.

angiography more problematic because of procedural or catheter-based emboli or further root injury. A potential role for CCT is to provide coronary angiography for patients with complicated aortic endocarditis who are to undergo valve replacement or reparative surgery.

CARDIAC CT PRE–VALVE REPLACEMENT SURGERY

Preliminary series have investigated the utility of CCT in the pre–valve replacement scenario, using the test for its negative predictive value. Predictably, studies have focused on aortic valve disease, which is generally spared from atrial fibrillation. Using both 16-CCT[15-17] and 64-CT,[18] both the negative predictive value of low calcium scores and the absence of significant CTA-detected coronary artery disease have been investigated, with the evolution clearly moving toward CTA and away from the use of calcium scoring alone. Larger series are needed to confirm that the negative predictive value remains excellent in a broader patient population.[17]

PAPILLARY FIBROELASTOMA

A papillary fibroelastoma is a primary tumor of the heart that typically involves one of the valves of the heart. Ninety percent of these tumors occur on valve surfaces; the aortic valve is the most common site, followed in order of decreasing frequency by the mitral, tricuspid, and pulmonary valves. Equal incidence is seen in males and females, with a mean age at presentation of 60

Text continued on page 285

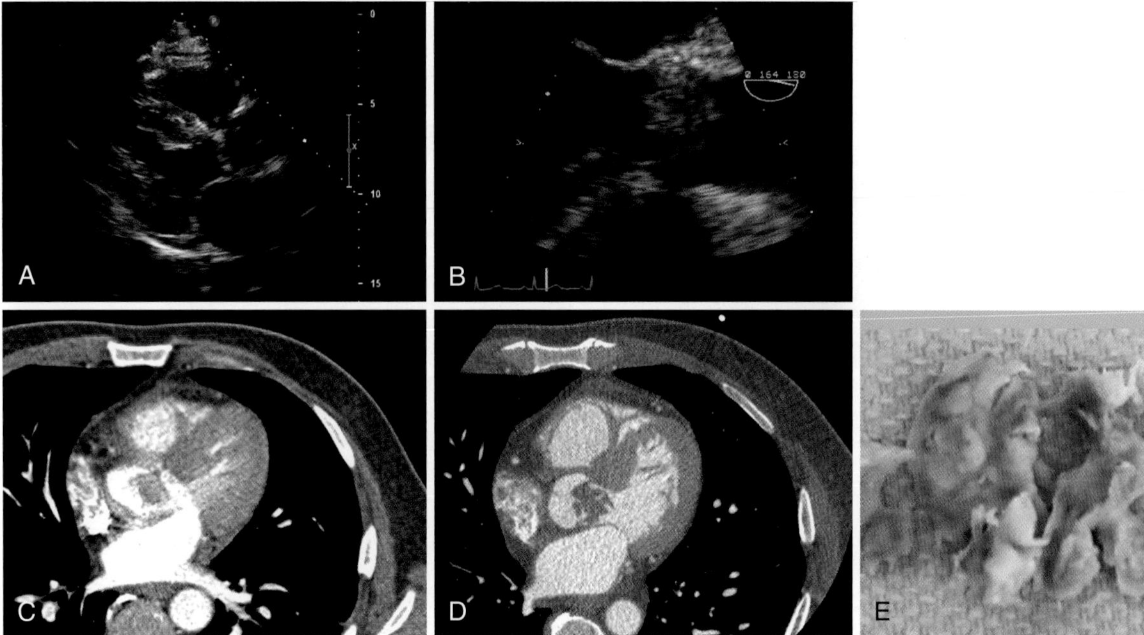

Figure 18-1. A 48-year-old man presented with chest pain, fever, and chills, and a 20-pound weight loss over 6 weeks following prostatectomy. His troponins were elevated. **A,** Transthoracic echocardiography revealed a shaggy soft tissue mass on the aortic valve, which appeared to dome. **B,** Transesophageal echocardiography revealed the shaggy mass in detail. **C,** A chest CT showed the large mass on the aortic valve (and no pulmonary embolism). An ECG-gated cardiac CT scan (**D**), performed to assess CT coronary angiography, revealed in clear detail the shaggy aortic valve lesion. Blood cultures were heavily positive for *Enterococcus faecalis*. These images illustrate the relative spatial resolution/image clarity of the four different modalities for detection of large vegetations. **E,** The surgically excised vegetation fragments.

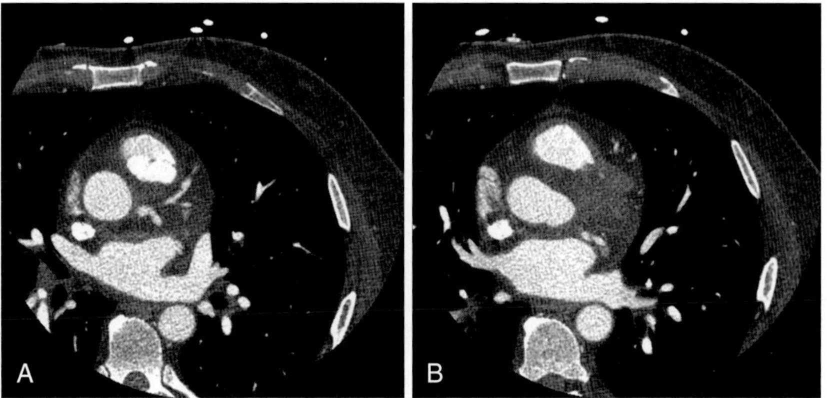

Figure 18-2. Same patient as Figure 18-1. Contrast-enhanced cardiac CT short-axis axial images at the level of the aortic root. Variation in the attenuation of the soft tissue is seen at the root and lower ascending aortic valve level, suggestive of inflammation.

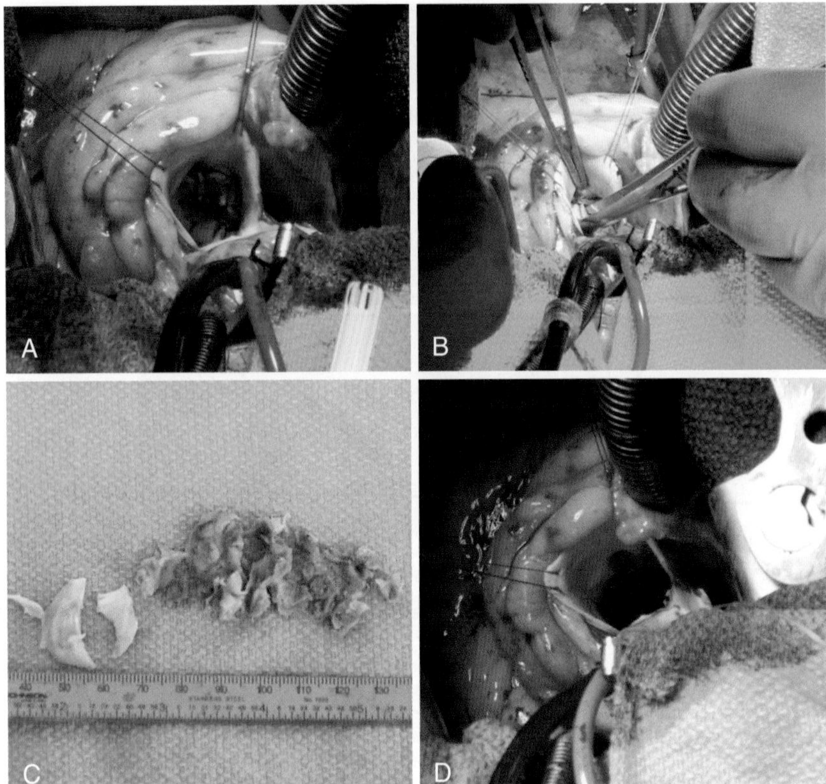

Figure 18-3. Same patient as Figure 18-1 and 18-2. Intraoperative images during resection of a large aortic valve vegetation. A 5-mm abscess/false aneurysm was seen at the root level, corroborating the impression of the CT scan obtained 4 days earlier that the aortic wall was inflamed.

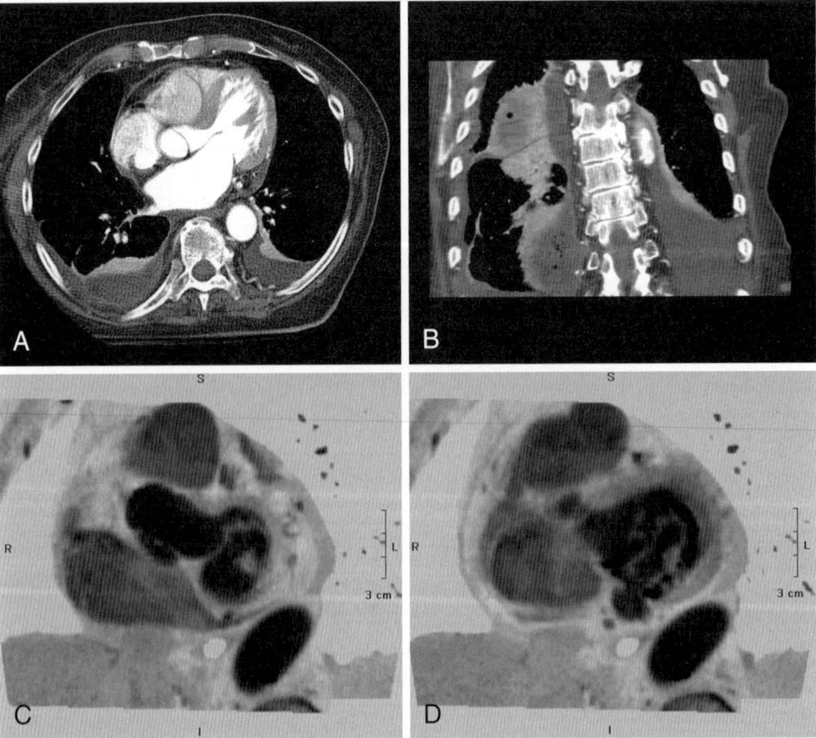

Figure 18-4. Mitral valve endocarditis (vegetation and abscess) likely secondary to empyema. Composite images from a cardiac CT study demonstrate small-to-moderate bilateral pleural effusions with a mild amount of pleural reaction (thickening and enhancement) involving the right pleural reflection. A small amount of pleural gas also is noted. No pleural tap had been performed. Inverted CT cine images demonstrate a soft tissue mass larger than 1 cm along the free edge of the posterior mitral valve leak, consistent with a vegetation. An extension of the blood pool (an abscess) also is seen on the medial aspect of the mitral annulus. **See Video 18-1.**

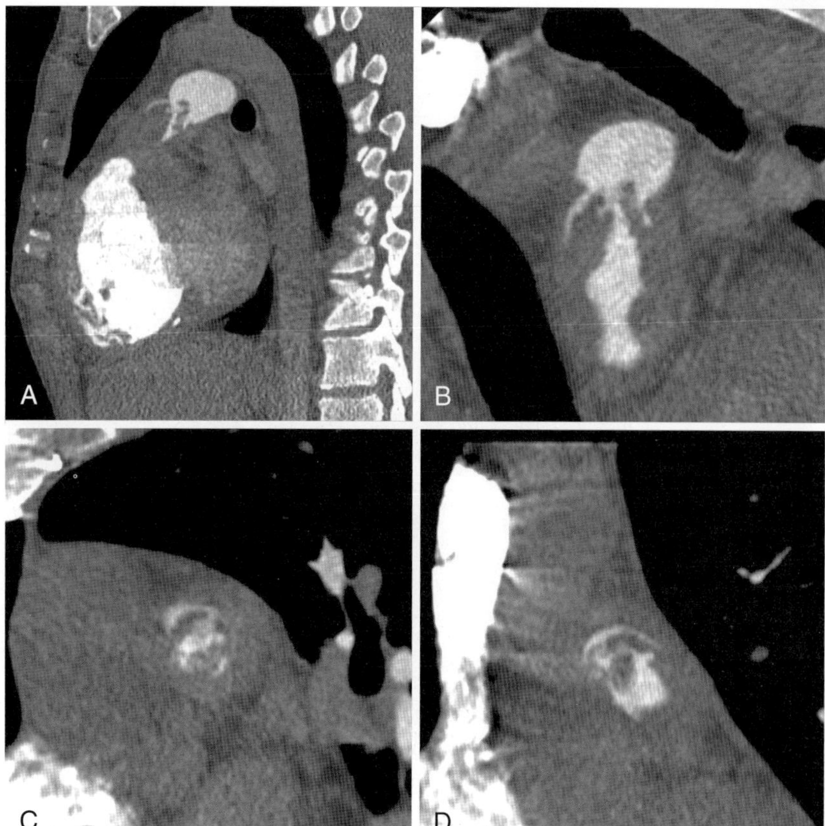

Figure 18-5. Contrast-enhanced ECG-gated CT scans of a 23-year-old patient with a prior Ross procedure, presenting with fevers and *Staphylococcus aureus* bacteremia. Transthoracic and transesophageal echocardiography suggested the presence of pulmonic valve vegetations but were inconclusive. Cardiac CT imaging revealed and confirmed vegetations on the pulmonic valve. **A** and **B,** Long-axis/outflow views. **C** and **D,** Cross-sectional/short-axis views of the pulmonic valve.

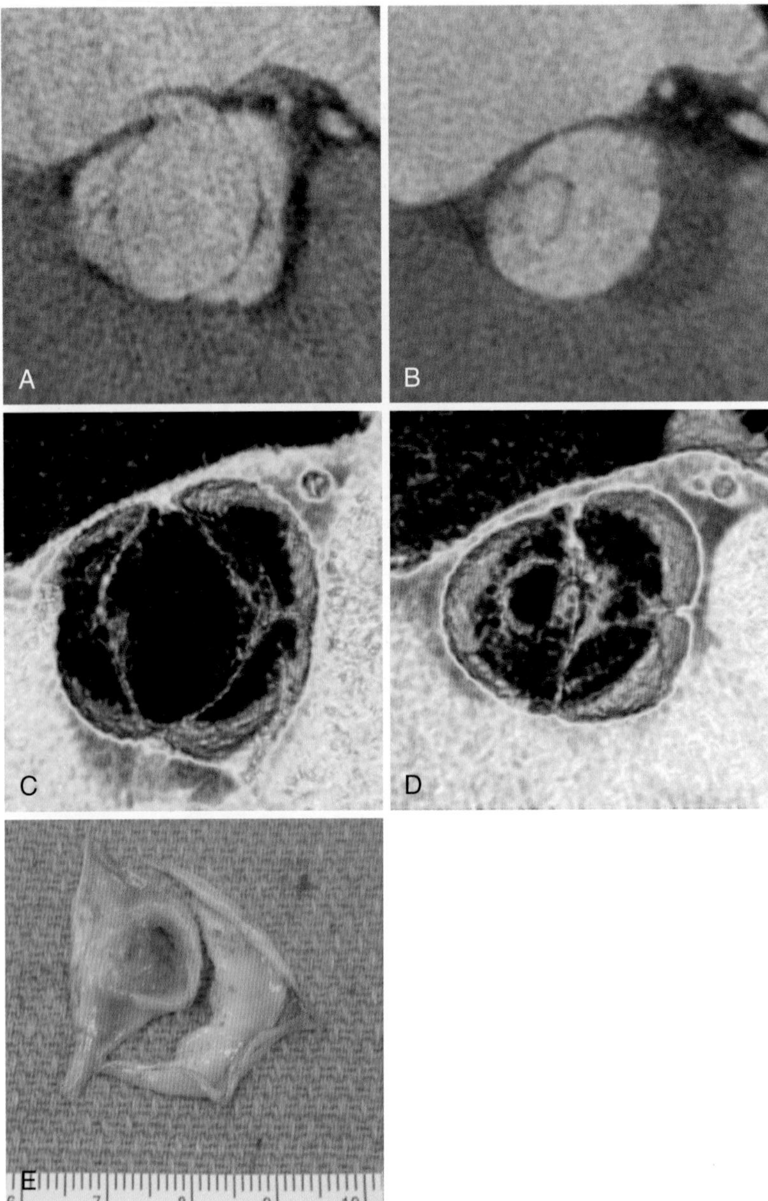

Figure 18-6. Oblique multiplanar reformatted images show a cross section through the aortic valve in the open position (**A**) and immediately below the valve in the closed position (**B**). **C** and **D**, The corresponding thin-slab three-dimensional (3D) volumetric reconstructions with the blood pool inverted to better display valvular anatomy. Note the functionally bicuspid valve in **A** and **C.** With the valve closed (**D**) there is clear delineation of the commissural fusion of the right and left cusps, the median raphe, and a 5-mm perforation of the noncoronary cusp, all best shown on the 3D volumetric reconstruction. **E,** Operative specimen showing a 5-mm perforation of the noncoronary cusp of the bicuspid aortic valve. (Reprinted with permission from Entrikin DW, Ntim WO, Kon ND, Carr JJ. Endocarditis with perforation of a bicuspid aortic valve as shown by cardiac-gated multidetector computed tomography. *J Cardiovasc Comput Tomogr.* 2007;1(3):177-180.)

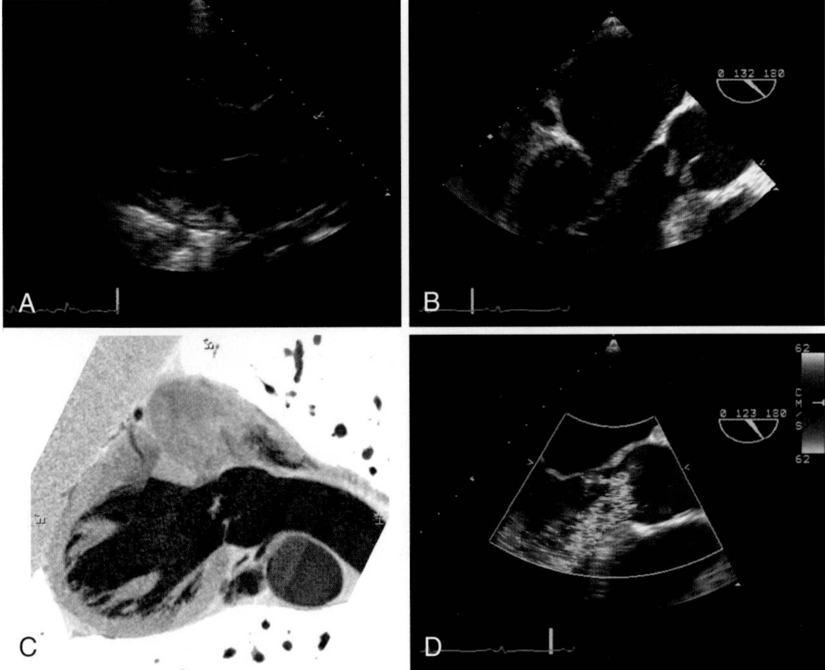

Figure 18-7. A 55-year-old man presented with fever and fatigue 2 months after a transurethral prostatectomy. A murmur of aortic insufficiency was detected, and *Staphylococcus aureus* grew in multiple blood cultures. The patient underwent transthoracic (TTE) and transesophageal echocardiography (TEE), both of which depicted vegetations on the aortic valve and a Gerbode defect (i.e., a fistula from the left ventricular outflow tract to the right atrium). The patient was referred for cardiac CT to assess coronary lesions before planned valve replacement surgery and correction of the Gerbode defect. **A,** TTE revealed thickened aortic valve leaflets consistent with vegetations. **B,** TEE conclusively identified aortic valve vegetations. **C,** Cardiac CT depicted the aortic valve lesions similarly to TEE. **D,** TEE with color Doppler conclusively and positively established the functional consequence of the aortic valve endocarditis—severe aortic insufficiency (AI), confirming the findings of TTE. The size of the regurgitant orifice, as depicted by cardiac CT, indirectly established the presence of severe AI. **See Videos 18-2 through 18-4.**

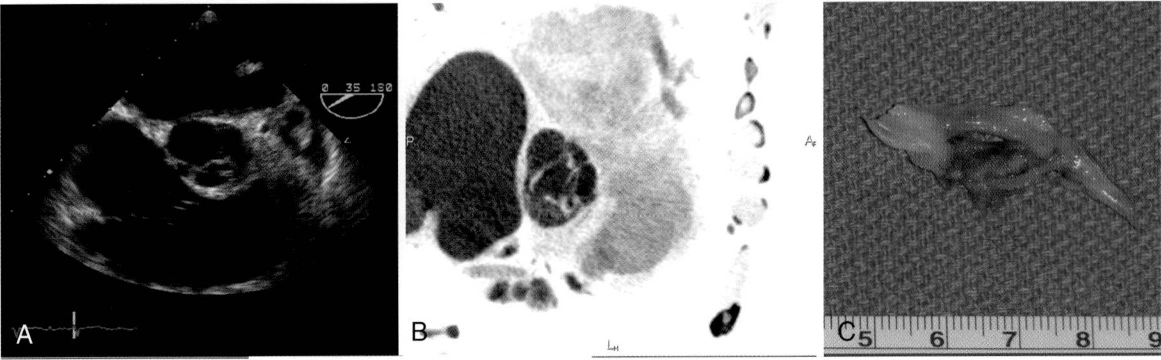

Figure 18-8. Corresponding transesophageal echocardiographic image (**A**), blood-pool inverted cardiac CT image (**B**), and surgical specimen photo (**C**) depicting a perforation of the right coronary leaflet due to *Staphylococcus aureus* endocarditis. **See Video 18-5.**

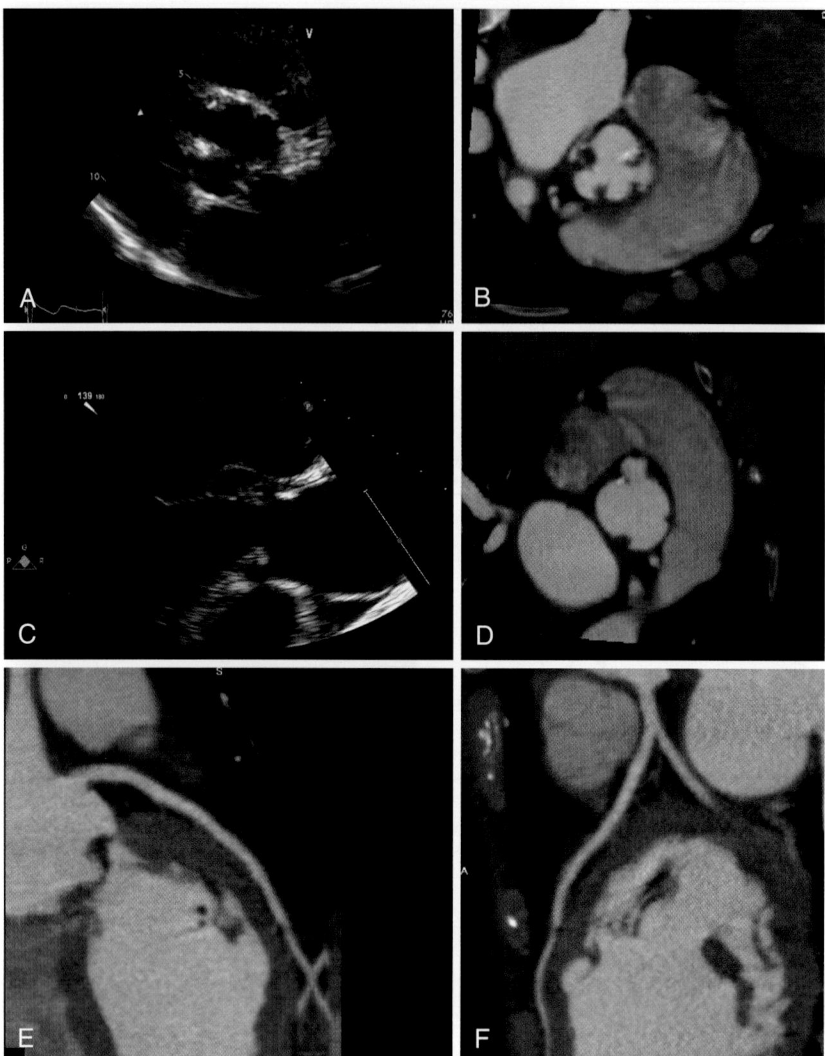

Figure 18-9. Composite of images in a patient with suspected aortic valve endocarditis. Echocardiographic and multiplanar and curved reformatted images demonstrate thickening and calcification of the aortic valve leaflets with a small perivalvular collection. The preoperative CT study also demonstrated normal coronary arteries, precluding the necessity for preoperative diagnostic conventional coronary arteriography. **See Video 18-6.**

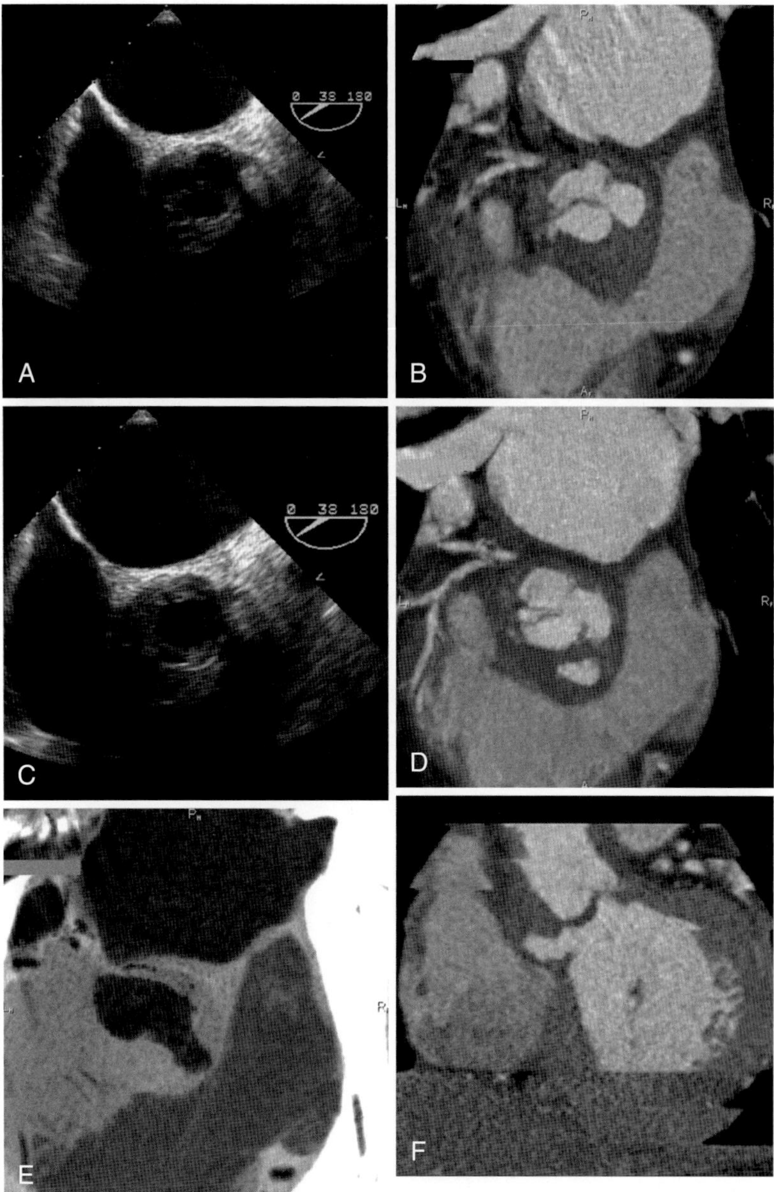

Figure 18-10. A 56-year-old man who presented with strokes with an embolic-type distribution was found to have *Staphylococcus aureus* bacteremia. He had a stentless aortic valve. **A,** Transesophageal echocardiography (TEE) reveals slightly thickened aortic valve leaflets, minimal nonspecific posterior root thickening, and possible anterior root thickening or reverberation artifact. **B,** Corresponding contrast-enhanced CT image reveals more extensive posterior root thickening and definite anterior root thickening. **C,** TEE image at a slightly lower level reveals circumferential thickening at the base of the leaflet, and, again, ambiguous depiction of the anterior root. There is a focal area of echolucency, indicating either less reverberation artifact or a cavity within thickened tissue. **D,** CT at approximately the same level clearly demonstrates a cavity within thickened, abscess-like tissue. **E** and **F,** The cavity into the tissue extended from the left ventricular outflow tract toward the right atrium, and appeared to be an impending Gerbode defect. The findings of circumferential vegetations at the base of the leaflets, and an anterior root abscess extending into the septum with an extension extending toward the right atrium, were confirmed at surgery. **See Videos 18-7 through 18-11.**

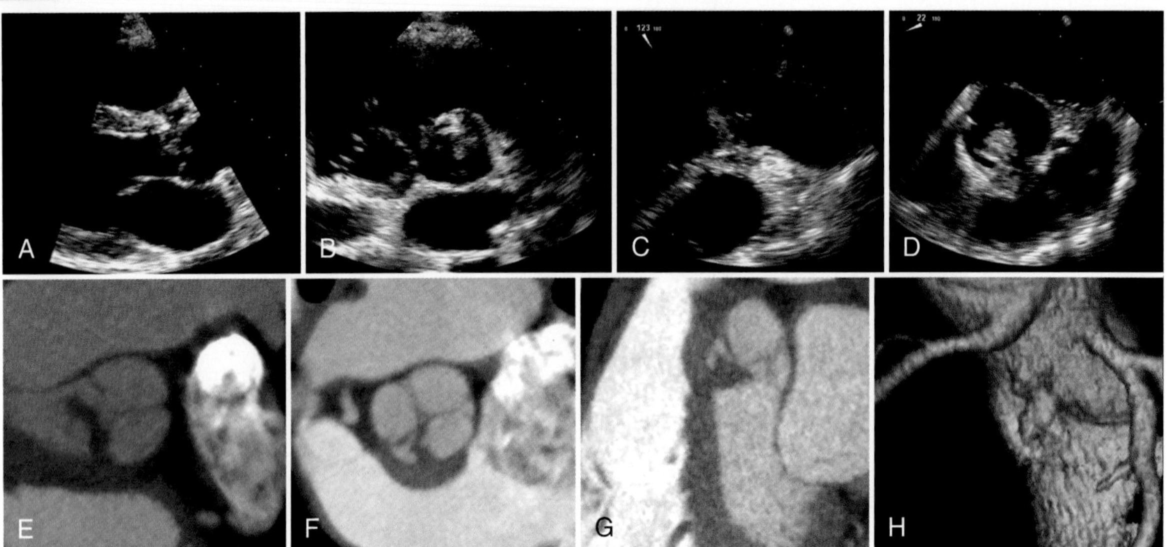

Figure 18-11. A 67-year-old woman presented with a transient ischemic attack (TIA). The patient underwent transthoracic echocardiography (TEE; **A** and **B**), which demonstrated a large amount of soft tissue involving the aortic valve leaflets, consistent with infective endocarditis. **A,** A small focal lucency is seen within the basal septum, suspicious for extension of the infectious/inflammatory process into the aortic root. The patient underwent TEE (**C** and **D**) demonstrating similar findings and increasing suspicion for an aortic root abscess. A cardiac CT study was undertaken to rule out any significant coronary artery disease to mitigate the risk of systemic embolization of aortic valve vegetation from conventional coronary angiography. No significant coronary artery disease was seen (not shown). **E** and **F,** Soft tissue thickening of the aortic valve leaflets, consistent with aortic valve vegetations and an increased rind-like region of soft tissue anterior to the aorta, extending into the basal septum. **G** and **H,** Focal nipple-like outpouchings of contrast from the aortic root into the basal septum consistent with a developing aortic root abscess. The diagnosis was infective endocarditis of the aortic valve with aortic root abscess, surgically confirmed.

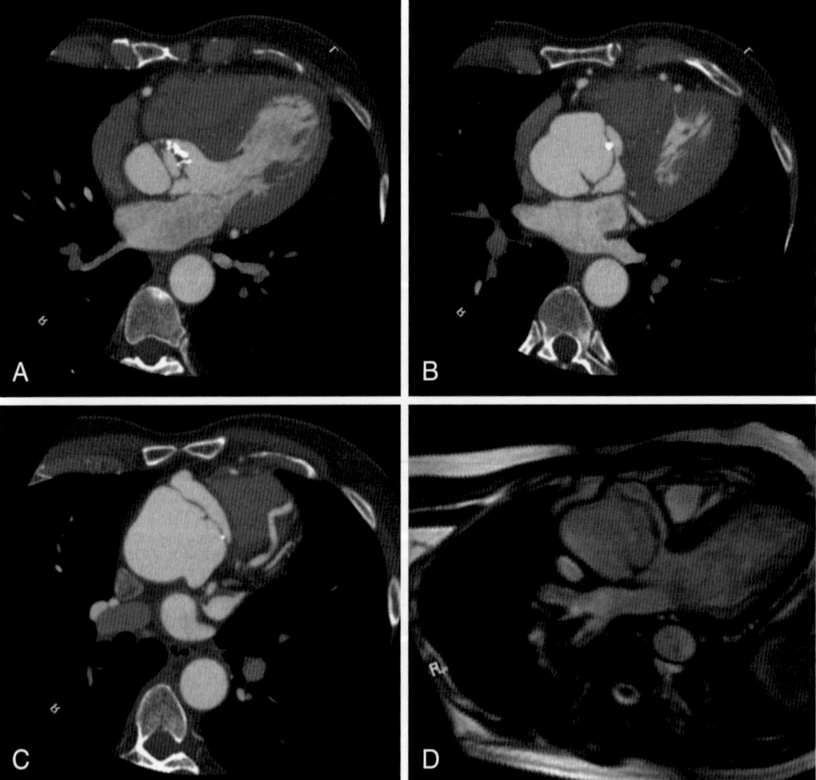

Figure 18-12. A 52-year-old man with a prior history of treated bacterial endocarditis. **A,** Thickening and extensive calcification is seen involving the aortic valve leaflets. **B,** A communication from the left ventricular outflow tract to a perivalvular collection is identified. **C,** The extent of this perivalvular collection is identified anterior to the ascending aorta. **D,** Cardiac MR steady-state free precession image through the left ventricular outflow tract confirms the communication between the left ventricular outflow tract and the perivalvular collection. This is likely the sequela of the patient's previous bacterial endocarditis.

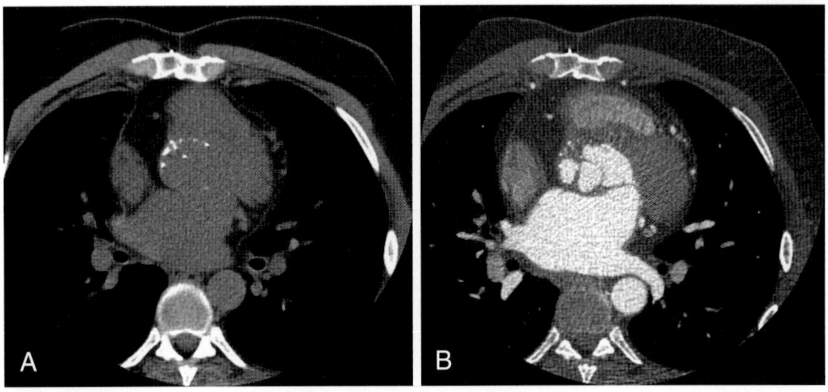

Figure 18-13. Non–contrast-enhanced and contrast-enhanced axial CT images at the aortic root level. Stippled calcification at the root level is apparent on the non–contrast-enhanced images. The contrast-enhanced image reveals that the calcification is of the outer wall of a partially thrombosed false aneurysm/lumen.

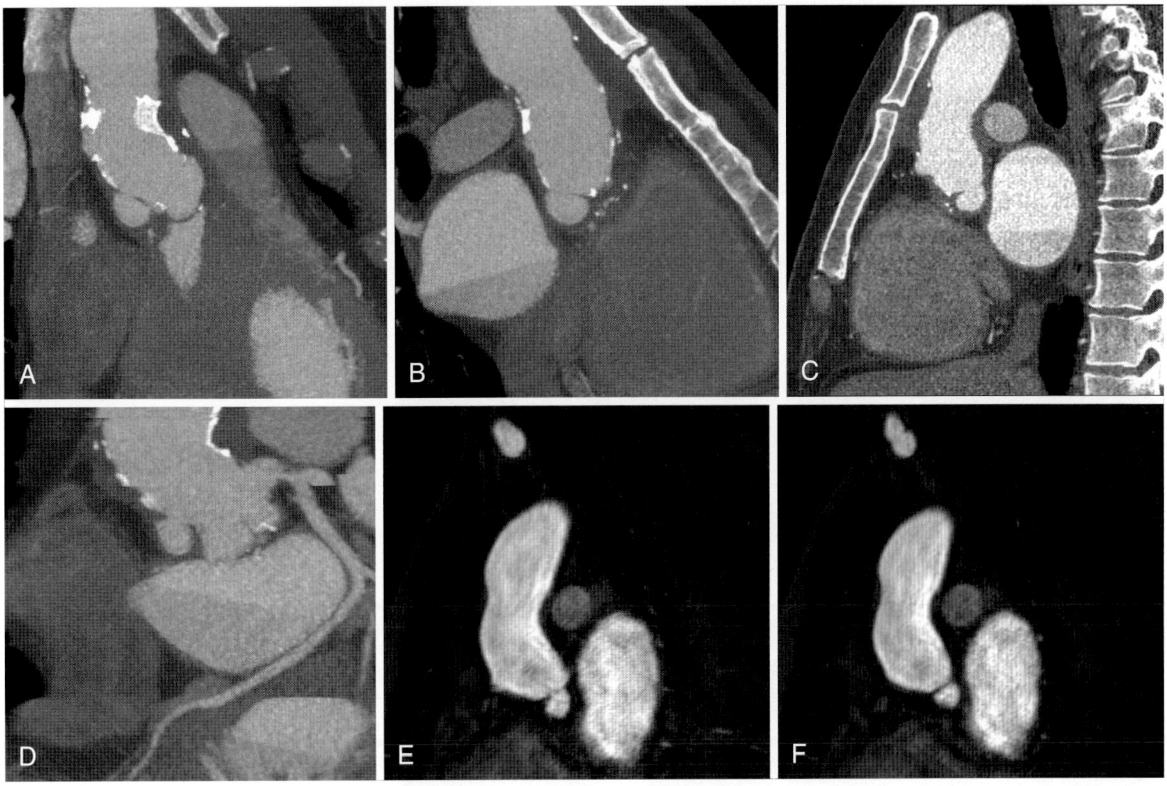

Figure 18-14. A–D, Contrast-enhanced CT images of a patient with a small false aneurysm off the aortic root, resulting from Q-fever endocarditis. **E** and **F**, Cardiac MRI SSFP images revealing the some small false aneurysm.

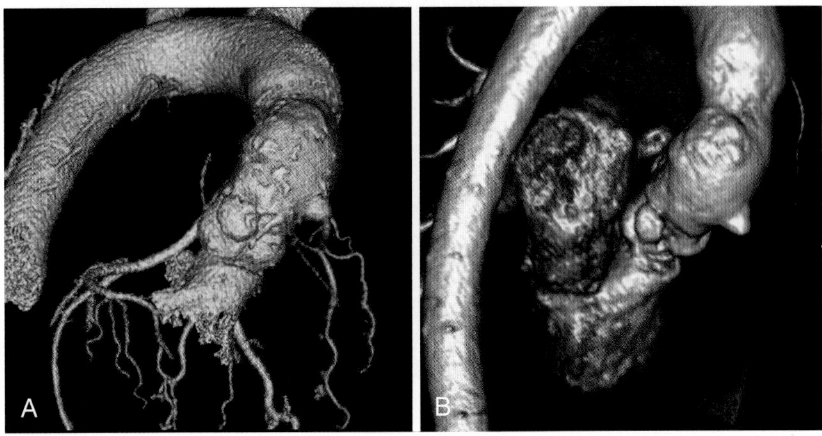

Figure 18-15. Same patient as Figure 18-14. Three-dimensional volume-rendered contrast-enhanced CT scan (**A**) and cardiac MR (**B**) images of a small "button-like" false aneurysm off the aortic root resulting from Q-fever endocarditis. Both modalities depict the lesion well; arguably, the CT image is clearer.

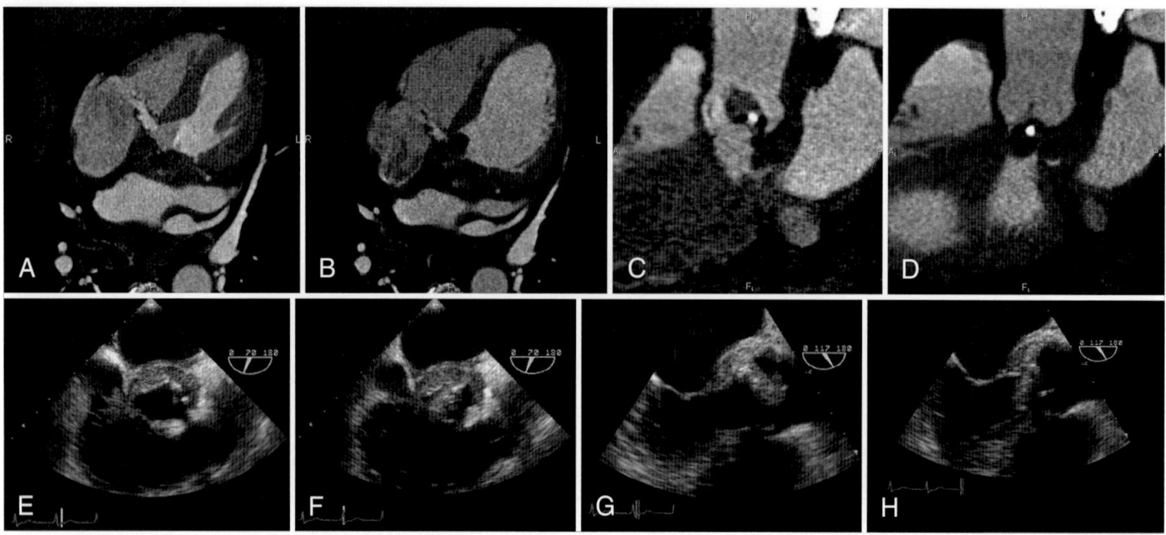

Figure 18-16. Cardiac CT and transesophageal echocardiography (TEE) revealed a large bulk of vegetations on the aortic valve, which prolapsed down into the left ventricular outflow tract (LVOT) in diastole. **A** through **D,** Cardiac CT systole (**A**) and in diastole (**B**). Differential attenuation within the left (LV) and right ventricular (RV) cavities reveals left-to-right LV-to-RA shunting of blood, and the prolapsing of the aortic valve vegetations onto the Gerbode defect orifice in diastole. Cardiac CT images in systole (**C**) and diastole (**D**) reveal the prolapsing of the aortic valve with its vegetations into the LVOT in diastole. In addition, a soft-tissue thickening of the left-sided aspect of the aortic root is clearly depicted, consistent with an aortic ring/root abscess. **E** through **H,** TEE images of the aortic valve and its vegetations, and the aortic ring abscess, with prolapsing of the aortic valve vegetations into the LVOT in diastole. Cardiac CT depicts left-to-right blood flow through the LV to RA fistula of the Gerbode defect. See also Figures 18-17 through 18-20; **Videos 18-12 and 18-13.**

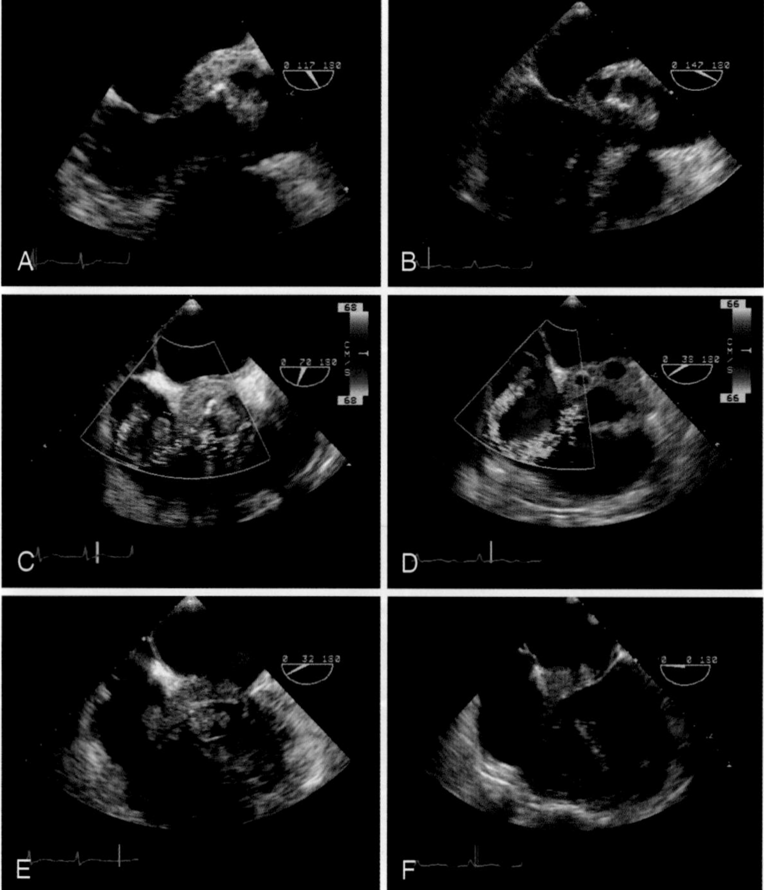

Figure 18-17. **A, C,** and **E** show transesophageal echocardiographic images obtained 3 days before those shown in **B, D,** and **F.** Note the rapid evolution of the abscess within a short period of time. See also Figures 18-16 and 18-18 through 18-20; **Videos 18-12 and 18-13.**

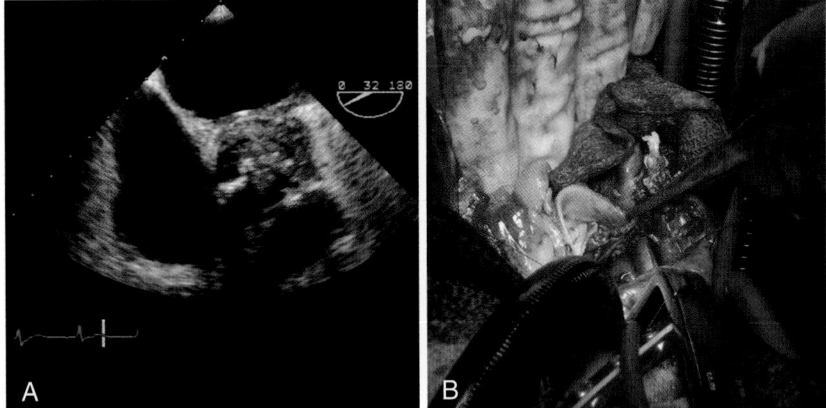

Figure 18-18. **A,** Transesophageal cross-sectional view of the large aortic valve vegetation. **B,** The vegetation being removed at surgery. See Figures 18-16, 18-17, 18-19, and 18-20; **Videos 18-12 and 18-13.**

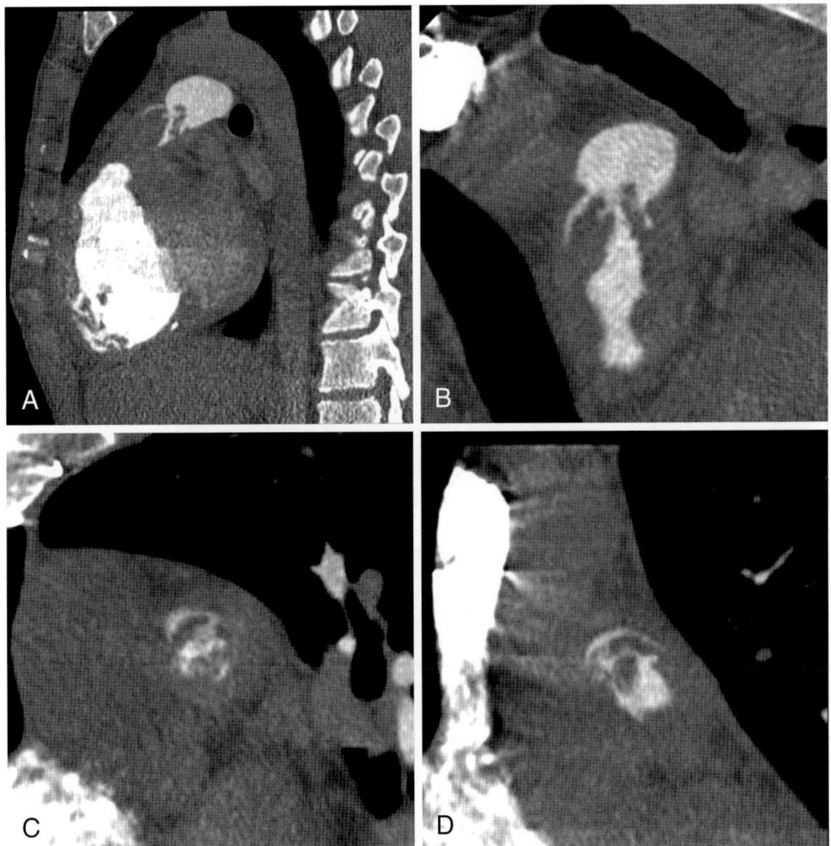

Figure 18-19. **A,** Cardiac CT reveals the abscess of the aortic root, but does provide a good depiction of the septal abscess. **B,** Transesophageal echocardiographic (TEE) view of the aortic root abscess with extension into the annulus fibrosus and into the septum. The abscess had resulted in first-degree atrioventricular (AV) block by this time. **C,** TEE spectral Doppler display of the left atrial appendage contraction during first-degree heart block. Atrial emptying is very early in diastole, just after the T wave. **D,** M-mode of the mitral valve during first-degree AV block. The mitral valve closes well before the onset of systole ("pre-closure")—a false-positive sign of severe aortic insufficiency. See Figures 18-16 through 18-18, 18-20; **Videos 18-12 and 18-13.**

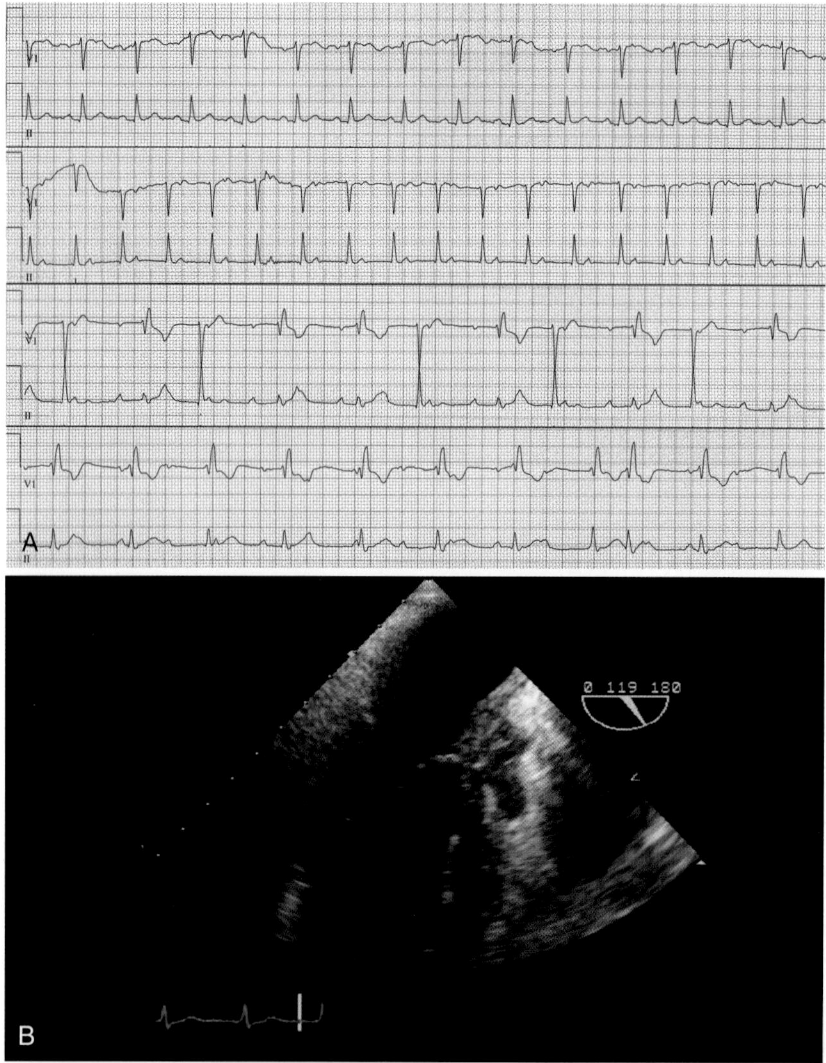

Figure 18-20. **A,** Serial rhythm strips revealing progressive complications of the septal abscess. *Top row:* Sinus rhythm/normal conduction; *second row:* marked first-degree atrioventricular (AV) block, *third row:* second-degree AV block with intermittent right bundle branch block; *bottom row,* complete heart block during sinus rhythm, with right bundle branch block. **B**, TEE oblique view revealing a large abscess that arose from the aortic value annulus and that has extended into the septum, resulting in the observed AV block. See Figures 18-16 through 18-19; **Videos 18-12 and 18-13.**

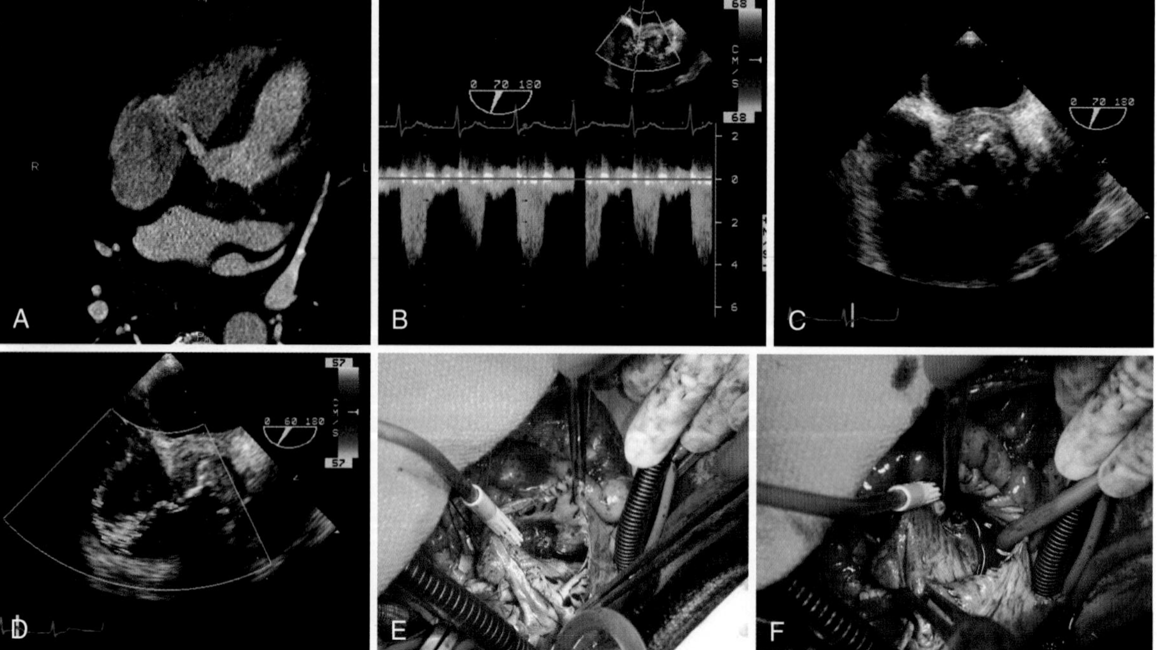

Figure 18-21. **A,** Cardiac CT reveals, by differential contrast/attenuation of the left and right blood pools, a Gerbode defect of the septum between the left ventricle and right atrium (RA). **B,** Spectral Doppler display of high-velocity flow between the left ventricular outflow tract (LVOT) and RA. **C** and **D,** Grayscale and grayscale with color Doppler flow mapping of the LVOT to the right atrial defect and flow. **E** and **F,** Surgical findings. **E,** The large fulgating vegetations into the right atrium are first seen. **F,** After removal of the vegetations, the defect communicating the LVOT to the RA is apparent (at the tip of the forceps).

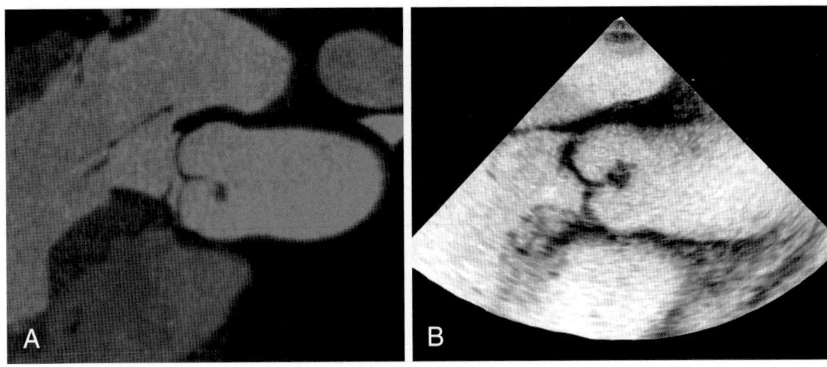

Figure 18-22. A frondular nodule seen extending from the aortic valve superiorly was identified on a short-thickness CT maximum intensity projection image through the left ventricular outflow tract/aortic valve plane (**A**) with excellent echocardiographic correlation. **B**, Corresponding TEE image with black-white inversion.

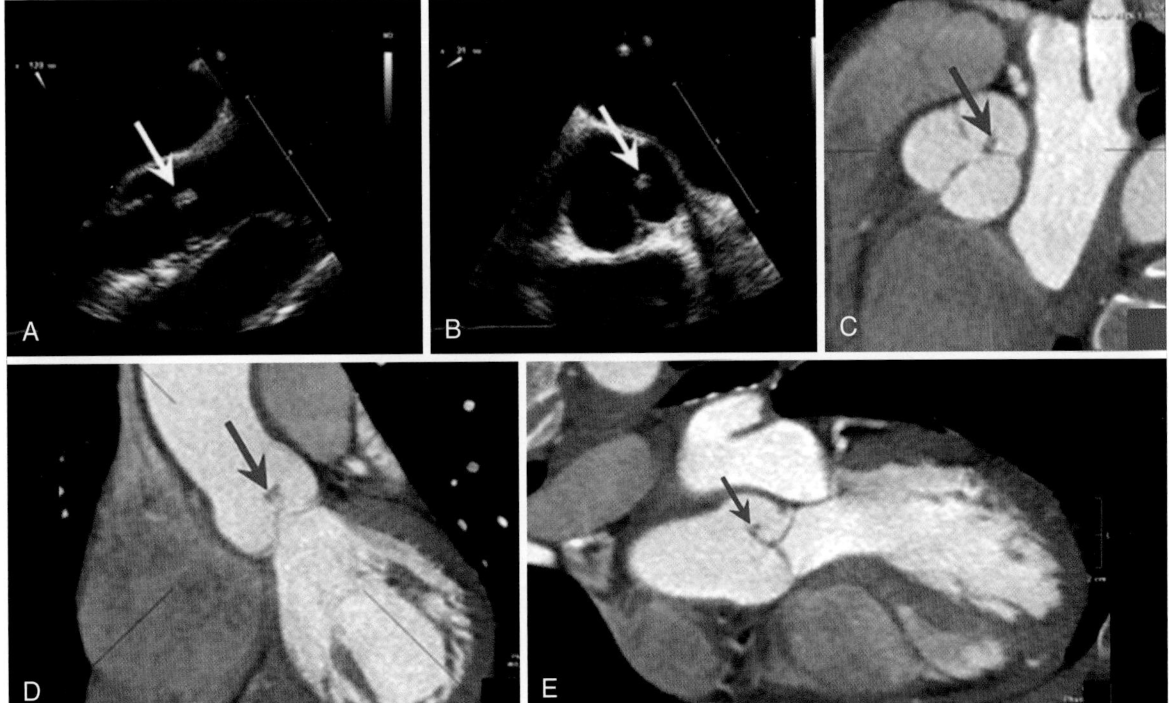

Figure 18-23. Transesophageal echocardiogram shows a mobile mass attached to the aortic valve in the parasternal long- (**A**) and short-axis (**B**) views. Contrast-enhanced 320-multidetector CT confirms the presence of a mass located between the noncoronary and left cusps as seen in the cross section of the aortic valve (**C**), the left ventricular outflow tract (**D**), and the three-chamber view (**E**). Arrows indicate a papillary fibroelastoma. (Reprinted with permission from Barbier G, Vazquez Figueroa JG, Rinehart S, et al: Tissue characterization of a papillary fibroelastoma on the aortic valve by contrast-enhanced 320-detector row computed tomography. *J Cardiovasc Comput Tomogr*. 2010;4(5):345-347.)

years. Papillary fibroelastomas, while generally considered rare, make up about 10% of all primary tumors of the heart.[19] They are the third most common type of primary tumor of the heart, behind cardiac myxomas and cardiac lipomas.[20]

Fibroelastomas usually are isolated and rarely are multiple. They can be difficult to visualize on MR imaging because they often are very small (<1 cm). Because the spatial resolution of CMR is less than that of CT, these small lesions may in fact be better visualized on CT. For images of fibroelastomas, see Figures 18-22 to 18-25; **Videos 18-14 through 18-21.**

CCT PROTOCOL POINTS

- The standard CCT protocol is utilized.
- Helical scanning should be considered to better evaluate valve morphology and perivalvular collections as well as to optimize for preoperative coronary artery assessment if moderate to severe valvular insufficiency precludes adequate beta blockade. This can be done in a low-dose, dose-modulated fashion.
- See Table 18-3.

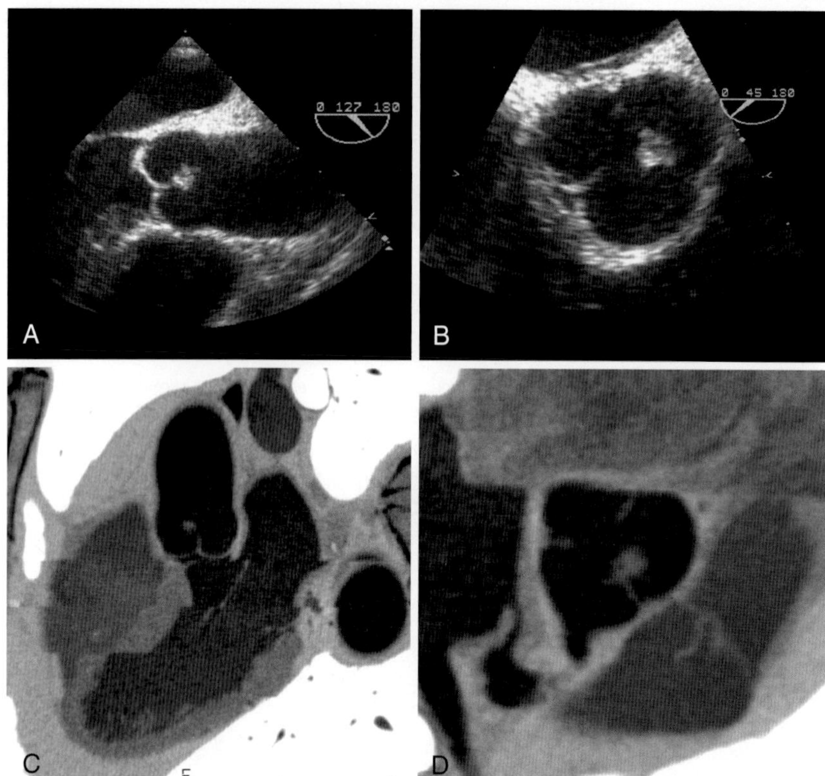

Figure 18-24. Grayscale echo images demonstrating a small fibroelastoma arising from the right coronary leaflet. Companion CT angiography (CTA) images demonstrate a similar appearance. CT images were post-processed in an inverted fashion, better demonstrating the lesion on a background relief of inverted contrast density (black). **See Videos 18-14 through 18-16.**

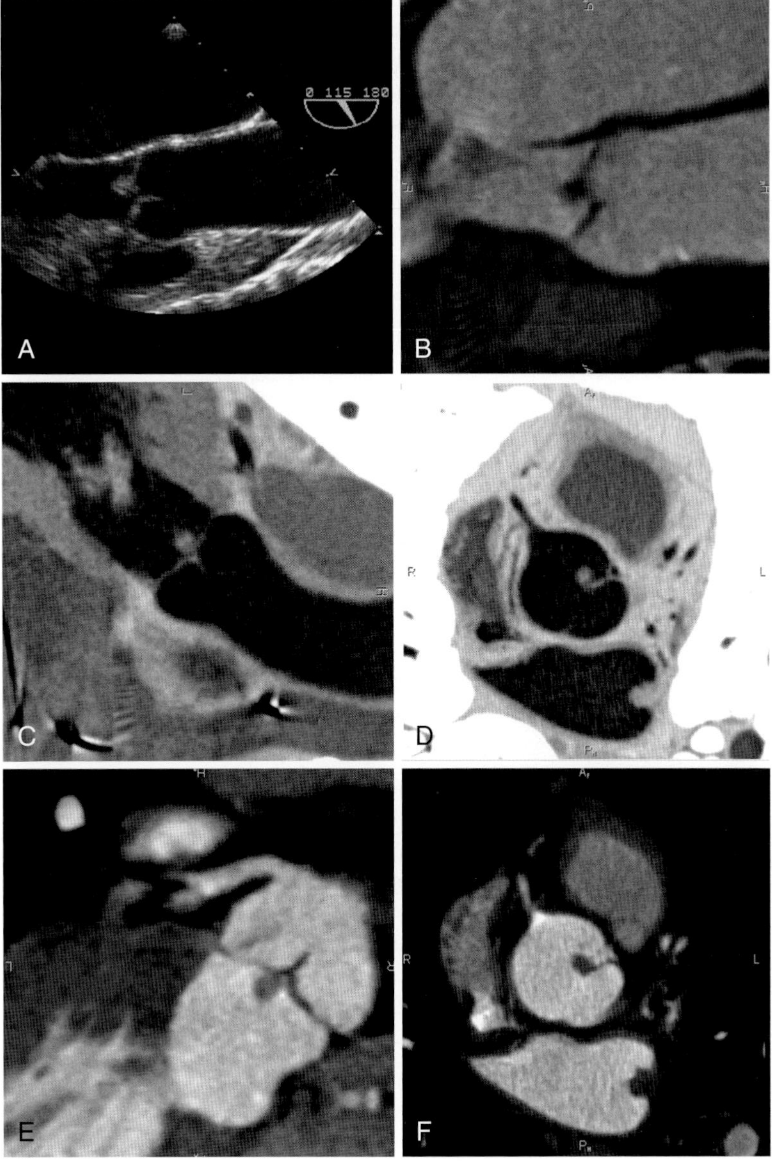

Figure 18-25. Multiple composite images from an echocardiogram and a cardiac CT demonstrate a nodular mass extending off the undersurface of the aortic valve. Postsurgical pathology showed it to be a small fibroelastoma. **See Videos 18-17 through 18-21.**

TABLE 18-3 ACCF 2010 Appropriateness Criteria for the Use of Cardiac Computed Tomography to Evaluate Infective Endocarditis and Valve Tumors

	APPROPRIATENESS RATING	INDICATION	MEDIAN SCORE
Evaluation of intra- and extracardiac structures	Appropriate	Characterization of native cardiac valves Suspected clinically significant valvular dysfunction Inadequate images from other noninvasive methods	8
		Characterization of prosthetic cardiac valves Suspected clinically significant valvular dysfunction Inadequate images from other noninvasive methods	8
		Evaluation of cardiac mass (suspected tumor or thrombus) Inadequate images from other noninvasive methods	8
		Coronary evaluation before noncoronary cardiac surgery Intermediate pretest probability of coronary artery disease	7
	Uncertain	None listed	
	Inappropriate	Initial evaluation of cardiac mass (suspected tumor or thrombus)	3

Data from Taylor AJ, Cerqueira M, Hodgson JM, et al. ACCF/SCCT/ACR/AHA/ASE/ASNC/NASCI/SCAI/SCMR 2010 appropriate use criteria for cardiac computed tomography. A report of the American College of Cardiology Foundation Appropriate Use Criteria Task Force, the Society of Cardiovascular Computed Tomography, the American College of Radiology, the American Heart Association, the American Society of Echocardiography, the American Society of Nuclear Cardiology, the North American Society for Cardiovascular Imaging, the Society for Cardiovascular Angiography and Interventions, and the Society for Cardiovascular Magnetic Resonance. *J Am Coll Cardiol.* 2010;56(22): 1864–1894.

References

1. Mendoza DD, Wang Z, Gaglia MA, Taylor AJ. Gerbode defect. *J Cardiovasc Comput Tomogr.* 2009;3(4):279-281.
2. Jeang MK, Fuentes F, Gately A, Byrnes J, Lewis M. Aortic root abscess. Initial experience using magnetic resonance imaging. *Chest.* 1986;89(4):613-615.
3. Feuchtner GM, Stolzmann P, Dichtl W, et al. Multislice computed tomography in infective endocarditis: comparison with transesophageal echocardiography and intraoperative findings. *J Am Coll Cardiol.* 2009;53(5):436-444.
4. Cowan JC, Patrick D, Reid DS. Aortic root abscess complicating bacterial endocarditis. Demonstration by computed tomography. *Br Heart J.* 1984;52(5):591-593.
5. Herrera CJ, Chaudhry FA, DeFrino PF, et al. Value and limitations of transesophageal echocardiography in evaluating prosthetic or bioprosthetic valve dysfunction. *Am J Cardiol.* 1992; 69(6):697-699.
6. Seward JB, Khandheria BK, Oh JK, Freeman WK, Tajik AJ. Critical appraisal of transesophageal echocardiography: limitations, pitfalls, and complications. *J Am Soc Echocardiogr.* 1992;5(3): 288-305.
7. Blanchard DG, Dittrich HC, Mitchell M, McCann HA. Diagnostic pitfalls in transesophageal echocardiography. *J Am Soc Echocardiogr.* 1992;5(5):525-540.
8. Mohr-Kahaly S, Kupferwasser I, Erbel R, et al. Value and limitations of transesophageal echocardiography in the evaluation of aortic prostheses. *J Am Soc Echocardiogr.* 1993;6(1):12-20.
9. Come PC. Pitfalls in the diagnosis of periprosthetic valvular regurgitation by pulsed Doppler echocardiography. *J Am Coll Cardiol.* 1987;9(5):1176-1179.
10. Ronderos RE, Portis M, Stoermann W, Sarmiento C. Are all echocardiographic findings equally predictive for diagnosis in prosthetic endocarditis? *J Am Soc Echocardiogr.* 2004;17(6):664-669.
11. Graupner C, Vilacosta I, SanRoman J, et al. Periannular extension of infective endocarditis. *J Am Coll Cardiol.* 2002;39(7): 1204-1211.
12. San Roman JA, Vilacosta I, Sarria C, et al. Clinical course, microbiologic profile, and diagnosis of periannular complications in prosthetic valve endocarditis. *Am J Cardiol.* 1999;83(7):1075-1079.
13. Vilacosta I, Graupner C, San Roman JA, et al. Risk of embolization after institution of antibiotic therapy for infective endocarditis. *J Am Coll Cardiol.* 2002;39(9):1489-1495.
14. Faletra F, Constantin C, De Chiara F, et al. Incorrect echocardiographic diagnosis in patients with mechanical prosthetic valve dysfunction: correlation with surgical findings. *Am J Med.* 2000;108(7): 531-537.
15. Reant P, Brunot S, Lafitte S, et al. Predictive value of noninvasive coronary angiography with multidetector computed tomography to detect significant coronary stenosis before valve surgery. *Am J Cardiol.* 2006;97(10):1506-1510.
16. Manghat NE, Morgan-Hughes GJ, Broadley AJ, et al. 16-detector row computed tomographic coronary angiography in patients undergoing evaluation for aortic valve replacement: comparison with catheter angiography. *Clin Radiol.* 2006;61(9):749-757.
17. Gilard M, Cornily JC, Pennec PY, et al. Accuracy of multislice computed tomography in the preoperative assessment of coronary disease in patients with aortic valve stenosis. *J Am Coll Cardiol.* 2006;47(10):2020-2024.
18. Meijboom WB, Mollet NR, van Mieghem CA, et al. Pre-operative computed tomography coronary angiography to detect significant coronary artery disease in patients referred for cardiac valve surgery. *J Am. Coll. Cardiol.* 2006;48(8):1658-1665.
19. Palecek T, Lindner J, Vitkova I, Linhart A. Papillary fibroelastoma arising from the left ventricular apex associated with nonspecific systemic symptoms. *Echocardiography.* 2008;25(5):526-528.
20. Matsumoto N, Sato Y, Kusama J, et al. Multiple papillary fibroelastomas of the aortic valve: case report. *Int J Cardiol.* 2007;122(1):e1-e3.

19 Assessment of Left Ventricular Function, Infarction, Perfusion, and Viability

Key Points

- Helical cardiac CT scanning is able to accurately determine the volumes of the cardiac chambers and ventricular ejection fraction.
- The high spatial resolution of CCT is a useful attribute in chamber quantification; the limited number of phase segmentations of the cardiac cycle, however, is detrimental.
- Unlike cardiac MR, CCT can quantitatively assess ejection fraction in hearts with pacemakers.

ASSESSMENT OF LEFT VENTRICULAR VOLUMES AND SYSTOLIC FUNCTION

The excellent spatial resolution of contrast-enhanced cardiac CT (CCT) permits the delineation of accurate endocardial and epicardial borders to a degree exceeding that of cardiac MRI. The avoidance of epicardial chemical shift artifact and the clear distinction between blood pool and myocardium (due to less blurring from partial volume effects and elimination of flow artifacts on cine gradient echo and steady-state free precession images in regions of increased trabeculation or slow flow) facilitates the straightforward quantification of left ventricular (LV) volumes and function.

By reconstructing retrospectively gated images, CCT is able to depict the regional and global systolic and diastolic phases of the heart and also to:

- ❒ Run as a cine-loop that allows for regional and overall wall motion assessment
- ❒ Calculate, using biplane Simpson's method applied to four- and two-chamber views, or the method of disks applied to a short-axis stack:
  - Diastolic volume
  - Systolic volume
  - Stroke volume
  - Ejection fraction
- ❒ Calculate and display:
  - Diastolic wall thickness
  - Systolic wall thickness
  - Systolic wall thickening
  - Systolic regional motion

Use of automatic edge detection and chamber segmentation algorithms and Simpson's method enables determination of LV end-diastolic volume from a selected diastolic reconstruction and LV end-systolic volume from a selected systolic reconstruction.

Selection of End-systole and End-diastole

End-systole

Although end-systole often is 35% or 40% of the R-R interval, that is not always the case, especially when the heart rate is elevated. Changing the reconstruction by even 1% can influence the determination of end-systolic volume.[1] To define end-systole optimally (given contemporary imaging temporal resolution of the acquisition, which determines the number of required phases needed),[1] more rather than fewer phases should be used, because the volumetric assessment depends on the number of cardiac cycles. Misidentification of end-systole increases measured end-systolic volume, by up to 20%.[2] At least 20 reconstructed phases should be used.

End-diastole

Use of 0% R-R interval should achieve an accurate end-diastole representation.

Use of mid-diastole as for coronary CT imaging is not an accurate determination of end-diastole, except possibly in atrial fibrillation, because the atrial contribution to ventricular filling would not yet have occurred.[1]

Segmentation Algorithms

Many algorithms have been developed that assist with chamber or infarct segment delineation, based on attenuation differences. Chamber identification/segmentation algorithms are based on the expected shape of the cavities of the cardiac chambers and great vessels and reduce the time to yield quantitation. At the same time, however, these algorithms increase variability when compared with manually traced short-axis slices. Often some manual adjustment still is required to obtain accurate chamber delineation. Typically, semiautomated quantification of LV volumes and function takes about 5 minutes with contemporary post-processing software. Post-processing time can also be reduced by segmenting only end-diastolic and end-systolic images instead of data from the entire cardiac cycle, as is usually done in cardiac MR (CMR). Semiautomated segmentation also may be improved by reconstructing the functional data set at an increased slice thickness (1.2–3 mm). This may reduce the amount of manual adjustment that may subsequently be needed.

Segmentation of infarct territory using a delayed enhancement technique is based on an arbitrary number of standard deviations above sampling of non-infarct territory.

As with all imaging modalities, navigating the complexities of the basal anatomy of the ventricles, especially the shape of the atrioventricular valve and of the outflow tract, is a challenge and generally requires manual editing.

TUBE MODULATION AND EXCESS NOISE

The original technique to determine ejection fraction was retrospective gating with constant (unmodulated) x-ray tube output. Although this gave optimal image quality, it did so at maximized radiation output. Contemporary techniques employ modulation of tube output to reduce radiation exposure, with peak output targeted to diastole for coronary imaging needs. However, such dose modulation, by reducing output through systole, improves the systolic noise-to-signal ratio and image quality. Although inter- and intraobserver variability of systolic images is greater when tube modulation is used, the variabilities are still within acceptable ranges.[1]

DEPENDENCE OF THE VOLUMETRIC ASSESSMENT ON THE NUMBER OF SHORT-AXIS SLICES

Twenty rather than ten short-axis 5-mm slices are needed to optimally assess the LV volume, because ten slices may leave interslice distances that will require volumetric interpolation and thus permit the introduction of measurement error.[1,2]

Validation of CT (versus Cardiac MR Standard)

CT is validated against the CMR standard for cardiac volumes and ejection fraction and shows good agreement and correlation[1]:

- CT end-systolic volume (ESV) versus CMR ejection fraction: −1.2% ± 4.6%; r = 0.96 (bias; correlation)
- CT end-diastolic volume (EDV) versus CMR EDV: −3.5 mL ± 15.2; r = 0.97 (bias; correlation)

CT is validated against the CMR[1] and echocardiography[2] standards for mass%:

- Myocardial mass versus MRI: 2.5 mL ± 15.0; r = 0.96

Standard deviation of EF difference:

- Is less between CCT and CMR than between echocardiography and CMR ($P < .001$)[1]
- Is less between CCT and CMR than between single-photon emission CT(SPECT) and CMR ($P < .001$)[1]

By CMR imaging, inclusion of the trabeculae in the cavitary volume improves inter- and intraobserver reproducibility of assessment of EDV and LV mass.[3]

Inclusion or exclusion of trabeculae causes the determination of LV mass to vary by up to 17% and the ejection fraction by 3%.[4,5]

- For plots of the regression and limits of agreement of CCT determinations of LV EDV, ESV, stroke volume, ejection fraction, and intraobserver variability compared with those yielded from CMR, see Figures 19-1 and 19-2.
- For CCT images of chamber quantification, see Figures 19-3 and 19-4
- For plots of CCT determinations of LV mass compared with those yielded from CMR, see Figure 19-5
- For CCT images of LV mass calculation see Figures 19-6 and 19-7
- Fine detail of the LV, such as the apical thin-point,[3] is apparent by CT.

The principal problem is that reconstructing images from data sets at 10% intervals will not necessarily catch (true) end-systole. There tends to be more variability for CT estimations of EDV than for ESV, because trabecular topography is more variable at end-diastole.

For the validation of CCT for the assessment of LV volumes and ejection fraction, see Table 19-1.

The variability of CCT determinations of cardiac volume and systolic function is approximately half of that of real-time three-dimensional echocardiography and of CMR.[16]

Current guidelines have classified the appropriateness of CT for evaluation of LV function post-MI or in heart failure as "uncertain" (in the context that echocardiography is technically limited). Otherwise, as a stand-alone indication, it is classified as "inappropriate," given the availability of techniques that do not require radiation. From a clinical standpoint, in the setting of contraindications to CMR (e.g., permanent pacemakers or implantable cardioverter defibrillators) and inadequate echocardiographic imaging, cardiac CT may be particularly useful.

Assessment of wall motion is feasible. The AHA 17-segment model[4] of the LV should be used. Cine CT is able to compile images of the heart at 10% phase intervals and to run dynamic loops (Figs. 19-8 and 19-9).

The sensitivity for detection of akinesis is better than for hypokinesis, illustrating the limitations of depicting systolic function in an insufficient number of phases.

Realistically, the utility of CT-determined wall motion is generally less than that of echocardiography, CMR, or catheterization, because the temporal resolution is lower than that with these other modalities. However, assessment of wall motion is possible and the technique continues to evolve (Table 19-2).

RIGHT HEART AND LEFT ATRIAL VOLUMES

CCT is able to quantify other cardiac chamber dimensions and their systolic function.

Right Ventricular Volumes

Right ventricular volumes can be quantified by CCT, although inadequate right ventricular (RV) contrast opacification renders about one quarter of studies inadequate.[18] The precise evaluation of RV volumes and RV function is of significant import in the setting of adult congenital heart disease, often in the postoperative state. While CMR is the accepted gold standard modality for evaluating the RV in these patients, many of them have contraindications to MR imaging, often the placement of an intra-cardiac device. In these patients CCT should be thought of as secondary choice for RV evaluation. Dose can be significantly mitigated

Text continued on page 296

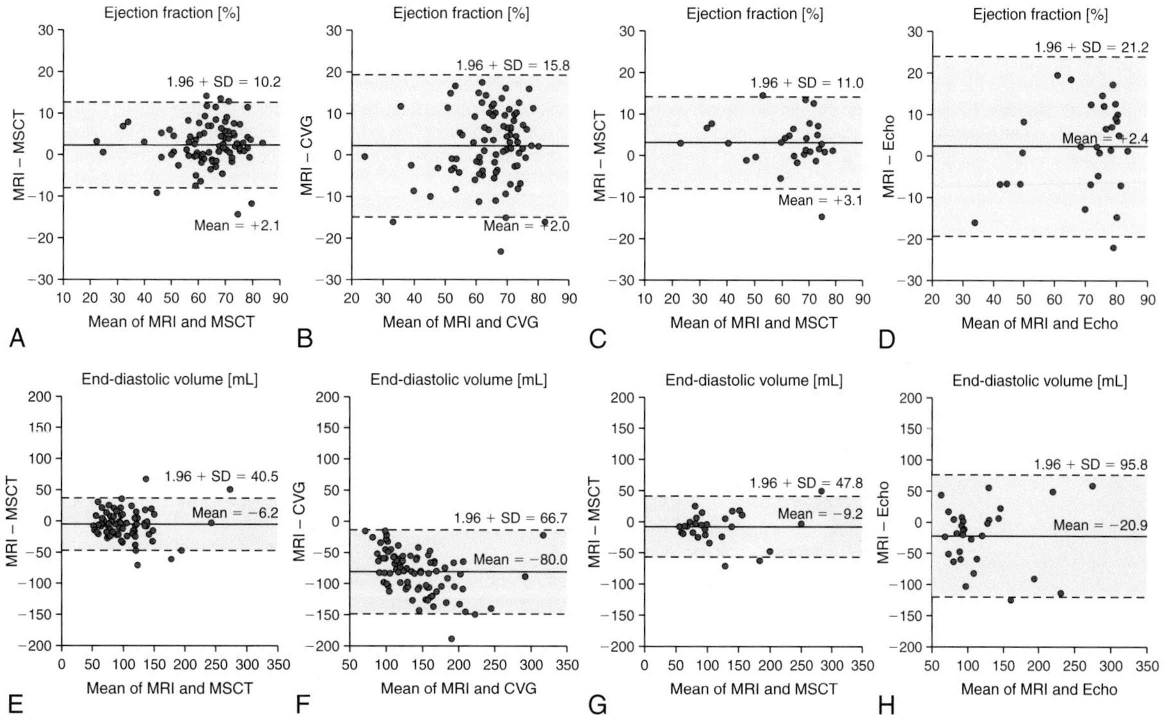

Figure 19-1. Assessment of ejection fraction: agreement between magnetic resonance imaging (MRI) and 16-slice multislice CT (MSCT) (**A**) and MRI and biplane cineventriculography (CVG) (**B**) in 88 patients. The agreement also is compared with the reference standard (MRI) for MSCT and transthoracic echocardiography (Echo) (**C** and **D**) in the subset of 30 patients who underwent echocardiography. The mean of the two methods compared is always plotted against the difference of the two. The *solid line* is the mean of the differences, whereas the *dashed lines* mark the limit of agreement (95% confidence intervals = 1.96 × SD) according to Bland and Altman. There were significantly larger limits of agreement for the comparison of CVG and Echo with MRI (**B** and **D**) than for the comparisons of MSCT with MRI (**A** and **C**). Agreement for assessment of end-diastolic volume between MRI and 16-slice MSCT (**E**) and MRI and CVG (**F**) in 88 patients. The agreement also is compared with the reference standard (MRI) for MSCT and Echo (**G** and **H**) in the subset of 30 patients according to Bland and Altman as described in Figure 20-13. There were significantly larger limits of agreement for the comparison of CVG and Echo with MRI (**F** and **H**) than for the comparisons of MSCT with MRI (**E** and **G**), and there was also a significantly larger overestimation of the end-diastolic volume with CVG than with MSCT (**E** and **F**).

Continued

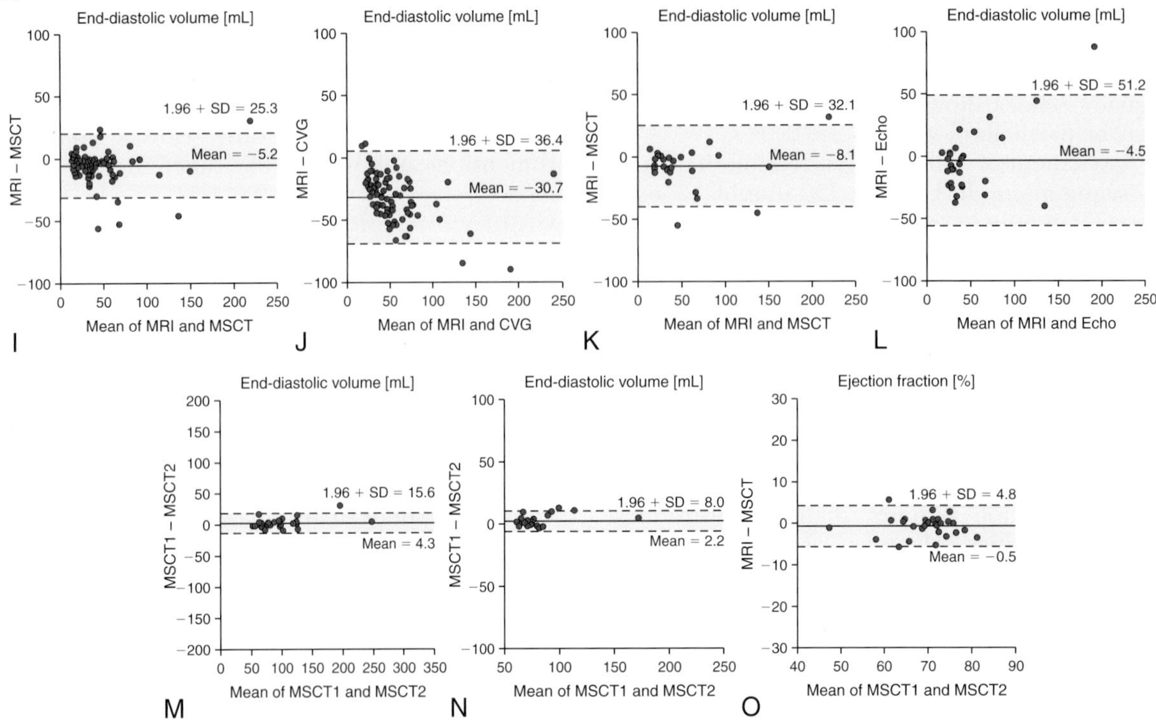

Figure 19-1, cont'd Agreement for assessment of end-systolic volume between MRI and 16-slice MSCT (**I**) and MRI and CVG (**J**) in 88 patients. The agreement is also compared with the reference standard (MRI) for MSCT and Echo (**K** and **L**) in the subset of 30 patients according to Bland and Altman as described in Figure 20-13. There were significantly larger limits of agreement for the comparison of CVG and Echo with MRI than for the comparisons of MSCT with MRI, and there was also a significantly larger overestimation of the end-systolic volume with CVG than with MSCT. Intraobserver agreement for assessment of ejection fraction (**M**), and end-systolic volume (**O**) with 16-slice MSCT in 29 patients randomly selected from the entire patient cohort. For all intraobserver analyses, the limits of agreement and the deviations from 0 were significantly smaller than for the comparison of MSCT with MRI (all $P < .004$) in the same 29 patients, demonstrating a low variability with MSCT. (Reprinted with permission from Dewey M, Muller M, Eddicks S, et al. Evaluation of global and regional left ventricular function with 16-slice computed tomography, biplane cineventriculography, and two-dimensional transthoracic echocardiography: comparison with magnetic resonance imaging. *J Am Coll Cardiol.* 2006;48(10):2034-2044.)

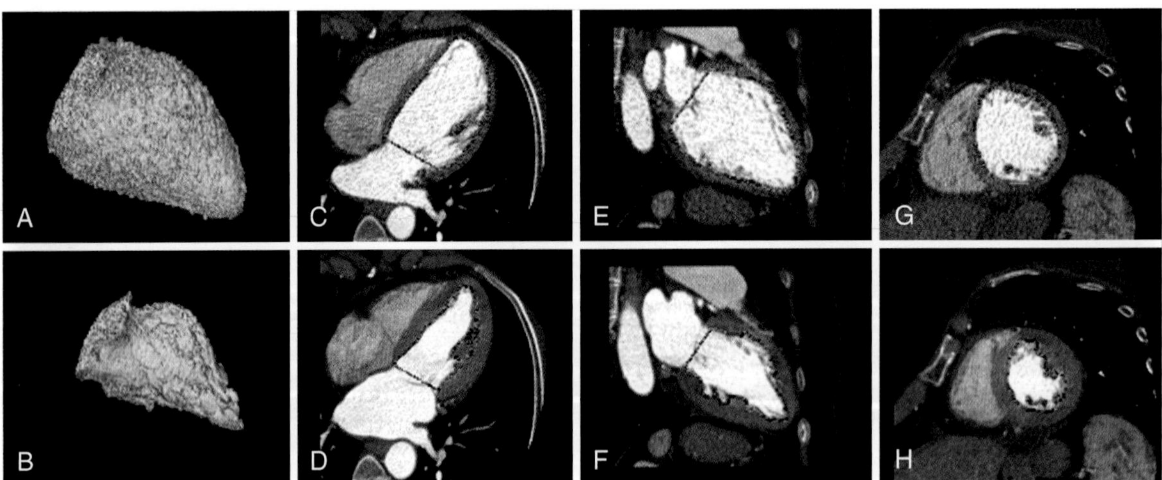

Figure 19-2. Automated cavitary delineation algorithms (unedited): diastole (**A, C, E, G**) and systole (**B, D, F, H**). Note the crisp delineation of the cavity/blood pool to the myocardium. **See Video 19-1.**

Figure 19-3. Multiple reconstructed images, helically acquired CT angiogram in patient with dilated cardiomyopathy pre-CRT therapy. **A,** Volume-rendered image. **B** through **D,** Automated planimetry of the LV blood volume. Because cardiac CT data sets were acquired in a four-dimensional isotropic fashion, reconstructions of various planes through the heart could easily be performed. Due to CT's high spatial resolution and high attenuation differences between the blood pool and myocardium, automated and semiautomatic segmentation was straightforward. This patient has a severely dilated left ventricle with an end-diastolic (ED) volume of 472 mL, indexed for body surface area to 248 mL/m^2. The left ventricular ejection fraction (LVEF) is severely decreased at 23%. ES, end-systole.

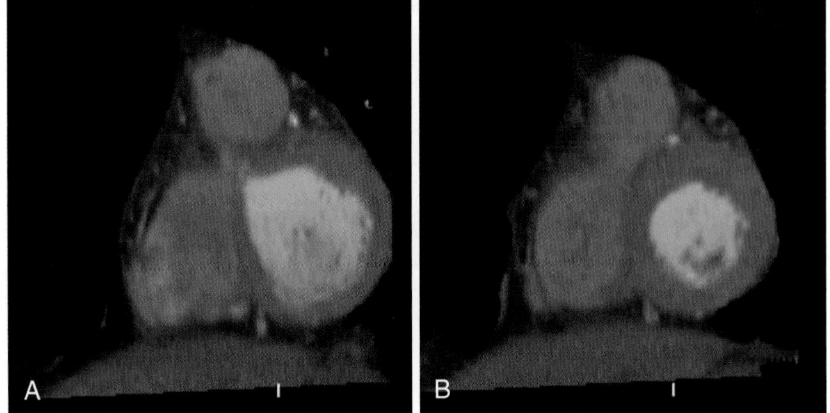

Figure 19-4. Reconstructed short-axis cine from a retrospective cardiac CT study shows an example of semi-automated left ventricular (LV) volume segmentation. Note that the mid- to distal septum demonstrates hypokinesis and corresponding hypodensity. **See Video 19-2.**

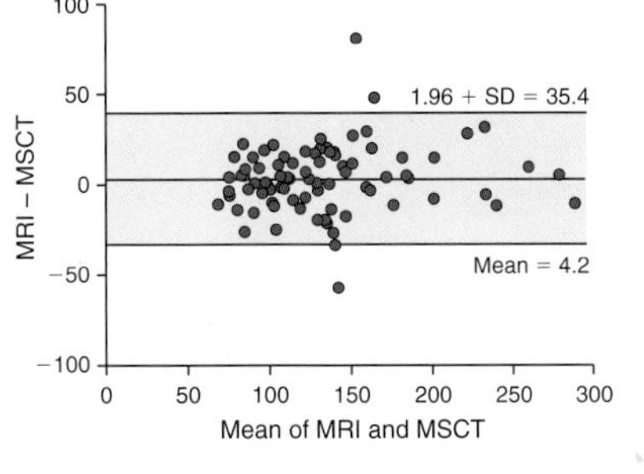

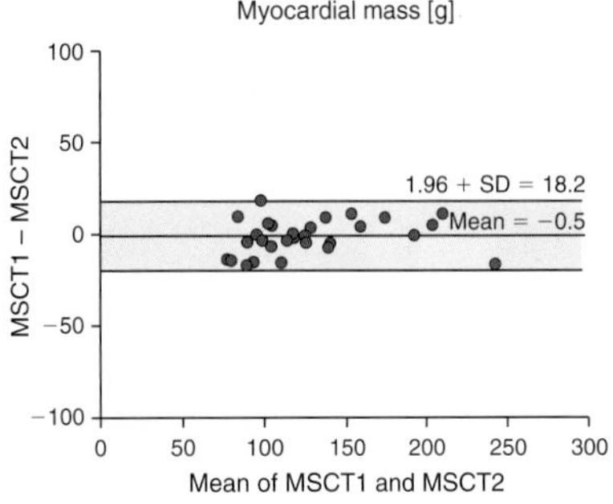

Figure 19-5. **A,** Agreement for assessment of myocardial mass between MRI and 16-slice multislice CT (MSCT). **B,** Intraobserver agreement for MSCT. (Reprinted with permission from Dewey M, Muller M, Eddicks S, et al. Evaluation of global and regional left ventricular function with 16-slice computed tomography, biplane cineventriculography, and two-dimensional transthoracic echocardiography: comparison with magnetic resonance imaging. *J Am Coll Cardiol.* 2006;48(10):2034-2044.)

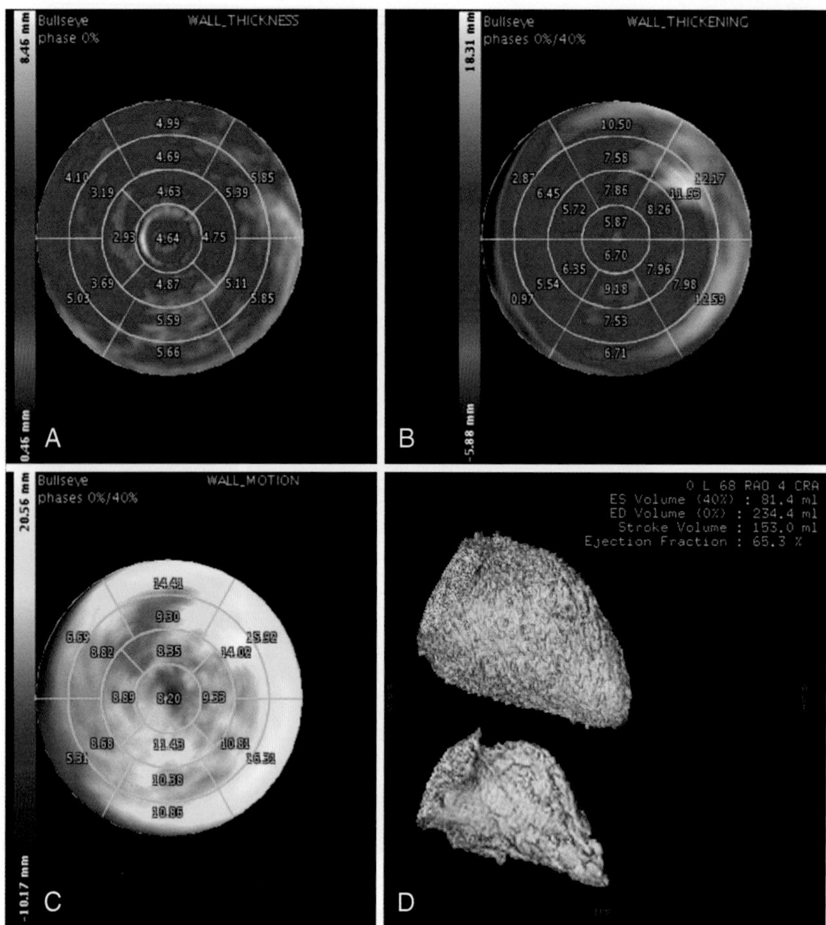

Figure 19-6. Automated calculation/plots of left ventricular wall thickness (**A**), left ventricular wall thickening (**B**), left ventricular wall motion (**C**), and left ventricular ejection fraction (**D**). 3D volume-rendered segmented reconstructions, in diastole (**D**, *upper image*: 234 mL) and in systole (**D**, *lower image*: 81 mL), yielding an ejection fraction of 6570. ED, end-diastolic; ES, end-systolic.

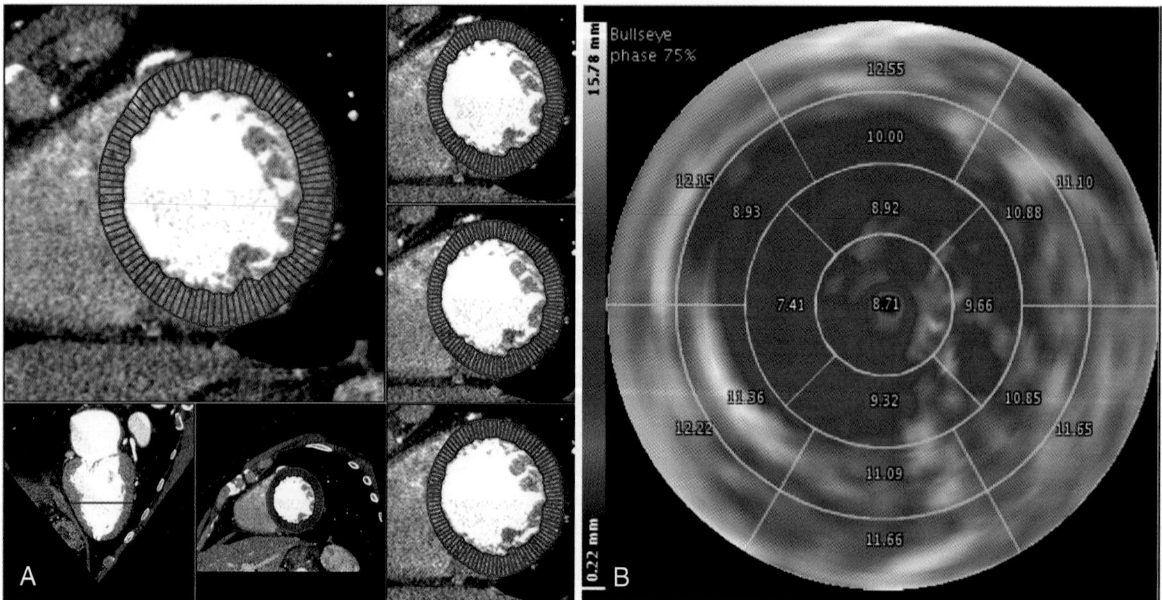

Figure 19-7. **A,** Automated quantification of left ventricular wall thickness. **B,** Segmented radial plot of wall thickness.

TABLE 19-1 Validation of 64-slice Cardiac CT Assessment of Left Ventricular Volumes and Ejection Fraction

AUTHOR	NO. OF PATIENTS	VALIDATION	BLAND-ALTMAN ANALYSIS: BIAS (95% LIMITS OF AGREEMENT)		
			LVEDV	LVESV	LVEF (%)
Schepis et al., 2006[6]	60 (known/ suspected CAD)	SPECT	34 mL (±52 mL)	9 mL (±32 mL)	1(±15)
Schlosser et al., 2007[7]	21 (suspected CAD)	CMR	19.9 mL (±20.3 mL)	13.4 mL ±10.3 mL	3.9 ±7.5
Wu et al., 2008[8]	63 (known/ suspected CAD)	CMR	−0.6 mL (±29.8 mL)	1.1 mL (±20.8 mL)	−0.2 (±8.2)
Nakamura et al., 2008[9]	71 (known/ suspected CAD)	CVG	5.4 mL (±56.1 mL)	7.8 mL (±29.4 mL)	−5.2 (±14.7)
Wu et al., 2008[10]	41 (referred for CT angiography)	CMR	−1.0 mL (±43.6 mL)	0.9 mL (±28.2 mL)	−0.1 (±12.0)
Abbara et al., 2008[11]	22 (SPECT within 3 months)	SPECT	—	—	0.0 (±12.5)
Busch et al., 2008[12] (dual-source CT)	15	CMR	3.7 mL (±49.9 mL)	−2.6 mL (±34.mL)	3.8 (±18.5)
Brodoefel et al., 2007[13] (dual-source CT)	20 (suspected/ known CAD)	CMR	−2.2 mL (±10 mL)	−1.4 mL (±5 mL)	0.7 (±5)
Bastarrika et al., 2008[14] (dual-source CT)	12 (heart transplant)	CMR	16.6 mL (±36.5 mL)	4.9 mL (±13.5 mL)	−0.3 (±6.2)
Spoeck et al., 2008[15]	20 (endoscopic CABG)	CVG	—	—	0.2 (±18.5%)

CABG, coronary artery bypass grafting; CAD, coronary artery disease; CMR, cardiac magnetic resonance; CVG, cineventriculography; LVEDV, left ventricular end-diastolic volume; LVEF, left ventricular ejection fraction; LVESV, left ventricular end-systolic volume; SPECT, single-photon emission computed tomography.

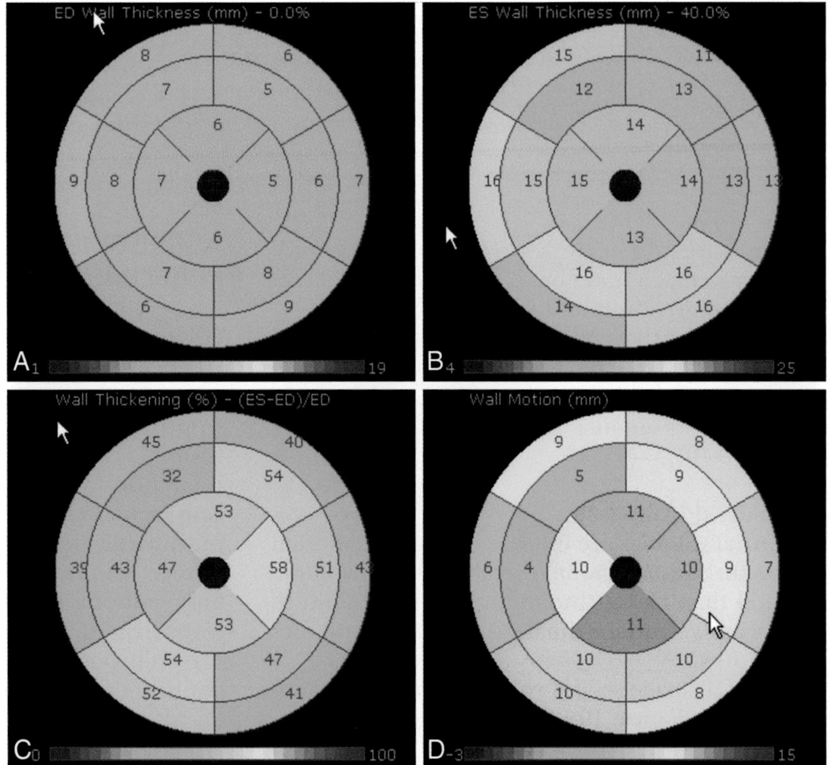

Figure 19-8. **A** and **B**, Plots of automatically traced left ventricular end-diastolic (ED) and end-systolic (ES) wall thicknesses. **C** and **D**, Plots of automatically traced and calculated left ventricular systolic wall thickening (%) and wall motion.

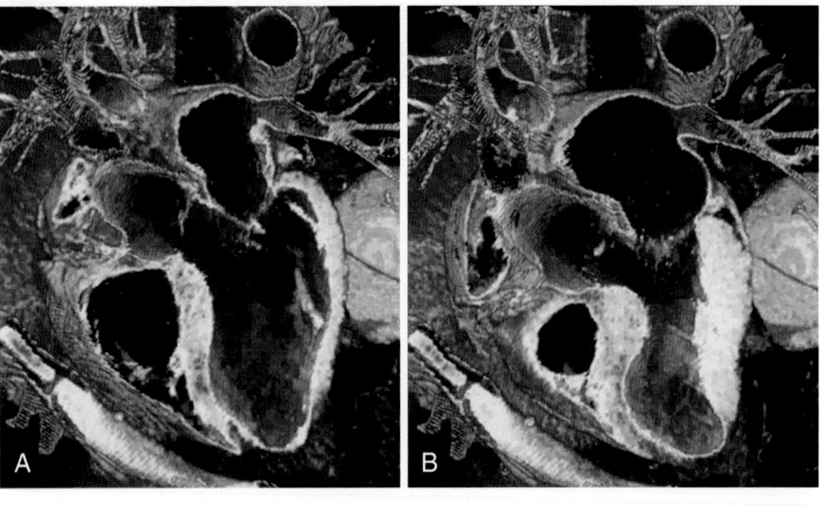

Figure 19-9. Three-dimensional volume-rendered views (three-chamber view) of diastole (**A**) and systole (**B**), demonstrating akinesis and an aneurysm of the distal anterior septum, apex, and inferior apex.

TABLE 19-2 Identification of Wall Motion Abnormalities by 64-Slice Cardiac CT Compared with Cardiac MR

	SENSITIVITY (%)	SPECIFICITY (%)	PPV (%)	NPV (%)
Hypokinesis	71	91	68	93
Akinesis	84	97	81	98

NPV, negative predictive value; PPV, positive predictive value.
Data from Sarwar A, Shapiro MD, Nasir K, et al: Evaluating global and regional left ventricular function in patients with reperfused acute myocardial infarction by 64-slice multidetector CT: a comparison to magnetic resonance imaging. *J Cardiovasc Comput Tomogr.* 2009;3(3):170-177.

TABLE 19-3 Right and Left Ventricular Volume Assessment by 16-Slice CT versus Cardiac MR

	END-DIASTOLIC VOLUME	END-SYSTOLIC VOLUME	EJECTION FRACTION	MASS
Left ventricle	$r = 0.97$	$r = 0.97$	$r = 0.97$	$r = 0.95$
Right ventricle	$r = 0.97$	$r = 0.94$	$r = 0.86$	

Data from Raman SV, Shah M, McCarthy B, Garcia A, Ferketich AK. Multi-detector row cardiac computed tomography accurately quantifies right and left ventricular size and function compared with cardiac magnetic resonance. *Am Heart J.* 2006;151(3):736-744.

by aggressive tube current modulation and low KV imaging so that a functional/retrospective data set can be acquired in under 6 mSv (Table 19-3).

For plots of the regression and limits of agreement of CCT determinations of RV volumes compared with those yielded from CMR, and for CCT images of RV volume chamber quantification, see Figure 19-10.

Left Atrial Volumes

Left atrial volumes are more accurately quantified by the three-dimensional threshold-based volume method than by biplane methods, which tend to significantly underestimate left atrial volumes (Table 19-4).[19]

For CCT images of LA volume chamber quantification, see Figure 19-11.

ASSESSMENT OF MYOCARDIAL PERFUSION

CT has been used to detect perfusion defects (seen as low-attenuation enhancement on acute arterial phase imaging) on first-pass imaging.[20] Approximately 1% of cardiac CT scans are performed during unsuspected acute myocardial infarction (MI).[21] Assessment of myocardial perfusion by contrast CT is experimental, and estimates of myocardial perfusion correlate with microsphere estimates of perfusion.[22] Lower kilovolts and smoother kernels are used. Nonperfused myocardium has a lower attenuation coefficient (i.e., it hypoenhances) than contrast-perfused and contrast-enhanced normal myocardium. Typically, an attenuation of 20 HU is used to distinguish

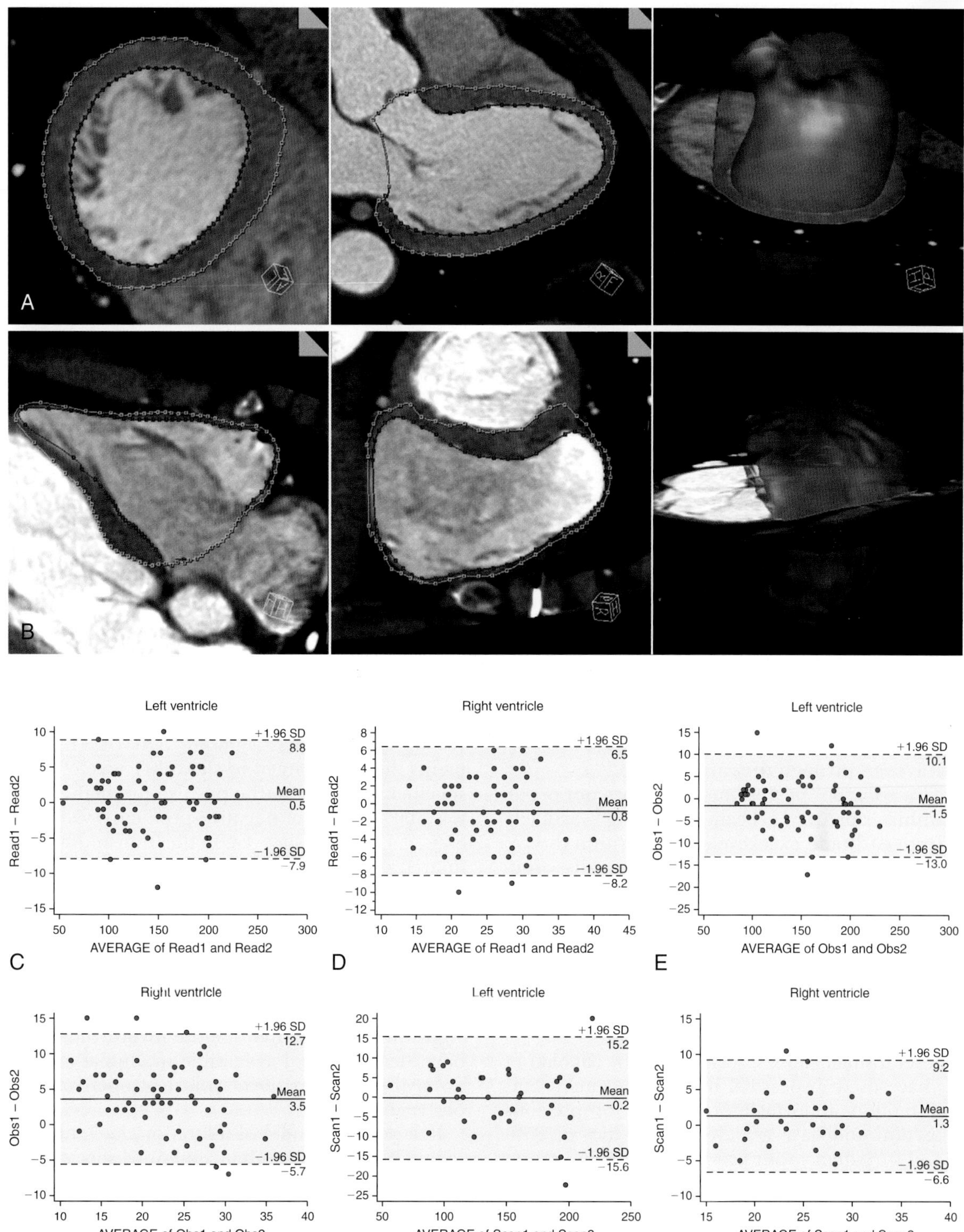

Figure 19-10. Left ventricular (LV; **A**) and right ventricular (RV; **B**) cavities are recognized semiautomatically. The software then determines the borders of the ventricular walls, which can be modified by the user. Note that the interventricular septum must be excluded from the RV wall manually. Plots: Bland-Altman plots of intra-observer (**C** and **D**), inter-observer (**E** and **F**), and inter-test differences (**G** and **H**). (Reprinted with permission from Schwarz F, Takx R, Schoepf UJ, et al. Reproducibility of left and right ventricular mass measurements with cardiac CT. *J Cardiovasc Comput Tomogr.* 2011;5(5):317-324.)

TABLE 19-4 Left Atrial Volumes by Three-Dimensional Threshold-based Volume Method versus Two-Plane Methods

			AREA	
	3D THRESHOLD-BASED VOLUME	***P* VALUE**	**LENGTH METHOD**	**PROLATE ELLIPSOID METHOD**
Interobserver variability	8%	<.001	13%	16%
Mean LA volume	Maximum: 90 ± 25 mL Minimum: 53 ± 18 mL			
Difference vs 3D threshold method (maximum and minimum LA volumes)		.001	−17%, −22%	−43%, −46%

3D, Three-dimensional; LA, left atrium

Data from Mahabadi AA, Samy B, Seneviratne SK, et al. Quantitative assessment of left atrial volume by electrocardiographic-gated contrast-enhanced multidetector computed tomography. *J Cardiovasc Comput Tomogr.* 2009;3(2):80-87.

normal from hypodense myocardium, because the attenuation coefficients of normal myocardium and hypodense myocardium typically are 102 ± 9 HU and 30 ± 11 HU, respectively.

Drastic changes in myocardial perfusion, as seen in acute infarction, can be imaged, both experimentally and clinically.[23,24]

An apparent perfusion defect is more likely to be true if:

- It is associated with a wall motion abnormality whose severity corresponds to the extent of hypoperfusion.
- It is seen through the cardiac cycle.
- The apparent perfusion defect does not occur within apparent "beam-hardening" artifacts from early and excessive contrast within the LV or the descending aorta, the chest wall—especially the anterior ribs, as well as motion-related artifacts. The effects of this attenuating artifact is to decrease myocardial attenuation, often in two specific locations: the basal inferolateral wall (due to high-density contrast in the adjacent descending aorta), and the antero-apical LV wall (due to the anterior ribs).

Several small studies, such as that by Nikolau et al., have used myocardial hypoenhancement and wall motion abnormalities as signs of previous infarction and have achieved sensitivities of 85% (23 of 27 patients with previous infarction among 106 patients).[25] Other studies, such as that by Gosalia et al., have used hypoenhancement alone and achieved sensitivity of 83%, specificity of 95%, positive predictive value of 94%, and negative predictive value of 86%.[26] Much larger studies are needed.

For examples of CCT images of myocardial perfusion defects, plots, and mapping, see Figures 19-12 through 19-18.

Myocardial Viability

CCT is following the (considerable) lead of MRI in the use of models of the kinetics of contrast effect to establish early hypoenhancement and late or delayed hyperenhancement dynamics, as with gadolinium. Preliminary and limited studies suggest that correlation with MRI is good, and follow-up studies in patients have validated that CCT demonstrates excellent agreement with CMR for assessing infarct size and transmurality/viability after acute MI (Table 19-5).[27]

Using the criteria of no hyperenhancement or only subendocardial hyperenhancement to predict viability, where there was a high degree (97%) of agreement, among 576 (A.S.E.) segments the sensitivity of 64-slice CCT was 92%, the specificity was 100%, the positive predictive value was 100%, and the negative predictive value was 85%.[28] Using 64-slice CCT, the transmurality of infarction (when >75%), as depicted by CT enhancement, predicts remodeling.[29] Infarcted myocardium typically has twice the attenuation (peak attenuation) when scanned about 5 minutes after contrast infusion.[30,31] The spatial extent of acute and healed infarction can be determined by CCT.[30] Use of a semi-automated signal intensity algorithm (>2 SD SI vs. remote myocardium) has been demonstrated as feasible in animal models, as has been the pattern typical of microvascular obstruction.[31]

In a porcine model of infarction, late-enhancement CMR and late-enhancement 64-slice cardiac CT demonstrated excellent correlation with tetrazolium staining for infarction (Table 19-6).[32]

For CCT images of myocardial late enhancement, see Figure 19-19.

SPECT, SPECT versus CTCA, Hybrid SPECT-CT, and PET-CT Systems

The comparative value of CT coronary angiography (CTCA) versus myocardial perfusion imaging (MPI) is not fully established. When compared to each other, they appear to afford similar overall event rates. Among 541 patients referred for coronary

Text continued on page 303

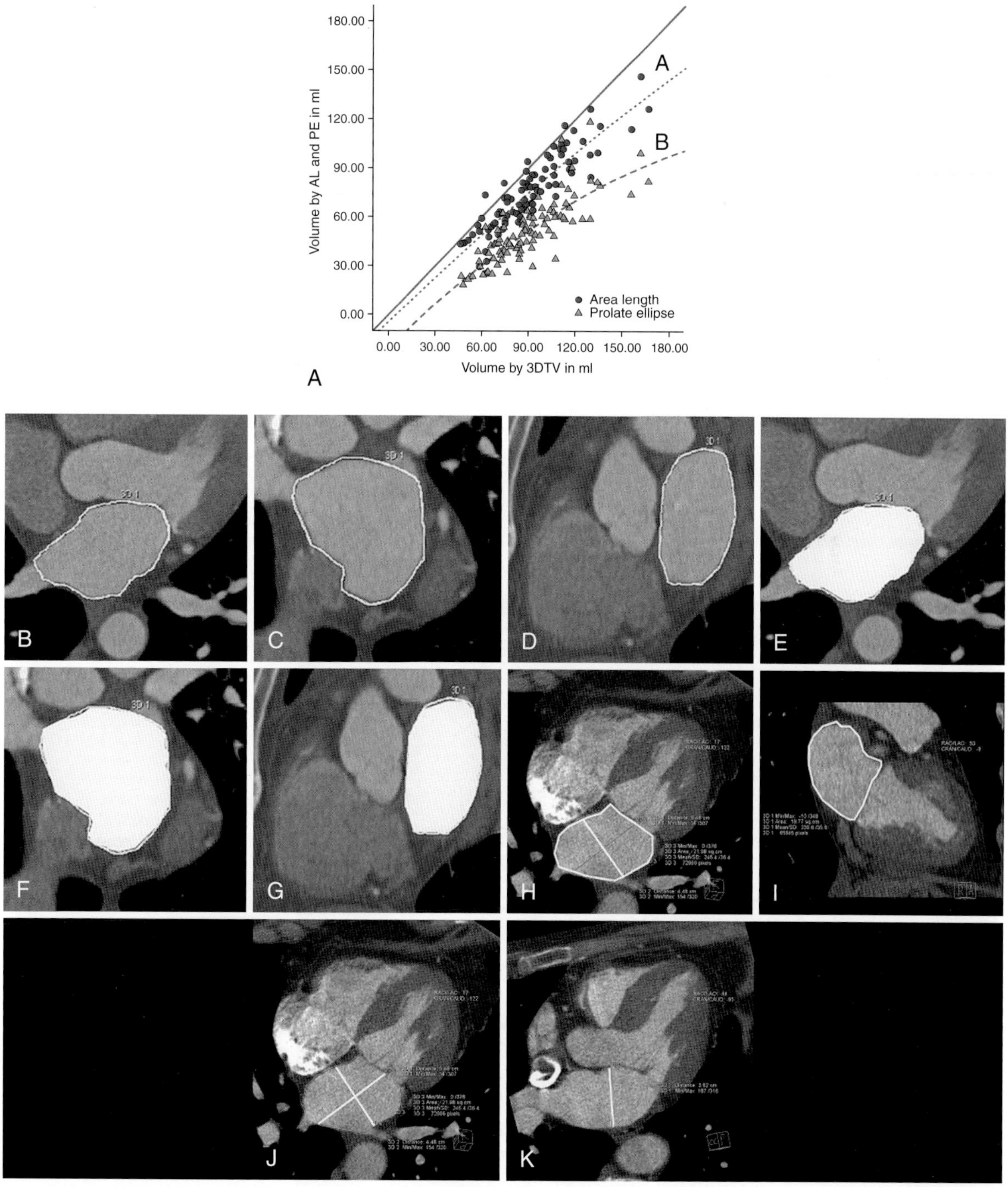

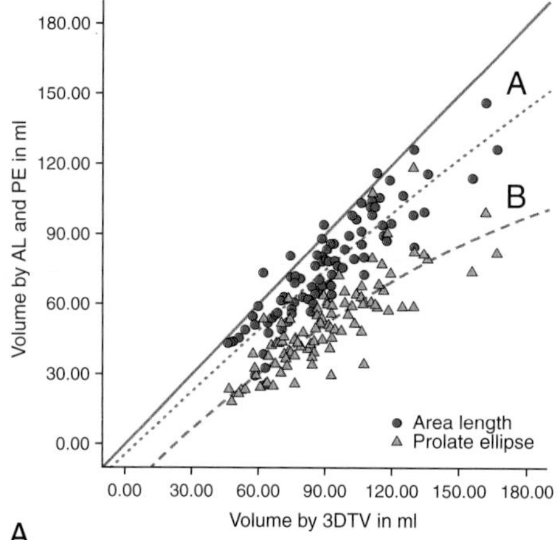

Figure 19-11. A, End-diastolic volumes of the left atrium (LA) by three-dimensional (3D) threshold-based volume (TV) compared with two-dimensional (2D)-based area length (AL) and prolate ellipse (PE) methods showing significant underestimation of LA volume by the 2D methods compared with 3D TV ($P < .001$ for both). Boundaries of the left atrium are traced in an axial slice (**B**) and the 3D reconstruction of the region of interest in coronal (**C**) and sagittal (**D**) views. After manual delineation, the volume is automatically calculated by summation of pixels inside the region of interest within a window width of 100 to 1000 Hounsfield units (*white pixels,* **E** through **G**). **H** through **K,** LA volume by area length method and prolate ellipse technique. **H** and **I,** For area length, the area of the left atrium was determined by manual drawings of the boundaries in both four- and two-chamber views. **H,** The anterior-posterior diameter of the left atrium was measured in four-chamber view. For prolate ellipse, the anterior-posterior and the medial-lateral diameter of the left atrium in four-chamber view (**J**) and the anterior-posterior diameter in three-chamber view (**K**) were measured. (Reprinted with permission from Mahabadi AA, Samy B, Seneviratne SK, et al. Quantitative assessment of left atrial volume by electrocardiographic-gated contrast-enhanced multidetector computed tomography. *J Cardiovasc Comput Tomogr.* 2009;3(2):80-87.)

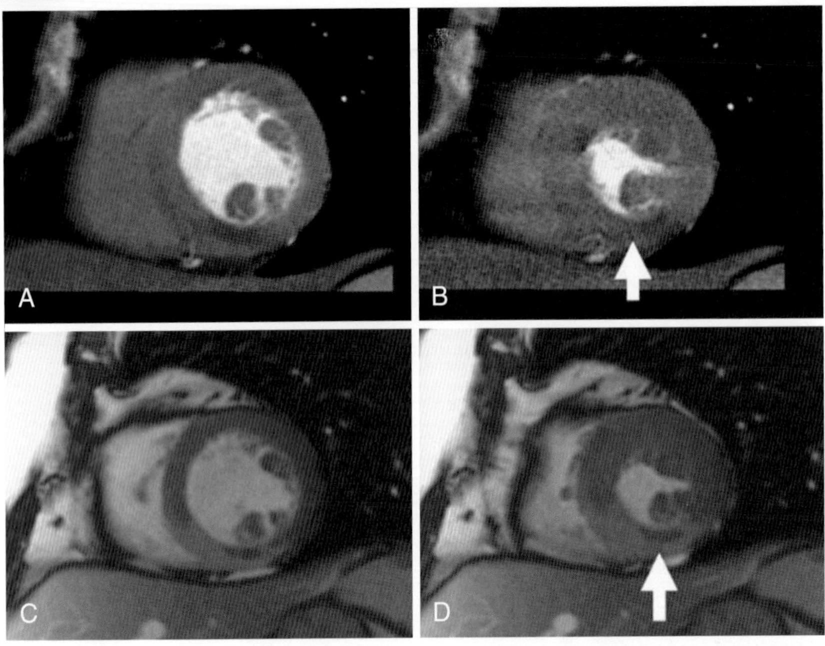

Figure 19-12. Gated cardiac CT scans (**A** and **B**) and cardiac MRI images (**C** and **D**). **A** and **C,** Diastole. **B** and **D,** Systole. Note the area of inferior hypokinesis on both, and of lower attenuation on CT scanning (*white arrow*) and lower signal on steady-state free precession (SSFP) cine images (*white arrow*). (Reprinted with permission from Sarwar A, Shapiro MD, Nasir K, et al. Evaluating global and regional left ventricular function in patients with reperfused acute myocardial infarction by 64-slice multidetector CT: a comparison to magnetic resonance imaging. *J Cardiovasc Comput Tomogr.* 2009;3(3):170-177.)

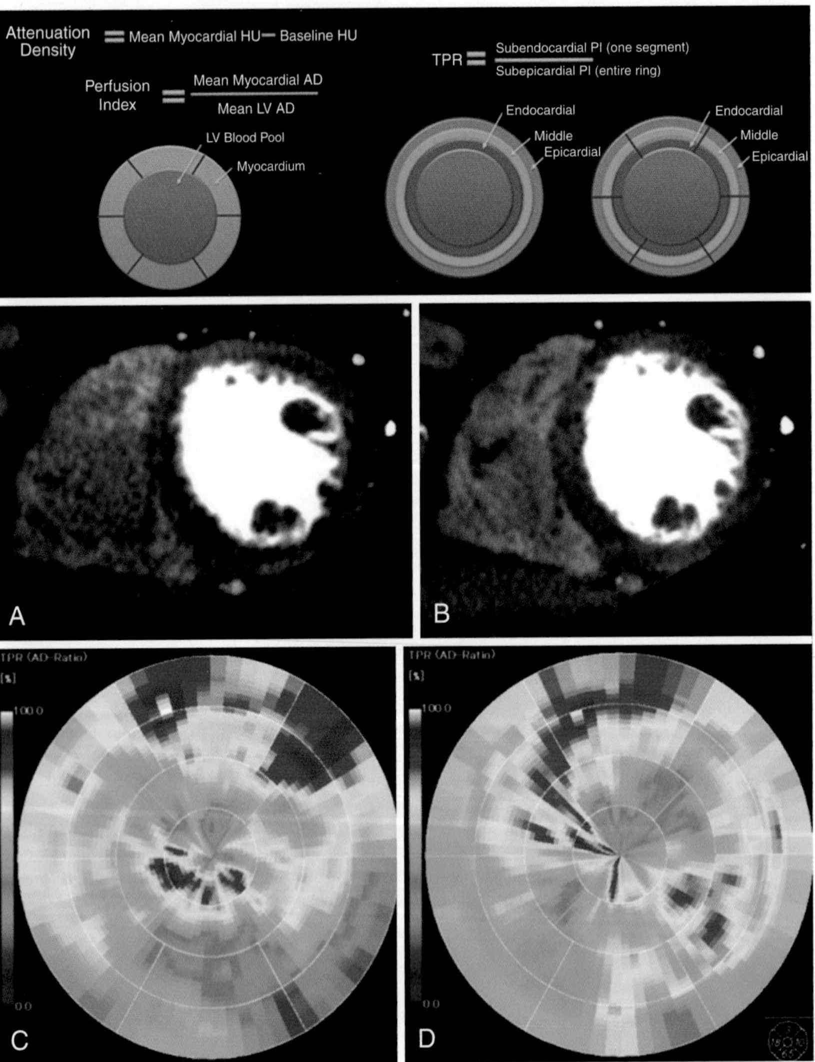

Figure 19-13. Top panel, A transmural perfusion ratio is calculated as the subendocardial attenuation density (AD) over the subepicardial attenuation density, where subendocardial attenuation density is the sector-specific subendocardial attenuation, and the subepicardial attenuation density is the mean attenuation of the entire subepicardial layer of any given short-axis slice. **A** and **B**, First pass contrast-enhanced CT scan short-axis images reveal reduced subendocardial attenuation of the basal anterior wall. **C** and **D,** Color coding and polar map demonstration of differences in attenuation within the myocardium. The same data set has been processed using Vital Images software (Minnetonka, MN), and advantage Windows General Electric software. These images in a patient with an occlusion of the left anterior descending artery (LAD) demonstrate different methodologies of color coding contrast attenuation differences within the myocardium. Polar maps based on a 17-segment American Heart Association model also visually help to characterize segments of decreased myocardial attenuation, which acts as a surrogate marker for decreased myocardial perfusion. In this case a large region of altered attenuation in the anterior wall is noted. These images also demonstrate the ongoing challenges of CT perfusion imaging, where motion artifact and beam-hardening artifact can cause variations in attenuation of the myocardium. LV, left ventricle; PI, pixel intensity.

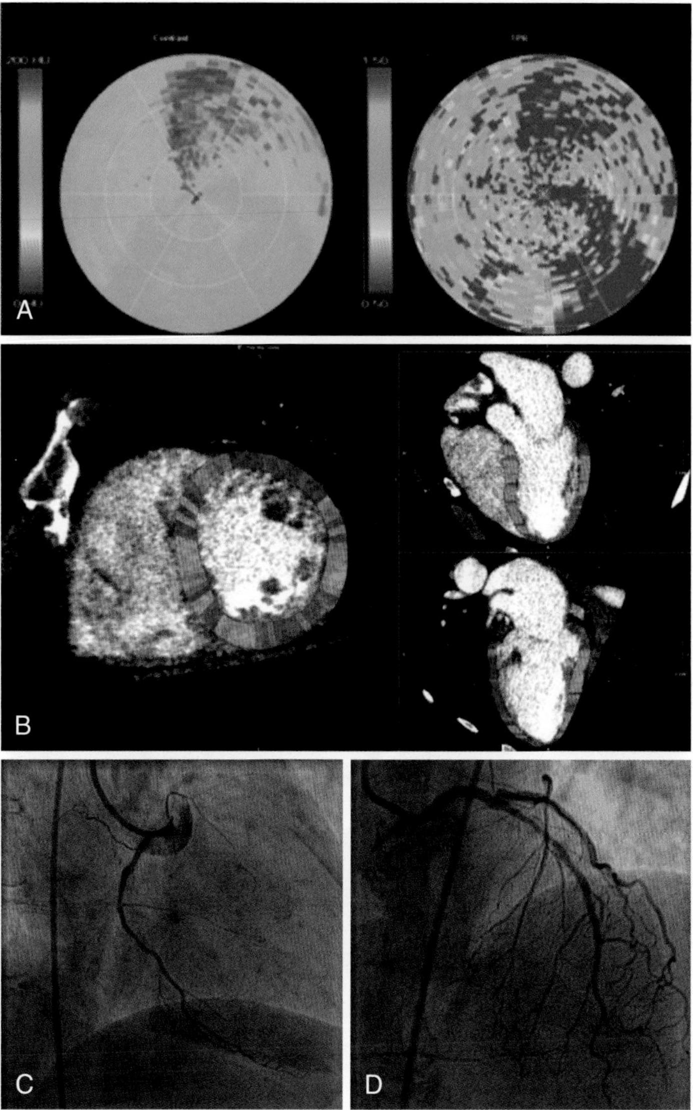

Figure 19-14. Myocardial perfusion. **A,** Polar maps at rest and with stress. **B,** Plots of transmural myocardial perfusion ratio (subendocardial attenuation density over subepicardial perfusion density). Note the lesser transmyocardial perfusion ratio of the inferoposterior wall. **C** and **D,** Right coronary artery occlusion at the mid-portion, responsible for the observed CT findings.

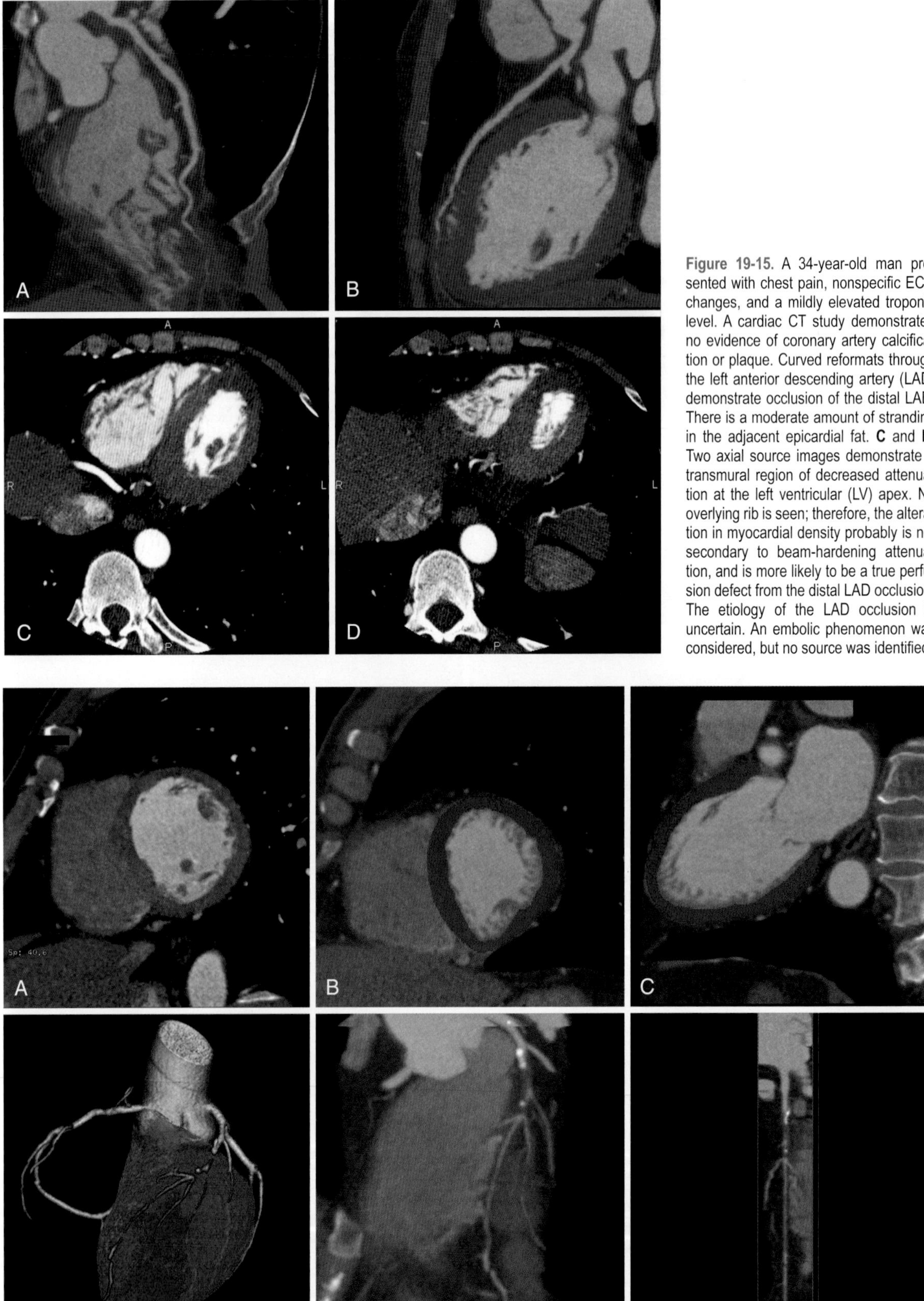

Figure 19-15. A 34-year-old man presented with chest pain, nonspecific ECG changes, and a mildly elevated troponin level. A cardiac CT study demonstrated no evidence of coronary artery calcification or plaque. Curved reformats through the left anterior descending artery (LAD) demonstrate occlusion of the distal LAD. There is a moderate amount of stranding in the adjacent epicardial fat. **C** and **D,** Two axial source images demonstrate a transmural region of decreased attenuation at the left ventricular (LV) apex. No overlying rib is seen; therefore, the alteration in myocardial density probably is not secondary to beam-hardening attenuation, and is more likely to be a true perfusion defect from the distal LAD occlusion. The etiology of the LAD occlusion is uncertain. An embolic phenomenon was considered, but no source was identified.

Figure 19-16. Multiple images in a patient presenting with chest pain. **A,** A short-axis reconstruction of the CT angiogram data set demonstrates low attenuation within the anterior wall. **B–D,** Color coding of the attenuation differences within the left ventricular myocardium demonstrates a geographic area of low attenuation within the anterior wall subtended by the left anterior descending artery (LAD). Low-attenuation areas (color-coded in blue) within the basal anterior and inferior walls represent artifact primarily from beam hardening. The basal inferior wall is an especially common location for beam-hardening attenuation artifact, which occurs due to high-density contrast within the descending thoracic aorta, which resides adjacent to the basal inferior wall (**C**). **E** and **F,** Complex high-grade stenosis/occlusion of the mid-LAD just distal to the takeoff of the D1 branch. The mid- to distal LAD does reconstitute, presumably by collaterals. A linear defect in the distal LAD represents a registration artifact in this prospectively acquired study.

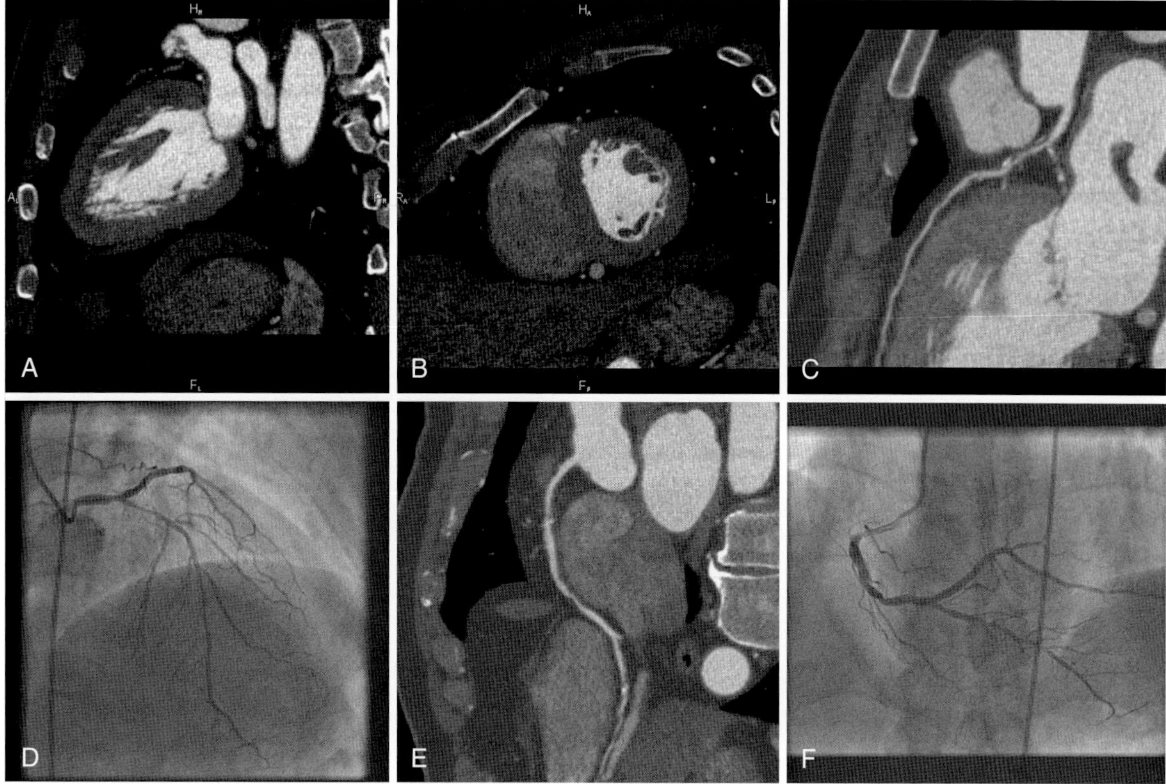

Figure 19-17. A 52-year-old man presented with acute chest pain, no ECG changes, and borderline troponin rise. **A** and **B,** Reconstructed long- and short-axis views through the left ventricle demonstrate a moderate-sized subendocardial hypodense zone within the anterolateral wall and a subtle similar hypodense zone in the inferior wall. There was no evidence of fatty metaplasia in these regions on the noncontrast calcium study, suggesting that these represent zones of hypoperfusion. CT angiographic (CTA) images demonstrate a severe proximal stenosis in the left anterior descending artery (LAD; **C** and **D**) and a tight stenosis in the mid–patent ductus arteriosus (PDA; **E** and **F**).

angiography who also underwent MPI and 64-slice CTCA, the annualized hard event rate (all cause mortality and nonfatal infarction) over a median of 672 days of follow-up were as presented in Table 19-7.[33]

There appears to be synergism between 64-CTCA and MPI results that improves prediction ($P < .005$).[33] This has been illustrated in a study of 180 patients presenting with chest pain who underwent both 64-slice CTCA and MPI; normal MPI and interpretable CTCA scans occurred in 97 patients. Among these normal MPI scans, certain coronary artery disease (CAD) patterns were identified, establishing that a normal MPI can be associated with a wide range of underlying CAD (Table 19-8).[34]

Hybrid single-photon emission CT (SPECT)-CT and positron emission tomography (PET)-CT scanning systems are able to obtain PET and CT scans with a very short interval between scans, using first PET and then CCT. PET and CT scans are obtained sequentially, not simultaneously, and then are superimposed after acquisition to facilitate anatomic determination of PET abnormalities. This has not yet been clearly shown to be superior to non-CT image superimposition, however.

The problem of breast and diaphragmatic attenuation of cardiac imaging, and also of liver and gut counts superimposed onto cardiac images, may be amenable to "correction" based on tissue depth and other details determined from the CT scan, but this also has yet to be established (Table 19-9).

CARDIAC CT PROTOCOL POINTS

- To evaluate systolic function, helical/retrospective scanning is needed.
- To evaluate myocardial perfusion:
  - Follow standard protocol for CCT.
  - Ensure review of noncontrast images to exclude the presence of fatty metaplasia.
- To evaluate delayed enhancement:
  - Obtain delayed (second) acquisition at 5 to 10 minutes after contrast administration. Slice thickness can be increased to 3 mm and kVp reduced (80–100 kVp).
- See Table 19-10.

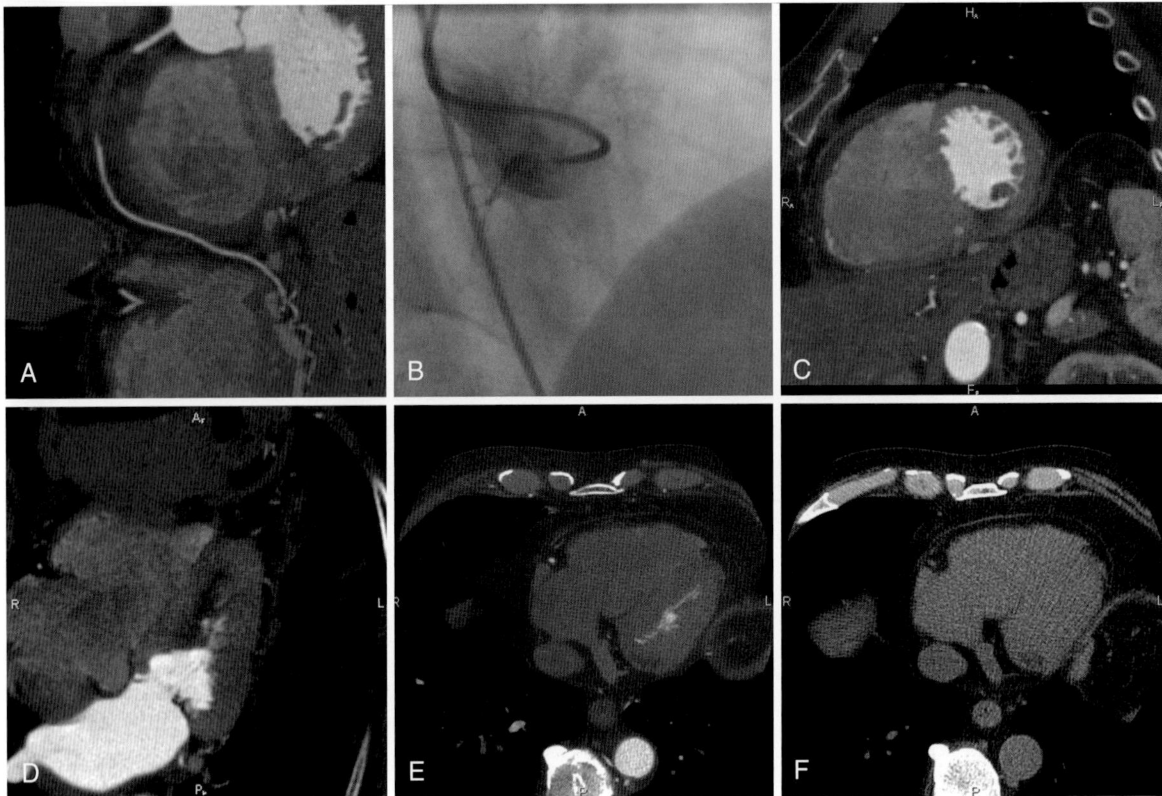

Figure 19-18. **A** through **D,** A 74-year-old woman presented with acute chest pain and borderline troponin rise. CT angiography (**A**) and corresponding conventional angiography (**B**) demonstrate an occlusion in the proximal right coronary artery. Reconstructed short- (**C**) and long-axis (**D**) left ventricular images demonstrate hypodensity in the basal to mid-inferoseptum, consistent with a perfusion defect. Coronary angiography demonstrated a complete occlusion of the right coronary artery. **E** and **F,** A 68-year-old man presented with atypical chest pain and an abnormal nuclear medicine study. Contrast-enhanced CTA images demonstrate an area of decreased attenuation within the basal inferolateral wall. Although this mimics a regional perfusion defect, the precontrast calcium score image demonstrates fatty attenuation as the cause of the apparent hypoperfusion zone.

TABLE 19-5 Myocardial Viability by CMR and CCT

	LE-CMR	LE-CCT	EARLY PERFUSION DEFICIT CCT
Mean infarct size	31.2 ± 22.5%	33.3 ± 23.8%	24.5 ± 18.3%

LE-CCT, late enhancement cardiac CT; LE-CMR, late enhancement cardiac magnetic resonance imaging.

Data from Mahnken AH, Koos R, Katoh M, et al. Assessment of myocardial viability in reperfused acute myocardial infarction using 16-slice computed tomography in comparison to magnetic resonance imaging. *J Am Coll Cardiol.* 2005;45(12):2042-2047.

TABLE 19-6 Experimental Correlation of Myocardial Infarction Late Enhancement by CMR and by CCT

PARAMETER	LE-CMR	LE-CCT
Correlation		
Infarct size with TTC	r^2 = 0.96; P <.001	r^2 = 0.93; P <.001
With LE-CCT	r^2 = 0.96; P <.001	
Signal difference of infarcted myocardium versus remote myocardium	554 ± 156%	191 ± 18%

LE-CCT, late enhancement cardiac CT; LE-CMR, late enhancement cardiac magnetic resonance imaging; TTC, triphenyltetrazolium chloride.
Data from Baks T, Cademartiri F, Moelker AD, et al. Multislice computed tomography and magnetic resonance imaging for the assessment of reperfused acute myocardial infarction. *J Am Coll Cardiol.* 2006;48(1):144-152.

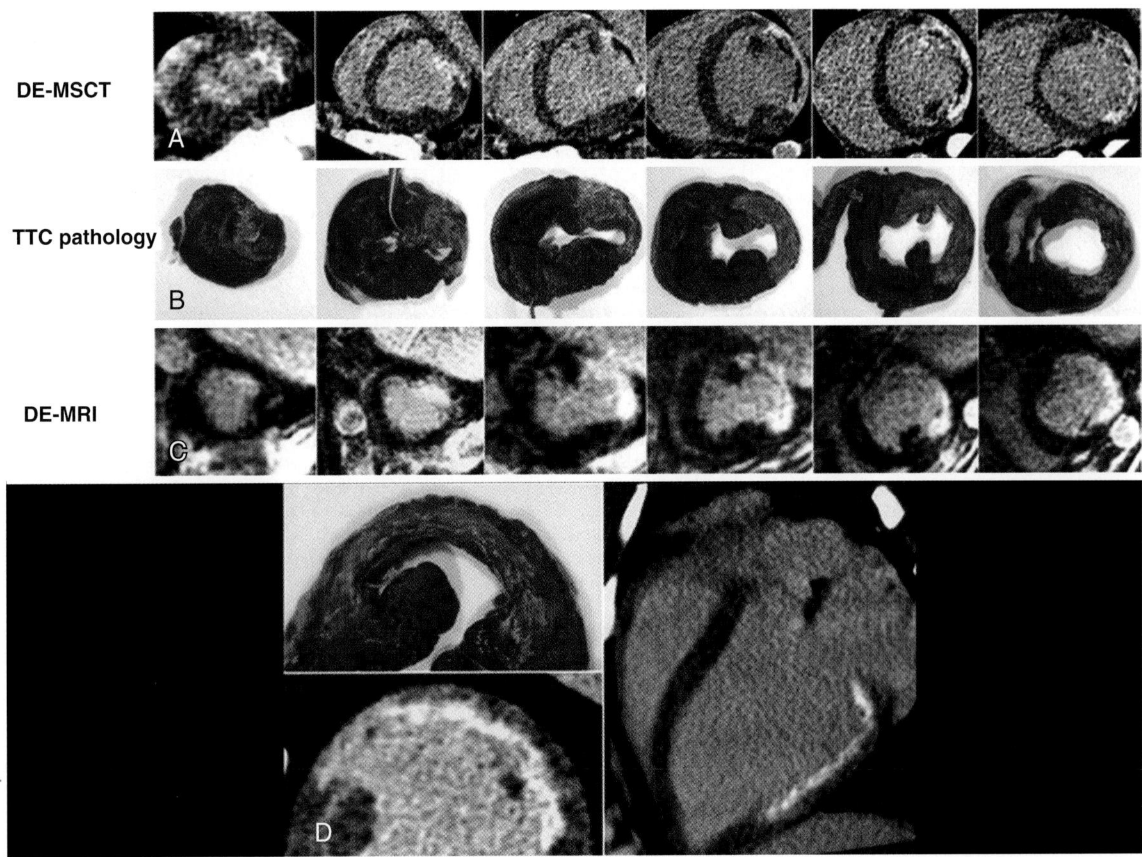

Figure 19-19. Acute reperfused myocardial infarction can be assessed accurately with delayed-enhancement multislice CT (DE-MSCT) (**A**) and delayed-enhancement magnetic resonance imaging (DE-MRI) (**C**) compared with postmortem triphenyltetrazolium chloride (TTC) pathology (**B**). The left ventricle is shown from base to apex. The MSCT images represent 1-mm slices compared with the photographed TTC pathology slices and the 8-mm MRI slices. **D,** In this pig with subendocardial infarction, the transmural differentiation of viable and nonviable myocardium is demonstrated with DE-MSCT in short-and long-axis views with TTC pathology as standard of reference.

Continued

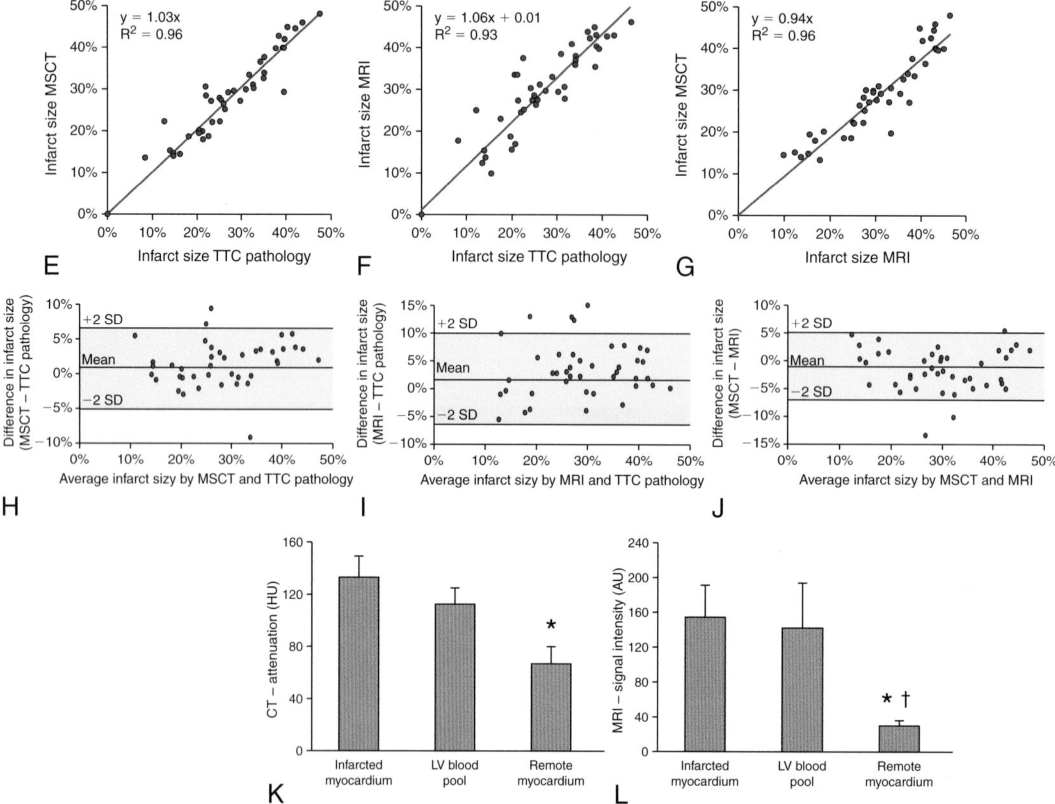

Figure 19-19, cont'd **E** through **G,** The relation between infarct size assessed with DE-MSCT, DE-MRI, and postmortem TTC pathology. **H** through **J,** Bland-Altman analyses show the excellent agreement between infarct size assessed with DE-MSCT, DE-MRI, and postmortem TTC pathology. **K** and **L,** Mean CT attenuation value for infarcted myocardium is significantly higher compared with noninfarcted myocardium. Mean magnetic resonance (MR) signal intensity value of infarcted myocardium is significantly higher compared with noninfarcted myocardium. *$P < .001$ compared with infracted myocardium; $P < .001$ compared with left ventricular (LV) blood pool. (Reprinted with permission from Baks T, Cademartiri F, Moelker AD, et al. Multislice computed tomography and magnetic resonance imaging for the assessment of reperfused acute myocardial infarction. *J Am Coll Cardiol.* 2006;48(1):144-152.)

TABLE 19-7 CT Coronary Angiography versus Myocardial Perfusion Imaging

	ANNUALIZED HARD EVENT RATES (%)
CTCA negative (≤50% stenosis)	1.8
CTCA positive (≤50% stenosis)	4.8
MPI Negative (SSS<4)	1.1
MPI Positive (SSS>4)	3.8

CTCA, computed tomographic coronary angiography; MPI, myocardial perfusion imaging.
Data from van Werkhoven JM, Schuijf JD, Gaemperli O, et al. Prognostic value of multislice computed tomography and gated single-photon emission computed tomography in patients with suspected coronary artery disease. *J Am Coll Cardiol.* 2009;53(7):623-632.

TABLE 19-8 Underlying Coronary Artery Disease Associated with a Normal Myocardial Perfusion Scan

Normal/no CAD	39%
Nonsignificant CAD (<50% stenosis)	38%
Significant CAD (>50% stenosis)	19%
Significant CAD (>50% stenosis); high risk: LMS	2%
Significant CAD (>50% stenosis); high risk: 3VD	2%

CAD, coronary artery disease; LMS, left main stem; 3VD, three-vessel disease.

TABLE 19-9 CT Coronary Angiography versus Hybrid Single-Photon Emission Computed Tomography

	NO. OF PATIENTS	SENSITIVITY (%)	SPECIFICITY (%)	PPV (%)	NPV (%)
CTCA	56 patients; 224 coronary segments; 23% excluded from analysis	96	63	31	99
Hybrid SPECT-CT		96	95	77	99

CTCA, computed tomographic coronary angiography; NPV, negative predictive value; PPV, positive predictive value.
Data from Rispler S, Keidar Z, Ghersin E, et al. Integrated single-photon emission computed tomography and computed tomography coronary angiography for the assessment of hemodynamically significant coronary artery lesions. *J Am Coll Cardiol.* 2007;49(10):1059-1067.

TABLE 19-10 ACCF 2010 Appropriateness Criteria for the Use of Cardiac Computed Tomography to Evaluate Ventricular Function

	APPROPRIATENESS RATING	INDICATION	MEDIAN SCORE
Evaluation of cardiac structure and function—evaluation of ventricular morphology and systolic function	Appropriate	Evaluation of left ventricular function Following acute MI or in HF patients Inadequate images from other noninvasive methods	7
		Quantitative evaluation of right ventricular function	7
		Assessment of right ventricular morphology Suspected arrhythmogenic right ventricular dysplasia	7
	Uncertain	Assessment of myocardial viability Prior to myocardial revascularization for ischemic left ventricular systolic dysfunction Other imaging modalities are inadequate or contraindicated	5
	Inappropriate	None listed	

HF, heart failure; MI, myocardial infraction.
Data from Taylor AJ, Cerqueira M, Hodgson JM, et al. ACCF/SCCT/ACR/AHA/ASE/ASNC/NASCI/SCAI/SCMR 2010 appropriate use criteria for cardiac computed tomography. A report of the American College of Cardiology Foundation Appropriate Use Criteria Task Force, the Society of Cardiovascular Computed Tomography, the American College of Radiology, the American Heart Association, the American Society of Echocardiography, the American Society of Nuclear Cardiology, the North American Society for Cardiovascular Imaging, the Society for Cardiovascular Angiography and Interventions, and the Society for Cardiovascular Magnetic Resonance. *J Am Coll Cardiol.* 2010;56(22):1864-1894.

References

1. Halliburton SS. Measurement of left ventricular volume and ejection fraction with computed tomography: small steps toward clinical utility. *J Cardiovasc Comput Tomogr.* 2008;2:231-233.
2. Bardo DME, Kachenoura N, Newby B, Lang RM, Mor-Avi V. Multidetector computed tomography evaluation of left ventricular volumes: sources of error and guidelines for their minimization. *J Cardiovasc Comput Tomogr.* 2008;2:222-230.
3. Papavassiliu T, Kuhl HP, Schroder M, et al. Effect of endocardial trabeculae on left ventricular measurements and measurement reproducibility at cardiovascular MR imaging. *Radiol.* 2005; 236(1):57-64.
4. Weinsaft JW, Cham MD, Janik M, et al. Left ventricular papillary muscles and trabeculae are significant determinants of cardiac MRI volumetric measurements: effects on clinical standards in patients with advanced systolic dysfunction. *Int J Cardiol.* 2008; 126(3):359-365.
5. Olivotto I, Maron MS, Autore C, et al. Assessment and significance of left ventricular mass by cardiovascular magnetic resonance in hypertrophic cardiomyopathy. *J Am Coll Cardiol.* 2008;52(7): 559-566.
6. Schepis T, Gaemperli O, Koepfli P, et al. Comparison of 64-slice CT with gated SPECT for evaluation of left ventricular function. *J Nucl Med.* 2006;47(8):1288-1294.
7. Schlosser T, Mohrs OK, Magedanz A, Voigtlander T, Schmermund A, Barkhausen J. Assessment of left ventricular function and mass in patients undergoing computed tomography (CT) coronary angiography using 64-detector-row CT: comparison to magnetic resonance imaging. *Acta Radiol.* 2007;48(1):30-35.
8. Wu YW, Tadamura E, Yamamuro M, et al. Estimation of global and regional cardiac function using 64-slice computed tomography: a comparison study with echocardiography, gated-SPECT and cardiovascular magnetic resonance. *Int J Cardiol.* 2008;128(1):69-76.
9. Nakamura K, Funabashi N, Uehara M, et al. Quantitative 4-dimensional volumetric analysis of left ventricle in ischemic heart disease by 64-slice computed tomography: a comparative study with invasive left ventriculogram. *Int J Cardiol.* 2008;129(1):42-52.
10. Wu YW, Tadamura E, Kanao S, et al. Left ventricular functional analysis using 64-slice multidetector row computed tomography: comparison with left ventriculography and cardiovascular magnetic resonance. *Cardiology.* 2008;109(2):135-142.
11. Abbara S, Chow BJ, Pena AJ, et al. Assessment of left ventricular function with 16- and 64-slice multi-detector computed tomography. *Eur J Radiol.* 2008;67(3):481-486.
12. Busch S, Johnson TR, Wintersperger BJ, et al. Quantitative assessment of left ventricular function with dual-source CT in comparison to cardiac magnetic resonance imaging: initial findings. *Eur Radiol.* 2008;18(3):570-575.
13. Brodoefel H, Kramer U, Reimann A, et al. Dual-source CT with improved temporal resolution in assessment of left ventricular function: a pilot study. *AJR Am J Roentgenol.* 2007;189(5): 1064-1070.
14. Bastarrika G, Arraiza M, De Cecco CN, Mastrobuoni S, Ubilla M, Rabago G. Quantification of left ventricular function and mass in heart transplant recipients using dual-source CT and MRI: initial clinical experience. *Eur Radiol.* 2008;18(9):1784-1790.
15. Spoeck A, Bonatti J, Friedrich GJ, Schachner T, Bonaros N, Feuchtner GM. Evaluation of left ventricular function by 64-multidetector computed tomography in patients undergoing totally endoscopic coronary artery bypass grafting. *Heart Surg Forum.* 2008;11(4):E218-E224.
16. Sugeng L, Mor-Avi V, Weinert L, et al. Quantitative assessment of left ventricular size and function: side-by-side comparison of real-time three-dimensional echocardiography and computed tomography with magnetic resonance reference. *Circulation.* 2006; 114(7):654-661.
17. Sarwar A, Shapiro MD, Nasir K, et al. Evaluating global and regional left ventricular function in patients with reperfused acute myocardial infarction by 64-slice multidetector CT: a comparison to magnetic resonance imaging. *J Cardiovasc Comput Tomogr.* 2009;3(3):170-177.
18. Raman SV, Shah M, McCarthy B, Garcia A, Ferketich AK. Multi-detector row cardiac computed tomography accurately quantifies right and left ventricular size and function compared with cardiac magnetic resonance. *Am Heart J.* 2006;151(3):736-744.
19. Mahabadi AA, Samy B, Seneviratne SK, et al. Quantitative assessment of left atrial volume by electrocardiographic-gated contrast-enhanced multidetector computed tomography. *J Cardiovasc Comput Tomogr.* 2009;3(2):80-87.
20. Ruzsics B, Lee H, Powers ER, Flohr TG, Costello P, Schoepf UJ. Images in cardiovascular medicine. Myocardial ischemia diagnosed by dual-energy computed tomography: correlation with single-photon emission computed tomography. *Circulation.* 2008; 117(9):1244-1245.
21. Hecht HS, Bhatti T. Multislice coronary computed tomographic angiography in emergency department presentations of unsuspected acute myocardial infarction. *J Cardiovasc Comput Tomogr.* 2009;3(4):272-278.
22. Weiss RM, Otoadese EA, Noel MP, DeJong SC, Heery SD. Quantitation of absolute regional myocardial perfusion using cine computed tomography. *J Am Coll Cardiol.* 1994;23(5):1186-1193.
23. Paul JF, Dambrin G, Caussin C, Lancelin B, Angel C. Sixteen-slice computed tomography after acute myocardial infarction: from perfusion defect to the culprit lesion. *Circulation.* 2003;108(3):373-374.
24. Koyama Y, Mochizuki T, Higaki J. Computed tomography assessment of myocardial perfusion, viability, and function. *J Magn Reson Imaging.* 2004;19(6):800-815.
25. Nikolaou K, Knez A, Sagmeister S, et al. Assessment of myocardial infarctions using multidetector-row computed tomography. *J Comput Assist Tomogr.* 2004;28(2):286-292.
26. Gosalia A, Haramati LB, Sheth MP, Spindola-Franco H. CT detection of acute myocardial infarction. *AJR Am J Roentgenol.* 2004; 182(6):1563-1566.
27. Mahnken AH, Koos R, Katoh M, et al. Assessment of myocardial viability in reperfused acute myocardial infarction using 16-slice computed tomography in comparison to magnetic resonance imaging. *J Am Coll Cardiol.* 2005;45(12):2042-2047.
28. Habis M, Capderou A, Ghostine S, et al. Acute myocardial infarction early viability assessment by 64-slice computed tomography immediately after coronary angiography: comparison with low-dose dobutamine echocardiography. *J Am Coll Cardiol.* 2007;49(11): 1178-1185.
29. Sato A, Hiroe M, Nozato T, et al. Early validation study of 64-slice multidetector computed tomography for the assessment of myocardial viability and the prediction of left ventricular remodelling after acute myocardial infarction. *Eur Heart J.* 2008;29(4):490-498.
30. Lardo AC, Cordeiro MA, Silva C, et al. Contrast-enhanced multidetector computed tomography viability imaging after myocardial infarction: characterization of myocyte death, microvascular obstruction, and chronic scar. *Circulation.* 2006;113(3):394-404.
31. Ruzsics B, Suranyi P, Kiss P, et al. Automated multidetector computed tomography evaluation of subacutely infarcted myocardium. *J Cardiovasc Comput Tomogr.* 2008;2:26-32.
32. Baks T, Cademartiri F, Moelker AD, et al. Multislice computed tomography and magnetic resonance imaging for the assessment of reperfused acute myocardial infarction. *J Am Coll Cardiol.* 2006; 48(1):144-152.
33. van Werkhoven JM, Schuijf JD, Gaemperli O, et al. Prognostic value of multislice computed tomography and gated single-photon emission computed tomography in patients with suspected coronary artery disease. *J Am Coll Cardiol.* 2009;53(7):623-632.
34. van Werkhoven JM, Schuijf JD, Jukema JW, et al. Anatomic correlates of a normal perfusion scan using 64-slice computed tomographic coronary angiography. *Am J Cardiol.* 2008;101(1):40-45.

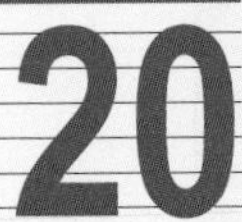

20 Assessment of Left Ventricular Structural Abnormalities

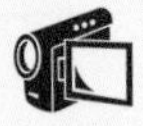

Key Point

- The high spatial resolution and excellent field of view of CCT enables it to depict a range of myocardial, septal, and other structural lesions.

MYOCARDIAL CRYPTS

Myocardial crypts (or clefts) have been defined as discrete V-shaped extensions of the blood pool inserting more than 50% into the compact myocardial wall that tend to be less visible during systole and are not associated with local hypokinesis or dyskinesia.[1] Increased prevalence of crypts has been reported in carriers of the gene for hypertrophic cardiomyopathy (as much as 81%).[2] However, myocardial crypts also are seen in normal subjects, so their precise significance has yet to be determined.[1]

For CCT images of myocardial crypts, see Figures 20-1 and 20-2; **Video 20-1**.

MYOCARDIAL DIVERTICULUM

Congenital left ventricular (LV) diverticula are rare cardiac malformations characterized as outpouchings of the myocardium and can be fibrous or muscular.[3] The prevalence has been reported between 0.02% and 0.04%.[4] They are associated with other congenital abnormalities in about 70% of cases. Muscular diverticula typically are apical and have a full-thickness myocardial wall with preserved systolic contraction. Diverticula can be differentiated from crypts or clefts by a narrow mouth but a wide outpouching extending beyond the normal LV margins. Cardiac CT (CCT) has been proposed as useful for differentiating aneurysm from pseudoaneurysm by exclusion of coronary artery disease, visualization of the LV wall layers, and dynamic assessment of regional wall function (Fig. 20-3).[5]

POST-INFARCTION VENTRICULAR PSEUDOANEURYSMS, SEPTAL RUPTURE, AND INTRAMYOCARDIAL HEMATOMA

Pseudoaneurysms are an uncommon complication of acute myocardial infarction, occurring in less than 1% of cases.[5] Cardiac surgery, penetrating or other trauma, and infection also can lead to the development of these abnormalities. The excellent spatial resolution of CT should be ideal for identifying the myocardial wall disruption. Single case reports have demonstrated the ability of CCT to depict post-infarction ventricular pseudoaneurysms, and coronary anatomy.[5-7]

- Post-infarction septal rupture and intramyocardial hematoma also have been noted in single case reports.
- For CCT images of post-infarction pseudoaneurysms, see Figure 20-4.
- For CCT images of post-infarction septal rupture, see Figures 20-5 and 20-6; **Videos 20-2 and 20-3.**

POST-INFARCTION LEFT VENTRICULAR ANEURYSM

True aneurysms of the LV most commonly are secondary to myocardial infarction but can (rarely) be congenital in origin or secondary to inflammatory (e.g., Kawasaki disease and sarcoidosis) or infectious (e.g., Chagas) disease. Occasionally changes associated with right ventricular dysplasia or hypertrophic cardiomyopathy also can be associated with LV aneurysm formation.

For CCT images of ventricular aneurysms, see Figures 20-7 through 20-10; **Videos 20-4 and 20-5.**

Text continued on page 317

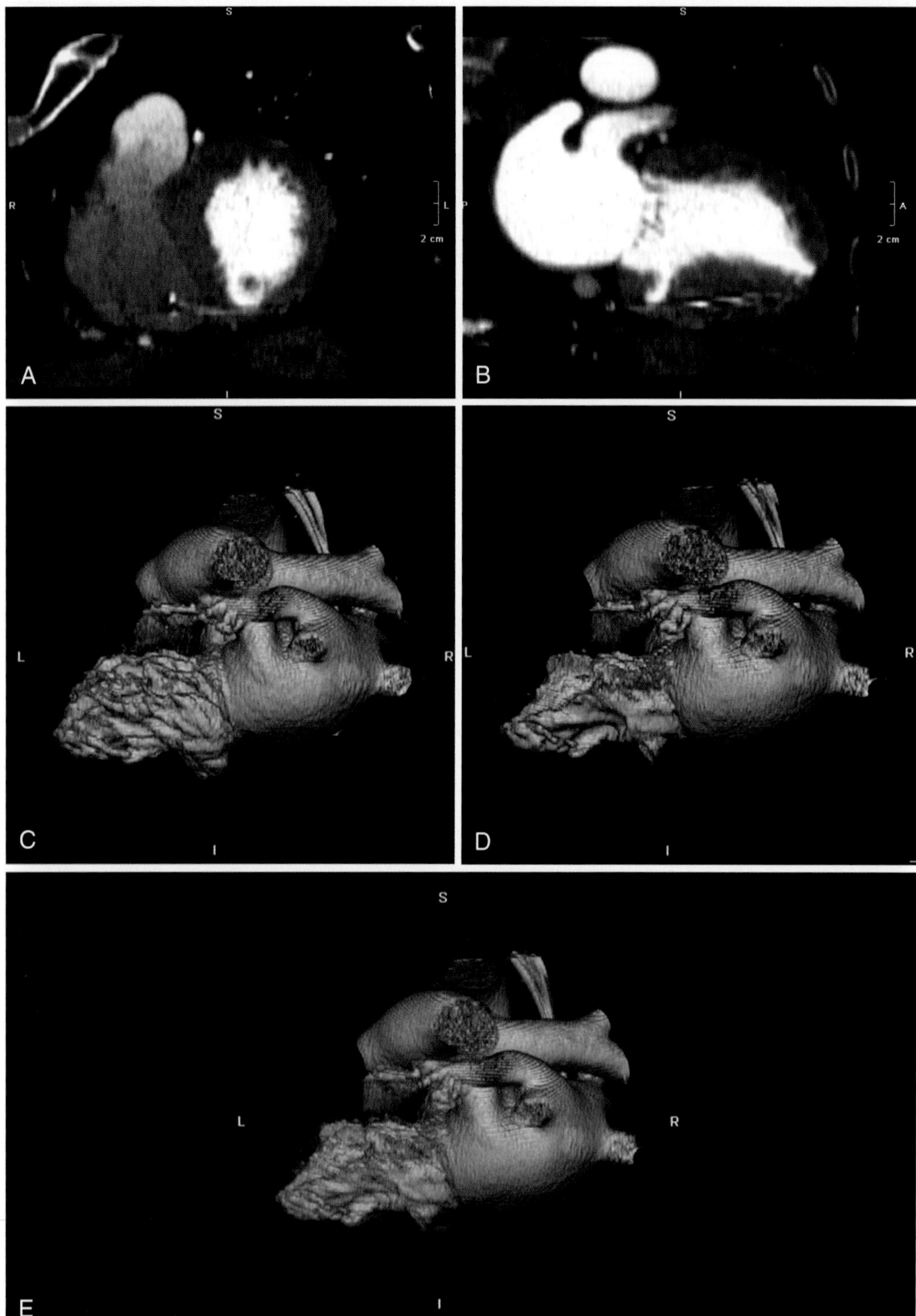

Figure 20-1. Multiple composite images from a cardiac CT study in a patient with hypertrophic cardiomyopathy demonstrating a basal inferior crypt and an enlarged left atrium.

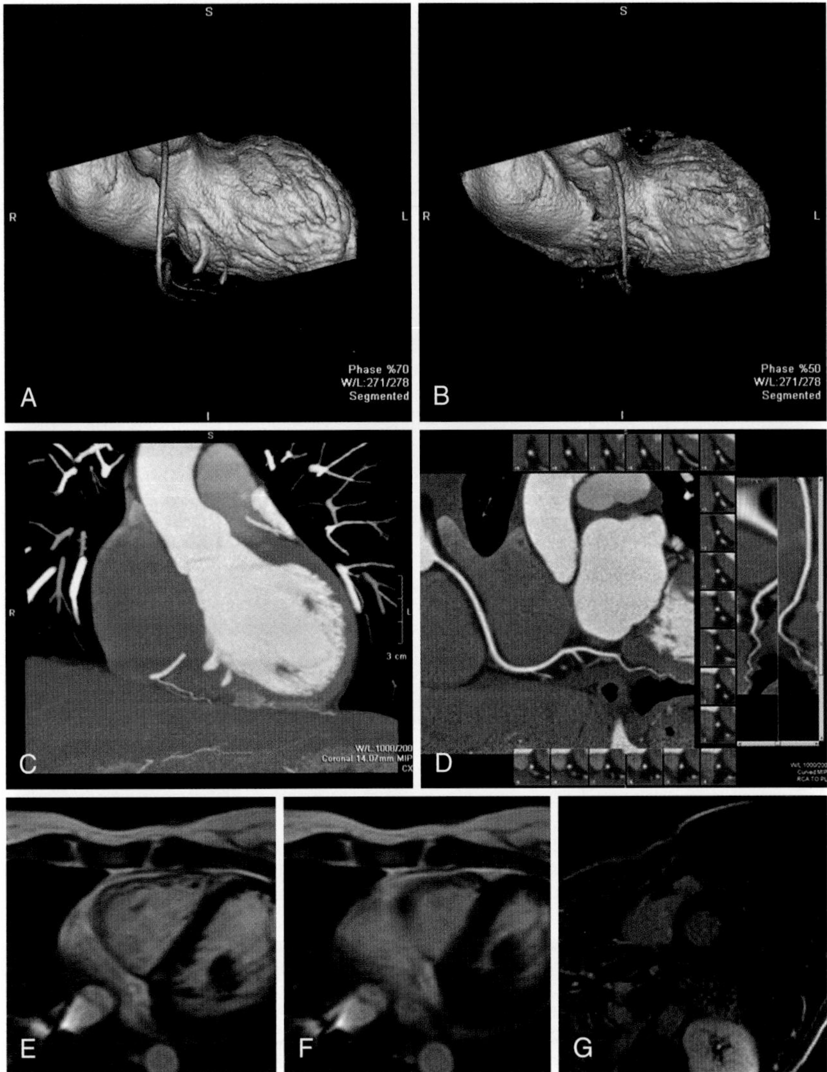

Figure 20-2. Composite images from a cardiac CT and cardiac MRI (CMR) demonstrate small crypt-like formations involving the inferior basal wall of the left ventricle. The underlying coronary arteries are normal. There was no history of hypertrophic cardiomyopathy. Similar findings were confirmed on CMR, with no delayed enhancement. **See Video 20-1.**

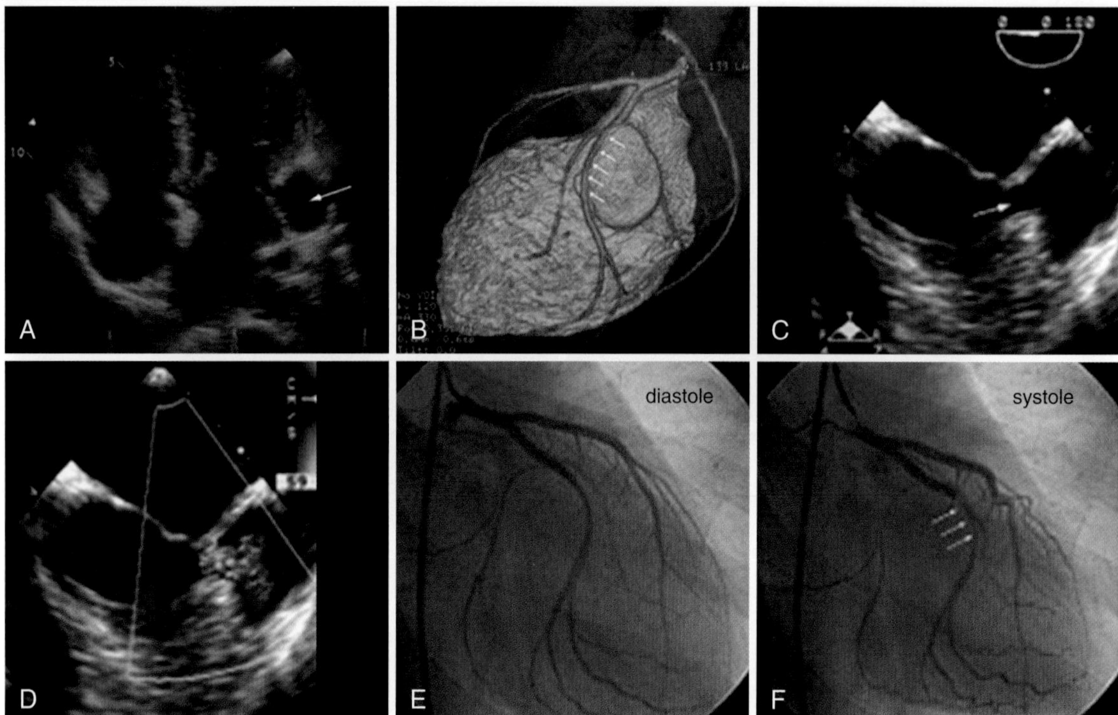

Figure 20-3. A 29-year-old asymptomatic man was referred for treatment of Crohn's disease. Before commencing treatment, the patient underwent cardiac assessment. **A,** An echocardiogram showed a localized low-echoic cavity with a discontinuity in the basal part of the left ventricular (LV) lateral wall close to the atrioventricular groove. **B,** Reconstructed multidetector CT clearly showed the spatial relationship between the coronary artery and the pseudoaneurysm (*arrows*). **C** and **D,** Color Doppler imaging showed bidirectional blood flow between the LV and the cavity through a narrow communication, consistent with a diagnosis of LV pseudoaneurysm. Coronary angiography showed no atherosclerotic stenosis. **E** and **F,** Remarkably, the proximal part of the left circumflex coronary artery (*arrows*) became very thin during systole due to a dyskinetic expansion of the pseudoaneurysm, indicating a myocardial bridging-like squeeze (Reprinted with permission from Katayama T, Murata M, Iwanaga S, et al. Left ventricular pseudoaneurysm with peculiar coronary artery collapse. *J Am Coll Cardiol.* 2009;53(19):1823.)

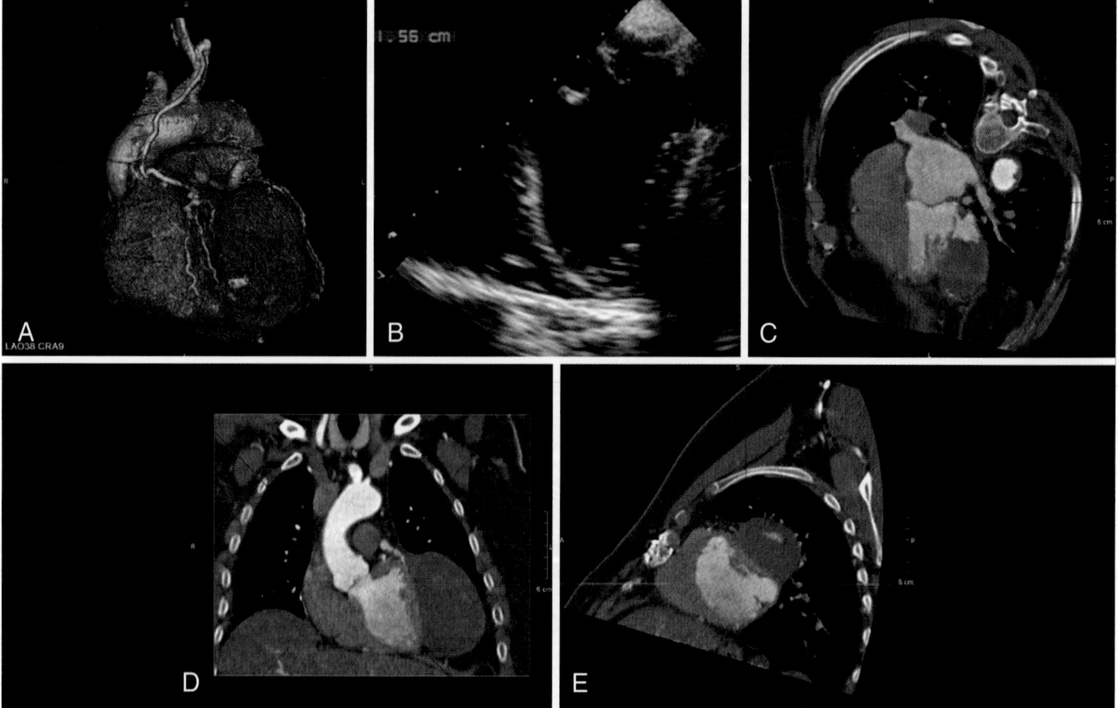

Figure 20-4. **A,** Three-dimensional volume-rendered image shows the patent left internal mammary to left anterior descending artery graft in relation to the left ventricular pseudoaneurysm (LVPA). **B,** Transesophageal image shows the large LVPA arising from the lateral wall below the mitral valve and reveals the abrupt myocardial discontinuity marking the neck of the LVPA. Cardiac CTA modified four-chamber (**C**), horizontal long-axis (**D**), and two-chamber (**E**) views of the heart show the posterobasal opening of the LVPA and its relation to adjacent cardiac structures. (Reprinted with permission from Yavari A, Sriskandan N, Khawaja MZ, et al. Computed tomography of a broken heart: chronic left ventricular pseudoaneursym. *J Cardiovasc Comput Tomogr.* 2008; 2:120.)

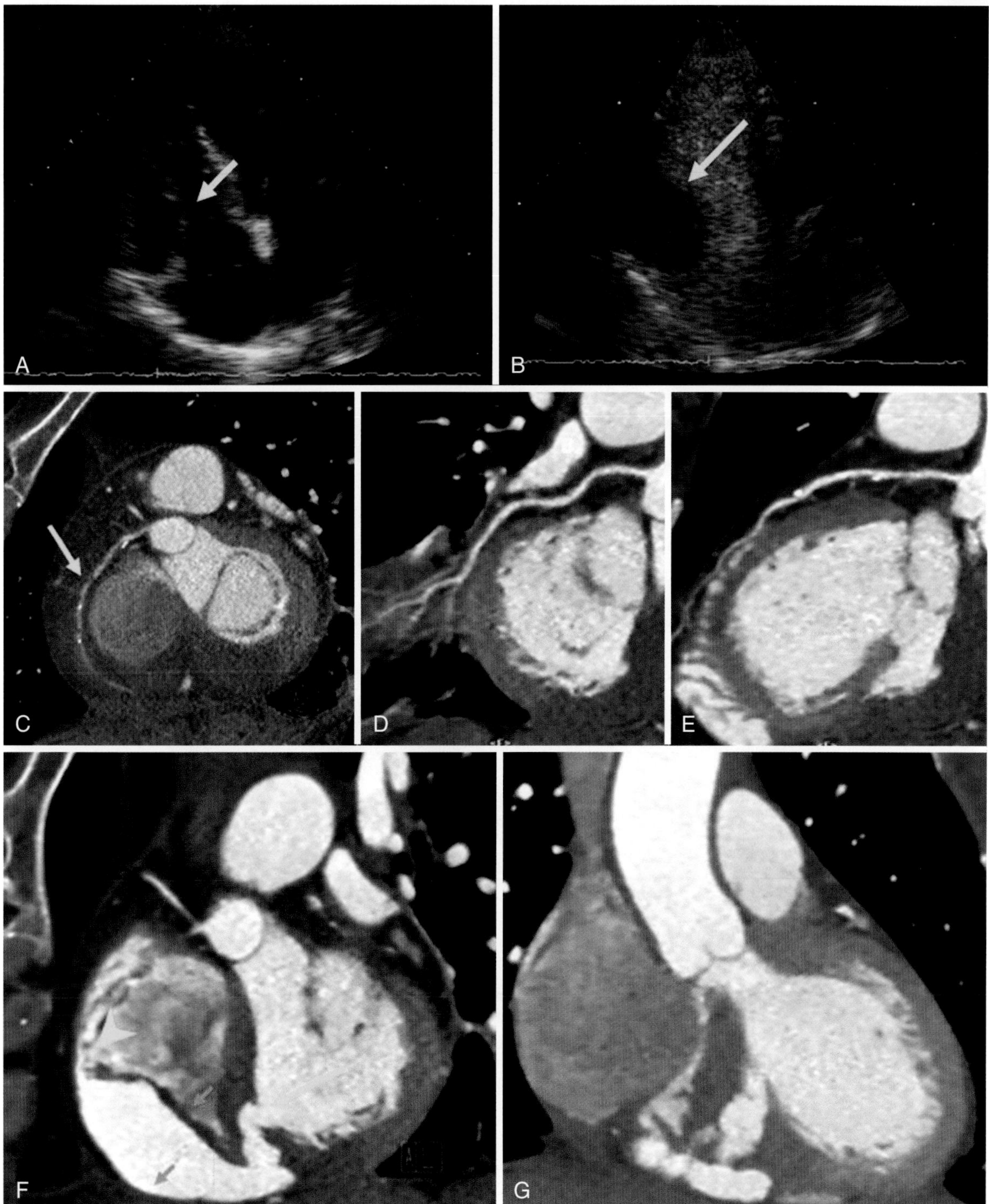

Figure 20-5. A, Four-chamber view echocardiogram with a cavity by the right ventricle (*arrow*). **B,** Four-chamber view after intravenous contrast, showing no enhancement of the structure (*arrow*). Curved multiplanar reconstructions show that the right coronary artery (**C**) has a high-grade lesion (*arrow*) and poor contrast opacification in the distal portion of the artery, and that there is nonsignificant stenosis of the left circumflex artery (**D**) and of the left anterior descending artery (**E**). **F,** Short-axis view shows the ventricular septal rupture (*larger arrow*), the myocardial dissection (*two small arrows* at both sides of the right ventricular wall), and the re-entry orifice on the right ventricle (*arrowhead*). **G,** Multiple orifices document the complex anatomy of the ventricular septal rupture. (Reprinted with permission from Bittencourt MS, Seltmann M, Muschiol G, Achenbach S. Ventricular septal rupture and right ventricular intramyocardial dissection secondary to acute inferior myocardial infarction. *J Cardiovasc Comput Tomogr.* 2010;4(5): 342-344.) **See Video 20-2.**

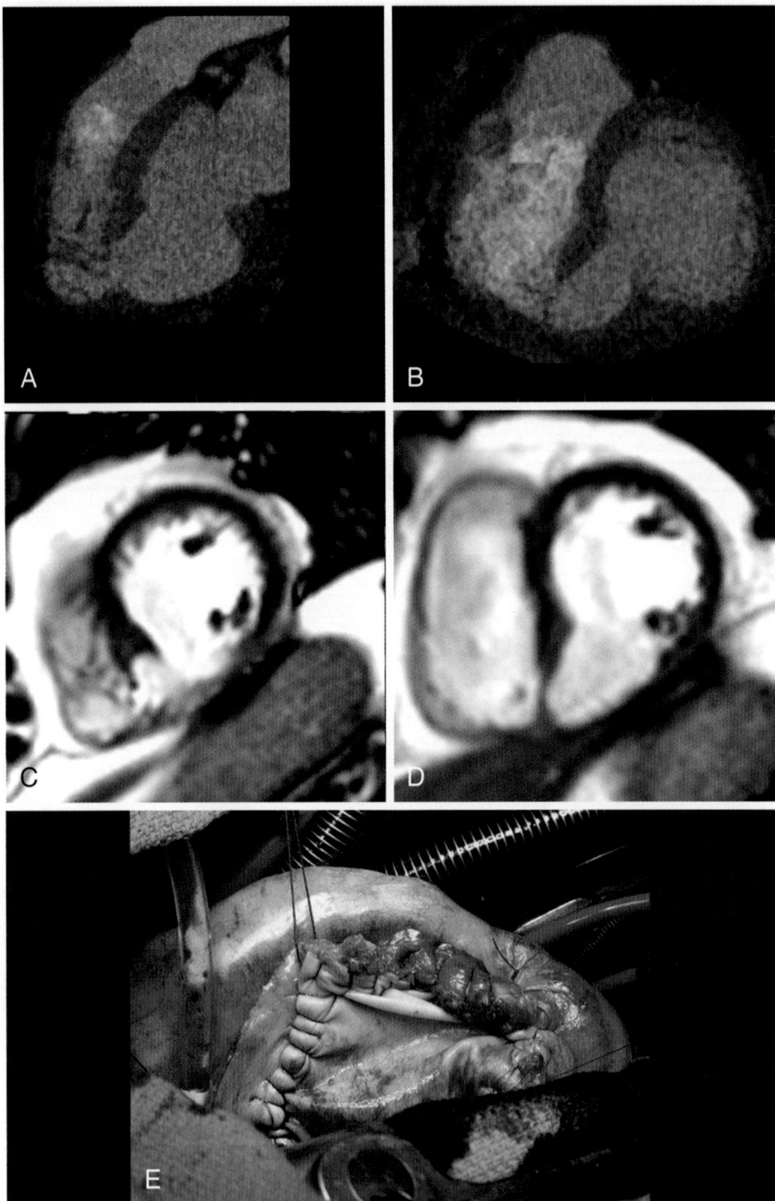

Figure 20-6. ECG-gated contrast-enhanced CT images (**A** and **B**), steady-state free precession cardiac MR (CMR) images (**C** and **D**), and photo (**E**) of the surgical repair of a post-infarction septal rupture. The CT and CMR images reveal the aneurysmal deformation of the inferior septum as well as the inferior wall. The CT images in particular reveal the detail of the septal rupture (fenestrations of the thinned aneurysmal septum). The thinness of the aneurysmal inferior septum and inferior wall is most obvious on the CMR images. The surgical photo shows the thinness of the aneurysmal septum, adjacent to the pericardial patch. **See Video 20-3.**

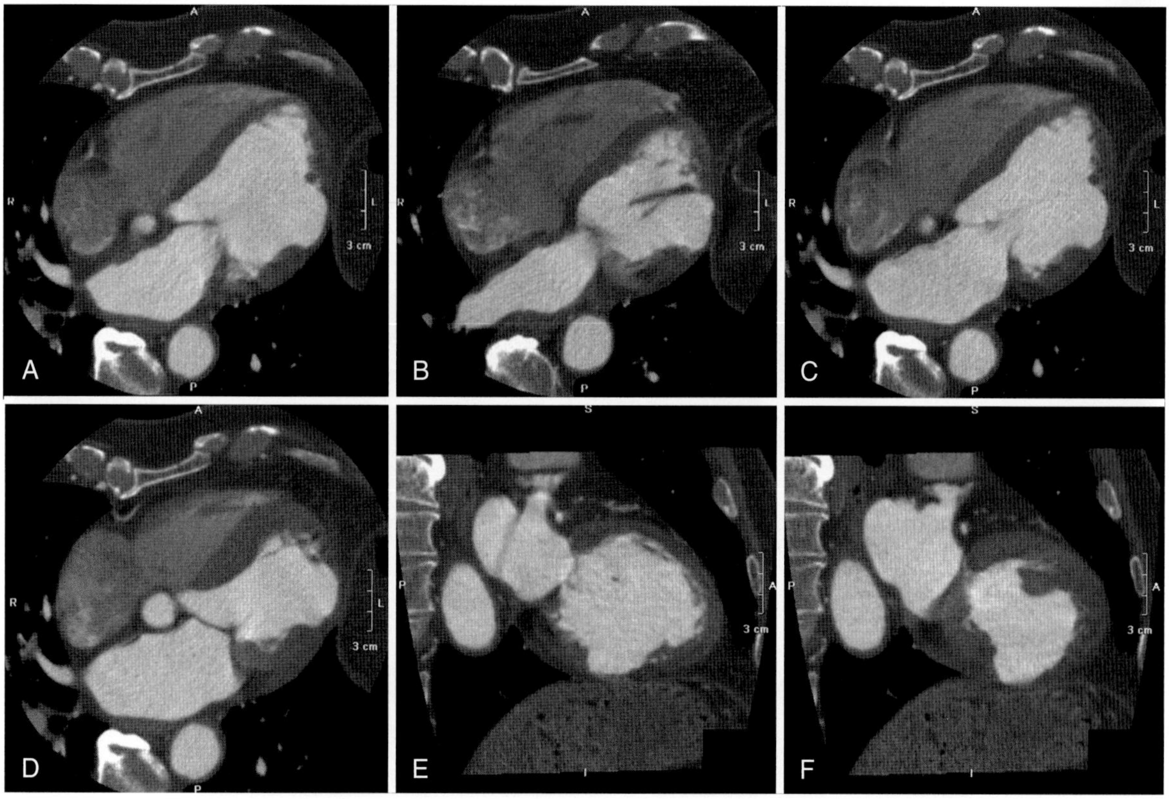

Figure 20-7. Composite image from a cardiac CT study in a 64-year-old man, previously healthy, with an episode of chest pain 6 weeks prior. Echocardiography performed on the same day, prior to the cardiac CT study, suggested a false aneurysm of the left ventricle. Multiple reformatted images of the left ventricle demonstrate a focal area of thinning and dyskinesis involving the inferolateral wall. The mouth of the aneurysm is larger than the mid-portion of the aneurysm. No evidence is seen of a pericardial effusion, or stranding of the pericardial fat. These findings all favor a true aneurysm. **See Video 20-4.**

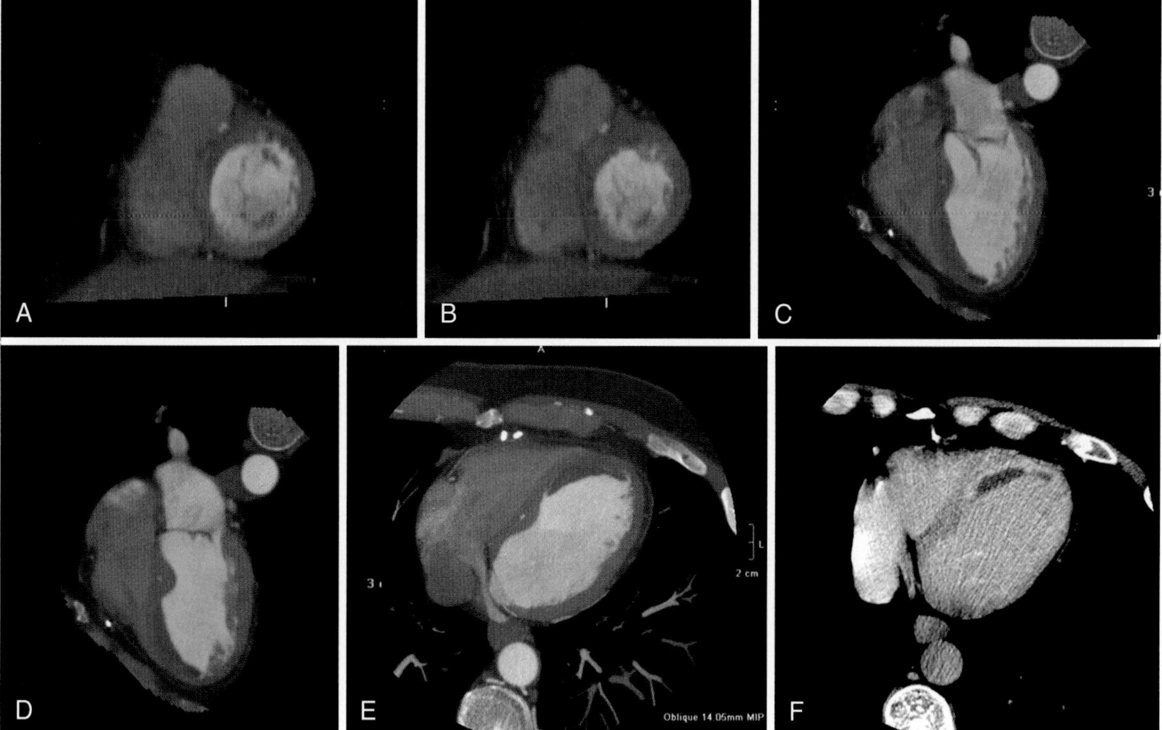

Figure 20-8. Evaluation of the left ventricle in the same patient as in Figure 20-7 demonstrates reduced left ventricular ejection fraction of 32%. A moderate area of laminated thrombus is noted adjacent to the septum in the mid- to distal portion of the left ventricle. Delayed imaging demonstrates an underlying region of delayed enhancement consistent with prior infarction in this area.

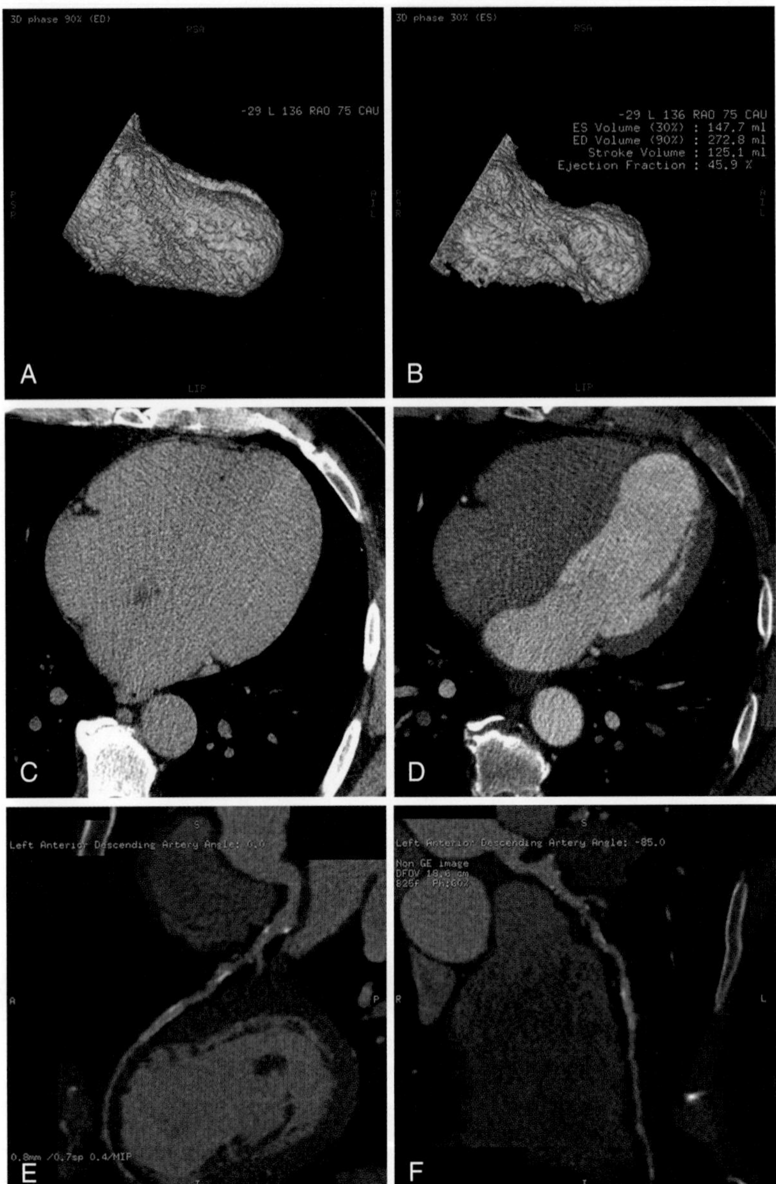

Figure 20-9. **A** and **B,** Volume-rendered representations of the entire ventricular volume. The study was acquired in a dose-modulated healed helical fashion. **A,** End diastole; **B,** end systole. These images demonstrate akinesis of the distal portion of the left ventricle consistent with a myocardial infarction in the left anterior descending artery (LAD) area. Functional analysis generates an indexed end-diastolic volume of 129 mL/m^2, moderately dilated. There is mild reduction in overall ejection fraction with a left ventricular ejection fraction of 46%. **C,** Precontrast calcium score study demonstrates a small amount of fatty metaplasia within the distal septum. **D,** The companion post-contrast image demonstrates focal thinning of the distal septum extending into the apex. Curved multiplanar reformations (**E**) and maximum intensity projection (MIP) (**F**) images through the left anterior descending coronary artery demonstrate moderate to severe disease within the proximal to mid-LAD. A 70% proximal LAD lesion consisting of mixed plaque is present. There has been prior stenting of a mid-LAD lesion (best seen on **A**). No evidence of in-stent restenosis is seen.

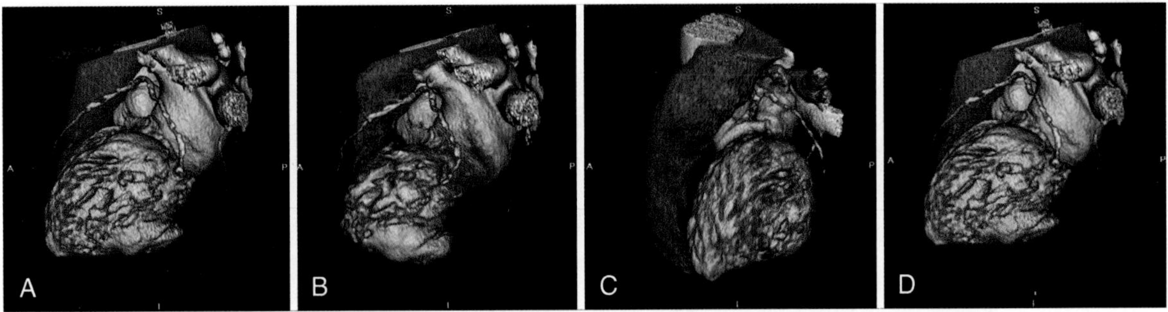

Figure 20-10. Multiple volume-rendered images demonstrate a focal aneurysm involving the inferolateral wall of the left ventricle. There is extensive coronary artery calcification involving the left anterior descending and circumflex arteries. **A** and **B**, diastole; **C** and **D**, systole. **See Video 20-5.**

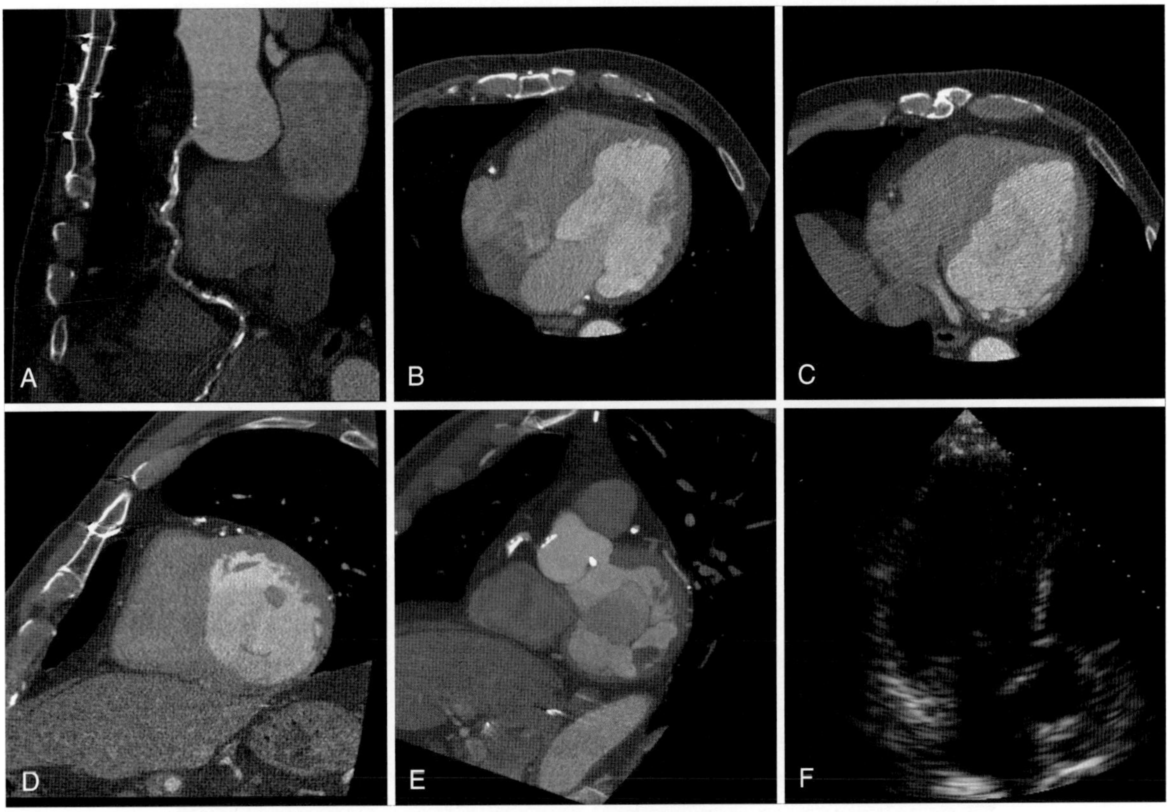

Figure 20-11. Multiple images from a cardiac CT study in a 62-year-old man with chest pain and ECG findings suggestive of a prior inferior wall infarct. **A,** Curved planar reformation through the right coronary artery demonstrates extensive calcification and a severe patent ductus arteriosus lesion. **B,** Moderate to severe thinning of the basal to mid inferolateral wall. **C,** Another image demonstrating the extensive thinning in the basal inferolateral wall. A small focus of soft tissue thickening also is seen within the left ventricle basally. **D,** Marked thinning of the basal inferolateral wall, a finding that indicates a previous myocardial infarction. The posterolateral papillary muscle is not identified, and has likely become atrophic post–myocardial infarction. **E,** A thin-section maximum intensity projection through the basal portion of the left ventricle demonstrates a soft tissue nodule within the basal-most portion of the left ventricle, and within the suspected infarct territory. The diagnosis was basal to mid-chronic inferolateral myocardial infarction with a small basal left ventricular thrombus.

THROMBUS

Intracavitary thrombus is a relatively common finding after late-presentation myocardial infarction. Typically, it is seen as a laminated low-attenuation lesion in a region of thin myocardial wall and often is associated with the presence of LV aneurysm.[8]

For CCT images of post-infarction left ventricular thrombi, see Figures 20-11 through 20-17; **Video 20-6.**

POST-INFARCTION FATTY METAPLASIA

Imaging of myocardial adipose tissue by CCT is feasible, and such tissue is a common concomitant finding in the setting of prior infarction, occurring in as many as 62% of such patients.[9] In this setting, the presence of myocardial adipose tissue is associated with the chronicity of infarction. However, it should be remembered that intramyocardial fat can be seen in individuals

Text continued on page 322

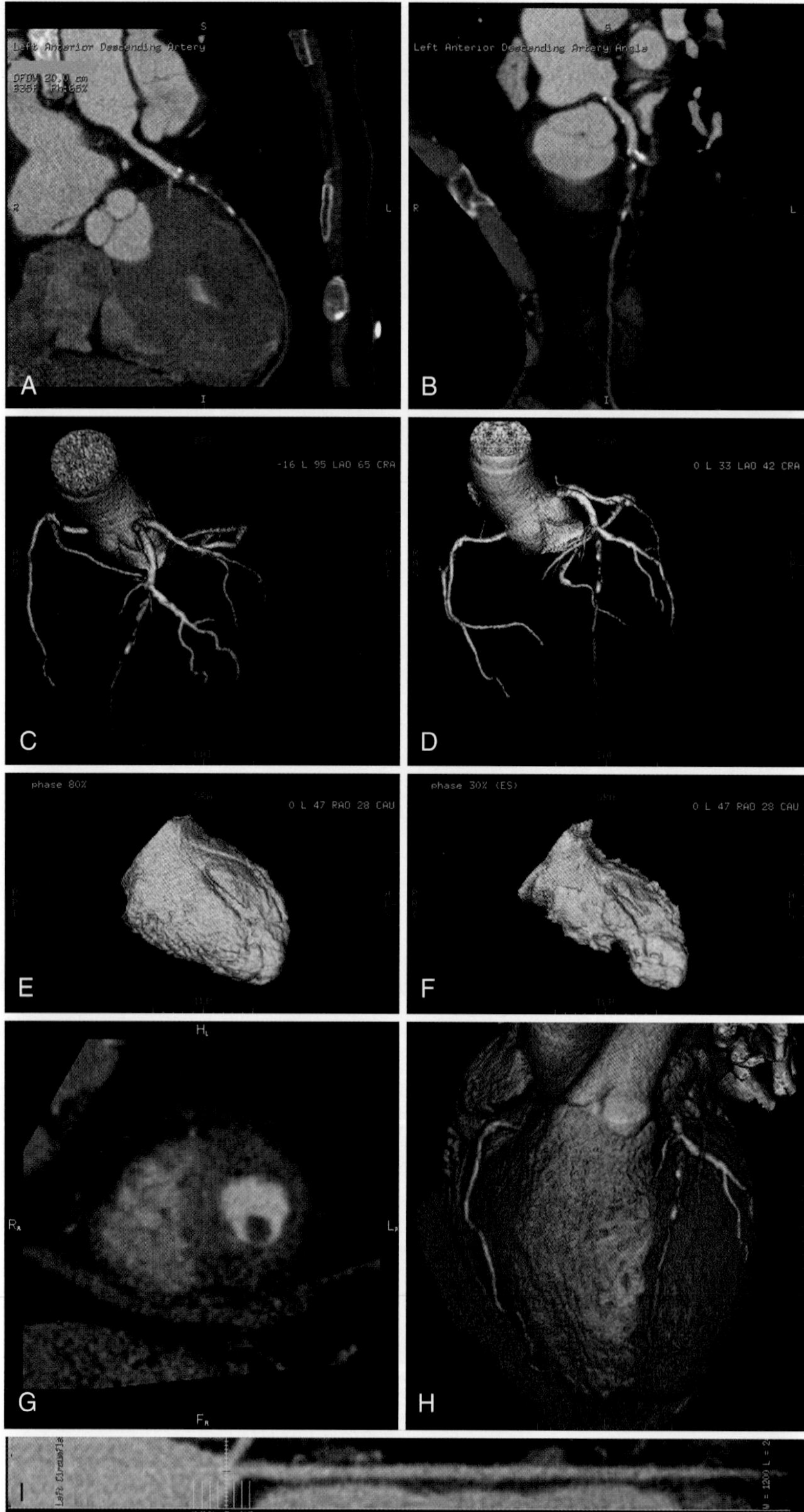

Figure 20-12. Multiple composite images demonstrate an occlusion of the mid–left anterior descending artery (LAD) with mid-distal reconstitution. An aneurysm is noted involving the apex of the left ventricle with a small free thrombus within the apex of the left ventricle. **See Video 20-6.**

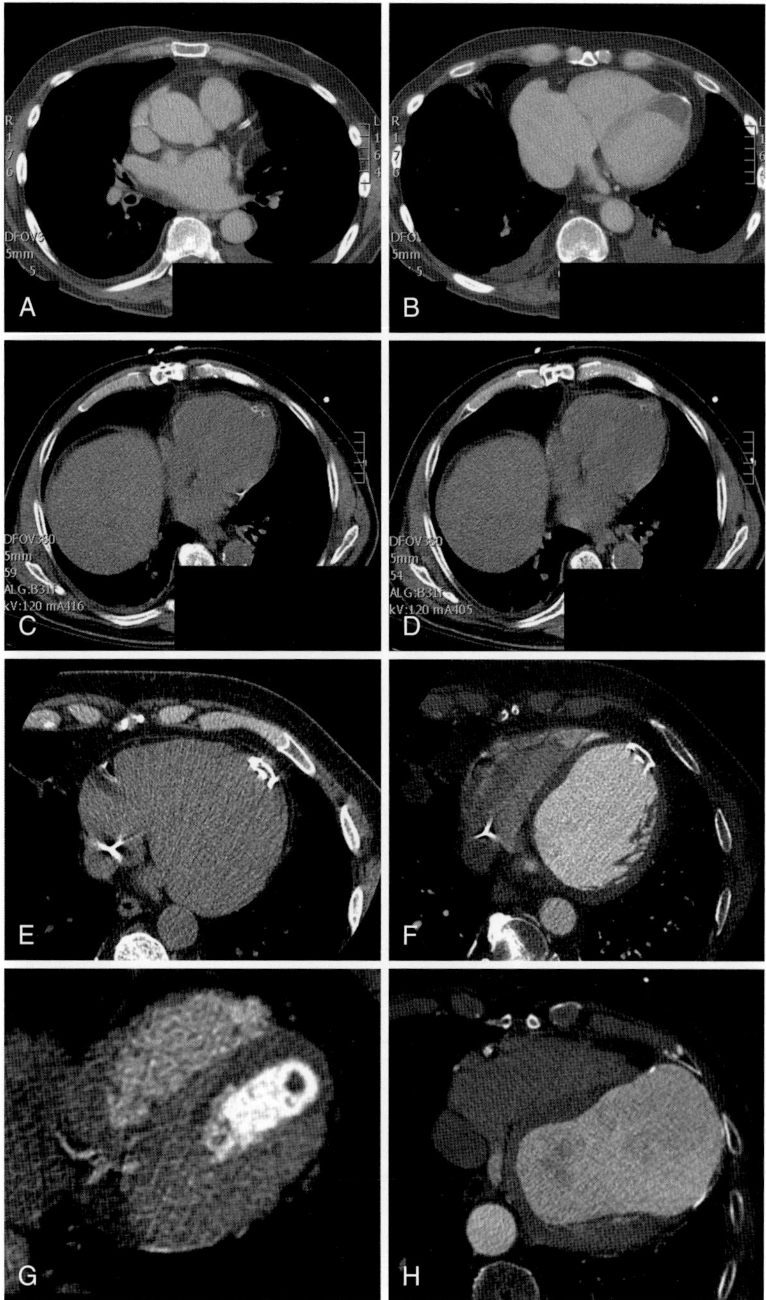

Figure 20-13. Calcified thrombi and calcified chronic infarctions. **A,** Contrast-enhanced chest CT scan image depicts a stent in the left anterior descending artery. **B,** Contrast-enhanced chest CT scan image depicts calcified myocardium and a large apical thrombus in this patient with prior anterior ST-elevation myocardial infarction and direct percutaneous intervention. **C** and **D,** Two noncontrast images obtained in a patient with a history of severe abdominal pain. The patient had a history of chronic renal failure, and contrast was not administered. The patient was subsequently diagnosed with small bowel ischemia. At the time of surgery, small emboli were seen within the superior mesenteric arterial tree. **C** and **D**, The patient's CT scan of the abdomen demonstrated a small partially calcified left apical thrombus, which may have been the source of the emboli. Non–contrast- (**E**) and contrast-enhanced (**F**) images depicting calcified myocardium and overlying calcified thrombus. **G,** Contrast-enhanced CT scan reveals an apical thrombus. **H,** Contrast-enhanced CT scan reveals an apical aneurysm with calcified myocardium.

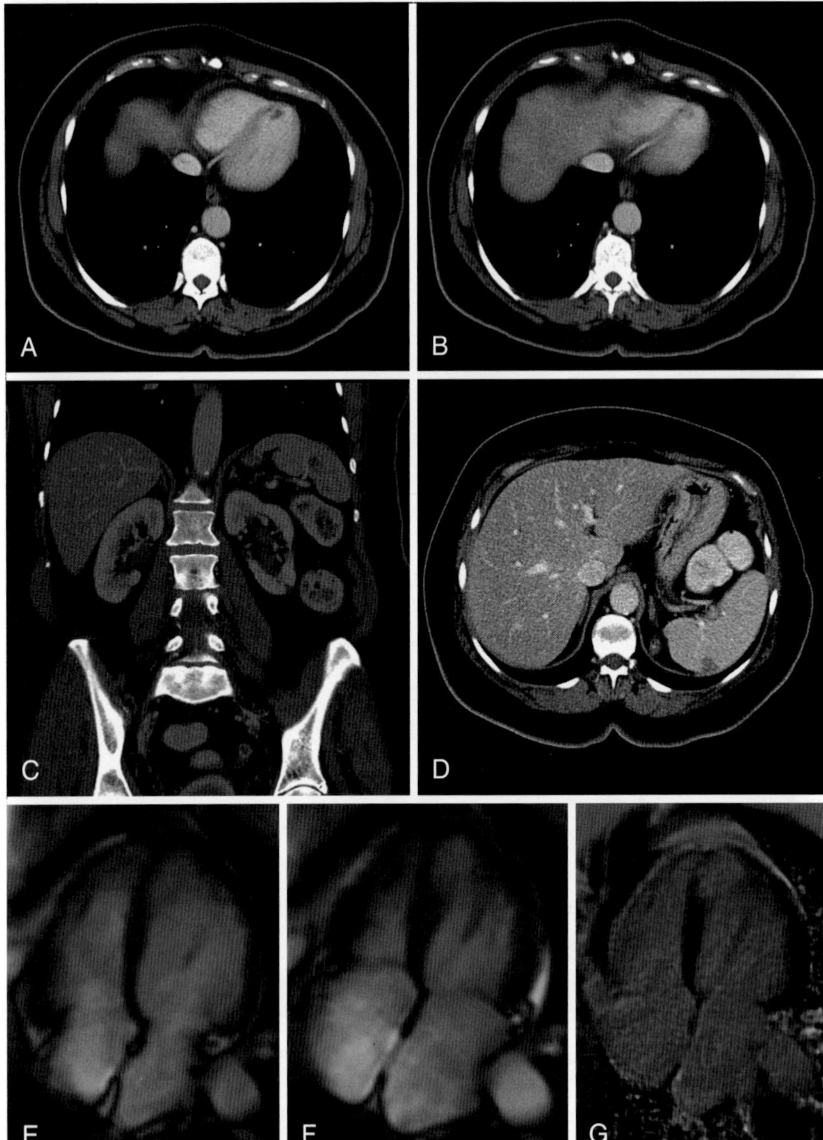

Figure 20-14. **A** through **D,** Composite non-gated images from a 72-year-old woman with left abdominal pain; diverticulitis was suspected. No evidence of diverticulitis was seen, however. **A** and **B,** A small thrombus was noted with a small left ventricular (LV) apical aneurysm. The clot is not intimately associated with the underlying LV wall, and a small amount of IV contrast has been insinuated between the clot and the adjacent LV wall. **C** and **D** depict prior left renal infarction with peripheral wedge-shaped focal defects, as well as a recent splenic infarct, seen as a peripheral hypodensity within the posterior portion of the spleen (**D**). **E** through **G,** Follow-up studies. A cardiac magnetic resonance study 2 months post–anticoagulation therapy shows a small focal apical aneurysm on gated steady-state free precession images (**E**, diastole and **F**, systole). The steady-state free precession and late gadolinium-enhanced images (**G**) reveal no evidence of a residual clot within the apical aneurysm.

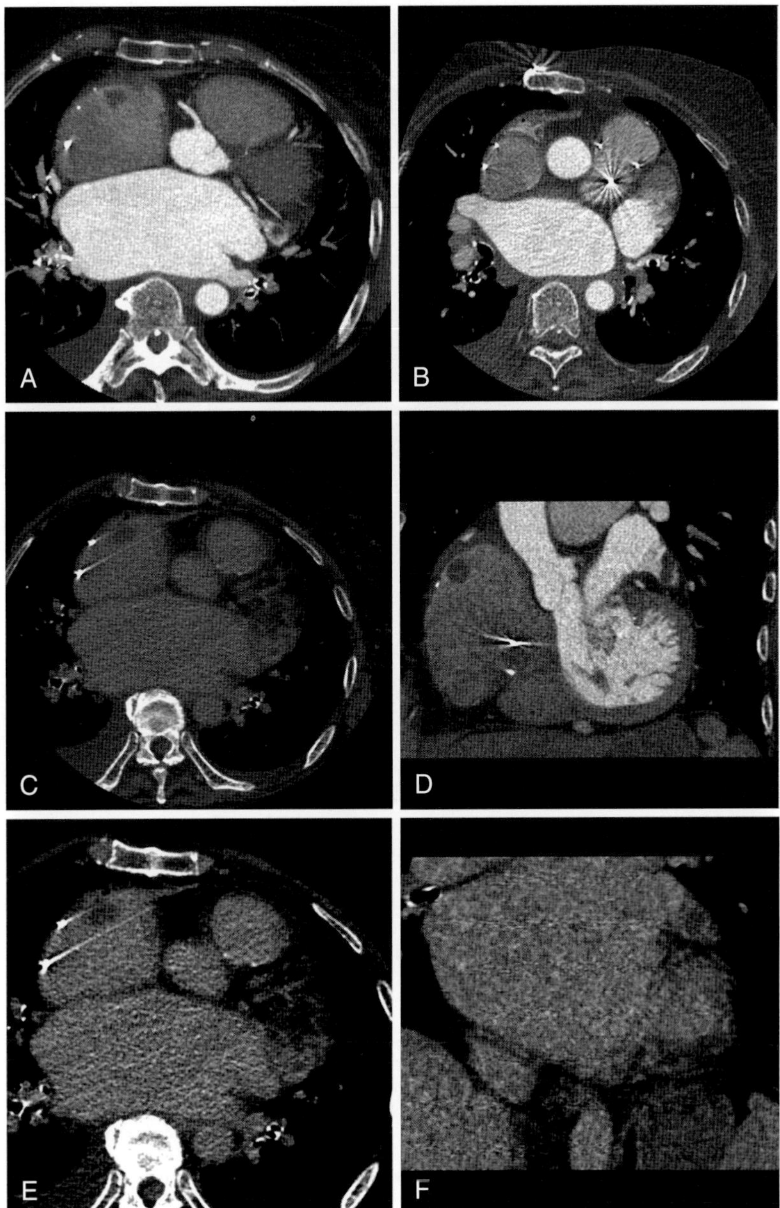

Figure 20-15. Multiple cardiac CT images in a patient with stroke. The patient had a prior history of anterior septal defect repair and pulmonic valve surgery. The patient also had a history of atrial fibrillation, but had recently ceased her anticoagulation therapy. **A,** A focal nodular filling defect within the inferior tip of the left atrial appendage. Two additional filling defects also are faintly seen within a poorly opacified right atrium. **B,** Hazy areas of low attenuation are seen within the tip of the dilated left atrial appendage. This was believed to represent unopacified blood, confirmed on delayed imaging. **E,** Image obtained 40 seconds after the first-pass acquisition confirms the filling defects within the inferior tip of the left atrial appendage, as well as anteriorly within the right atrium. **F,** Reconstructed image also demonstrates the right atrial and left atrial thrombi. Contrast is seen around the thrombi in both atria. The presence of contrast around these thrombi increases the potential for embolization.

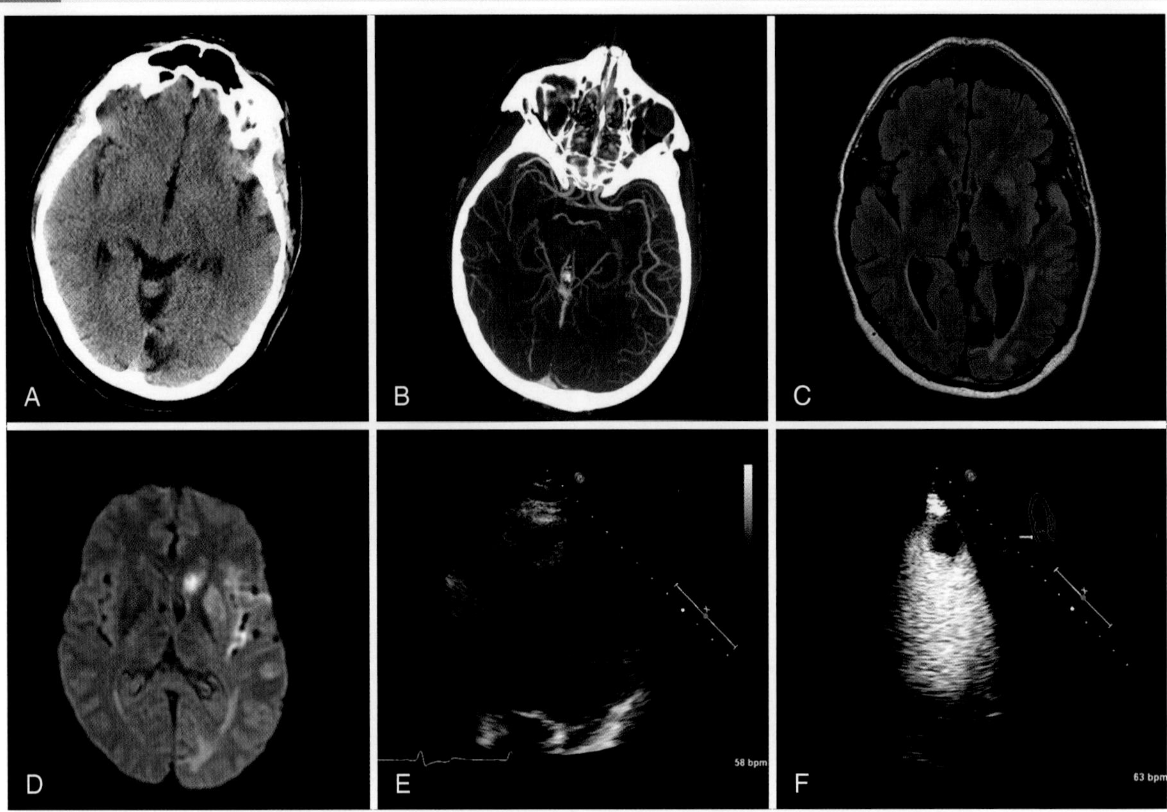

Figure 20-16. **A** 62-year-old man presented with left middle cerebral artery syndrome. **A,** Non-contrast head CT demonstrates subtle loss of gray:white matter differentiation at the insular cortex and left superior temporal lobe. **B,** A maximum intensity projection image of a cerebral CT angiogram demonstrates a corresponding short-segment incomplete occlusion of the distal left M1 middle cerebral artery. **C,** Fluid attenuation inversion recovery (FLAIR) MRI image shows a likely acute infarct in the left caudate head and left insular region. **D,** Diffusion-weighted image confirmed findings in **C. E** and **F,** Transthoracic echocardiography: apical chamber views. **E,** Technical difficulty was encountered; an apical thrombus was suggested but not proved. **F,** Image obtained after injection of IV contrast for left ventricular opacification. An apical thrombus is present, the presumed source of the stroke.

without coronary disease, with the RV affected more commonly than the LV. In normal subjects, RV fat is most commonly seen in the anterolateral and inferolateral segments, whereas LV deposits may be more common in basal segments.

For CCT images of post-infarction myocardial fatty metaplasia, see Figures 20-18 through 20-21; **Video 20-7.**

LEFT VENTRICULAR APICAL VENTS AND VALVOTOMY SCARS

Older cardiac surgery techniques employed trans-apical punctures to vent the left ventricle or to insert valvotomy forceps. The residuum is apparent as a localized scar. For CCT images of postoperative (non-infarction) apical scars, see Figure 20-22.

MYOCARDIAL CALCIFICATION

CCT is superbly able to image myocardial calcification, the most common cause of which, at the left ventricular level, is remote myocardial infarction. Other causes include remote rheumatic infection, hyperparathyroidism, and trauma. Extensive myocardial calcification is sometimes referred to as "porcelain heart."

For CCT images of rheumatic myocardial calcification, see Figures 20-23 and 20-24.

CARDIAC CT PROTOCOL POINTS

The standard CCT protocol is followed (Table 20-1).

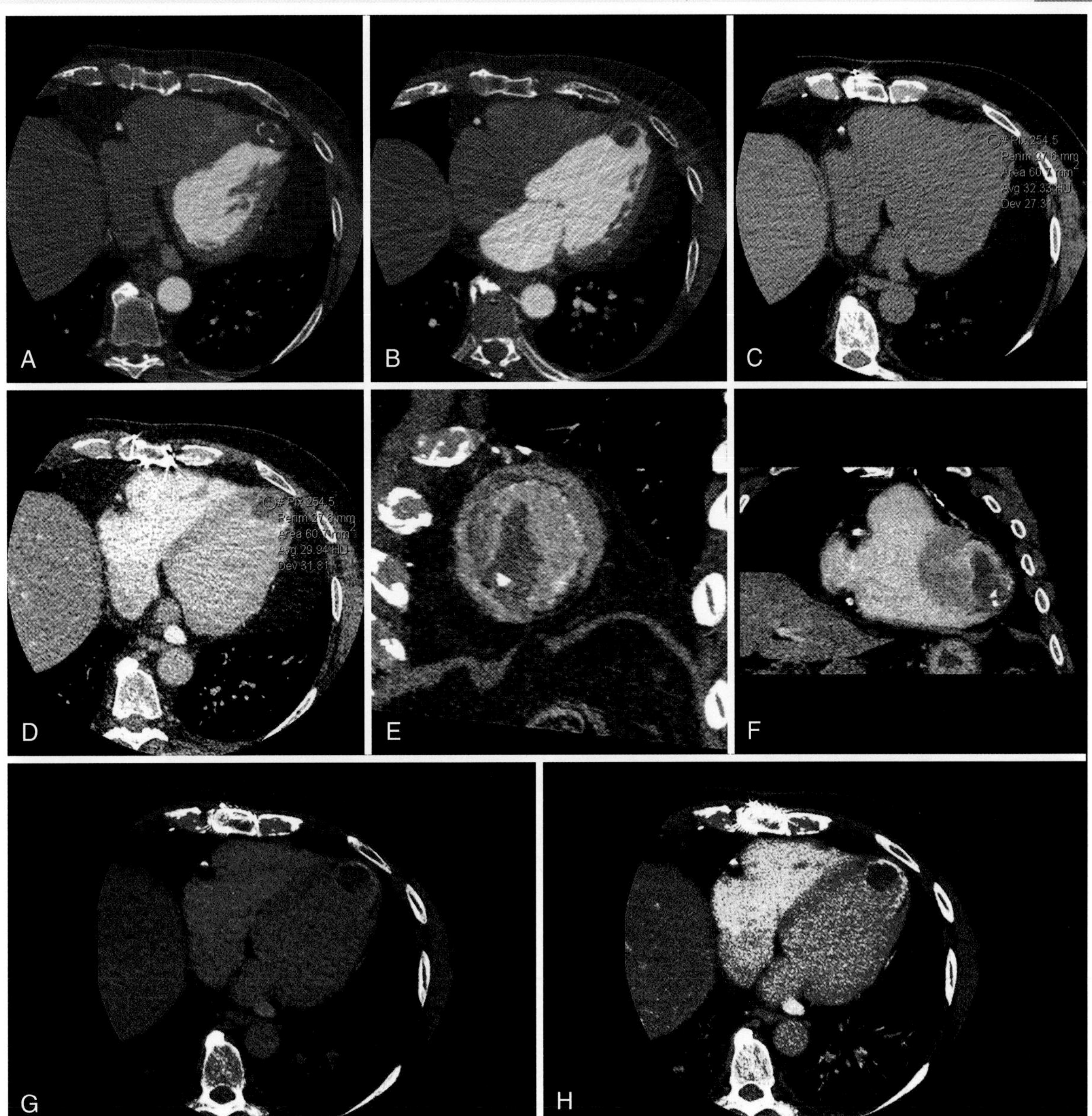

Figure 20-17. **A** 62-year-old man presented with a left hemispheric stroke. Imaging was done to rule out a cardiac source for the embolism. The patient had previously undergone coronary artery bypass grafting. **A** and **B,** ECG-gated arteriographic images through the heart demonstrate a soft tissue–density mass, likely thrombus within the apex of the left ventricle (LV). The inferior portion of the mass (**A**) contains calcification, suggesting that this component of the mass is chronic in nature. The calcification within the thrombus is in proximity to the adjacent thinned-walled LV apex, which is likely an old apical infarct/aneurysm. **C** and **D,** ECG-gated images pre-contrast (**C**) and delayed, post-contrast (**D**) at the same slice location confirm no evidence of enhancement within the apical mass, making thrombus the most likely diagnosis. **E** and **F,** ECG-gated delayed images in short-axis (**E**) and obliqued long-axis (**F**) planes demonstrate a partially calcified thrombus within the LV apex. The more superior portion of the thrombus is removed from the adjacent LV wall, suggesting an increased likelihood of embolic potential. The delayed images also demonstrate a fatty metaplasia within the apical infarct as well as late iodine enhancement subendocardially, as can be seen on late gadolinium-enhanced imaging with MRI. **G** and **H,** Spectral ECG-gated CT acquisition on the delayed phase. These monochromatic representations using a color map of the delayed acquisition show that the late iodine enhancement within the chronic LV apical infarct can be better identified with a keV of 65 (**H**) as opposed to a keV of 95 (**G**).

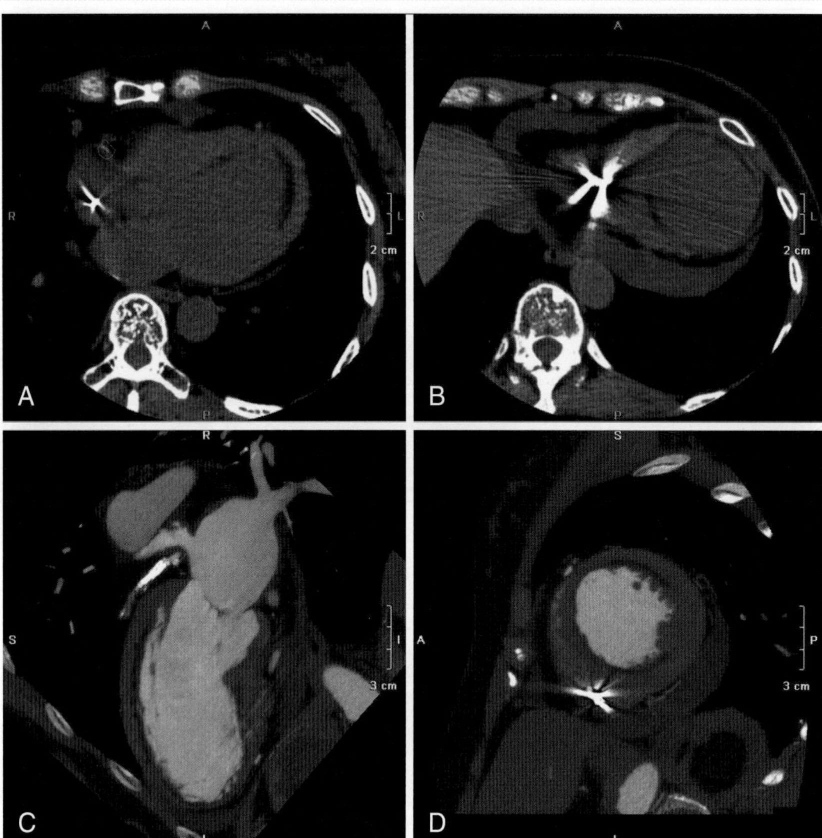

Figure 20-18. Composite images from a cardiac CT study demonstrate extensive fatty metaplasia involving the septum, anterior wall, and entire left ventricular apex. Fatty metaplasia is primarily subendocardial, with near full-thickness extent at the true left ventricular apex. Clinically, the patient has had prior left anterior descending artery territory infarction, with stenting of the proximal left anterior descending artery. There is an implantable cardiac defibrillator lead, and a moderate pericardial effusion is present. **See Video 20-7.**

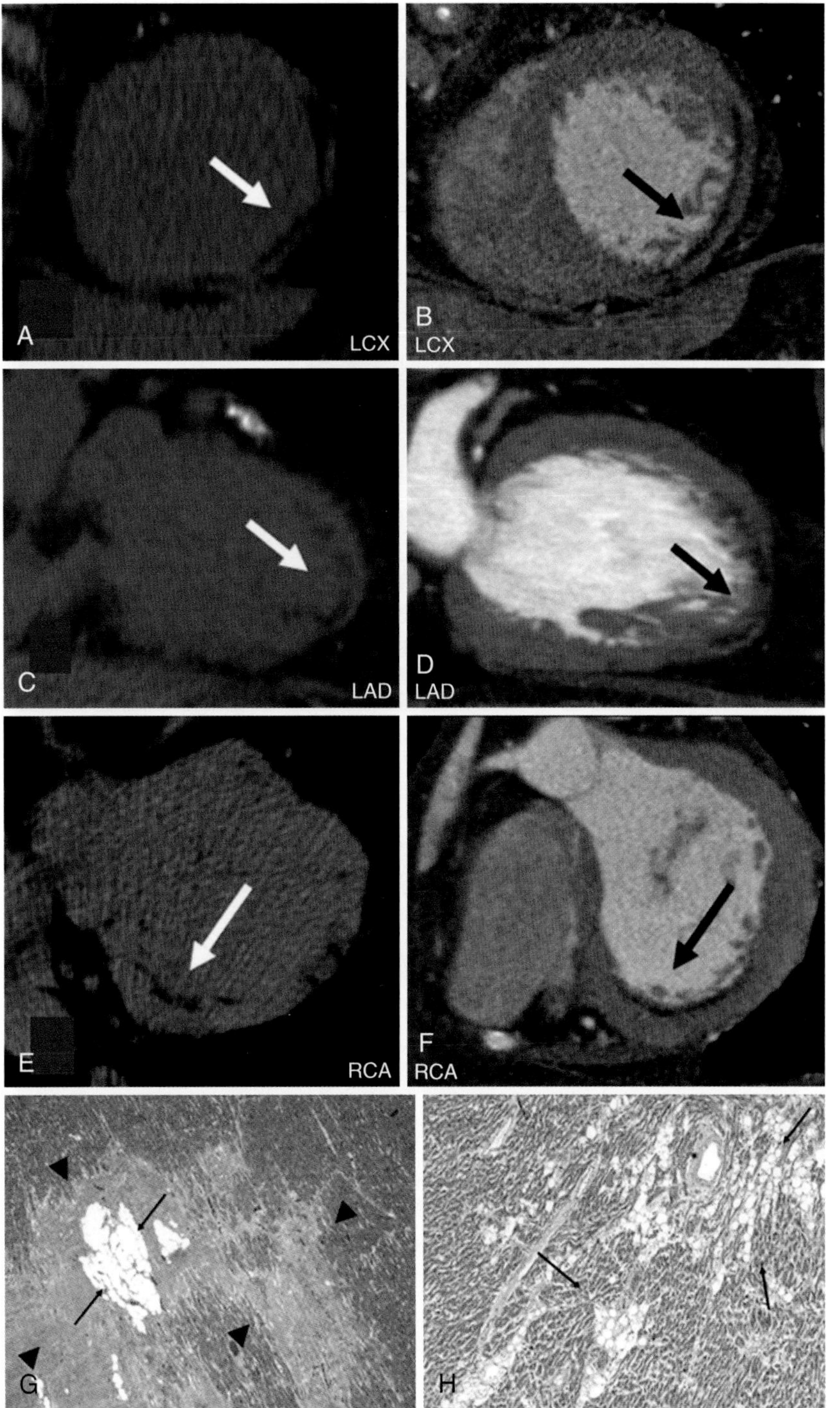

Figure 20-19. Fat deposition in infarcted myocardium. Pre- and post-contrast images of the heart in the left circumflex (LCx; **A** and **B**) artery; left anterior descending (LAD; **C** and **D**) artery; and right coronary artery (RCA; **E** and **F**) distribution are shown (each pair of images is from a different patient). Fat deposition typically is subendocardial and large enough to cover a significant portion of infarcted myocardium. Associated findings included thinning of myocardium (**A** through **D**), abnormal myocardial function, and corresponding coronary artery disease (not shown but present in all three persons). The findings help differentiate fat deposition of infarct scar from fat deposition as a normal variant . **G** and **H,** Fat deposition of infarcted myocardium (**G**) compared with healthy myocardium (**H**). Microphotograph of a myocardial specimen (original magnification, ×2; hematoxylin & eosin stain) from a 67-year-old man with severe triple-vessel coronary artery disease show fat deposition in an area of healed infarct (*long arrows*). This patient had multiple areas of patchy replacement fibrosis (*arrowheads*) in the distribution of the left anterior descending artery (not included in present study). Some of these foci show entrapped fat. **G,** Photomicrograph of myocardial specimen (original magnification, ×4) from a remote area shows the presence of fat in the interstitial area (*arrows*) between cardiomyocytes without accompanying interstitial or replacement fibrosis. (Reprinted with permission from Raney AR, Saremi F, Kenchaiah S, et al. Multidetector computed tomography shows intramyocardial fat deposition. *J Cardiovasc Comput Tomogr*. 2008; 2(3):152-163.)

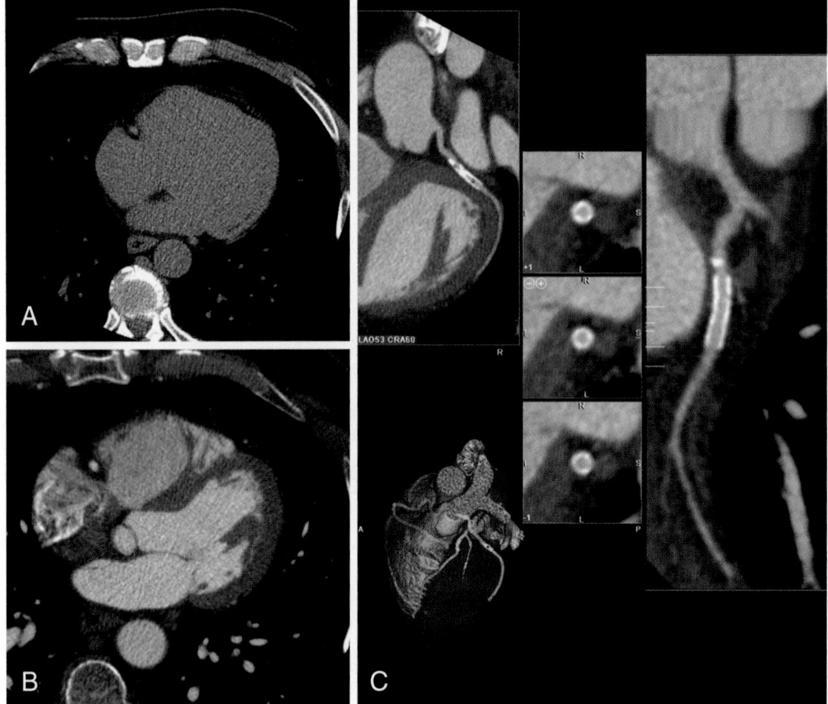

Figure 20-20. **A** and **B,** Subendocardial low attenuation along the lateral wall. **C,** A patent stented mid–left circumflex artery.

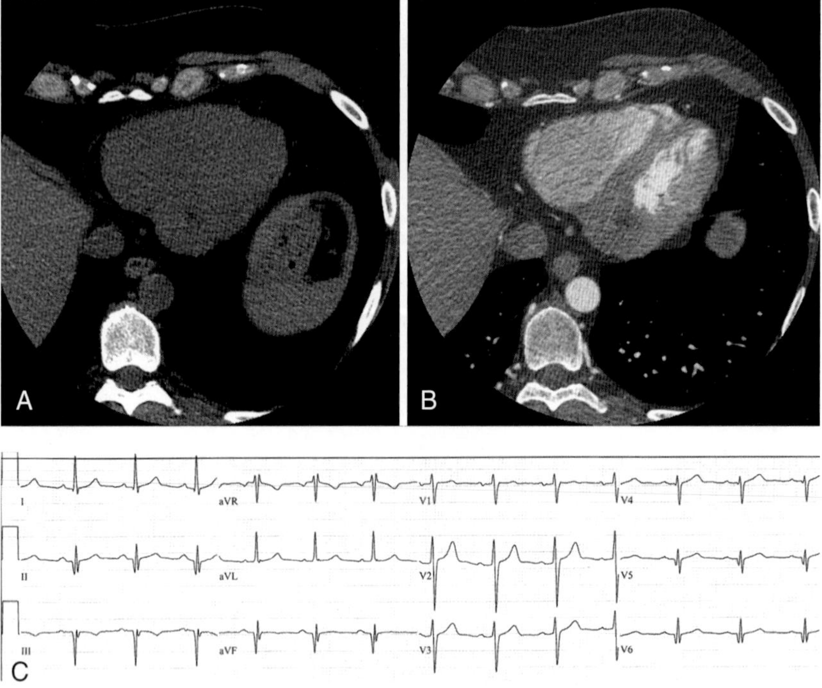

Figure 20-21. **A,** Precontrast CT image demonstrates subendocardial fat within the basal inferior wall of the left ventricle. This finding can also be appreciated on the contrast-enhanced study in **B. C**, The 12-lead ECG demonstrates Q waves within the inferior leads, consistent with a prior inferior infarct. While the distribution of the fatty metaplasia identified on the cardiac CT study is subendocardial and would seem to suggest that the infarction was subendocardial, the infarction actually was transmural.

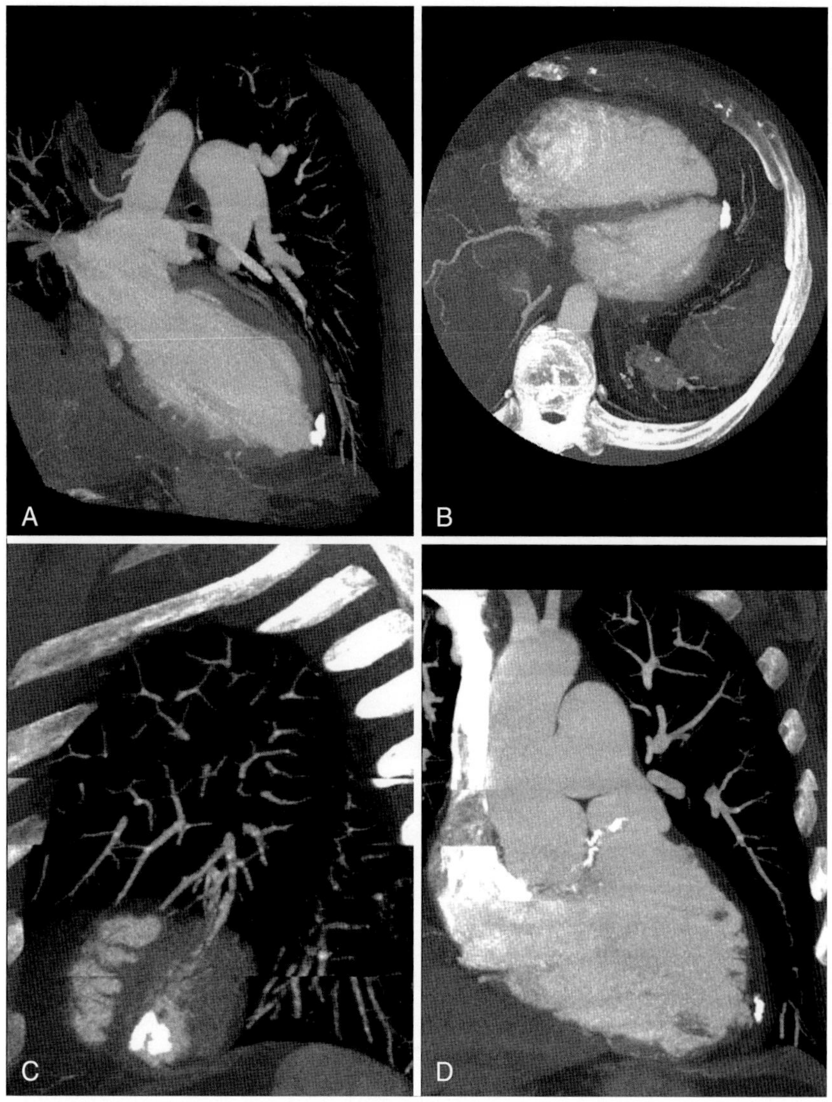

Figure 20-22. Multiple maximum intensity projection images in a patient with a history of repaired tetralogy of Fallot. These images illustrate a historical complication of open heart surgery. The focal thinning and calcification seen at the tip of the true apex represent the prior apical vent site for the patient's previous cardiac surgery. In this case the vent site is calcified myocardium. (Reprinted with permission from Hajsadeghi F, Ahmadi N, Eshaghian S, Budoff M. Porcelain heart. *J Cardiovasc Comput Tomogr*. 5(3):183-185.)

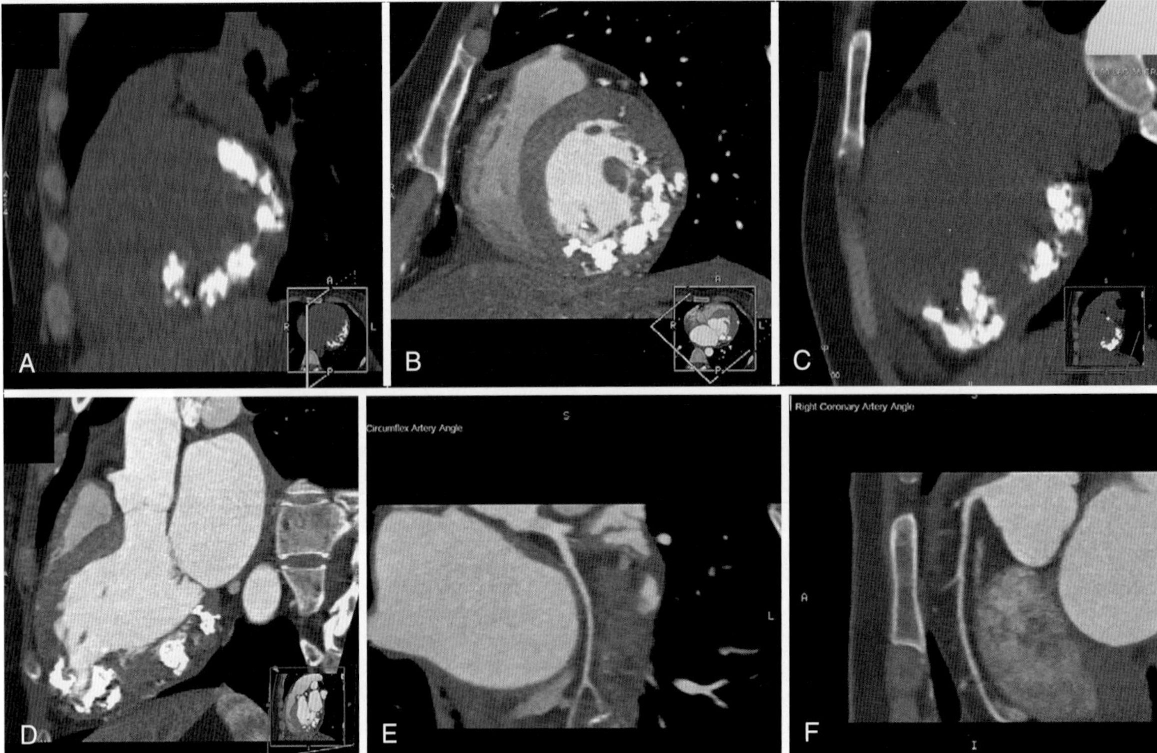

Figure 20-23. "Porcelain heart": extensive myocardial calcification. Cardiac CT angiography. Non–contrast- (**A** and **C**) and contrast-enhanced (**B** and **D**) images, in the short-axis orientation (**A** and **B**) and three-chamber orientation (**C** and **D**). Note the clumpy focal subendocardial to midwall myocardial calcification. **E** and **F,** Normal coronary arteries (curved multiplanar reformats) of the (A) left anterior descending, (B) left circumflex coronary artery, and (E) right coronary artery. (Reprinted with permission from Hajsadeghi F, Ahmadi N, Eshaghian S, Budoff M. Porcelain heart. *J Cardiovasc Comput Tomogr.* 5(3):183-185.)

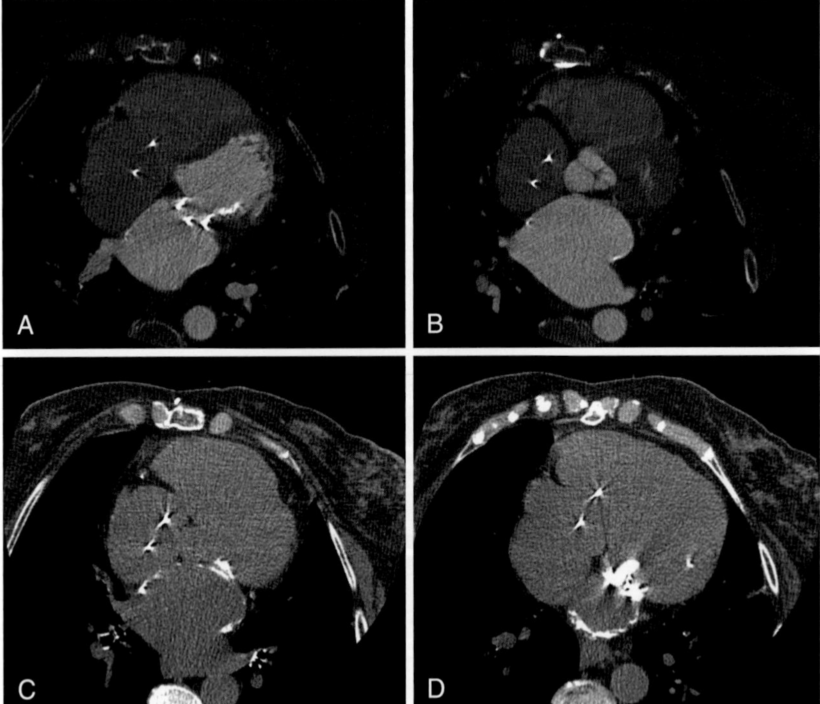

Figure 20-24. Multiple images from a cardiac CT data set in a patient with prior mitral valve surgery and atrial fibrillation. **A** and **B,** Contrast-enhanced images. **C** and **D,** Non–contrast-enhanced images. These images demonstrate an enlarged left atrium, as well as extensive curvilinear calcification within the left atrial wall. Diffuse calcification of the left atrial wall, as in this case, can be seen in the setting of chronic rheumatic mitral valve stenosis and atrial fibrillation.

TABLE 20-1 ACCF 2010 Appropriateness Criteria for the Use of Cardiac Computed Tomography to Evaluate Ventricular Morphology

	APPROPRIATENESS RATING	INDICATION	MEDIAN SCORE
Evaluation of cardiac structure and function—evaluation of ventricular morphology and systolic function	Appropriate	Evaluation of left ventricular function Following acute MI or in HF patients Inadequate images from other noninvasive methods	7
		Quantitative evaluation of right ventricular function	7
		Assessment of right ventricular morphology Suspected arrhythmogenic right ventricular dysplasia	7
	Uncertain	None listed	
	Inappropriate	Initial evaluation of left ventricular function Following acute MI or in HF patients	2

HF, heart failure; MI, myocardial infarction.

Data from Taylor AJ, Cerqueira M, Hodgson JM, et al. ACCF/SCCT/ACR/AHA/ASE/ASNC/NASCI/SCAI/SCMR 2010 appropriate use criteria for cardiac computed tomography. A report of the American College of Cardiology Foundation Appropriate Use Criteria Task Force, the Society of Cardiovascular Computed Tomography, the American College of Radiology, the American Heart Association, the American Society of Echocardiography, the American Society of Nuclear Cardiology, the North American Society for Cardiovascular Imaging, the Society for Cardiovascular Angiography and Interventions, and the Society for Cardiovascular Magnetic Resonance. *J Am Coll Cardiol.* 2010;56(22):1864-1894.

References

1. Johansson B, Maceira AM, Babu-Narayan SV, Moon JC, Pennell DJ, Kilner PJ. Clefts can be seen in the basal inferior wall of the left ventricle and the interventricular septum in healthy volunteers as well as patients by cardiovascular magnetic resonance. *J Am Coll Cardiol.* 2007;50(13):1294-1295.
2. Germans T, Wilde AA, Dijkmans PA, et al. Structural abnormalities of the inferoseptal left ventricular wall detected by cardiac magnetic resonance imaging in carriers of hypertrophic cardiomyopathy mutations. *J Am Coll Cardiol.* 2006;48(12):2518-2523.
3. Afonso L, Kottam A, Khetarpal V. Myocardial cleft, crypt, diverticulum, or aneurysm? Does it really matter? *Clin Cardiol.* 2009;32(8): E48-E51.
4. Ohlow MA. Congenital left ventricular aneurysms and diverticula: definition, pathophysiology, clinical relevance and treatment. *Cardiol.* 2006;106(2):63-72.
5. Ghersin E, Kerner A, Gruberg L, Bar-El Y, Abadi S, Engel A. Left ventricular pseudoaneurysm or diverticulum: differential diagnosis and dynamic evaluation by catheter left ventriculography and ECG-gated multidetector CT. *Br J Radiol.* 2007;80(957):e209-e211.
6. Yavari A, Sriskandan N, Khawaja MZ, Walker DM, Giles JA, McWilliams ET. Computed tomography of a broken heart: chronic left ventricular pseudoaneurysm. *J Cardiovasc Comput Tomogr.* 2008;2: 120-122.
7. Katayama T, Murata M, Iwanaga S, Kawamura A, Yoshikawa T, Ogawa S. Left ventricular pseudoaneurysm with peculiar coronary artery collapse. *J Am Coll Cardiol.* 2009;53(19):1823.
8. Hoey ET, Mansoubi H, Gopalan D, Tasker AD, Screaton NJ. MDCT features of cardiothoracic sources of stroke. *Clin Radiol.* 2009;64(5): 550-559.
9. Ichikawa Y, Kitagawa K, Chino S, et al. Adipose tissue detected by multislice computed tomography in patients after myocardial infarction. *JACC Cardiovasc Imaging.* 2009;2(5):548-555.

21 Myopathies

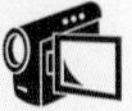

Key Points

- Cardiac CT's ability to depict fine structural detail within the heart enables it to characterize the morphologic features of cardiomyopathies such as wall thickness, left ventricular mass, mass distribution, and chamber dimensions.
- CCT's inability of to provide functional data beyond ejection fraction limits the functional characterization of cardiomyopathies, which would need to include characterization of atrioventricular valve insufficiency, pulmonary pressures, and outflow obstruction.
- CCT can contribute to the evaluation of undifferentiated dilated cardiomyopathy by identification or exclusion of underlying coronary artery disease.
- CCT, unlike CMR, is able to image hearts with pacemakers and implantable cardioverter defibrillators.

Recent technical advances in cardiac CT (CCT) have been driven largely by the requirements for accurate noninvasive coronary angiography. As a consequence of improved image quality and temporal resolution, attention has also turned to the broader application of cardiac CT assessment to other disease entities. The role of CT in the assessment of cardiomyopathy has, to date, been largely restricted to the measurement of left ventricle (LV) size and function. Other modalities such as echocardiography, cardiac MR (CMR), and nuclear techniques usually are favored for work-up of these patients, with additional information often obtainable with regard to concurrent disturbances such as mitral insufficiency, pulmonary hypertension, and left ventricular outflow tract obstruction. However, disease-specific morphologic features and the potential for CT-derived tissue characterization are increasing opportunities for the assessment of nonischemic myocardial disease by this rapidly evolving modality.

Limitations of noncoronary CCT at this stage include challenges in temporal resolution for functional assessment and the significant radiation exposure often incurred with the use of retrospective reconstruction techniques. Subsequently, comparatively little has been published on the assessment of cardiomyopathies by CCT. Dose modulation can play a role in radiation reduction. For morphology and tissue characterization purposes, prospective ECG-gating, multisegment acquisition/reconstruction, and wide-range detector systems allow dynamic volume assessment with significantly reduced radiation exposures. Furthermore, the development of dual-source/spectral energy imaging holds significant potential for the refinement of tissue characterization techniques with CT.

EPIDEMIOLOGY IN CLINICAL PRACTICE

Nonatherosclerotic cardiovascular abnormalities of potential clinical relevance are seen in 4.4% of patients referred for suspected coronary artery disease (CAD).[1] Of these, incidental hypertrophic cardiomyopathy is the most common myopathy identified (12%).

DILATED CARDIOMYOPATHY

There is no established routine role yet for cardiac CT in the evaluation of dilated cardiomyopathies, and little role in the assessment of LV function in general, given the other means to establish it.

A potential role may arise for the negative predictive value of CCT in regard to the presence of coronary disease in cases of probable idiopathic dilated cardiomyopathy. Validation has begun in selected patients. In a single-center study, among 61 patients with dilated cardiomyopathy (DCM) and 139 patients undergoing coronary angiography, 16-slice CT yielded 99.8% negative predictive value for significant (>50%) coronary stenoses.[2] Feasibility was 97%. The most common artifact observed in this series was a hypertrophied coronary venous system in proximity to the coronary arteries. Given the increased size of hearts with

DCM and the greater spatial dispersion of the coronary tree, as well as frequent coexistence of atrial fibrillation, wide-detector CCT with the potential for single cardiac cycle acquisition may have an advantage over 64-slice CT.

A further application may be the use of CCT before consideration of cardiac resynchronization therapy (CRT) as a single-modality assessment of cardiac function, coronary venous anatomy, regional wall motion, and scar.[3] The presence of myocardial dyssynchrony has been assessed with CCT and shown to be reproducible and to correlate with two- and three-dimensional echocardiography measures.[4] However, the clinical application of these techniques still must be prospectively evaluated (Fig. 21-1; **Videos 21-1 through 21-3**).

HYPERTROPHIC CARDIOMYOPATHY

Cardiac CT is able to depict the distribution of hypertrophy in hypertrophic cardiomyopathy (HCM)[5] and quantify it, as can CMR, although with the risk of radiation exposure, contrast allergy, and nephropathy. Validated by CMR, myocardial

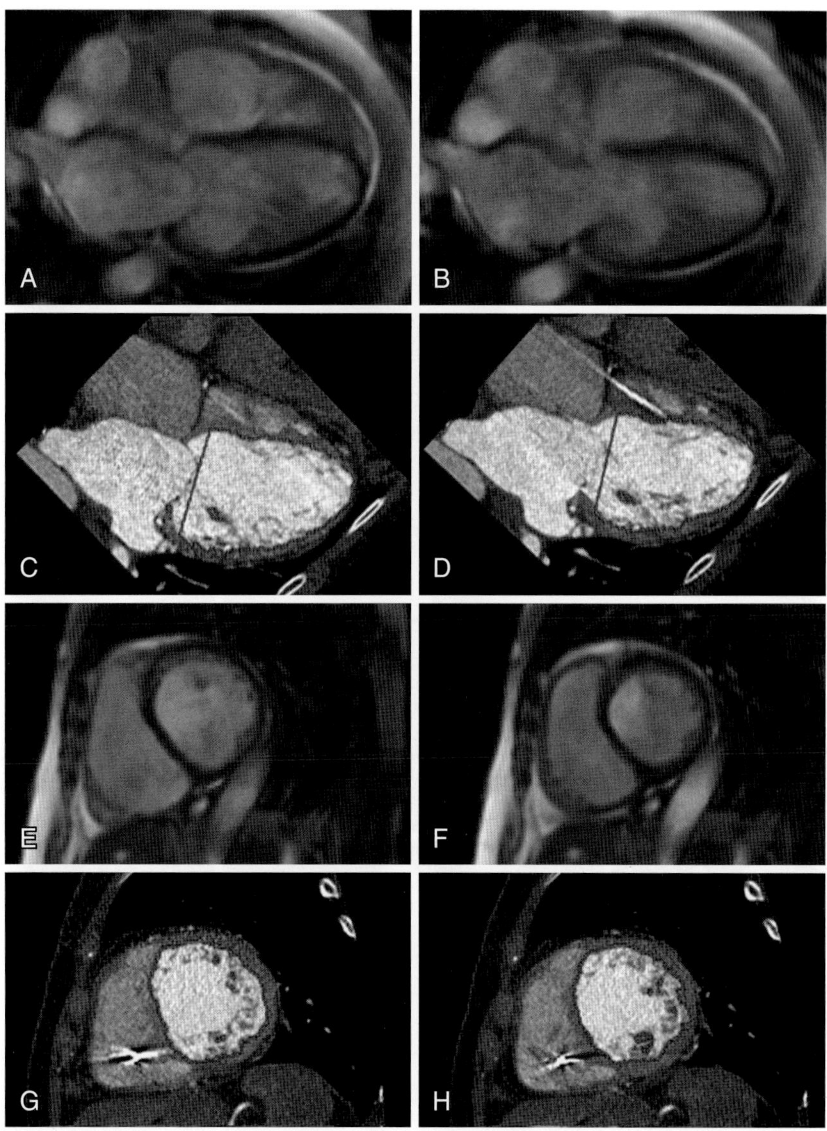

Figure 21-1. Cardiac MRI and cardiac CT images in a 50-year-old woman with dilated cardiomyopathy and heart failure. **A** and **B,** Cardiac MRI cine steady-state free precession (SSFP) images in the four-chamber orientation with end-diastole (**A**) and end-systole (**B**). **C** and **D,** Four-chamber reconstructions from a helically acquired cardiac CT study, with end-systole (**C**) and end-diastole (**D**). Severe left ventricular dilatation is seen, with severe systolic left ventricular dysfunction. **E** and **F,** Cardiac MRI cine SSFP images in the short-axis projection with end-diastole (**E**) and end-systole (**F**). **G** and **H,** Short-axis reconstructions from a helically acquired cardiac CT study, with end-systole (**G**) and end-diastole (**H**). Severe left ventricular dilatation is seen, with severe systolic left ventricular dysfunction. The studies were obtained 2 weeks apart. There was no significant change in the patient's medication between the two studies. Left ventricular indices are as follows: MR study: LVEDV: 272 mls, LVESV: 216 mls, LVEF: 20%; CT study: LVEDV: 274 mls, LVESV: 226 mls, LVEF: 17%. **See Videos 21-1 through 21-3.**

mass in HCM appears to be at least as good a predictor of cardiovascular mortality as wall thickness greater than 30 mm.[6] Notably, 20% of phenotype HCM cases may have normal myocardial mass. Although echocardiography still is the mainstay of assessment of HCM and hypertrophic obstructive cardiomyopathy (HOCM), especially because of its versatile Doppler capabilities, some cases of HCM are difficult to image, especially at the apex, which is relevant when evaluating possible apical variant HCM. The excellent spatial resolution of CT also may facilitate the identification of myocardial crypts, which have been suggested as an early sign of underlying cardiomyopathy in patients who carry an HCM mutation.[7] CMR or cardiac CT may thus complement echocardiographic assessment. The potential of CCT to plan and then assess the myocardial response to percutaneous transluminal septal ablation for HOCM also has been reported.[8] Currently, myocardial fibrosis assessment by late gadolinium CMR is well documented and may play a role in risk stratification in the future. While its validation is currently limited to case reports, the potential for characterization of myocardial fibrosis by delayed contrast CT may demonstrate a similar utility.[9]

Coronary CT angiography (CTA) in persons with HCM is likely to be relatively straightforward, because many are taking β-blockers to control their HCM. Feasibility of chest pain evaluation in HCM has been suggested (Figs. 21-2 through 21-10; **Videos 21-4 and 21-5).**

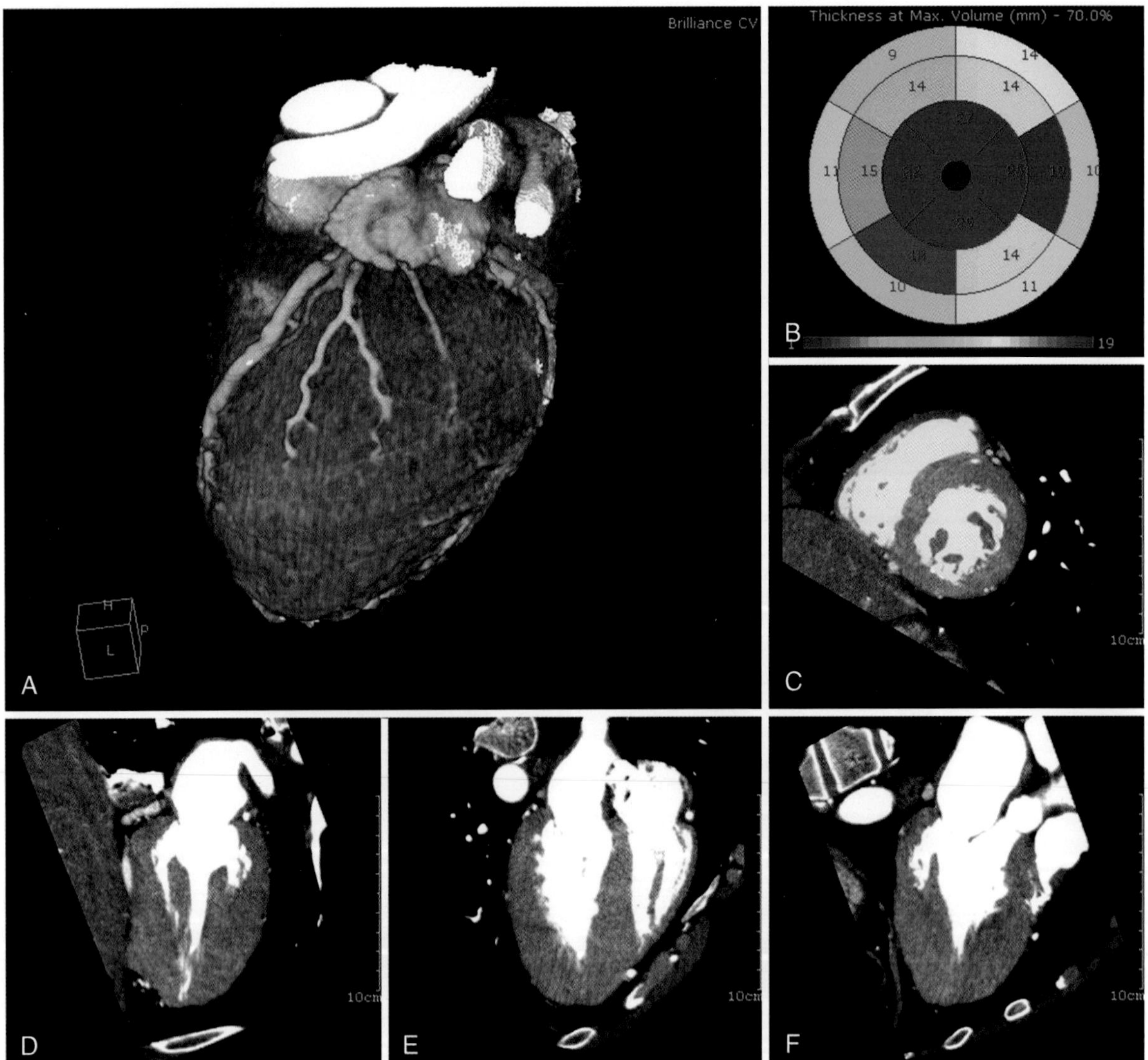

Figure 21-2. A, Three-dimensional volume-rendered view from a left anterior oblique position in a patient with hypertrophic cardiomyopathy with a predominant apical distribution. From the outside, the heart is not remarkable. Contrast-enhanced four-chamber, short axis, three-chamber, and two-chamber views (in diastole) also are shown. The distribution of hypertrophy is predominantly apical and anterior, and notably spares the base of the septum/left ventricular outflow tract. Using automatic segmentation algorithms, the wall thickness in diastole is displayed, and is color-coded according to the severity of the thickening (**B**). The greatest thickening is apical. **C,** The automatic segmentation depiction of the left and right ventricular walls and cavities.

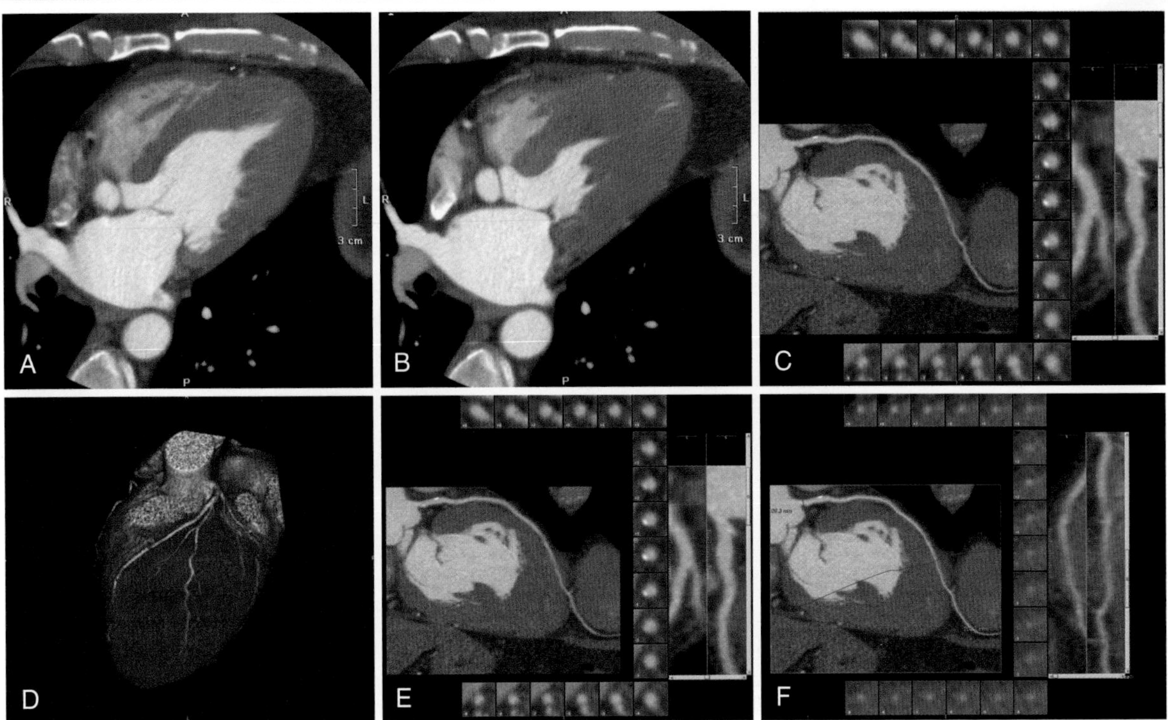

Figure 21-3. Composite images from a cardiac CT study demonstrate marked nonobstructive, predominantly apical hypertrophic cardiomyopathy. There is apical and mid-cavitary obliteration at end-systole with associated mild thinning of the left ventricular apex. Mild atherosclerotic coronary artery disease is seen. A mid-left anterior descending artery intramyocardial bridge also is present. **See Video 21-4.**

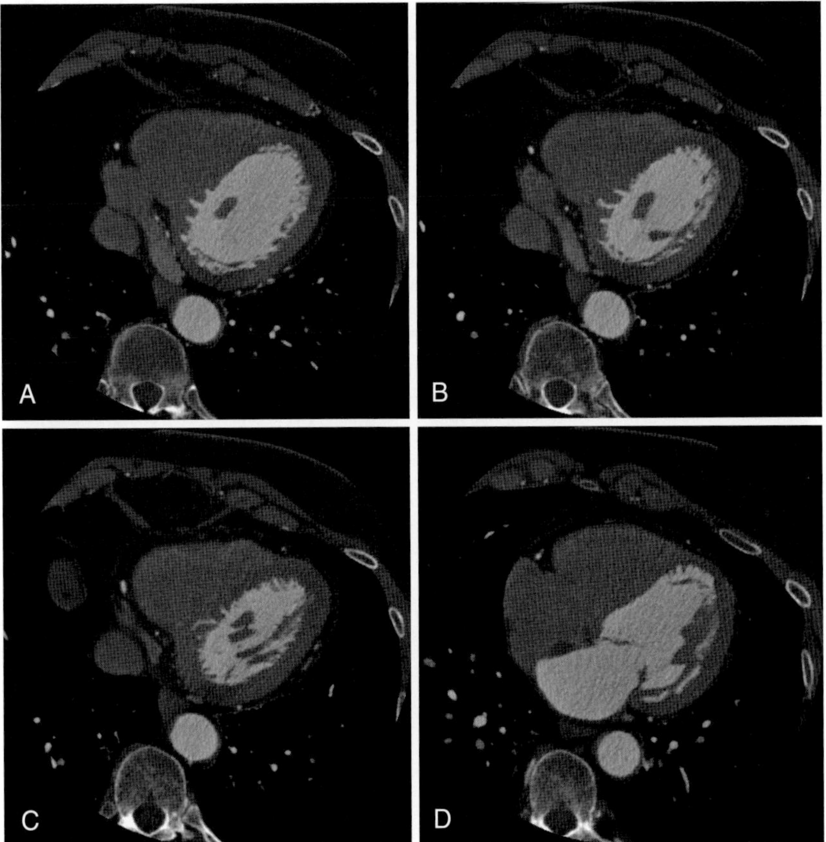

Figure 21-4. Axial images from a cardiac CT demonstrate subtle asymmetric left ventricular hypertrophy of the left ventricular apex, as well as numerous crypt-like extensions of contrast into the basal inferior left ventricular wall. These findings are suspicious for hypertrophic cardiomyopathy.

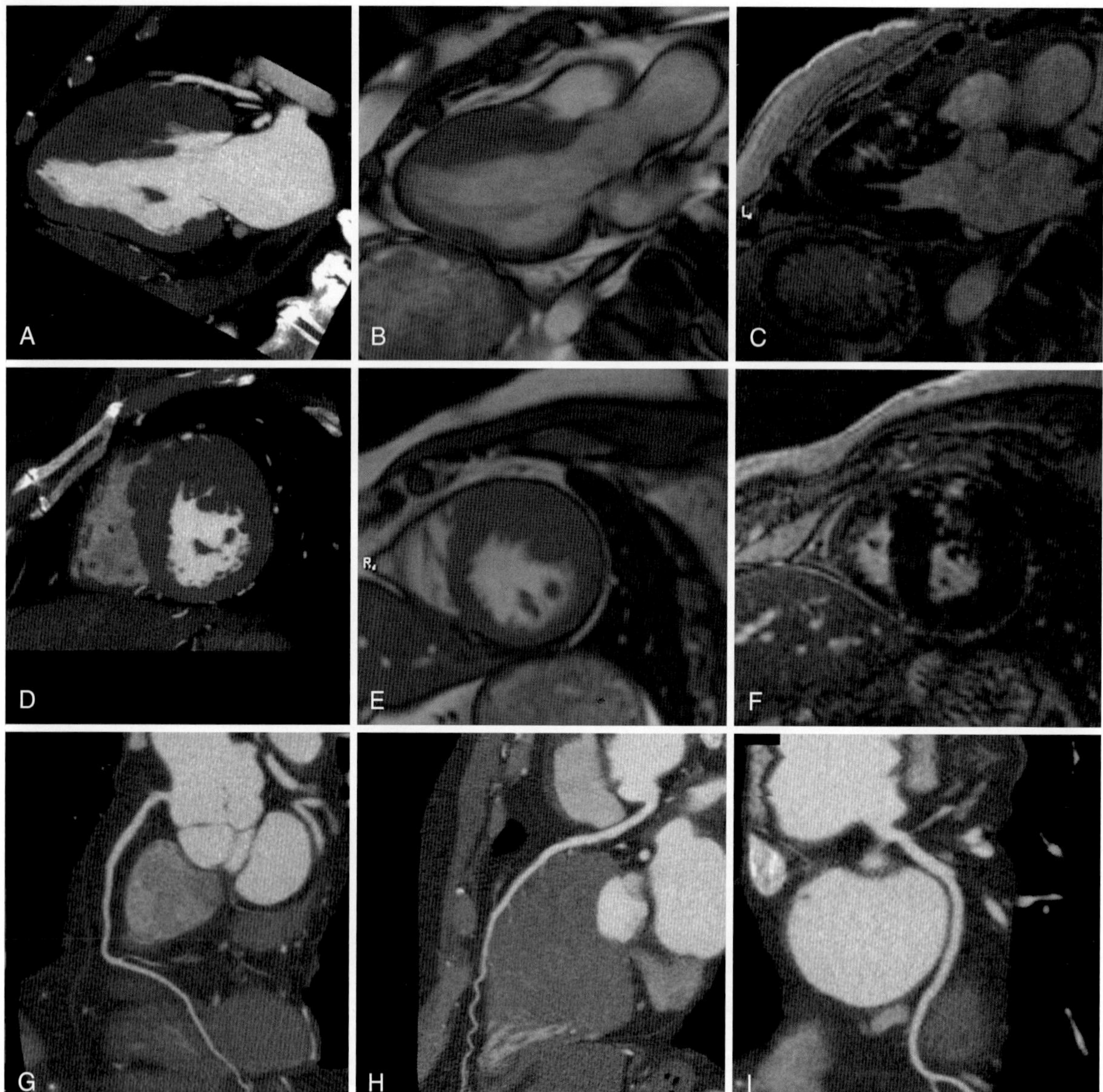

Figure 21-5. Composite panel of cardiac CT and CMR images in a 64-year-old patient with an abnormal ECG and chest pain. A cardiac CT study (**A, D, G–I**) in this patient demonstrates marked asymmetric septal and anterior wall hypertrophy, very suggestive of hypertrophic cardiomyopathy (HCM). Coronary CTA (**G–I**) was normal. A corresponding follow-up CMR study confirms the diagnosis of HCM with asymmetric left ventricular hypertrophy (**B** and **E**). Note the punctuate foci of late gadolinium enhancement within the anterior wall (**C** and **F**), not seen on the single arterial phase CT study.

INFILTRATIVE CARDIOMYOPATHY AND TISSUE CHARACTERIZATION

Tissue characterization previously has been possible only with CMR sequences to demonstrate the following:

- Scar (late enhancement)
- Inflammation (early relative enhancement)
- Edema (increased T2 signal)
- Intramyocardial fat (suppressible T1 signal)
- Iron overload (short T2* time).

Cardiac CT late enhancement (5 to 10 minutes after contrast injection) techniques are beginning to evolve.

Using a definition of intramyocardial fat as attenuation of −30 to −190 Hounsfield units (without histologic validation), fat has been observed in both left and right normal healthy ventricles, as well as within areas of prior infarction.[10] Dystrophic myocardial calcification diagnosed by CT in the absence of significant coronary disease also has been reported as a rare cause of congestive heart failure.[11]

SARCOIDOSIS

Using 64-slice CT and scanning immediately and 10 minutes after contrast injection, delayed enhancement has been shown in a case of sarcoidosis, with a nonischemic pattern similar to that seen with CMR, and colocalizing to areas of myocardial chronic sarcoidosis thinning.[12] Fusion single-photon emission CT (SPECT)/CT may improve diagnostic accuracy compared with SPECT alone (Figs. 21-11 through 21-13; **Video 21-6**).[13]

AMYLOIDOSIS

In cases of amyloidosis, delayed phase scanning (10 minutes) has been shown to yield late enhancement patterns that correspond to those seen in CMR late enhancement scanning (Fig. 21-14).[14]

FABRY DISEASE

Although Fabry disease, a disorder of α-galactosidase deficiency, is most commonly assessed with cardiac MRI and echocardiography, the characteristic findings of LV hypertrophy and associated delayed contrast enhancement patterns consistent with myocardial fibrosis have also been appreciated with CCT (Figs. 21-15 through 21-17).[15]

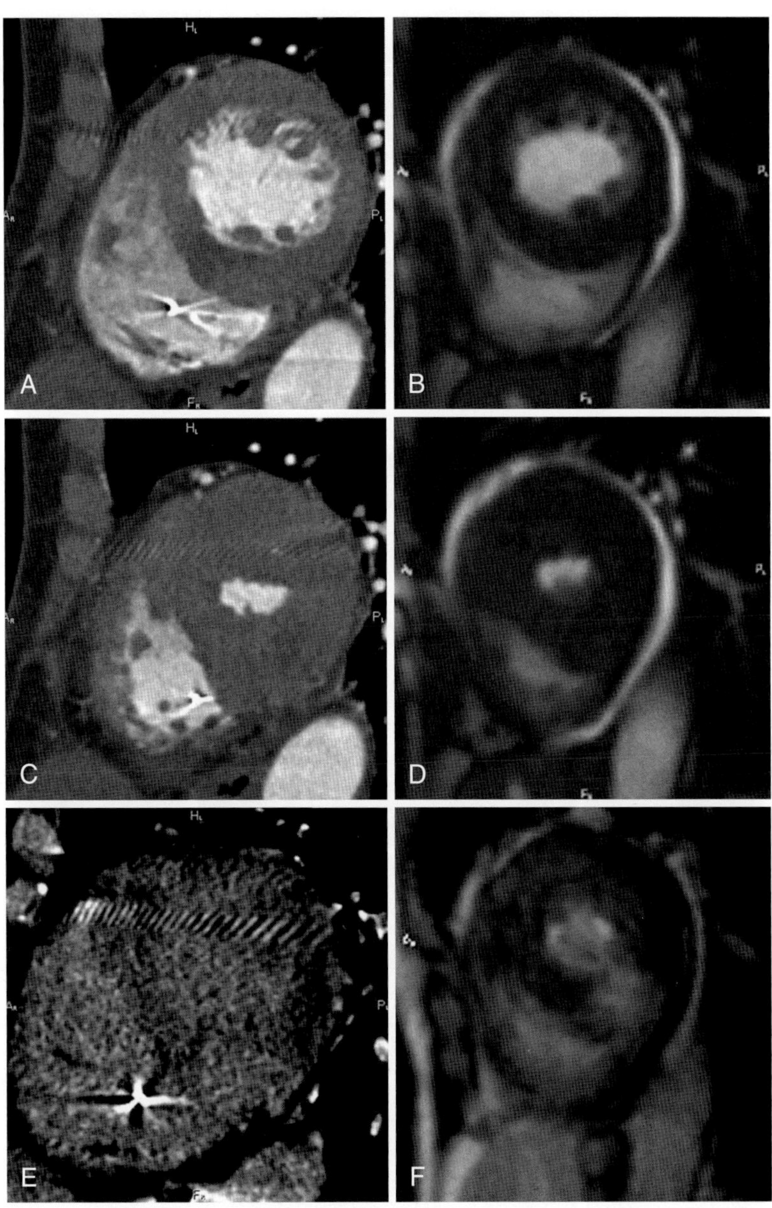

Figure 21-6. Composite panel of images from a cardiac CT (**A, C,** and **E**) and MRI (**B, D,** and **F**) in a patient with hypertrophic obstructive cardiomyopathy (HOCM). The patient had a history of ventricular tachycardia. **A** through **D**, Concentric left ventricular hypertrophy, more prominent in the septum, as well as right ventricular hypertrophy (CT). CT images also demonstrate a moderate-sized region of lower attenuation (likely hypoperfusion) in the mid- to inferior basal septum, with a moderate-sized focus of delayed enhancement of the inferoseptum/inferior wall. This correlates well with the late gadolinium MR image (**F**) and suggests a localized myocardial fibrosis.

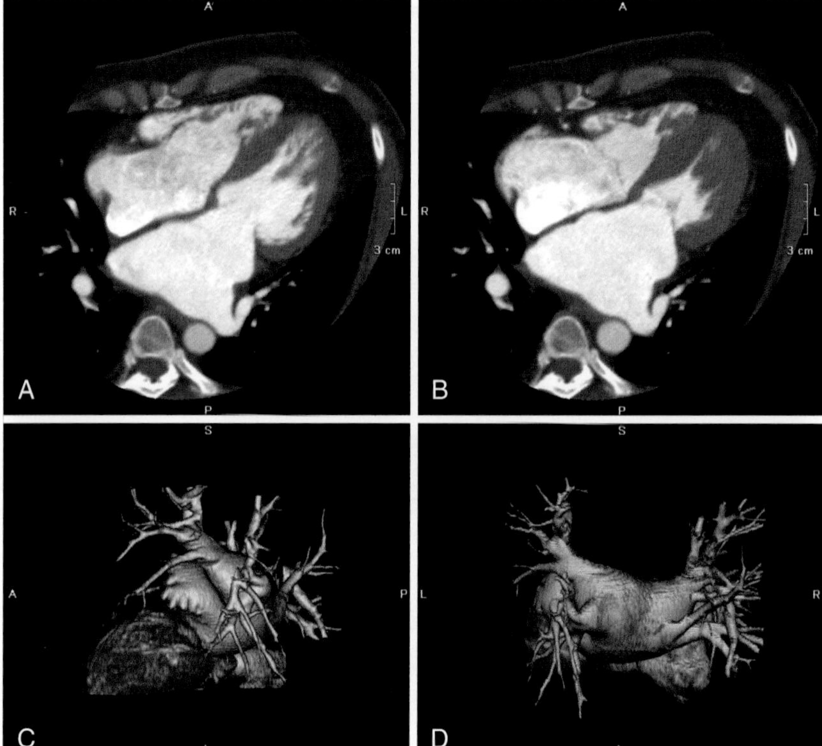

Figure 21-7. Composite images in a patient with hypertrophic cardiomyopathy demonstrate a small-volume left ventricle and marked enlargement of the left atrium (diastole, **A**; systole, **B**) The patient has underlying atrial fibrillation, which may be related to associated diastolic dysfunction.

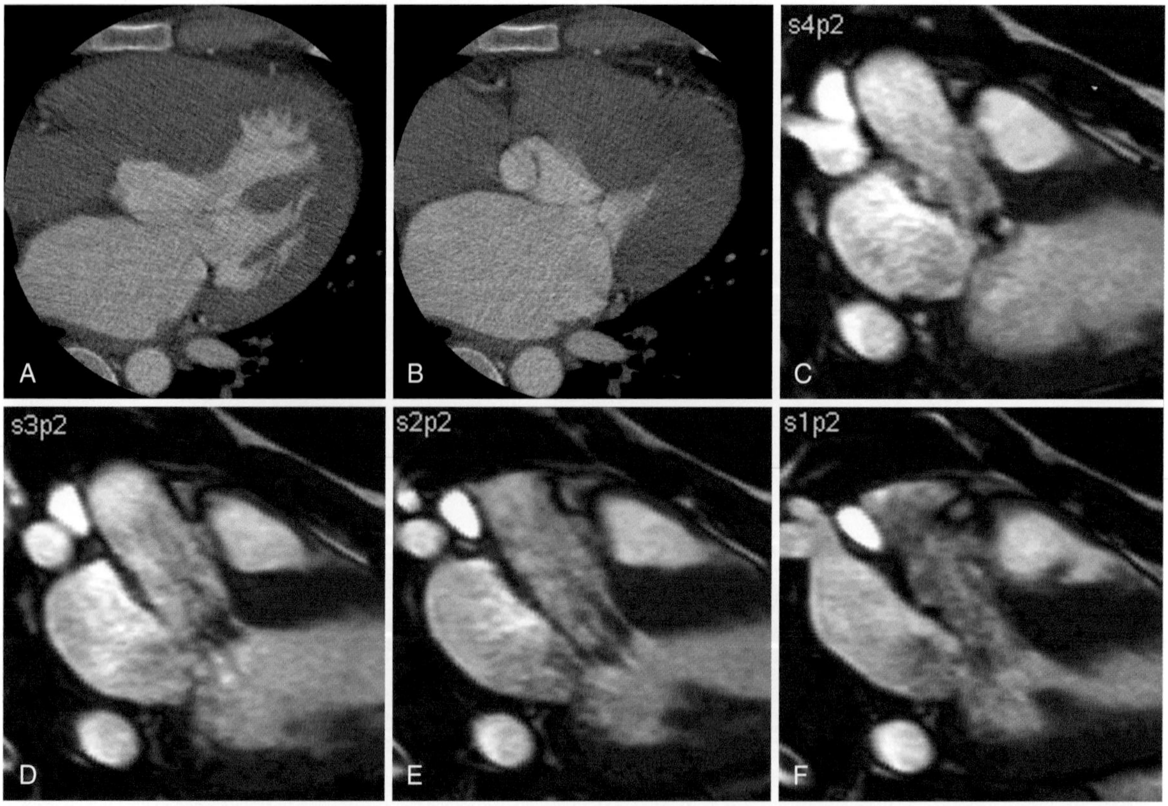

Figure 21-8. Composite images from cardiac CT and MRI studies in a patient with obstructive hypertrophic cardiomyopathy. CT images demonstrate systolic anterior motion (SAM) of the anterior mitral valve leaflet with SAM–septal contact. Left ventricular outflow tract CMR images demonstrate a moderate amount of intervoxel dephasing within the left ventricular outflow tract, extending into the ascending aorta and across the mitral valve plane into the left atrium. **See Video 21-5.**

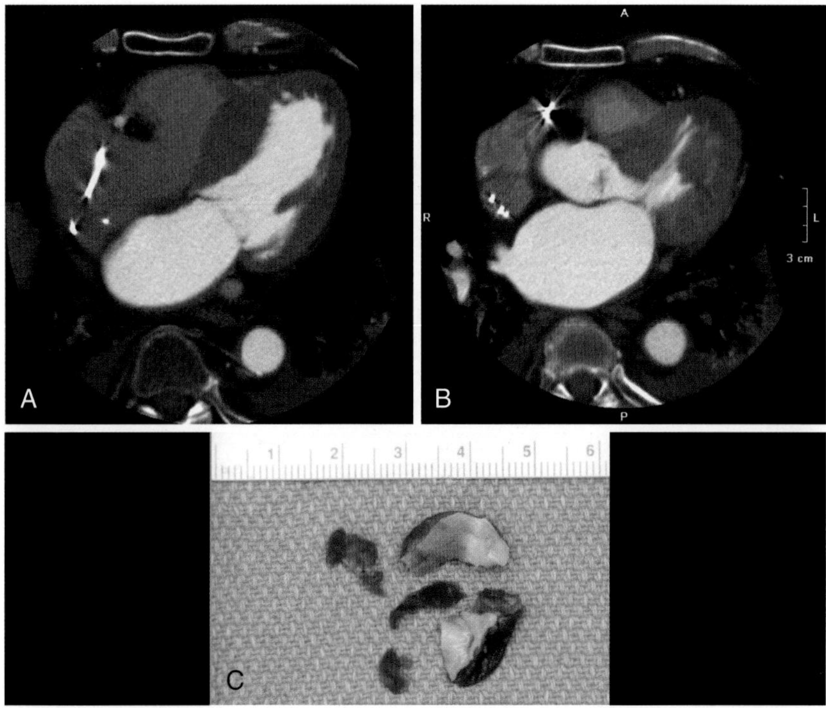

Figure 21-9. **A** and **B,** Two axial images from a cardiac CT data set demonstrate marked hypertrophy of the intraventricular septum. Note: right ventricular apical thickening is also present. Moderate left atrial enlargement also is present. The patient underwent subsequent myomectomy for relief of obstruction (**C**).

VENTRICULAR NONCOMPACTION

Echocardiography and CMR are the usual tests to assess for isolated left ventricular noncompaction (ILVN), but a case report of 64-slice CT demonstrated the characteristic morphologic and functional features of ILVN.[16] The achievable spatial resolution and blood pool to myocardial definition of CCT make it a promising alternative modality to echocardiography and CMR (Figs. 21-18 through 21-22).

STRESS (TAKOTSUBO) CARDIOMYOPATHY

History, echocardiography, and conventional coronary angiography are the usual tests to establish a diagnosis of stress cardiomyopathy. There are few data on the role of CCT, but single case reports have demonstrated the findings of apical ballooning and normal coronary arteries.[17] Because typically less coronary disease is present, the negative predictive value of CCT appears to be useful for such cases (Fig. 21-23).

ARRHYTHMOGENIC RIGHT VENTRICULAR DYSPLASIA/ CARDIOMYOPATHY

Evaluation for the morphologic features suggestive of arrhythmogenic right ventricular dysplasia/cardiomyopathy (ARVD/C) is a relatively common reason for referral for noninvasive imaging, but assessment is difficult and is most commonly done by CMR. Abnormalities of the thin wall of the right ventricle (RV) and the presence of intramyocardial fat often are sought but are notoriously difficult to assess. The excellent spatial resolution of CCT and its ability to detect intramyocardial fat may prove CT to be a useful adjunct for the identification of ARVD/C, particularly in the presence of contraindications to CMR (such as the presence of an ICD).[18] CCT can assess RV volumes and ejection fraction (EF). Case reports and small series have demonstrated the ability of 64-slice CCT to detect abnormalities of the RV, including trabeculations, intramyocardial fat, localized aneurysms, and scalloping of the free wall.[19,20] However, the presence of ICDs may increase the prevalence of misregistration of data sets and streak artifacts.[20] Senescent fatty infiltration can be seen in normal individuals, especially with ageing, and should be differentiated from changes associated with ARVD/C.[21]

Arrhythmogenic right ventricular cardiomyopathy or dysplasia is a specific form of fibrofatty degeneration of the RV wall that renders the RV regionally dilated, hypokinetic, thinned, and arrhythmogenic (with premature ventricular contractions and ventricular tachycardia). The morphologic findings of ARVD enable the diagnosis to be supported by imaging, to some extent.

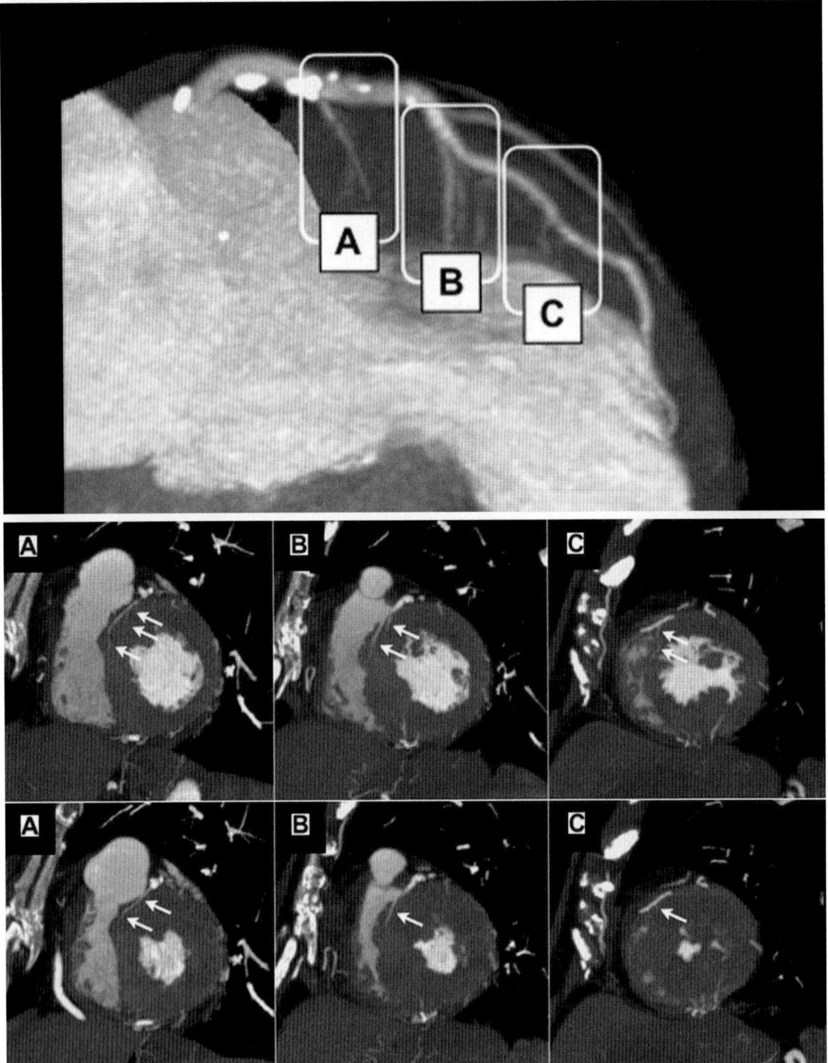

Figure 21-10. Alcohol septal ablation. Three septal arteries of the left anterior descending artery on septal plane maximum intensity projection images in diastole. Positions of the first (*A*), second (*B*), and third (*C*) septal branches are marked on the large image on the left. The upper (diastolic images) and lower (systolic images) show left ventricular short-axis maximum intensity projection images, corresponding to the first (*A*), second (*B*) and third (*C*) septal branches as seen in short-axis views (*arrows*). Each septal branch is wide and long in diastole, but narrow and short in systole. Diastolic images show the first septal branch arborized into two end-arteries in the myocardium and perfused entire hypertrophic myocardium at the basal interventricular septum (A). (Reprinted with permission from Okayama S, Uemura S, Soeda T, et al. Role of cardiac computed tomography in planning and evaluating percutaneous transluminal septal myocardial ablation for hypertrophic obstructive cardiomyopathy. *J Cardiovasc Comput Tomogr.* 2010;4(1):62-65.)

Contrary to conventional wisdom, there is no gold standard test for the diagnosis of ARVD. MRI conventionally has been considered the best available test; however, diagnosis by MRI has limited interobserver agreement. In addition, MRI image acquisition is particularly disadvantaged by frequent premature ventricular contractions, which are extremely common in ARVD.

Current CT scanning is able to depict most of the anatomic features used as diagnostic criteria for ARVD and offers a handier means to obtain the same information.[20] Correlation between MRI and CT findings has not been widely published. CT electron beam CT (EBCT) has been shown to image features of ARVD. In the series of 14 patients with ARVD reported by Tada et al.,[22] the incidence of findings was as follows:

- Abundant epicardial fat: 86%
- Conspicuous trabeculations with low attenuation: 71%
- Scalloped surface of the RV free wall: 79%
- Intramyocardial fat:
  - RV only: 30%
  - RV and LV: 5%
  - LV only: 5%

Finding fat among 1 mm of myocardium when there are several millimeters of adjacent epicardial fat is improbable.

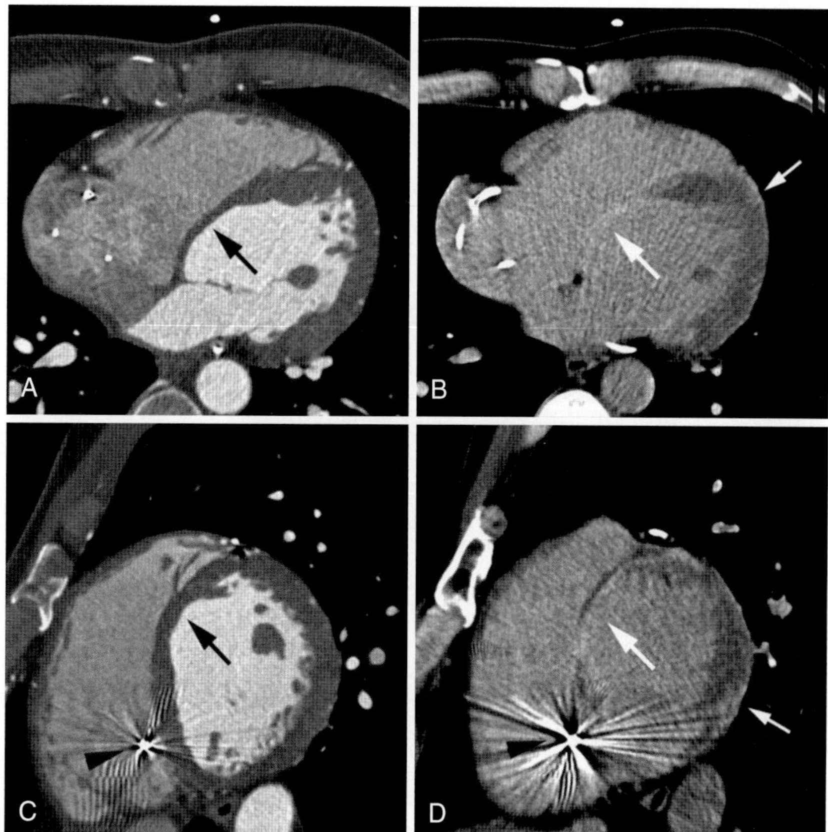

Figure 21-11. First-pass CT angiographic and delayed enhancement images obtained by dual-source CT (DSCT) after injection of 100 mL contrast agent. First-pass images are reconstructed with a 0.75-mm slice thickness. Delayed images were acquired 10 minutes after contrast injection and are reconstructed as 3-mm thick multiplanar reconstruction to decrease image noise. **A** and **B,** Corresponding first-pass (**A**) and delayed (**B**) images in transaxial orientation. **C** and **D,** Corresponding short-axis reformats. In a pattern typical for cardiac sarcoidosis, thinning of the basal anterior septum with corresponding transmural enhancement in the delayed scan is clearly detectable (*large arrows*). *Small arrows* point to additional areas of late myocardial enhancement in the apical (**B**) and lateral (**D**) regions. The *arrowheads* point to the right ventricular implantable cardioverter defibrillator (ICD) electrode, which causes streak artifacts. In addition, sections of ICD electrodes are visible in the right atrium. (Reprinted with permission from Muth G, Daniel WG, Achenbach S. Late enhancement on cardiac computed tomography in a patient with cardiac sarcoidosis. *J Cardiovasc Comput Tomogr*. 2008;2:272-273.)

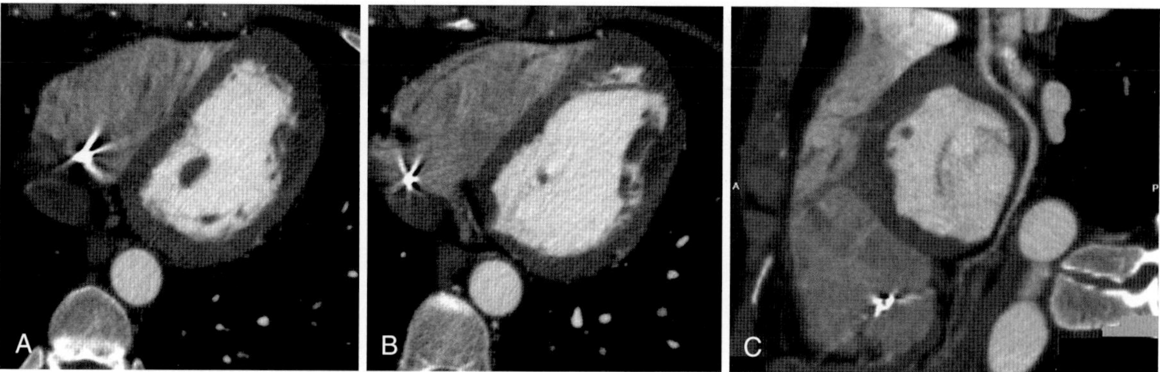

Figure 21-12. A 39-year-old woman presented with heart block. A pacemaker was inserted. Echocardiography demonstrated moderate hypokinesis with regional variability and an apical aneurysm. As MRI was contraindicated, she came for a cardiac CT examination, which demonstrated multifocal areas of myocardial thickening associated with focal hypodensity and hypokinesis. A small inferoapical aneurysm also was noted. CT angiography demonstrated a normal left anterior descending artery and left circumflex coronary artery. The right coronary artery was partially obscured by moderate beam-hardening artifact from the pacemaker. No mediastinal lymphadenopathy was noted on the cardiac CT. The differential diagnoses based on the CT were sarcoid or myocarditis, or—less likely—myocardial metastases. A myocardial biopsy yielded a diagnosis of cardiac sarcoidosis.

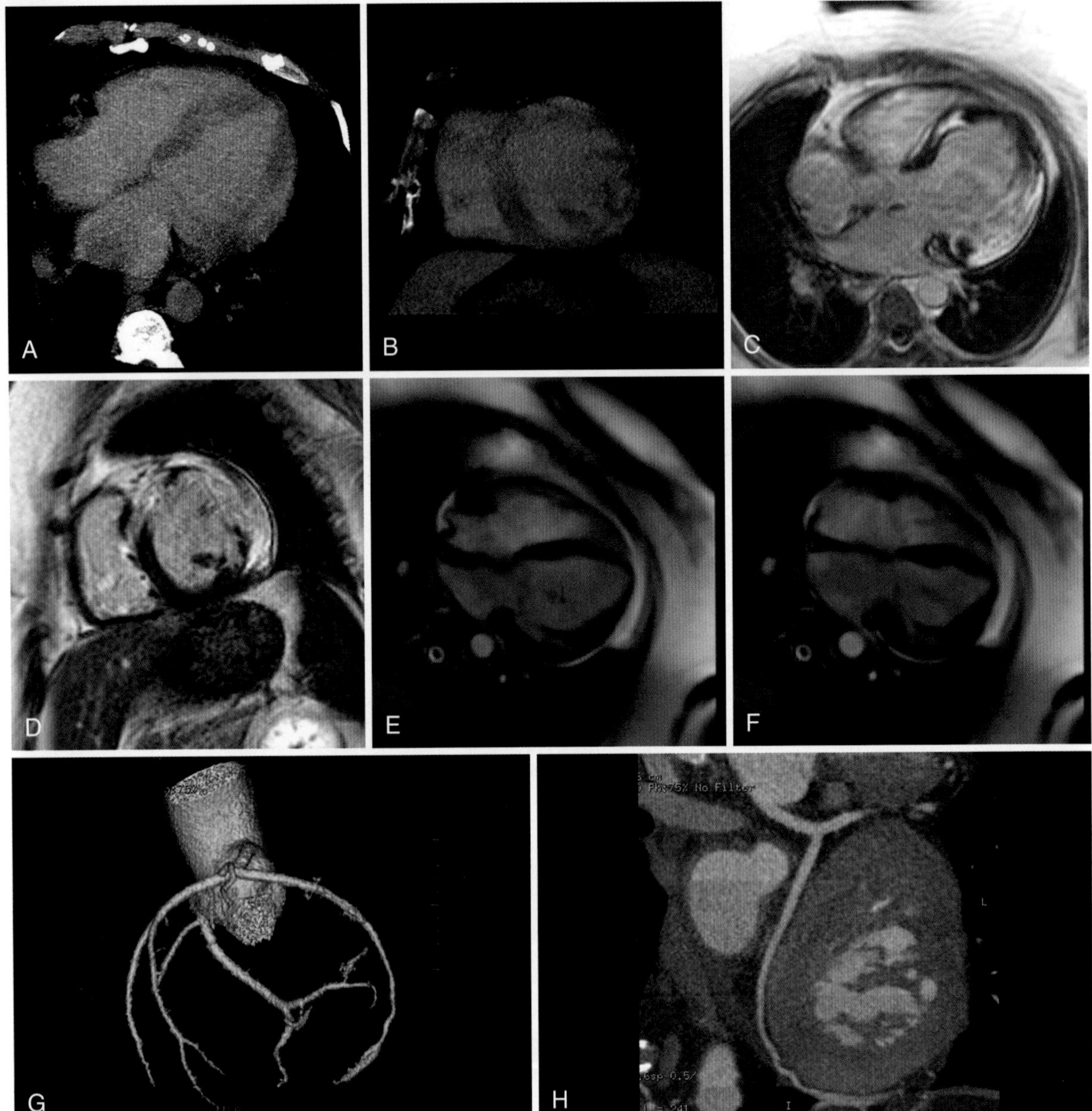

Figure 21-13. Cardiac sarcoidosis. Contrast-enhanced axial (**A**) and short-axis oblique cardiac CT images (**B**). High attenuation/contrast enhancement is present in the mid-septum and the mid-anterior and lateral walls. **C** and **D,** CMR imaging reveals late gadolinium enhancement of the mid- and anterior septum and lateral walls. **E** and **F,** CMR steady-state free precession imaging demonstrates akinesis and local aneurysm of the dilation of the lateral wall segment that exhibits late enhancement. **G** and **H,** Coronary CTA demonstrates absence of coronary disease. **See Video 21-6.**

MRI-BASED CRITERIA FOR DIAGNOSIS OF ARVD

The MRI-based criteria for the diagnosis of ARVD, borrowed by CCT, include:

- Dilated RV[23]
- Low right ventricular ejection fraction (<35%) with normal left ventricular ejection fraction (LVEF)
- Segmental dilation, or "scalloping" (aneurysm) of the RV free wall
- Ectasia of the right ventricular outflow tract[23]
- Segmental hypokinesis of the RV
- Dyskinetic bulges[23]
- Excess trabeculation of the right ventricle
- Enlargement of the right atrium[23]

Proposed Modified Task Force Criteria

According to Modified Task Force Criteria, the diagnosis of ARVD is based on a combination of major and minor criteria. A diagnosis of ARVD requires satisfaction of either two major criteria *or* one major and two minor criteria *or* four minor criteria (Table 21-1).[24]

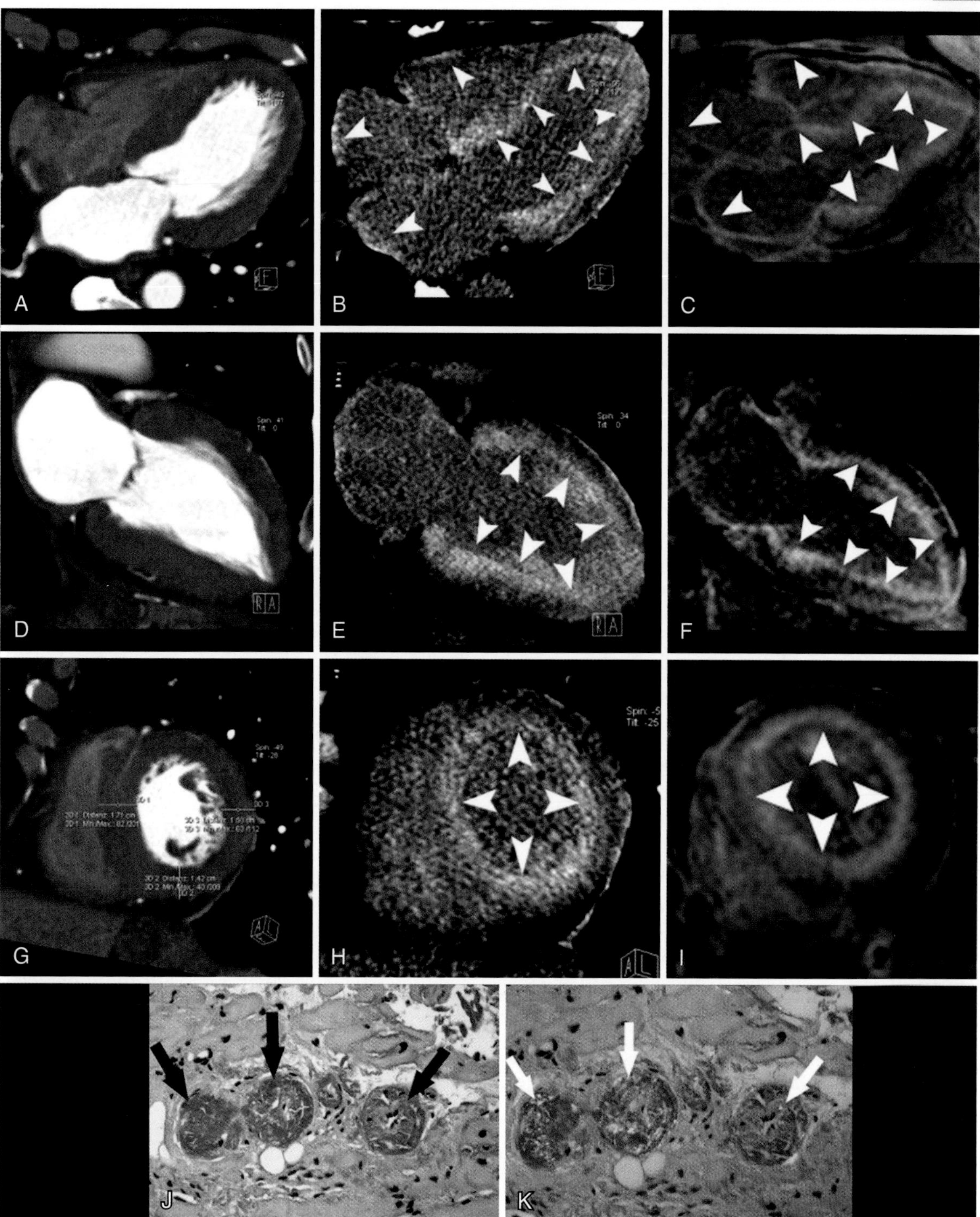

Figure 21-14. Composite illustration of cardiac CT in systemic amyloidosis. Multiplanar reconstructions of the early-phase CT scan using 5-mm-thick slices in a four-chamber view (**A**) show left ventricular hypertrophy. Delayed scan in a similar projection (**B**) shows late enhancement at multiple locations (*arrows*). The finding of cardiac amyloidosis was confirmed by right ventricular endomyocardial biopsy (Congo red stain, **J**) showing green birefringence under polarized light (**K**). The delayed CT scan enhancement was confirmed by cardiac magnetic resonance late-enhancement imaging (inversion recovery turbo-FLASH; **C, F**). (Reprinted with permission from Marwan M, Pflederer T, Ropers D, et al. Cardiac amyloidosis imaged by dual-source computed tomography. *J Cardiovasc Comput Tomogr.* 2008;2(6):403-405.)

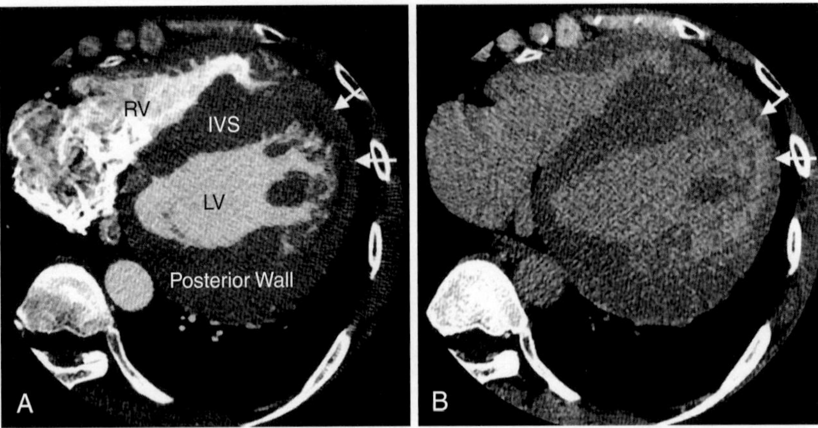

Figure 21-15. Axial source images of enhanced multislice CT acquired 30 seconds (**A**) and 8 minutes (**B**) after the injection of the contrast material. Images show extreme hypertrophy of the interventricular septum (IVS) and posterior wall compared with the apical and lateral walls of the left ventricle (LV). The apical and lateral portions revealed lower CT intensity than the IVS in the early phase (*arrows*). Conversely, in the late phase, the apical and lateral portions of the LV (*arrows*) were abnormally enhanced compared with the extremely hypertrophic IVS, suggesting more fibrotic changes in the apical and lateral myocardium. RV, right ventricle. (Reprinted with permission from Funabashi N, Toyozaki T, Matsumoto Y, et al. Images in cardiovascular medicine. Myocardial fibrosis in Fabry disease demonstrated by multislice computed tomography: comparison with biopsy findings. *Circulation*. 2003;107(19):2519-2520.)

Assessment of ARVD by CCT is feasible, and CCT in this context appears to have its best application as a screening test for ARVD. If findings are negative for ARVD (as discussed earlier), the patient may be considered to be free of ARVD. If those features are positive, however, further testing with cine MRI may be undertaken to confirm findings and offer a superior means to assess for fatty infiltration (Figs. 21-24 through 21-28; **Video 21-7**).

CHAGAS DISEASE

About one third of people infected with *Trypanosoma cruzi* will develop Chagas heart disease. The disease may present with LV dysfunction, ventricular aneurysms, conduction abnormalities, or ventricular tachycardia.[25] Myocardial fibrosis is common in these patients and correlates with LV function. When present, myocardial fibrosis has been reported as subepicardial or midwall in 47% of patients and subendocardial or transmural in 53% of patients—making differentiation from CAD-related infarction difficult in some cases.[26] The demonstration of typical myocardial findings in the presence of normal coronary arteries and seropositivity for *T. cruzi* is suggestive of the diagnosis (Fig. 21-29; **Video 21-8**).

MYOCARDITIS

Myocarditis typically is diagnosed by excluding CAD and obtaining corroborative imaging such as CMR (late enhancement of a nonischemic pattern) or by achieving definitive diagnosis with a positive endomyocardial biopsy. Few studies or case reports have been performed to date on the imaging findings of cardiac CT in suspected or proven myocarditis cases, but those that have been reported described patchy late enhancement in a typically nonischemic pattern that is similar to the late enhancement seen in corresponding CMR studies. CTA, unlike CMR, is able to offer high negative predictive value of CAD, which often is clinically needed information.[27,28] In a series of 12 cases of acute myocarditis, CCT (first pass) demonstrated an absence of CAD, and a late enhancement (5 minutes) demonstrated areas of focal (6 patients) or multifocal (6 patients) hyperenhancement. The extent and location of hyperenhancement by CCT correlated well with those depicted by CMR ($r = 0.92$, $P = .0004$) (Fig. 21-30).[29]

CCT PROTOCOL POINTS

- To evaluate systolic function, helical/retrospective scanning is needed.
- To evaluate myocardial perfusion:
  - The standard protocol for CCT is followed.
  - Ensure review of noncontrast images to exclude the presence of fatty metaplasia.
- To evaluate delayed enhancement:
  - Delayed (second) acquisition at 5 to 10 minutes after contrast administration. Slice thickness can be increased to 3 mm and kVp reduced (80 to 100 kVp).
- See Table 21-2.

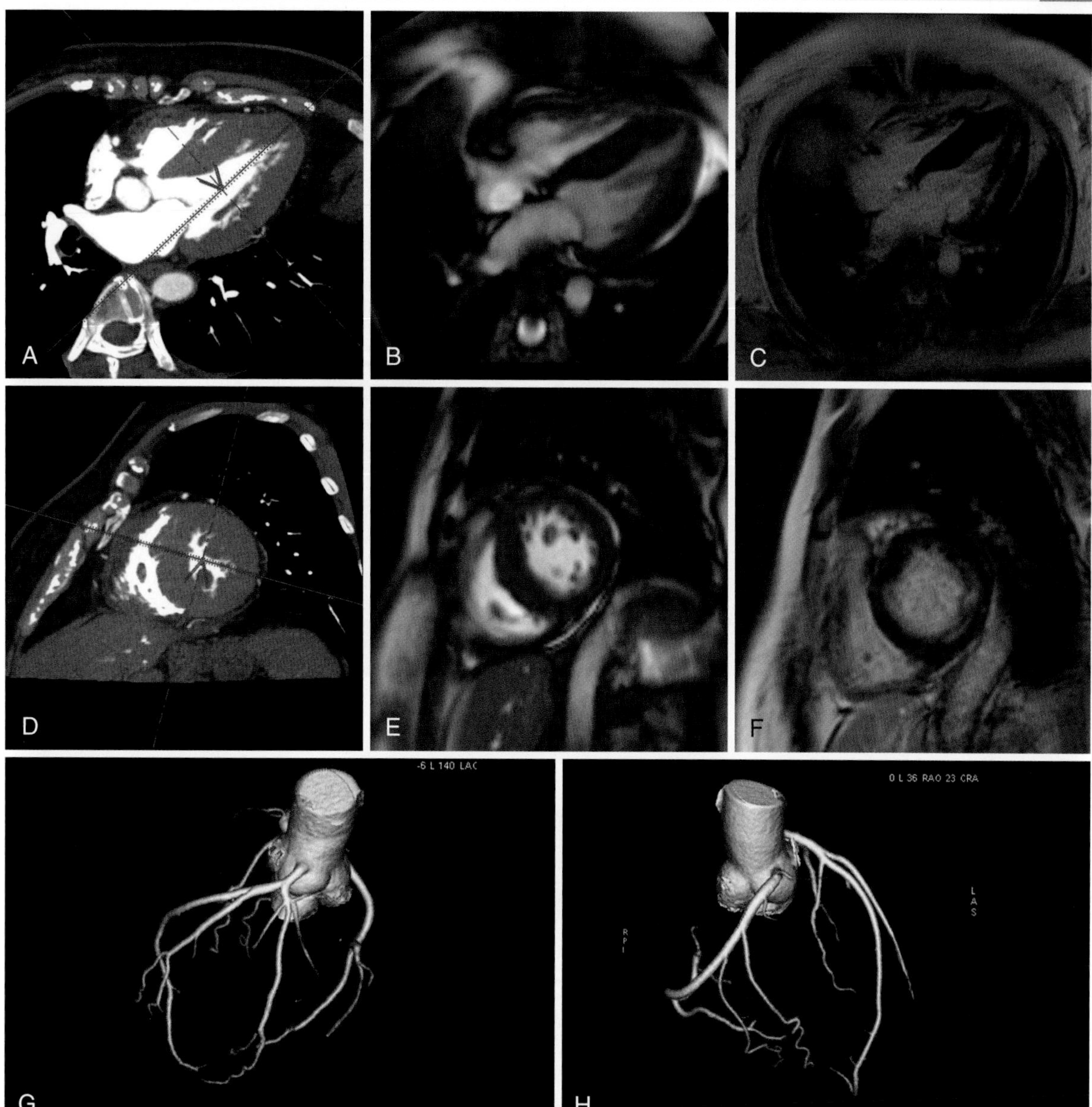

Figure 21-16. Cardiac CT and corresponding cardiac MRI images of a 42-year-old woman with chest pain. Four-chamber CCT (**A**), CMR SSFP (**B**), and CMR LGE (**C**), and short-axis oblique CCT (**D**), CMR SSFP (**E**), and CMR LGE (**F**) reformatted cardiac CT images through the heart. These images demonstrate concentric left and right ventricular hypertrophy. **G** and **H,** Volume-rendered images. The coronary arteries in this patient were normal, with no evidence of coronary artery disease. Given the diffuse ventricular hypertrophy, a cardiomyopathy process was considered in the differential. The patient subsequently underwent a cardiac MRI study. **D–F** demonstrate a four-chamber and short-axis abscess at PMH through the heart confirming biventricular hypertrophy. The right most compatible demonstrates mid-wall late enhancement within the lateral wall of the left ventricle. The slight enhancement is in a nonischemic pattern. Given this pattern, one of the considerations for this patient was Fabry disease, which was confirmed by genetic testing.

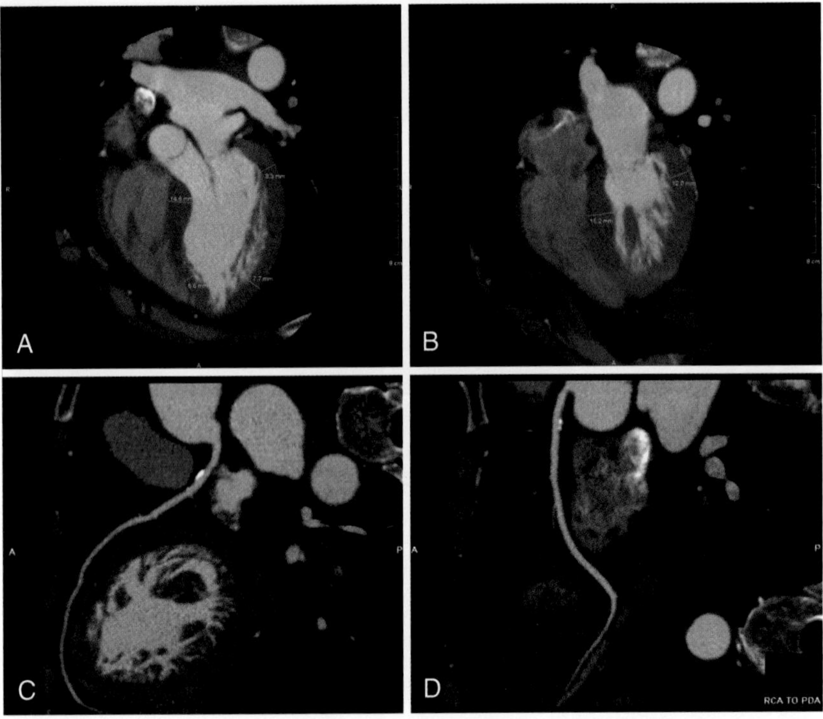

Figure 21-17. Composite images from a 54-year-old woman with known Fabry disease (heterozygous) who presented with an abnormal ECG and nonspecific chest pain. As this condition has an increased risk of early coronary artery disease, a CTA was performed and demonstrated only mild disease in the proximal left anterior descending artery (**C**) and right coronary artery (**D**). The ventricular reconstructions (**A** and **B**) showed moderate diffuse increase in myocardial thickness, consistent with Fabry-associated cardiac involvement.

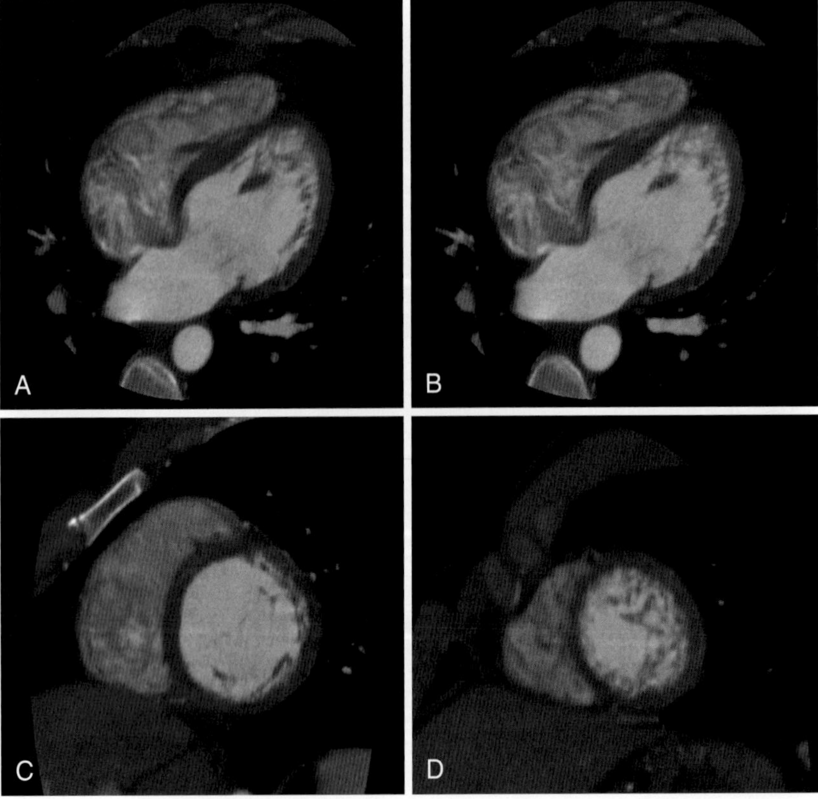

Figure 21-18. A 56-year-old man with multiple coronary risk factors, an indeterminant myocardial perfusion imaging (MPI) study, an echocardiogram demonstrating mild left ventricular (LV) systolic dysfunction, and mild LV dilation. A cardiac CT study demonstrated normal coronary arteries. The cardiac CT study additionally demonstrated mild LV dilation EDV (114 mL/m^2) and a mild reduction in LV systolic function (ejection fraction 50%). Note was made of a progressive increase in fine trabeculations toward the apex of the left ventricle. A left ventricular apical ratio of noncompacted to compacted myocardium of 3.1 to 1 was established, consistent with a diagnosis of noncompaction cardiomyopathy.

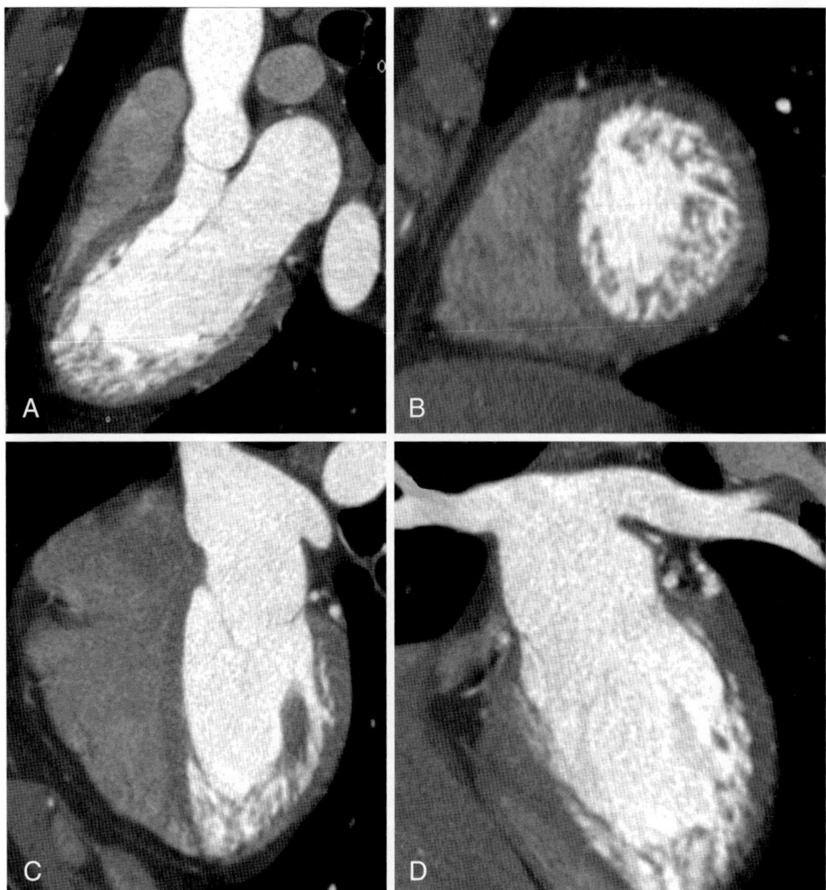

Figure 21-19. Modified long-axis (**A**), short-axis (**B**), four-chamber (**C**), and two-chamber (**D**) views of the heart show the distribution of the noncompacted myocardium. The base and the midportions of the antero- and inferoseptal walls are relatively spared, whereas the remainder of the myocardium is contiguously involved, with an average noncompacted-to-compacted ratio of 2.4 to 1. (Reprinted with permission from Carlson DW, Sullenberger LE, Cho KH, et al. Isolated ventricular noncompaction. *J Cardiovasc Comput Tomogr*. 2007;1:108-109.)

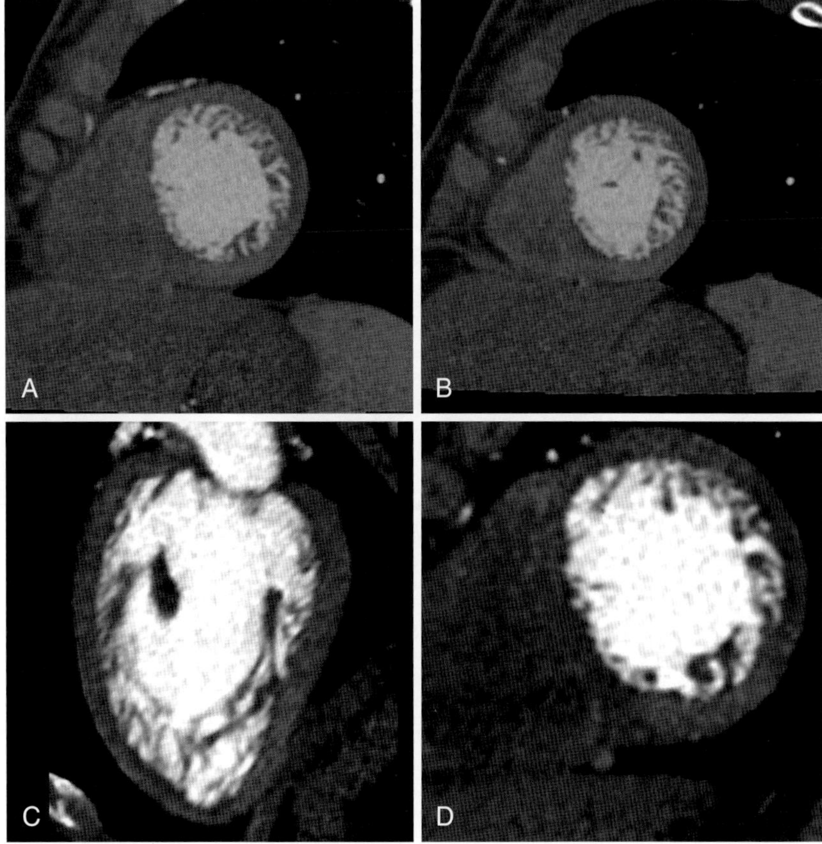

Figure 21-20. Multiplanar reconstructions through the left ventricle in a 52-year-old woman presenting with shortness of breath and atypical chest pain. Images were obtained prospectively over a single heartbeat using a 320-detector scanner. Moderate hypertrophic lesion is seen in the left ventricle, more prominently in the view of the apex. The noncompacted-to-compacted layer ratio was 2.6 to 1, borderline abnormal. The long-axis projection demonstrates a subtle fine subendocardial decrease in attenuation involving most of the left ventricle. This may reflect subtle hypoperfusion of the subendocardium in the setting of small vessel disease, or compaction cardiomyopathy.

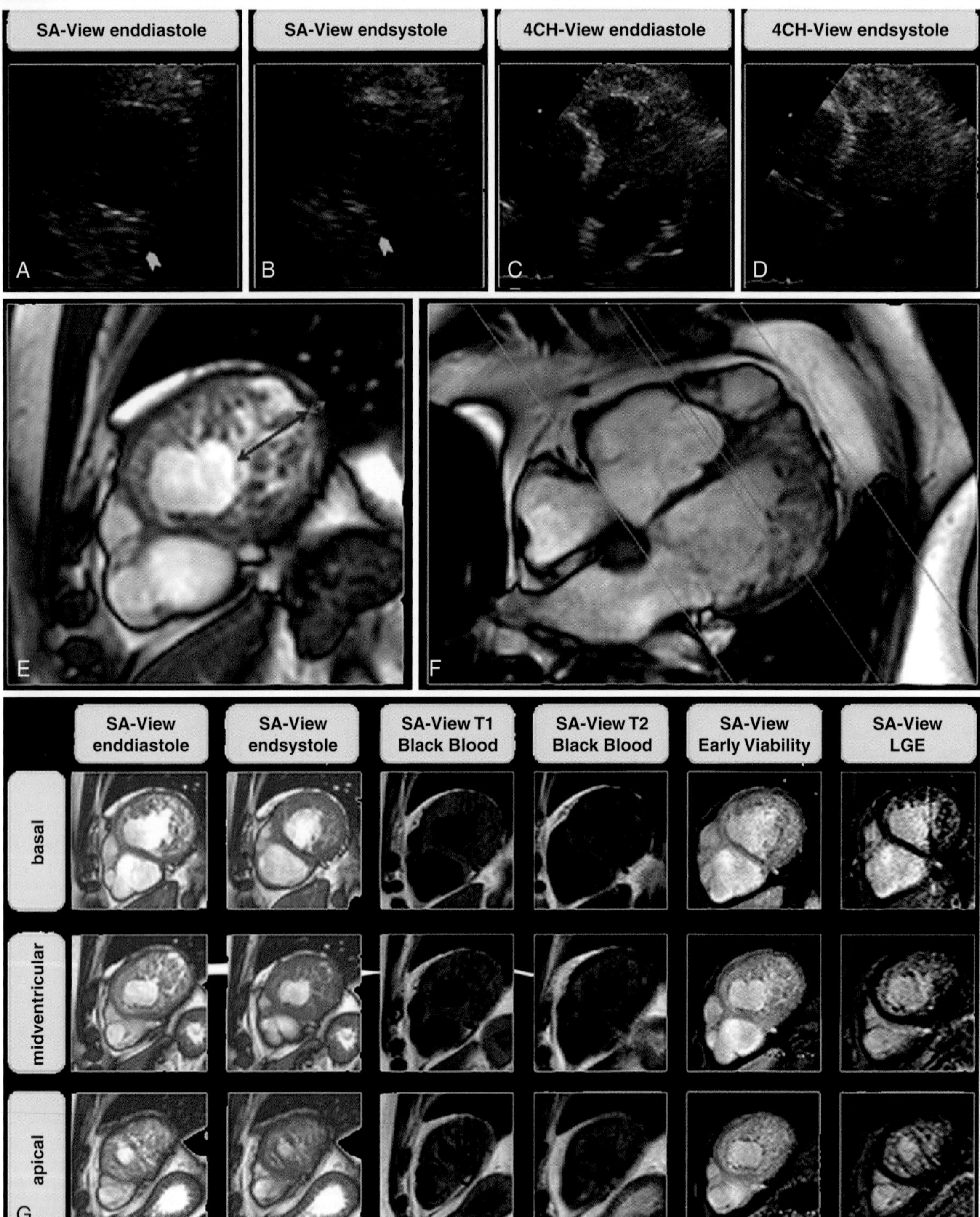

Figure 21-21. **A** through **F,** A 61-year-old man was referred for cardiovascular magnetic resonance (CMR) imaging after a star-shaped inferior intramural mass thought to be a malignancy was discovered on a routine echocardiogram (**A–D**). The CMR images showed significant noncompacted myocardium predominantly of the left ventricle (LV). The ratio of noncompacted (**E,** *red arrow*) to compacted area (**E,** *green arrows*) was 4 to 1 (pathological is defined as 2.5 to 1). The LV was mildly dilated with preserved systolic function. The noncompacted areas were hypokinetic, and the septum was thinned and akinetic with paradoxical motion. Noncompaction of the myocardium is a congenital cardiomyopathy characterized by deep intertrabecular recesses connected to the ventricular cavity resulting from arrest of normal embryogenesis. This case highlights the diagnostic benefits of CMR imaging over echocardiography. CMR accurately characterizes tissue, with trabeculation more clearly visualized and assessed. This has significant clinical implications, because complications of noncompaction include heart failure, thromboembolism, and ventricular arrhythmia. (Reprinted with permission from Schuster A, Duckett SG, Hedstrom E, et al. Noncompaction of the myocardium: the value of cardiovascular magnetic resonance imaging. *J Am Coll Cardiol.* 2001;58(13):e25.)

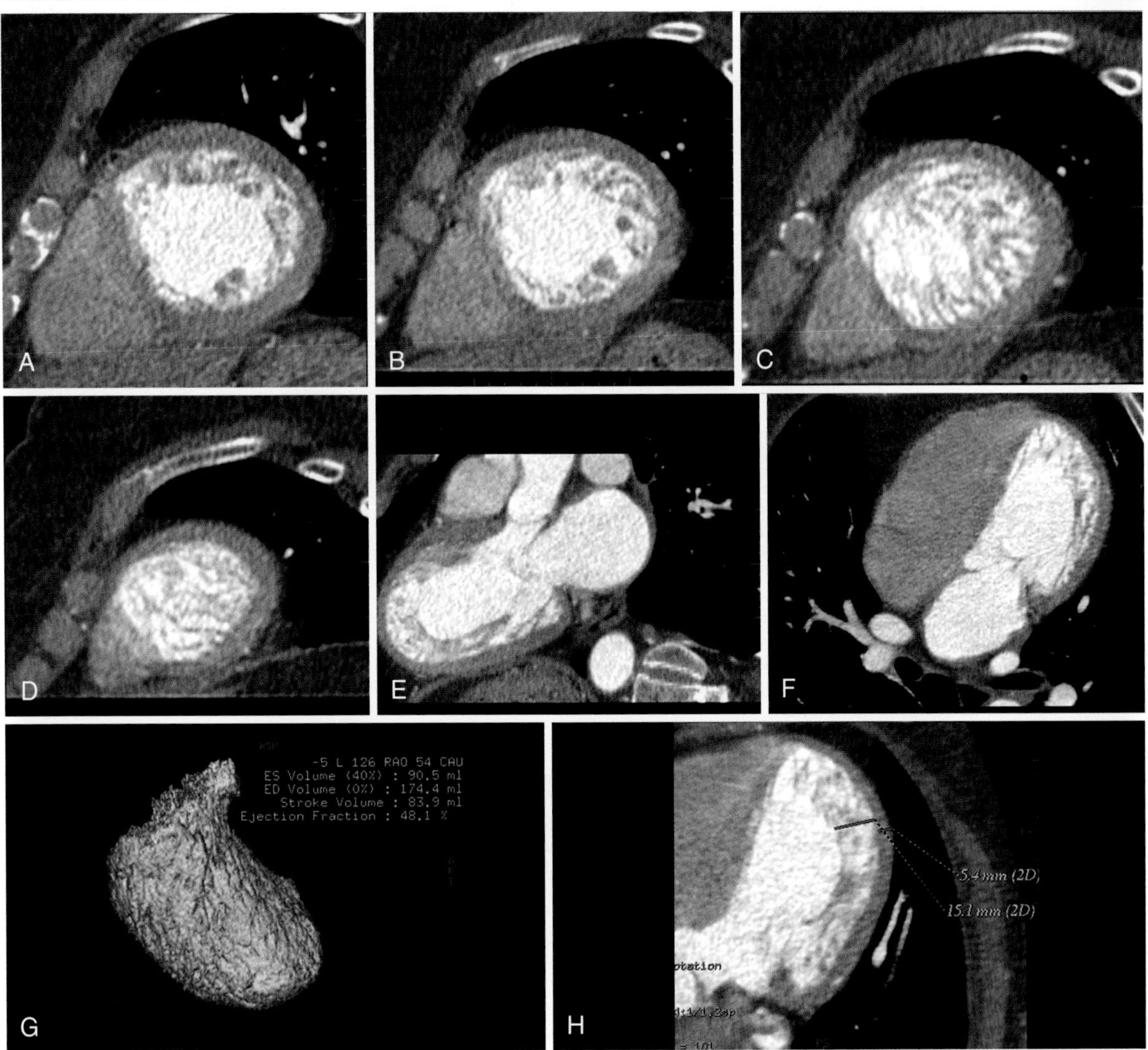

Figure 21-22. A 47-year-old woman presented with shortness of breath and atypical chest pain. Despite attempts at beta blockade, the patient's heart rate remained elevated at 75 beats per minute. A low-dose helically acquired cardiac CT study was performed to rule out coronary artery disease. The patient's overall radiation dose was 5.4 mSvs. No coronary artery disease was identified (images not shown). Short-axis reconstructions (**A–D**) demonstrated increased trabeculations from the mid- to apical portion of the left ventricle. An end-diastolic noncompacted-to-compacted ratio of 2.81 was obtained. Functional evaluation of the left ventricle demonstrated a mildly dilated left ventricle with a corrected left ventricular (LV) end-diastolic volume of 104 mL/m^2. The LV ejection fraction was mildly reduced at 48%. This constellation of findings is suspicious for noncompaction cardiomyopathy.

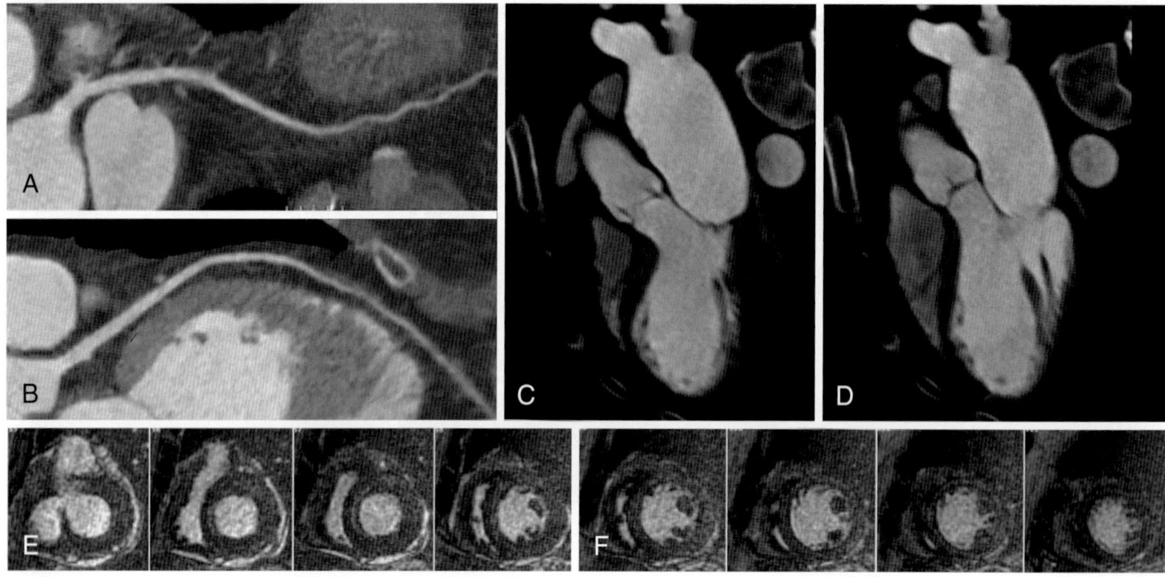

Figure 21-23. A 71-year-old woman with Takotsubo cardiomyopathy presented with acute chest pain and nonspecific ST-T changes in leads V_2-V_5 on electrocardiogram after an emotional conversation with her son. **A** and **B,** Reconstructed images of the left anterior descending (LAD) artery by coronary CT angiography showed no obstructive lesions. Three-chamber cardiac CT images acquired during end-systole (**C**) and end-diastole (**D**) demonstrated the characteristic apical ballooning pattern of regional dilatation and hypokinesis. **E** and **F,** Delayed gadolinium enhancement MR images in short-axis orientation did not demonstrate significant late enhancement. (Reprinted with permission from Maroules CD, Linz NA, Boswell GE. Recurrent Takotsubo cardiomyopathy. *J Cardiovasc Comput Tomogr*. 2009;3(3):187-189.)

TABLE 21-1 Modified Task Force Criteria for the Diagnosis of Arrhythomogenic Right Ventricular Cardiomyopathy

	ORIGINAL TASK FORCE CRITERIA	REVISED TASK FORCE CRITERIA
I. Global or regional dysfunction and structural alterations*		
Major		
	Severe dilatation and reduction of RV ejection fraction with no (or only mild) LV impairment Localized RV aneursyms (akinetic or dyskinteic areas with diastolic bulging) Severe segmental dilatation of the RV	**By 2D echo:** Regional RV akinesia, dyskinesia, or aneursym *and* 1 of the following (end diastole): — PLAX RVOT ≥32 mm (corrected for body size [PLAX/BSA] ≥19 mm/m^2) — PSAX RVOT ≥36 mm (corrected for body size [PSAX/BSA] ≥21 mm/m^2) — *or* fractional area change ≤33%
		By MRI: Regional RV akinesia or dyskinesia or dyssynchronous RV contraction *and* 1 of the following: — Ratio of RV end-diastolic volume to BSA ≥110 mL/m^2 (male) or ≥100 mL/m^2 (female) — *or* RV ejection fraction ≤40%
		By RV angiography: Regional RV akinesia, dyskinesia or aneurysm
Minor		
	Mild global RV dilatation and/or ejection fraction reduction with normal LV Mild segmental dilatation of the RV Regional RV hypokinesia	**By 2D echo:** Regional RV akinesia, or dyskinesia *and* 1 of the following (end diastole): — PLAX RVOT ≥29 to <32 mm (corrected for body size [PLAX/BSA] ≥16 to <19 mm/m^2) — PSAX RVOT ≥32 to <36 mm (corrected for body size [PSAX/BSA] ≥18 to <21 mm/m^2) — *or* fractional area change >33% to ≤40%

TABLE 21-1 Modified Task Force Criteria for the Diagnosis of Arrhythomogenic Right Ventricular Cardiomyopathy—cont'd

	ORIGINAL TASK FORCE CRITERIA	REVISED TASK FORCE CRITERIA
		By MRI: Regional RV akinesia or dyskinesia or dyssynchronous RV contraction *and* 1 of the following: — Ratio of RV end-diastolic volume to BSA ≥100 to <110 mL/m^2 (male) or ≥90 to <100 mL/m^2 (female) — *or* RV ejection fraction >40% to ≤45%
II. Tissue characterization of wall		
Major		
	Fibrofatty replacement of myocardium on endomyocardial biopsy	Residual myocytes <60% by morphometric analysis (or <50% if estimated), with fibrous replacement of the RV free wall myocardium in ≥1 sample, with or without fatty replacement of tissue on endomyocardial biopsy
Minor		
		Residual myocytes 60% to 75% by morphometric analysis (or <50% to 65% if estimated), with fibrous replacement of the RV free wall myocardium in ≥1 sample, with or without fatty replacement of tissue on endomyocardial biopsy
III. Repolarization abnormalities		
Major		
		Inverted T waves in right precordial leads (V_1, V_2 and V_3) or beyond in individuals >14 years of age (in the absence of complete right bundle-branch block QRS ≥120 msec)
Minor		
	Inverted T waves in right precordial leads (V_2 and V_3) (people age >12 years, in absence of right bundle-branch block)	Inverted T waves in leads V_1 and V_2 in individuals >14 years of age (in the absence of complete right bundle-branch block) or in V_4, V_5, or V_6 Inverted T waves in leads V_1, V_2, V_3, and V_4 in individuals >14 years of age in the presence of complete right bundle-branch block
IV. Depolarization/conduction abnormalities		
Major		
	Epsilon waves or localized prolongation (>110 ms) of the QRS complex in right precordial leads (V_1 to V_3)	Epsilon wave (reproducible low-amplitude signals between end of QRS complex to onset of the T wave) in the right precordial leads (V_1 to V_3)
Minor		
	Late potentials (SAECG)	Late potentials by SAECG in ≥1 of 3 parameters in the absence of a QRS duration of ≥110 msec on the standard ECG Filtered QRS duration (fQRS) ≥114 msec Duration of terminal QRS <40 µV (low-amplitude signal duration) ≥38 msec Root mean-square voltage of terminal 40 msec ≤ 20 µV Terminal activation duration of QRS ≥ 55 msec measured from the nadir of the S wave to the end of the QRS, including R′, in V_1, V_2, or V_3, in the absence of complete right bundle-branch block

Continued

TABLE 21-1 Modified Task Force Criteria for the Diagnosis of Arrhythmogenic Right Ventricular Cardiomyopathy—cont'd

	ORIGINAL TASK FORCE CRITERIA	REVISED TASK FORCE CRITERIA
V. Arrhythmias		
Major		
		Nonsustained or sustained ventricular tachycardia of left bundle-branch morphology with superior axis (negative or indeterminate QRS in leads II, III, and aVF and positive in lead aVL)
Minor		
	Left bundle-branch block-type ventricular tachycardia (sustained and nonsustained) (ECG, Holter, exercise)	Nonsustained or sustained ventricular tachycardia of RV outflow configuration, left bundle-branch block morphology with inferior axis (positive QRS in leads II, III, and aVF and negative in lead aVL) or of unknown axis
	Frequent ventricular extrasystoles (>1000 per 24 hr) (Holter)	>500 ventricular extrasystoles per 24 hr (Holter)
VI. Family history		
Major	Familial disease confirmed at necropsy or surgey	ARVC/D confirmed in a first-degree relative who meets current Task Force criteria ARVC/D confirmed pathologically at autopsy or surgery in a first-degree relative Identification of a pathogenic mutation[†] categorized as associated or probably associated with ARVC/D in the patient under evaluation
Minor		
	Family history of premature sudden death (<35 years of age) due to suspected ARVC/D	History of ARVC/D in a first-degree relative in whom it is not possible or practical to determine whether the family member meets current Task Force criteria
	Familial histroy (clinical diagnosis based on present criteria)	Premature sudden death (<35 years of age) due to suspected ARVC/D in a first-degree relative ARVC/D confirmed pathologically or by current Task Force criteria in second-degree relative

2D, two-dimensionsal; ARVC, arrhythmogenic right ventricular cardiomyopathy; ARVD, arrhythmogenic right ventricular dysplasia; aVF, augmented voltage unipolar left foot lead; aVL, augmented voltage unipolar left arm lead; BSA, body surface area; LV, left ventricle/ventricular; PLAX, parasternal long-axis view; PSAX, parasternal short-axis view; RV, right ventricle/ventricular; RVOT, right ventricular outflow tract; SAECG, signal-averaged electrocardiography.

Diagnostic terminology for original criteria: This diagnosis is fulfilled by the presence of 2 major, or 1 major plus 2 minor criteria, or 4 minor criteria from different groups. Diagnostic terminology for revised criteria: definite diagnosis: 2 major, or 1 major and 2 minor criteria, or 4 minor criteria from different categories: borderline. 1 major and 1 minor, or 3 minor criteria from different categories; possible: 1 major or 2 minor criteria from different categories.

*Hypokinesis is not included in this or subsequent definitions of RV regional wall motion abnormalities for the proposed modified criteria.

[†]A pathogenic mutation is a DNA alteration associated with ARVC/D that alters or is expected to alter the encoded protein, is unobserved or rare in a large non-ARVC/D control population and either alters or is predicted to alter the structure or function of the protein or has demonstrated linkage to the disease phenotype in a conclusive pedigree.

Reprinted with permission from Marcus FI, McKenna WJ, Sherrill D, et al. Diagnosis of arrhythmogenic right ventricular cardiomyopathy/dysplasia: proposed modification of the Task Force criteria. *Circulation*. 2010;121(13):1533–1541.

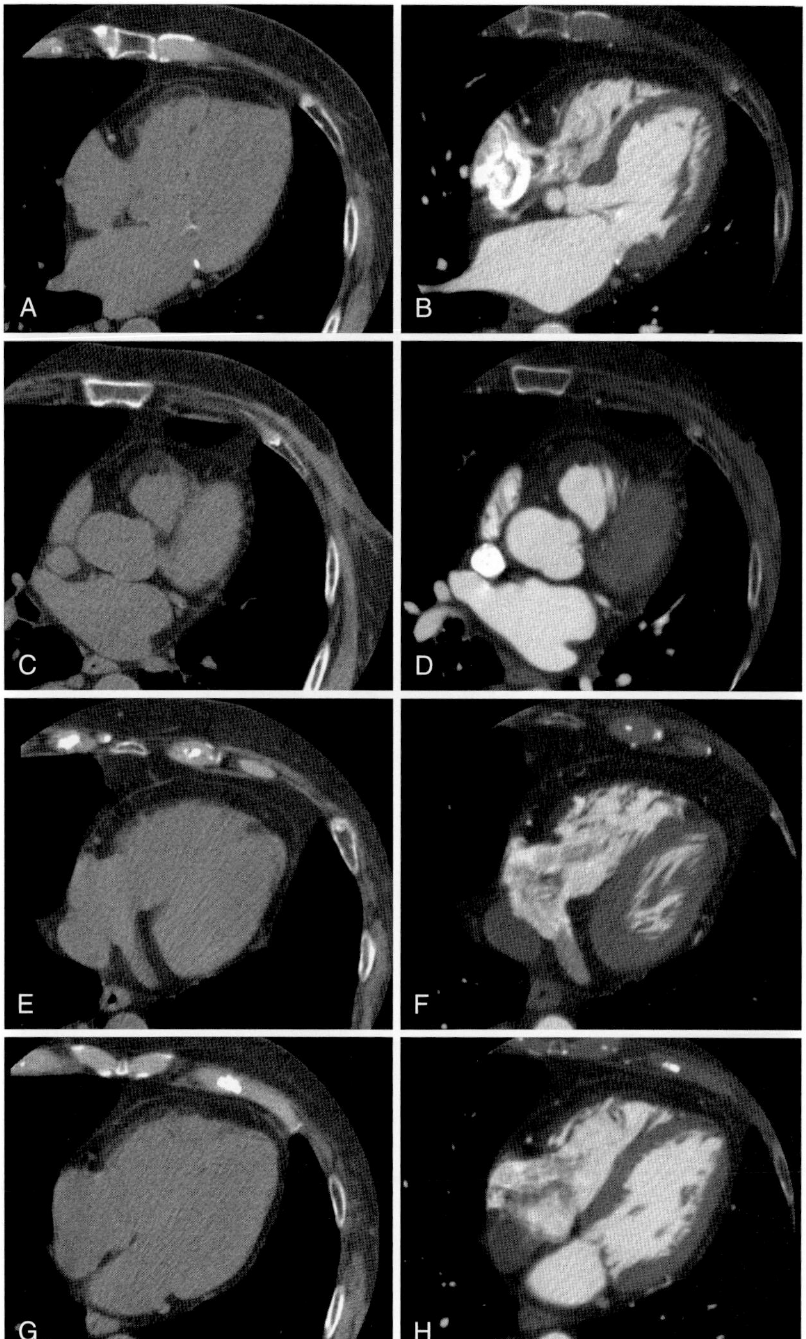

Figure 21-24. Composite images from a cardiac CT study performed to rule out coronary artery disease. This study demonstrates extensive fatty infiltration involving the free wall of the right ventricle, as well as a small focal area of fatty infiltration in the apex of the right ventricle, extending into the apex of the left ventricle. There is normal left and right ventricular function. No underlying flow-limiting coronary artery disease was identified, and there was no history of arrhythmia in this patient. It is thought that these findings likely represent senescent fatty infiltration of primarily the right ventricle.

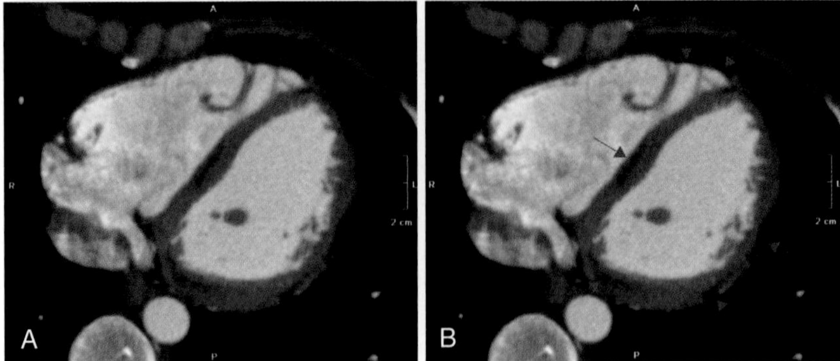

Figure 21-25. Axial images from a cardiac CT study in a young woman with ventricular arrhythmias. Note is made of multiple areas of streaky focal fatty infiltration involving the left ventricle and right ventricular apex (*arrowheads*) as well as the right ventricular side of the midseptum (*arrow*). A focal area of thinning involving the mid-portion of the lateral wall of the left ventricle also is noted. The underlying coronary arterial tree was normal with no evidence of atherosclerotic coronary artery disease.

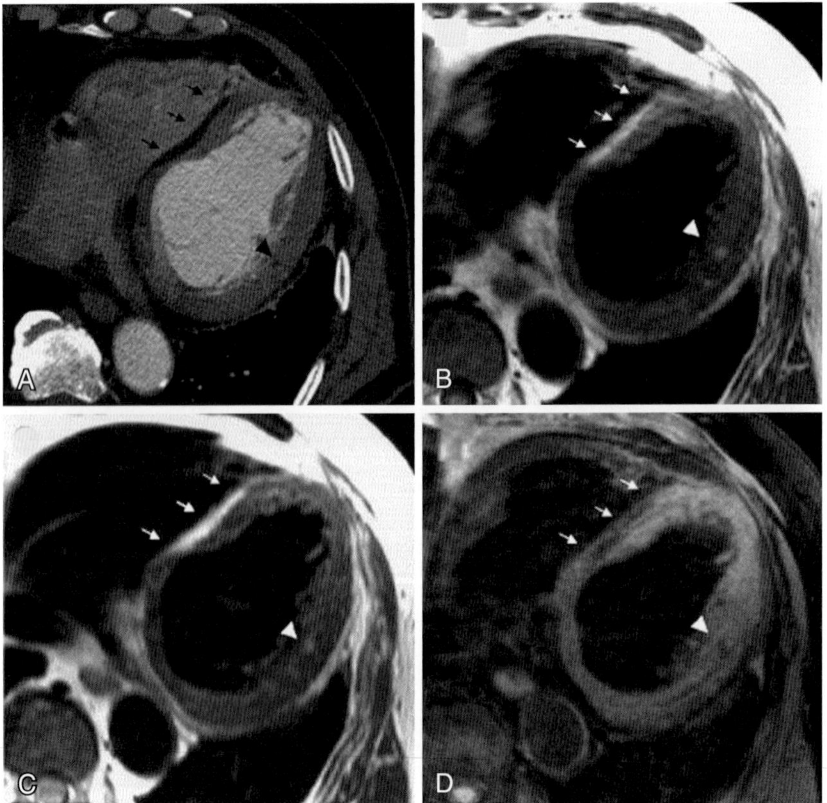

Figure 21-26. **A,** Contrast-enhanced CT image in transverse-axis illustrates low-density areas (–20 to about –50 HU), suggesting fat infiltration along the right ventricular (RV) side of the interventricular septum (*arrows*) and in the left ventricular (LV) myocardium (*arrowhead*). **B,** Dark-blood T1-weighted turbo spin-echo image discloses hyperintensity in the areas mentioned above. **C,** Dark-blood T2-weighted image demonstrates high signals in the corresponding areas, indicative of fatty infiltration of biventricular myocardium. **D,** In a dark-blood T1-weighted turbo spin-echo image with fat saturation, the areas of hyperintensity along the RV side of the septum (*arrows*) and LV wall (*arrowhead*) become low-signal. (Reprinted with permission from Wu YW, Tadamura E, Kanao S, et al. Structural and functional assessment of arrhythmogenic right ventricular dysplasia/cardiomyopathy by multi-slice computed tomography: comparison with cardiovascular magnetic resonance. *Int J Cardiol.* 2007;115(3):e118-e121.)

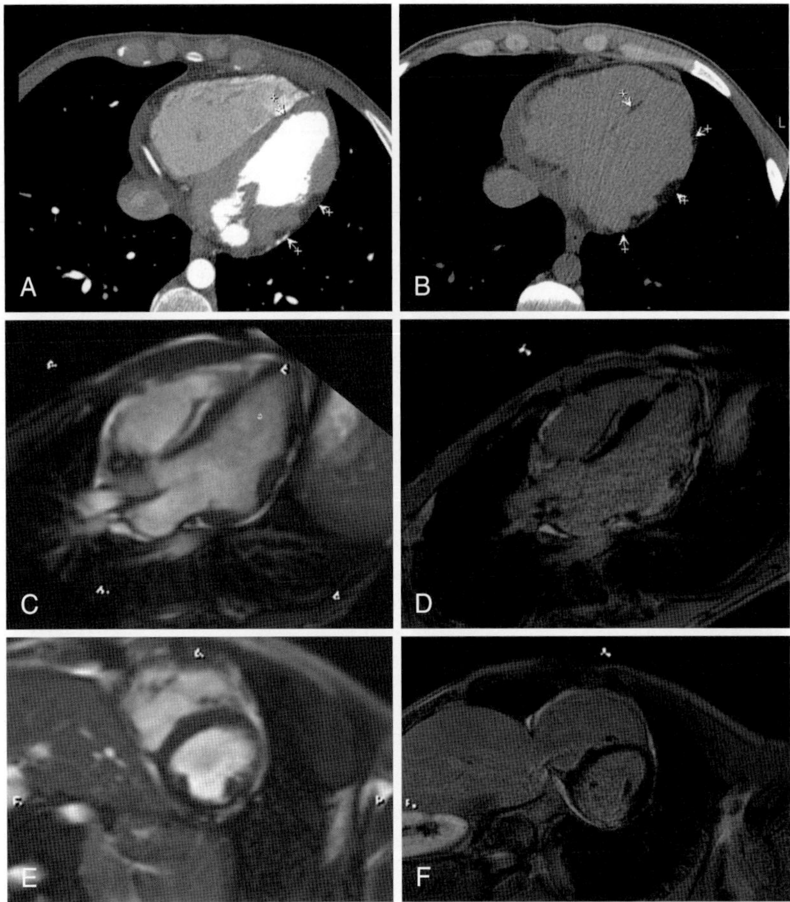

Figure 21-27. **A,** Contrast-enhanced CT axial image reveals an aneurysm of the inferolateral wall, right ventricular dilation, and intramyocardial low-attenuation fat within the left ventricle focally, and near globally within the right ventricle. The right ventricle also is dilated. **B,** The intramyocardial fat is even more obvious. **C** through **F,** Steady-state free precession (SSFP) CMR and late-enhancement CMR four-chamber and short-axis images reveal focal thinning of the left ventricle and matching late enhancement, and dilation of the right ventricle and global late enhancement. This patient had a strong family history of sudden cardiac death. The diagnosis was arrhythmogenic right ventricular cardiomyopathy (ARVC).

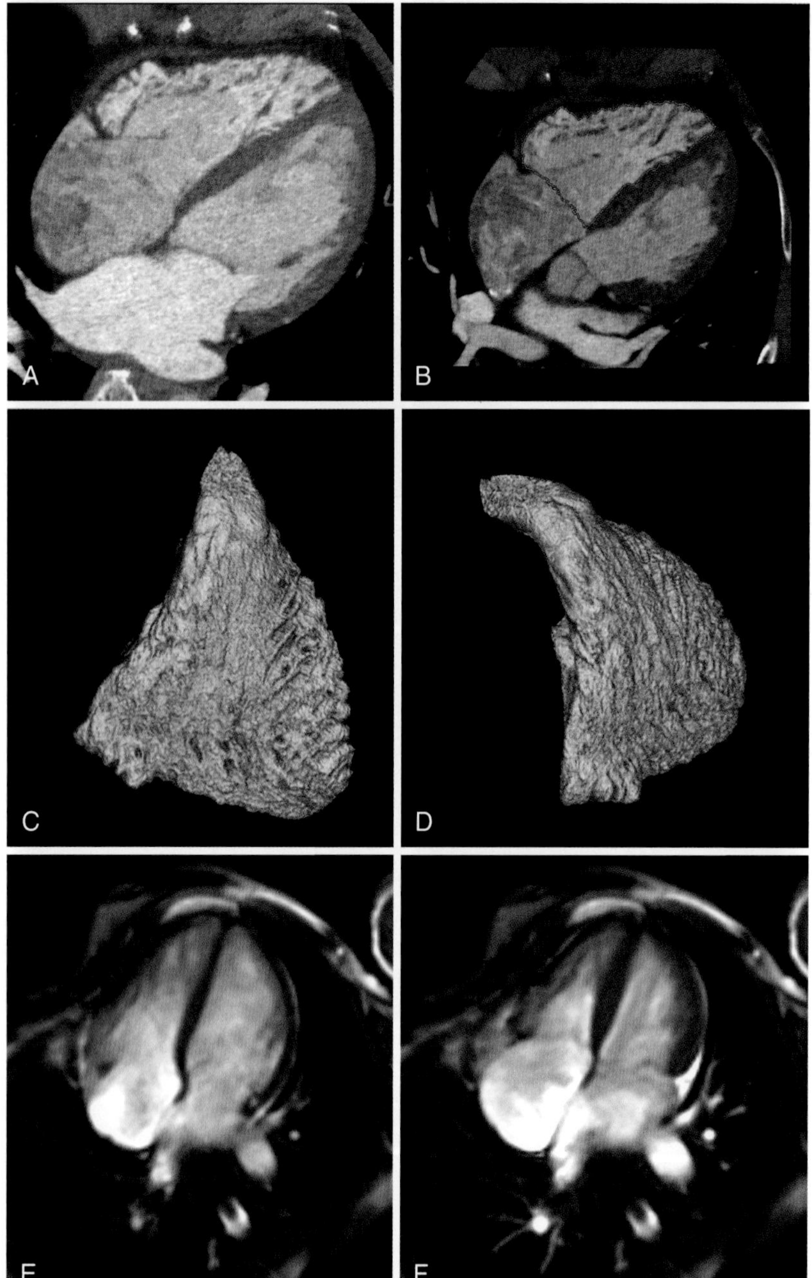

Figure 21-28. A 42-year-old man presented with multiple premature ventricular contractions (PVCs), and a history of syncopal episodes. A cardiac CT examination was performed because of an indeterminant myocardial perfusion imaging (MPI) study. No coronary artery disease was seen on the cardiac CT study (not shown). The study was acquired prospectively, and therefore images have been obtained in mid-diastole. **A,** Short-thickness MIP image in a four-chamber orientation. **B,** A four-chamber reformation of this source data set used for right ventricular (RV) telemetry. A focal area of outpouching and a mild increase in trabeculation are seen in the basal subtractions portion of the right ventricle. **C** and **D,** Volume-rendered images demonstrate this basal focal outpouching of the right ventricle. As the study was obtained in a nonhelical fashion, further evaluation of the right ventricle with an MRI study was suggested. This confirmed the area of focal outpouching, and hypokinesis in the basal portion of the free wall of the right ventricle. While the MRI study demonstrated a normal RV volume and ejection fraction, the patient was referred for electrophysiologic assessment. **See Video 21-7.**

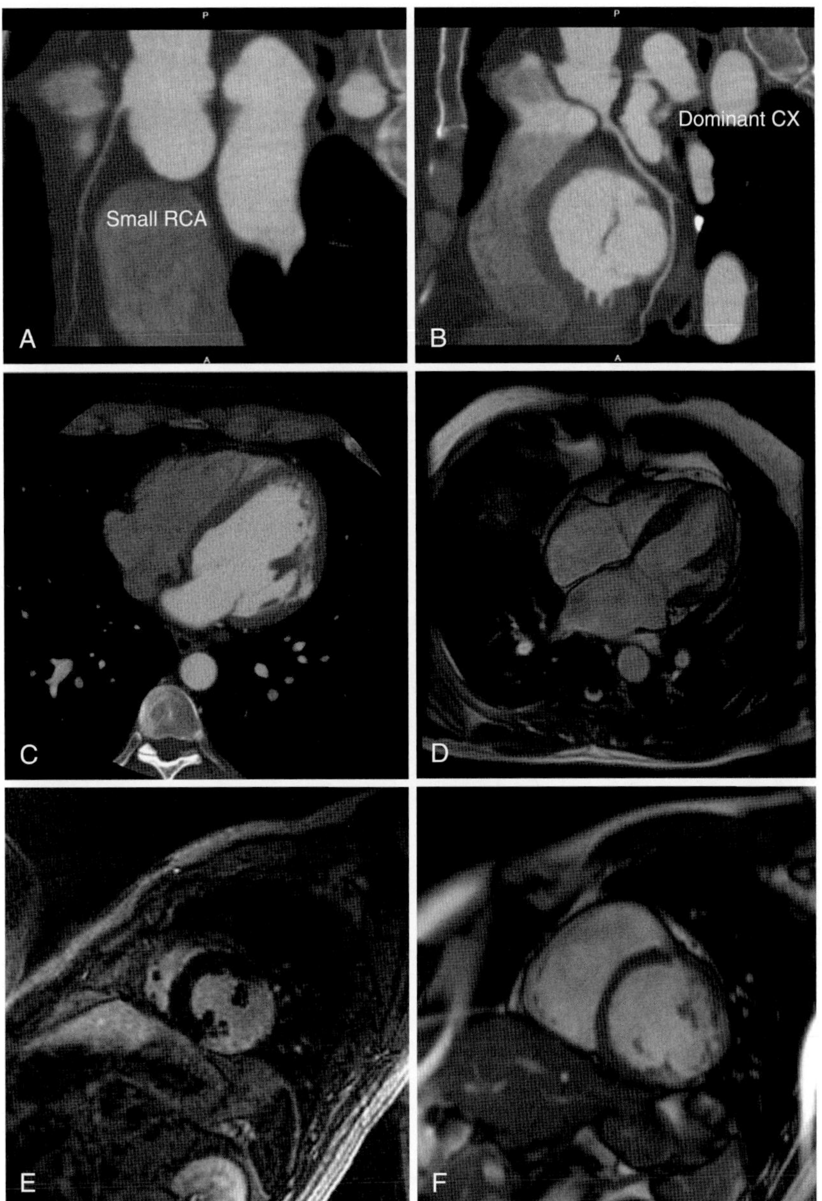

Figure 21-29. Composite images from a cardiac CT and cardiac MRI study in a 44-year-old man with ventricular tachycardia. Cardiac CT was done to rule out underlying coronary artery disease. No evidence of coronary artery disease was identified, including no evidence of soft or hard plaque. There is a focal area of aneurysmal thinning involving the mid-lateral wall. CMR confirmed delayed enhancement in this region. Clinical history and serology was highly suggestive of Chagas disease. Successful ablation of this focal area of aneurysmal thinning was undertaken. The focal area of aneurysmal thinning was believed to reflect a focal area of Chagas myocarditis. **See Video 21-8.** RCA, right coronary artery. (Adapted from Sparrow P, Merchant N, Provost Y, et al. Cardiac MRI and CT features of inheritable and congenital conditions associated with sudden cardiac death. *Eur Radiol.* 2009;19(2):259-270.)

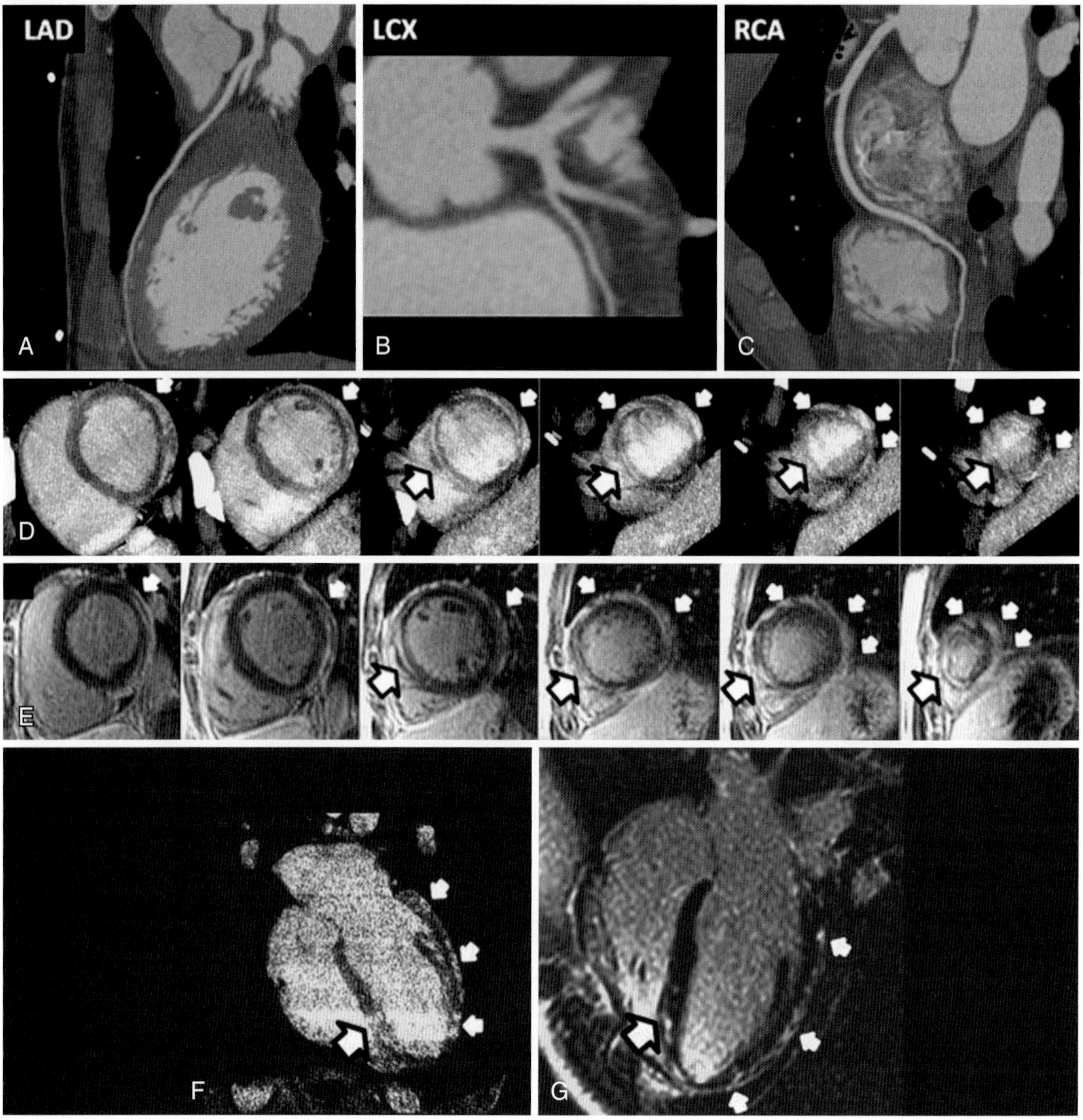

Figure 21-30. Myocarditis. **A** through **C,** Normal epicardial coronary arteries shown by coronary CT angiography. LAD, left anterior descending artery; LCX, left circumflex coronary artery; RCA, right coronary artery. **D,** Short-axis reconstructions of delayed-enhancement cardiac CT show intramyocardial layers of hyperenhancement within the septum (*black arrows*) and epicardial and near-transmural hyperenhancement of the anterior, lateral, and apical walls (*white arrows*). Short-axis views of the delayed-enhancement CMR study (**E**) show identical patterns of myocardial hyperenhancement in the septum (*black arrows*) and anterior, lateral, and apical walls (*white arrows*). **F** and **G,** Four-chamber reconstruction of delayed-enhancement cardiac CT (**F**) shows delayed hyperenhancement within the septum (*black arrow*) and anterolateral and apical walls (*white arrow*). Short-axis views of the delayed-enhancement CMR study (**G**) show identical patterns of myocardial hyperenhancement in the septum (*black arrow*) and anterolateral and apical walls (*white arrows*). (Reprinted with permission from Axsom K, Lin F, Weinsaft JW, Min JK. Evaluation of myocarditis with delayed-enhancement computed tomography. *J Cardiovasc Comput Tomogr*. 2009;3(6):409-411.)

TABLE 21-2 ACCF 2010 Appropriateness Criteria for the Use of Cardiac Computed Tomography to Evaluate Cardiomyopathy

	APPROPRIATENESS RATING	INDICATION	MEDIAN SCORE
Evaluation of cardiac structure and function—evaluation of ventricular morphology and systolic function	Appropriate	Evaluation of left ventricular function Following acute MI or in HF patients Inadequate images from other noninvasive methods	7
		Quantitative evaluation of right ventricular function	7
		Assessment of right ventricular morphology Suspected arrhythmogenic right ventricular dysplasia	7
	Uncertain	None listed	
	Inappropriate	None listed	

HF, heart failure; MI, myocardial infarction.
Data from Taylor AJ, Cerqueira M, Hodgson JM, et al. ACCF/SCCT/ACR/AHA/ASE/ASNC/NASCI/SCAI/SCMR 2010 appropriate use criteria for cardiac computed tomography. A report of the American College of Cardiology Foundation Appropriate Use Criteria Task Force, the Society of Cardiovascular Computed Tomography, the American College of Radiology, the American Heart Association, the American Society of Echocardiography, the American Society of Nuclear Cardiology, the North American Society for Cardiovascular Imaging, the Society for Cardiovascular Angiography and Interventions, and the Society for Cardiovascular Magnetic Resonance. *J Am Coll Cardiol.* 2010;56(22):1864-1894.

References

1. Knickelbine T, Lesser JR, Haas TS, et al. Identification of unexpected nonatherosclerotic cardiovascular disease with coronary CT angiography. *JACC Cardiovasc Imaging.* 2009;2(9):1085-1092.
2. Andreini D, Pontone G, Pepi M, et al. Diagnostic accuracy of multidetector computed tomography coronary angiography in patients with dilated cardiomyopathy. *J Am Coll Cardiol.* 2007;49(20):2044-2050.
3. Truong QA, Hoffmann U, Singh JP. Potential uses of computed tomography for management of heart failure patients with dyssynchrony. *Crit Pathw Cardiol.* 2008;7(3):185-190.
4. Truong QA, Singh JP, Cannon CP, et al. Quantitative analysis of intraventricular dyssynchrony using wall thickness by multidetector computed tomography. *JACC Cardiovasc Imaging.* 2008;1(6):772-781.
5. Stolzmann P, Scheffel H, Bettex D, et al. Subvalvular aortic stenosis: comprehensive cardiac evaluation with dual-source computed tomography. *J Thorac Cardiovas Surg.* 2007:240-241.
6. Olivotto I, Maron MS, Autore C, et al. Assessment and significance of left ventricular mass by cardiovascular magnetic resonance in hypertrophic cardiomyopathy. *J Am Coll Cardiol.* 2008;52(7):559-566.
7. Germans T, Wilde AA, Dijkmans PA, et al. Structural abnormalities of the inferoseptal left ventricular wall detected by cardiac magnetic resonance imaging in carriers of hypertrophic cardiomyopathy mutations. *J Am Coll Cardiol.* 2006;48(12):2518-2523.
8. Okayama S, Uemura S, Soeda T, Horii M, Saito Y. Role of cardiac computed tomography in planning and evaluating percutaneous transluminal septal myocardial ablation for hypertrophic obstructive cardiomyopathy. *J Cardiovasc Comput Tomogr.* 2010;4(1):62-65.
9. Shiozaki AA, Santos TS, Artega E, Rochitte CE. Images in cardiovascular medicine. Myocardial delayed enhancement by computed tomography in hypertrophic cardiomyopathy. *Circulation.* 2007;115(17):e430-e431.
10. Raney AR, Saremi F, Kenchaiah S, et al. Multidetector computed tomography shows intramyocardial fat deposition. *J Cardiovasc Comput Tomogr.* 2008;2:152-163.
11. El-Bialy A, Shenoda M, Saleh J, Tilkian A. Myocardial calcification as a rare cause of congestive heart failure: a case report. *J Cardiovasc Pharmacol Ther.* 2005;10(2):137-143.
12. Muth G, Daniel WG, Achenbach S. Late enhancement on cardiac computed tomography in a patient with cardiac sarcoidosis. *J Cardiovas Comput Tomogr.* 2008;2(4):272-273.
13. Momose M, Kadoya M, Koshikawa M, Matsushita T, Yamada A. Usefulness of 67Ga SPECT and integrated low-dose CT scanning (SPECT/CT) in the diagnosis of cardiac sarcoidosis. *Ann Nucl Med.* 2007;21(10):545-551.
14. Marwan M, Pflederer T, Ropers D, et al. Cardiac amyloidosis imaged by dual-source computed tomography. *J Cardiovasc Comput Tomogr.* 2008;2(6):403-405.
15. Funabashi N, Toyozaki T, Matsumoto Y, et al. Images in cardiovascular medicine. Myocardial fibrosis in Fabry disease demonstrated by multislice computed tomography: comparison with biopsy findings. *Circulation.* 2003;107(19):2519-2520.
16. Carlson DW, Sullenberger LE, Cho KH, Feuerstein IM, Taylor AJ. Isolated ventricular noncompaction. *J Cardiovas Comput Tomogr.* 2007;1:108-109.
17. Maroules CD, Linz NA, Boswell GE. Recurrent Takotsubo cardiomyopathy. *J Cardiovasc Comput Tomogr.* 2009;3(3):187 189.
18. Sparrow P, Merchant N, Provost Y, Doyle D, Nguyen E, Paul N. Cardiac MRI and CT features of inheritable and congenital conditions associated with sudden cardiac death. *Eur Radiol.* 2009;19(2):259-270.
19. Wu YW, Tadamura E, Kanao S, et al. Structural and functional assessment of arrhythmogenic right ventricular dysplasia/cardiomyopathy by multi-slice computed tomography: comparison with cardiovascular magnetic resonance. *Int J Cardiol.* 2007;115(3):e118-e121.
20. Bomma C, Dalal D, Tandri H, et al. Evolving role of multidetector computed tomography in evaluation of arrhythmogenic right ventricular dysplasia/cardiomyopathy. *Am J Cardiol.* 2007;100(1):99-105.
21. Raney AR, Saremi F, Kenchaiah S, et al. Multidetector computed tomography shows intramyocardial fat deposition. *J Cardiovasc Comput Tomogr.* 2008;2(3):152-163.
22. Tada H, Shimizu W, Ohe T, et al. Usefulness of electron-beam computed tomography in arrhythmogenic right ventricular dysplasia. Relationship to electrophysiological abnormalities and left ventricular involvement. *Circulation.* 1996;94(3):437-444.
23. Midiri M, Finazzo M, Brancato M, et al. Arrhythmogenic right ventricular dysplasia: MR features. *Eur.Radiol.* 1997;7(3):307-312.
24. Marcus FI, McKenna WJ, Sherrill D, et al. Diagnosis of arrhythmogenic right ventricular cardiomyopathy/dysplasia: proposed modification of the task force criteria. *Circulation.* 2010;121(13):1533-1541.
25. Marcu CB, Beek AM, van Rossum AC. Chagas' heart disease diagnosed on MRI: the importance of patient "geographic" history. *Int J Cardiol.* 2007;117(2):e58-e60.

26. Rochitte CE, Oliveira PF, Andrade JM, et al. Myocardial delayed enhancement by magnetic resonance imaging in patients with Chagas' disease: a marker of disease severity. *J Am Coll Cardiol.* 2005; 46(8):1553-1558.
27. Brooks MA, Sane DC. CT findings in acute myocarditis: 2 cases. *J Thorac Imaging.* 2007;22(3):277-279.
28. Axsom K, Lin F, Weinsaft JW, Min JK. Evaluation of myocarditis with delayed-enhancement computed tomography. *J Cardiovasc Comput Tomogr.* 2009;3(6):409-411.
29. Dambrin G, Laissy JP, Serfaty JM, Caussin C, Lancelin B, Paul JF. Diagnostic value of ECG-gated multidetector computed tomography in the early phase of suspected acute myocarditis. A preliminary comparative study with cardiac MRI. *Eur Radiol.* 2007;17(2): 331-338.

22 Electrophysiologic Applications of Cardiac CT

Key Points

- Cardiac CT is an excellent means of depicting pulmonary venous anatomy to plan pulmonary venous isolation procedures and of anticipating several potential complications of pulmonary venous isolation procedures.
- CCT is an excellent means of depicting coronary venous anatomy to plan cardiac resynchronization procedures.
- CCT yields superb detail of the atrial appendages in sinus rhythm; in atrial fibrillation, however, because of higher heart rates, irregular cardiac cycle length, and slow filling of the appendage, depiction of thrombi is poor.

CARDIAC CT IMAGING IN PATIENTS WITH ATRIAL FIBRILLATION

Cardiac CT (CCT) scanning remains problematic in atrial fibrillation (AF) in several ways because of inadequate temporal resolution:

- The heart rate tends to be higher in patients with AF (Table 22-1).
- The cardiac cycle length is always irregular.
- The increment in heart rate is greater during contrast injection and during image acquisition.
- Opacification of the left atrial appendage (LAA), which usually is dilated and nearly effectively stagnant, is delayed well beyond that of the left heart cavities and coronary arteries, potentially resulting in pseudothrombus in the left atrium, the result of incomplete opacification of the LAA due to enlargement of the LAA and altered flow characteristics in the left atrium due to AF (Table 22-2).[2]

With different cardiac cycle lengths, multicycle/segmented acquisition image quality is seriously compromised. Using 64-slice CCT, overall only half (54%) of coronary CT angiography (CTA) image studies of AF are of adequate or good quality.[1] Use of retrospective imaging at full tube output increases radiation exposure. Although feasible, cardiac/coronary imaging during AF with CT scanning requires further development to obtain increased yield and to lessen radiation exposure.

Structural noncoronary studies such as pulmonary venous and coronary venous anatomy studies are more likely than coronary CTA studies to be adequate.

However, using 320-slice CCT, the large majority of cases can be adequately imaged despite the presence of AF (Table 22-3).[3]

The distal left circumflex artery appears to pose the most problems in evaluating for the presence and severity of coronary artery disease (CAD).[4]

IDENTIFICATION OF LEFT ATRIAL OR LEFT ATRIAL APPENDAGE THROMBUS

The presence of underlying AF challenges the accurate detection of atrial appendage thrombi. In contrast to patients in sinus rhythm, the variable cardiac cycle length and greater and more variable heart rate increase in response to the stimuli of scanner acceleration and contrast injection of patients in AF excessively tax the ability of 64-slice CT scanners to accurately assess the LAA. The left atrium, whose imaging is less affected by AF than is that of the appendage, is more readily assessed for the presence[5] or absence of thrombus. The stagnation of flow within the LAA necessitates a delayed scan at 2 or more minutes post-injection, with additional radiation exposure.

Stagnation of flow within the LAA is a major confounder of assessment of the LAA for thrombosis. The delayed clearance of non–contrast-enhanced blood within the LAA has established the high incidence of false positive studies without delayed images. For example, Martinez et al. [6] found that in 402 consecutive patients undergoing non–ECG-gated CCT and transesophageal echocardiographic (TEE) pre-pulmonary venous isolation, CCT identified 40 LAA filling defects, of which only 9 were confirmed by TEE. False negatives also are common; for example in Tang

TABLE 22-1 CTA Characteristics of Patients in Sinus Rhythm and in Atrial Fibrillation

	ATRIAL FIBRILLATION (n = 24)	SINUS RHYTHM (n = 119)	P
Pre-scan heart rate	54 ±14 bpm	62 ±112 bpm	<.01
Postinjection heart rate	103 ± 30 bpm	71±17 bpm	<.01
Nondiagnostic CTA studies	8%	10%	ns
Good or excellent CTA image quality	54%	79%	.01
Radiation exposure	26 ± 8 mSv	8 ± 4 mSv	<.01

Data from Wolak A, Gutstein A, Cheng VY, et al. Dual-source coronary computed tomography angiography in patients with atrial fibrillation: initial experience. *J Cardiovasc Comput Tomogr.* 2008;2(3):172-180.

TABLE 22-2 Left Atrial Appendage Volume and the Incidence of Pseudothrombus

	ATRIAL FIBRILLATION	SINUS RHYTHM	
Left atrial appendage volume	15 ± 7 mL	7 ± 3 mL	0.02
(Proven) pseudothrombus in the left atrial appendage during CTA without delayed imaging	71%	0	

Data from Saremi F, Channual S, Gurudevan SV, Narula J, Abolhoda A. Prevalence of left atrial appendage pseudothrombus filling defects in patients with atrial fibrillation undergoing coronary computed tomography angiography. *J Cardiovasc Comput Tomogr.* 2008;2(3):164-171.

TABLE 22-3 Diagnostic Performance of CTA in the Context of Atrial Fibrillation

AUTHOR	SENSITIVITY (%)	SPECIFICITY (%)	PPV (%)	NPV (%)	EVALUABLE SEGMENTS (NO.)	DOSE (mSv)
Xu et al.[3]	90	99	86	99	97	13 ± 5
Pasricha et al.[4]					99	19

et al.'s study, only 4 of 10 thrombi seen on TEE were seen on CCT.[7] Some false-positive defects persist even after delay.[8]

There are few data to this point, but small early studies have shown correlation between TEE and contrast cardiovascular CT (CVCT) measurements of LAA size and correlation of findings of thrombi larger than 7 mm.[9] Higher heart rates and irregular rhythm (the norm in AF) challenge feasibility at this point. ECG gating is important. CVCT is unable to show left atrial or appendage spontaneous contrast.

Small accessory LAAs are recognized by 64-slice CCT, but these, due to their novel recognition, are still of unknown significance.[10] Accessory LAAs have been reported in 10% to 15% of the adult population undergoing cardiac CT (Figs. 22-1 through 22-4).[11]

PRE-PROCEDURE CARDIAC MAPPING: ASSESSMENT OF PULMONARY VEIN ANATOMY FOR PLANNING OF PULMONARY VEIN ABLATION FOR ATRIAL FIBRILLATION

Atrial fibrillation usually is initiated by ectopic activity within the proximal pulmonary veins. Catheter-based techniques, in which access to the left atrium occurs via a transseptal puncture of the interatrial septum, are able to deliver radiofrequency current (or cryotherapy) to the sites that have been identified by mapping techniques as responsible for AF, electrically isolating them from the remainder of the atria. The usual success rate in achieving sinus rhythm at 1 year with two or three attempts is 75% to 85%—a marked improvement compared to medical therapy, which affords about 20% success.

Anatomic features are not adequate to identify the site responsible for AF.

Conventionally, real-time retrograde injection of contrast dye into the left atrium has been used during the procedure to visually guide catheter placement. However, opacification of the right inferior pulmonary vein is difficult to achieve by reflux venography. Other modalities such as intracardiac echocardiography and TEE are less robust than reflux venography, which is less robust than CCT in detecting normal and variant anatomy (e.g., supernumerary and common ostia and branch variation) (Table 22-4).[12,13]

Variations in pulmonary venous anatomy are fairly common. The most common variant is a

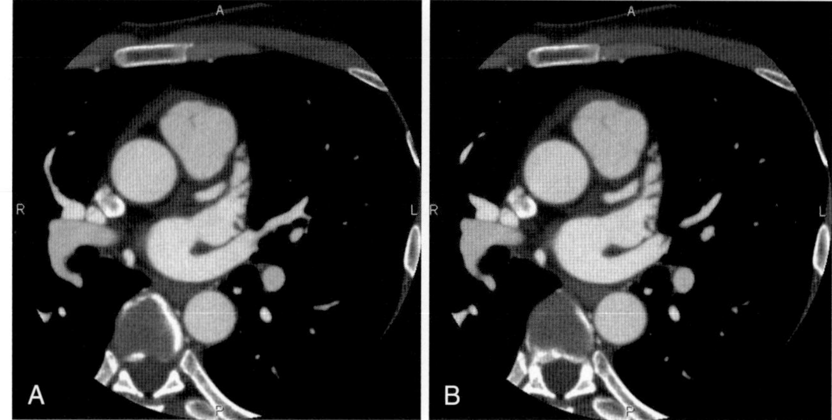

Figure 22-1. Two axial images from a cardiac CT study pre–pulmonary vein ablation demonstrate a normal-appearing left atrial appendage (LAA) with small pectinate muscular bands within the LAA.

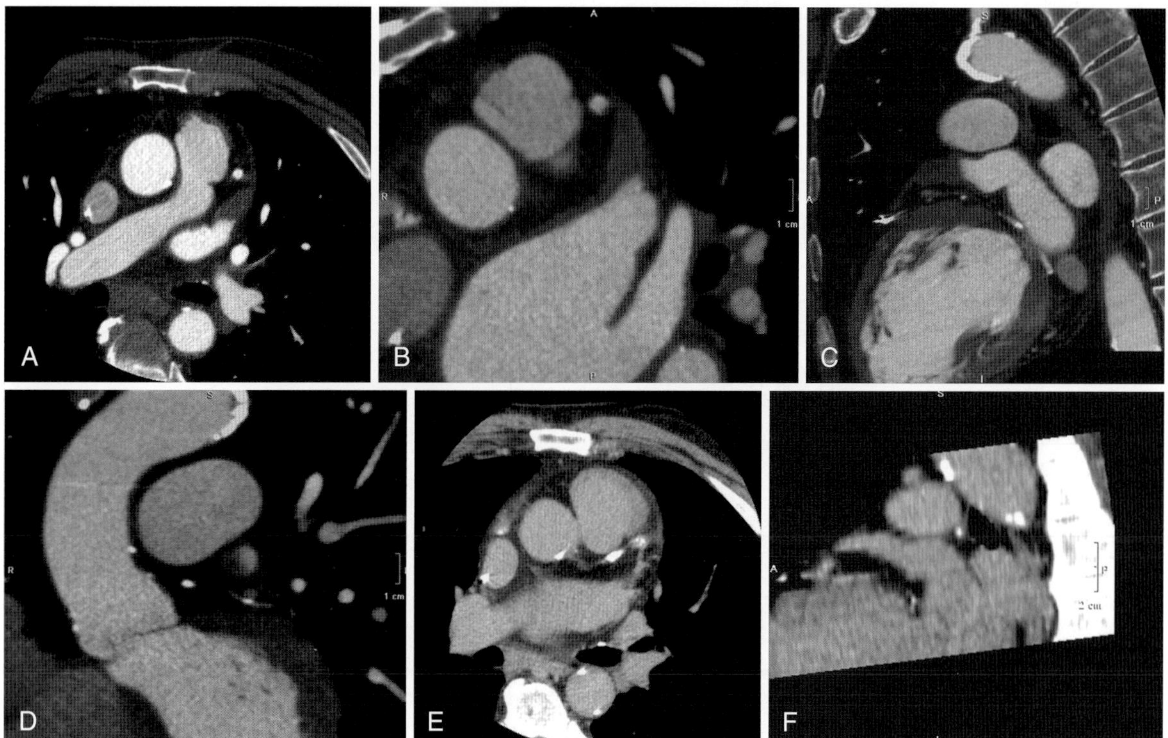

Figure 22-2. Multiple cardiac CT images in a patient being considered for pulmonary vein ablation. Initial phase images demonstrate a region of decreased attenuation within the tip of the left atrial appendage (LAA). This has a very linear demarcation with the adjacent contrast-enhanced portion of the LAA. This linear configuration is suspicious for a meniscus effect, with non-opacified blood as opposed to thrombus sitting anteriorly within the LAA tip. This is confirmed on delayed phase imaging (**E** and **F**), where normal uniform enhancement is seen throughout the LAA.

separate right middle pulmonary vein. Pulmonary venous variants include:

- Three to five right-sided ostia (28%)[14]
- One or two separate middle lobe pulmonary venous ostia (26%)[14]
- A single right ostium on the right side (2%)[14]
- A single left-sided ostium (14%)[14]
- A right superior supranumerary pulmonary vein (2.2%), which passes behind the bronchus intermedius and drains mainly the posterior segment of the right upper lobe, but also receives a few subsegmental branches from the superior segment of the right lower lobe (mean diameter: 5.1 mm)[15]

Anomalous Variants

- Right pulmonary vein to the superior vena cava
- Right pulmonary vein to the right atrium
- Right pulmonary vein to the inferior vena cava or a hepatic vein (i.e., scimitar syndrome)
- Left pulmonary vein to the innominate vein (i.e., vertical vein)

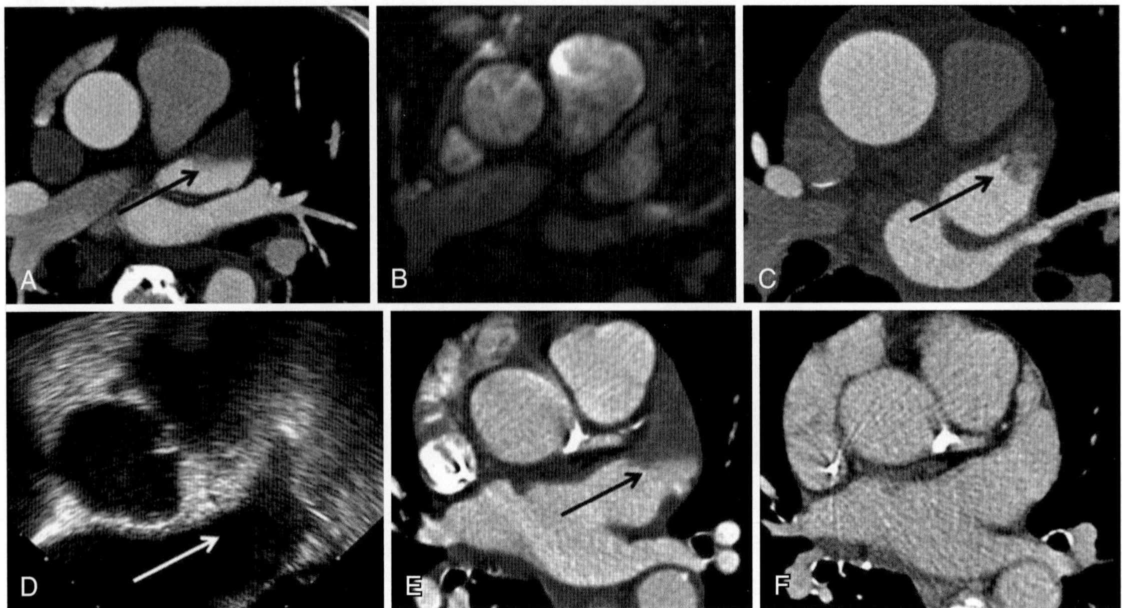

Figure 22-3. Axial images of cardiac CTAs from three patients with atrial fibrillation at the time of scanning (**A, C,** and **E**). Filling defects in the LAA are shown by the black arrows, which include fluid–fluid levels (**A** and **E**) and multiple round defects (**C**). Corresponding follow-up images of each patient are shown (**B, D,** and **F**) to rule out thrombosis of the LAA, including a 60-second MR angiogram (**B**) and a transesophageal echocardiographic (TEE) study (**D**), which were performed the next day, and a 2-minute delayed CT (**F**). Follow-up images were all negative for real thrombus. TEE showed low-level echoes (spontaneous echo contrast; *white arrow*). False filling defects are common in the LAA of patients with atrial fibrillation and are most likely related to stasis of blood in a noncontractile atrium. (Reprinted with permission from Saremi F, Channual S, Gurudevan SV, et al. Prevalence of left atrial appendage pseudothrombus filling defects in patients with atrial fibrillation undergoing coronary computed tomography angiography. *J Cardiovasc Comput Tomogr*. 2008;2(3):164-171.)

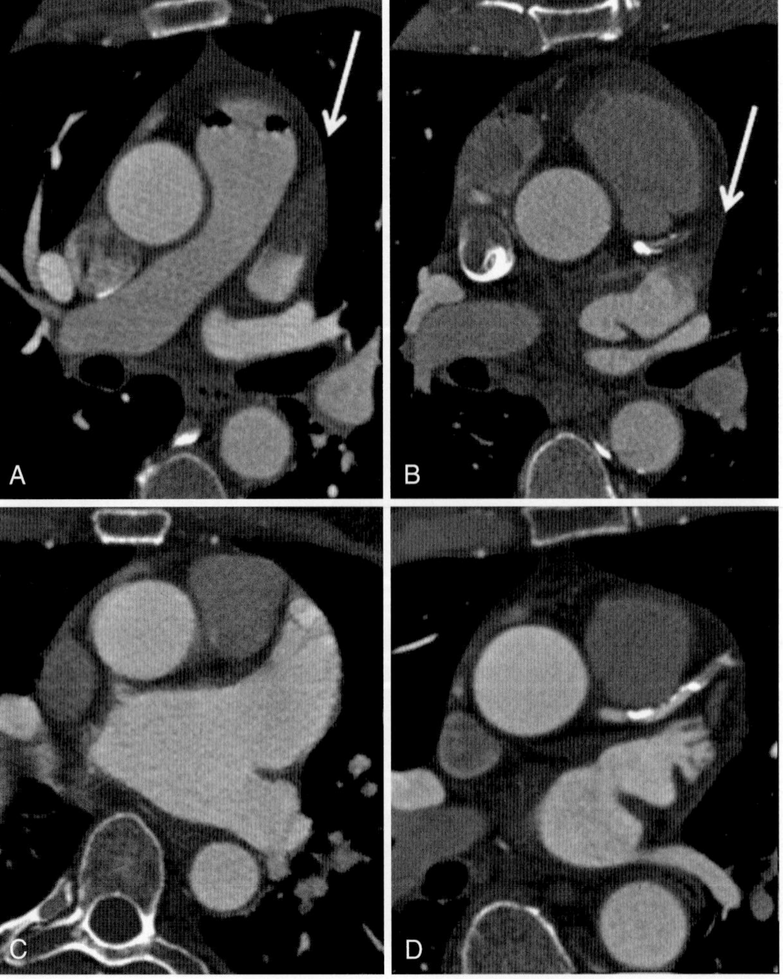

Figure 22-4. Axial images of cardiac CTAs from four patients with atrial fibrillation at the time of scanning. Filling defects (*white arrows*) in the left atrial appendage include fluid–fluid levels (**A**) and irregular or round defects (**B**). **C** and **D** show a completely filled left atrium with filling defects. Follow-up transesophageal echocardiography (TEE; **A, B,** and **D**) and MR angiography (**C**) did not show thrombus. (Reprinted with permission from Saremi F, Channual S, Gurudevan SV, et al. Prevalence of left atrial appendage pseudothrombus filling defects in patients with atrial fibrillation undergoing coronary computed tomography angiography. *J Cardiovasc Comput Tomogr*. 2008;2(3):164-171.)

Factors Affecting Pulmonary Venous Size

The size (diameter) of pulmonary veins depends on:

- Volume status
- Respiratory phase (inspiration decreases pulmonary venous return and size).[16] Expiratory phase images provide a better match to MRI depiction of pulmonary veins.
- The phase of the cardiac cycle (by 25%–45%):[17]
  - Maximal size of pulmonary veins: 35%[17]
  - Minimal size of pulmonary veins: 85%[17]

The use of image guidance during pulmonary venous isolation/ablation procedures reduces fluoroscopy times and increases success.

CCT has become the principal noninvasive diagnostic test to depict venous anatomy of the heart for the following reasons:

- Especially when compared with TEE, intracardiac echocardiography, and reflex venography, it is less operator dependent.
- Unlike cardiac MR (CMR), it can be performed on patients with pacemakers and implantable cardioverter defibrillators.
- Its results are reproducible.
- It can depict the thickness of the wall of the pulmonary veins.
- It can characterize the lung parenchyma for complications such as pulmonary edema and infarction.
- It can image the mediastinum both before and after ablation. This can assist in visualizing the relation of the esophagus to the left atrium and in detecting the presence of large intrathoracic hiatus hernias.

TABLE 22-4 Detection of All Pulmonary Ostia by Imaging Modality

IMAGING MODALITY	PERCENTAGE DETECTION OF ALL FOUR PULMONARY VENOUS OSTIA (*n* = 24)
Cardiac CT	98
ICE	93
TEE	81
Reflux venography	71

ICE, intracardiac echocardiography; TEE, transesophageal echocardiography. From Wood MA, Wittkamp M, Henry D, et al. A comparison of pulmonary vein ostial anatomy by computerized tomography, echocardiography, and venography in patients with atrial fibrillation having radiofrequency catheter ablation. *Am J Cardiol.* 2004;93(1):49-53.

CCT can offer several forms of depiction of pulmonary venous and left atrial anatomy that may be useful to interventional electrophysiologists before they undertake catheter-based ablation procedures and to interventional cardiologists:

- Three-dimensional (3D) reconstruction of surface views depicting the coronary venous structures on the myocardium
- "Endoscopic" views to depict pulmonary veins from a perspective within the left atrium
- 3D views of pulmonary veins and the left atrium, with or without the remainder of the heart
- Diagnostic imaging of pulmonary vein stenosis, achieved with multiplanar reconstructions, maximal intensity projections, and volume-rendered images

Examples of normal pulmonary veins are shown in Figures 22-5 and 22-6.

The size of pulmonary veins is variable and is influenced by several factors (Table 22-5).

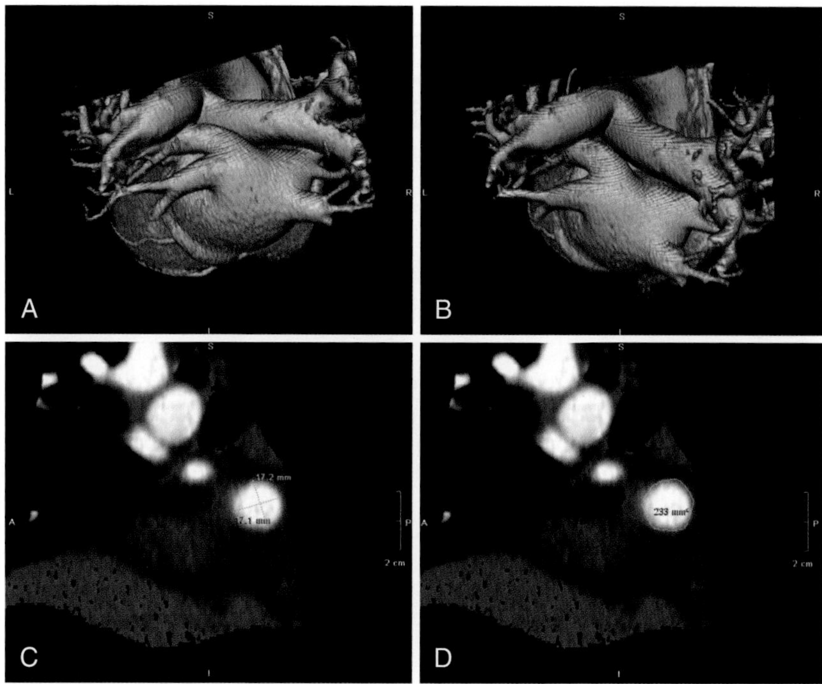

Figure 22-5. Composite images from a pre–pulmonary vein ablation cardiac CT study demonstrating an enlarged left atrium and enlarged pulmonary veins. Double-oblique reformations (**C**, **D**) across the pulmonary vein ostia allow for accurate orthogonal measurements, as well as an area measurement of the pulmonary vein ostium.

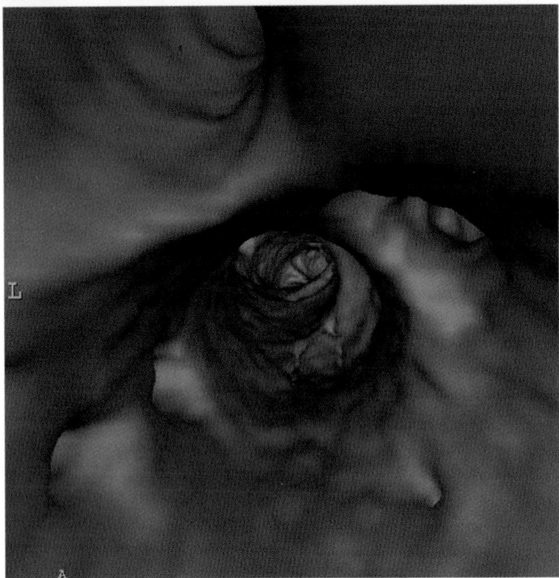

Figure 22-6. An endoluminal view of pulmonary veins.

TABLE 22-5 Factors Influencing Size of Pulmonary Veins

LARGER	SMALLER
Chronic long-term atrial fibrillation	Chronic short-term atrial fibrillation
Chronic atrial fibrillation	Paroxysmal atrial fibrillation
Larger LA	Smaller LA
Mitral disease	No mitral disease
LV disease	No LV disease
Volume loaded	Volume depleted
Male	Female

LA, left atrium; LV, left ventricle.

There is a wide range of variant pulmonary venous anatomy, and image examples of variant pulmonary venous anatomy are seen in Figures 22-7 through 22-12.

Impact of respiration on pulmonary venous morphology:

- Inspiration:
  - Increases the intervein distance (2–4 mm)
  - Increases the angle between ("splays") the veins
  - Decreases the diameter of the veins

Impact of the cardiac cycle on pulmonary venous ostia:

- Enlarges at end-systole versus end-diastole (35–45%)
- Maximum diameter, on average, at 35% RR interval
- Minimum diameter, on average, at 85% of RR interval (atrial contraction post–early diastolic emptying into the LV)

In pre-ablation cases, CCT affords more imaging information than does CMR, albeit at the expense of increased radiation exposure (Table 22-6).

REGISTRATION OF CT-GENERATED THREE-DIMENSIONAL IMAGES OF THE LEFT ATRIUM

Registration of CT-generated 3D images of the left atrium, cavae, pulmonary veins, and coronary sinus allows for accurate catheter navigation and catheter ablation.[18] Fluoroscopic position is superimposed on 3D CT images. In limited but promising studies, the mean average registration error is 1.4 mm (0.9–2.3 mm).[18] CT reconstructions usually are performed at 75% of the cardiac cycle.

Inherent problems and assumptions include[19]:

- Variation in LA size according to volume (filling pressure)
- Variation in LA size according to phase of cardiac cycle
- Variation in LA size according to phase of respiration
- Distortion of LA shape by catheter pressure

Examples of coregistered mapping of pulmonary veins are seen in Figure 22-13.

An example of LA volume reduction after successful pulmonary venous isolation is seen in Figure 22-14.

Studies on larger numbers of patients are needed to understand more broadly the range of contribution and risks of this technology.[19]

PRE-PROCEDURE CARDIAC MAPPING: BIVENTRICULAR PACEMAKER LEAD INSERTION

Biventricular pacing of failed ventricles with wide QRS complexes, most often left bundle branch block, is an accepted but expensive intervention both to alleviate symptoms of heart failure[20,21] and to reduce mortality.[22] The technique involves the insertion of pacer leads into the right ventricular (RV) apex and via the coronary sinus into a target coronary sinus tributary vein. The optimal site for left ventricular (LV) lead placement is variable but most often is a posterolateral tributary or lateral marginal branch, both of which allow pacing of the lateral wall of the LV.

Routinely, coronary venous anatomy is defined intraoperatively during biventricular lead implantation by retrograde coronary sinus venography, which offers real-time guidance and the use of a relatively small amount of dye (10–15 mL). Visualization of all branches, especially second-generation branches, may be challenging, especially if the heart has assumed nonstandard orientation

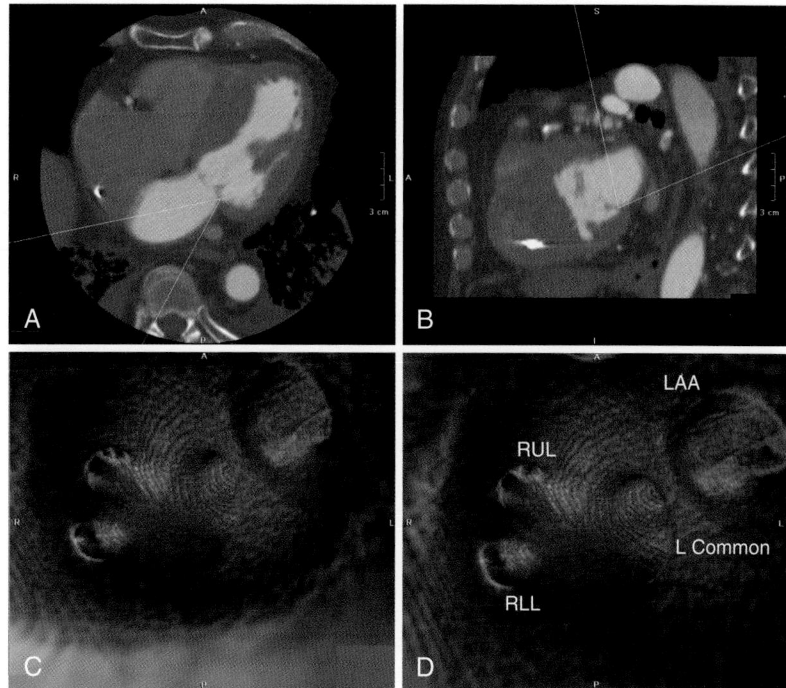

Figure 22-7. Composite data set from a pre–pulmonary vein ablation cardiac CT study in a patient with hypertrophic cardiomyopathy and atrial fibrillation. Left atrial angioscopic views demonstrate a normal variant of pulmonary venous anatomy with a conjoint common left pulmonary vein ostium, and separate right upper/right lower lobe pulmonary venous ostia. LAA, left atrial appendage; L Common, left common pulmonary vein; RLL, right lower lobe vein; RUL, right upper lobe vein.

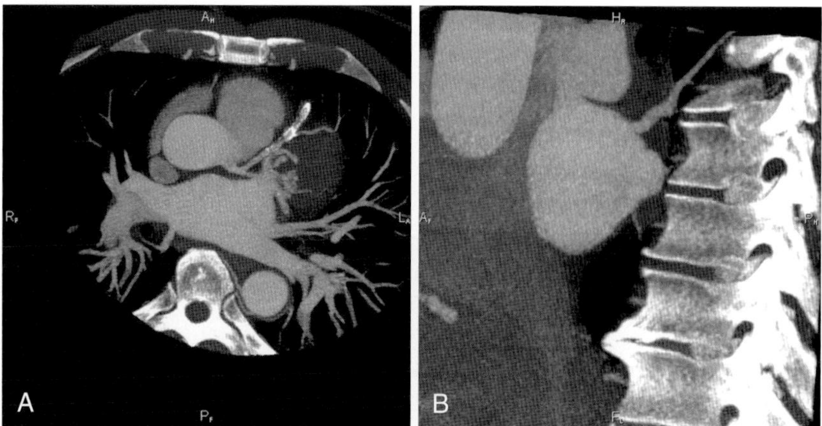

Figure 22-8. Two maximum intensity projection images from a cardiac CT examination demonstrate a common variation of normal pulmonary vein anatomy: an accessory vein separately draining the superior segment of the right lower lobe.

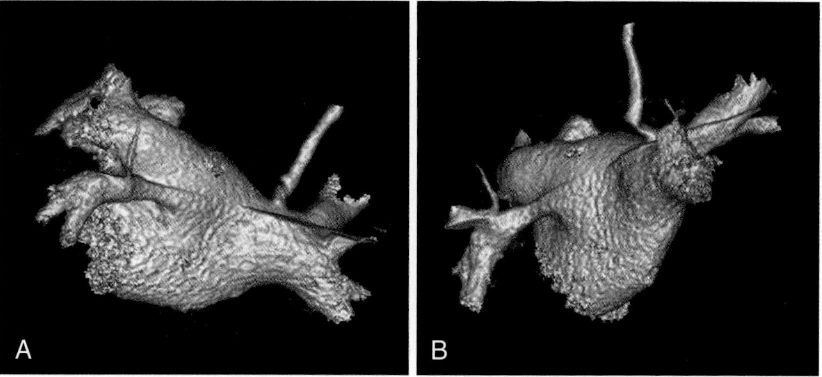

Figure 22-9. Two volume-rendered images from a cardiac CT study in a patient with atrial fibrillation, pre–pulmonary vein ablation. An accessory pulmonary vein is seen draining the superior segment of the right lower lobe. This vein drains into the roof of the left atrium. Just proximal to the confluence of the accessory vein into the left atrium, there is a bandlike moderate stenosis of the accessory vein. Careful evaluation of the CT data sets does not demonstrate a motion artifact at this site. The underlying lung parenchyma is unremarkable. There has been no prior intervention in this patient. The diagnosis was congenital stenosis of an accessory pulmonary vein.

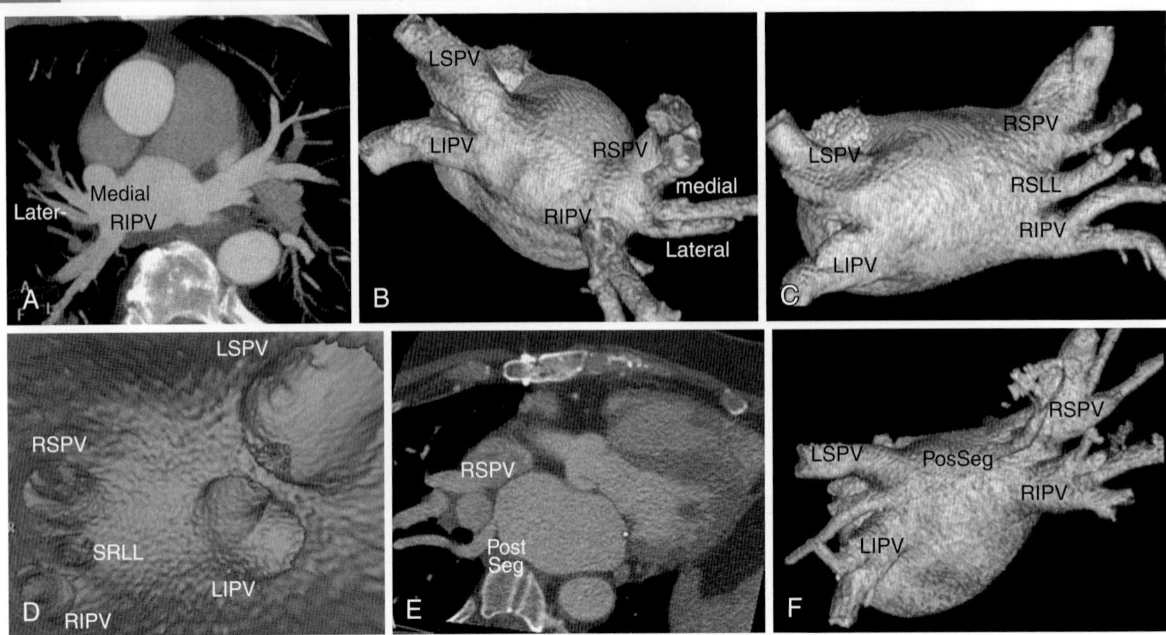

Figure 22-10. **A** and **B,** Separate ostia for the medial and lateral segmental branches of the right middle lobe. Transverse maximum intensity projection (MIP) (**A**) and three-dimensional (3D) volume-rendered images of the left atrium (**B**) show separate ostia for the medial and lateral segmental branches of the right middle lobe. **C** and **D,** Separate ostium for the right lower lobe superior segmental vein. **C,** The 3D volume-rendered image of the left atrium shows direct drainage of the superior segmental vein of the right lower lobe into the left atrium. **D,** Endocardial view shows the accessory ostium opening superior to the RIPV. **E** and **F,** Separate ostium for the posterior segmental branch of the right upper lobe. Transverse oblique contrast-enhanced CT image (**E**) and 3D volume-rendered image of the left atrium (**F**) show direct drainage of the posterior segmental branch of right upper lobe (PosSeg) into the left atrium. There is also an accessory ostium for the right middle lobe vein. Note the normal drainage of the RSPV. Later, lateral; LIPV, left inferior pulmonary vein; LSPV, left superior pulmonary vein; PosSeg, posterior segmental branch of right upper lobe; RIPV, right inferior pulmonary vein; RSLL, right superior lower lobe artery; RSPV, right superior pulmonary vein; SRLL, superior segmental vein from the right lower lobe. (Reprinted with permission from Rajiah P, Kanne JP. Computed tomography of pulmonary venous variants and anomalies. *J Cardiovasc Comput Tomogr*. 2010;4(3):155-163.)

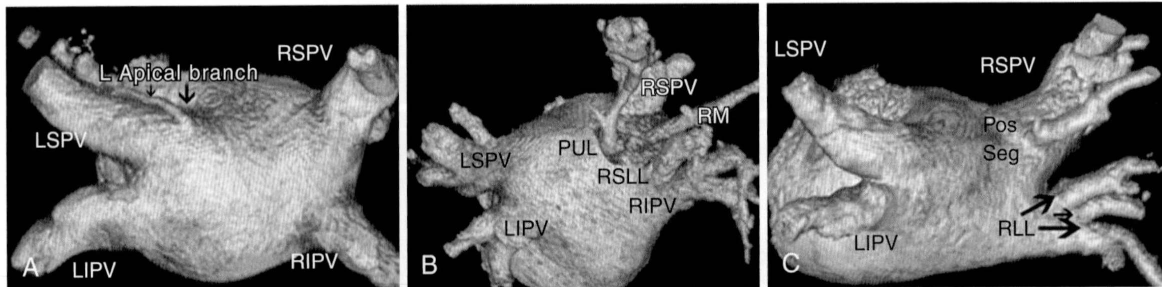

Figure 22-11. **A,** Separate ostium for the apicoposterior vein of the left upper lobe. The three-dimensional (3D) volume-rendered image of the left atrium shows direct drainage of the apicoposterior segmental vein of the left upper lobe (L apical branch) into the left atrium. There is a separate ostium for LSPV. **B** and **C,** Multiple accessory ostia. **B,** The 3D volume-rendered image of a patient with seven pulmonary venous ostia shows separate ostia for the right middle lobe vein (RM), superior segment of the right lower lobe (RSLL), and posterior segment vein from the right upper lobe (PUL), in addition to RSPV, RIPV, LSPV, and LIPV. **C,** The 3D volume-rendered image in another patient with seven pulmonary venous ostia shows three separate ostia for the right lower lobe veins (RLL; *arrows*) and a separate ostium for the vein to the posterior segment of the right upper lobe (Pos Seg), in addition to the RSPV, LSPV, and LIPV. LIPV, left inferior pulmonary vein; LSPV, left superior pulmonary vein; RIPV, right inferior pulmonary vein; RSPV, right superior pulmonary vein. (Reprinted with permission from Rajiah P, Kanne JP. Computed tomography of pulmonary venous variants and anomalies. *J Cardiovasc Comput Tomogr*. 2010;4(3):155-163.)

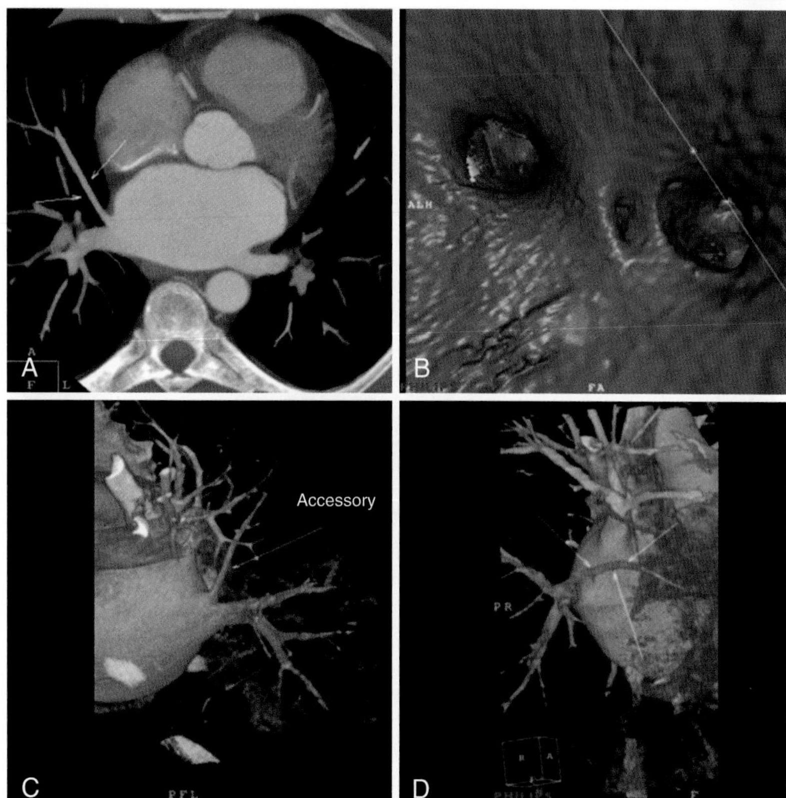

Figure 22-12. Multiple images from a cardiac CTA study in a patient with atrial fibrillation, pre–pulmonary vein isolation. These images demonstrate a common normal variant of pulmonary vein anatomy. An accessory right middle lobe pulmonary vein is seen draining via a separate ostium into the left atrium. The virtual angioscopic view (**B**) demonstrates a right upper lobe pulmonary vein, the right lower lobe pulmonary vein, and interposed between the two, closer to the right lower lobe pulmonary vein, is a separate right middle lobe pulmonary vein ostium. Art, artery.

TABLE 22-6 Comparison of CMR and CT Pulmonary Venograpphy

	CMR	CTA
Radiation dose (mSv)	0	0.7–6
Spatial resolution (mm)	1.5–3	0.5–0.7
Gating/motion compensation	None	May be ECG-gated
Evaluation of lungs	Limited	Excellent, within the obtained FOV
Evaluation of mediastinum	Limited	Excellent, within the obtained FOV
Evaluation of coronary artery anatomy	Poor	If gated, especially if 320-slice CCT, excellent
Evaluation of sinoatrial coronary branch	None	If gated, and heart rate is low, can be imaged

CCT, cardiac computed tomography; CMR, cardiac magnetic resonance; CTA, computed tomographic angiography; ECG, electrocardiographically, FOV, field of view.

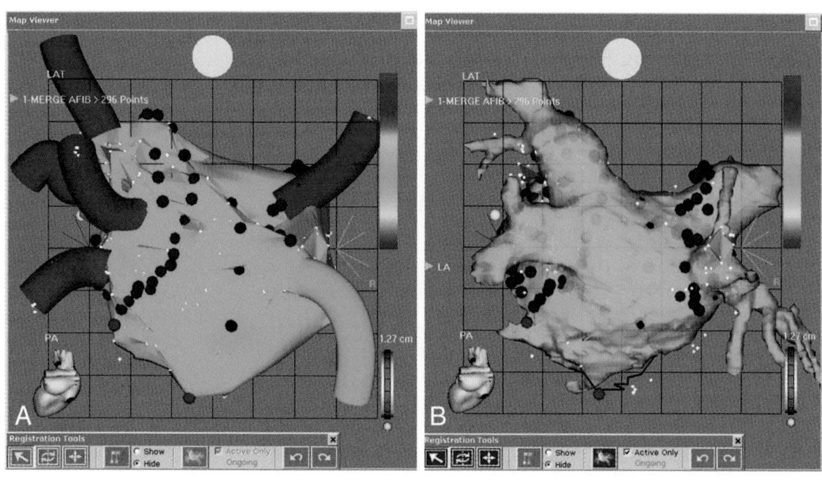

Figure 22-13. **A,** Coregistration of multidetector CT (MDCT) three-dimensional (3D) volume-rendered image and catheter navigation sites of the left atrium and pulmonary veins. The individual pulmonary veins are colored differently. **B,** Coregistration of MDCT 3D volume-rendered LA and pulmonary veins image, and catheter navigation sites. Some catheter position sites appear on either side of the surface of the left atrium (brighter indicates within; darker indicates on).

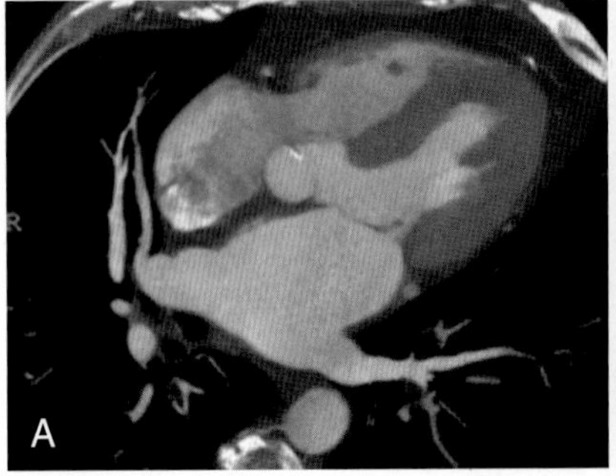

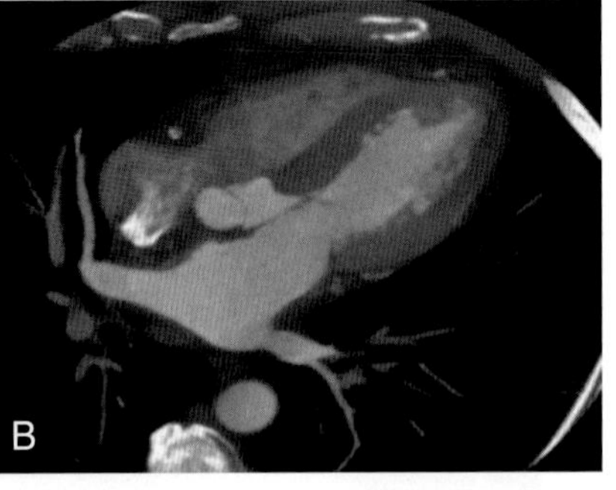

Figure 22-14. Images pre– (**A**) and post– (**B**) pulmonary venous ablation, demonstrating left atrial volume reduction following pulmonary venous atrial fibrillation ablation. The keen observer will see that they are in different phases of the cycle, reducing the credibility of the images.

in the chest.[23] There are variants of coronary sinus tributary anatomy such that target tributaries may arise off the main body of the coronary sinus at widely different distances from the coronary sinus os. Furthermore, in ischemic heart disease, vascular territories with significant obstructive coronary artery disease may have a paucity of coronary sinus venous drainage. Such significant variation in coronary sinus and coronary venous anatomy renders preoperative imaging studies useful.

In most patients 64-slice CT can visualize the coronary venous anatomy. The coronary sinus and posterior interventricular (middle) vein can be seen in almost all patients, and the posterior vein of the left ventricle can be seen in 82% to 96% of cases. In addition, CCT depicts the frequent anatomic variants of the coronary venous system. Previous infarction slightly reduces visualization of the posterior vein of the left ventricle and significantly reduces the visualization of the left marginal vein.[24] Determination of cardiac venous anatomy is feasible by CCT, using volume-rendering reconstructions,[25] and also is feasible using electron beam CT technology.[26]

Preoperative assessment of the coronary sinus anatomy provides the following advantages for the implanter:

- Definition of the precise location, orientation, and size of the coronary sinus os in the right atrium. Such knowledge may assist in the selection of coronary sinus access equipment and guide catheters.
- Definition of the initial course of the coronary sinus, which may assist in both coronary sinus access technique and the selection of an appropriate coronary sinus guide catheter.
- Definition of the presence of optimal target tributaries and suitable secondary options for LV lead placement. This may reduce intraprocedural contrast administration.
- Precise definition of the distance of the target tributaries from the coronary sinus os, the size of the os of the target vessel, and the detailed course and change in caliber of the target vessel. Such knowledge assists in selection of coronary sinus guide catheters, inner coronary sinus guides, and LV leads.
- In rare instances, assessment of coronary sinus anatomy by CT may demonstrate a paucity of target tributaries and may lead to a decision not to perform LV lead implantation due to lack of suitable target tributaries.
- CT scan imaging may make it possible to distinguish between viable and nonviable areas of myocardium, and this may assist in CS lead placement.
- Identification of a Thebesian valve at the ostium of the coronary sinus, which, if large, may obstruct introduction of a pacing lead into the coronary sinus[27] (prevents reflux of RA blood into the coronary sinus during right atrial systole)

Disadvantages of preoperative coronary sinus CT assessment include the radiation exposure to the patient and the amount of contrast that must be administered (80–100 mL), which may put patients with pre-existing renal dysfunction at risk for worsening renal function.

REVIEW OF CORONARY VENOUS ANATOMY

- Anterior interventricular vein
- Great cardiac vein
- Lateral (marginal) LV branch
- Posterior (marginal) LV branch
- Middle (posterior) cardiac vein
- Thebesian veins ("venae cordis minimae") are diminutive and drain directly into all cardiac cavities.
- Variants of coronary venous anatomy are extremely common:
  - Number of branches, especially of the anterior and middle cardiac veins[6]
  - Size of branches
  - Location of branches
  - Distances between branches
  - Presence of a large (and potentially obstructive) valve at the ostium to the coronary sinus (Thebesian valve)
  - Presence of valves at the ostia of the branches (Vieussens valves)[6]
  - The location of the ostia[7]
  - Intramural versus epicardial courses[6]
  - Collateralization between branches[6]

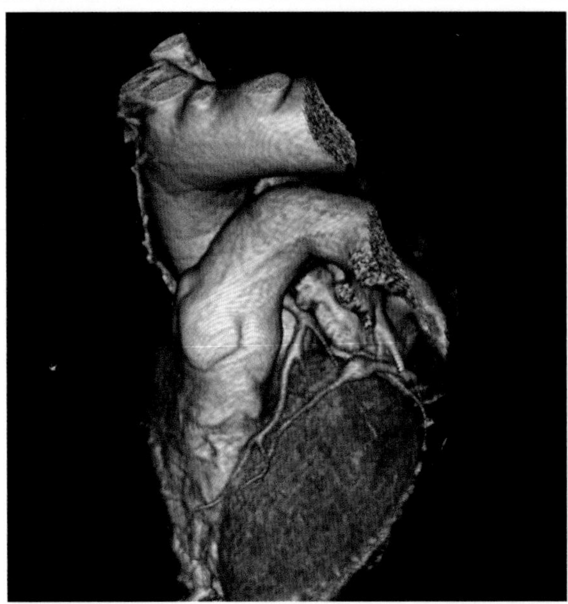

Figure 22-15. A varix of the great cardiac vein as it joins the anterior cardiac vein.

The great cardiac and middle cardiac veins are the most consistent branches of the coronary venous system.[23] The anterior and middle cardiac veins are seen in 90% of individuals, but the lateral and posterior veins (together) are seen in less than 50% of individuals.[23] The most common variant seen on CT is separate ostia of the coronary sinus and of the small cardiac vein.

The presence of a vein branch of sufficient size (the lead is up to 3 mm in diameter), in the correct location to enable electrical "resynchronization," is not invariable; for example, absence of a left marginal (lateral) branch may occur.[25]

Hence, verification of the coronary venous anatomy may be useful in planning the procedure (Figs. 22-15 through 22-19).

ASSESSMENT OF POST-PROCEDURE COMPLICATIONS

Potential complications of pulmonary venous ablation that can be assessed by CVCT include:

- Pulmonary venous stenosis at the site of ablation
- Formation of left atrial to esophageal fistulas

DEVELOPMENT OF PULMONARY VEIN STENOSIS, OBSTRUCTION, AND INFARCTION

The incidence of pulmonary venous stenosis depends on both the definition and the ablative technique used. Initial incidence was reported to be as high as 42%,[28] but substantial procedural changes and device advances have reduced the risk to approximately 1.3% if ablations are performed at the ostia rather than within the vein. Pulmonary venous stenosis most commonly affects the left-sided pulmonary veins: left upper pulmonary vein (LUPV), 43%; left lower pulmonary vein, 41%; right upper pulmonary vein, 13%; right lower pulmonary vein, 3%.[29] Clinically, patients may be asymptomatic, but if more than one vein to one lung is involved, most patients are symptomatic with cough, 89%; hemoptysis, 63%; dyspnea on exertion, 58%; pleuritic chest pain, 58%; wheezing, 42%; dyspnea at rest, 37%; or orthopnea, 32%.[29] The percentage of stenosis has a reasonable correlation with gradient across the stenosis.[30] The average onset of time before symptoms develop is 3 months.[30]

Severe pulmonary vein stenosis may be said to be present when the luminal narrowing is 70%.[31]

Obstruction and pulmonary venous infarction may occur.[32]

Helpful adjunctive signs leading to a diagnosis of pulmonary vein stenosis, in addition to luminal narrowing, include:

- Thickening of the wall of the vein
- A shelflike appearance

False-positive diagnosis of pulmonary vein stenosis may occur with:

- Draping of the LUPV over the aorta
- Prominent folds (the "Q-tip" of the LUPV as seen on TEE)
- Thin slices that do not depict the full diameter

CCT tends to overrepresent the occurrence of pulmonary venous occlusion. Saad et al.[31] found that of 15 patients with apparent occlusion of a pulmonary vein after ablation, only 7 had occlusion on angiography (Figs. 22-20 through 22-25; **Videos 22-1 and 22-2**).

The current treatment for pulmonary vein stenosis is balloon angioplasty with or without stenting, which, although usually successful (mean stenosis of 80 ± 13% and gradient of 12 ± 5 mm Hg pre-procedure to a stenosis of 9 ± 8% and gradient of 3 ± 4 mm Hg post-procedure), has a considerable restenosis rate of more than 50%.[30]

Pulmonary Venous to Esophageal Fistulas

A rare (<0.5%) and disastrous (dominant mortality) complication of pulmonary venous radiofrequency[33-35] ablation is breakdown of tissue of the wall of the pulmonary vein and the adjoining wall of the esophagus, with fistula formation, which usually occurs 3 to 7 days post-procedure.[36] Cardiac CT can image the relation of the pulmonary veins to the aorta.[36] Direct apposition of a left

Text continued on page 376

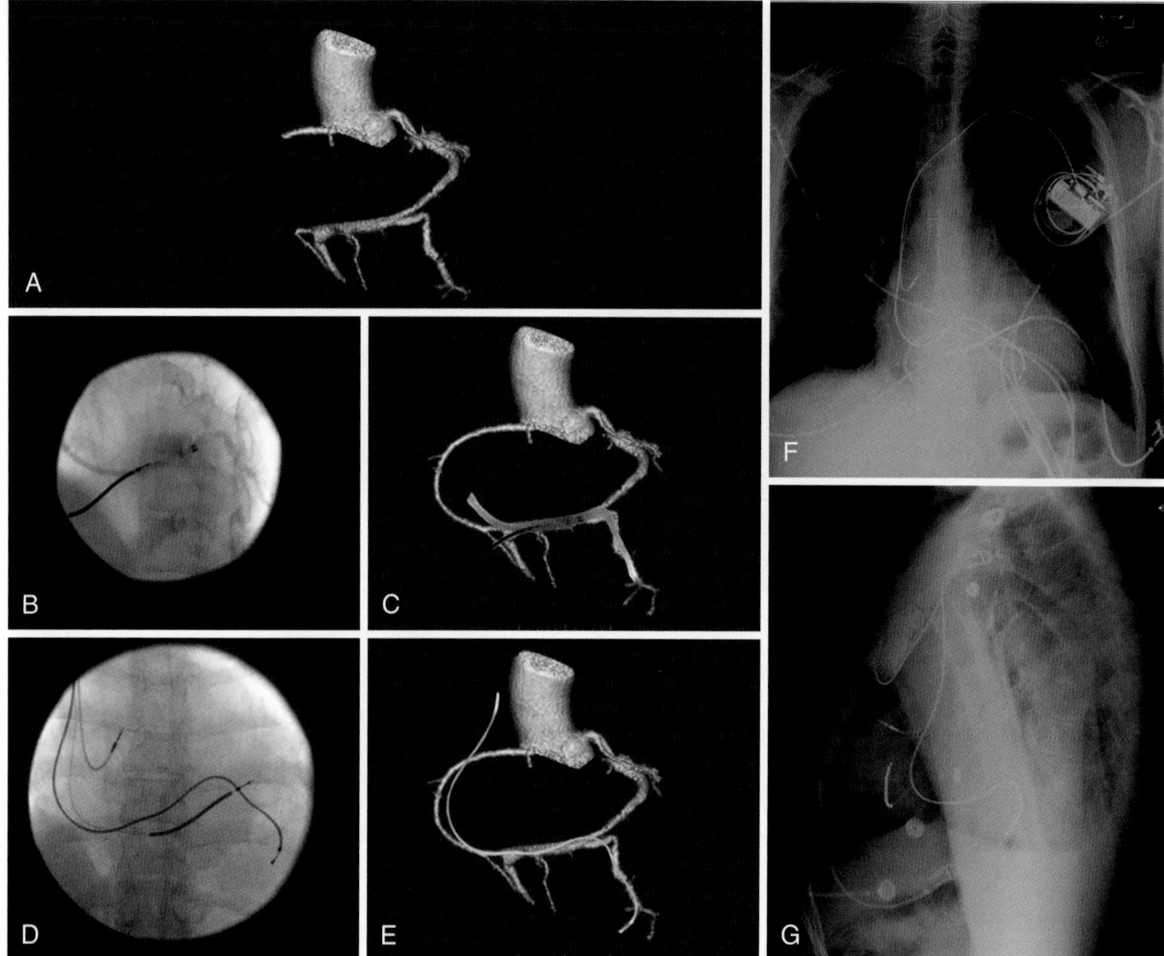

Figure 22-16. A 45-year-old man with familial dilated cardiomyopathy (LVEF 17%), left bundle branch block, and class III symptoms according to the New York Heart Association classification. Preoperative CT (three-dimensional reconstruction) shows a suitable, single, large posterolateral coronary sinus tributary target. In this case, knowledge of the size of the target vessel (5 mm at takeoff from the main body of the coronary sinus) allowed planning of lead selection. Also, note that the preoperative CT examination demonstrates a "kink" in the target vessel approximately 2 to 3 cm into it. This knowledge allowed selection of the anticipated needed delivery technique—a stylet rather than a guidewire, because the stylet is relatively stiffer. As anticipated, a first attempt with the (gentler) guidewire failed, because of the kink, not because of a decrease in vessel size. The coronary sinus guide and venogram imaging balloon were placed just proximal to the ostium of the target vessel in the coronary sinus, based on anatomic knowledge derived from the CT scan. The stylet-driven coronary sinus lead is relatively large. Final coronary sinus lead position is depicted by intraoperative fluoroscopic imaging (**D**), and postoperative postero-anterior (**F**) and lateral (**G**) chest radiographs.

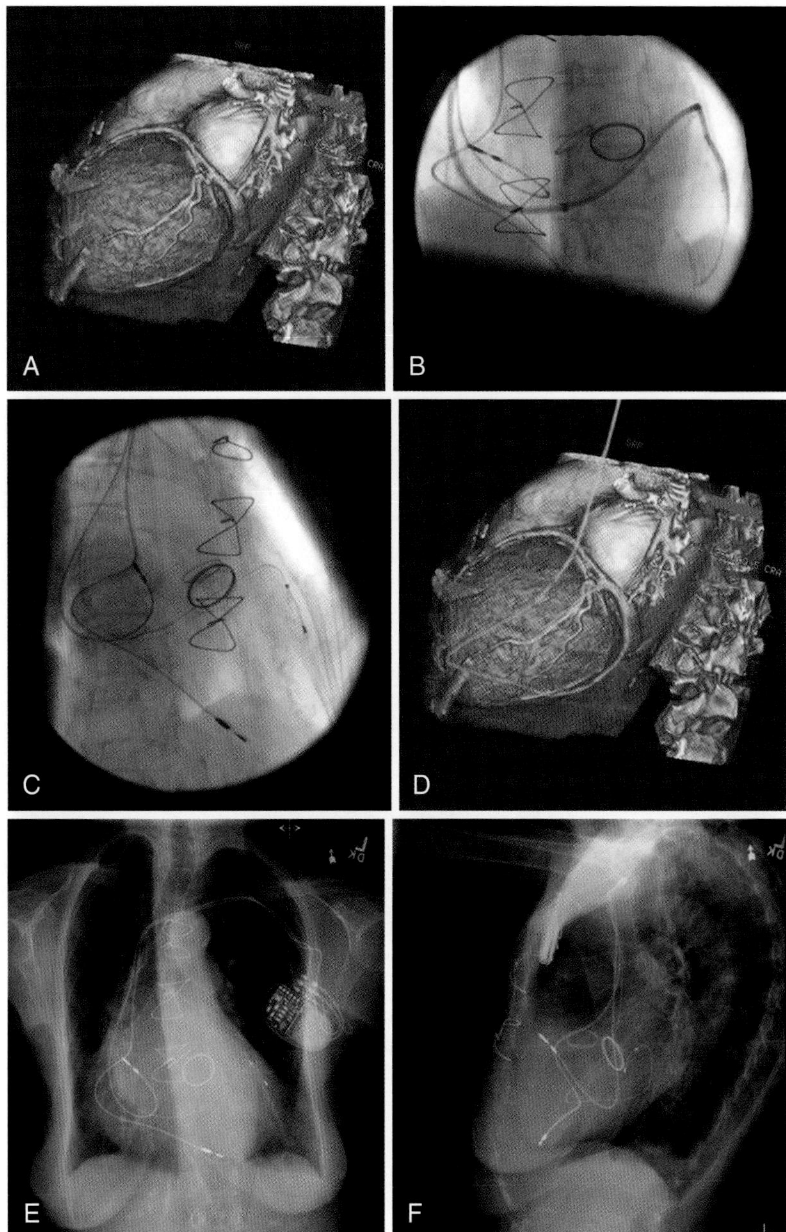

Figure 22-17. A 79-year-old woman with rheumatic heart disease and permanent atrial fibrillation/flutter status developed progressive left ventricular dysfunction post–atrioventricular node ablation and forced right ventricular pacing. She had New York Heart Association level III heart failure and (**A**) wide left bundle branch block with pacing. Her pacemaker was upgraded to cardiac resynchronization therapy with a pacemaker (CRT-PM). The preoperative CT examination showed two potential targets; the preferred target was the lateral marginal vein, shown on CT and then corroborated with selective coronary sinus venography. The final coronary sinus lead position is depicted by intraoperative fluoroscopic imaging (**C**) and postoperative posteroanterior (**E**) and lateral (**F**) chest radiographs.

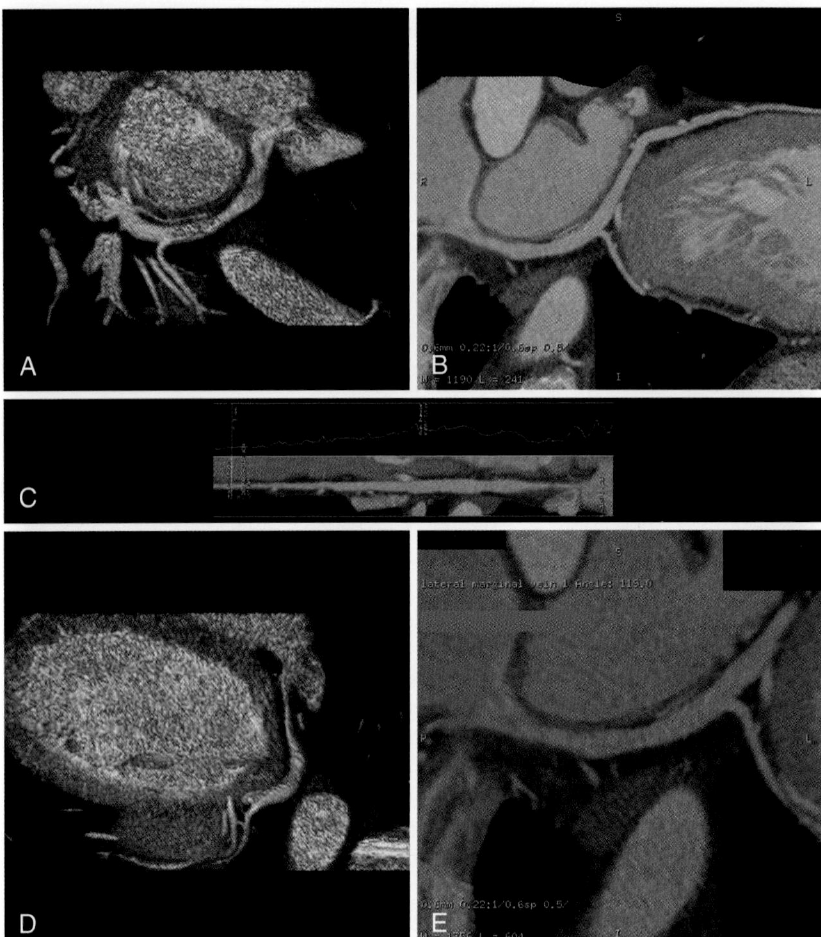

Figure 22-18. ECG-gated CT coronary venography. **A,** Three-dimensional (3D) volume-rendered image of the coronary sinus and the middle cardiac vein. **B,** Multiplanar reconstruction of the coronary sinus and the anterior cardiac vein, also demonstrating the lateral marginal vein. **C,** Straightened multiplanar reconstruction of the coronary venous system from the coronary sinus to the anterior cardiac vein. Note the narrowing of the proximal part of the coronary sinus. **D,** 3D volume-rendered image of the coronary sinus and a lower lateral marginal vein, close to an obtuse marginal artery branch. This projection demonstrates the narrowed proximal coronary sinus, which is not apparent on the upper images. **E,** A curved multiplanar reconstruction of the coronary sinus and large lower lateral marginal vein.

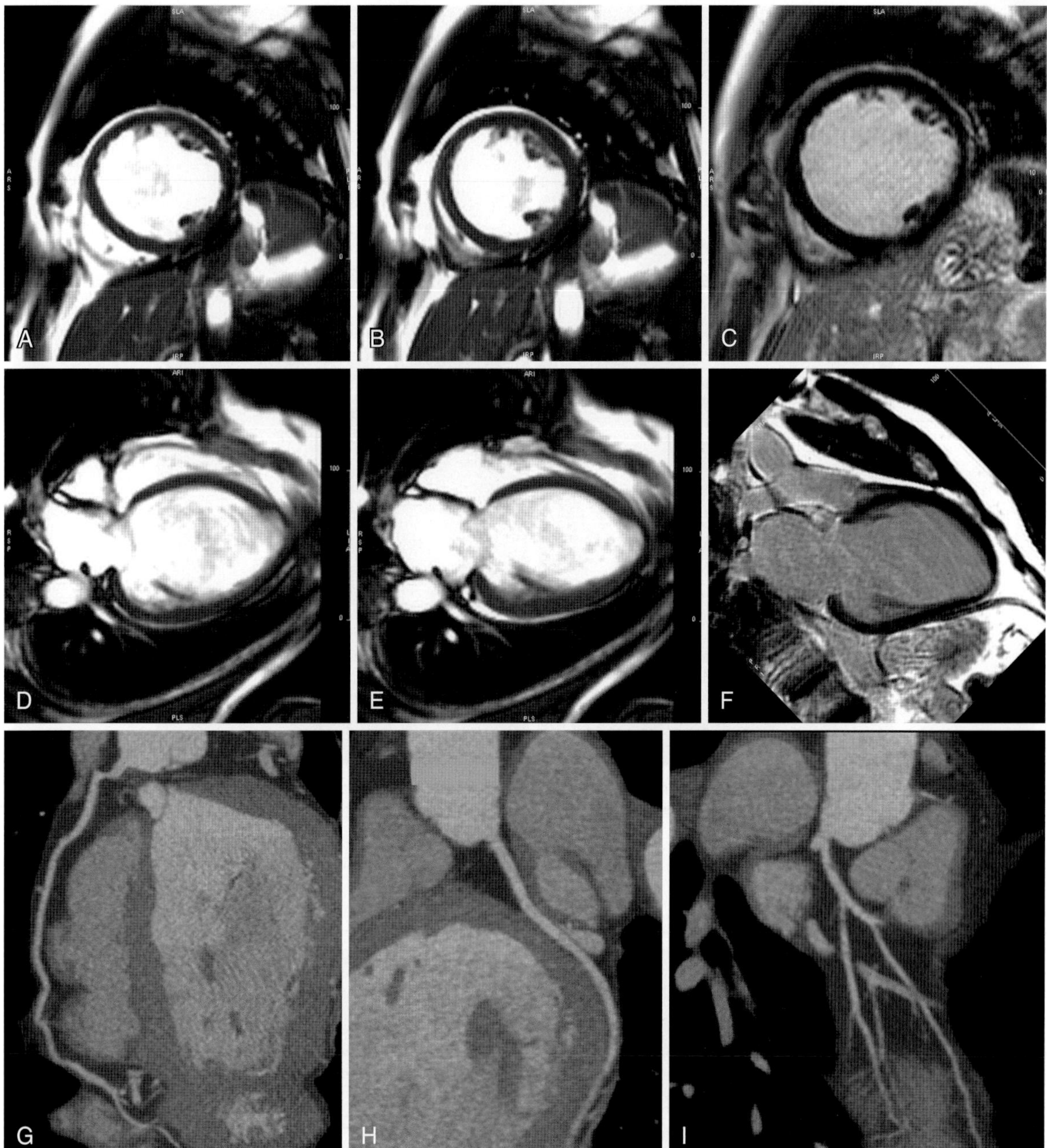

Figure 22-19. Dilated cardiomyopathy with a left bundle branch block and dyssynchrony. **A** through **F**, CMR images: SSFP images in diastole (**A** and **D**); SSFP images in systole (**B** and **E**); and late gadolinium enhancement (**C** and **F**). The ejection fraction was 15%; note how much better the right ventricular contraction is than that of the left ventricle. The dyssynchronous contraction changes the orientation of the long axis of the left ventricle. There was no late enhancement, consistent with a nonischemic basis to the cardiomyopathy. **G** through **I,** ECG-gated contrast-enhanced CT coronary angiography demonstrating a normal right coronary artery (**G**), a normal left circumflex artery (**H**), and a normal left anterior descending coronary artery (**I**), confirming the nonischemic basis of the dilated cardiomyopathy.

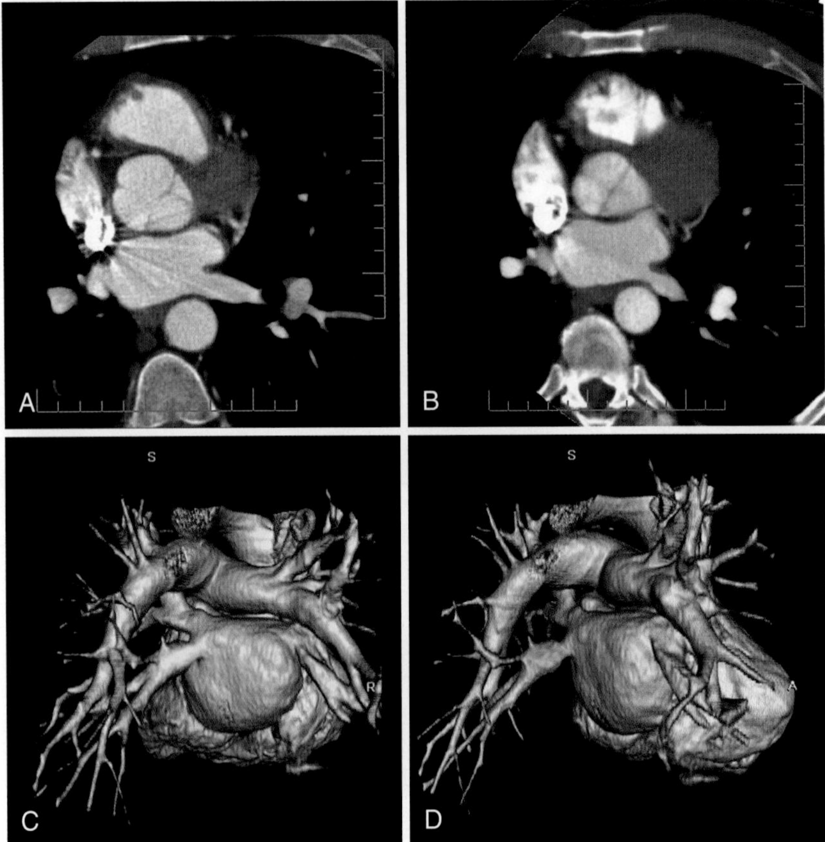

Figure 22-20. Images from a cardiac CT study done prior to (**A, C**) and post–pulmonary vein (**B, D**) ablation. Note the moderate pulmonary vein ostial stenosis involving the left lower lobe pulmonary vein. **See Videos 22-1 and 22-2.**

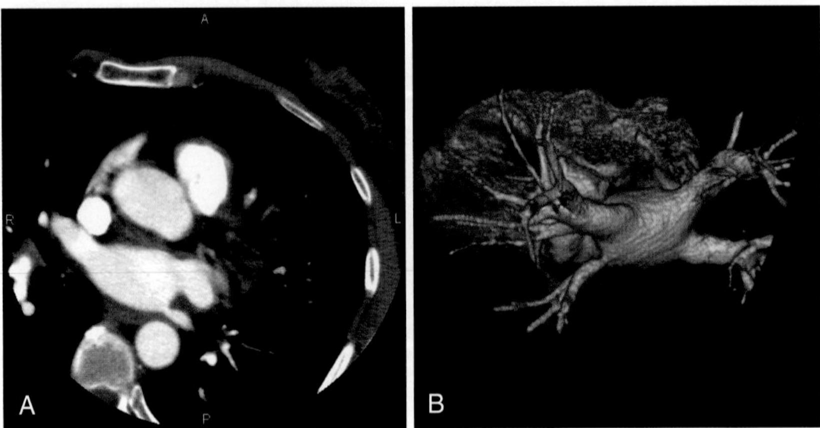

Figure 22-21. Axial source image (**A**) and volume-rendered image (**B**) depicting a 50% stenosis of the left lower lobe juxta-ostial pulmonary vein.

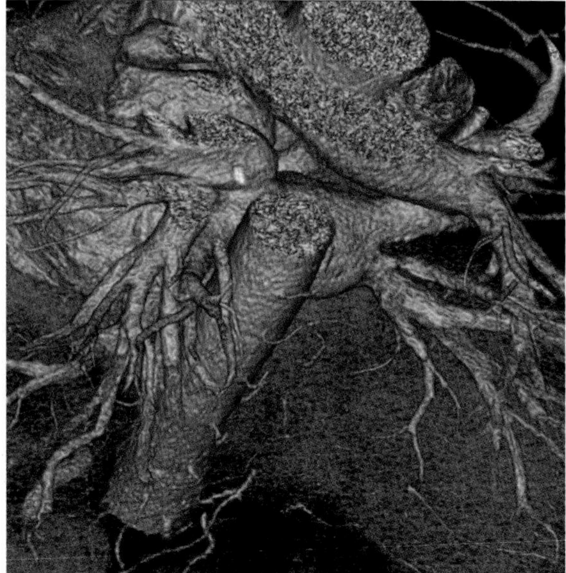

Figure 22-22. A volume-rendered image in a patient with chest pain starting 4 days post–pulmonary vein isolation for atrial fibrillation. No cause for the patient's chest pain was identified. Incidental note is made of a moderate stenosis of one of the right lower lobe pulmonary venous branches at its confluence with the right common lower lobe pulmonary vein. A mild amount of narrowing of the right lower lobe pulmonary vein itself also is identified.

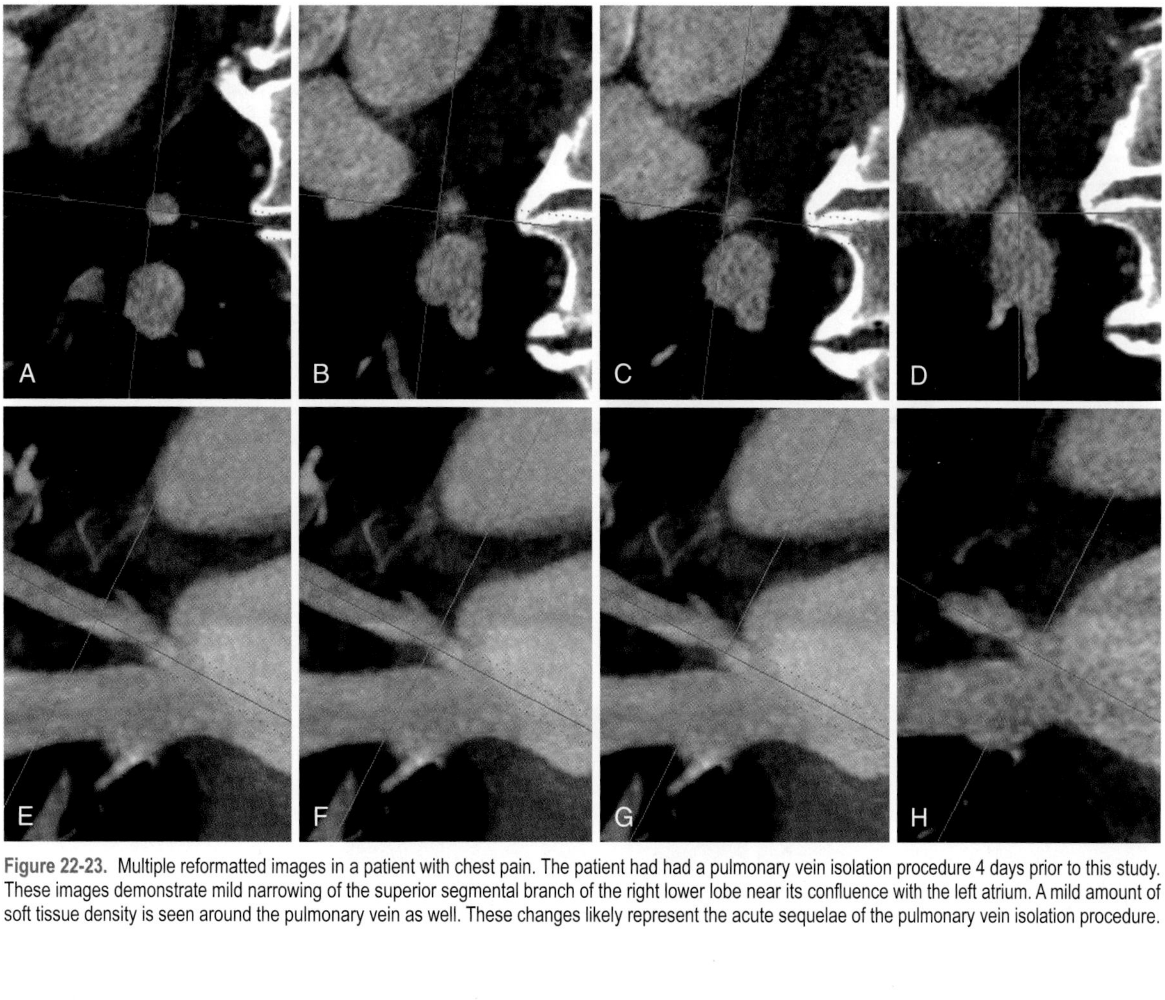

Figure 22-23. Multiple reformatted images in a patient with chest pain. The patient had had a pulmonary vein isolation procedure 4 days prior to this study. These images demonstrate mild narrowing of the superior segmental branch of the right lower lobe near its confluence with the left atrium. A mild amount of soft tissue density is seen around the pulmonary vein as well. These changes likely represent the acute sequelae of the pulmonary vein isolation procedure.

pulmonary vein against the esophagus underlies this complication. Local discontinuity of the fat layer between the LA and the esophagus is believed to underlie the complication.[36] It has been demonstrated that radiofrequency ablation of the left atrium as it overlies the esophagus results in a higher temperature in the esophagus.[37,38]

Among the most common presentations of left atrial to esophageal fistulas are fever and chest pain. Stroke results from embolization of air in the left atrium.

CCT ECG gating is not required. Particular attention should be paid to the mediastinum to identify stranding of the fat, localized fluid collection adjacent to the esophagus, and the presence of mediastinal, intrapericardial, and left atrial air (Table 22-7).

For images of left atrial to esophageal fistulas, see Figures 22-26 and 22-27.

SINOATRIAL NODAL ARTERY

See Figure 22-28.

POST-ABLATION THROMBUS

See Figure 22-29.

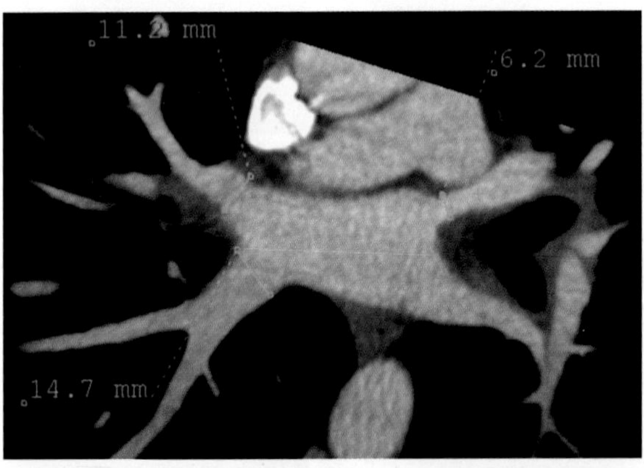

Figure 22-24. Multiplanar reconstructed image from a cardiac CT scan post-ablation demonstrates soft tissue around the ostium of the left superior and inferior pulmonary veins, causing a moderate stenosis of the left superior vein ostium.

IDENTIFICATION OF PACEMAKER OR IMPLANTABLE CARDIOVERTER DEFIBRILLATOR MALPOSTION

Pacemaker and implantable cardioverter defibrillator malposition and perforation may be imaged by CCT (Figs. 22-30 and 22-31).

ASSESSMENT OF ARRHYTHMOGENIC RIGHT VENTRICULAR CARDIOMYOPATHY

See Chapter 21, Myopathies.

CCT PROTOCOL POINTS

- ❒ Standard CCT protocol is followed (Table 22-8).

TABLE 22-7 Summary of Clinical Findings in Cases of Reported Atrial-Esophageal Fistulas

No. of patients	49
Time to diagnosis (days)	3–41
Symptoms/presentation	
Neurologic	69%
Fever	75%
Sepsis	33%
Chest pain	28%
Leukocystosis	25%
No. of patients with bacteremia	
Monomicrobial	2
Polymicrobial	2
Mortality	67%

Data from Siegel MO, Parenti DM, Simon GL. Atrial-esophageal fistula after atrial radiofrequency catheter ablation. *Clin Infect Dis.* 2010;51(1):73-76.

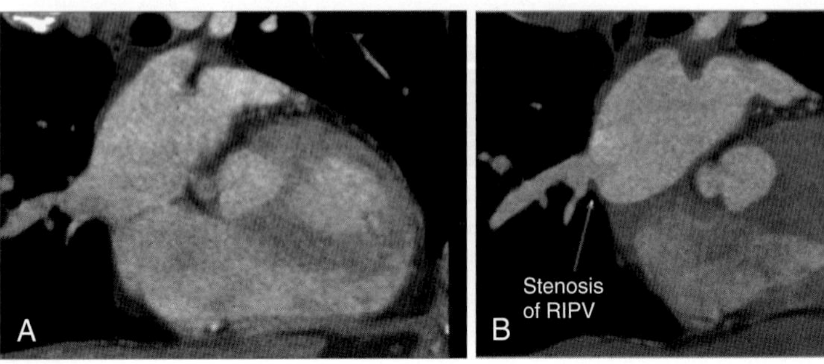

Figure 22-25. Two multiplanar reconstructed images from a cardiac CT scan pre– (**A**) and post– (**B**) pulmonary vein ablation demonstrate an inferior ridge of soft tissue causing a mild stenosis of the right inferior pulmonary vein (RIPV).

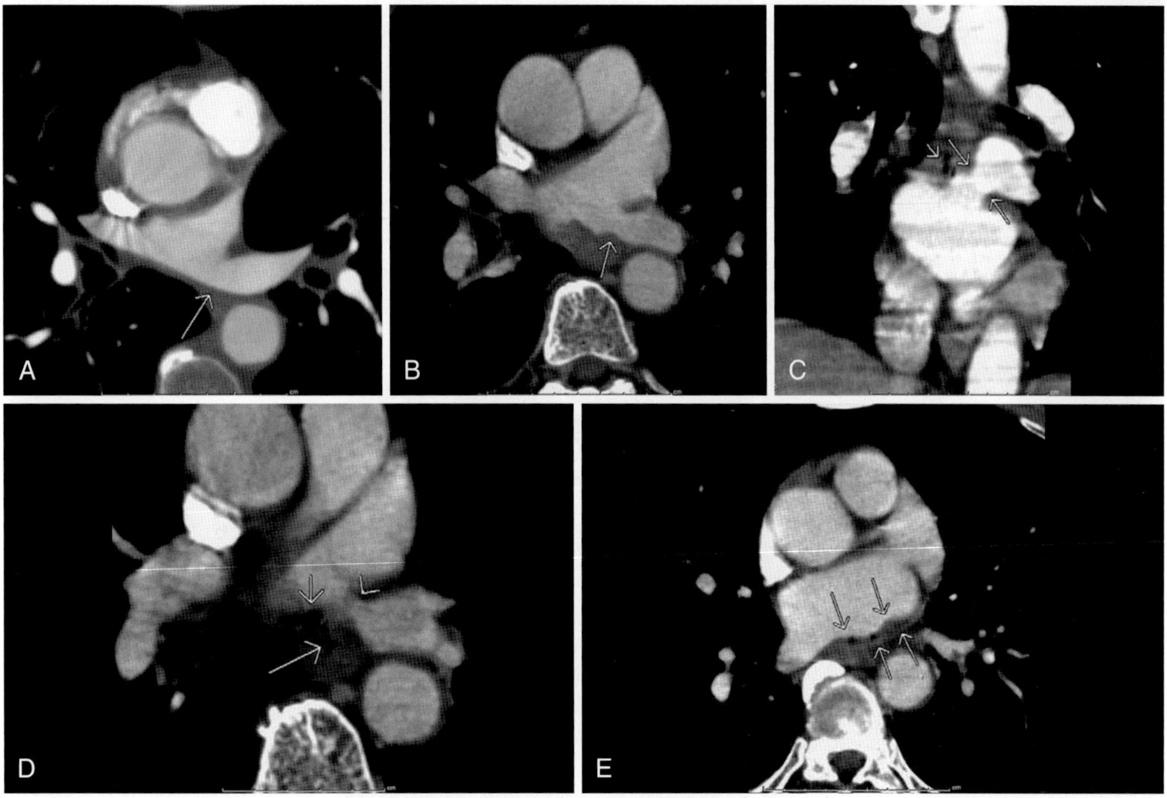

Figure 22-26. Left atrial to esophageal fistula. A 59-year-old man presented with altered mental status, fever, and peripheral petechiae 5 weeks post–pulmonary venous isolation. **A,** A pre–radiofrequency catheter ablation (RFCA) axial CT scan of the chest with IV contrast was performed as part of a routine preoperative examination for atrial fibrillation 6 weeks before the emergent or post-RFCA examination. This earlier scan showed a smooth-contoured normal variant single left common pulmonary vein (*large arrow*). **B,** Post-RFCA axial CT chest scan with IV contrast showed a narrowed, irregular, and ulcerated single left common pulmonary vein (*large arrow*). New, irregular soft tissue was seen inseparable/indistinguishable to the adjacent esophagus, which was causing mass effect and lobulated contour abnormality on the posterior left atrium (LA) adjacent to and involving the left common pulmonary vein/LA junction. **C,** Post-RFCA coronal CT of the chest with IV contrast showed a narrowed, irregular, and ulcerated single left common pulmonary vein (*large arrows*). Small pockets of extraluminal air suggested pneumomediastinum (*small arrow*). **D,** Post-RFCA axial CT scan of the chest with IV contrast showed a curvilinear lucency traversing the esophageal wall, suggesting a transmural fistulous tract (*large arrow*). Small extraluminal air pockets compatible with localized rupture are seen (*small arrow*), as is an ulcerated and narrowed single left common pulmonary vein (*arrowhead*). **E,** Post-RFCA axial CT scan of the chest with IV contrast revealed left atrial posterior wall thickening, posterior mediastinal fat induration, and pneumomediastinum or questionable air within the LA (*large arrows*). (Reprinted with permission from Malamis AP, Kirshenbaum KJ, Nadimpalli S. CT radiographic findings: atrio-esophageal fistula after transcatheter percutaneous ablation of atrial fibrillation. *J Thorac Imaging.* 2007;22(2):188-191.)

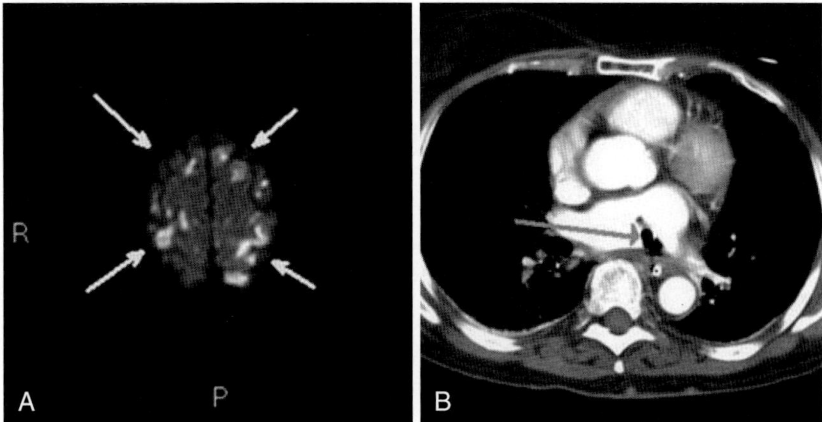

Figure 22-27. Left atrial to esophageal fistula. A 72-year-old woman presented 2 weeks post–pulmonary venous isolation with leukocytosis, dyspnea, and a seizure. **A,** Diffusion-weighted MRI of the head demonstrates extensive bilateral infarcts (*arrows*). **B,** CT scan of the chest with IV contrast demonstrates air in the left atrium (*arrow*). (Reprinted with permission from Vassileva CM, Shawgo T, Shabosky J, et al. Repair of left atrial-esophageal fistula following percutaneous radiofrequency ablation for atrial fibrillation. *J Card Surg.* 2011;26(5):556-558.)

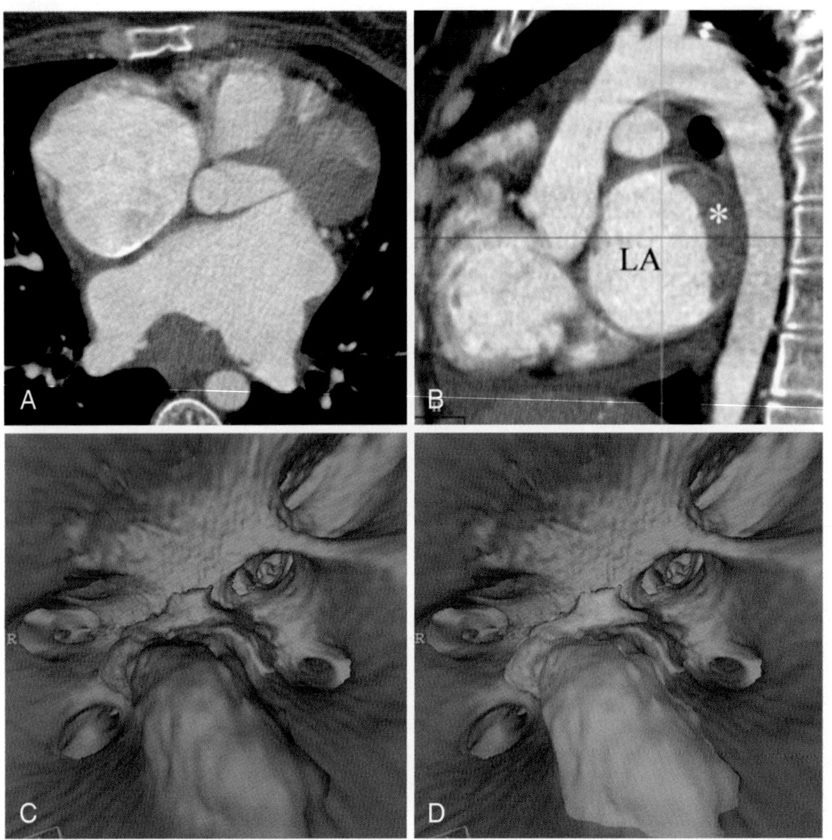

Figure 22-28. Reformatted and volume-rendered images from a cardiac CT study in a patient complaining of chest pain post–pulmonary vein isolation procedure. A large soft tissue density is seen within the posterior wall of the left atrium (LA). A small amount of increased density also is seen posterior to the left atrium within the posterior mediastinum. There is no evidence of any mediastinal air. The diagnosis was intra-atrial and mediastinal hematoma post–pulmonary vein/left atrial ablation.

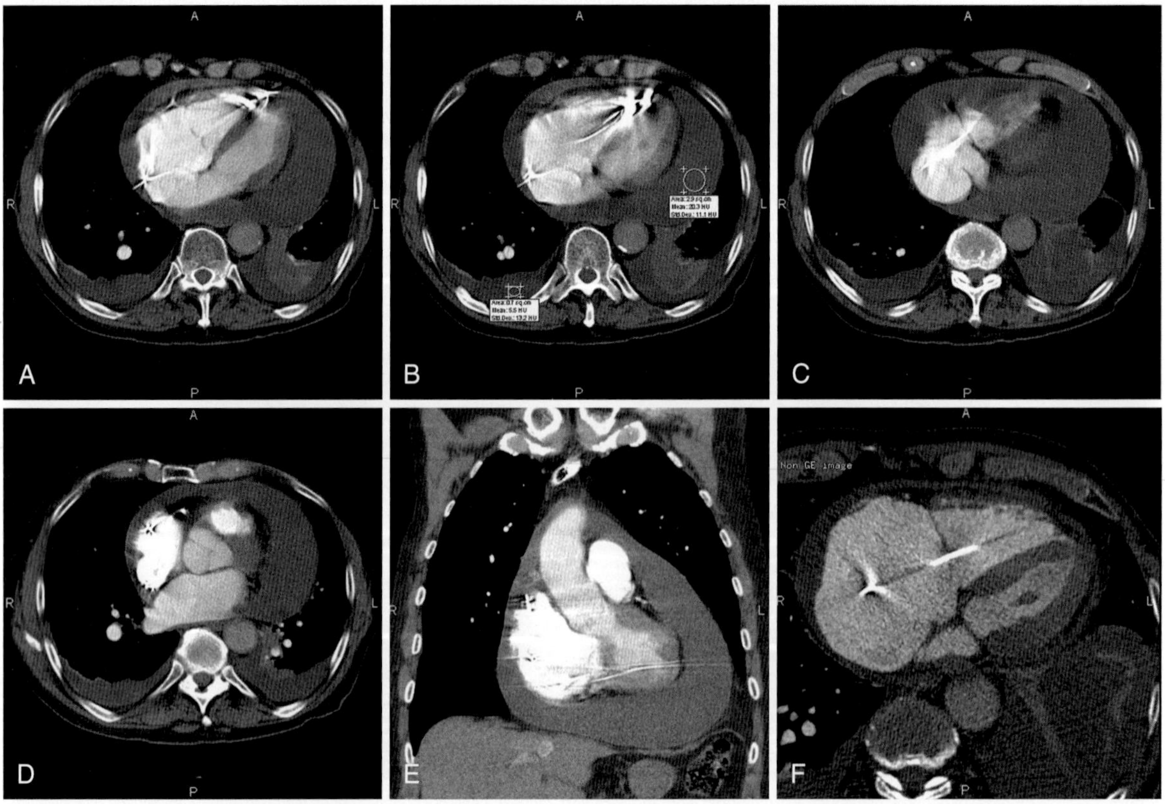

Figure 22-29. Composite series of images from a cardiac CT examination in a patient with pericardial tamponade post–pacemaker insertion. There is a moderate-to-large pericardial effusion with a Hounsfield measurement (20 HU) higher than what would be acceptable for water (normal fluid). Despite blooming artifact, there is suspicion that the pacemaker tip extends beyond the confines of the right ventricular apex. Additional note is made of small bilateral pleural effusions. **F** has been obtained post-pericardiocentesis, during which a large amount of bloody pericardial fluid was withdrawn. The pacemaker was removed, and a new pacemaker was placed.

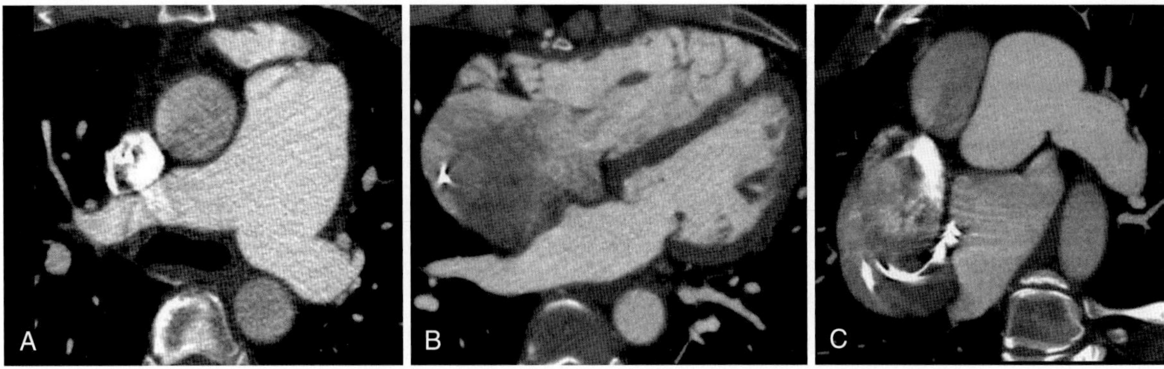

Figure 22-30. Multiple images from a cardiac CT study in a patient with underlying congenital heart disease. Transgression of pacemaker wires across a patent foramen ovale into the left atrium has occurred. The main and central pulmonary arteries are markedly enlarged, and there is straightening of the intraventricular septum, consistent with ongoing pulmonary arterial hypertension.

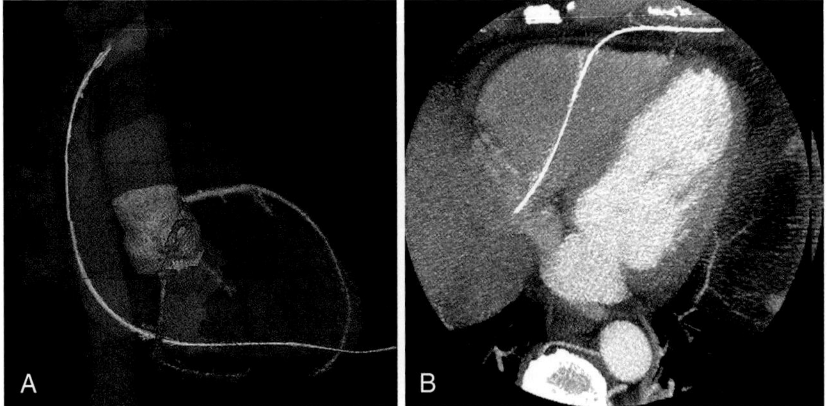

Figure 22-31. ECG-gated cardiac CT images in a patient post-pacemaker insertion. The tip of the right ventricular lead extends through the right ventricular apex and into the epicardial fat. There is no evidence of a pericardial effusion.

TABLE 22-8 ACCF 2010 Appropriateness Criteria for the Use of Cardiac Computed Tomography to Evaluate Cardiac Electrophysiologic Matters

	APPROPRIATENESS RATING	INDICATION	MEDIAN SCORE
Evaluation of cardiac structure and function—evaluation of ventricular morphology and systolic function, and intra- and extracardiac structures	Appropriate	Evaluation of pulmonary vein anatomy Prior to radiofrequency ablation for atrial fibrillation	8
		Noninvasive coronary vein mapping Prior to placement of biventricular pacemaker	8
		Assessment of right ventricular morphology Suspected arrhythmogenic right ventricular dysplasia	7
	Uncertain	None listed	
	Inappropriate	None listed	

Data from Taylor AJ, Cerqueira M, Hodgson JM, et al. ACCF/SCCT/ACR/AHA/ASE/ASNC/NASCI/SCAI/SCMR 2010 appropriate use criteria for cardiac computed tomography. A report of the American College of Cardiology Foundation Appropriate Use Criteria Task Force, the Society of Cardiovascular Computed Tomography, the American College of Radiology, the American Heart Association, the American Society of Echocardiography, the American Society of Nuclear Cardiology, the North American Society for Cardiovascular Imaging, the Society for Cardiovascular Angiography and Interventions, and the Society for Cardiovascular Magnetic Resonance. *J Am Coll Cardiol.* 2010;56(22):1864-1894.

References

1. Wolak A, Gutstein A, Cheng VY, et al. Dual-source coronary computed tomography angiography in patients with atrial fibrillation: initial experience. *J Cardiovasc Comput Tomogr.* 2008;2(3):172-180.
2. Saremi F, Channual S, Gurudevan SV, Narula J, Abolhoda A. Prevalence of left atrial appendage pseudothrombus filling defects in patients with atrial fibrillation undergoing coronary computed tomography angiography. *J Cardiovasc Comput Tomogr.* 2008;2(3):164-171.
3. Xu L, Yang L, Fan Z, Yu W, Lv B, Zhang Z. Diagnostic performance of 320-detector CT coronary angiography in patients with atrial fibrillation: preliminary results. *Eur Radiol.* 2011;21(5):936-943.
4. Pasricha SS, Nandurkar D, Seneviratne SK, et al. Image quality of coronary 320-MDCT in patients with atrial fibrillation: initial experience. *AJR Am J Roentgenol.* 2009;193(6):1514-1521.
5. Oncel D, Oncel G. Dual-source computed tomography imaging in a patient with atrial fibrillation and left atrial thrombus. *J Cardiovasc Comput Tomogr.* 2007;1(3):170-171.
6. Martinez MW, Kirsch J, Williamson EE, et al. Utility of nongated multidetector computed tomography for detection of left atrial thrombus in patients undergoing catheter ablation of atrial fibrillation. *JACC Cardiovasc Imaging.* 2009;2(1):69-76.
7. Tang RB, Dong JZ, Zhang ZQ, et al. Comparison of contrast enhanced 64-slice computed tomography and transesophageal echocardiography in detection of left atrial thrombus in patients with atrial fibrillation. *J Interv Card Electrophysiol.* 2008;22(3):199-203.
8. Martinez MW, Williamson EE, Lin G, Brady PA. Multidetector computed tomography with delay imaging for detection of left atrial thrombus. *J Cardiovasc Comput Tomogr.* 2009;3(5):354-355.
9. Jaber WA, White RD, Kuzmiak SA, et al. Comparison of ability to identify left atrial thrombus by three-dimensional tomography versus transesophageal echocardiography in patients with atrial fibrillation. *Am J Cardiol.* 2004;93(4):486-489.
10. Lee WJ, Chen SJ, Lin JL, Huang YH, Wang TD. Images in cardiovascular medicine. Accessory left atrial appendage: a neglected anomaly and potential cause of embolic stroke. *Circulation.* 2008;117(10):1351-1352.
11. Duerinckx AJ, Vanovermeire O. Accessory appendages of the left atrium as seen during 64-slice coronary CT angiography. *Int J Cardiovasc Imaging.* 2008;24(2):215-221.
12. Wood MA, Wittkamp M, Henry D, et al. A comparison of pulmonary vein ostial anatomy by computerized tomography, echocardiography, and venography in patients with atrial fibrillation having radiofrequency catheter ablation. *Am J Cardiol.* 2004;93(1):49-53.
13. Jongbloed MR, Bax JJ, Lamb HJ, et al. Multislice computed tomography versus intracardiac echocardiography to evaluate the pulmonary veins before radiofrequency catheter ablation of atrial fibrillation: a head-to-head comparison. *J Am Coll Cardiol.* 2005;45(3):343-350.
14. Marom EM, Herndon JE, Kim YH, McAdams HP. Variations in pulmonary venous drainage to the left atrium: implications for radiofrequency ablation. *Radiol.* 2004;230(3):824-829.
15. Arslan G, Dincer E, Kabaalioglu A, Ozkaynak C. Right top pulmonary vein: evaluation with 64 section multidetector computed tomography. *Eur J Radiol.* 2008;67(2):300-303.
16. Noseworthy PA, Malchano ZJ, Ahmed J, Holmvang G, Ruskin JN, Reddy VY. The impact of respiration on left atrial and pulmonary venous anatomy: implications for image-guided intervention. *Heart Rhythm.* 2005;2(11):1173-1178.
17. Choi SI, Seo JB, Choi SH, et al. Variation of the size of pulmonary venous ostia during the cardiac cycle: optimal reconstruction window at ECG-gated multi-detector row CT. *Eur Radiol.* 2005;15(7):1441-1445.
18. Sra J, Krum D, Malloy A, et al. Registration of three-dimensional left atrial computed tomographic images with projection images obtained using fluoroscopy. *Circulation.* 2005;112(24):3763-3768.
19. Triedman J. Virtual reality in interventional electrophysiology. *Circulation.* 2005;112(24):3677-3679.
20. Abraham WT, Fisher WG, Smith AL, et al. Cardiac resynchronization in chronic heart failure. *N Engl J Med.* 2002;346(24):1845-1853.
21. Bristow MR, Saxon LA, Boehmer J, et al. Cardiac-resynchronization therapy with or without an implantable defibrillator in advanced chronic heart failure. *N Engl J Med.* 2004;350(21):2140-2150.
22. Cleland JG, Daubert JC, Erdmann E, et al. The effect of cardiac resynchronization on morbidity and mortality in heart failure. *N Engl J Med.* 2005;352(15):1539-1549.
23. Singh JP, Houser S, Heist EK, Ruskin JN. The coronary venous anatomy: a segmental approach to aid cardiac resynchronization therapy. *J Am Coll Cardiol.* 2005;46(1):68-74.
24. Van de Veire NR, Schuijf JD, De Sutter J, et al. Non-invasive visualization of the cardiac venous system in coronary artery disease patients using 64-slice computed tomography. *J Am Coll Cardiol.* 2006;48(9):1832-1838.
25. Jongbloed MR, Lamb HJ, Bax JJ, et al. Noninvasive visualization of the cardiac venous system using multislice computed tomography. *J Am Coll Cardiol.* 2005;45(5):749-753.
26. Mao S, Shinbane JS, Girsky MJ, et al. Coronary venous imaging with electron beam computed tomographic angiography: three-dimensional mapping and relationship with coronary arteries. *Am Heart J.* 2005;150(2):315-322.
27. Shinbane JS, Budoff MJ. Computed tomographic cardiovascular imaging. *Stud Health Technol Inform.* 2005;113:148-181.
28. Chen SA, Hsieh MH, Tai CT, et al. Initiation of atrial fibrillation by ectopic beats originating from the pulmonary veins: electrophysiological characteristics, pharmacological responses, and effects of radiofrequency ablation. *Circulation.* 1999;100(18):1879-1886.
29. Qureshi AM, Prieto LR, Latson LA, et al. Transcatheter angioplasty for acquired pulmonary vein stenosis after radiofrequency ablation. *Circulation.* 2003;108(11):1336-1342.
30. Packer DL, Keelan P, Munger TM, et al. Clinical presentation, investigation, and management of pulmonary vein stenosis complicating ablation for atrial fibrillation. *Circulation.* 2005;111(5):546-554.
31. Saad EB, Rossillo A, Saad CP, et al. Pulmonary vein stenosis after radiofrequency ablation of atrial fibrillation: functional characterization, evolution, and influence of the ablation strategy. *Circulation.* 2003;108(25):3102-3107.
32. Ravenel JG, McAdams HP. Pulmonary venous infarction after radiofrequency ablation for atrial fibrillation. *AJR Am J Roentgenol.* 2002;178(3):664-666.
33. Doll N, Borger MA, Fabricius A, et al. Esophageal perforation during left atrial radiofrequency ablation: is the risk too high? *J Thorac Cardiovasc Surg.* 2003;125(4):836-842.
34. Sonmez B, Demirsoy E, Yagan N, et al. A fatal complication due to radiofrequency ablation for atrial fibrillation: atrio-esophageal fistula. *Ann Thorac Surg.* 2003;76(1):281-283.
35. Pappone C, Oral H, Santinelli V, et al. Atrio-esophageal fistula as a complication of percutaneous transcatheter ablation of atrial fibrillation. *Circulation.* 2004;109(22):2724-2726.
36. Lemola K, Sneider M, Desjardins B, et al. Computed tomographic analysis of the anatomy of the left atrium and the esophagus: implications for left atrial catheter ablation. *Circulation.* 2004;110(24):3655-3660.
37. Cummings JE, Schweikert RA, Saliba WI, et al. Assessment of temperature, proximity, and course of the esophagus during radiofrequency ablation within the left atrium. *Circulation.* 2005;112(4):459-464.
38. Siegel MO, Parenti DM, Simon GL. Atrial-esophageal fistula after atrial radiofrequency catheter ablation. *Clin Infect Dis.* 2010;51(1):73-76.

23 Cardiac and Paracardiac Masses

Key Points

- The initial evaluation of cardiac masses should be performed using echocardiography.
- Cardiac CT scanning is able to image cardiac masses and can contribute to their evaluation. The superior field of view of CCT compared with both transthoracic echocardiography and TEE may assist with the assessment of paracardiac masses.
- From the pathology point of view, it is important to recall that imaging and histology are distinct entities.
- The goal of CCT should be to determine whether a mass demonstrates malignant features such as tissue plane violation.

Although CCT is able to image most lesions within the heart, especially larger ones,[1,2] its role is secondary to those of echocardiography and MRI in the evaluation of lesions within the heart. CCT's greatest contribution is to evaluate the thorax in detail for complex cardiac masses (both those extending into the heart and those located elsewhere). Neither transthoracic nor transesophageal echocardiography has sufficient field of view to see beyond the heart into the chest cavity or even entirely around the heart. For example, a pericardial cyst often is not apparent by echocardiography (unless the cyst abuts the chest wall).

Lesions that are atypical for myxomas should be further evaluated by CT scanning to ensure that there are no signs of malignant disease elsewhere within the chest or abdomen.[3]

CT scanning is unparalleled in its ability to identify calcification within lesions, such as pericardial masses or thickening.

Although CCT is able to image small and mobile structures within the heart, such as vegetations, echocardiography, by virtue of having vastly superior temporal resolution, is the preferred test for imaging small and mobile lesions within the heart itself. For any mass lesion other than the most obvious myxoma, it would be unwise not to perform a CT scan of the chest and abdomen to exclude signs of malignancy elsewhere.

CCT may assist with surgical planning in cases such as the younger patient with presumed atrial myxoma by confirming lesional characteristics as seen by echocardiography and by excluding significant coronary artery disease.[4]

CCT can image a wide range of intra- and paracardiac structures:

- ❐ Intracardiac masses and lesions
  - Vegetations
  - Thrombi
  - Tumors/masses
  - Abscesses
- ❐ Paracardiac masses and lesions
  - Cysts
  - Tumors/masses

CARDIAC MASSES

Cardiac masses can be categorized with respect to nature:

- ❐ Thrombus
- ❐ Cysts
- ❐ Abscesses
- ❐ Neoplasms

Thrombus

Thrombus, the most common type of intracardiac mass, is most often located within the left atrial appendage. It is often associated with mitral valve disease and underlying atrial dysrhythmias.

In the left ventricle, thrombi usually are apical in location and usually are associated with prior myocardial infarct. This may occur in an area of associated severe hypokinesis, or within a left ventricular aneurysm. Left ventricular thrombi can be laminar, more rounded and mass-like, or pedunculated. Long-standing thrombi can calcify. Pre–contrast-enhanced and delayed imaging can be used to aid in differentiating between a non-enhancing thrombus and an enhancing tumor.

If a thrombus is suspected within the right atrium, in the absence of an instigating factor such as a central line or pacing wire, one must attempt to exclude tumor or tumor thrombus from an intra-abdominal source such as renal cell carcinoma or hepatocellular carcinoma.

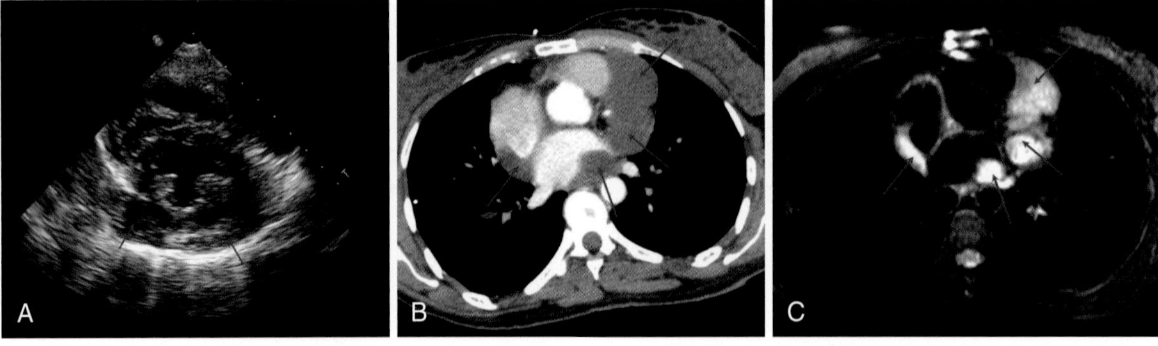

Figure 23-1. Echinococcus of the heart. **A,** Transthoracic echocardiography in the short-axis view demonstrates the presence of a pericardial cyst in the inferior and posterior basal part of the left ventricle (*red arrows*). **B,** Contrast-enhanced CT in the axial view demonstrates four pericardial cysts (*red arrows*). **C,** T2-weighted turbo spin magnetic resonance confirms the liquid nature of the structures by a homogeneous hyperintense signal (*red arrows*). (Reprinted with permission from Gerber BL, Pasquet A, El Khoury G, et al. Echinococcosis of the heart and ascending aorta. *Circulation.* 2012;125(1):185-187.)

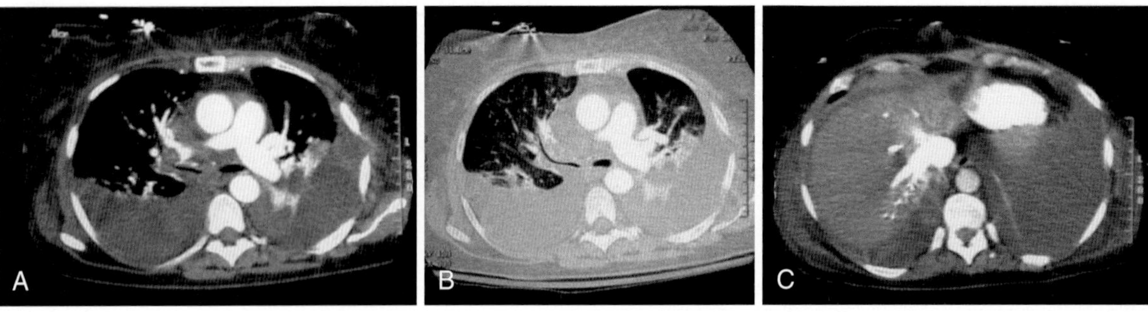

Figure 23-2. **A,** Contrast-enhanced CT at the level of the pulmonary arteries. The patient presented with shock and right-sided heart failure. An echocardiogram (*not shown*) had shown a large pericardial effusion, which was drained with only partial improvement. CT scanning shows bilateral effusions and soft tissue masses around the pulmonary arteries as well as soft tissue within the pulmonary arteries. Deep venous thrombosis was present. **B,** Contrast-enhanced CT at the level of the pulmonary arteries. The right pulmonary artery is nearly entirely obliterated and both bronchi are compressed; the right bronchus is slit-like. The patient's shortness of breath was multifactorial. **C,** Contrast-enhanced CT at the level of the liver. The inferior vena cava (IVC) is severely dilated, as are the hepatic veins, and there is reflux into the IVC of contrast dye infused from the upper extremities, consistent with severe right-sided heart failure. There is a rim of ascites. The diagnosis was adenocarcinoma of lung with pleural effusions, tamponade, pulmonary artery obstruction from extrinsic compression, angioinvasion, and pulmonary thromboembolism.

Cysts

Pericardial Cysts

For discussion and examples of pericardial cysts, see Chapter 17.

Echinococcosis

Echinococcosis of the heart, also known as hydatid disease or echinococccal disease, is the result of parasitic infection with the tapeworm *Echinococcus granulosus.* The parasite is shared in its life cycle with another mammal such as a dog or sheep, and the disease is endemic in sheep-ranching areas. The incubation period is months to years. Echinococcus eggs lead to the growth of cysts of 5 to10 cm in size that characterize the disease and may involve the heart (Fig. 23-1).

Abscesses

For a discussion and examples of cardiac abscesses, see Chapter 20.

Cardiac Neoplasms

Cardiac neoplasms are rare. They include, in order of frequency:

1. Metastases (the most common, by 20- to 40-fold)
2. Malignant primary neoplasms
3. Benign primary neoplasms

In a consecutive autopsy series of 12,485 cases, the prevalence of primary cardiac tumors was 0.056% and of cardiac metastases 1.23%.[5]

Metastases

Metastatic cardiac disease spreads to the heart by four pathways:

- Retrograde lymphatic extension: lung, breast, lymphoma
- Hematogenous spread: melanoma, breast, lymphoma
- Direct contiguous extension: lung, esophagus, breast, lymphoma, thymoma
- Transvenous extension: kidney, liver (up the inferior vena cava), bronchogenic (down a pulmonary vein)

The most common primary sources for cardiac metastases include lung bronchogenic carcinoma, breast adenocarcinoma, lymphoma, melanoma, and sarcomas (Figs. 23-2 through 23-6).

Thymoma. A thymoma is a tumor of epithelial cell origin that arises from the thymus gland. The incidence of thymomas increases with age, with

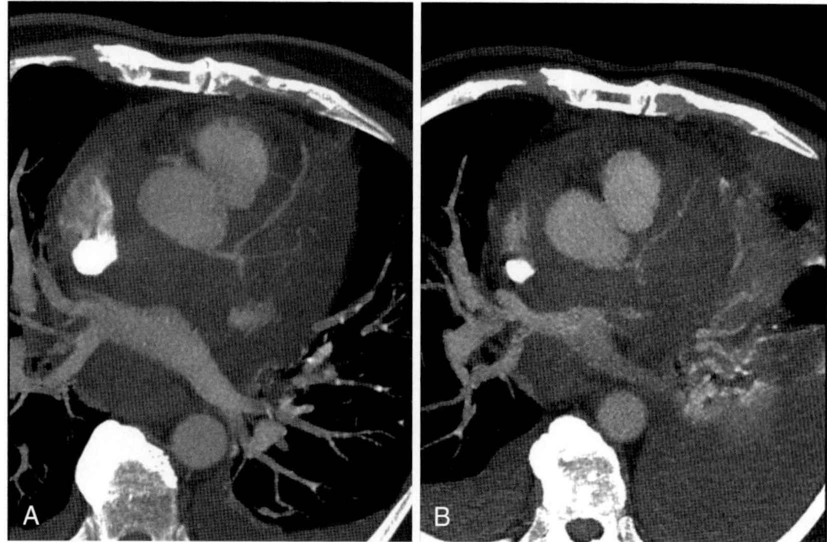

Figure 23-3. Images in a patient with metastatic bronchogenic carcinoma. **A,** Extensive soft tissue infiltration of the mediastinum. The soft tissue insinuates between the left atrium and the aorta, and courses around the left main and left anterior descending (LAD) arteries. Contrast also is seen within a ramus branch. The circumflex system was patent, but not imaged on this generated maximum intensity projection. Absence of an epicardial fat plane around the coronary arteries is suspicious for invasion of the epicardial fat, and tumor encasement of the coronary arteries. A follow-up study 3 months later demonstrates faint contrast within the proximal portion of the ramus, but occlusion of the ongoing ramus branch. The LAD and circumflex artery show, however, a slightly more irregular appearance. Arterial infarction occurred, believed to be due to coronary artery compression by bronchogenic carcinoma.

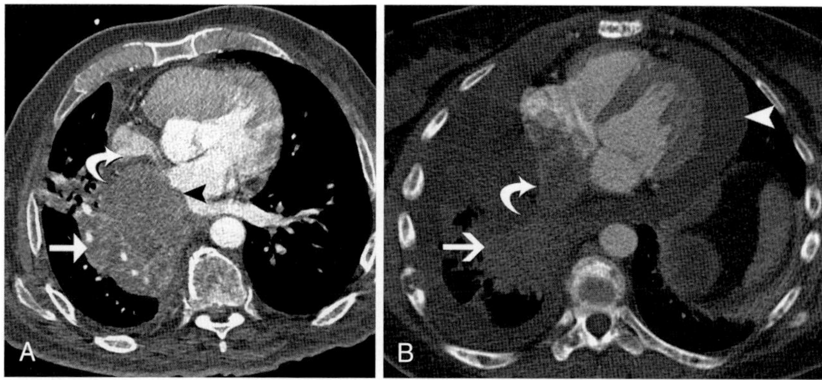

Figure 23-4. **A,** CT image of a 72-year-old man shows a large non-small cell lung carcinoma (*white arrow*) infiltrating the right atrium (*curved arrow*) and the left atrium (*black arrowhead*). **B,** Transverse CT image of a 63-year-old woman shows a large spiculated mass in the right lower lobe (*white arrow*), pathologically proven to be squamous cell carcinoma, extending to the right atrium (*curved arrow*). There is also a malignant pericardial effusion (*arrowhead*). (Reprinted with permission from Rajiah P, Kanne JP, Kalahasti V, Schoenhagen P. Computed tomography of cardiac and pericardiac masses. *J Cardiovasc Comput Tomogr*. 2011;5(1):16-29.)

a mean age at diagnosis of about 40 years. About 30% to 40% of patients with thymoma present with one of a number of parathymic syndromes, most commonly myasthenia gravis, pure red cell aplasia, or hypogammaglobulinemia. About 30% of patients present with symptoms caused by compression of surrounding structures, including the superior vena cava and esophagus, and approximately 30% to 40% of patients have no symptoms at all. Thymomas may arise centrally within the anterior mediastinum, but are more commonly eccentric in location. On noncontrast imaging, thymomas have Hounsfield unit attenuation similar to that of muscle (40–60 HU). Areas of cystic degeneration calcification also can be seen. Contrast-enhancement of these tumors may be inhomogeneous or heterogeneous in appearance. A well-defined CT appearance may suggest the presence of a fibrous capsule. Ill-defined margins, extracapsular extension of soft tissue, and obliteration of surrounding fat planes should raise concern for invasive or malignant thymoma, and thymic carcinoma.

Malignant Primary Cardiac Neoplasms

Malignant primary tumors can be classified by tissue type:

- Mesenchymal: sarcoma
- Lymphoid: lymphoma
- Rare others: inflammatory myofibroblastic

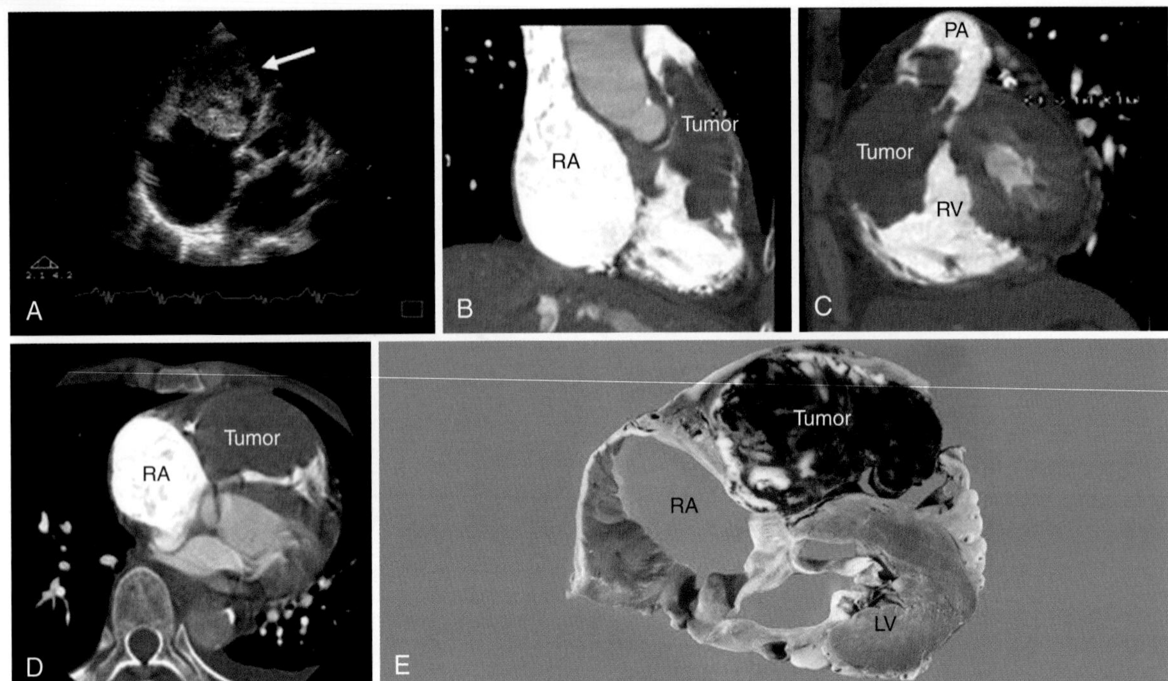

Figure 23-5. A 62-year-old female dialysis patient presented with intermittent fever, dyspnea, and hoarseness (due to a diagnosed thyroid tumor). While she was treated for fever of unknown origin, transthoracic echocardiography (**A**) showed a solid high-echoic mass (*arrow*) extending into the main pulmonary artery (PA) and obliterating the right ventricular outflow tract. **B, C,** and **D,** A 64-multislice CT scan demonstrated a large ellipsoid mass (59 × 55 × 35 mm) extensively involving the right ventricular (RV) wall. Transvenous biopsy confirmed undifferentiated thyroid carcinoma. At 20 days after admission, the patient died of decompensated heart failure. **E,** An autopsy confirmed the findings of transthoracic echocardiography, multislice CT scan, and the biopsy. Right ventricular outflow tract obstruction from metastatic thyroid cancer is extremely rare. We speculate that the patient's immunosuppression therapy as well as the fact that she was a dialysis patient may have contributed to the tumor's progression. LV, left ventricle; RA, right atrium. (Reprinted with permission from Yanagisawa S, Suzuki Y, Yuasa T, Tanaka T. Right ventricular outflow tract obstruction: metastatic thyroid carcinoma. *J Am Coll Cardiol.* 2010;55(11):1159.)

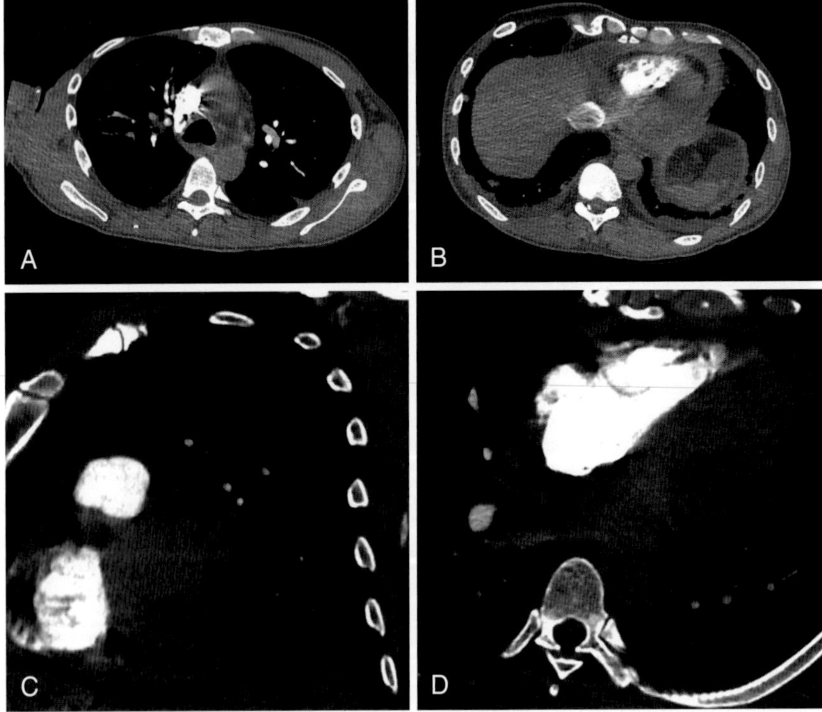

Figure 23-6. Multiple images from a CT pulmonary embolism study in a 48-year-old man with prior history of chest wall sarcoma who presented with chest pain and shortness of breath. **A,** Thinning of the right anterior chest wall from prior tumor resection. The heart appears encased by the pericardium, suspicious for pericardial metastatic disease. **B,** Marked thickening of the pericardium, with primarily soft tissue attenuation material. **C** and **D,** These images have been generated in a lower window width level to better appreciate a large 3.7-cm low-density mass involving the posterior lateral wall of the left ventricle, and extending into the ventricular cavity. This finding is suspicious for a myocardial metastatic deposit.

These types are discussed in the following sections.

Primary Cardiac Sarcoma. Sarcomas are the most common primary malignant cardiac neoplasms and the second most common primary cardiac neoplasm. They occur most commonly in adults and are very rare in infants and children. If presenting in a child, they usually are rhabdomyosarcomas.

Multiple sarcoma cell types exist, in approximately the following proportions:

- Angiosarcoma: 35%
- Undifferentiated: 25%
- Malignant fibrous histiocytoma: 15% to 20%
- Leiomyosarcoma: 5% to 10%
- Osteosarcoma: 5%
- Rhabdomyosarcoma: 5%

Angiosarcoma and osteosarcoma have a male-to-female predominance of 2:1. Approximately 80% of angiosarcomas occur in the right side of heart, often with distant metastases at initial presentation (Figs. 23-7 through 23-10).[5]

Primary Cardiac Lymphoma. Primary cardiac lymphoma can be defined as lymphoma mostly confined to the heart or pericardium. Almost all of these tend to be aggressive B-cell lymphomas. They can involve any chamber, but seem to favor the right atrium. Multifocal presentation is common, with involvement of two chambers seen at presentation approximately 75% of the time. Because lymphatic obstruction occurs as part of the infiltrative process, cardiac lymphoma also may present with large pericardial or pleural effusions (Figs. 23-11 and 23-12).[5]

Inflammatory Myofibroblastic Tumor. Inflammatory myofibroblastic tumors are rare tumors of unclear nature but are believed to be malignant, with a prominent fibrotic component. They may arise in different sites, of which the most common is the lung (Fig. 23-13).

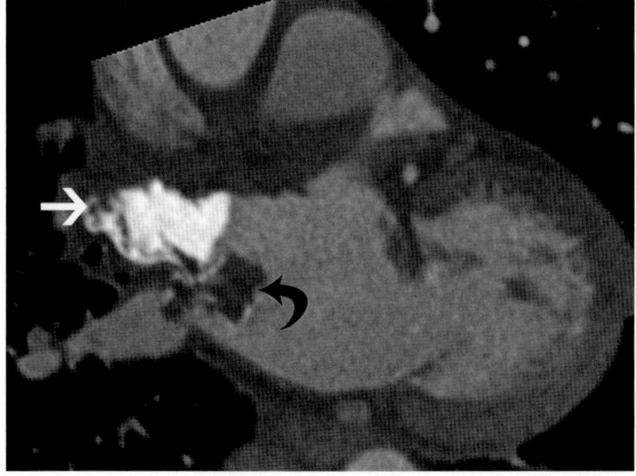

Figure 23-7. Coronal oblique reformatted CT image shows a heterogeneous mass in the left atrium containing soft tissue (*curved arrow*) and calcified (*arrow*) components. Extension into the right superior pulmonary vein suggests malignancy. The biopsy showed osteosarcoma. (Reprinted with permission from Rajiah P, Kanne JP, Kalahasti V, Schoenhagen P. Computed tomography of cardiac and pericardiac masses. *J Cardiovasc Comput Tomogr.* 2011;5(1):16-29.)

Benign Primary Cardiac Neoplasms

Benign neoplasms may be intracavitary, mural, or epicardial focal masses.

These can be classified pathologically according to histologic features and cellular differentiation as arising from:

- Muscle: rhabdomyoma
- Fibrous tissue: fibroma
- Vascular: hemangioma
- Fat: lipoma
- Nervous system: pheochromocytoma
- Ectopic: teratoma
- Others:
  - myxoma
  - papillary fibroelastoma

The more common benign neoplasms are described in the following sections.

Myxoma. Myxomas are the most commonly occurring primary cardiac neoplasms, accounting for approximately 50% of all primary cardiac tumors. Myxomas have a slight female predilection. Most patients present at between 30 and 60 years of age. Myxomas usually are sporadic, but autosomal dominant inheritance can be seen in persons with Carney complex. Ninety percent of lesions are solitary, intracavitary, and atrial in location. The left atrium is far more commonly involved than the right (70–80% versus 10–20%). Myxomas have a predilection for the fossa ovalis,

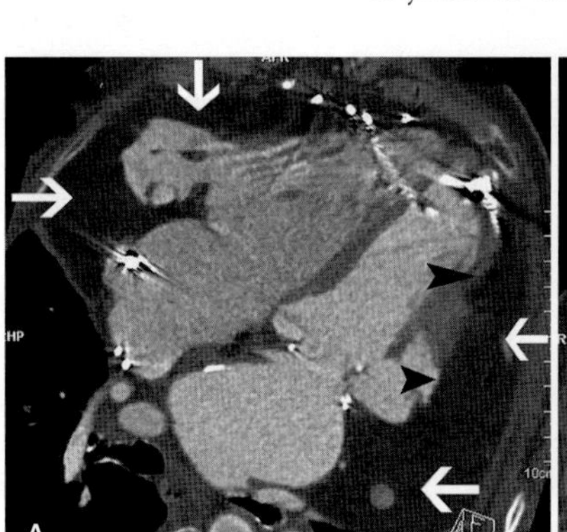

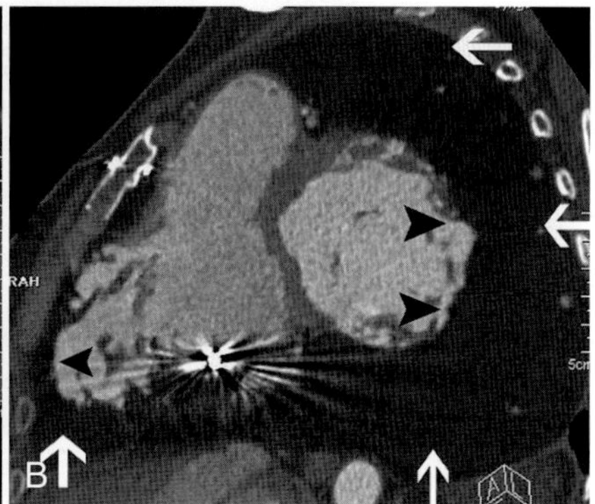

Figure 23-8. Transverse (**A**) and short-axis reformatted (**B**) CT images of a 74-year-old man with a large liposarcoma show a large fatty mass (*arrows*) encasing and infiltrating the heart, as evidenced by irregular margins, particularly along the lateral wall of the left ventricle (*arrowheads*). (Reprinted with permission from Rajiah P, Kanne JP, Kalahasti V, Schoenhagen P. Computed tomography of cardiac and pericardiac masses. *J Cardiovasc Comput Tomogr.* 2011;5(1):16-29)

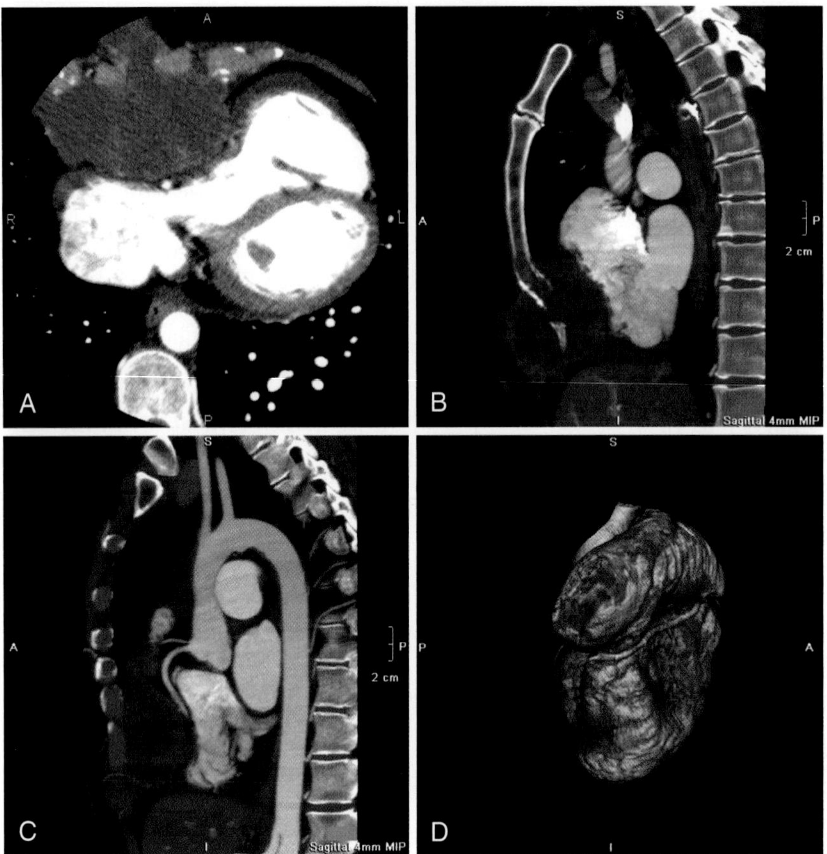

Figure 23-9. Right heart dilation due to a secundum atrial septal defect. A large soft tissue mass has eroded the xiphisternum and is compressing the anterior aspect of the right ventricle. The diagnosis was Ewing sarcoma.

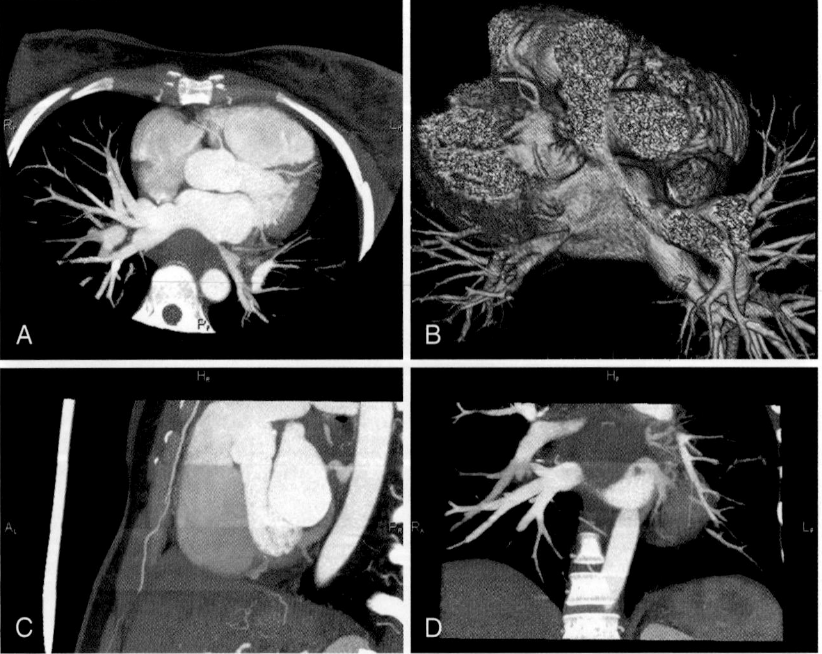

Figure 23-10. Composite images from a cardiac CT study demonstrate a mass posterior to the left atrium. This mass also insinuates around the left inferior pulmonary vein, causing a marked left inferior pulmonary vein stenosis. The diagnosis was sarcoma.

Figure 23-11. Contrast-enhanced chest CT scans at the level of the heart before (**A**) and after (**B**) treatment. The patient initially was thought, on the basis of an echocardiogram, to have a myxoma, because a mobile mass was seen within the right atrium. The left image provides important additional information: there is also mass involvement of the right posterior aspect of the right atrium, and soft tissue behind the left atrium—far more extensive masses than could be explained by myxoma. There are pulmonary infiltrates, and pleural effusion. Biopsy established that the patient had a B-cell lymphoma. He was treated with chemotherapy, without complication. The right image shows a follow-up scan at the same level. The masses have nearly entirely disappeared. He is disease free 6 years later.

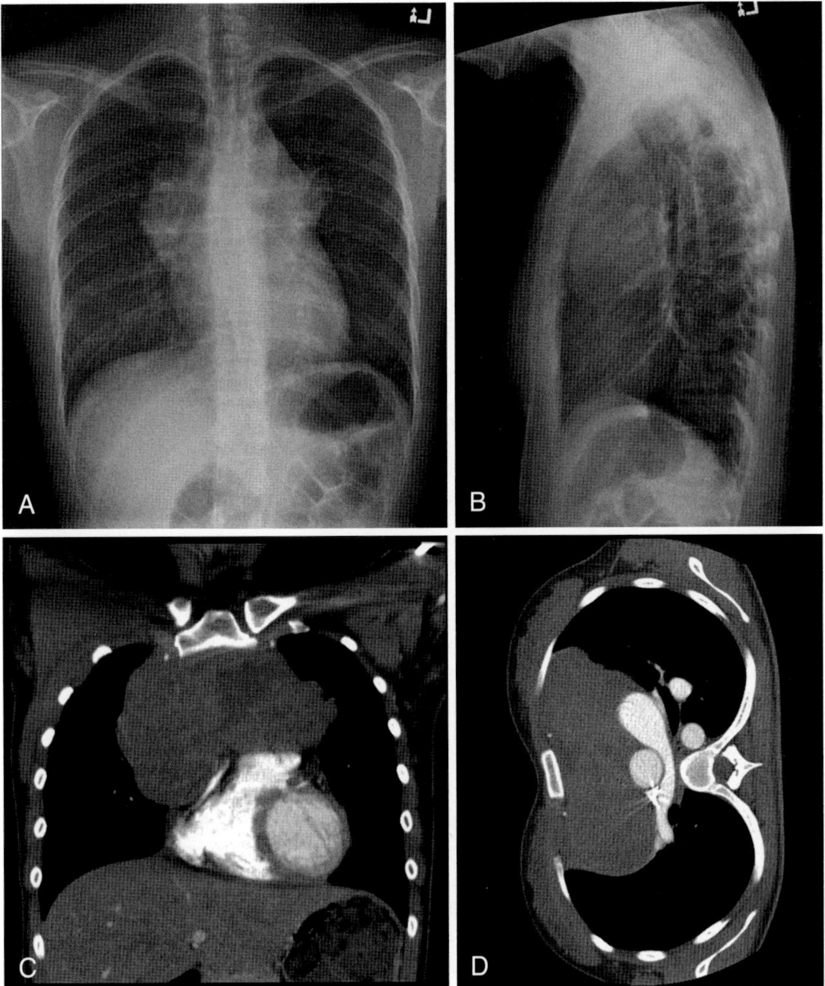

Figure 23-12. A 28-year-old woman presented with shortness of breath. The posteroanterior (**A**) and lateral (**B**) chest radiographs demonstrate a large lobulated anterior mediastinal mass. No definite calcifications are seen. The CT images confirm a large heterogeneous soft tissue mass within the anterior mediastinum. Areas of lower attenuation likely reflect intralesional necrosis. No evidence is seen of calcification or fat. There is loss of the fat plane around the ascending aorta and main pulmonary artery, raising the possibility of great vessel involvement. The mass also compresses along the superior margin of the right coronary artery (**C**). Tissue sampling confirmed a diagnosis of large diffuse B-cell lymphoma.

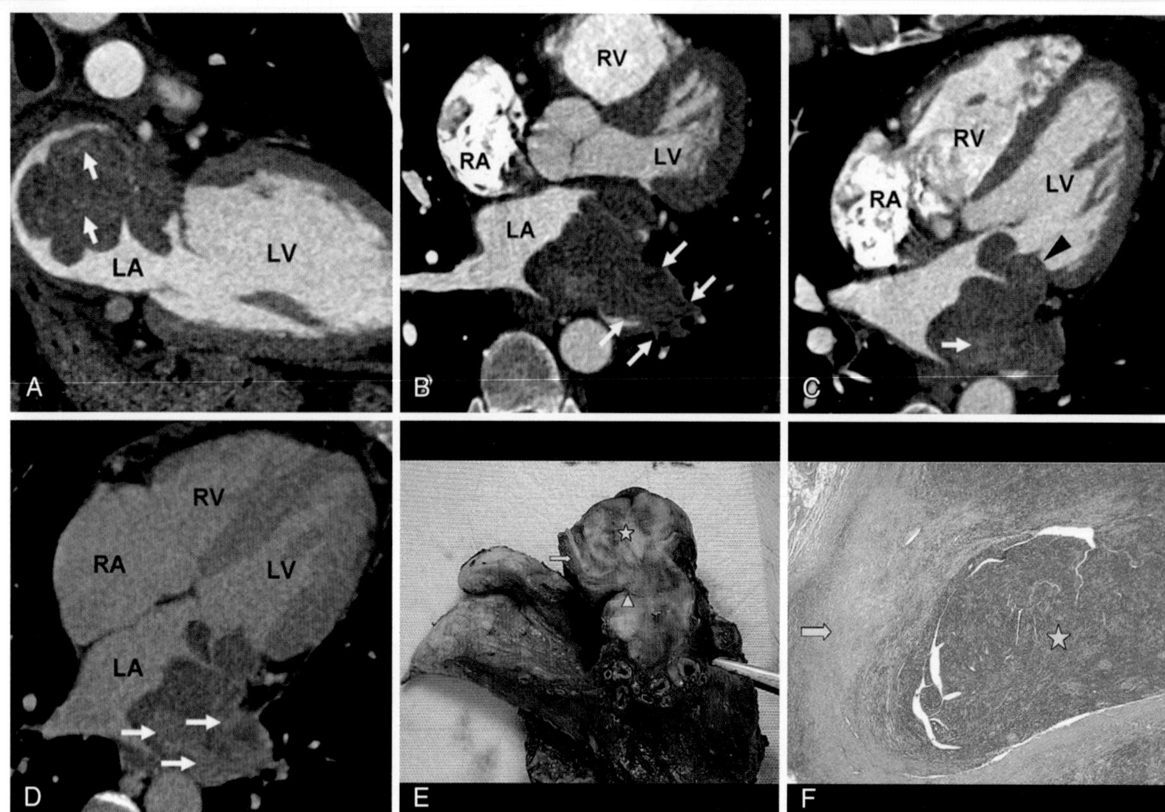

Figure 23-13. Inflammatory myofibroblastic tumor. **A,** Two-chamber view through the left atrium and ventricle. A lobulated, low-attenuation mass is seen attached to the roof of the left atrium. It contains some subtle patchy areas of enhancement (*arrows*). A frond of tissue is seen prolapsing through the mitral valve orifice in diastole. CT value within the central portion of the mass was measured at 65 HU. CT dose-length product for the first-pass scan was 1200 mGy cm. **B,** Axial oblique reconstruction through the origin of the left inferior pulmonary vein shows the mass extending into the proximal portion of this vessel (*arrows*). **C,** Four-chamber view. A lobulated mass is seen attached to the left lateral wall of the left atrium. It extends into the left inferior pulmonary vein and breaches the pericardium. Some subtle central patchy enhancement (*arrow*) can be seen. The posterior mitral valve leaflet is involved (*arrowhead*) and shows restricted motion. **D,** Delayed image acquired after 2 minutes. Four-chamber view shows persistent patchy central enhancement within the left atrial mass (*arrows*). CT value within the central portion of the mass was measured at 98 HU. The patient underwent surgical excision. **E** and **F,** Histopathology specimens. **E,** Gross cut resection specimen shows the lobulated surface architecture of this tumor (*star*) extending from the left atrium (*arrow along left atrial wall*) into the lung. The arrowhead points to the junction of the left inferior pulmonary vein with the left atrium. **F,** Hematoxylin & eosin–stained photomicrograph (magnification ×16) shows sheets of poorly cellular fibrous tumor (*arrow*) intermixed with numerous chronic inflammatory cells and fibroblasts (*star*). LA, left atrium; LV, left ventricle; RV, right ventricle; RA, right atrium (Reprinted with permission from Hoey ET, Ganesh V, Gopalan D, Screaton NJ. Cardiac inflammatory myofibroblastic tumor: evaluation with dual-source CT. *J Cardiovasc Comput Tomogr.* 2009;3(2):114-116.)

and generally have a narrow stalk rather than a broad base attachment.

Gated CT imaging in the setting of atrial myxoma can demonstrate the location of the mass and its motion through the cardiac cycle relative to the mitral valve and pulmonary veins. In addition, the presence of calcification within the mass can be well demonstrated on CT. If there is concern regarding the possibility of thrombus as opposed to myxoma, precontrast and delayed enhanced imaging can be performed to confirm delayed enhancement within the tumor (Figs. 23-14 through 23-17).[6]

Cardiac Lipoma. Lipomas are common intra- and extracardiac tumors that can present at any age. They occur equally in males and females.[5]

Although they often arise from the epicardial surface and grow into epicardial fat, cardiac lipomas can arise from the endocardial surface of any chamber. For example, fat often can be seen on the interatrial septum with cardiac CT. This may represent isolated lipomatosis of the interatrial septum, but it also may be associated with more generalized lipomatosis within the mediastinum. It can be difficult to distinguish lipomatosis from an atrial septal lipoma. In general, a lipoma tends to demonstrate a mass-like appearance with focality, as opposed to a more uniform deposition of fat with the interatrial septum.

In general, CT depicts fat very well, with fatty structures and lesions demonstrating a low negative Hounsfield unit value. No soft tissue component should be associated with a benign lipoma. If soft tissue density is present within a lipoma, although this could represent internal hemorrhage, the possibility of malignant degeneration into a liposarcoma should be strongly considered.

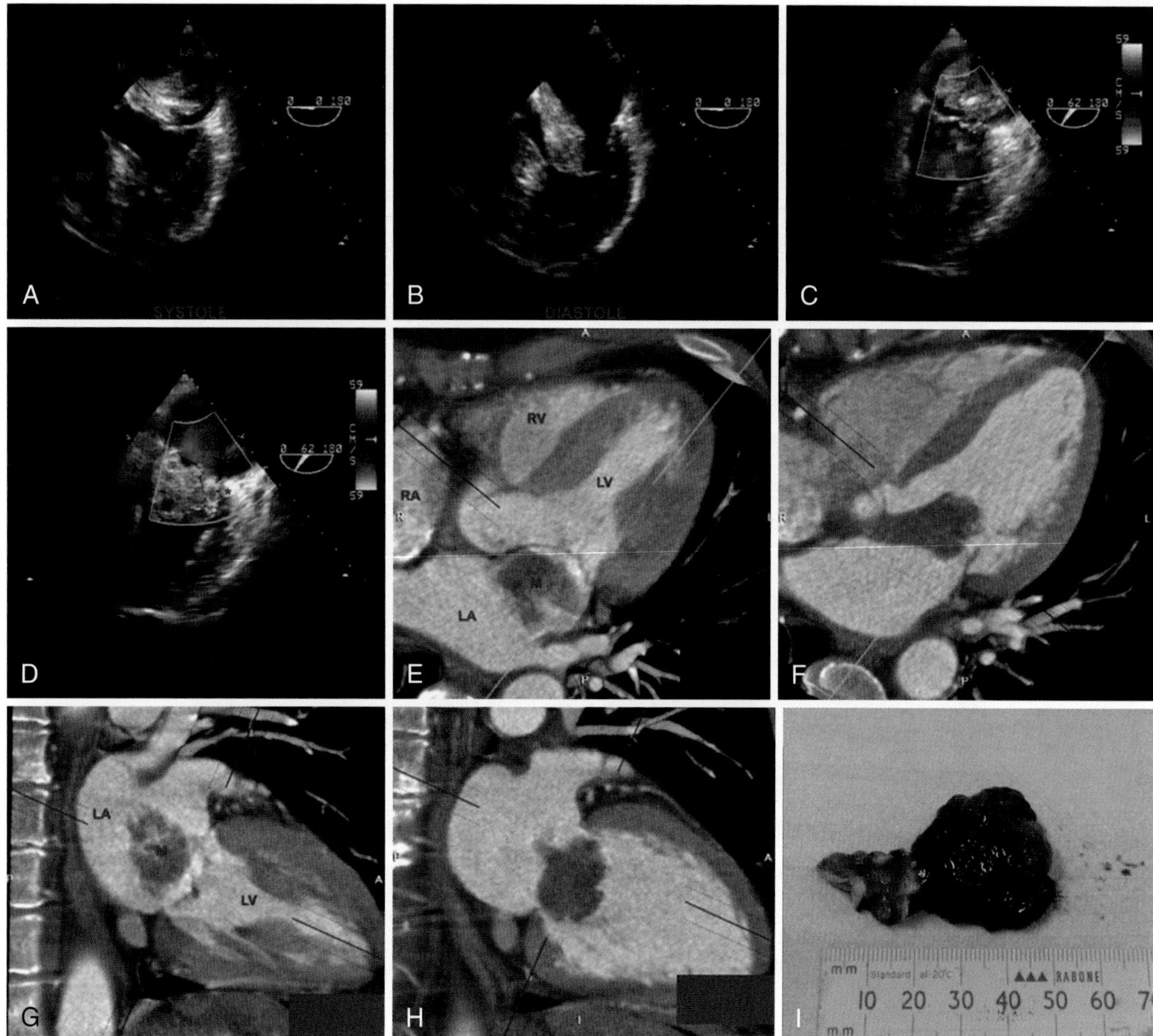

Figure 23-14. **A** through **D,** Transesophageal echocardiographic (TEE) images. **A,** Four-chamber view: end-systolic frame. The mass is fully retracted into the left atrium. Note the irregular front of the mass as well as echolucent areas consistent with areas of internal hemorrhage or necrosis. **B,** Four-chamber view: end-diastolic frame. The myxomatous mass has prolapsed fully through the mitral valve into the left ventricle. **C,** Two-chamber two-dimensional TEE view with superimposed Doppler color flow at systole. The myxoma is fully within the left atrium. **D,** Diastolic frame of the same view as **C.** The myxoma has prolapsed across the mitral valve into the left ventricle. Within the left atrium there is homogenous blood flow toward the left ventricle (*blue*). At the level of the mitral valve, the blood accelerates and becomes turbulent, seen as Doppler color aliasing (level marked with red *) with velocities suggestive of dynamic mitral valve obstruction by the prolapsing myxomatous mass. **E** through **H,** ECG-gated multidetector cardiac CT images. **E,** Four-chamber view in end-systole. The mass can be clearly seen within the LA, clear of the mitral valve leaflets just below. **F,** Four-chamber view in end-diastole. The mass has prolapsed through the mitral valve into the LV. Note the irregular lobulated front of the mass and the pedunculated stalk attachment to the interatrial septum. **G,** Two-chamber view in end-systole. **H,** Two-chamber view in end-diastole. **I,** Photograph of excised myxoma. LA, left atrium; LV, left ventricle; M, myxoma; RA, right atrium; RV, right ventricle. (Reprinted with permission from Kakouros N, McWilliams E, Giles J. Left atrial myxoma. *J Cardiovasc Comput Tomogr.* 2008;2(3):188-190.)

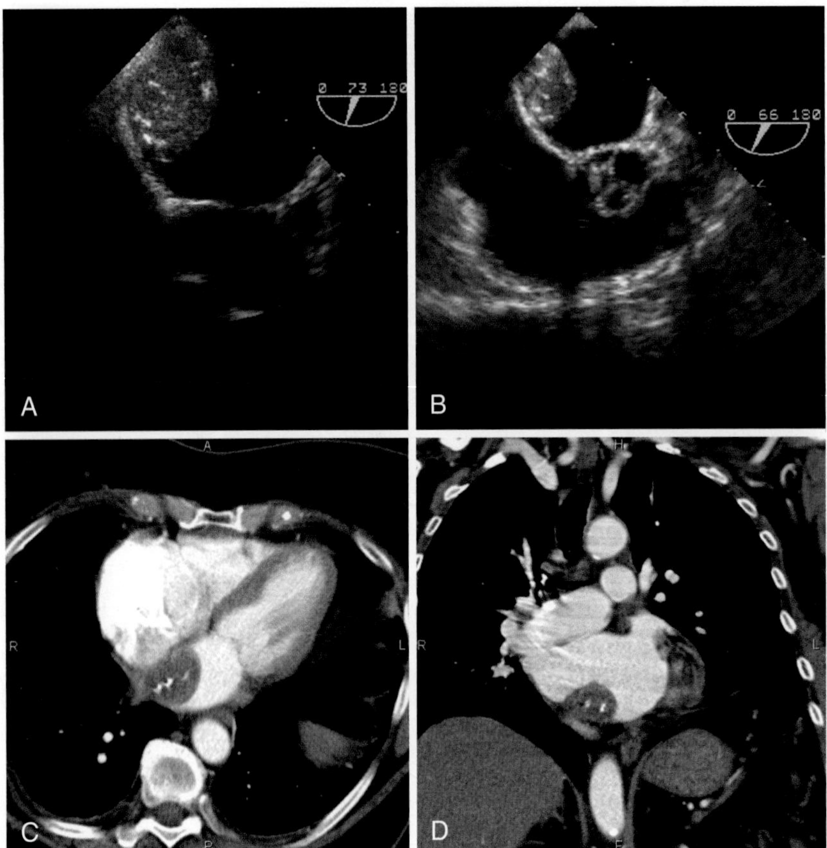

Figure 23-15. Transesophageal echocardiography demonstrates a soft tissue mass within the left atrium contiguous with the intra-atrial septum. The mass demonstrates internal heterogeneity with apparent multiple punctate foci of increased echogenicity. A non-gated CT scan of the thorax confirms the soft tissue mass within the posterior aspect of the left atrium, contiguous with the interatrial septum, and extending into the ostium of the right lower pulmonary vein. The CT images confirm that there are multiple punctate foci of calcification within the mass, as suggested by the regions of increased echogenicity seen on the echocardiogram. These imaging features and the location of this lesion are typical for a left atrial myxoma, which was surgically proven.

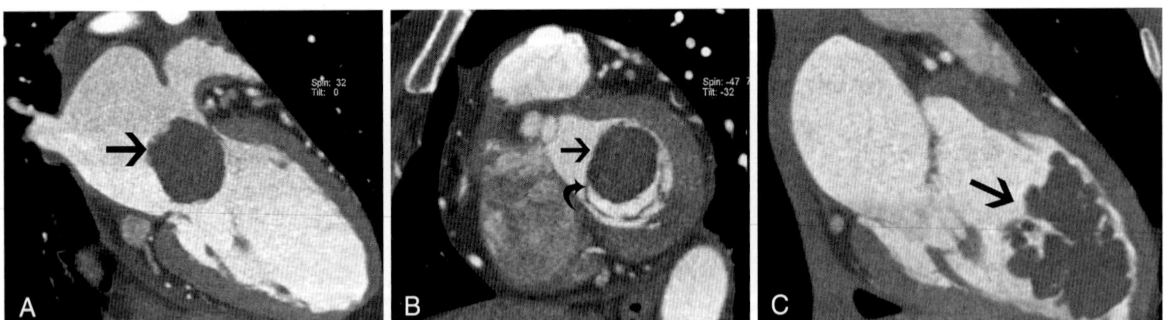

Figure 23-16. Vertical long-axis (**A**) and short-axis (**B**) reformatted CT images of a 65-year-old woman with a myxoma show a well-defined, mobile mass (*arrow*) attached to the anterior mitral valve leaflet (*curved arrow*). Vertical long-axis image (**C**) of another patient shows a left ventricular myxoma (*arrow*) with papillary fronds and faint contrast enhancement. (Reprinted with permission from Rajiah P, Kanne JP, Kalahasti V, Schoenhagen P. Computed tomography of cardiac and pericardiac masses. *J Cardiovasc Comput Tomogr*. 2011;5(1):16-29.)

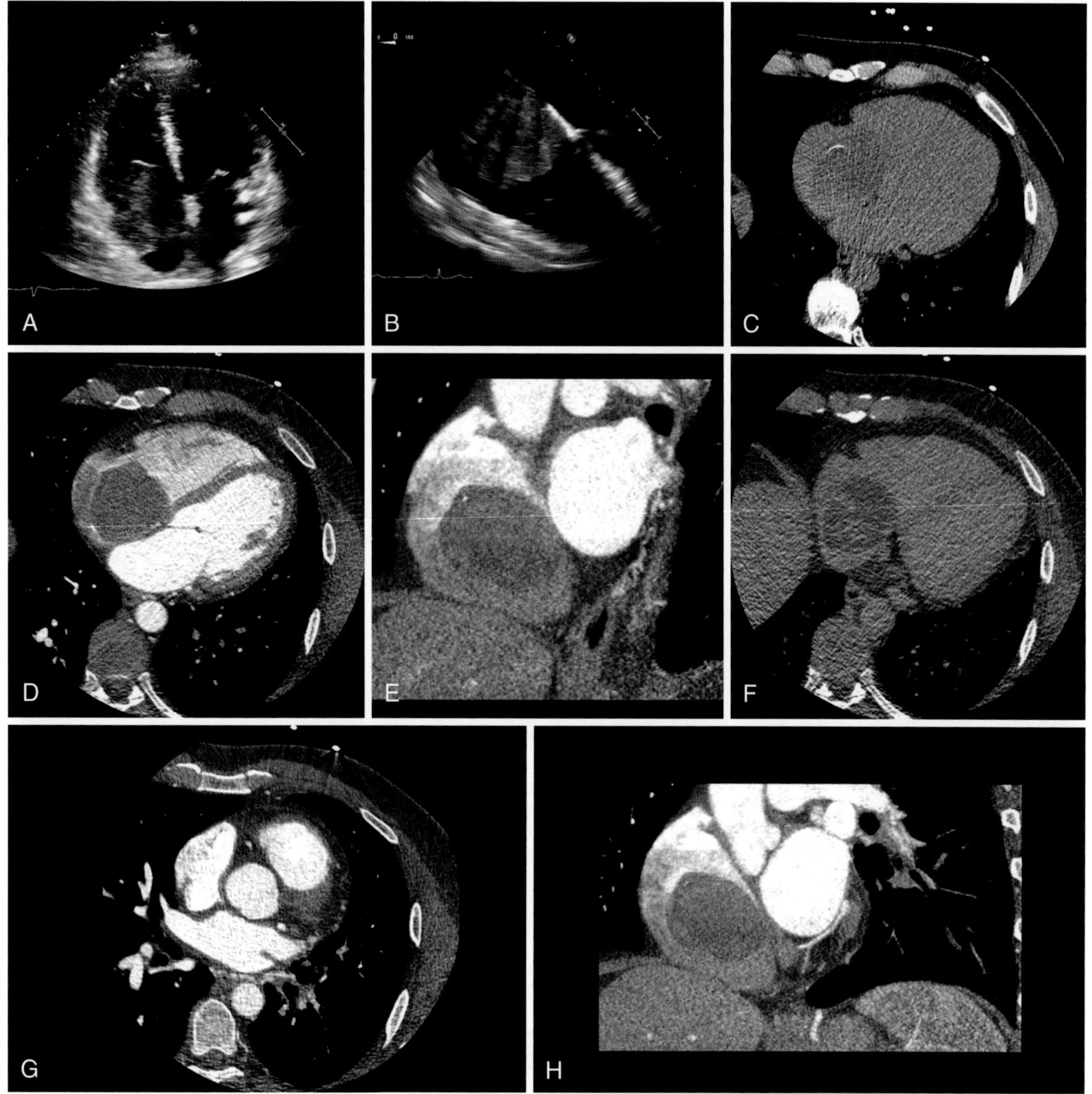

Figure 23-17. A 43-year-old man presented for preoperative evaluation of a right atrial mass, detected by transthoracic echocardiography (**A**), and confirmed as having an attachment to the lower interatrial septum by transesophageal echocardiography (**B**). The mass has the features of a myxoma. The right ventricle is dilated and has mild systolic dysfunction—a nonspecific finding, but consistent with tumor or other embolism into the pulmonary vasculature. **C** through **H,** Multiple ECG-gated cardiac CT images have been obtained. **C** and **D**, Images obtained pre-contrast show a subtle, slightly lower-attenuation mass within the right atrium. A small amount of intralesional calcium is seen. **D,** This image, obtained arteriographically, does not demonstrate any arterial enhancement. **E,** Attachment of the mass to the interatrial septum. **F,** A delayed image shows heterogeneous enhancement within the mass. **G** and **H,** An unexpected finding of occlusion of the left lower lobe pulmonary artery. No associated mass is seen. There are hypertrophied bronchial collaterals to the left lower lobe. Differential contrast enhancement is seen in the contralateral inferior pulmonary veins, indicating differential contrast filling. These findings likely relate to a prior, occluding pulmonary embolism, likely from the right atrial mass. Surgical resection and pathology confirmed a diagnosis of right atrial myxoma.

Myocardial fat can be seen in many nonneoplastic conditions, such as myocardial infarction[7,8] or arrhythmogenic cardiomyopathy,[9] and in fact may be a normal process within the heart.[10]

The morphology of nonneoplastic myocardial fat differs from that of a lipoma. Fatty metaplasia within an infarct usually follows the course of a vascular territory and may be associated with wall thinning and hypokinesis of the same segment (Fig. 23-18).

Papillary Fibroelastoma. See Chapter 20.

CCT PROTOCOL POINTS

- ❒ Coverage: Full thorax
- ❒ Additional scans
  - Precontrast
  - Delayed
- ❒ See Table 23-1.

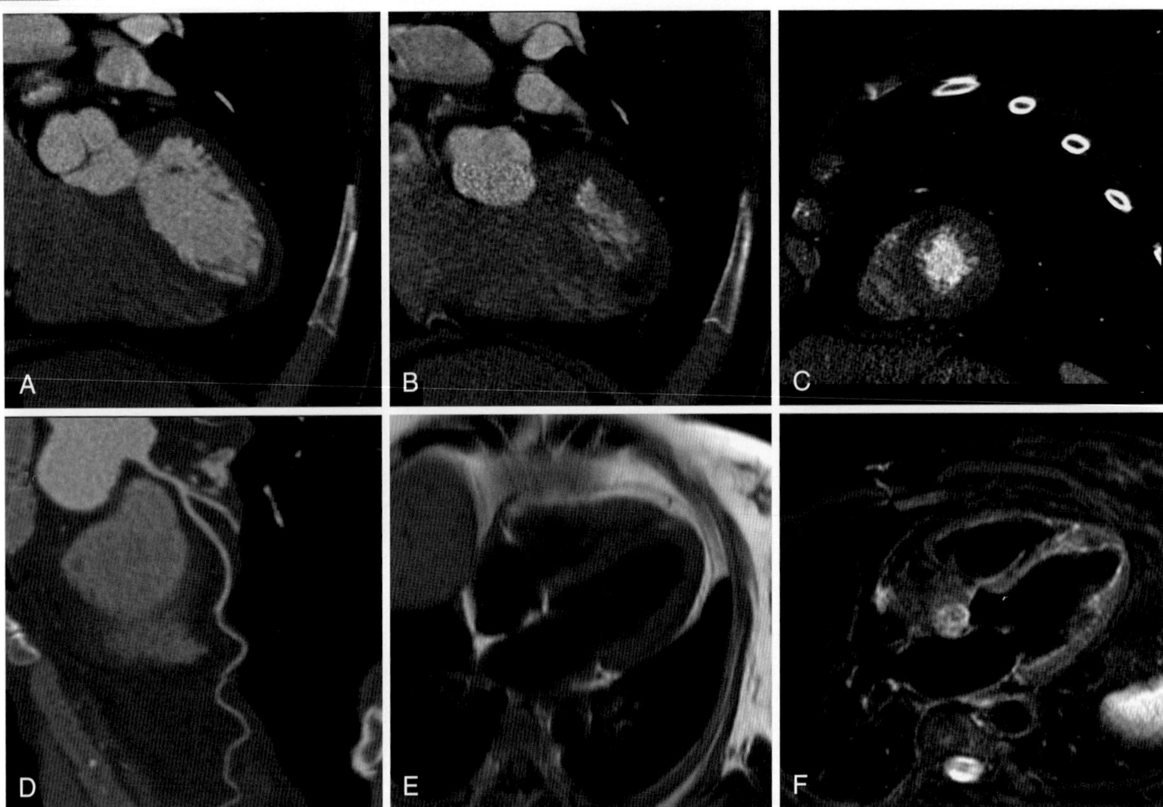

Figure 23-18. A 47-year-old woman presented with atypical chest pain and nonspecific ECG changes. **A** and **B,** Oblique long-axis reconstructions from a cardiac CT study through the apex of the left ventricle demonstrate a rounded area of low, fatty attenuation within the anteroapical wall of the left ventricle. **C,** The corresponding short-axis reconstruction also demonstrates the focal region of fatty infiltration. No associated thinning of the anteroapical wall is seen. **D,** Curved planar reformation through the left anterior descending artery (LAD) demonstrates a normal-appearing LAD with no evidence of underlying coronary artery disease or stenosis. This would argue against a prior infarct with fatty metaplasia. **E** and **F,** The patient went on to have a cardiac MRI study for further evaluation. **E,** An ECG-gated double inversion recovery fast spin-echo image of the heart demonstrates a small rounded mass-like focus of increased signal intensity suspicious for intramyocardial fat in the anteroapical wall of the left ventricle. **F,** A fat-suppressed spin-echo image demonstrates a corresponding region of decreased signal intensity within the left ventricular apex, confirming the presence of a focal region of intramyocardial fat. The diagnosis was a small intramyocardial lipoma.

TABLE 23-1 ACCF 2010 Appropriateness Criteria for the Use of Cardiac Computed Tomography to Evaluate Cardiac Masses

	APPROPRIATENESS RATING	INDICATION	MEDIAN SCORE
Evaluation of intra- and extracardiac structures	Appropriate	Evaluation of cardiac mass (suspected tumor or thrombus) Inadequate images from other noninvasive methods	8
	Uncertain	None listed	
	Inappropriate	Initial evaluation of cardiac mass (suspected tumor or thrombus)	3

Data from Taylor AJ, Cerqueira M, Hodgson JM, et al. ACCF/SCCT/ACR/AHA/ASE/ASNC/NASCI/SCAI/SCMR 2010 appropriate use criteria for cardiac computed tomography. A report of the American College of Cardiology Foundation Appropriate Use Criteria Task Force, the Society of Cardiovascular Computed Tomography, the American College of Radiology, the American Heart Association, the American Society of Echocardiography, the American Society of Nuclear Cardiology, the North American Society for Cardiovascular Imaging, the Society for Cardiovascular Angiography and Interventions, and the Society for Cardiovascular Magnetic Resonance. *J Am Coll Cardiol.* 2010;56(22):1864-1894.

References

1. Hoey ET, Ganesh V, Gopalan D, Screaton NJ. Cardiac inflammatory myofibroblastic tumor: evaluation with dual-source CT. *J Cardiovasc Comput Tomogr.* 2009;3(2):114-116.
2. Peters CM, Kalra N, Sorrell VL. Extensive recurrent cardiac lipoma. *J Cardiovasc Comput Tomogr.* 2009;3(4):282-283.
3. Joseph MX, Forrest QG, Hutchison SJ. Mass confusion. *Can J Cardiol.* 2001;17(9):977-981.
4. Kakouros N, McWilliams E, Giles J. Left atrial myxoma. *J Cardiovasc Comput Tomogr.* 2008;2(3):188-190.
5. Burke AP, Virmani R. Tumors and tumor-like conditions of the heart. In: Silver MD, Gottlieb AI, Schoen FR, eds. *Cardiovascular Pathology.* 3rd ed. Philadelphia: Churchill Livingston; 2001.
6. Vaideeswar P, Butany JW. Benign cardiac tumors of the pluripotent mesenchyme. *Semin Diagn Pathol.* 2008;25(1):20-28.
7. Su L, Siegel JE, Fishbein MC. Adipose tissue in myocardial infarction. *Cardiovasc Pathol.* 2004;13(2):98-102.
8. Baroldi G, Silver MD, De Maria R, Parodi O, Pellegrini A. Lipomatous metaplasia in left ventricular scar. *Can J Cardiol.* 1997;13(1):65-71.
9. Burke AP, Farb A, Tashko G, Virmani R. Arrhythmogenic right ventricular cardiomyopathy and fatty replacement of the right ventricular myocardium: are they different diseases? *Circulation.* 1998;97(16):1571-1580.
10. Raney AR, Saremi F, Kenchaiah S, et al. Multidetector computed tomography shows intramyocardial fat deposition. *J Cardiovasc Comput Tomogr.* 2008;2(3):152-163.

24 Simple Congenital Heart Disease

Key Points

- Although echocardiography plus MRI is still the best overall modality for the evaluation of complex congenital heart lesions, especially postoperatively, there are exceptions.
- As children and adults with congenital disease age, a growing number of them acquire contraindications to CMR, such as pacemakers and ICDs.
- Many surgical and interventional procedures use metallic components such as stents, occluded devices, and bioprosthetic valves, which often can confound MR imaging. In these cases, CT may be of benefit.
- While higher in radiation dose, retrospective imaging allows accurate measurement of right and left ventricular size and function.
- Using technique optimization, a number of complex congenital heart lesions can be well imaged with CTA.
- Surgical corrections for congenital heart disease can be well assessed with CTA. Upper and lower extremity contrast opacification may be necessary, as well as delayed imaging, especially if intracardiac thrombi are to be excluded.

The established tests for the assessment of congenital heart disease are transthoracic (TTE) and transesophageal echocardiography (TEE), cardiac MRI, and cardiac catheterization.

Cardiac CT (CCT) is an emerging alternative because of its rapid acquisition times and post-processing robustness, but the potential radiation risks are particularly relevant for children and younger adults. Nonetheless, its use has increased prominently in the assessment of congenital heart disease.[1]

Most intracardiac lesions can be assessed by echocardiography, and many procedures can be planned and guided with TTE, TEE, or intracardiac echocardiography, thus avoiding radiation risk and also providing Doppler assessment.

For patients with congenital heart disease, MRI is the established test for the evaluation of extracardiac surgical shunts, pulmonary vascular anomalies and complications, and aortic anomalies. This modality avoids the risk of radiation exposure and also provides flow information. Cardiac MRI also is the preferred test for quantifying right ventricular function and the degree of pulmonic insufficiency.

Clearly CCT is able to provide nonphysiologic but superb anatomic delineation of a wide range of congenital cardiac and thoracic vascular defects,[2-4] and its use has increased substantially during the past decade. However, it remains unclear which lesions should be assessed by CCT, given the radiation risk-free, and widespread availability of other established modalities[5] and the natural and proven complementarity of echocardiography and cardiac MRI.[1,6]

The greatest contribution of CCT, therefore, is likely to be:

- In patients who cannot undergo MRI or whose MRI images are insufficient in lesions such as extracardiac shunts
- For the assessment of coronary anatomy, such as identification of an anomalous left anterior descending coronary artery in patients with tetralogy of Fallot[7]

CT imaging is appropriate for a number of congenital pathologies. The most common of these are discussed in the following sections. It may be useful to categorize congenital lesions based on their level of simplicity rather than on physiology, as follows.

SIMPLE LESIONS

- Aorta
  - Bicuspid aortic valve (see Chapter 18)
  - Coarctation (see Chapter 28)
  - Sinus of Valsalva aneurysm (see Chapter 28)
- Shunts
  - Atrial septal defect (ASD)
  - Ventricular septal defect (VSD)
  - Patent ductus arteriosus (PDA)
  - Partial anomalous pulmonary venous return (PAPVR)
- Coronary artery
  - Anomalous origin (see Chapter 11)
  - Anomalous termination (see Chapter 12)

- Other
  - Cor triatriatum
  - Ebstein anomaly

Aorta

Bicuspid Aortic Valves

See Chapter 17.

Coarctation

Coarctation of the aorta, a congenital narrowing of the aorta, accounts for approximately 5% of all congenital heart disease. The narrowing is most commonly located just distal to the origin of the left subclavian artery. Traditionally, coarctations were classified as *infantile* (preductal) or *adult* (postductal) types, but this classification is often misleading, because age of presentation has been found to be related more to the degree of narrowing and the presence of associated abnormalities than to location. The diameter of the aortic arch in adults often is normal compared with children, in whom a hypoplastic arch commonly is observed. The presence of multiple collateral arteries also is a featured adult presentation. (Collaterals arise primarily from the internal mammary and intercostal arteries, usually between the third and eighth ribs). Historically, surgical corrections ranging from end-to end reanastomosis to subclavian flap repair have been employed. Percutaneous treatment with angioplasty and stent placement are newer options. Complications of both surgical and interventional procedures include pseudoaneurysms, aneurysms, and recoarctation.

See Chapter 24, Aortic Diseases.

Sinus of Valsalva Aneurysm

See Chapter 26, Aortic Diseases.

Shunts

Atrial Septal Defect

Atrial septal defects account for 6% to 14% of all congenital heart disease and as much as 30% to 40% of congenital heart disease in adults. There are three types of ASD[8]:

- Ostium secundum ASD (70%), the most common type, is located in the region of the fossa ovalis (Figs. 24-1 through 24-5).
- Sinus venosus ASD (15%) is located above the fossa ovalis, adjacent to the superior aspect of the atrial septum, near the entrance of the superior vena cava (SVC) into the right atrium. This form of ASD is commonly associated with PAPVR of the right upper lobe pulmonary vein into the SVC (Figs. 24-6 and 24-7; **Videos 24-1 through 24-4**).

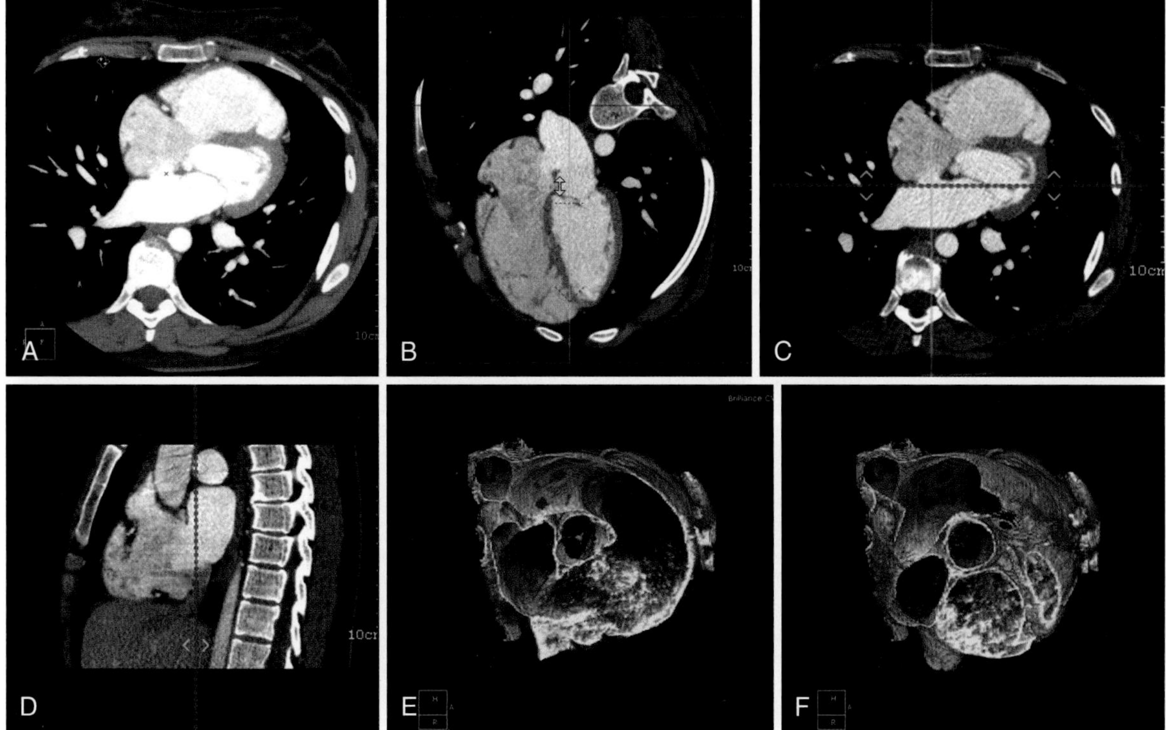

Figure 24-1. **A** through **D**, MIP contrast-enhanced four-chamber views. A secundum atrial septal defect (ASD) is present, as are right atrial and right ventricular dilation. The left heart contrast attenuation is greater than the right heart contrast due to a saline bolus passing through the right heart; the differential contrast happens to demonstrate left-to-right flow across the ASD. **E** and **F,** Three-dimensional volume-rendered views at the base of the heart. **E,** Absence of the mid-posterior interatrial septum, as well as dilation of the right atrium, right ventricle, and pulmonary artery. **F,** The interatrial septum is present at a more posterior level. There is right atrial and right ventricular dilation. Secundum ASD with right heart volume overload.

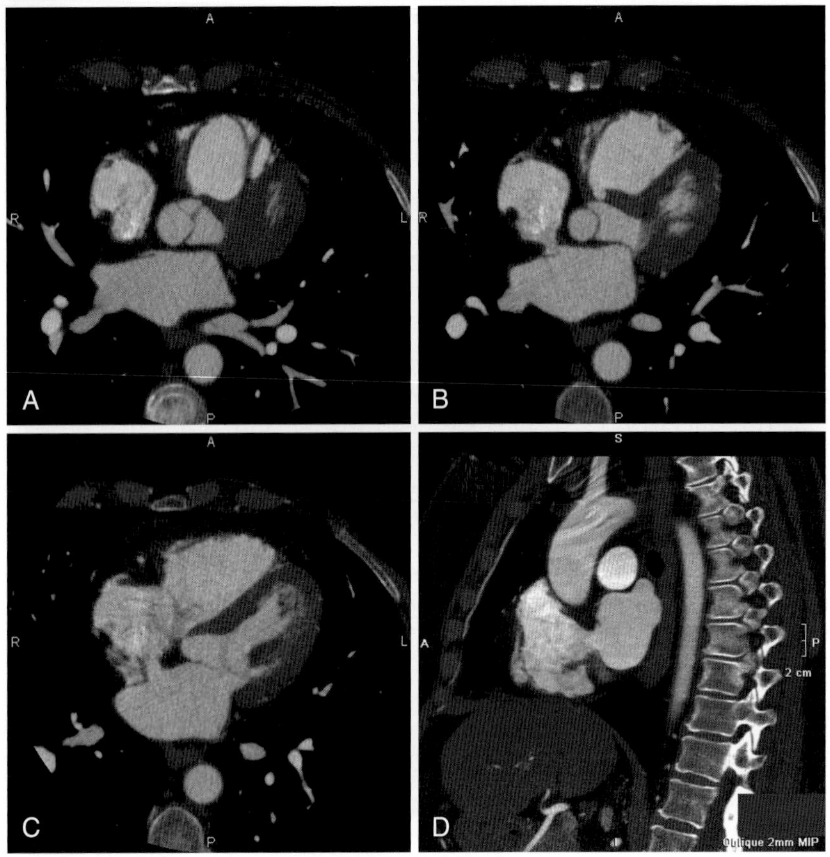

Figure 24-2. Multiple images from a cardiac CT study in a 54-year-old woman with shortness of breath on exertion and atypical chest pain. **A** and **B,** Axial source images from the CT data set. These images demonstrate an inadherent flaplike portion of the upper interatrial septum. A communication across this flap is seen (**B**) corresponding to a patent foramen ovale (PFO). **C** and **D,** Below the PFO in the midportion of the interatrial septum, a second defect which measures 1.3 cm is seen within the interatrial septum, with an appearance typical for a small to moderate-sized ostium secundum defect. The study was obtained in mid-diastole. The diagnosis was coexistent PFO and ostium secundum atrial septal defect.

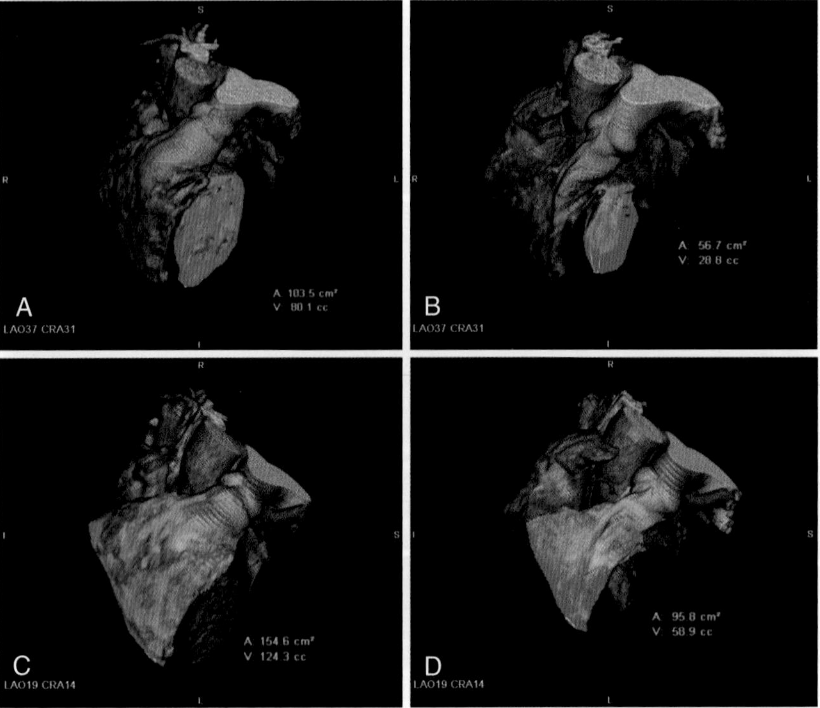

Figure 24-3. Same patient as Figure 24-2. Multiple volume-rendered images from a helically acquired cardiac CT study. **A** and **B,** Functional evaluation of the left ventricle. **C** and **D,** Functional evaluation of the right ventricle. End-diastolic images are seen in **A** and **C** and end-systolic images in **B** and **D.** In this patient with coexisting patent foramen ovale and ostium secundum atrial septal defect, stroke volumetry of the right and left ventricles generated a Qp/Qs of 1.3–1, a mild left-to-right shunt.

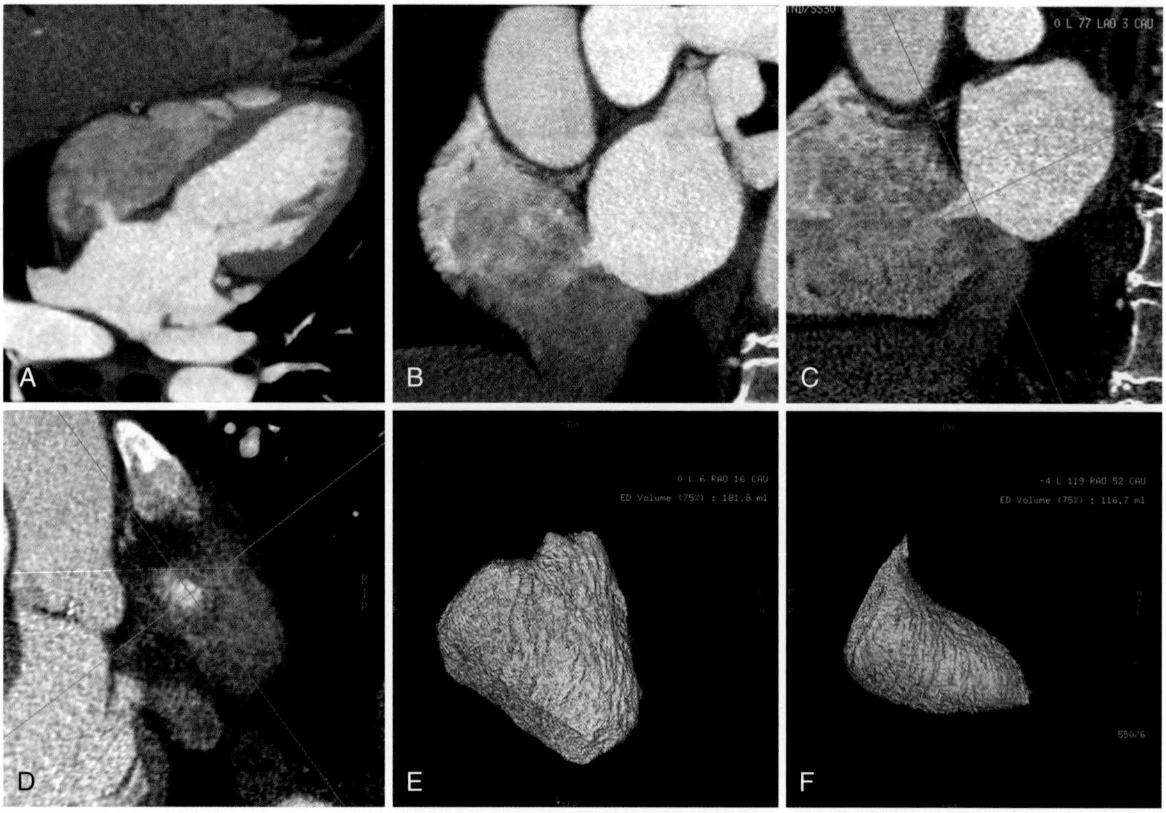

Figure 24-4. Multiple images from a cardiac CTA study demonstrate a small atrial septal defect (ASD). Four-chamber reconstruction (**A**) and a short-axis reconstruction across the interatrial septum (**B**). Contrast is seen shunting from left to right across the midportion of the interatrial septum. **C** and **D,** Cross-sectional localization of the ASD. On this diastolic phase prospectively acquired image, the cross-sectional measurement of the ASD is 11 × 11 mm. **E** and **F,** Volume-rendered representations of stroke-volumetry between the right ventricle (**E**) and the left ventricle (**F**). Although this study was acquired prospectively, and the latest phase within diastole was reconstructed at 80% of the R-R interval, these measurements still provide a reasonable measure of stroke volumetry. In this case a Qp/Qs by stroke volumetry was measured at 1.5 to 1.

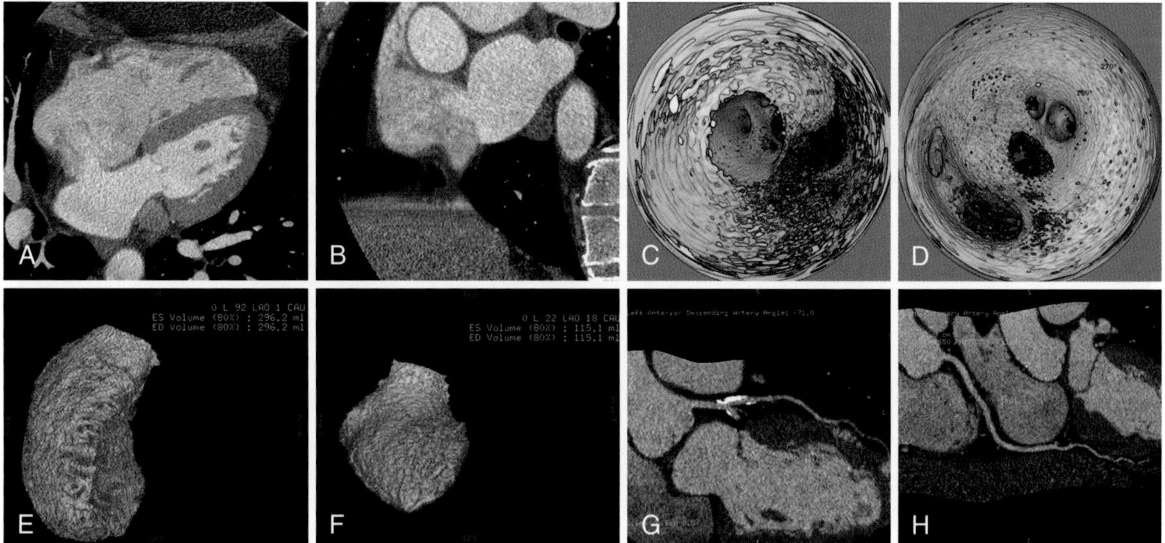

Figure 24-5. **A,** Four-chamber projection demonstrates a secundum atrial septal defect (ASD) with contrast extending across the ASD from left to right. **B,** Short-axis projection through the interatrial septum demonstrates the ASD, which measures 16 mm. **C,** Angioscopic projection from within the right atrium demonstrates the ASD with the pulmonary veins visualized through the ASD within the left atrium. **D,** Opposite angioscopic projection from within the left atrium demonstrates the ASD and the pulmonary veins. **E,** Volume-rendered image of the right ventricle demonstrates the right ventricular end-diastolic volume of 296 mL (enlarged). **F,** Volume-rendered image of the left ventricle with an end-diastolic volume of 115 mL. Assuming no valvular insufficiency, by the ratio of the end-diastolic volumes there is a flow ratio of 2.6:1. **G,** Curved reformation of the left anterior descending artery (LAD) demonstrates mild calcific plaque in the proximal LAD without significant stenosis. **H,** Curved reformation through the right coronary artery demonstrates no evidence of atherosclerosis or stenosis.

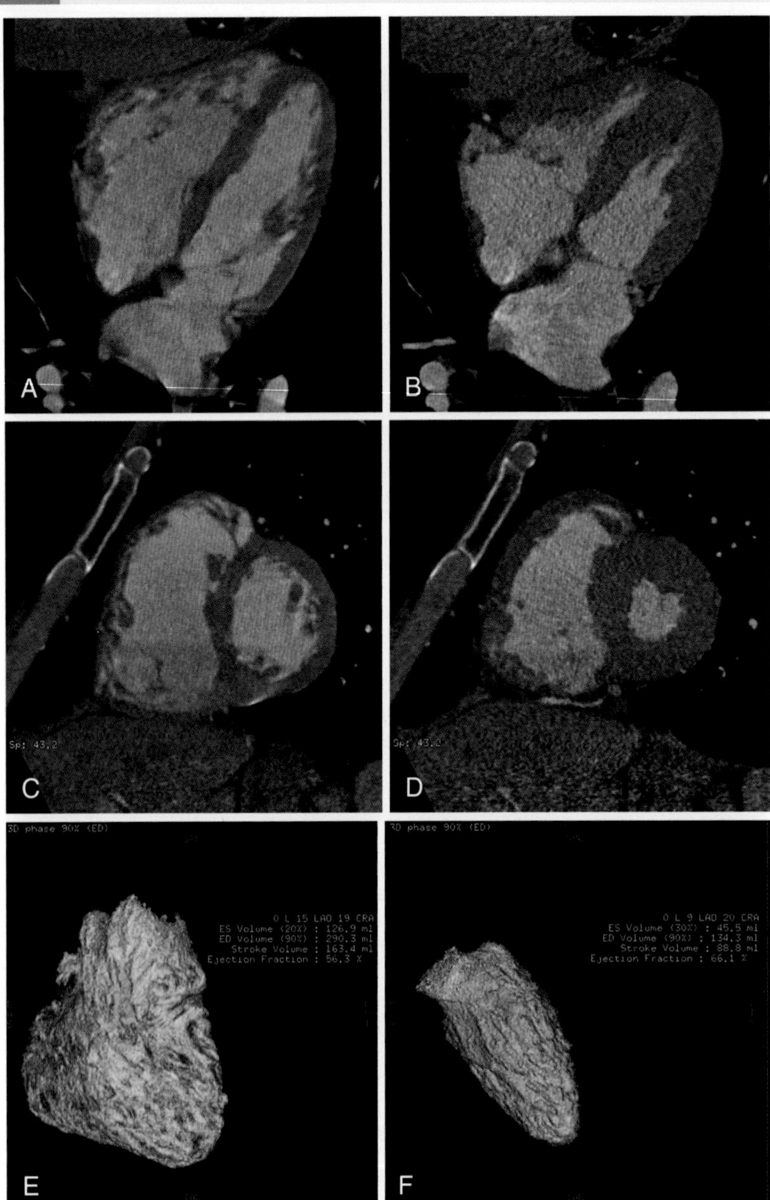

Figure 24-6. Multiple composite images from a cardiac CT study in a 52-year-old man with atypical chest pain and shortness of breath. Figure 24-7 demonstrates the presence of a sinus venosus defect, and multiple anomalous pulmonary veins The study was obtained retrospectively, in a low-dose, dose-modulated fashion. The patient's overall dose–length product (DLP) for the study was 398 (mGy cm). **A** and **B,** Images reconstructed into four-chamber and short-axis oblique projections. **A** and **C,** End-diastole; **B** and **D,** end-systole. These images demonstrate marked dilatation of the right ventricle, and moderate right ventricular hypertrophy. **E** and **F,** A functional assessment of both the right and left ventricles. The left ventricle demonstrates normal ejection fraction at 66%. The right ventricle (**E**) also demonstrates normal systolic function with an ejection fraction of 56%. Stroke volumetry, however, demonstrates a Qp/Qs of 2.1:1. **See Videos 24-1 and 24-2.**

- ❐ Ostium primum ASD (15%) is part of the spectrum of atrioventricular (AV) septal defects, which often are associated with incompetence of the AV valve.

Unroofed Coronary Sinus. The coronary sinus is a normal structure that is located posteriorly within the left AV groove. The confluence of the coronary sinus and the right atrium is located along the posterior inferior wall of the right atrium. In the normal state, no communication between the coronary sinus and the left atrium exists. An unroofed coronary sinus is a rare type of ASD in which the superior margin of the coronary sinus is deficient, allowing communication between the left atrium and coronary sinus to occur. This defect is commonly associated with a persistent left SVC, which is seen in approximately 0.1% to 0.5% of the general population. A small number of left SVCs (8%) drain directly into the left atrium. Associated unroofed coronary sinuses common, occurring over 70% of these patients.[9] The morphology of the coronary sinus defect can vary, ranging from total deficiency of the roof of the coronary sinus, to a well-defined single defect between the coronary sinus and the left atrium, as well as multiple small cribriform-like fenestrations between the coronary sinus and left atrium. Coronary sinus defects also can occur in the setting of other congenital heart diseases, including tetralogy of Fallot, PAPVR, cor triatriatum, and pulmonary atresia.[10]

The hemodynamic changes associated with ASDs depend on the size of the defect and the amount of shunting across the defect. Small ASDs with a small left-to-right shunt are well tolerated

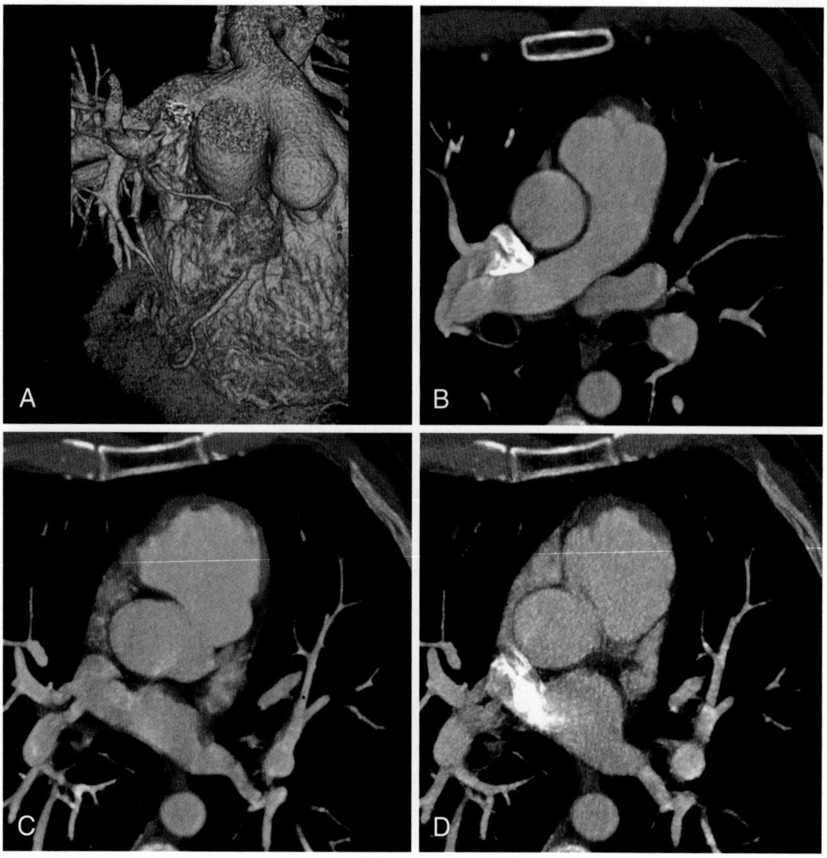

Figure 24-7. Same patient as Figure 24-6. **A** and **B,** Partial anomalous pulmonary venous return (PAPVR) from the right upper lobe into the superior vena cava. **C,** There is more complexity to this setting of PAPVR, with a right middle lobe branch as well as a more posteriorly oriented branch from the right lower lobe—likely the superior segment—also draining into the cavoatrial junction. **D,** Streaming of contrast across a high superior sinus stenosis defect. This contrast extends down from the superior vena cava, and across the atrial septal defect into the left atrium. While the association of PAPVR and a superior sinus venosus defect is well documented, it is important for the cardiac CT imager to look for the presence of more than one single anomalous vein, because multiple anomalous veins may be present. See **Videos 24-3 and 24-4.**

and produce few adverse hemodynamic consequences. When the ASD is large, right ventricular volume overload may occur, resulting in right atrial and right ventricular enlargement. After the age of 30, the incidence of pulmonary vascular disease increases in patients with ASDs. As pulmonary hypertension develops, a reversal of the shunt can occur, with blood flowing from the right to left across the ASD, a phenomenon known as Eisenmenger physiology.

In general, there are two ways to repair ASDs: a surgical approach with patching of the ASD and diversion of an anomalous vein if one is present. More recent advances of percutaneous occluder devices across the interatrial septum can also be used.

Although CCT is not primarily used as a diagnostic tool for ASDs, patients occasionally are unable to undergo TEE or MRI, and in this setting cardiac CT offers a valuable alternative. ASDs can be categorized and sized using CT. In addition, concomitant assessment of pulmonary vein anatomy and volumetric QP/QS quantification using right and left ventricular volumes can be derived from a single cardiac CT data set. Suitability for occluder device placement can be determined by identifying a rim of atrial tissue surrounding all margins of the ASD. Evaluation of the occluder device post-placement is better performed on CT than MRI, although small peridevice leaks are most likely best identified on TEE (Figs. 24-8 and 24-9; **Video 24-5**).

Patent Foramen Ovale/Aneurysm of the Interatrial Septum. A patent foramen ovale is a result of the failure of anatomic fusion of the septum primum over the limbus of the fossa ovalis, which normally occurs when left atrial pressures exceed right atrial pressures after birth. The lack of fusion of this so-called "flap valve" of the fossa ovalis can allow left-to-right shunting. (Right-to-left shunting occurs only when right atrial pressure is higher than that on the left.) A patent foramen ovale is a common finding, present in 25% of adults.[11]

Atrial septal aneurysms are a localized region of thinning of the interatrial septum that bulges into the right or left atrium. These are defined by bowing of the septum from the base of the interatrial septum by more than 10 or 15 mm.[12] Most of these aneurysms are believed to be congenital in origin. Some may be caused by postsurgical remodeling of the interatrial septum from prior atrial septal surgery. The prevalence of atrial septal aneurysms is about 1% based on autopsy series. Although they are generally felt to be a benign clinical entity, atrial septal aneurysms often are fenestrated and can be associated with interatrial shunting.[13] Cardiogenic embolism also

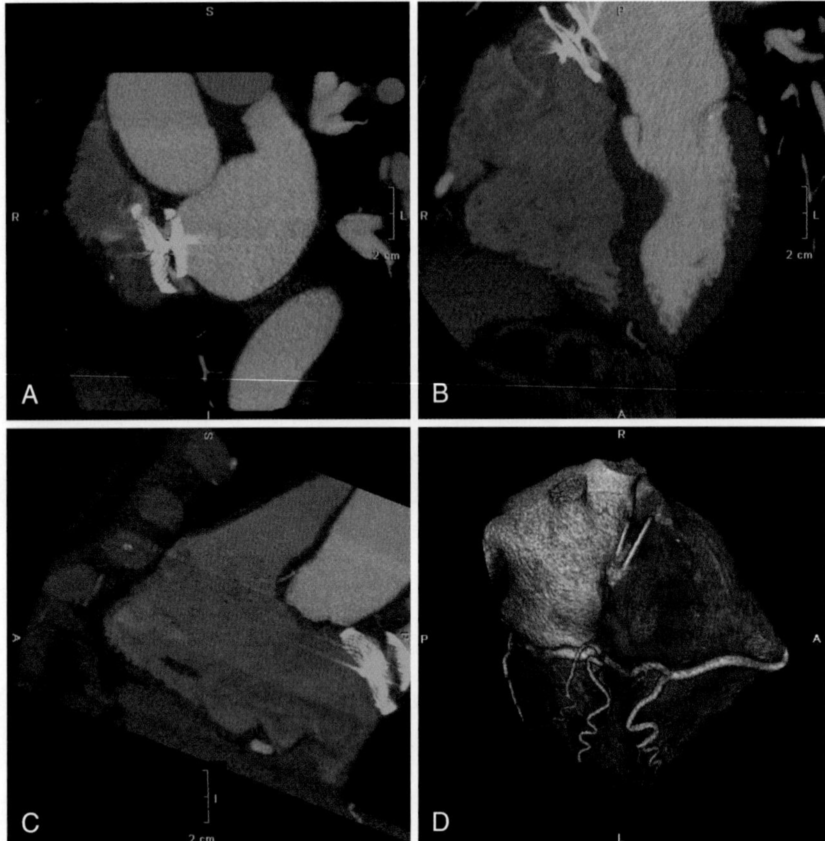

Figure 24-8. Multiple maximum intensity projection and volume-rendered images from a cardiac CT study in a patient with prior placement of an Amplatzer atrial septal occluder device demonstrates this device across the intra-atrial septum. No definite evidence of a residual shunt is seen. See **Video 24-5.**

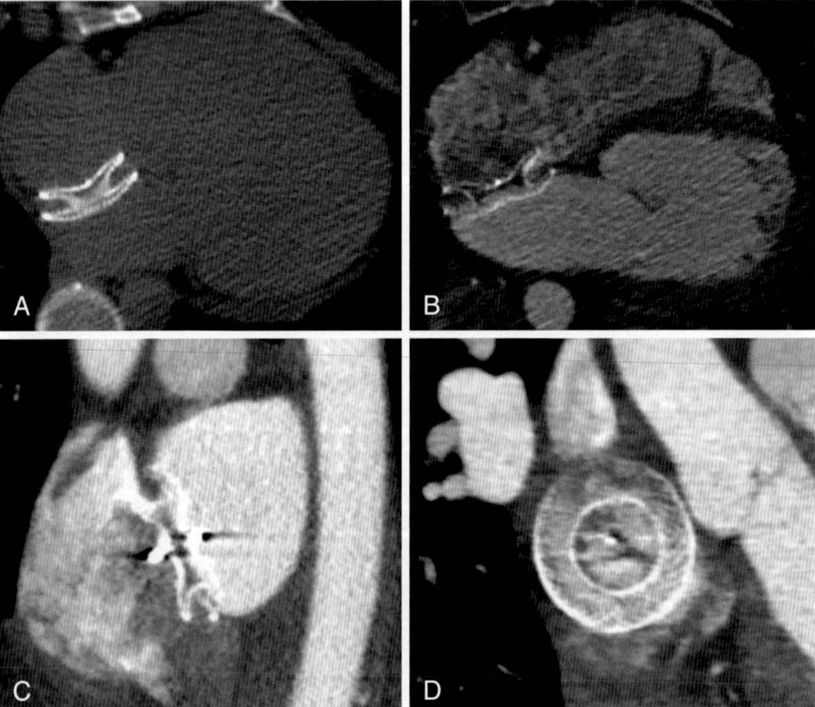

Figure 24-9. Composite images from a cardiac CT study pre- and post-contrast after placement of an Amplatzer atrial septal defect–occluding device. The Amplatzer device is well-seated.

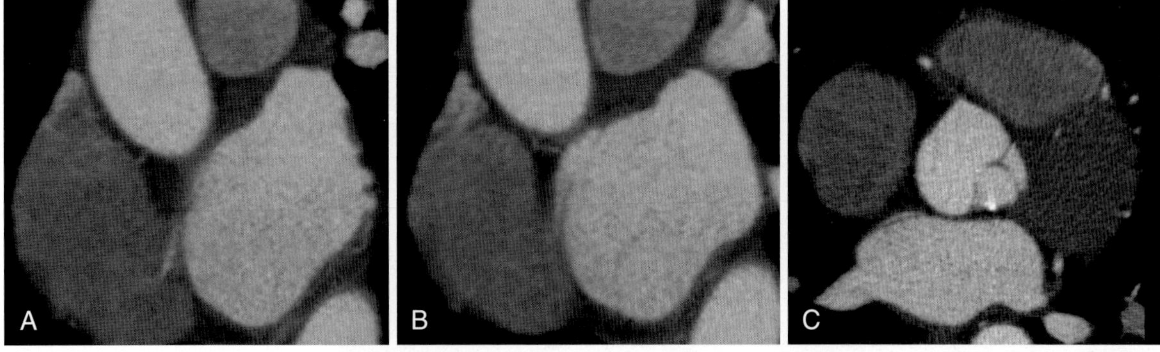

Figure 24-10. Composite images from a cardiac CT examination demonstrate a valve-incompetent patent foramen ovale, with a jet of contrast seen extending from the left atrium into the right atrium.

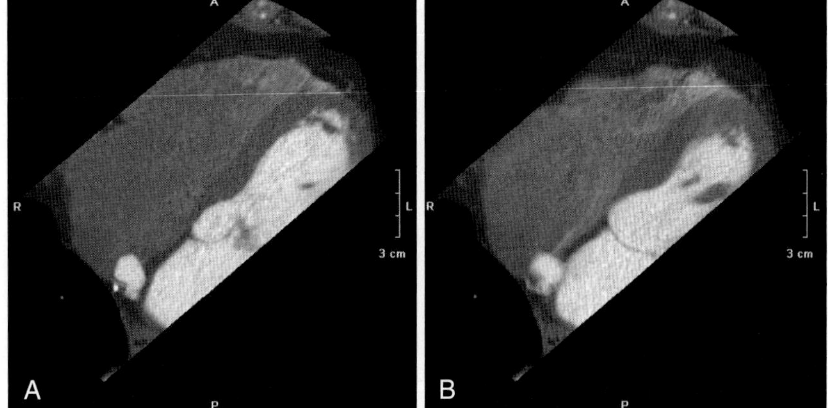

Figure 24-11. Composite images from a cardiac CT study demonstrate a moderate-sized intra-atrial septal aneurysm, with a small pinhole-like shunt. Systolic images from the cardiac CT study on the left (**A**) demonstrate a small jet of contrast extending from the intra-atrial septal aneurysm into the right atrium. **See Video 24-6.**

may occur as a result of thrombus formation within the aneurysm or as a paradoxical embolism. Other congenital lesions such as patent foramen ovale and atrial septal defects also may be associated with atrial septal aneurysms. Ventricular septal aneurysms are often discovered unexpectedly as part of a cardiac CT study and are generally not the primary reason for cardiac CT study. In a patient with cryptogenic stroke, or in whom echocardiography is suboptimal, cardiac CT may be used to further evaluate for an intracardiac source of embolization. Interatrial septal aneurysms and associated shunting can be identified on cardiac CT (Figs. 24-10 through 24-15; **Video 26-6**).

Ventricular Septal Defect

The term *ventricular septal defect* applies to any of a group of congenital malformations that are characterized by a hole in the ventricular septum. VSDs are the most common congenital cardiac defect, representing between 25% and 30% of all congenital heart lesions.[14]

VSDs are classified according to their location, as follows:

- ❒ Perimembranous VSD
  - Located close to the central fibrous body of the septum
  - These defects border the membranous septum and the tricuspid, mitral, and aortic valves (Fig. 24-16).
- ❒ Muscular VSD
  - Confined to the muscular portion of the septum
  - The entire circumference of the defect is within the muscular septum.
  - These lesions may be located in the inlet, trabecular, or outlet regions of the muscular septum.
  - A large defect may involve more than one region.
- ❒ Juxta- or subarterial VSD
  - Located superiorly, with the superior rim of the defect formed by both the aortic and pulmonary valve leaflets
- ❒ Atrioventricular septal defect (AVSD), including endocardial cushion and AV canal defects
  - This more complex form of intracardiac shunt encompasses a wide range of anatomic findings that relate primarily to:
    - Abnormal development of the endocardial cushions and related structures
    - Abnormal development of the atrioventricular valves
  - A number of different classifications for AVSD have been used, but most commonly

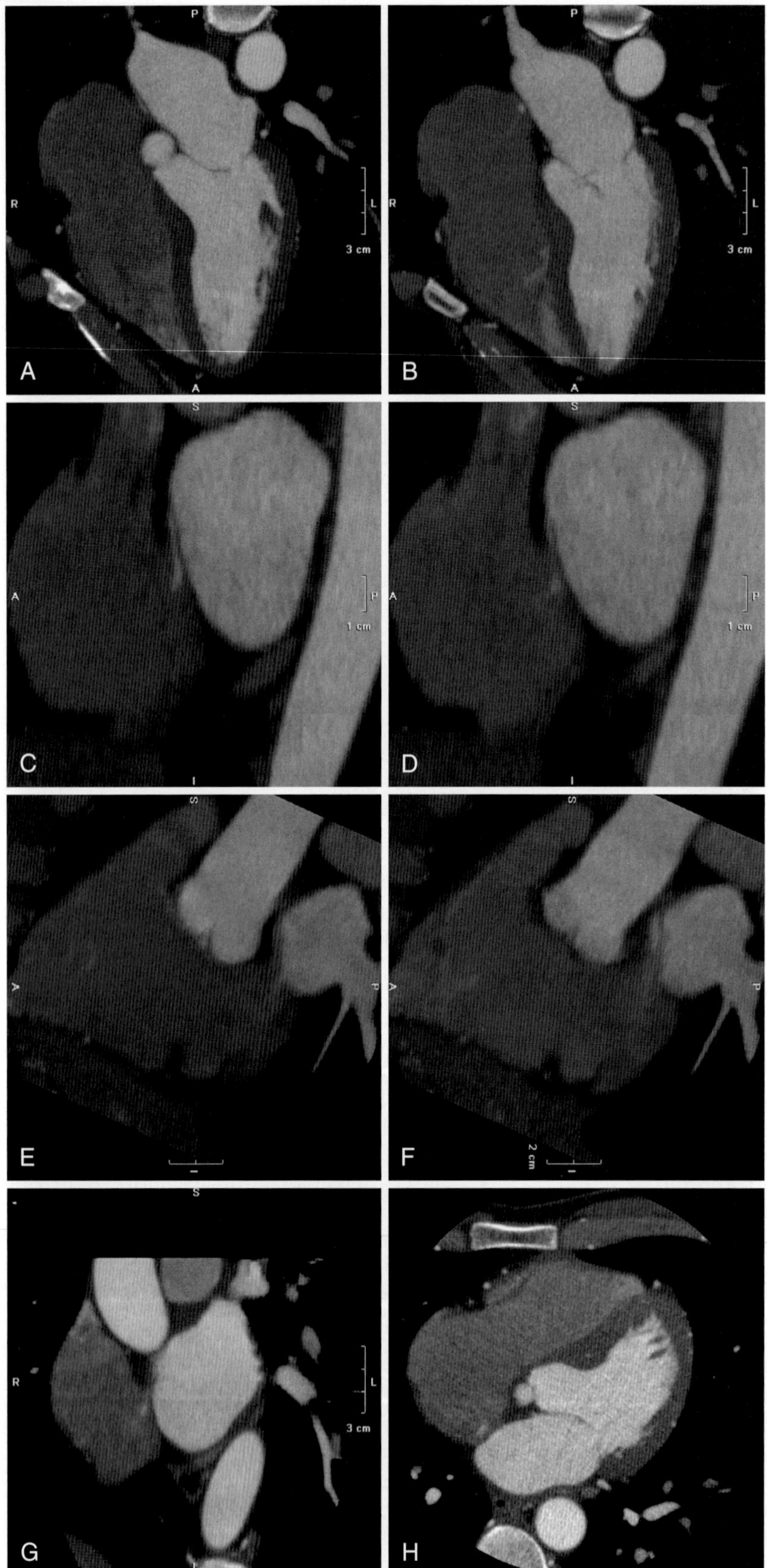

Figure 24-12. Reconstructed images from a cardiac CT data set of a patient with a PFO: four-chamber view (**A, B**) short-axis oblique (**C, D**), long-axis oblique (**E, F**), short axis at the atrial level (**G**), and standard axial projection (**H**). The interatrial septum components—septum primum and secundum—are inadherent, and there is passage of higher contrast left atrial blood via the PFO into the adjacent right atrium. Images with a vertical projection (**C–G**) depict the PFO along its course, whereas more horizontal or axial views do not and depict only the blush of high attenuation dye in the right atrium without displaying the passageway of the PFO along its length.

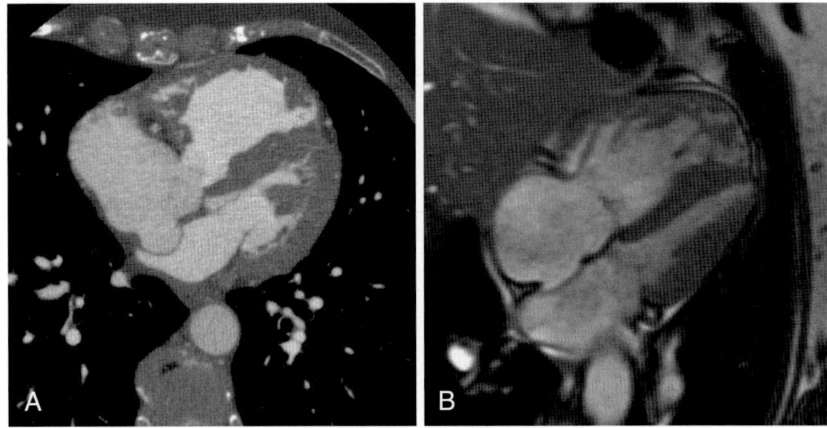

Figure 24-13. A 53-year-old woman presented with progressive shortness of breath. **A,** Image obtained from a prospectively acquired cardiac CT study. Images have been obtained at mid to end-diastole. Marked right ventricular hypertrophy is present. There is a focal area of thinning and aneurysmal development of the interatrial septum. The aneurysmal tissue is displaced into the left atrium, suggesting that the right atrial pressure is greater than that of the left atrium. A four-chamber steady-state free precession (SSFP) image (**B**) from a cardiac MRI study obtained in systole demonstrates similar, but less, displacement of the aneurysmal interatrial septal tissue to the left. No intra- or extracardiac shunt was identified. The diagnosis was interatrial septal aneurysm in a patient with idiopathic pulmonary arterial hypertension.

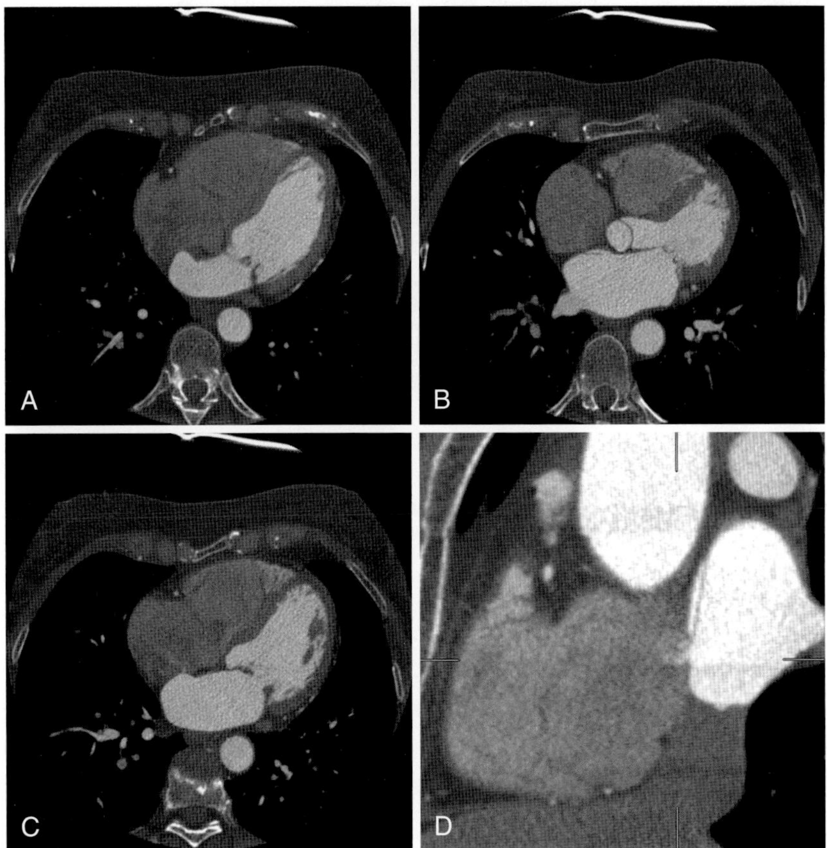

Figure 24-14. Cardiac CT study in a 55-year-old woman. **A,** A small focal outpouching of the interatrial septum. The length of this structure along its base in the orientation of the interatrial septum was 15 mm, with a depth of 10 mm, confirming it to be a small interatrial septal aneurysm. **B,** A small amount of contrast is seen beneath inadherent interatrial septum. **C** and **D,** A small pocket of contrast is seen extending from the left atrium into the right atrium. **D,** The inadherent interatrial flap, with a small puff of contrast extending from the left atrium to the right atrium inferior to the inferior edge of the interatrial flap. This most likely represents a small fenestration or ASD of the interatrial septal aneurysm.

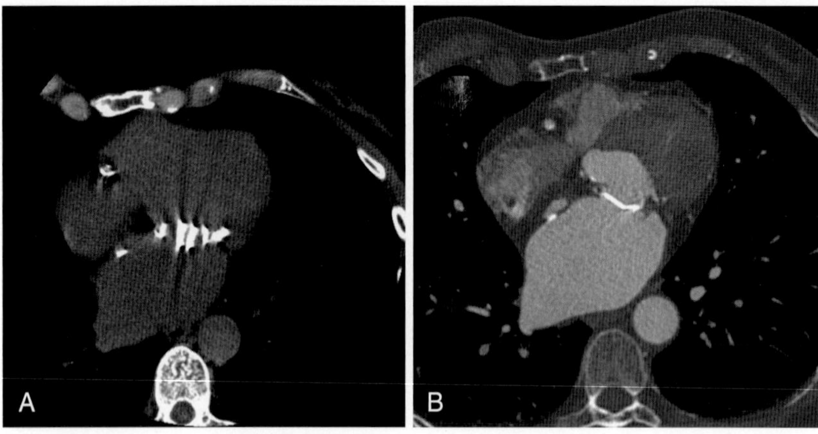

Figure 24-15. Cardiac CTA study a 62-year-old woman with a remote history of mitral valve surgery. An echocardiogram has identified an echogenic mass within the interatrial septum. **A,** The noncontrast image demonstrates a small focus of increased density along the course of the interatrial septum. There is a moderate amount of beam-hardening artifact at the level of the mitral valve plane from the patient's prior mitral valve replacement. **B,** The contrast-enhanced study demonstrates contrast extending underneath the foraminal ovale flap, but no evidence of any shunting across the interatrial septum. A small amount of high density is seen, associated with the inadherent interatrial flap. This most likely represents a small amount of calcification of the flap, or possibly a small surgical clip. No evidence is seen of an interatrial septal mass or tumor. The residual interatrial septum demonstrates a mild amount of lipomatosis.

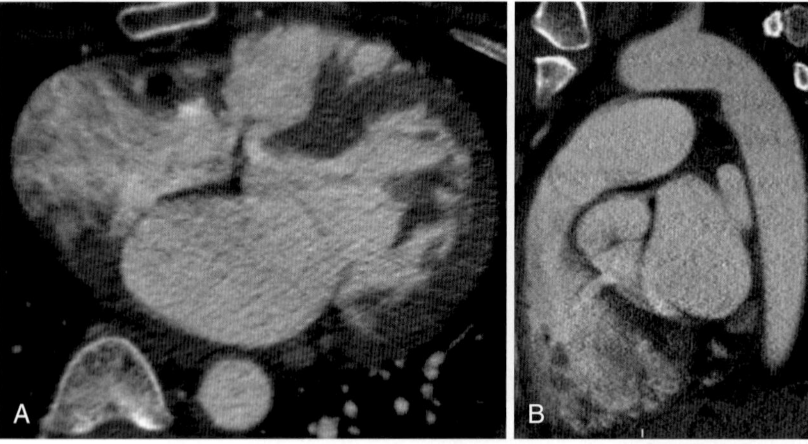

Figure 24-16. Cardiac CT study demonstrates a small, high intraventricular septal defect with left-to-right shunting. Note the moderate enlargement of the main pulmonary artery.

they are divided into partial and complete forms.
  - In the partial form of AVSD, the principal defect occurs in the atrial septum with a resultant ostium primum defect, but no associated malformation of the ventricular septum.
  - In the complete form of AVSD, a ventricular defect also is present. The defect may involve the entire junction of the atria and ventricles separating the atria from the ventricles.
- The atrioventricular valves can act as a common valve. The severity of the defect and resultant shunt depends on the integrity of the supporting structures of the AV valves and how much appropriately directed flow (RA to RV and LA to LV) occurs.
- Associated AV valve regurgitation also is common.
- The complete form of AVSD is common in trisomy 21 (Down syndrome): 45% of patients with Down syndrome have congenital heart disease, and about 40% of those have an AVSD.[15]

CT is not used for primary evaluation of VSDs but occasionally occult VSDs can be seen on CT, especially in the setting of complex congenital heart disease.

Ventricular Septal Aneurysm. The membranous septum is the thinnest, weakest portion of the intraventricular septum. Aneurysmal dilatation of this portion of the septum usually is small, ranging from 0.5 to 3.0 cm. Most membranous septal aneurysms are congenital in origin, and most likely relate to redundant septal tissue closure of a small VSD. Occasionally a small residual pinhole-like or cribriform-like residual VSD within the aneurysmal tissue persists. Aneurysms within the muscular portion of the intraventricular septum are rare and are more likely due to prior myocardial infarction. Ventricular septal aneurysms often are an unexpected finding as part of a cardiac CT study and

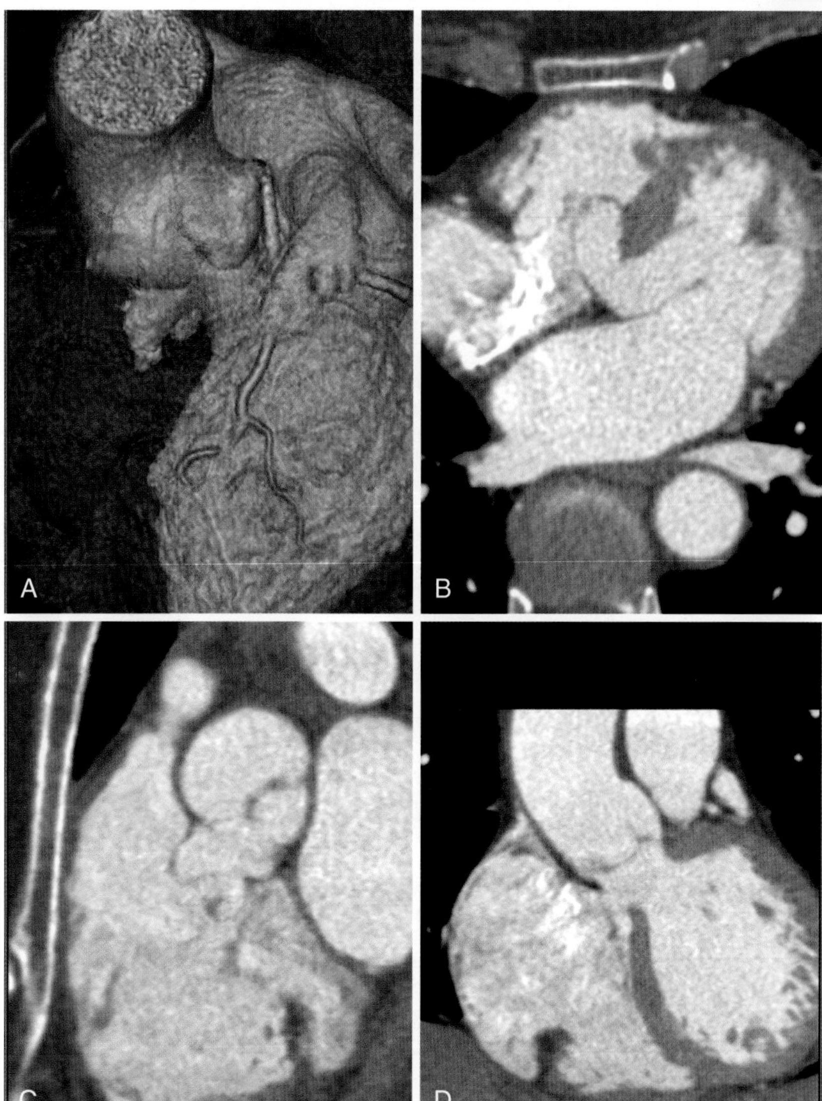

Figure 24-17. Reconstructed images from a cardiac CT data set. These images demonstrate a small, high-ventricular septal aneurysm. **A,** Volume-rendered image demonstrates a focal outpouching of contrast beneath the sinuses of Valsalva extending into the less well opacified right ventricle. Similar findings are seen on the other three reconstructed images. Unfortunately, due to the moderate amount of contrast within the right ventricle, the presence of a small fenestration or shunt across this ventricular septal aneurysm is not identifiable. There is, however, no evidence of a clot within the aneurysm sac.

usually are not the primary reason for cardiac CT study.

Similarly, single case reports have demonstrated the ability to depict an incidental membranous septal aneurysm.[16]

For CCT images of ventricular septal aneurysms, see Figures 24-17 and 24-18.

Partial Anomalous Pulmonary Venous Return

Normally the four pulmonary veins drain into the left atrium. In PAPVR, there is anomalous drainage of one or more of the pulmonary veins. Although this anomaly can involve any of the four pulmonary veins, it usually occurs on the right side. As with total anomalous pulmonary venous return, the pulmonary venous connection does not cross the midline—that is, a left pulmonary vein will never drain to a right-sided systemic venous structure. Anomalous drainage of the right upper lobe vein usually occurs directly into the SVC at a level just above the right atrium. There usually is an associated sinus venosus ASD. Anomalous connection of the right inferior pulmonary vein to the inferior vena cava (i.e., scimitar syndrome) often is associated with a hypogenetic right lung and an ostium secundum ASD. PAPVR of the left upper lobe usually is via a left vertical vein that drains into the brachiocephalic vein and then to the superior vena cava. This also can be associated with an ostium secundum ASD.

MRI is considered the gold standard test for evaluating for PAPVR. Occasionally occult PAPVR can be seen during a cardiac CT study obtained for other purposes; therefore, it is prudent to identify pulmonary vein anatomy in all cardiac CT studies as part of an overall study review (Figures 24-19 to 24-28; **Video 24-7**).

Text continued on page 411

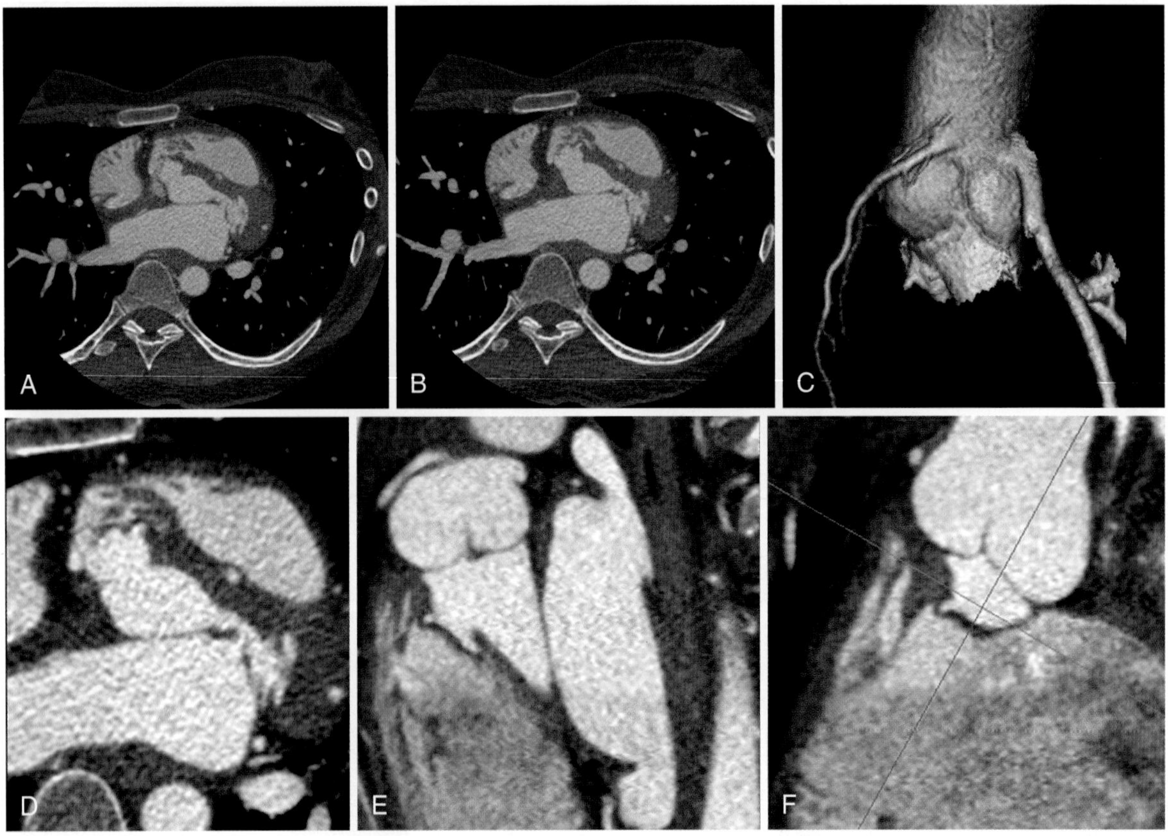

Figure 24-18. Multiple images from a cardiac CT study in a 32-year-old woman. **A** and **B,** Source axial CT images, which demonstrate a focal area of thinning and outpouching at the base of the interventricular septum. (This is seen in magnification in part **D.**) A small amount of redundancy and undulation is associated with this focal area of outpouching. There is a small nipple-like projection seen extending from this small aneurysm sac, best visualized on the volume-rendered image shown in **C** and in reformatted images **D** and **E.** Overall this appearance is very suggestive of a small membranous ventricular septal aneurysm. No evidence is seen of a fenestration or shunting, and there is no evidence of a thrombus within the aneurysm sac.

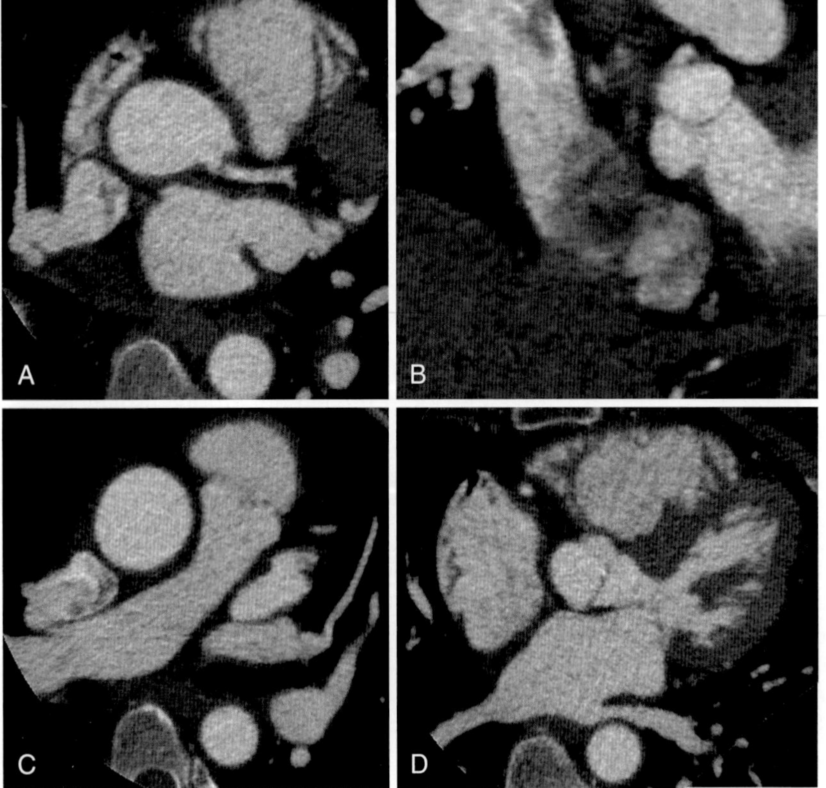

Figure 24-19. Multiple images from a cardiac CT study demonstrate right upper lobe partial anomalous pulmonary venous return to the superior vena cava. The central pulmonary arteries are not enlarged. No evidence of a concomitant sinus venosus atrial septal defect is present, which likely explains the lack of significant enlargement of the pulmonary arteries or of the right ventricle.

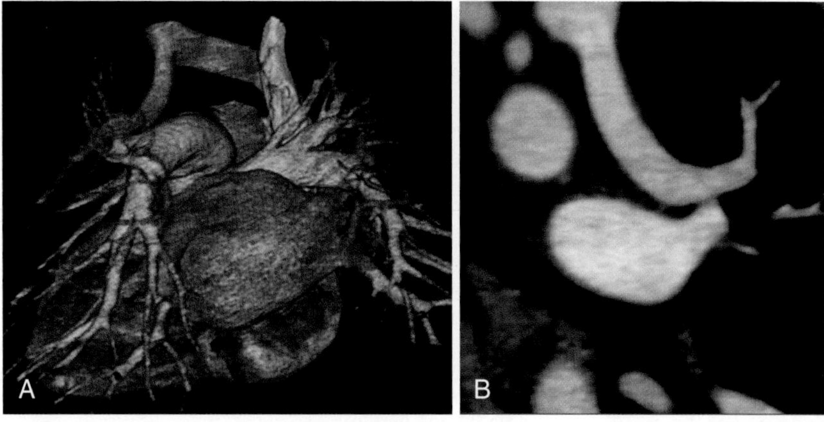

Figure 24-20. Cardiac CT study demonstrates a left vertical vein draining the left upper lobe pulmonary venous system superiorly into the innominate vein.

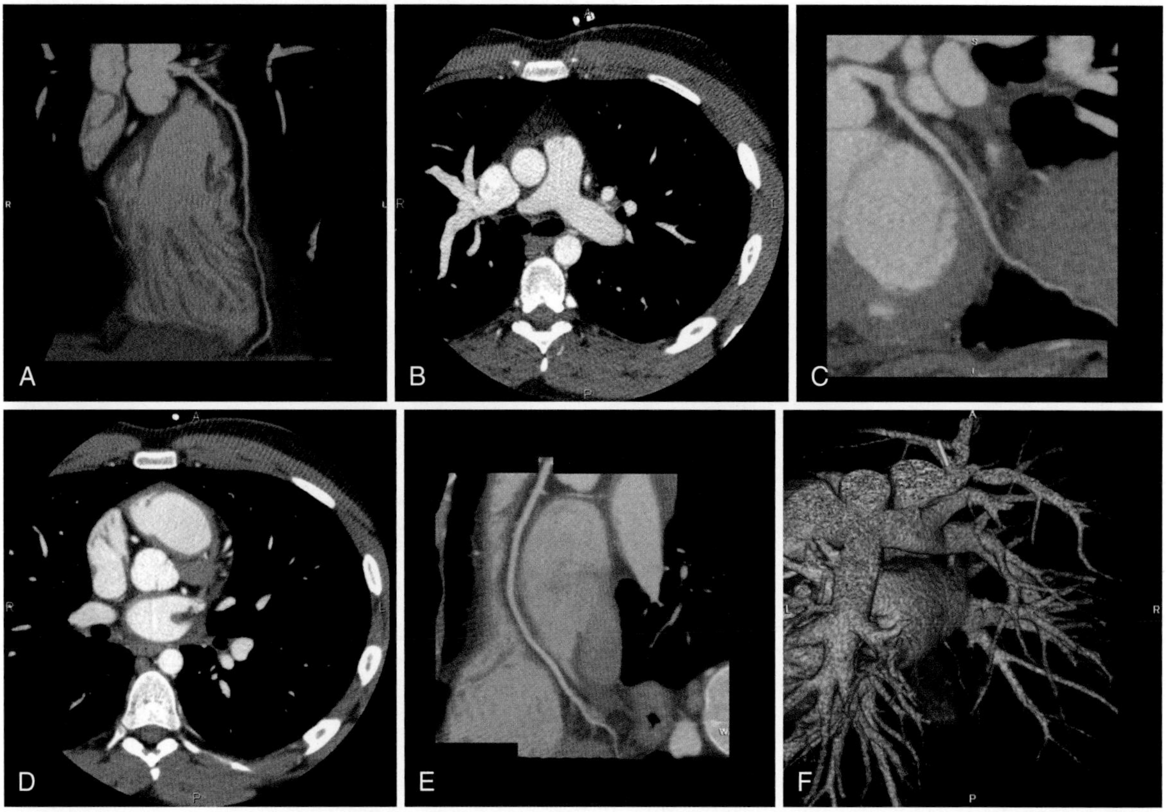

Figure 24-21. A 28-year-old man presented with chest pain and elevated troponin levels and underwent cardiac CT scanning. **A**, **C**, and **E**, Curved multiplanar reconstructions demonstrate normal coronary arteries. **B**, **D**, and **F**, An incidental finding of partial anomalous venous return of the right upper lobe veins into the superior vena cava. **B**, Axial source image reveals multiple veins draining into the superior vena cava. **D**, Axial source image demonstrates an intact sinus venosus and an enlarged right ventricular outflow tract due to the left-to-right shunt. **F**, A volume-rendered image demonstrates the anomalous pulmonary vein draining into the superior vena cava (*yellow arrow*).

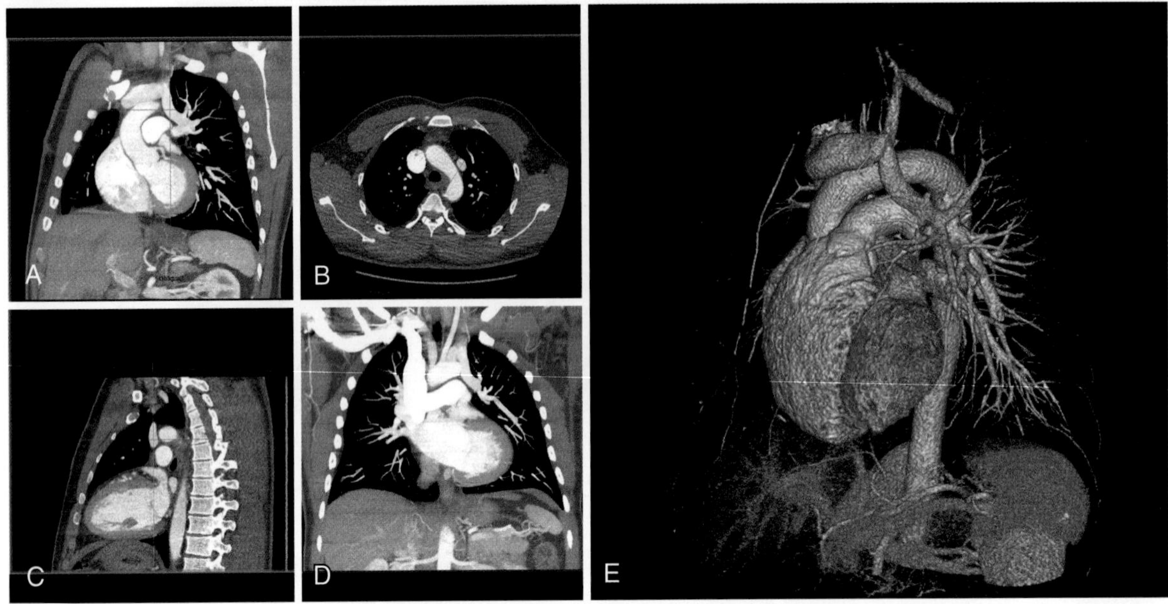

Figure 24-22. Note the vertical vein of left lung pulmonary venous drainage to the innominate vein. See **Video 24-7.**

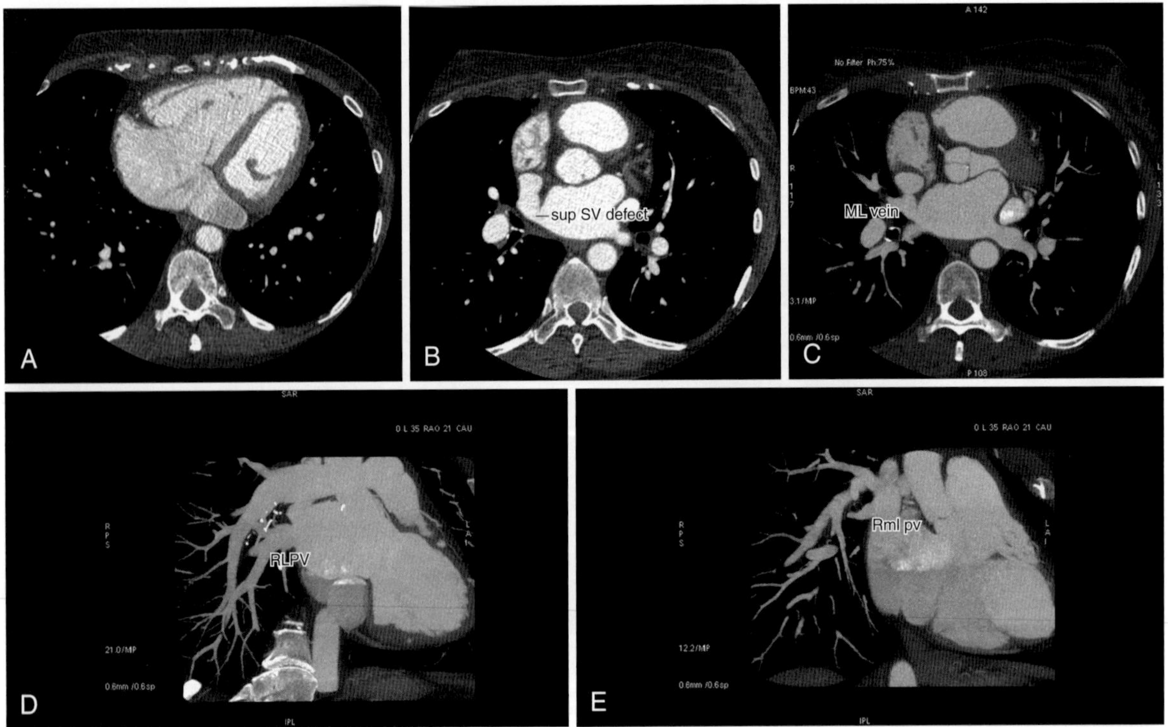

Figure 24-23. A composite of images from a cardiac CT study in a 32-year-old woman. **A,** Enlargement of the right ventricle, right atrium, and coronary sinus. **B,** A well-defined defect within the upper portion of the intra-atrial septum at the level of the superior vena cava. This location is typical for a superior sinus venosus (SV) defect. **C** and **D,** Right lower lobe pulmonary vein draining normally into the left atrium. **E,** The right upper and right middle lobe pulmonary veins demonstrate the right upper lobe and a branch of the right middle lobe vein draining into the superior vena cava, indicative of partial anomalous pulmonary venous return, in this case associated with the superior sinus venosus defect.

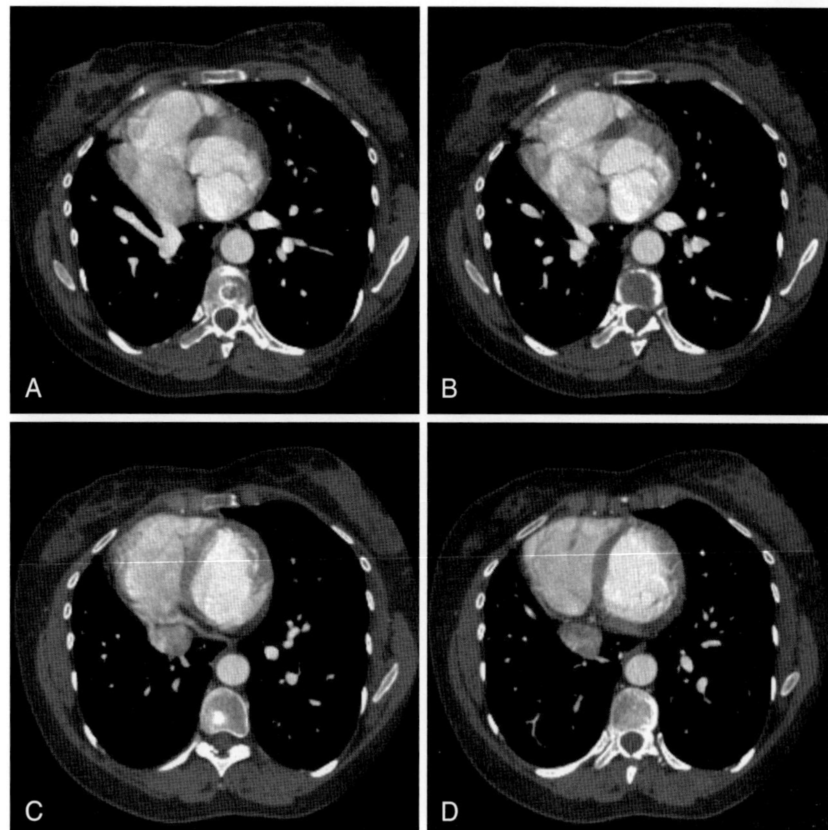

Figure 24-24. Partial anomalous venous return of the right upper lobe to the right atrium. Note the multiple pulmonary veins returning to the right atrium.

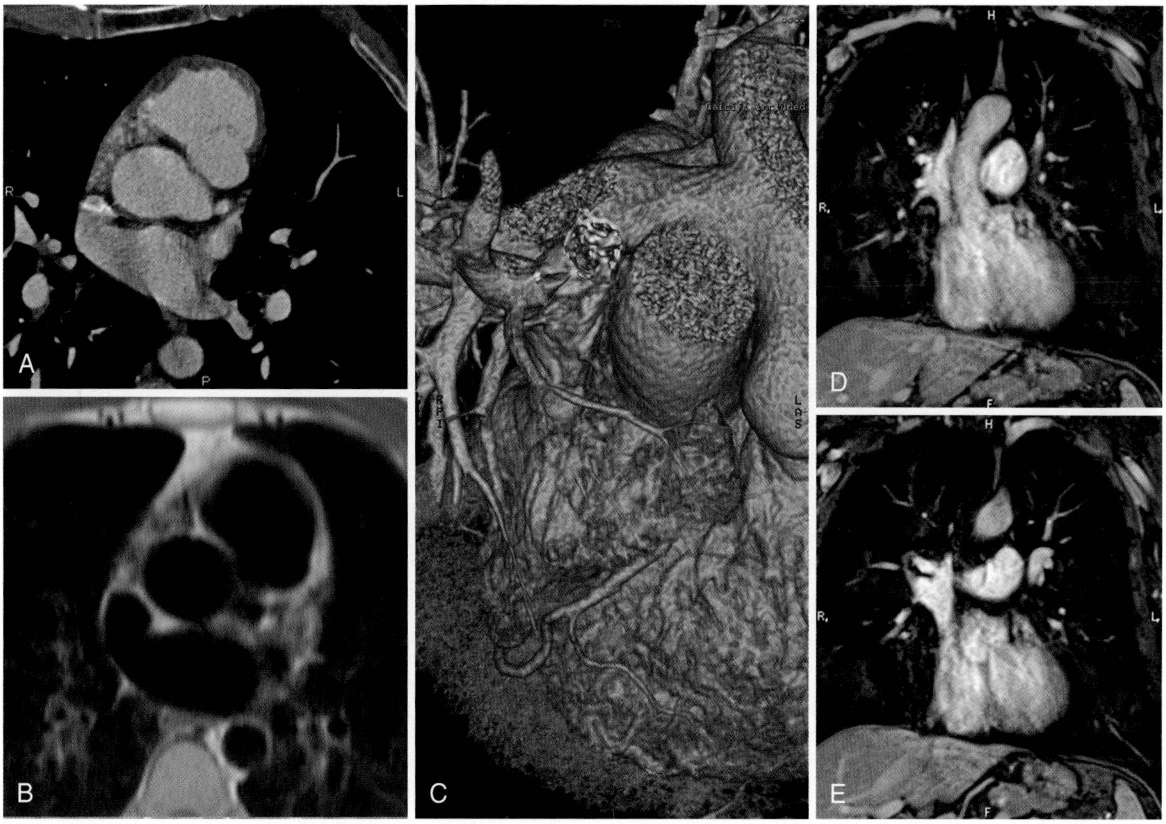

Figure 24-25. Correlative images from a preoperative cardiac CT study (**A,C**) and a cardiac MRI study (**B, D, E**) in a patient with sinus venosus defect and right upper lobe partial anomalous pulmonary venous return. The CT and MRI studies demonstrate concordance in evaluation of the sinus venosus defect. The volume-rendered CT data set (**C**) demonstrates multiple right upper and right middle lobe pulmonary veins with separate ostia entering into the superior vena cava.

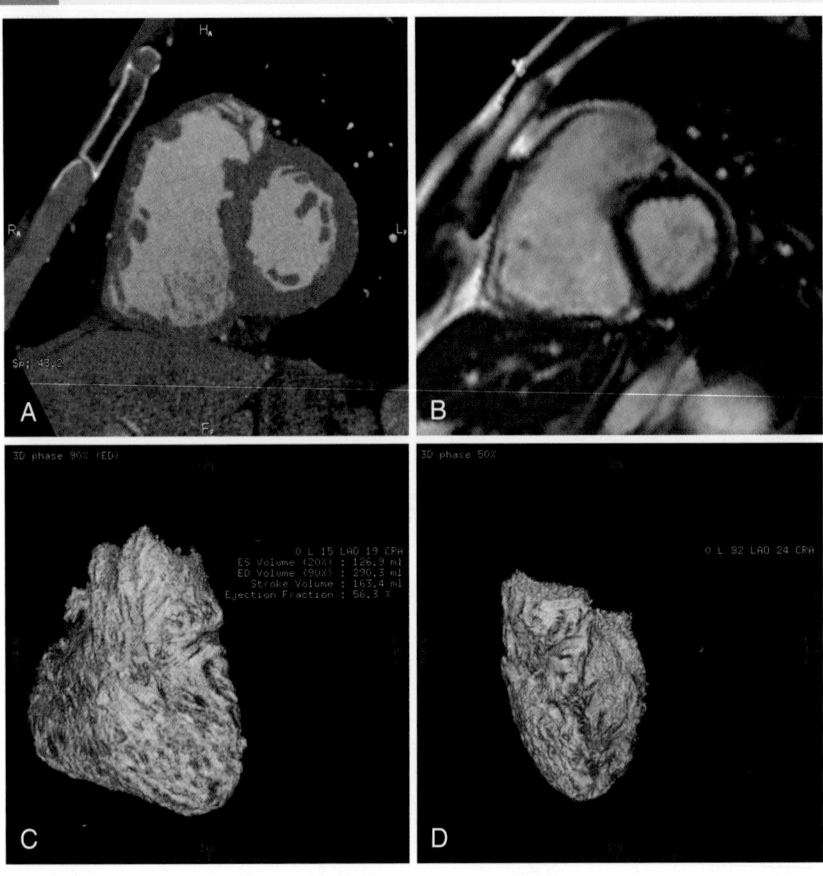

Figure 24-26. Short-axis oblique cardiac CT (**A**) and cardiac MRI (**B**) images of a patient with sinus venosus defect and partial anomalous pulmonary venous return. 3D-rendered cardiac CT depletions of the right ventricle in diastole (**C**) and systole (**D**). There is moderate-to-severe right ventricular dilatation and hypertrophy, the latter of which is better appreciated on the cardiac CT study.

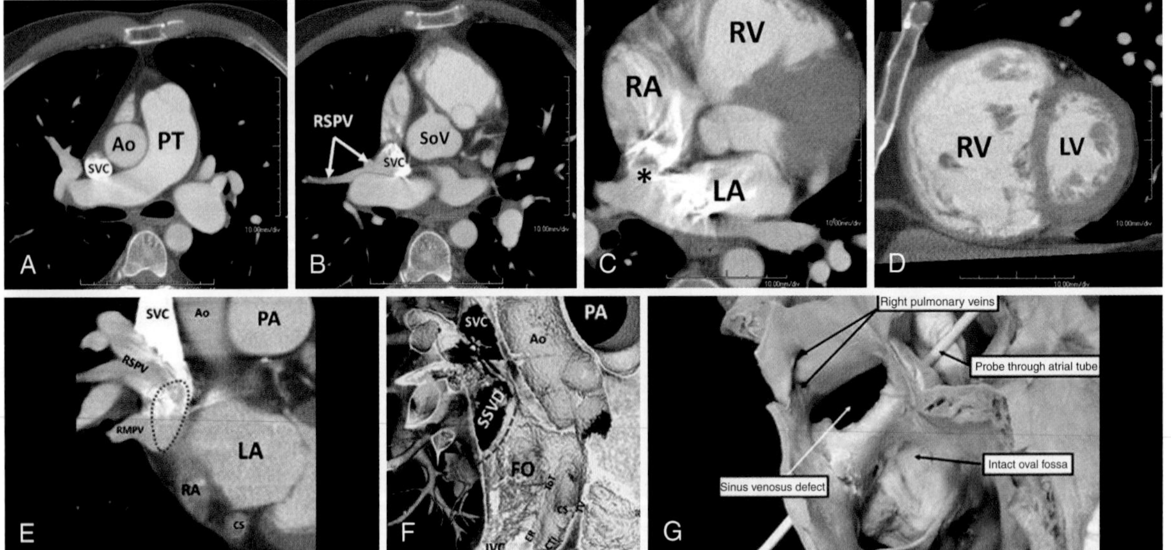

Figure 24-27. A 53-year-old man was diagnosed with a cardiac murmur by his primary care physician. Axial images were obtained at the level of the pulmonic trunk (**A**), the sinuses of Valsalva (**B**), and the superior cavoatrial junction (**C**). **E,** An oblique sagittal image through the superior cavoatrial junction demonstrates anomalous drainage of the right superior pulmonary vein (RSPV) into the distal superior vena cava (SVC) immediately before the atrial junction; the *red dotted oval* marks the SSVD position. **F,** Thick slab blood pool inversion volume-rendered image in a similar oblique sagittal plane demonstrates the anatomy of the interatrial septum from the right atrial perspective (as would be seen during right-sided atriotomy at surgery). Note the position of the superior sinus venosus defect, which is superior and posterior to the fossa ovalis. The *dotted blue line* indicates the inferior/anterior margin of the SSVD, which is actually formed by complete invagination of a portion of the superior interatrial fold, which forms a "tube" of extracardiac fat (see probe position in **C**). **G,** Anatomic specimen demonstrating a SSVD. Ao, ascending aorta; CS, coronary sinus; CTI, cavotricuspid isthmus; ER, Eustachian ridge; FO, fossa ovalis; IVC, inferior vena cava; LA, left atrium; PA, pulmonary artery; RA, right atrium; RMPV, right middle pulmonary vein; RSPV, right superior pulmonary vein; SSVD, superior sinus venosus defect; SVC, superior vena cava; ToT, tendon of Todaro; TV, tricuspid valve. (Reprinted with permission from Schreiber C, Horer J, Vogt M, et al. The surgical anatomy and treatment of interatrial communications. MMCTS 2007(1018):2386 and Shroff GS, Carr JJ, Gandhi S, Entrikin DW. Superior sinus venosus type defect demonstrated by cardiac computed tomographic angiography. *SCCT Case of the Month,* September 2011. Available at http://archive.constantcontact.com/fs027/1101901294184/archive/1107876096973.html.)

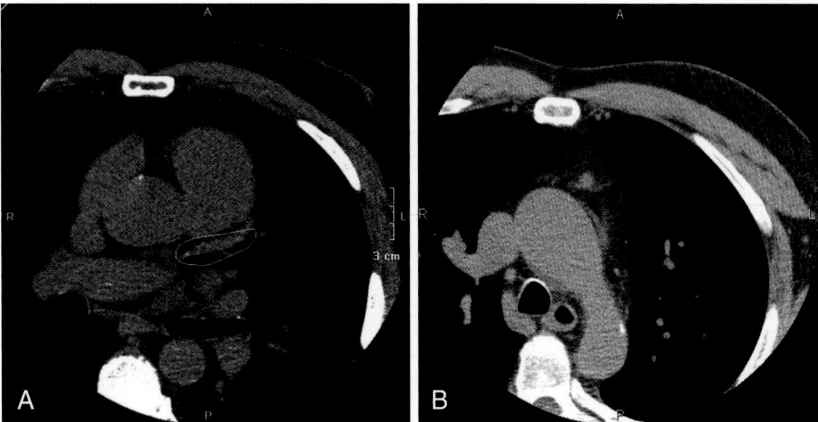

Figure 24-28. On a coronary calcium study (**A**), an anomalous pulmonary venous return to the IVC is incidentally revealed (**B**).

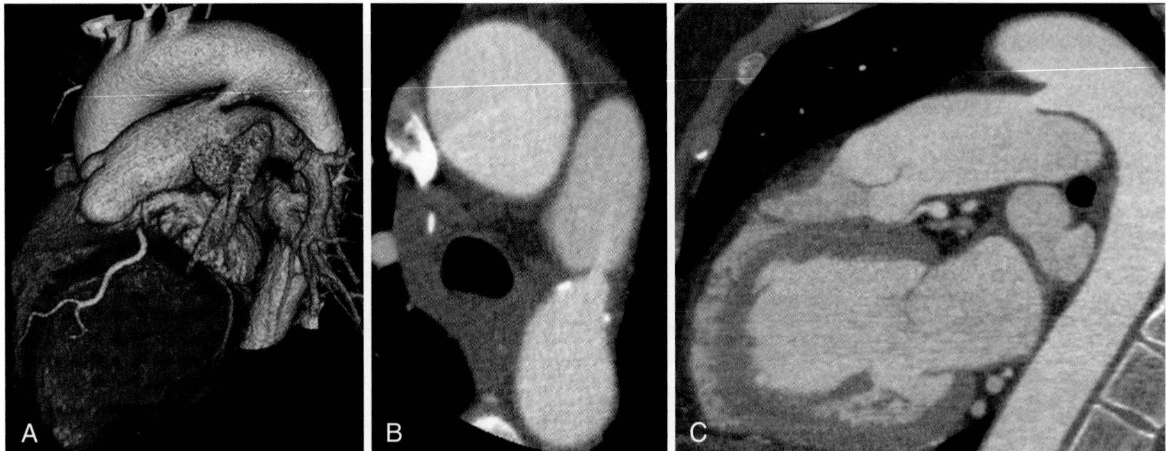

Figure 24-29. Multiple composite images from a cardiac CT scan in a patient with a murmur, and echocardiography demonstrating abnormal flow within the main pulmonary artery. A patent ductus arteriosus is present. A small amount of calcification along the undersurface of the aortic arch is noted, but no calcification involving the patent ductus arteriosus itself is apparent.

Patent Ductus Arteriosus

The ductus arteriosus is a vascular communication between the descending thoracic aorta and the main pulmonary artery, which closes functionally secondary to muscular contraction within 10 to 15 hours after birth and closes anatomically by fibrosis and thrombosis in 99% of infants by 1 year. In infants and children, patency of this vessel is an integral part of several complex congenital diseases such pulmonary atresia or aortic arch interruption. In adolescents and adults, however, a PDA is usually an isolated entity.

In children, a PDA often can be identified on echocardiography, and further evaluation is rarely required. In adolescents and adults, however, the appropriate acoustic window may not be present; in these patients, CTA or MRA allows accurate depiction of the PDA. The resolution of CTA allows for precise landmarking if interventional closure of the PDA is under consideration. The PDA appears as a tubular connection, usually between the undersurface of the aortic arch and the superior margin of the main or left pulmonary artery. Often the pulmonary artery receiving the aortic shunt becomes enlarged or aneurysmal (Figs. 24-29 through 24-31).

Coronary Artery

Anomalous origin of the coronary artery is discussed in Chapter 11. Anomalous termination of the coronary artery is discussed in Chapter 12.

Other

Cor Triatriatum

Cor triatriatum of the left atrium (i.e., cor triatriatum sinister) is a rare congenital anomaly in which the common pulmonary venous chamber is separated from the left atrium by a fibromuscular septum. This condition occurs in less than 0.5% of patients with congenital heart disease. The embryologic basis of cor triatriatum is uncertain. Theories include abnormal incorporation of the embryonic pulmonary vein into the left atrium; abnormal septation with a membrane

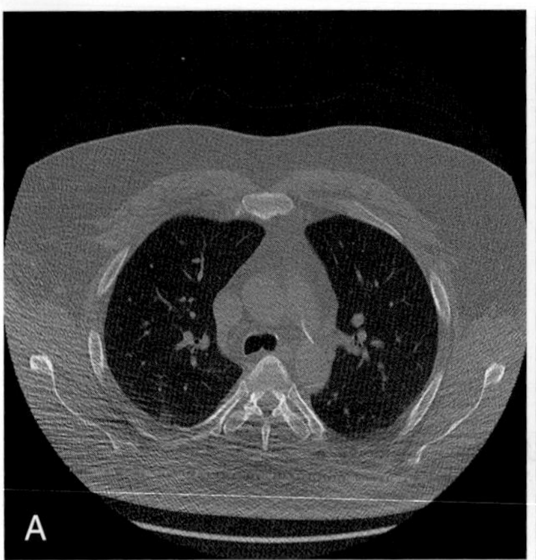

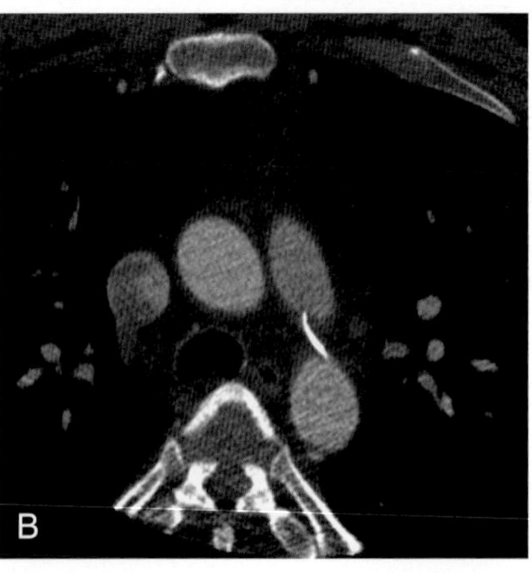

Figure 24-30. Contrast-enhanced CT scan axial images at the level of the proximal descending aorta reveal a prominently calcified ductus arteriosus extending from the descending aorta to the medial wall of the pulmonary artery.

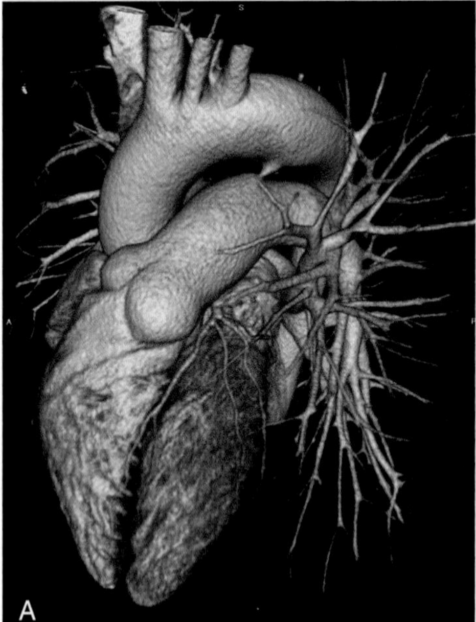

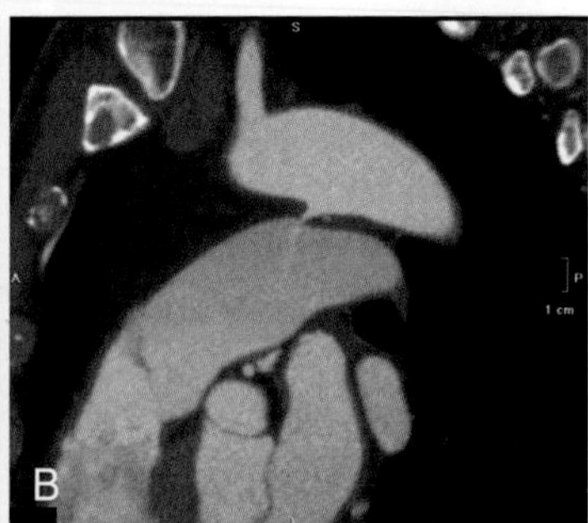

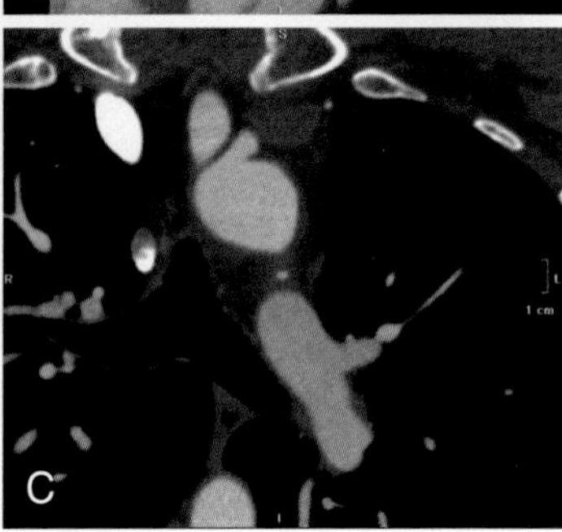

Figure 24-31. A, Three-dimensional volume-rendered image depicts patency of a ductus arteriosus between the isthmus portion of the aorta and the main pulmonary artery. **B,** There is communication between the aorta superiorly and the main pulmonary artery inferiorly. Note the positive contrast entering the pulmonary artery from the aorta. Note as well the calcium adjacent to the ductus. **C,** Axial source image demonstrates the patent ductus between the aorta and the pulmonary artery.

dividing the left atrium, representing an abnormal growth of the septum primum; and abnormal entrapment, in which the embryonic portion of the sinus venosus traps the common pulmonary vein. The outcome is an obstructive membrane at the junction of the common pulmonary vein of the left atrium. This creates two separate chambers within the left atrium: the distal chamber, consisting of the pulmonary veins and the confluence, and the proximal chamber, including the left atrium and left atrial appendage. The fibromuscular septum may be completely intact, causing severe pulmonary venous inflow obstruction into the left atrium, incompatible with life. In adults, the fibromuscular septum usually is fenestrated or incomplete. The degree of obstruction at the exit of the accessory chamber relates to the onset and severity of symptoms. Late presentation also can be due to the development of atrial fibrillation and left atrial thrombus formation. If pulmonary venous obstruction does exist, and evidence of pulmonary venous hypertension is present, surgical resection of the residual fibromuscular septum is performed (Figs. 24-32 and 24-33; **Video 24-8**).

Ebstein Anomaly

Ebstein anomaly is a condition of the tricuspid valve leaflet in which, often, all three valve leaflets are abnormal. The basal attachments of the septal and often the posterior leaflets are displaced apically within the right ventricle. Apical displacement of the septal tricuspid leaflet of greater than 8 mm/m^2 is felt to be diagnostic. The anterosuperior leaflet often is markedly enlarged and has an abnormal attachment to the

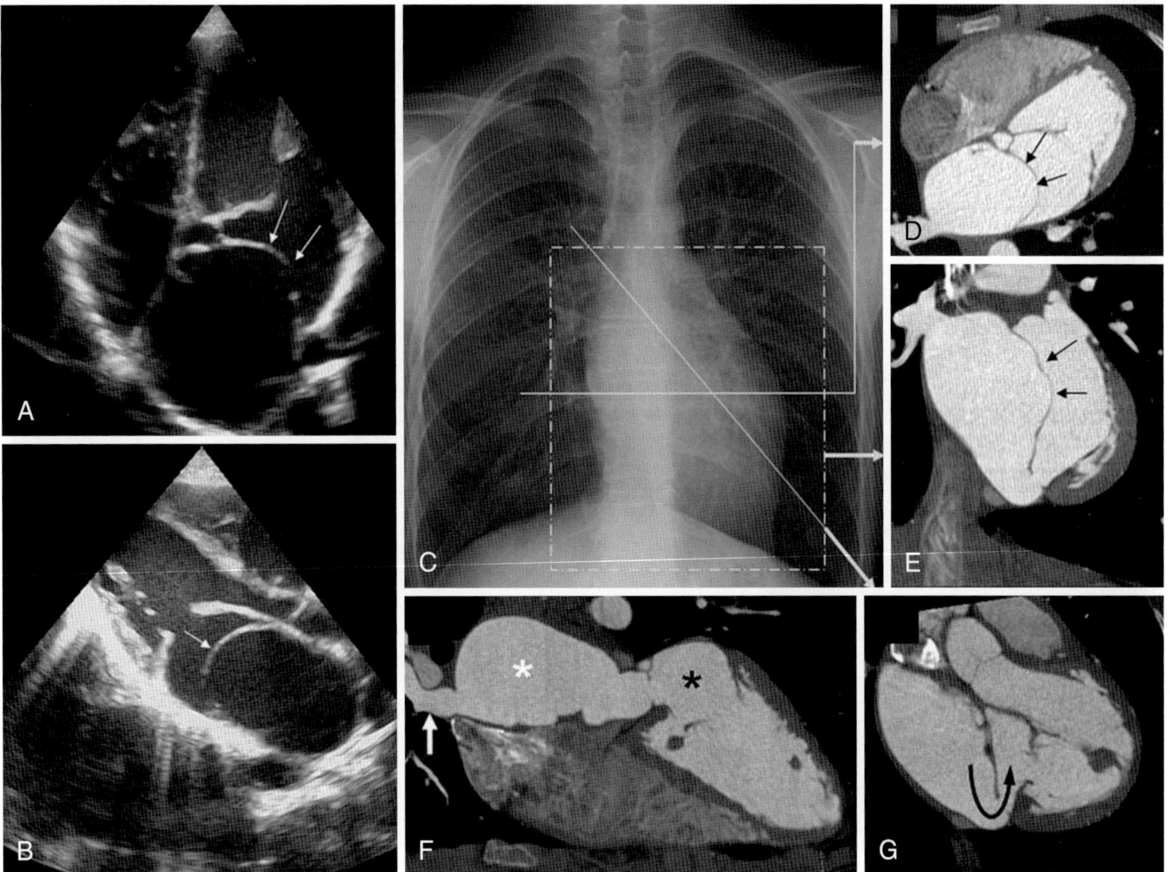

Figure 24-32. A 17-year-old patient was referred for recurrent syncopal episodes on exertion. He had no relevant past medical history. Peripheral blood pressure was 100/60 mm Hg. Electrocardiography showed a right bundle branch block. The transthoracic echocardiogram demonstrated a left atrium divided into two compartments by a membrane appearing as an almost-complete diaphragm (**A** and **B**). The mitral valve appeared dysplastic, with mild regurgitation. Pulmonary arterial pressure was estimated to be 50 mm Hg. A diagnosis of cor triatriatum sinistrum was achieved. Before surgery, a cardiac CT scan was performed. Cardiac CT scan reformations are represented by line drawings superimposed on the chest radiograph (**C**). Cardiac CT confirmed the diagnosis by showing an enlarged left atrium divided into 2 compartments by a thin membrane (**D** and **E**). This diaphragm presented with a small perforation in its inferolateral portion (**F** and **G**). No further cardiovascular anomaly was depicted. Cardiac surgery was performed to resect the accessory membrane and repair the mitral valve. (Reprinted with permission from Gahide G, Barde S, Francis-Sicre N. Cor triatriatum sinister: a comprehensive anatomical study on computed tomography scan. *J Am Coll Cardiol.* 2009;54(5):487). **See Video 24-8.**

free wall of the right ventricle. It can give the appearance of a large open "billowing sail." Due to the apical displacement of the septal and posterior leaflets, a component of the inlet portion of the right ventricle is functionally incorporated into the right atrium, characterized as the "atrialized" portion of the right ventricle. The remaining trabecular and outlet portions of the right ventricle then constitute the functional portion of the right ventricle. The degree of tricuspid insufficiency is variable, and about one third of patients have an associated PFO or ASD. Infrequently, other associated congenital lesions such as VSDs and tetralogy of Fallot also can occur (Fig. 24-34).

CCT PROTOCOL POINTS

- The usual CCT protocol is followed.
- Contrast: In the setting of a left-to-right shunt, "washing out" the right side of the heart by increasing the rate and amount of saline push (60 mL at 6 mL/sec) often can aid in identifying the shunt. If, however, evaluation of right and left ventricular size and function is needed (e.g., MR contraindicated, echocardiography suboptimal), then a low-dose helical acquisition with increased contrast enhancement of the right heart is needed, and a mixture of the saline push (30–50% contrast, 50–70% saline) is suggested.
- See Table 24-1

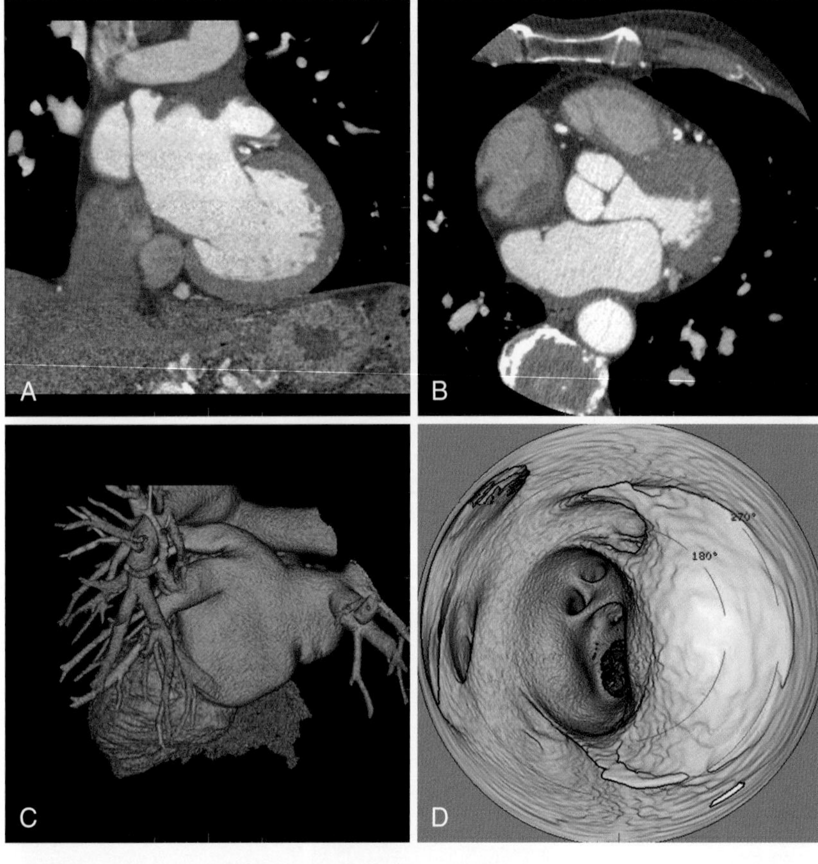

Figure 24-33. Multiple images from a cardiac CT study in a 54-year-old man with atypical chest pain. **A** and **B** demonstrate a thin but incomplete septum within the right aspect of the left atrium. **C,** The volume rendered image has been obtained from a posterior projection showing the right aspect of the left atrium as smaller than the left, with a waist-like appearance along the right, inferior margin of the left atrium. There is no evidence of pulmonary vein stenosis. **D,** A virtual endoscopic rendering within the left atrium. The right upper and right lower lobe pulmonary vein ostia are well-defined. A partial ridge through the medial/right aspect of the left atrium corresponds to the partial septum seen above. The diagnosis was forme fruste of cor triatriatum, with an incomplete septum. **See Video 24-8.**

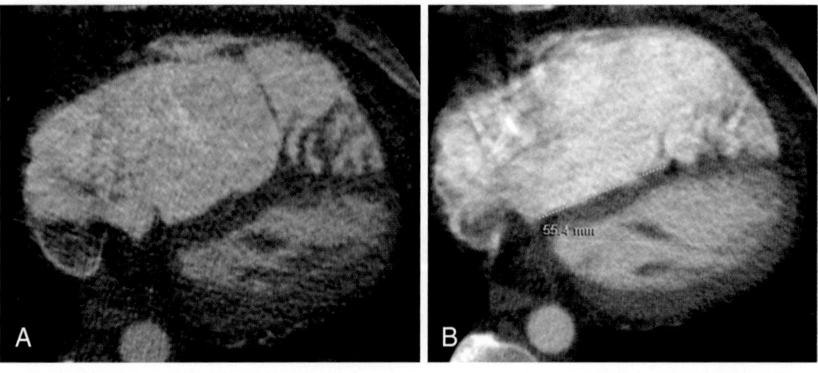

Figure 24-34. Cardiac CT study in a patient with Ebstein anomaly. The study demonstrates marked anterior displacement of the sub-tricuspid valve leaflet with a large atrialized portion of the right ventricle.

TABLE 24-1 ACCF 2010 Appropriateness Criteria for the Use of Cardiac Computed Tomography to Evaluate Adult Congenital Heart Disease

APPROPRIATENESS RATING	INDICATION	MEDIAN SCORE
Appropriate	Assessment of coronary arterial and other thoracic arteriovenous vessels	9
	Assessment of complex adult congenital heart disease	8
	Quantitative evaluation of right ventricular function	7
Uncertain	None listed	
Inappropriate	None listed	

Data from Taylor AJ, Cerqueira M, Hodgson JM, et al. ACCF/SCCT/ACR/AHA/ASE/ASNC/NASCI/SCAI/SCMR 2010 appropriate use criteria for cardiac computed tomography. A report of the American College of Cardiology Foundation Appropriate Use Criteria Task Force, the Society of Cardiovascular Computed Tomography, the American College of Radiology, the American Heart Association, the American Society of Echocardiography, the American Society of Nuclear Cardiology, the North American Society for Cardiovascular Imaging, the Society for Cardiovascular Angiography and Interventions, and the Society for Cardiovascular Magnetic Resonance. *J Am Coll Cardiol.* 2010;56(22):1864-1894.

References

1. Samyn MM. A review of the complementary information available with cardiac magnetic resonance imaging and multi-slice computed tomography (CT) during the study of congenital heart disease. *Int J Cardiovasc Imaging.* 2004;20(6):569-578.
2. Aggarwala G, Thompson B, van Beek E, Jagasia D. Multislice computed tomography angiography of Ebstein anomaly and anomalous coronary artery. *J Cardiovasc Comput Tomogr.* 2007;1(3):168-169.
3. Saremi F, Gurudevan SV, Narula J, Abolhoda A. Multidetector computed tomography (MDCT) in diagnosis of "cor triatriatum sinister." *J Cardiovasc Comput Tomogr.* 2007;1(3):172-174.
4. Cook SC, Raman SV. Multidetector computed tomography in the adolescent and young adult with congenital heart disease. *J Cardiovasc Comput Tomogr.* 2008;2(1):36-49.
5. Inglessis I. Editorial: Which diagnostic test modality for adult congenital heart disease? *J Cardiovasc Comput Tomogr.* 2007;2:23-25.
6. Hirsch R, Kilner PJ, Connelly MS, Redington AN, St John Sutton MG, Somerville J. Diagnosis in adolescents and adults with congenital heart disease. Prospective assessment of individual and combined roles of magnetic resonance imaging and transesophageal echocardiography. *Circulation.* 1994;90(6):2937-2951.
7. Achenbach S, Dittrich S, Kuettner A. Anomalous left anterior descending coronary artery in a pediatric patient with Fallot tetralogy. *J Cardiovasc Comput Tomogr.* 2008;2:55-56.
8. Kaplan S. Congenital heart disease in adolescents and adults. Natural and postoperative history across age groups. *Cardiol Clin.* 1993;11(4):543-556.
9. Ootaki Y, Yamaguchi M, Yoshimura N, Oka S, Yoshida M, Hasegawa T. Unroofed coronary sinus syndrome: diagnosis, classification, and surgical treatment. *J Thorac Cardiovasc Surg.* 2003;126(5): 1655-1656.
10. Gonzalez-Juanatey C, Testa A, Vidan J, et al. Persistent left superior vena cava draining into the coronary sinus: report of 10 cases and literature review. *Clin Cardiol.* 2004;27(9):515-518.
11. Hara H, Virmani R, Ladich E, et al. Patent foramen ovale: current pathology, pathophysiology, and clinical status. *J Am Coll Cardiol.* 2005;46(9):1768-1776. doi:10.1016/j.jacc.2005.08.038.
12. Mugge A, Daniel WG, Angermann C, et al. Atrial septal aneurysm in adult patients. A multicenter study using transthoracic and transesophageal echocardiography. *Circulation.* 1995;91(11):2785-2792.
13. Zhao BW, Mizushige K, Xian TC, Matsuo H. Incidence and clinical significance of interatrial shunting in patients with atrial septal aneurysm detected by contrast transesophageal echocardiography. *Angiol.* 1999;50(9):745-753.
14. Hoffman JI, Kaplan S. The incidence of congenital heart disease. *J Am Coll Cardiol.* 2002;39(12):1890-1900.
15. Al-Hay AA, MacNeill SJ, Yacoub M, Shore DF, Shinebourne EA. Complete atrioventricular septal defect, Down syndrome, and surgical outcome: risk factors. *Ann Thorac Surg.* 2003;75(2):412-421.
16. Ferreira AC, Rodriguez Y, Fishman JE, Ghersin E. Cardiac multidetector computed tomography incidental finding of a membranous septal aneurysm. *J Cardiovasc Comput Tomogr.* 2008;2(3):197-198.

25 Assessment of Complex and Repaired Congenital Heart Disease

Key Points

- Although echocardiography and MRI are still the best overall modalities for the evaluation of aortic and complex congenital heart lesions, especially postoperatively, there are exceptions.
- A growing number of children and adults with congenital disease acquire contraindications to cardiac MRI, such as pacemakers and implantable cardioverter defibrillators.
- Many surgical and interventional procedures use metallic components such as stents, occluder devices, and bioprosthetic valves, which often can confound MR imaging. In these cases CT may be beneficial.
- Although retrospective imaging is higher in radiation dose, it allows accurate measurement of right and left ventricular size and function.
- Using technique optimization, a number of complex congenital heart lesions can be well imaged with CT angiography.
- Surgical corrections for congenital heart disease can be well assessed with CT angiography. Upper and lower extremity contrast opacification may be necessary, as well as delayed imaging, especially if intracardiac thrombi are to be excluded.

The established tests for the assessment of congenital heart disease are transthoracic and transesophageal echocardiography, cardiac MRI, and cardiac catheterization.

Cardiac CT (CCT) is an emerging alternative, because of its rapid acquisition times and postprocessing robustness. The potential radiation risks are particularly relevant for children and younger adults, especially because its use has increased prominently in the assessment of congenital heart disease.[1]

Most intracardiac lesions can be assessed by echocardiography, and many procedures can be planned and guided with transthoracic, transesophageal, or intracardiac echocardiography, avoiding radiation risk and also providing Doppler assessment.

Among the patient population with congenital heart disease, MRI is the established test for the evaluation of extracardiac surgical shunts, pulmonary vascular anomalies and complications, and aortic anomalies. This modality avoids the risk of radiation exposure, and also provides flow information. Cardiac MRI also is the preferred test to quantify right ventricular (RV) function and the degree of pulmonic insufficiency.

CCT provides nonphysiologic but superb anatomic delineation of a very wide range of congenital cardiac and thoracic vascular defects,[2-4] and its use has substantially increased, but it remains unclear which lesions should be assessed by CCT, given the established, radiation risk–free, and widespread availability of other modalities,[5] and the proven complementarity of echocardiography and cardiac MRI.[1,6]

The greatest contribution of CCT, therefore, is likely to be:

- In patients who cannot undergo MRI, or those with lesions such as extracardiac shunts in whom MRI images are insufficient
- For the assessment of coronary anatomy, such as identification of anomalous left anterior descending (LAD) coronary artery in patients with tetralogy of Fallot[7]

A number of congenital pathologies are suited for CT imaging (see Table 25-1). The most common are discussed in the following sections. It may be useful to categorize congenital lesions based on their simplicity rather than on physiology.

COMPLEX LESIONS

Lesions that may be described as complex include the following:

- Tetralogy of Fallot
- Postsurgical tetralogy of Fallot
- Transposition of the great arteries
- Postsurgical transposition of the great arteries
  - Mustard baffles
  - Jatene's arterial switch operation

- ❒ Congenitally corrected transposition of the great arteries
- ❒ Fontan procedure
  - Glenn shunt
- ❒ Other commonly performed surgical repairs
  - Blalock-Taussig shunt
  - Waterston-Cooley shunt
  - Pott's shunt
  - Rastelli procedure

Tetralogy of Fallot

Tetralogy of Fallot is a common type of complex congenital heart disease. With an incidence of 0.1 per 1000 live births, it occurs in approximately 5.5% of all patients with congenital heart disease. The underlying abnormality is anterior displacement of the infundibular septum, which results in the three basic malformations that characterize this disorder:

- ❒ Severe stenosis of the right ventricular outflow tract (RVOT)
- ❒ An overriding aorta
- ❒ Infundibular venticular septal defect (VSD)

The fourth element of the tetralogy is hypertrophy of the right ventricle, which occurs as a consequence of the three basic defects just cited.

Over the years, the surgical approach to this condition has changed. There has been a move from a staged approach in favor of a primary repair, with a progressive lowering of the age at repair and a surgical technique that avoids or reduces the need for a ventriculotomy.

The goals of surgical correction of tetralogy of Fallot are to relieve the RVOT obstruction and to close the underlying VSD.

The RVOT obstruction can be relieved in one of three ways:

- ❒ Resection of a portion of the infundibular septum and other structures contributing to the outflow tract obstruction, such as prominent muscle bundles or muscular trabeculae
- ❒ Enlarging the pulmonary outflow tract by placement of a transannular patch, which is constructed from prosthetic material or from autologous pericardium. This patch is applied to the anterior aspect of the RVOT.
- ❒ Placement of an external conduit, usually involving a prosthetic pulmonary valve, between the right ventricle and the pulmonary trunk. This often is performed with a Dacron or Gore-Tex conduit and a bioprosthetic valve.

With all three methods, the VSD is closed with a patch of prosthetic material in such a way that the overriding aorta valve is exclusively committed to the left ventricular outflow tract.

Unfortunately, despite the improved surgical management, complications and residual sequelae after repair of tetralogy of Fallot are still common. Residual or recurrent VSD, RVOT obstruction or aneurysm formation, and pulmonary artery regurgitation and/or stenosis all lead to significant right ventricular dysfunction, resulting in significant morbidity and premature mortality.

MRI is currently the gold standard tool for postoperative evaluation of repaired tetralogy of Fallot. A number of patients, however, have relative contraindications to cardiac MRI, including pacemakers, claustrophobia, and underlying vascular stents, which can be difficult to image well due to susceptibility artifact.

Gated cardiac CT of postoperative tetralogy of Fallot patients allows:

- ❒ Demonstration of residual anatomic problems:
  - Residual VSD if present
  - Pulmonary arterial stenosis (with or without stenting), which can be central or peripheral
  - RVOT aneurysm
- ❒ Monitoring
  - Any underlying ascending aortopathy
  - Aortopulmonary collaterals
- ❒ Quantification of right/left ventricular size and function

See Figures 25-1 through 25-3; **Video 25-1.**

Postsurgical Tetralogy of Fallot

Most patients with tetralogy of Fallot will have had surgery. Corrective surgery for tetralogy of Fallot can include the following procedures:

- ❒ Placement of a ventricular septal patch, closing the high ventricular septal defect
- ❒ Resection of RVOT/infundibular muscle bundles, which usually are the cause of RVOT obstruction
- ❒ Pulmonic valvotomy. Pulmonic valve tissue often is dysplastic, thickened, and dysfunctional.
- ❒ Placement of an RVOT patch, often in conjunction with RVOT muscle bundle resection to increase the volume of the RVOT
- ❒ Transannular repair with placement of a transannular patch. This procedure is performed when the pulmonary valve annulus is small and restrictive. The surgery leaves the patient with free pulmonary insufficiency.
- ❒ Pulmonic valve implantation. A porcine bioprosthesis or human homograft usually is chosen. These can be utilized in adults undergoing late repair, and in patients with prior pulmonary valvotomy/transannular patch placement who have developed severe RV dilatation.

In patients who have severe hypoplasia, or atresia of the RVOT, an extracardiac conduit can be placed. This usually extends from the RVOT or the body of the RV to a central pulmonary artery.

Most imaging follow-up for tetralogy of Fallot repair is done with echocardiography and cardiac MRI. In patients with contraindications to cardiac MRI, such as a pacemaker, or the patient's inability to undergo an MRI study due to body habitus or claustrophobia, a CCT study can be of benefit.

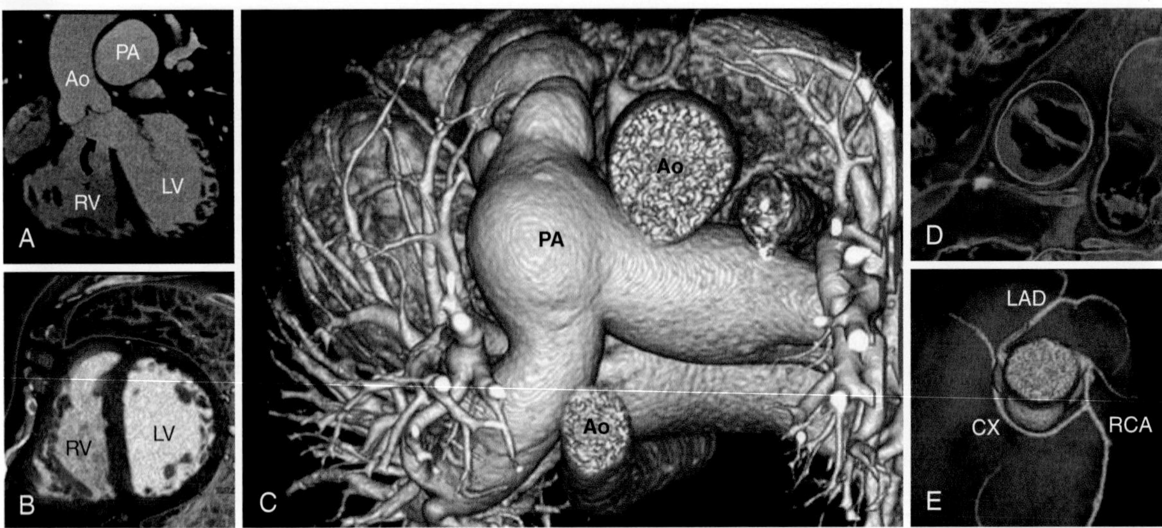

Figure 25-1. A 48-year-old man with unrepaired tetralogy of Fallot (ToF) was admitted with dyspnea on exertion and several episodes of cyanosis. The diagnosis of ToF had been established in early infancy, but surgical repair had been repeatedly refused. Retrospectively, ECG-gated 64-slice CT angiography (CTA) showed multiple abnormalities of cardiovascular morphology and function, and ruled out coronary artery disease and pulmonary embolism in a single noninvasive examination. The following findings of ToF were demonstrated on CTA: an overriding aorta (Ao); a large outlet ventricular septal defect (*arrow*); a dilated and hypertrophic right ventricle (RV) (**A**), with reduced left ventricular function (ejection fraction: 30%); and interventricular septum flattening (**B**). Right ventricular outflow tract obstruction was minimal (overlapping double outlet right ventricle anatomy). The pulmonary artery (PA) (**C**) was aneurysmal with a diameter of 47 mm. The pulmonary valve was bicuspid (**D**). There were no filling defects in the pulmonary arteries. The aortic root and ascending Ao were not dilated, with a nonstenotic tricuspid aortic valve. The coronary arteries were anomalous but not stenotic. The right coronary artery (RCA) and left anterior descending artery (LAD) arose from the tubular ascending Ao with a normal course subsequently. The left circumflex artery (CX) originated from the RCA and took a retro-aortic course, terminating in the atrioventricular groove (**E**). Owing to advanced heart failure and pulmonary hypertension, surgical correction was not feasible, and the patient was referred for heart–lung transplantation. (Reprinted with permission from Galea N, Noce V, Carbone I. Computed tomography angiography: uncommon findings in an adult patient with unrepaired tetralogy of Fallot. *Eur Heart J.* 2010;31(23):2843.)

While evaluation of pulmonic insufficiency and tricuspid insufficiency is, at best, limited with CT imaging, accurate morphologic evaluation of the right and left cardiac chambers, RV and LV volumes and ejection fractions, and central and peripheral pulmonary arterial anatomy can be obtained with high accuracy using a low-dose, dose-modulated helical acquisition. To assess the right ventricle as well as the left ventricle adequately on a CCT study, increased density of contrast is needed on the right side of the heart. This makes evaluation for intracardiac shunts such as an underlying patent foramen ovale or a VSD patch leak more challenging.

A CCT study for postoperative evaluation of a patient with tetralogy of Fallot repair would include the following:

- Determination of RV end-diastolic volume (EDV), RV end-systolic volume (ESV), RV ejection fraction (RVEF)
- Left ventricular EDV, left ventricular ESV, left ventricular EF
- Evaluation of the intraventricular septum for patch integrity
- Evaluation of the RVOT
- Evaluation of the native or bioprosthetic pulmonary valve
- Evaluation of an RV-to-PA conduit if one is present
- Evaluation of central right and left pulmonary arteries
- Evaluation of peripheral pulmonary arteries
- Evaluation of the ascending aorta, which can become dilated in the setting of tetralogy of Fallot
- **See** Figures 25-4 through 25-6; **Video 25-2.**

Transposition of the Great Vessels

Transposition of the great arteries (TGA) includes concordant atrioventricular connections and discordant ventriculoarterial connections. The aorta arises anterior to the pulmonary artery, from the morphologic right ventricle, and the main pulmonary artery arises from the morphologic left ventricle.

Before the arterial switch procedure was developed, patients with TGA required an atrial switch procedure such a Mustard or Senning procedure. This surgical correction creates an intra-atrial baffle separating systemic from pulmonary venous blood flow. The baffle redirects systemic blood from the inferior and superior venae cavae to the mitral valve and into the left ventricle. The pulmonary venous return is redirected to the tricuspid valve and the RV. The main difference between these two procedures is that the Mustard operation involves resection of atrial septal tissue in the formation of a baffle using either synthetic

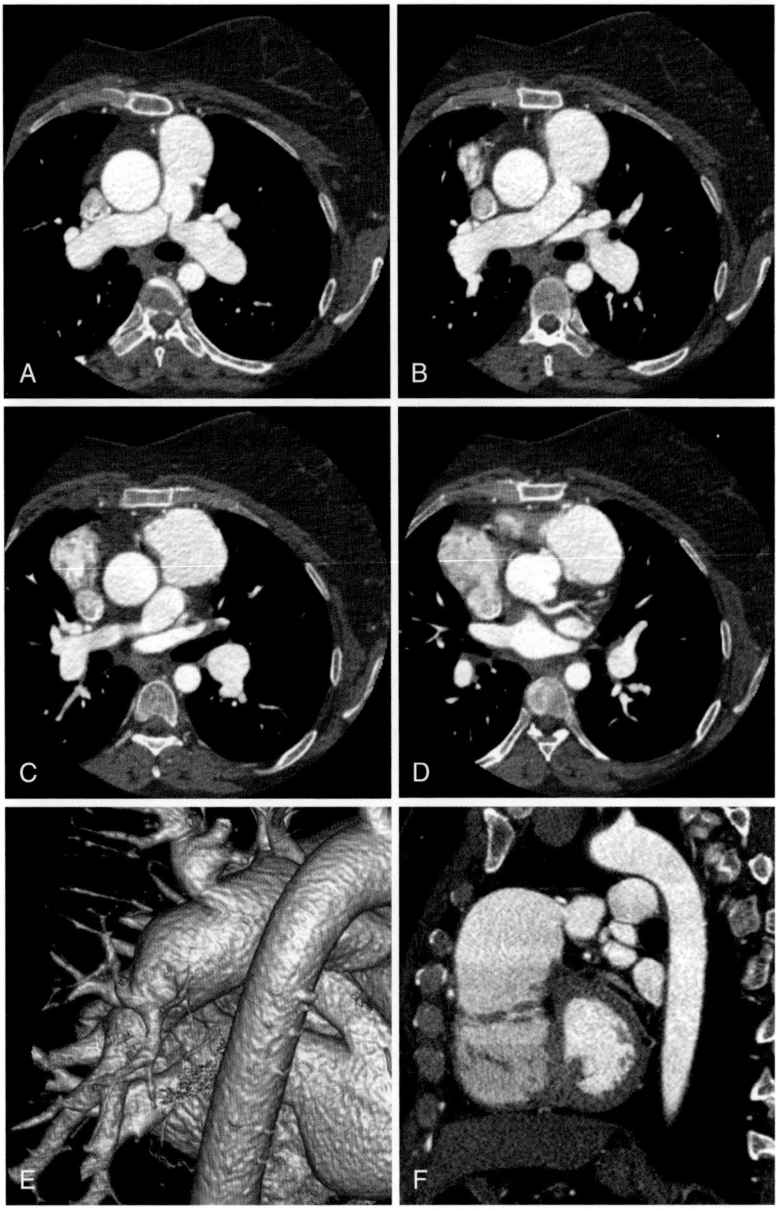

Figure 25-2. A 29-year-old woman post–repair for tetralogy of Fallot. The patient has had prior transannular repair. **A** and **B,** Enlargement of the main pulmonary artery post-transannular repair. **A,** Moderate narrowing at the origin of the left pulmonary artery, and a fine linear web within the origin of the right pulmonary artery. **C,** A small amount of calcification is present within the right ventricular outflow tract (RVOT) patch. There has been prior resection of right ventricular outflow tract muscle bundles. The right lower and left lower pulmonary arteries are moderately enlarged. **E,** The lateral basal segmental branch is seen to arise posteriorly from the left lower lobe pulmonary artery. Just inferior to this slice location, marked attenuation of the left lower lobe lateral basal segment is seen (**D**), demonstrating a site of peripheral pulmonary arterial stenosis in a patient with tetralogy of Fallot. **E,** The peripheral pulmonary arterial stenosis is also well demonstrated in a posteriorly projected volume rendered image of the left pulmonary artery. **F,** A complication of the transannular repair: RVOT patch dilatation, RV dilatation, and straightening of the intraventricular septum due to RV volume overload. **See Video 25-1.**

material, or autologous pericardium. The Senning procedure utilizes a baffle created from tissue from the right atrial wall and atrial septum, without the use of any extrinsic materials. In these procedures, however, the left ventricle remains the pulmonary ventricle, and the right ventricle the systemic ventricle. These operations usually were performed between the first month and first year of life.

MRI is the best modality to evaluate the integrity of the underlying surgical corrections, as well as to monitor the systemic right ventricle, which, in the long term, has a risk of failing. In patients with contraindications to MRI, evaluation of the postsurgical heart can be done using CCT.

Complications that can be assessed by cardiac CT include

- Progressive RV (systemic ventricle) dilatation and dysfunction due to long-term pumping against systemic pressures
- Evaluation of the superior and inferior baffles. The two major complications include baffle obstruction and baffle leak. Baffle stenoses are uncommon, but occur with greater frequency in the superior limb, with an incidence of 5% to 10% versus inferior limb obstruction, which occurs in only 1% to 2% of cases.

Baffle leaks may be present in up to 25% of patients,[8] but most are small, and usually not hemodynamically significant. In patients with

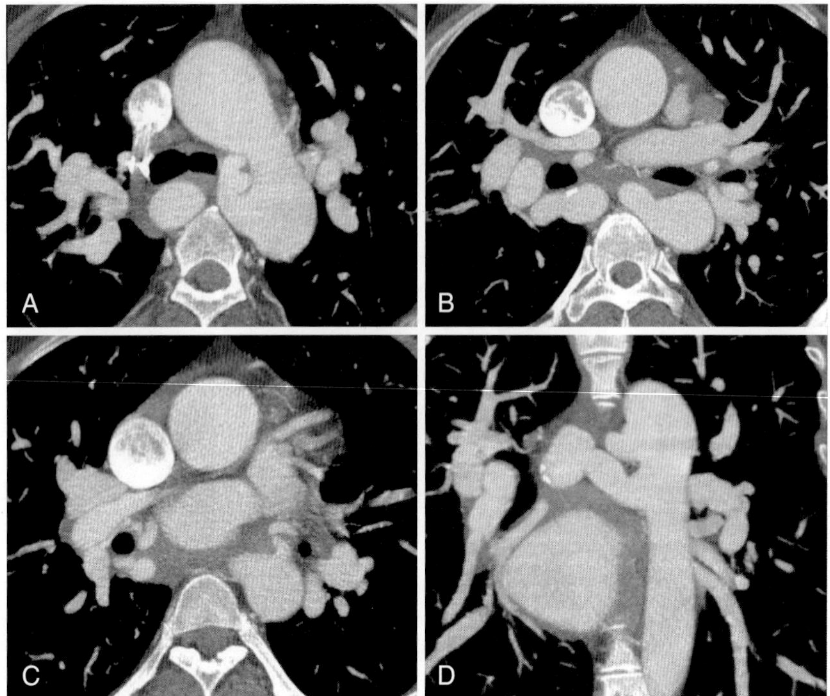

Figure 25-3. Multiple images from a cardiac CT examination in a patient with unrepaired tetralogy of Fallot. There are strikingly large major aorticopulmonary collateral arteries.

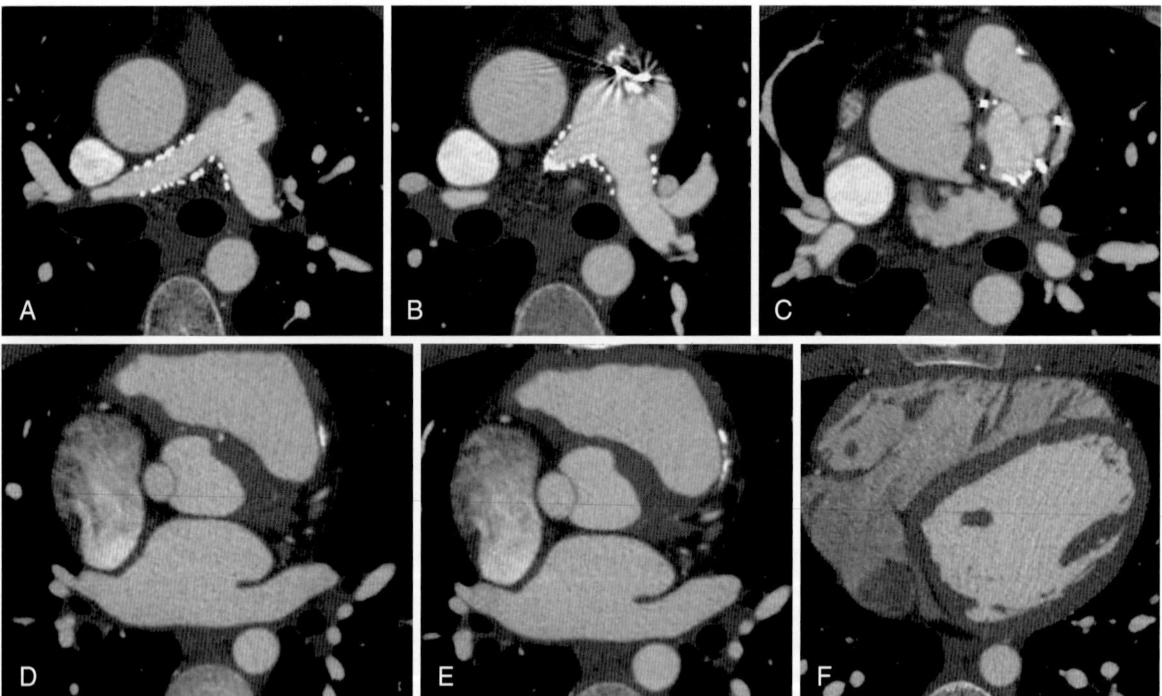

Figure 25-4. Multiple images from a cardiac CT study in a patient with tetralogy of Fallot repair. Right and left central pulmonary arterial stents have been placed for alleviation of central pulmonary arterial stenosis. The stents are patent, although a small amount of neointimal hyperplasia is seen within both stents. Biventricular enlargement is present.

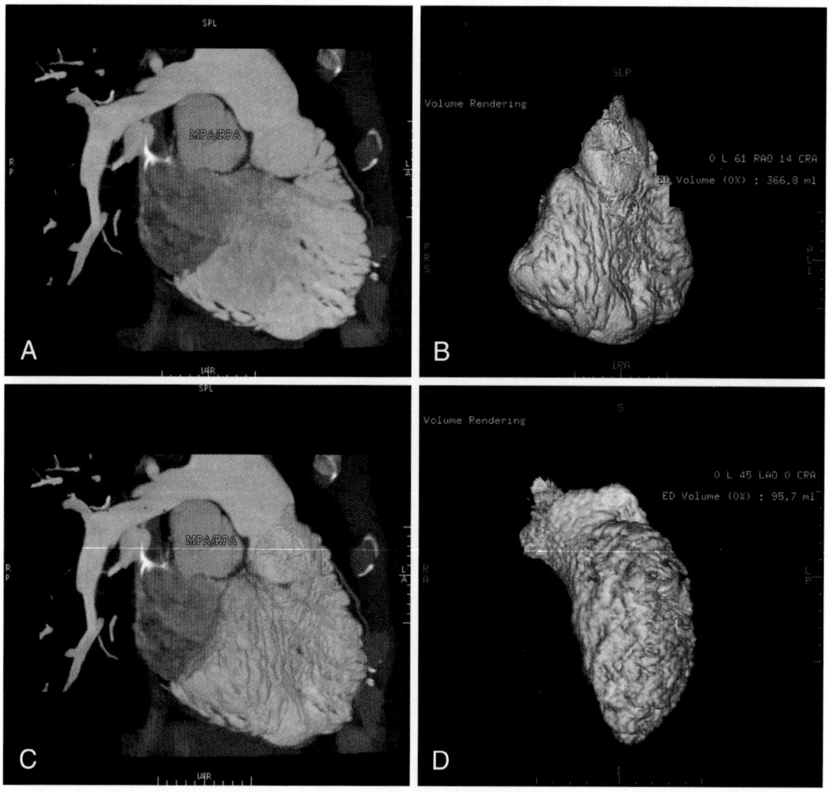

Figure 25-5. Reformatted and volume-rendered images from a 32-year-old man status post repair for tetralogy of Fallot (ToF). One of the most common complications of surgical repair for ToF is subsequent dilatation of the right ventricle, and this case demonstrates marked dilatation of the right ventricle. The RV end-diastolic volume on this study was calculated at 367 mL, 213 mL/m^2, severely dilated. In this case, a right ventricular outflow tract patch was not placed, and no aneurysm, or "denuding," of the right ventricular outflow tract is present.

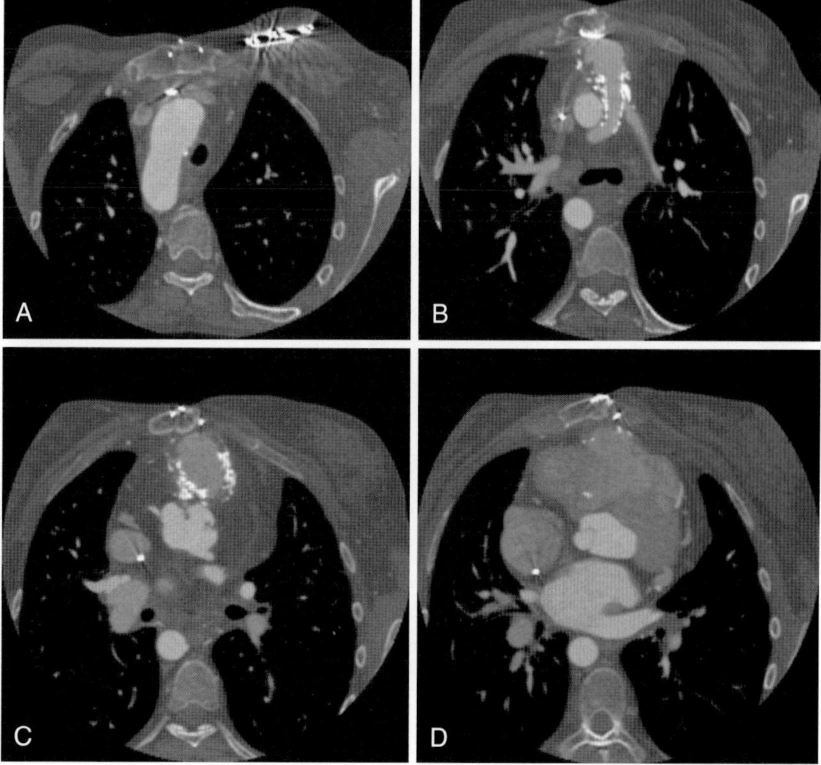

Figure 25-6. Multiple images from a cardiac CT study in a patient with transposition of the great arteries (TGA), post–Mustard procedure. **A,** The aorta anterior to the main pulmonary artery. Pacer wires are seen within the superior vena cava (SVC). The pacing wires extend from the SVC into the left atrial appendage and left ventricle. **B,** Moderate dilatation of the anterior right ventricle. **C** and **D,** Marked narrowing of the distal SVC and the superior limb of the Mustard baffle are seen. **C,** Coronal reformatted image through the superior baffle. **D,** A perpendicular cross-section through the distal portion of the superior baffle limb. A secondary sign of baffle obstruction seen in this image set is reflux of contrast down the azygos vein. The diagnosis was baffle stenosis/obstruction of the superior limb of the Mustard procedure in a patient with TGA. **See Video 25-2.**

large baffle leaks, right-to-left shunting can occur, resulting in systemic arterial desaturation, requiring surgical or percutaneous closure.

Postsurgical Transposition of the Great Vessels

Mustard/ Baffle Procedure

- Baffle stenosis and leaks. This evaluation by cardiac CT is more limited than MRI, because it often is challenging to obtain adequate contrast in both the superior baffle limb (SVC) and inferior baffle limb (IVC) simultaneously.[8]
- Superior baffle obstruction occurs in approximately 5% to10% of patients; inferior baffle stenosis is seen in about 1% to 2% of cases.
- Baffle leaks are more common and have been reported in up to 25% of cases. Most are not hemodynamically significant.
- Pulmonary vein stenosis occurs in about 2% of patients.
- See Figures 25-7 through 25-9.

Protocol Points in Patients Undergoing Mustard Procedure

- Coverage should include the lung apices to the upper abdomen. Most commonly the study should cover the thorax, to include the systemic thoracic veins, due to frequent venous occlusion/ stenosis, particularly if a pacemaker is in place
- Contrast: Automated trigger set: right pulmonary artery location, HU: 150
- Additional scans
  - Pre-contrast–like calcium score
  - Delayed acquisition if a clot in a baffle limb is suspected

Arterial Switch

In the arterial switch (also called the Jatene switch), the aorta and pulmonary arteries are transected above their respective valves and reoriented to their proper concordant ventricle. The coronary arteries are removed with a small buttonhole of aortic tissue and reimplanted into the

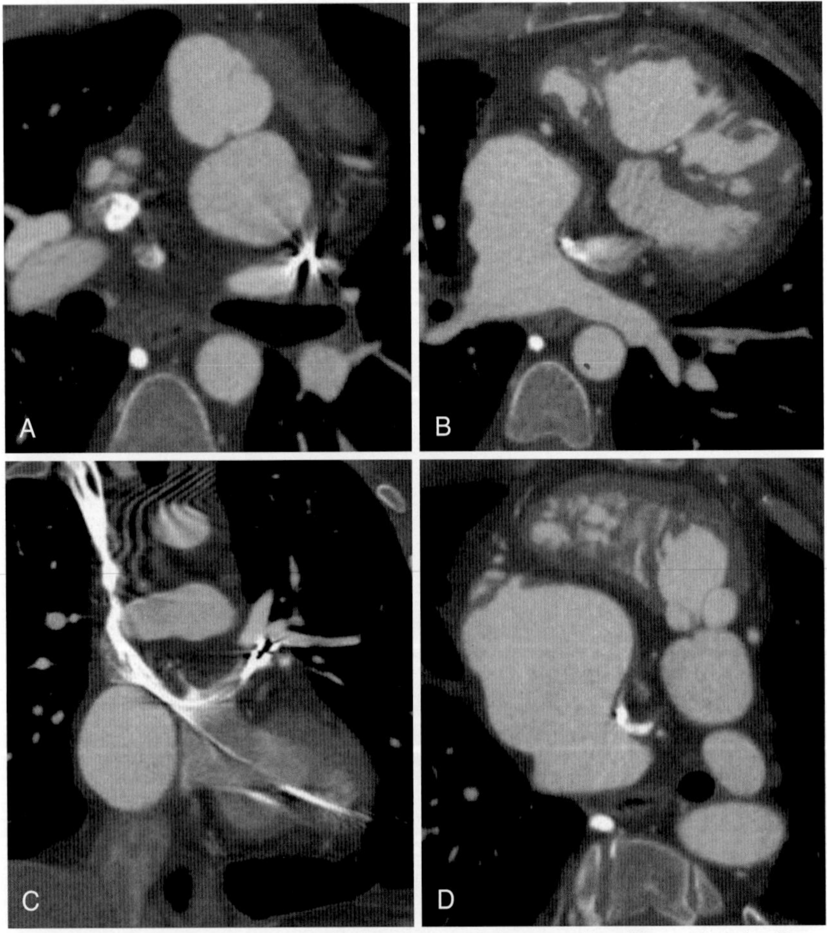

Figure 25-7. Multiple images from a cardiac CT study in a patient with a Mustard repair for transposition of the great arteries. Pacemaker wires through the superior baffle are noted. Moderate-to-severe stenosis of the superior baffle is also noted. Note enlargement of the azygos vein, with high-attenuation contrast within the azygos vein suggesting retrograde superior–to-inferior flow within the azygos vein. This is a surrogate marker for superior baffle obstruction.

aorta. The excised regions of the aorta usually are patched with pericardium.

Postoperative complications that are well delineated by cardiac CT include:

- Proximal pulmonary arterial stenosis (5–25% of cases, with incidence decreasing as surgical techniques and experience improve)
- Coronary artery stenosis (reported in 18% of cases, with 12% being significant)[9]

For images of cases with Jatene's arterial switch operation, see Figures 25-10 through 25-13; **Videos 25-3 and 25-4.**

Congenitally Corrected Transposition of the Great Arteries

Congenitally corrected transposition of the great arteries (CCTGA) is a condition in which the atria have a normal position, and receive appropriate venous return. The atria, however, are connected to the opposite ventricle. The ventricles, in turn, are connected to the "wrong" great artery. This results in atrioventricular discordance and ventricular arterial discordance. Systemic venous return from the SVC and the IVC flow into the right atrium, across the mitral valve, into the left atrium, and into the main pulmonary artery. Similarly, pulmonary venous return flows into the left atrium, across the tricuspid valve, into the right ventricle, and out into the aorta and the systemic arterial tree. Symptoms for this condition include double discordant transposition of the great arteries, and L-TGA due to the position of the aorta usually being posterior and to the left of the main pulmonary artery. The most common associated conditions with CCTGA include ventricular septal defects, tricuspid valve abnormalities, and pulmonary stenosis/LVOT obstruction. The coronary arteries in this condition usually are inverted. Childhood presentation with congestive heart failure usually relates to a large underlying VSD, or severe tricuspid regurgitation leading to medical management, and VSD closure. The complications include RV dysfunction and tricuspid regurgitation. In general, imaging follow-up for the patient with CCTGA is performed with echocardiography and MRI. The role for CCT in these patients is limited. One complication of this condition is an increasing rate over time in the development of heart block, which occurs at a rate of approximately 2% per year. An underlying pacemaker precludes evaluation of systemic RV function with an MRI, and a low-dose dose modulated CT examination can be considered to evaluate RV function in these patients (Figs. 25-14 through 25-16).

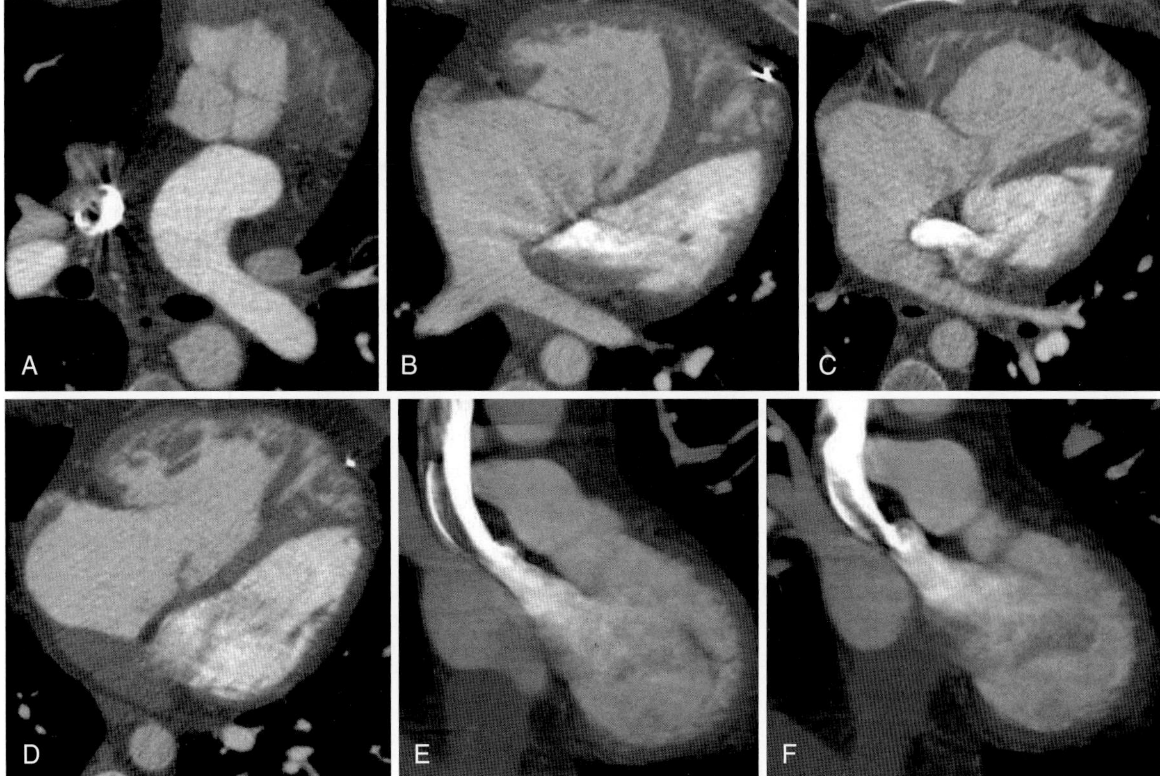

Figure 25-8. Multiple images from a cardiac CT study in a patient post–Mustard procedure for transposition of the great arteries. Note is made of a patent superior baffle, with no increased density in the azygos vein. There is enlargement and hypertrophy of the anterior right/systemic ventricle. Nonopacified blood is seen within the inferior baffle. A delayed imaging (60 seconds delay) CT scan would be required for complete evaluation (inclusive of opacification of the inferior baffle).

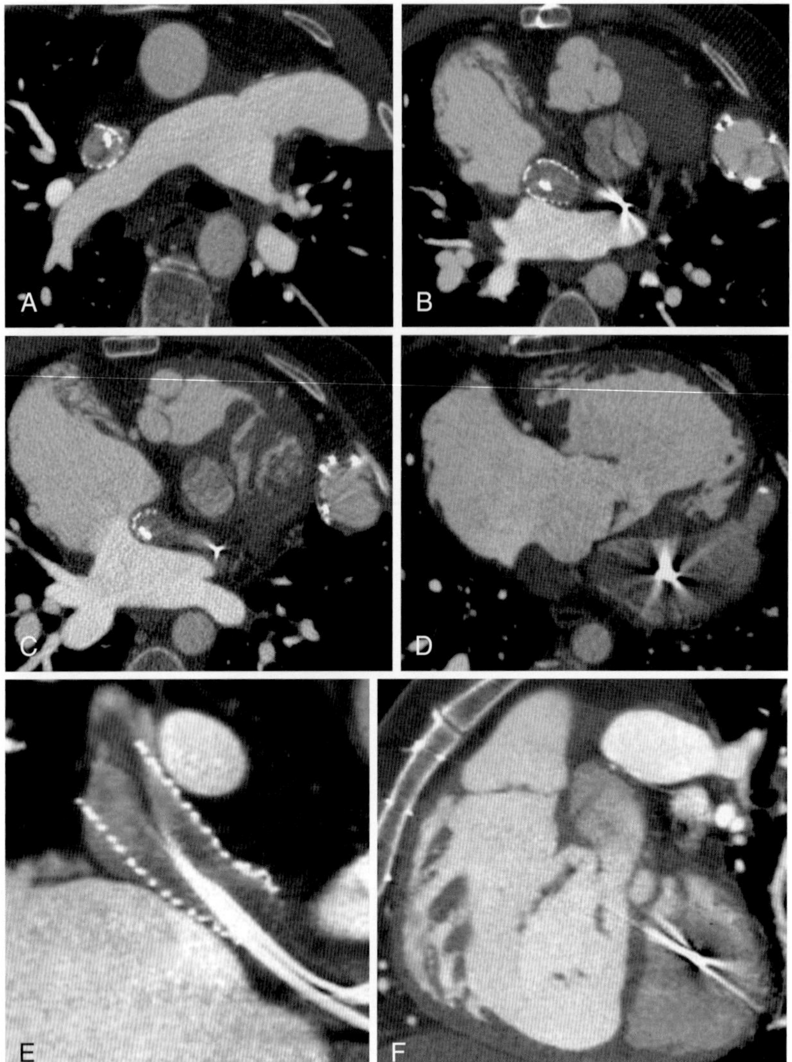

Figure 25-9. Multiple images from a cardiac CT study in a patient with complex congenital heart disease. This patient has transposition of the great vessels with the morphology of a double-outlet right ventricle (**A, B**). The aorta arises more anteriorly than usual and has a trileaflet valve. The main pulmonary segment has a bicuspid pulmonic valve (**B**). There has been a prior Mustard procedure. A stent is seen within the superior vena cava that extends into the superior baffle limb (**A–C**). Pacing wires are seen within the stented superior baffle limb, which maintains a normal caliber (**E**). The main pulmonary artery is disconnected from the central pulmonary artery (**F**), and an extracardiac conduit extends from the left ventricle apex to supply the main pulmonary artery (**A–D**).

Fontan Procedure

The Fontan procedure was first described in 1971 for bypass of the underdeveloped tricuspid valve.[10] It is performed principally in patients with tricuspid atresia and in varied congenital lesions where the primary abnormality relates to a single functioning ventricle. The goal of the procedure is to create a circulation in which the systemic venous blood returns directly to the pulmonary arteries. Many different modifications of the Fontan procedure have been employed. The most common procedure currently in use is the total cavopulmonary connection, in which IVC blood is channeled through the right atrium to the right or main pulmonary artery, and SVC blood is connected to the right pulmonary artery. This procedure is called a *Glenn shunt.*

Glenn Shunt

Complications of a Glenn shunt that can be assessed by cardiac CT include:

- **Clot formation in the Fontan circulation.** Thromboembolic events can occur within both the pulmonary and systemic circulation. The Fontan circuit itself is believed to represent a hypercoagulable state. Thrombus within the Fontan circuit can occur within the IVC, the Fontan conduit itself, the right atrium, and the pulmonary arteries.
- **Stenosis in the conduit.** Conduit stenosis is uncommon, and may relate to chronic thrombosis, calcification of the conduit, and narrowing of surgical anastomotic sites at the baffle and SVC/right pulmonary artery anastomoses.

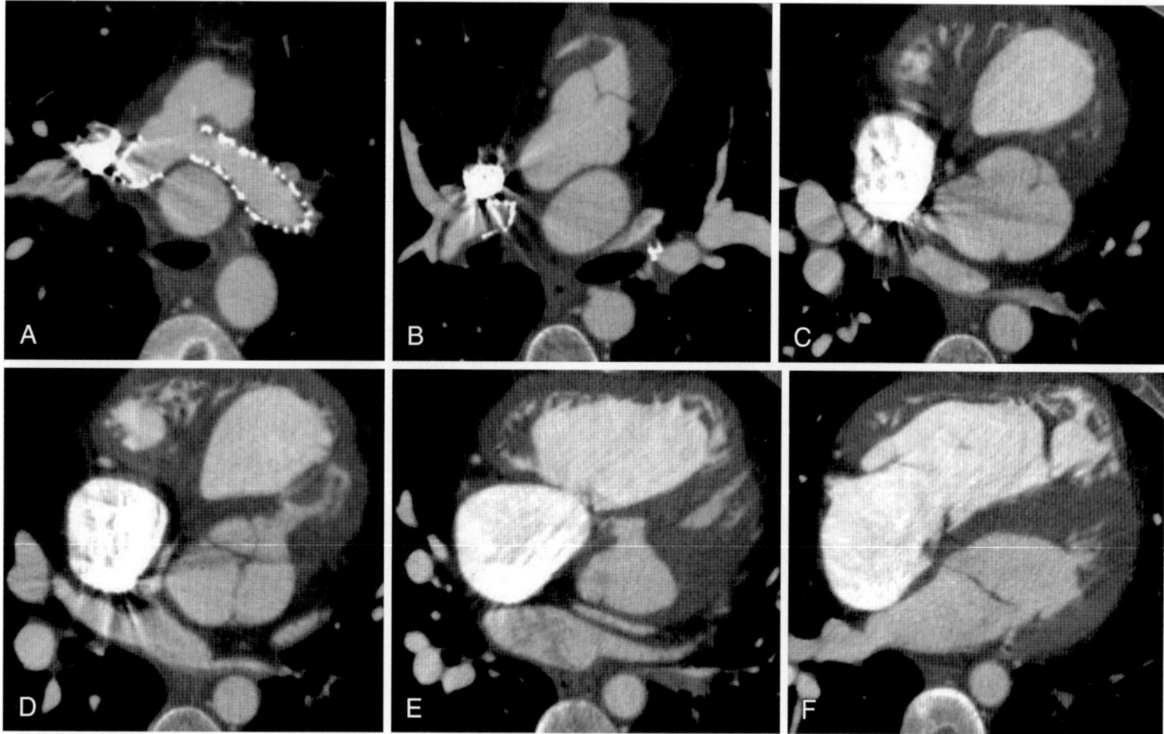

Figure 25-10. Multiple images from a cardiac CT study in a patient with complex congenital heart disease. A Jatene repair has been done for d-transposition, and there has been stenting of both the right and left pulmonary arteries post–Jatene repair. The stents are patent and without evidence of any underlying restenosis or thrombosis. The right ventricle is hypertrophied and dilated, consistent with prior pressure overload and strain.

- **Failure of the single ventricle.** Evaluation of ventricular function is better done with cardiac MRI and echocardiography. In patients for whom cardiac MRI is contraindicated, a low-dose, dose-modulated helical cardiac CT study can accurately assess and follow the size and function of the single ventricle.
- **Causes for cyanosis.** Most patients with non-fenestrated Fontan circulation do not have hypoxemia. If arterial oxygen saturations drop below 90%, the etiology of the hypoxemia should be sought. The following are common causes for hypoxemia in the setting of a Fontan procedure:
  - A persistently open surgical fenestration
  - The presence of pulmonary arterial malformations. The development of partial malformations may relate to the exclusion of the hepatic veins from IVC flow and from the pulmonary circulation. The etiology of this relationship is unclear, however. Small arteriovenous malformations (AVMs) may be difficult to evaluate using contrast-enhanced ultrasound or MRI. CT scanning and conventional angiography are preferred methods for AVM detection. The presence of pulmonary AVMs in these patients is a significant abnormality and relates to a worsening prognosis.
  - Systemic venous collateralization with connection to the pulmonary vein or pulmonary venous atrium. Systemic venous collaterals can be seen in approximately one third of patients with a bidirectional cavopulmonary connection.[11] The sites that can be identified on a CT scan as a potential site of systemic venous collateralization are reopening of the left SVC connecting to the coronary sinus, reopening of the left-sided cardinal vein, IVC flow into the portal vein, and thebesian veins connecting to the pulmonary venous atrium.

Some of these collaterals are amenable to percutaneous closure (Figs. 25-17 through 25-21; **Videos 25-5 and 25-6**).

Other Types of Fontan Procedure

The Fontan procedure is a palliative procedure for patients with a univentricular circulation. A number of variations exist, with a general principle of diversion of the systemic venous return to the pulmonary artery with the absence of a subpulmonic ventricle, or to the exclusion of the subpulmonic ventricle if it is significantly hypoplastic.

Variations of the Fontan procedure are as follows:

- **Classic Fontan:** A valve conduit or direct anastomosis between the right atrium and the pulmonary artery. This may involve the right atrial appendage or right atrium proper, and may extend to the main pulmonary artery or the right pulmonary artery.

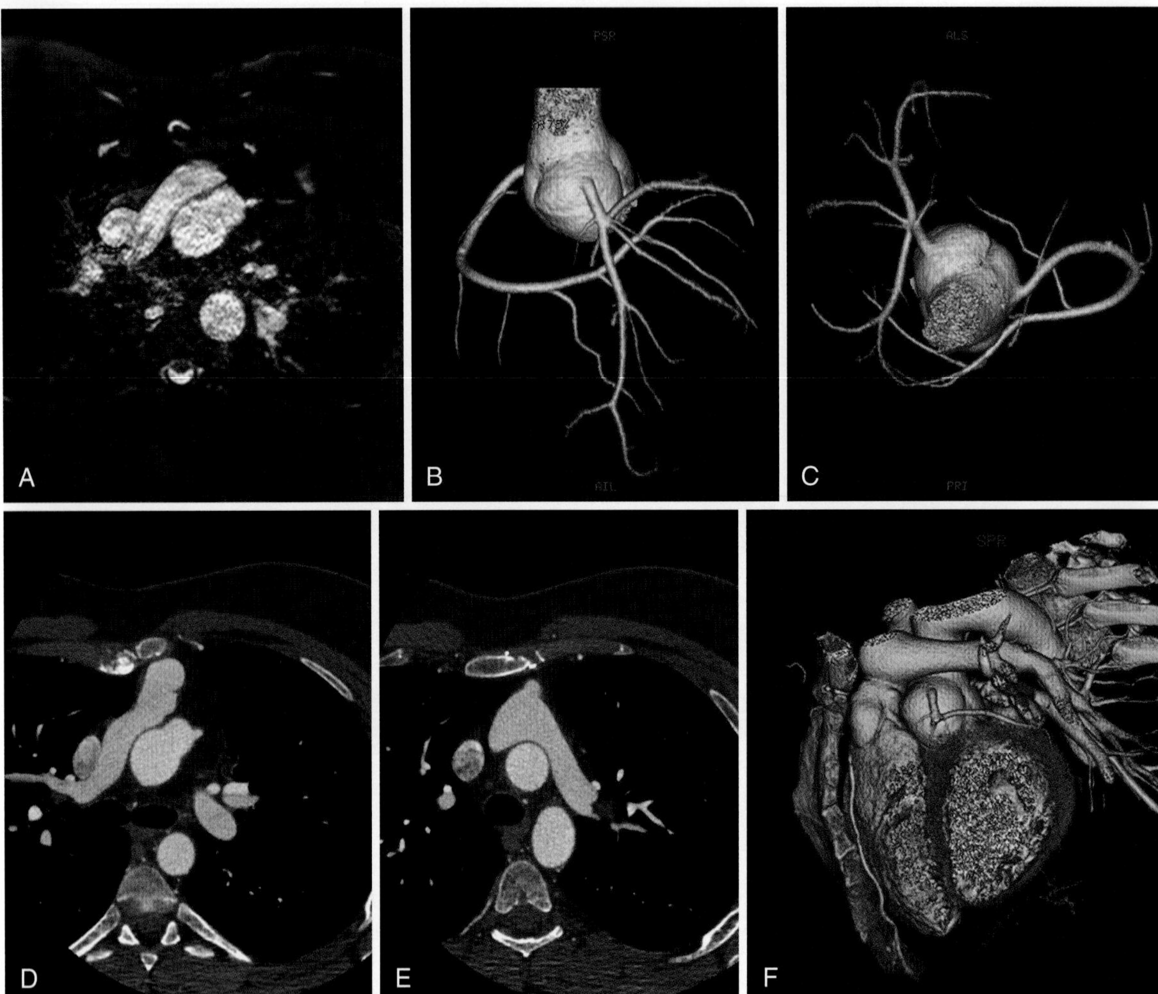

Figure 25-11. Multiple images in a patient with transposition of the great arteries, and a Jatene switch procedure. The patient initially underwent a cardiac MRI study, which suggested that the implanted left coronary artery might be stenosed at its origin (**A**). The patient subsequently underwent a cardiac CT study to evaluate pulmonary and coronary artery anatomy. **B** and **C,** Volume-rendered images demonstrate normal coronary artery origins with no evidence of a right or left coronary artery implantation stenosis. **D** through **F,** Multiple images through the pulmonary arteries. The main pulmonary artery is situated anterior to the aorta, with the central right and left pulmonary arteries draped around the descending aorta. No evidence is seen of a right or left pulmonary arterial stenosis. The main pulmonary artery is mild to moderately narrowed at its anastomosis at the level of the arterial switch procedure (**F**).

- **Extracardiac Fontan**: In this procedure, inferior vena cava blood is directed to the pulmonary artery—usually the right pulmonary artery—via an extracardiac conduit. A Glenn shunt, consisting of a communication from the SVC to the same pulmonary artery [RPA], also may be created.
- **Fenestrated Fontan**: The surgical creation of a hole within the Fontan connection to allow decompression of the Fontan circuit, usually from the Fontan connection into the right atrium. This reduces pressure within the Fontan circuit at the expense of a right-to-left shunt and resultant systemic hypoxemia, and usually is later closed.
- **RA to RV Fontan**: A conduit extends between the right atrium and right ventricle. It is extracardiac in location, and is often valved.
- **Total cavopulmonary connection (TCPC)/lateral tunnel**: In this procedure, inferior vena caval flow is directed a conduit, or baffle, within or lateral to the right atrium, into the superior vena cava. Along the superior margin of the SVC, a bidirectional Glenn shunt is created.

Cardiac CT Protocol Points in Fontan Procedures

- **Coverage:** Lung apices to upper abdomen. Most commonly the study should cover the thorax to include the systemic thoracic veins, due to frequent venous occlusion/stenosis, particularly if a pacemaker is in place. The examination must proceed with arm and leg injections. A femoral line is much preferred over a lower extremity (e.g., foot dorsum) IV.

Text continued on page 432

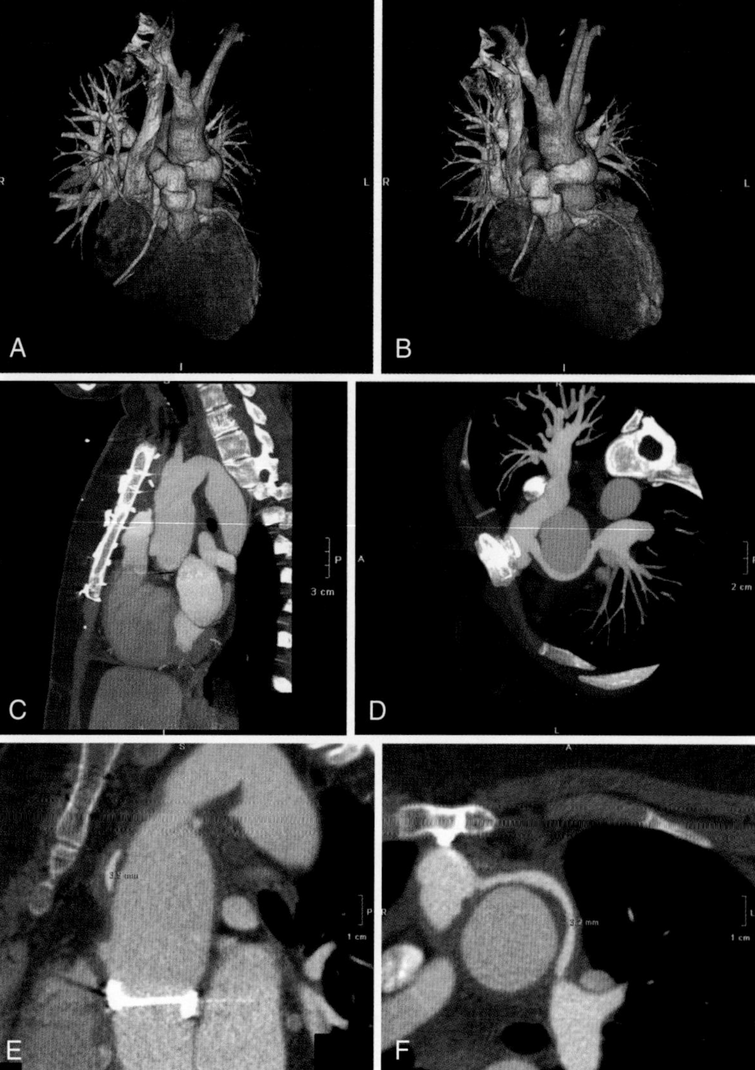

Figure 25-12. Composite image from a cardiac CT study in a patient with transposition of the great vessels, status post–Jatene arterial switch procedure. These images demonstrate one of the complications of this arterial switch procedure. In this procedure, the aorta and main pulmonary arteries are transected at a level above the valve sinuses, and switched. The coronary arteries are removed with a button of tissue, and are reimplanted into the aorta. The residual "buttonholes" in the native aorta (soon to be the main pulmonary artery after the arterial switch) are patched, usually with pericardium. After the surgical procedure the right and left pulmonary arteries have to course around the aorta. This can cause narrowing and kinking of the pulmonary arteries. On the series of images shown here, deformity of the main pulmonary artery segment is seen, likely from prior pericardial patching. This is best visualized in the volume-rendered images, **A** and **B.** There is also marked attenuation and narrowing of the left pulmonary artery as it courses around the aorta and irregularity and indentation of the right pulmonary artery as well. **E** and **F,** Soft tissue thickening around the ribbon-like left pulmonary artery. **See Video 25-3.**

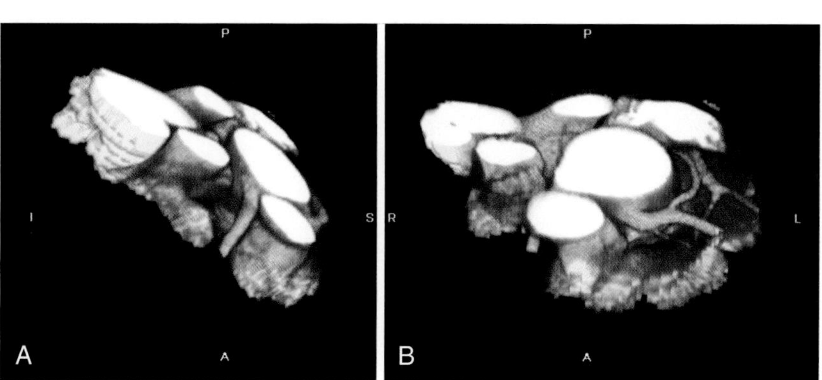

Figure 25-13. Volume-rendered images from a cardiac CT study in a patient with a Jatene arterial switch procedure. As part of the arterial switch procedure, the coronary arteries are removed with a small cuff/button of aortic tissue from the original aorta prior to the arterial switch. Small residual buttonhole defects are then subsequently matched, often with pericardium, because the original aorta will become the main pulmonary artery after the switch procedure is completed. The coronary arteries and their buttonholes are subsequently reimplanted into the aorta. One of the complications of this procedure is the development of coronary arterial stenoses post-reimplantation. These usually occur proximally in the reimplanted coronary arteries. On these images, the right coronary artery (**A**), and the left proximal coronary artery system (**B**) are normal in appearance. **See Video 25-4.**

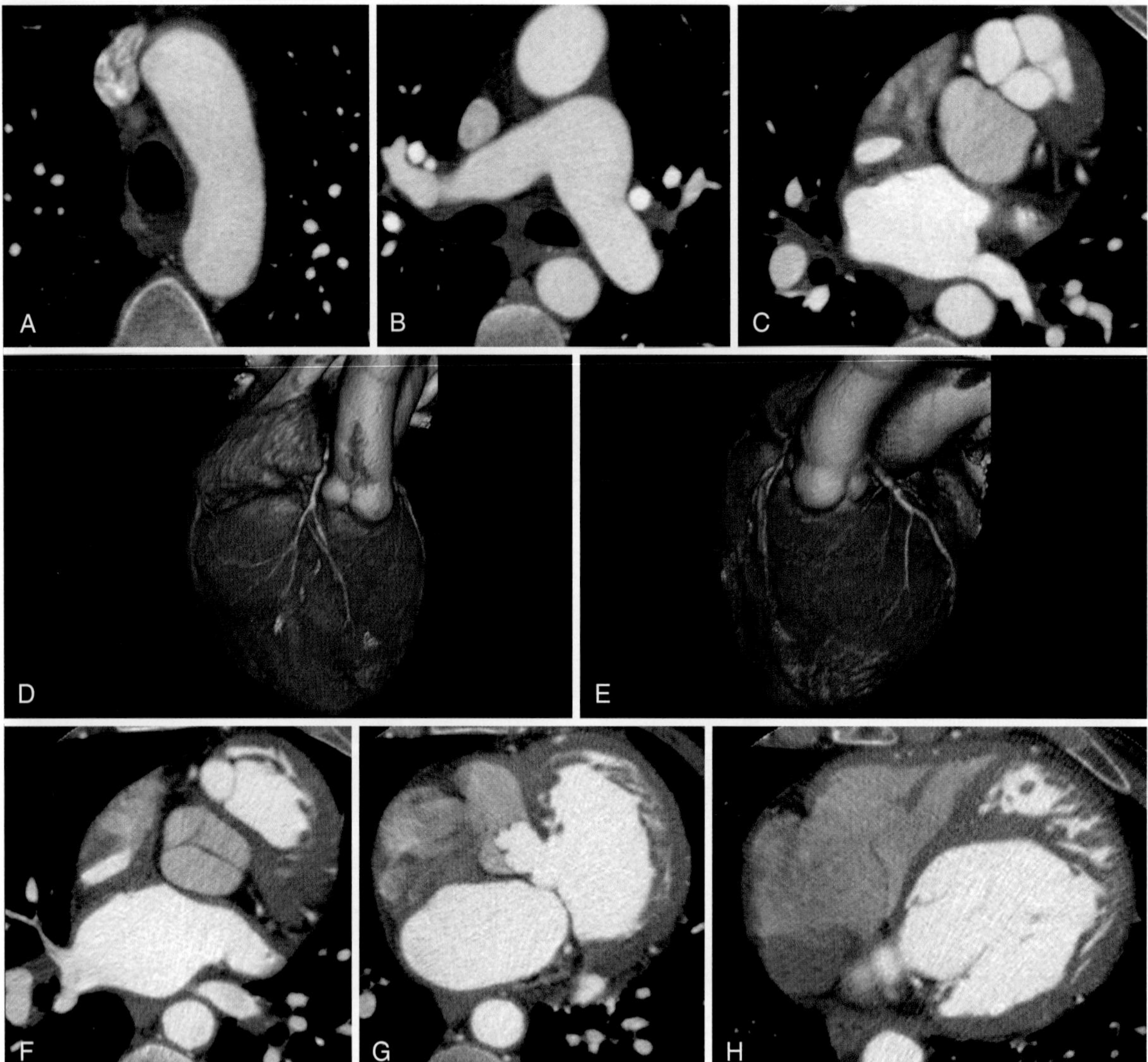

Figure 25-14. Multiple composite images from a cardiac CT examination in a patient with congenitally corrected transposition of the great arteries. There is arterial ventricular discordance, with the aorta arising anteriorly from a muscular conus, and a trabeculated right ventricle. There is ventriculoatrial discordance, with pulmonary venous blood entering into the left atrium, and from the left atrium across the tricuspid valve into the right ventricle. Moderate dilatation of the right/systemic ventricle is present.

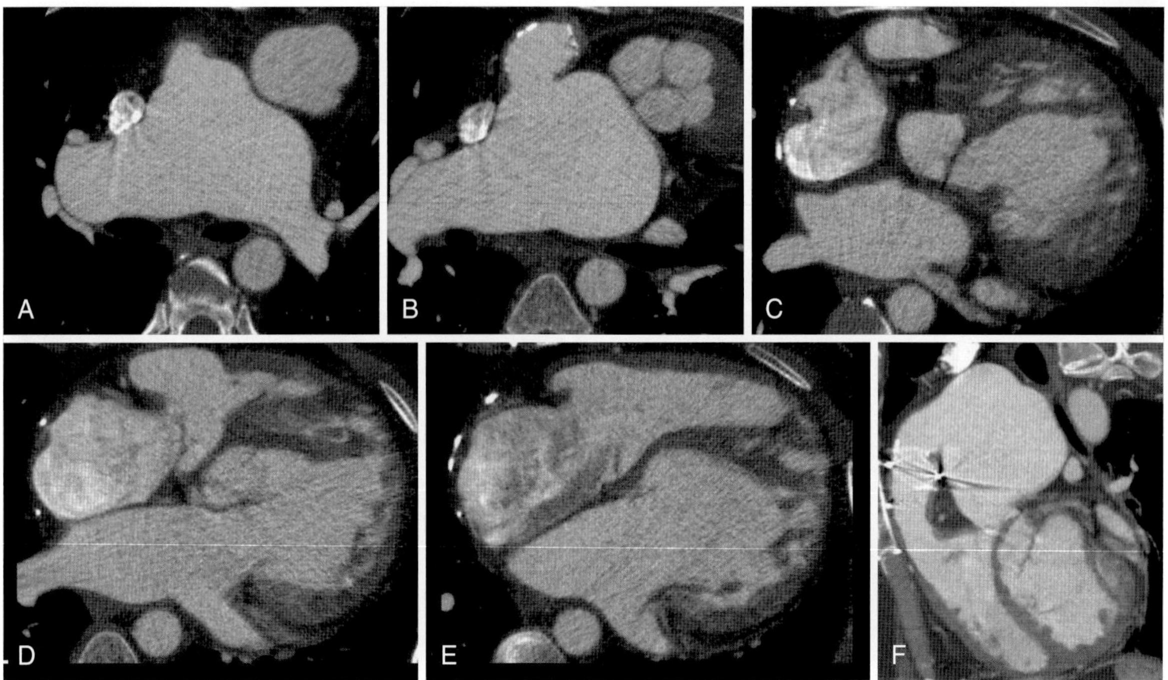

Figure 25-15. Multiple axial and reformatted images from a cardiac CT study in a patient with congenitally corrected transposition. This study focused on an external right ventricular-to-pulmonary artery conduit in a patient with severe subpulmonic right ventricular outflow tract obstruction. The conduit is patent, with aneurysmal enlargement of the main and right pulmonary arteries. There is calcification of the conduit.

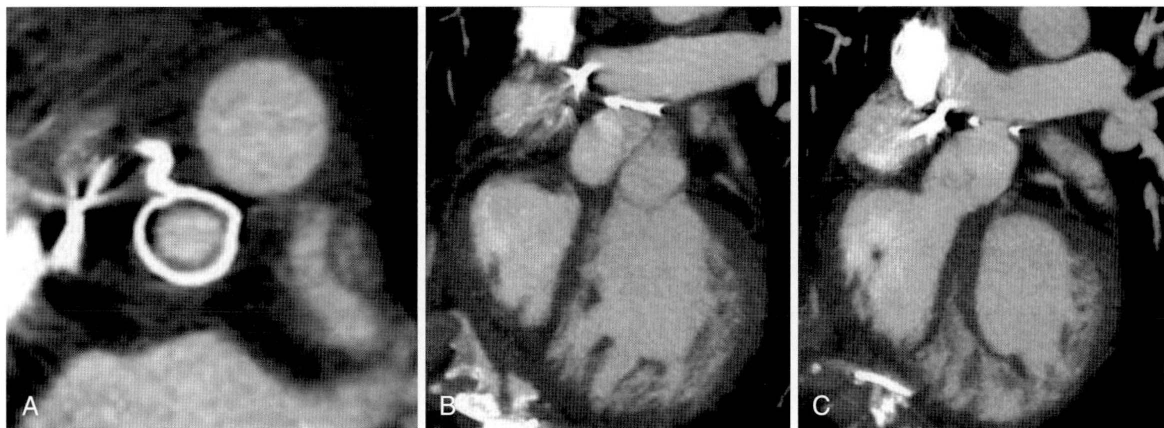

Figure 25-16. Composite images from a cardiac CT study in a patient with d-transposition and pulmonary arterial banding prior to Jatene switch surgery. The pulmonary artery segment is disconnected from the central mediastinal pulmonary arteries. There is a left ventricle-to-pulmonary artery conduit, which is patent and has moderate peripheral calcification. This patient also has had baffling from the superior (SVC) and inferior venae cavae to the systemic venous ventricle. The upper limb of this baffle demonstrated prior stenosis and has subsequently been stented. Pacemaker wires through the SVC baffle into the left ventricle are present. Delayed imaging demonstrates patency of the SVC limb of the baffle.

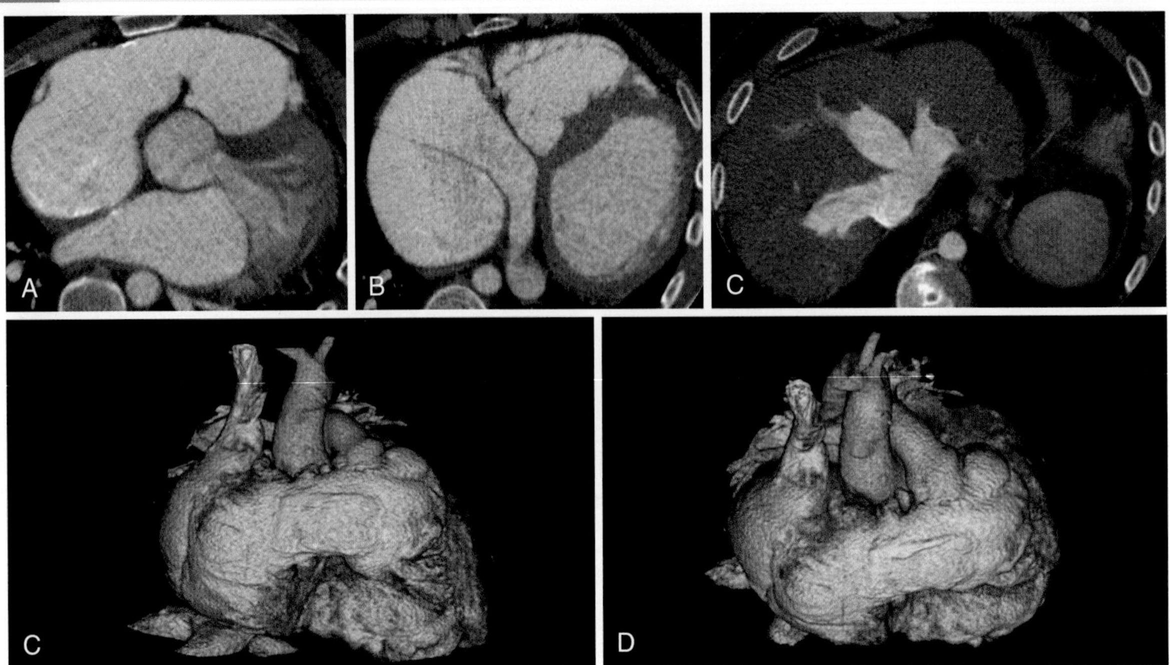

Figure 25-17. Multiple images from a cardiac CT study in a patient with complex congenital heart disease. This patient has underlying tricuspid atresia. There is a modified Fontan shunt, extending from the right atrium to the right ventricle. A small amount of calcification within the conduit is seen. No evidence of thrombus within the shunt is seen. The inferior vena cava is markedly distended, the eustachian valve is large and redundant, and there is marked enlargement of the intrahepatic veins.

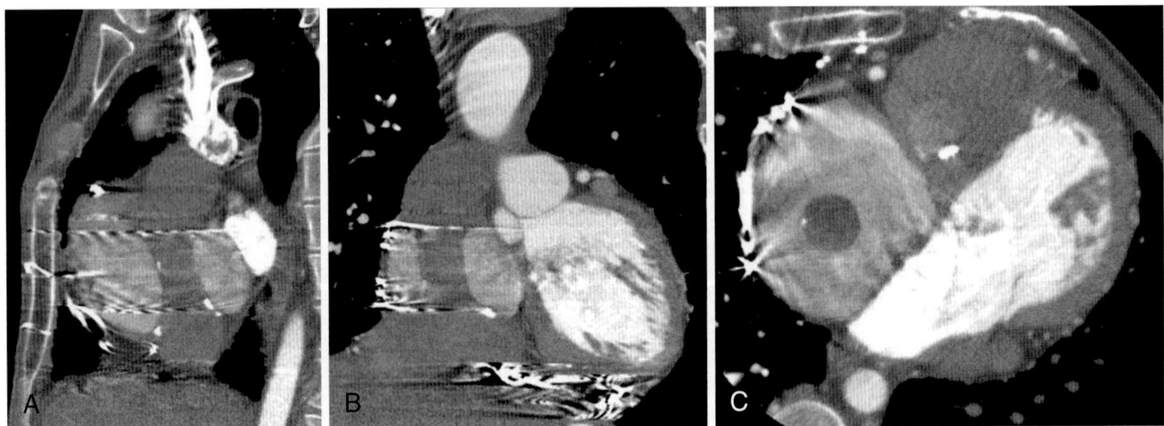

Figure 25-18. Multiple images from a cardiac CT study in an arterial phase in a patient with complex congenital heart disease. This study demonstrates a tubular structure extending within the right atrium in a patient with tricuspid atresia. This represents an intracardiac Fontan conduit extending from the inferior vena cava, through the right atrium, and anastomosing with the right pulmonary artery. A delayed phase is required to evaluate the patency of this conduit.

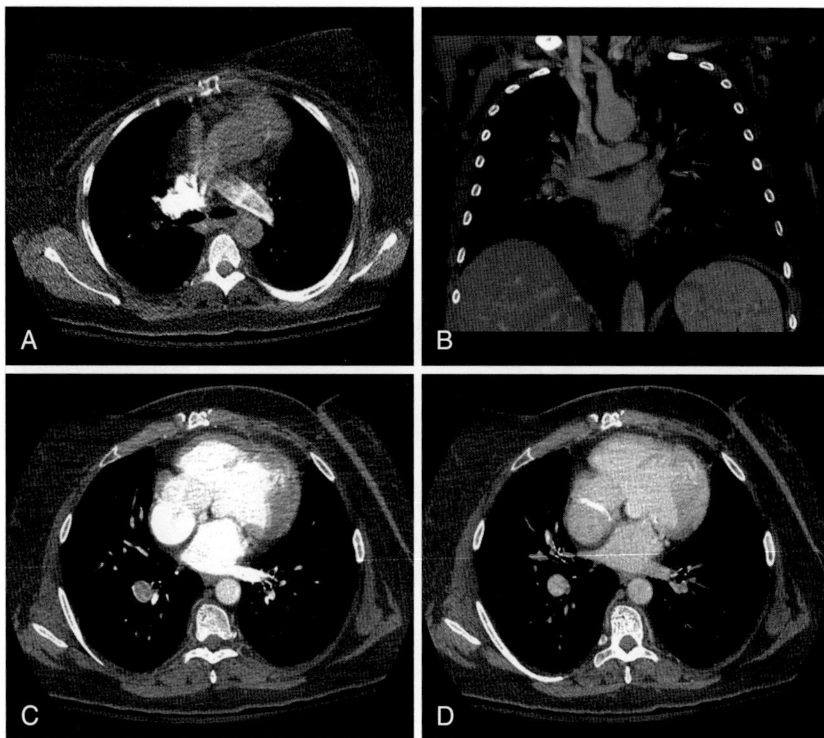

Figure 25-19. Multiple images from a chest CT study in a 52-year-old woman with a history of complex congenital heart disease and a prior Glenn anastomosis with a fenestrated lateral tunnel procedure. The patient presented with progressive shortness of breath and progressive desaturation. This study was performed with simultaneous injection of contrast into the right antecubital vein and the right common femoral vein. A bolus timing acquisition was also obtained from both the right upper extremity injection and the right leg injection, prior to the initial CT angiogram. A 45-second-delayed acquisition through the chest also was subsequently obtained. **A,** Single image obtained from a bolus timing injection from the right upper extremity demonstrates contrast extending into a bidirectional Glenn shunt. Most of the contrast material flows into the right pulmonary artery, but contrast also is seen extending into the left pulmonary artery. **B,** The coronal reconstruction from the delayed acquisition demonstrates mixing of contrast within the pulmonary arterial tree, making evaluation for thromboembolic disease problematic. **C,** An axial image acquired on the first-pass study demonstrates low attenuation within the right lower lobe pulmonary artery. **D,** The delayed study subsequently shows contrast opacification of the right lower lobe pulmonary artery, with no evidence of a filling defect, demonstrating that this is a flow artifact and not an embolism. **See Video 25-5 and 25-6**; **Figure 25-20.**

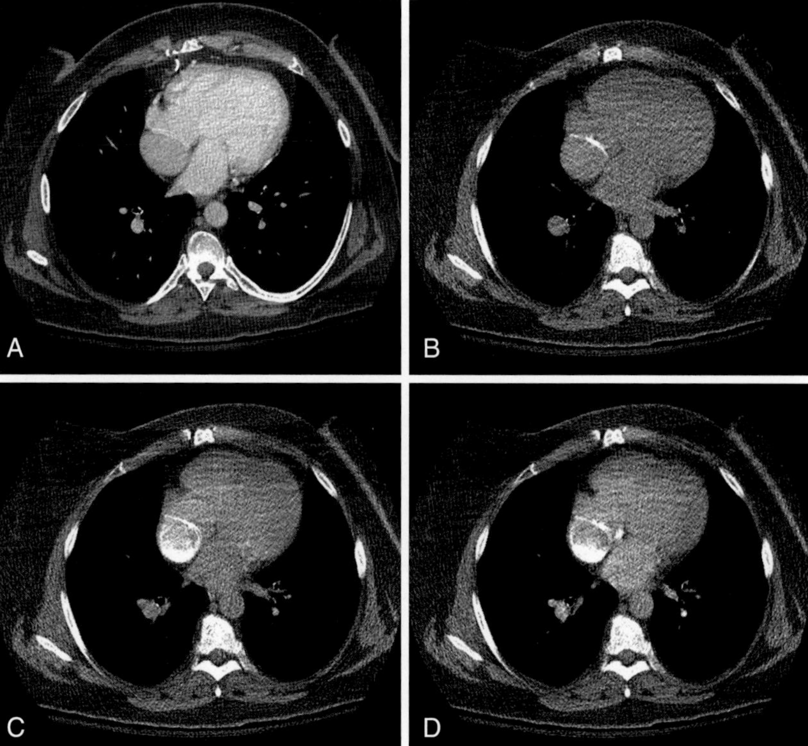

Figure 25-20. Same patient as in Figure 25-19. Multiple low-dose contrast-enhanced CT acquisitions at 2-second intervals have been obtained at the level of the lateral tunnel Fontan during the injection of contrast from the common femoral line. These images demonstrate contrast material entering into the inferior vena and lateral Fontan tunnel. A small amount of contrast medium is seen leaking across the lateral tunnel into the adjacent right atrium. This represents either the residual presence of a prior fenestration, or a leak that has subsequently developed between the lateral tunnel and the adjacent right atrium. This is likely one explanation for the patient's desaturation. **See Video 25-5 and 25-6.**

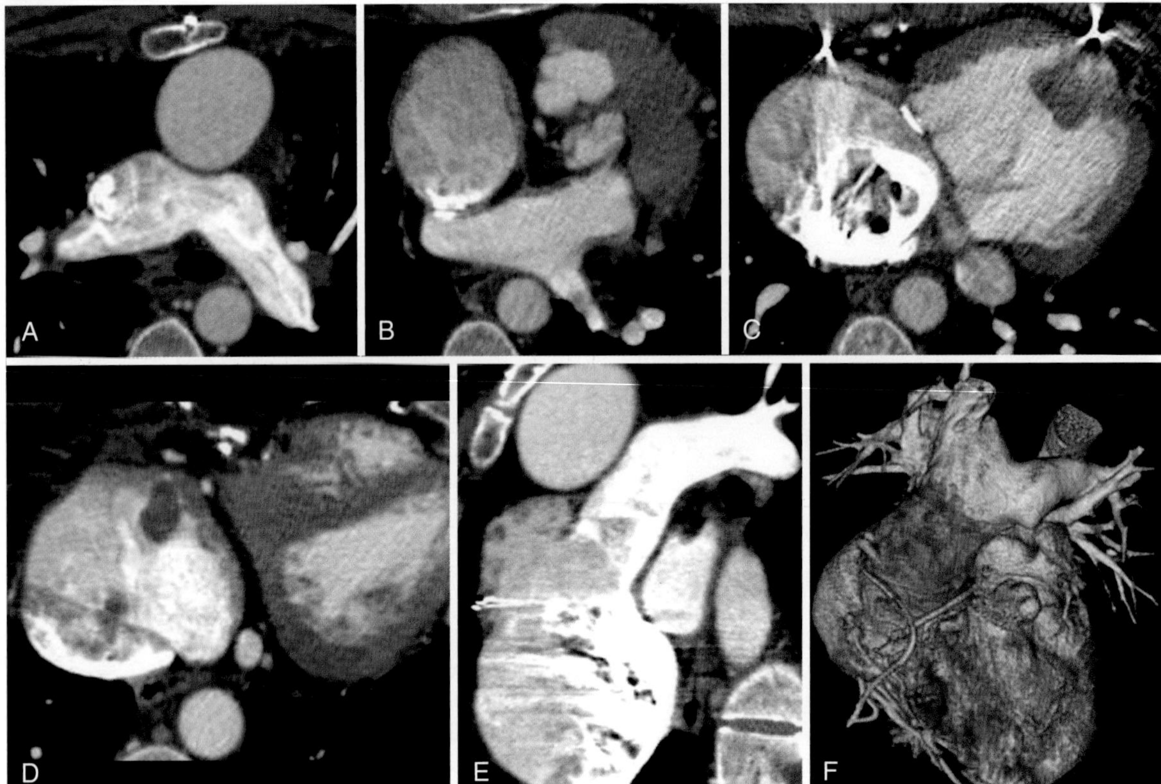

Figure 25-21. Multiple images from a cardiac CT study in a patient with transposition of the great arteries and tricuspid atresia. A Fontan shunt is identified, and is patent. A filling defect within the inferior aspect of the right atrium likely represents a small intra-atrial thrombus. A large ventricular septal defect is noted.

- ❐ **Contrast:** Start of injection: time 0 for arm line with a 5-second delay for the leg line. The leg injected should be elevated 30 to 60 degrees during or at the end of the injection. A dynamic scan should be performed each second through the Fontan connection during injection to monitor arrival of contrast and evaluate for any leaks. The start time of acquisition is at 70 seconds minus the scan time in seconds.
  - Arm line: right arm is preferred over left. Injection of contrast medium is as follows: 3 mL/sec × 20 sec = 60 mL of nondiluted contrast; followed by 2 mL/sec × 50 sec = 100 mL of diluted contrast (50% contrast/50% saline).
  - Leg line: a femoral line preferred over a peripheral line, using either the right or left leg. Injection of contrast medium is as follows: 2 mL/sec × 65 sec = 130 mL. If biphasic injection is possible, then 3 mL/sec × 25 sec = 75 mL, followed by 1 mL/sec × 42 sec = 42 mL.
- ❐ Additional scans: 1 minute delayed scan
- ❐ Post-processing: If RV/LV function assessment is needed, then helical acquisition is obtained with reconstruction of a functional data set.

OTHER COMMONLY PERFORMED SURGICAL REPAIRS

Blalock-Taussig Shunt

The Blalock-Taussig shunt, first successfully performed in 1944 for tetralogy of Fallot, is designed to direct flow from either subclavian artery to the ipsilateral pulmonary artery distal to the stenosis. It can be complicated by stenosis formation at the anastomosis. It is one of the easier systemic pulmonary shunts to correct once it is no longer required (Fig. 25-22).

Rastelli Procedure

The Rastelli procedure is performed in patients with TGA and associated pulmonary outflow tract obstruction and VSD. A baffle is created using the VSD, directing blood through the LVOT to the aorta. The subpulmonic region is oversewn, and an RVOT-to-pulmonary artery conduit is created. This conduit may or may not be valved (Fig. 25-23).

Waterston-Cooley Shunt

The Waterston-Cooley shunt directs flow from the ascending aorta to the right pulmonary artery.

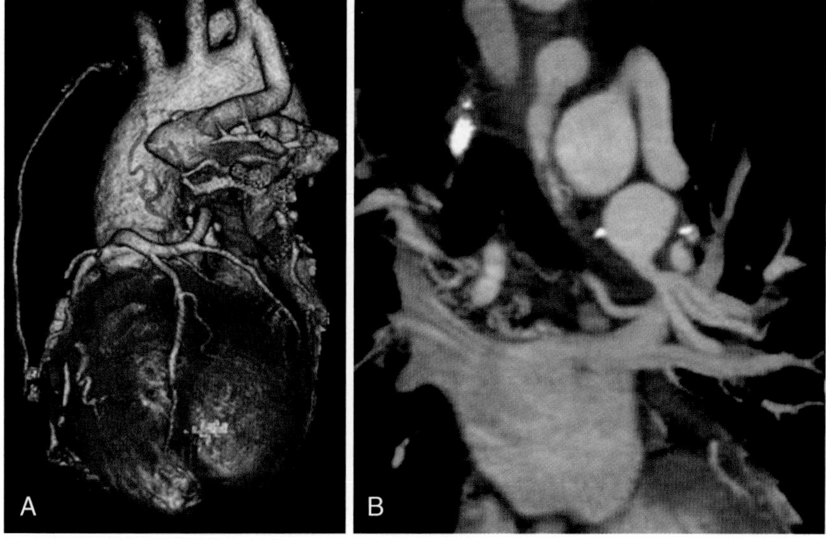

Figure 25-22. A patient with type IV truncus arteriosus who had previously undergone a modified left Blalock-Taussig shunt with a unifocalization procedure of aortopulmonary collaterals.

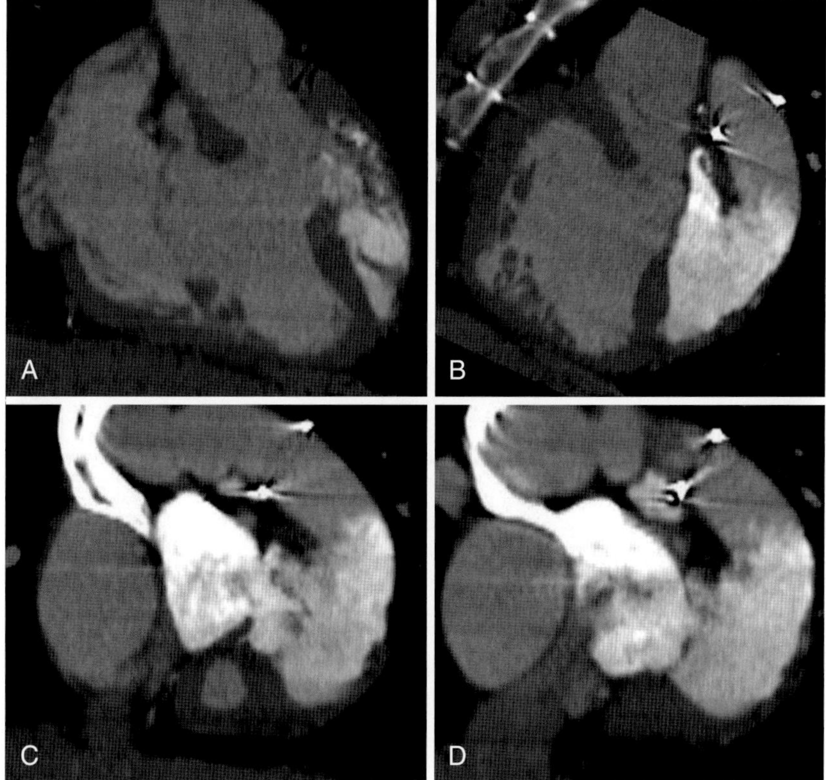

Figure 25-23. Multiple images from a cardiac CT study in a patient with transposition of the great arteries and subpulmonic obstruction. There has been interval surgical correction with a Rastelli procedure (right ventricular outflow tract to pulmonary artery conduit) that is valved. The conduit is well demonstrated and patent on this study. The superior baffle and inferior baffles are patent. The systemic venous return is directed to the mitral valve, out the right ventricular outflow tract conduit, and into the main pulmonary artery.

TABLE 25-1 ACCF 2010 Appropriateness Criteria for the Use of Cardiac Computed Tomography to Evaluate Adult Congenital Heart Disease

APPROPRIATENESS RATING	INDICATION	MEDIAN SCORE
Appropriate	Assessment of anomalies of coronary arterial and other thoracic arteriovenous vessels	9
	Assessment of complex adult congenital heart disease	8
	Quantitative evaluation of right ventricular function	7
Uncertain	None listed	
Inappropriate	None listed	

Data from Taylor AJ, Cerqueira M, Hodgson JM, et al. ACCF/SCCT/ACR/AHA/ASE/ASNC/NASCI/SCAI/SCMR 2010 appropriate use criteria for cardiac computed tomography. A report of the American College of Cardiology Foundation Appropriate Use Criteria Task Force, the Society of Cardiovascular Computed Tomography, the American College of Radiology, the American Heart Association, the American Society of Echocardiography, the American Society of Nuclear Cardiology, the North American Society for Cardiovascular Imaging, the Society for Cardiovascular Angiography and Interventions, and the Society for Cardiovascular Magnetic Resonance. *J Am Coll Cardiol.* 2010;56(22):1864-1894.

The size of the shunt is of prime importance, because too large a shunt will cause pulmonary edema.

Pott's Shunt

Pott's shunt, first described in 1945, is used primarily for treating tricuspid atresia. The shunt directs flow from the descending aorta to the left pulmonary artery. One advantage of this shunt is that it avoids the potential for kinking and obstruction of the arterial segment as in the Blalock-Taussig shunt. However, this shunt is the most difficult to correct once the underlying anomaly has been corrected.

Bilateral Glenn Shunts

The Glenn shunt is a palliative procedure performed to increase pulmonary blood flow. A direct connection between the SVC and the pulmonary artery—usually between a right SVC and the right pulmonary artery—is created. A common complication of the Glenn shunt is the development of pulmonary AVMs and associated systemic arterial desaturation. In the setting of bilateral SVCs, bilateral Glenn shunts are created, usually from the right SVC to the right PA and the left SVC to the left PA.

References

1. Samyn MM. A review of the complementary information available with cardiac magnetic resonance imaging and multi-slice computed tomography (CT) during the study of congenital heart disease. *Int J Cardiovasc Imaging.* 2004;20(6):569-578.
2. Aggarwala G, Thompson B, van Beek E, Jagasia D. Multislice computed tomography angiography of Ebstein anomaly and anomalous coronary artery. *J Cardiovasc Comput Tomogr.* 2007;1(3):168-169.
3. Saremi F, Gurudevan SV, Narula J, Abolhoda A. Multidetector computed tomography (MDCT) in diagnosis of "cor triatriatum sinister.". *J Cardiovasc Comput Tomogr.* 2007;1(3):172-174.
4. Cook SC, Raman SV. Multidetector computed tomography in the adolescent and young adult with congenital heart disease. *J Cardiovasc Comput Tomogr.* 2008;2(1):36-49.
5. Inglessis I. Editorial: Which diagnostic test modality for adult congenital heart disease? *J Cardiovasc Comput Tomogr.* 2007;2:23-25.
6. Hirsch R, Kilner PJ, Connelly MS, Redington AN, St John Sutton MG, Somerville J. Diagnosis in adolescents and adults with congenital heart disease. Prospective assessment of individual and combined roles of magnetic resonance imaging and transesophageal echocardiography. *Circulation.* 1994;90(6):2937-2951.
7. Achenbach S, Dittrich S, Kuettner A. Anomalous left anterior descending coronary artery in a pediatric patient with Fallot tetralogy. *J Cardiovasc Comput Tomogr.* 2008;2:55-56.
8. Park SC, Neches WH, Mathews RA, et al. Hemodynamic function after the Mustard operation for transposition of the great arteries. *Am J Cardiol.* 1983;51(9):1514-1519.
9. Bonhoeffer P, Bonnet D, Piechaud JF, et al. Coronary artery obstruction after the arterial switch operation for transposition of the great arteries in newborns. *J Am Coll Cardiol.* 1997;29(1):202-206.
10. Fontan F, Baudet E. Surgical repair of tricuspid atresia. *Thorax.* 1971;26(3):240-248.
11. Magee AG, McCrindle BW, Mawson J, Benson LN, Williams WG, Freedom RM. Systemic venous collateral development after the bidirectional cavopulmonary anastomosis. Prevalence and predictors. *J Am Coll Cardiol.* 1998;32(2):502-508.

26 Aortic Diseases

Key Points

- CT scanning is the dominant imaging test for the assessment of acute aortic diseases.
- Without ECG-gating, motion artifacts are still a problem for assessment of the ascending aorta and root; ECG-gating obviates such artifacts and provides superlative imaging detail for what was formerly a problem area for CT imaging.
- Knowledge of the range of aortic lesions and their complications is imperative.

CT scanning has emerged as the de facto test of choice for the identification of diseases of the aorta. As a result of its widespread and 24-hour availability, its suitability to evaluate critically ill patients (as long as they can be moved), and the appropriateness of its spatial and temporal resolution to the needs of most aortic pathologies, CT scanning has become the principal test for the evaluation of diseases of the aorta.[1,2] Although CT scanning is the leading test to diagnose structural disease of the aorta, it is less able to diagnose the functional consequences of such disease. Often, therefore, CT scanning is combined with another modality to establish both the anatomic and functional disturbances of aortic disease. For example, although both CT scanning and echocardiography are strong tests to identify dissection of the aorta, most patients are managed with both, because CT identifies a far greater extent of the aorta than echocardiography does, but echocardiography is better for identifying cardiac complications (e.g., aortic insufficiency, cardiac tamponade and myocardial ischemia). Integrated imaging strategies remain the most clinically solid approach.

The only issues limiting the use of CT are the risks of radiation and of contrast-related renal insufficiency. To reduce the risks of radiation where they are most harmful, therefore, evaluation of aortic congenital malformations (such as coarctation) in very young patients is performed by magnetic resonance imaging or angiography (MRI/MRA).

Sixteen-slice CCT was already such a powerful modality for the diagnosis of the structural aspects of aortic disease that the improvements that occurred as 40- and 64-slice CCT were developed to assess cardiac (coronary) disease only enhanced CCT's dominance. Imaging techniques that struggle with coronary artery imaging are generally more successful with aortic imaging because the aorta is almost a logarithm greater in size and is subject to less motion than the coronary arteries.

Normal thoracic aortic diameters overall and by gender are presented in Table 26-1.

CT ARTIFACTS AND AORTIC DISEASES

Although CT is the principal diagnostic test for diseases of the aorta, CT artifacts may confound assessment of aortic diseases. The older the CT scanner, the greater the number of artifacts (at least half of CT studies on scanners from 1999 or earlier have significant artifacts over the ascending aorta).

Potentially problematic artifacts include:

- ❒ Streak artifacts off the brachiocephalic vein (from contrast), confounding assessment of the aortic arch behind it
- ❒ Streak artifacts off the superior vena cava (from contrast or pacer wires), confounding assessment of the ascending aorta beside it
- ❒ Streak artifacts off the spine, confounding assessment of the descending aorta beside it
- ❒ Older scanners (slow, or without cardiac gating) may generate "pulsation" artifacts of superimposed images of the aorta in different positions due to translation from cardiac motion, conferring the impression of an intimal flap. There is almost 1 cm of translational motion of the ascending aorta through the cardiac cycle.
- ❒ Motion artifacts
- ❒ See Figure 26-1.

ATHEROSCLEROTIC CALCIFICATION

Atherosclerotic plaques in the aorta are extremely common. The two sites most often involved are the abdominal aorta and the distal floor of the arch. Although there is general correlation between the extent of aortic and coronary atherosclerosis, many

TABLE 26-1 Normal Thoracic Aortic Diameters Overall and by Gender

	OVERALL (n = 103), MEAN (SD)	WOMEN (n = 44), MEAN (SD)	MEN (n = 59), MEAN (SD)	P VALUE
Aortic Root				
Diameter, short-axis ED (cm)	3.1 (0.3)	2.9 (0.2)	3.2 (0.3)	<.001
Area, short-axis ED (cm^2)	7.9 (1.6)	6.9 (1.4)	8.5 (1.7)	<.001
Ascending Aorta				
Diameter, short-axis ED (cm)	2.8 (0.4)	2.8 (0.4)	2.8 (0.3)	.61
Diameter, short-axis ES (cm)	3.0 (0.3)	2.9 (0.4)	3.0 (0.3)	.40
Diameter, axial ES (cm)	3.0 (0.3)	3.0 (0.4)	3.1 (0.3)	.46
Descending Thoracic Aorta				
Diameter, short-axis ED (cm)	2.1 (0.2)	2.0 (0.2)	2.2 (0.2)	.005
Diameter, short-axis ES (cm)	2.2 (0.2)	2.2 (0.2)	2.3 (0.2)	.011
Diameter, axial ES (cm)	2.3 (0.2)	2.1 (0.1)	2.3 (0.3)	<.001

ED, end-diastolic; ES, end-systolic.
Data from Lin FY, Devereux RB, Roman MJ, et al. Assessment of the thoracic aorta by multidetector computed tomography: age- and sex-specific reference values in adults without evident cardiovascular disease. *J Cardiovasc Comput Tomogr.* 2008;2(5):298-308.

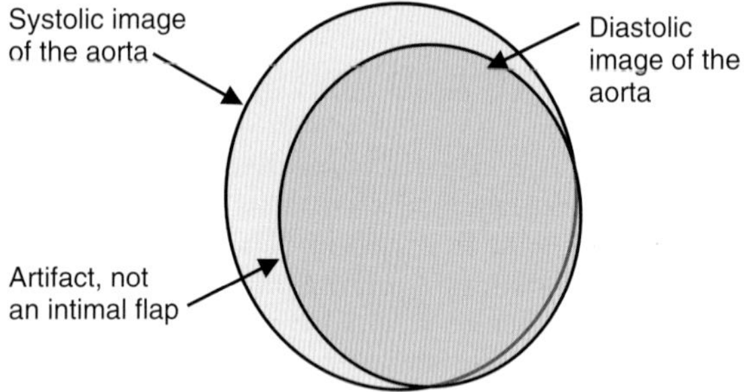

Figure 26-1. The systolic motion (translation and pulsation) of the aorta on non–ECG-gated imaging may render a superimposition image artifact to suggest an intimal flap.

patients will have small flecks of aortic calcification without having significant coronary disease.

Intimal calcification is a marker of intimal position. "Intimal displacement" (into the lumen) is a convenient sign of mural thickening due to either occurrence of a false lumen within the wall of the aorta or development of intramural hematoma. If there is thickening over (i.e., on the luminal side of) intimal calcification, it usually is from thrombus, particularly if the aorta is dilated at that site.

For images of calcification of the aorta, see Figures 26-2 and 26-3.

AORTIC DISSECTION

CT is the principal modality used to diagnose acute aortic dissection (AAD).[3] CCT has emerged as the initial diagnostic modality to identify or exclude AAD by virtue of:

- Imaging both the thoracic and abdominal aorta (vs. echocardiography), which has far more limited field-of-view
- Its speed (vs. MRI)
- Its very high degree of accuracy (vs. angiography)
- Its ability to image the majority of side branches (vs. echocardiography)
- Its ability to image important variants of dissection such as intramural hematoma (vs. angiography)
- The fact that most referring physicians are comfortably familiar with it

Studies comparing CT to other modalities were numerous 12 to 15 years ago; however, few studies have been done involving the current generation of CT equipment. Studies from a decade ago cannot depict the relative accuracy of any test that has developed as much as CCT has in the past 5 years. To further complicate comparisons, TEE and MRI also have evolved over the last decade.

Findings of aortic dissection that CCT is able to image include:

- Intimal flap
- False lumen. The false lumen generally arises off the outer curvature of the aorta (as the tear is usually located on the outside curvature).
- Thrombosis within the false lumen (suggests/consistent with chronicity or healing)
- Entry tear. The two most common sites of entry tears are 2 cm above the aortic valve and 1 cm distal to the left subclavian artery.
- Exit (re-entry) tear
- Pleural effusion
- Pericardial effusion
- Mediastinal hematoma
- Branch vessel involvement. The finding that a branch vessel arises from the false lumen does not establish that its vascular bed is underperfused, only that it is jeopardized. One of the few signs of vascular bed hypoperfusion that is clinically

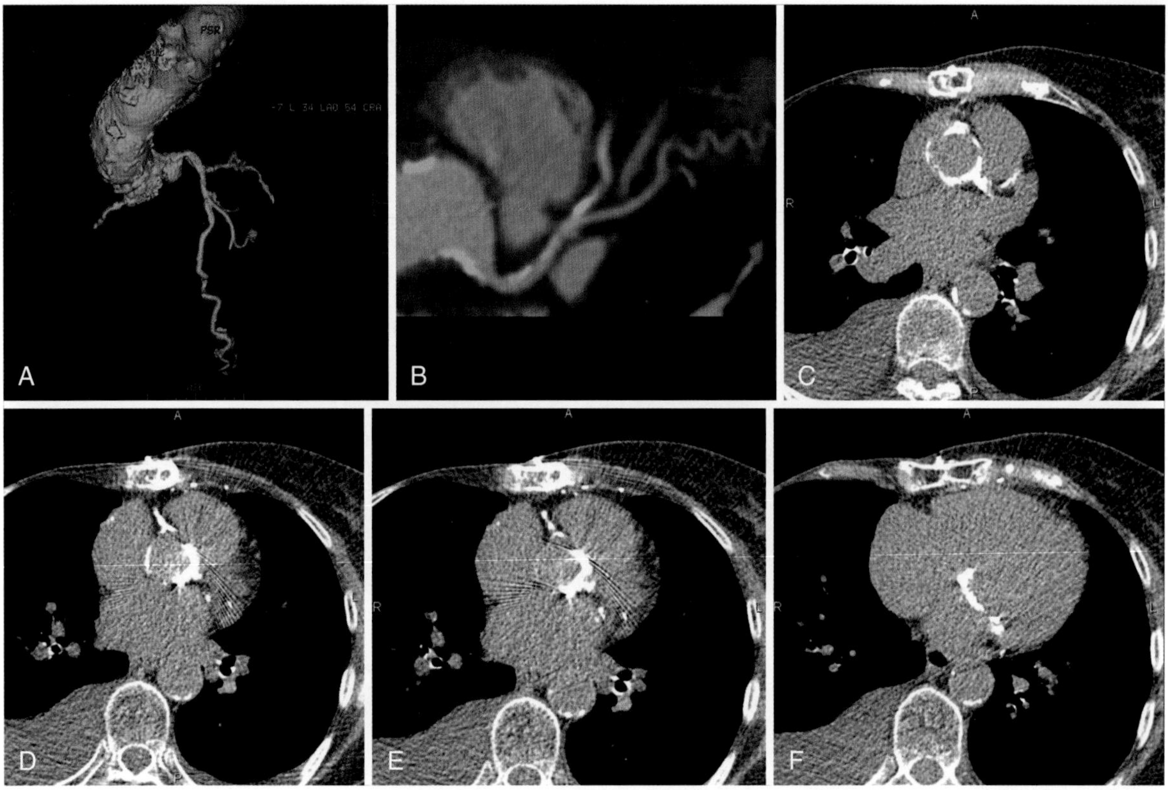

Figure 26-2. Porcelain aorta—unclampable in the ascending segment. **A,** Three-dimensional volume-rendered image of the aortic root and ascending aorta reveals extensive contiguous and circumferential calcification of the aorta well into the ascending portion. Above that, the calcification is spotty. **B,** Calcification at the ostium of the left main stem coronary artery and in a plaque in the left anterior descending artery. All the coronary arteries had extensive "hard" plaques. **C** and **D,** Non–contrast-enhanced axial CT images reveal nearly circumferential calcification of the aortic root and calcification down the proximal left coronary artery (**C**) and down the proximal right coronary artery (**D**). **E** and **F**, Extensive aortic valve and annular calcification (**E**) and mitral annular calcification (**F**).

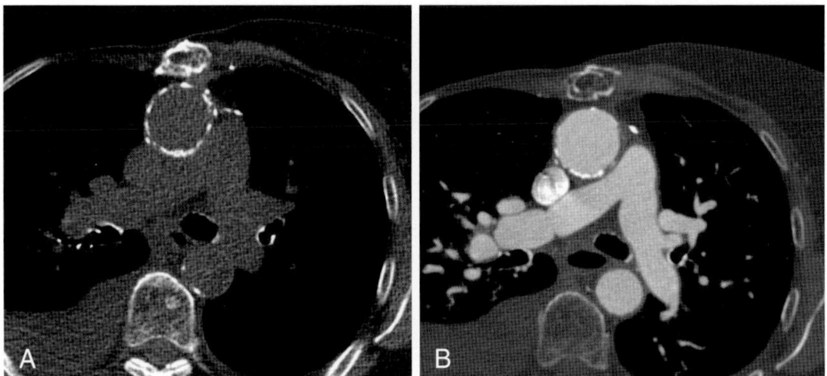

Figure 26-3. Cardiac CT images of a 78-year-old man being assessed for a redo coronary artery bypass graft (CABG). **A,** The precontrast image demonstrates extensive—almost circumferential—calcification around the ascending aorta. This configuration can be termed a *porcelain aorta.* **B,** Administration of intravenous contrast somewhat decreases the conspicuity of the underlying extensive aortic calcification. An evaluation of the extent of calcification and atherosclerotic disease of the ascending aorta is available to the cardiothoracic surgeon in the planning of the patient's redo CABG by noncontrast CT scanning.

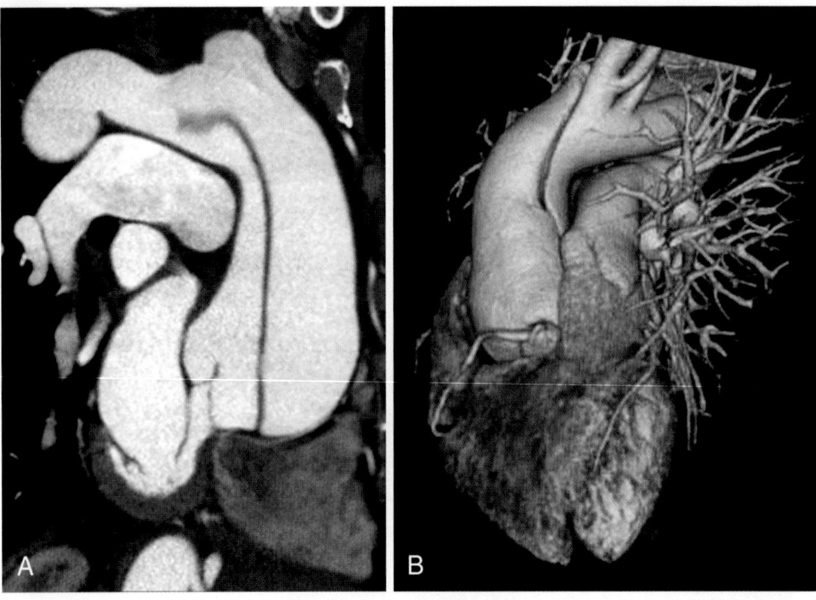

Figure 26-4. Composite images from a cardiac CT study in a patient with Marfan syndrome demonstrate a type A dissection with an associated ascending aortic aneurysm. No extension of this flap into either coronary artery was present.

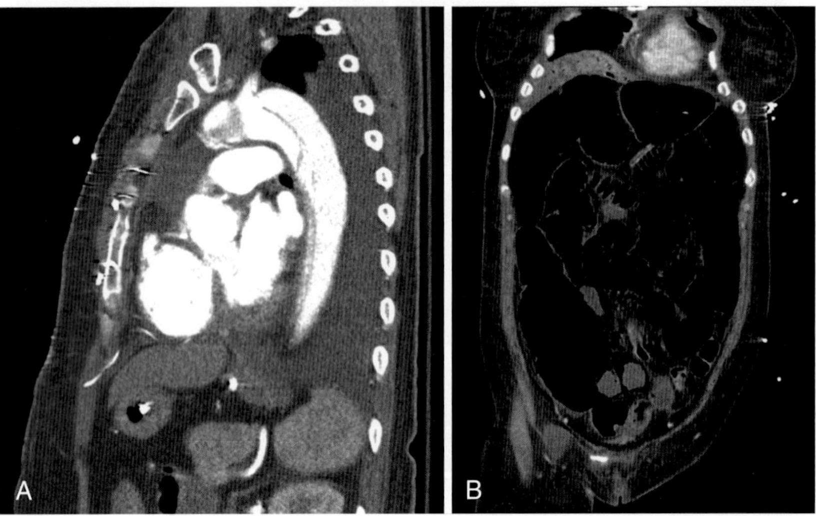

Figure 26-5. **A,** The left sagittal view displays an intimal tear immediately distal to the left subclavian artery, and a flap extending distally. There are sternal wires from a recent aortocoronary bypass grafting operation. **B,** The right coronal abdominal view reveals gross distention with air, due to mesenteric ischemia malperfusion from the dissection flap.

supported is that of pallor of the kidneys during a contrast-enhanced scan.

- Coronary artery involvement, especially if ECG gating is employed

The diagnosis of a dissection is made when an intimal flap is identified. Lack of thrombosis within the false lumen supports acuity of the dissection, while thrombosis supports chronicity.

Potential false positives that may occur include streak artifact from residual contrast in the SVC across the ascending aorta appearing as linear artifact masquerading as an intimal flap. The linearity of the line artifact across the ascending aorta, the presence of multiple lines, the presence of nearby bright lines, and the traversing of tissue planes by the lines indicate that these are artifact. Intimal flaps are not straight in their entirety.

CCT is the most commonly used modality for following aortic diameter in patients with aortic dissection in the chronic phase and is able to identify progressive enlargement as well as persistence of flow in the false lumen.[4] Aortic diameter of type B (distal) dissection cases increases in 37% of cases with a thrombosed false lumen and in 90% of cases with a persistent false lumen. Growth rate has been noted to be 4 ± 7 mm/year in the ascending aorta, 2 ± 9 mm/year in the arch, and 1 ± 6 mm/year in the descending aorta.[5]

For images of acute aortic dissection, see Figures 26-4 through 26-13 and **Video 26-1.**

Text continued on page 443

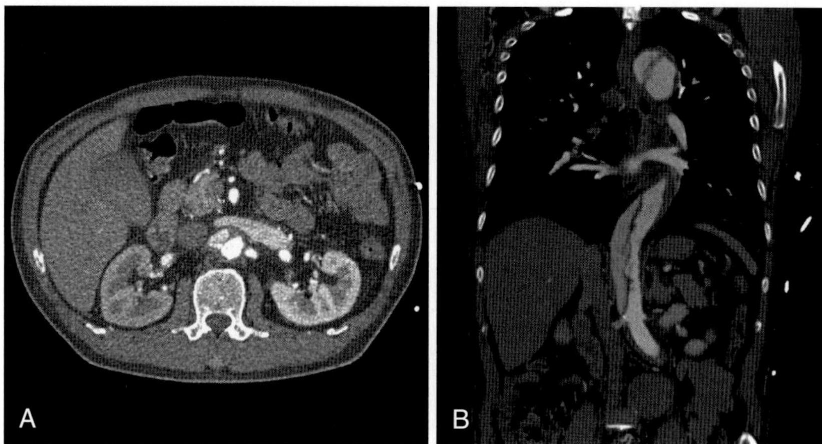

Figure 26-6. Acute type B aortic dissection with protracted hypertensive crisis. The intimal flap can be seen to the right renal ostium and may continue past the calcified plaque into the proximal renal artery. The right kidney enhances less than the left one. The diagnosis was renal ischemia and refractory hypertension.

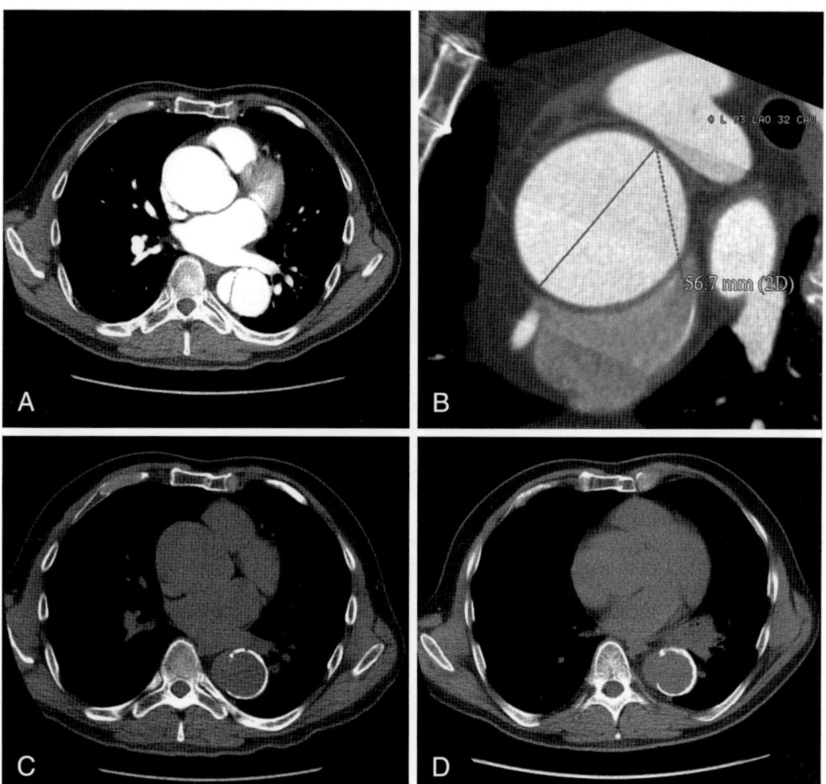

Figure 26-7. Aneurysm of the ascending aorta in chronic type B/distal dissection of the aorta. Note the extensive calcification of the free wall of the false lumen of the type B dissection, which is perfectly seen on the noncontrast images (**C**, **D**) and poorly seen on the contrast-enhanced images (**A**).

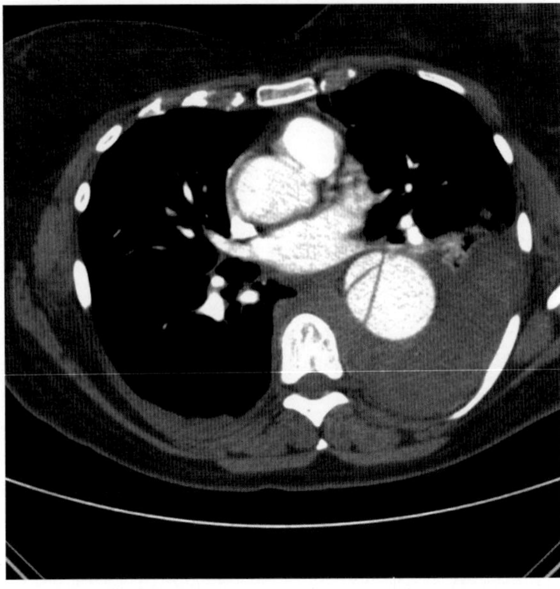

Figure 26-8. Triple lumen: a "triple-barreled" aorta due to recurrent dissection of the aorta. Note the pleural effusion, which was hemorrhagic.

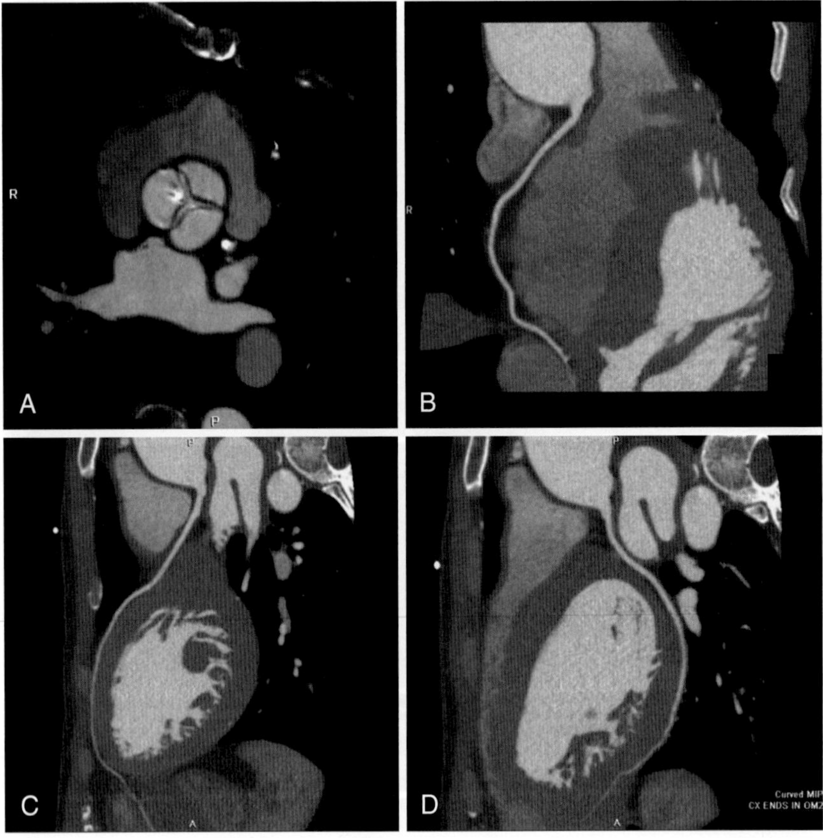

Figure 26-9. A 44-year-old man with severe aortic stenosis. This study was done preoperatively prior to aortic valve surgery to rule out any underlying significant coronary artery disease. **A,** Moderate aortic valve thickening, calcification, and restriction of the aortic valve leaflets. Curved multiplanar reformations through the right coronary artery (**B**), left anterior descending artery (**C**), and circumflex/OM1 (**D**) are normal.

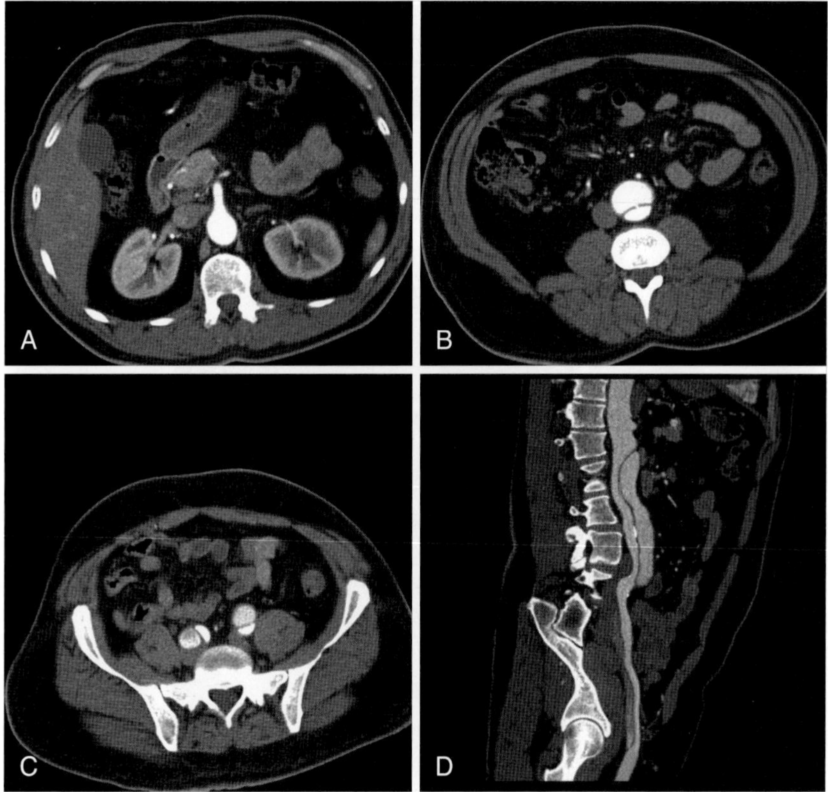

Figure 26-10. An abdominal level–only type B dissection, in a patient with a family history of the same.

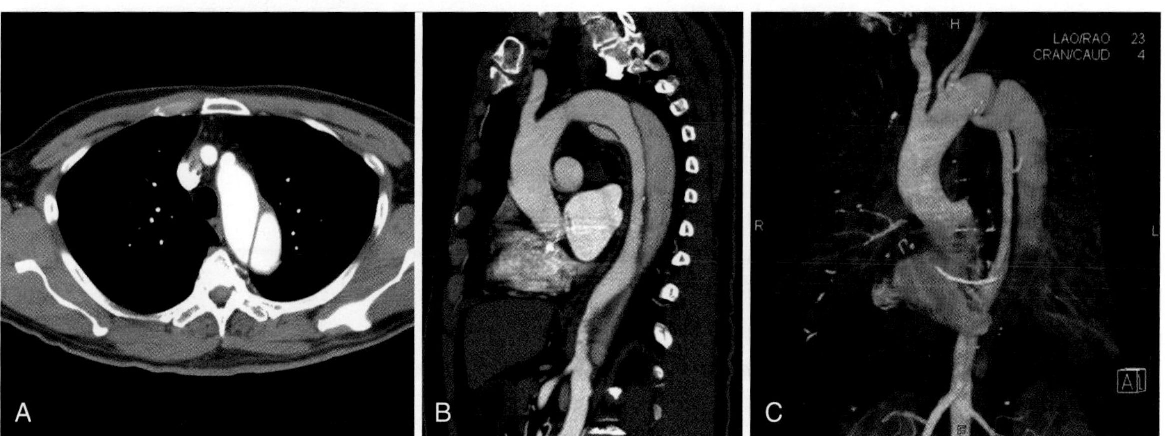

Figure 26-11. Contrast-enhanced CT aortography images of a patient with a chronic type B aortic dissection. The intimal flap is well visualized because it has become stiff and immobile.

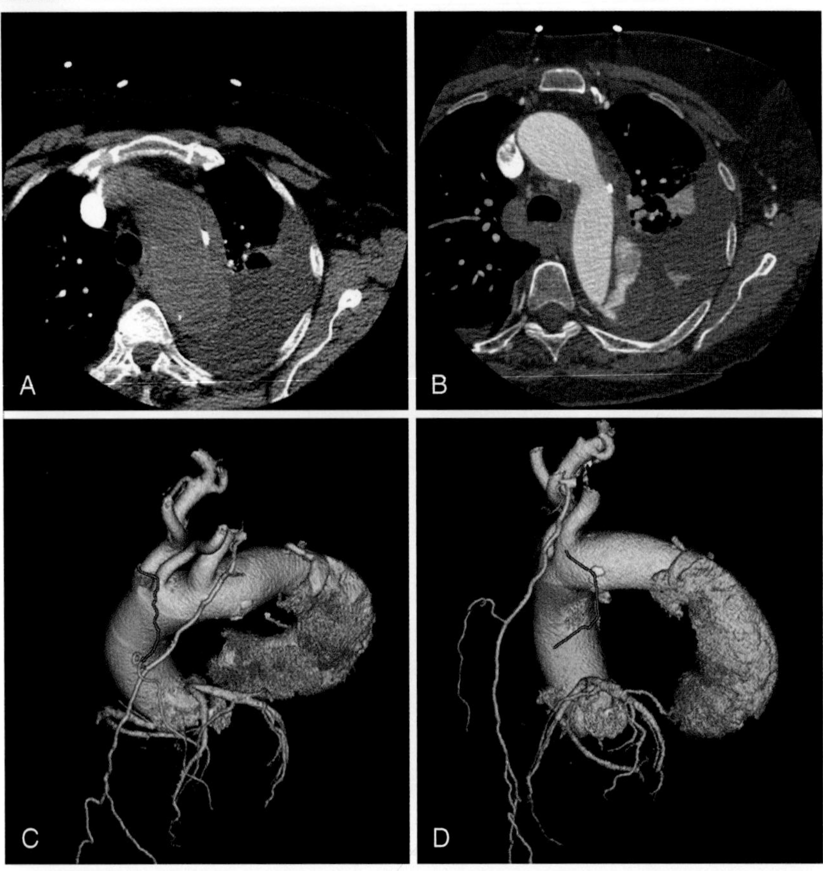

Figure 26-12. Non-contrast and contrast-enhanced CT scan images of a patient with a chronic type B aortic dissection. **A,** Non-contrast axial image reveals intimal displacement by the false lumen, marked by the inward displacement of calcified intimal plaques, and indicating either aortic dissection or intramural hematoma. **B,** Contrast-enhanced axial image at the lower arch level reveals intimal displacement, an intimal flap, an entry intimal tear in the proximal descending aorta, as well as partial thrombosis of the false lumen. **C** and **D,** Three-dimensional volume-rendered images of the irregularities of the distal false lumen. See **Video 26-1.**

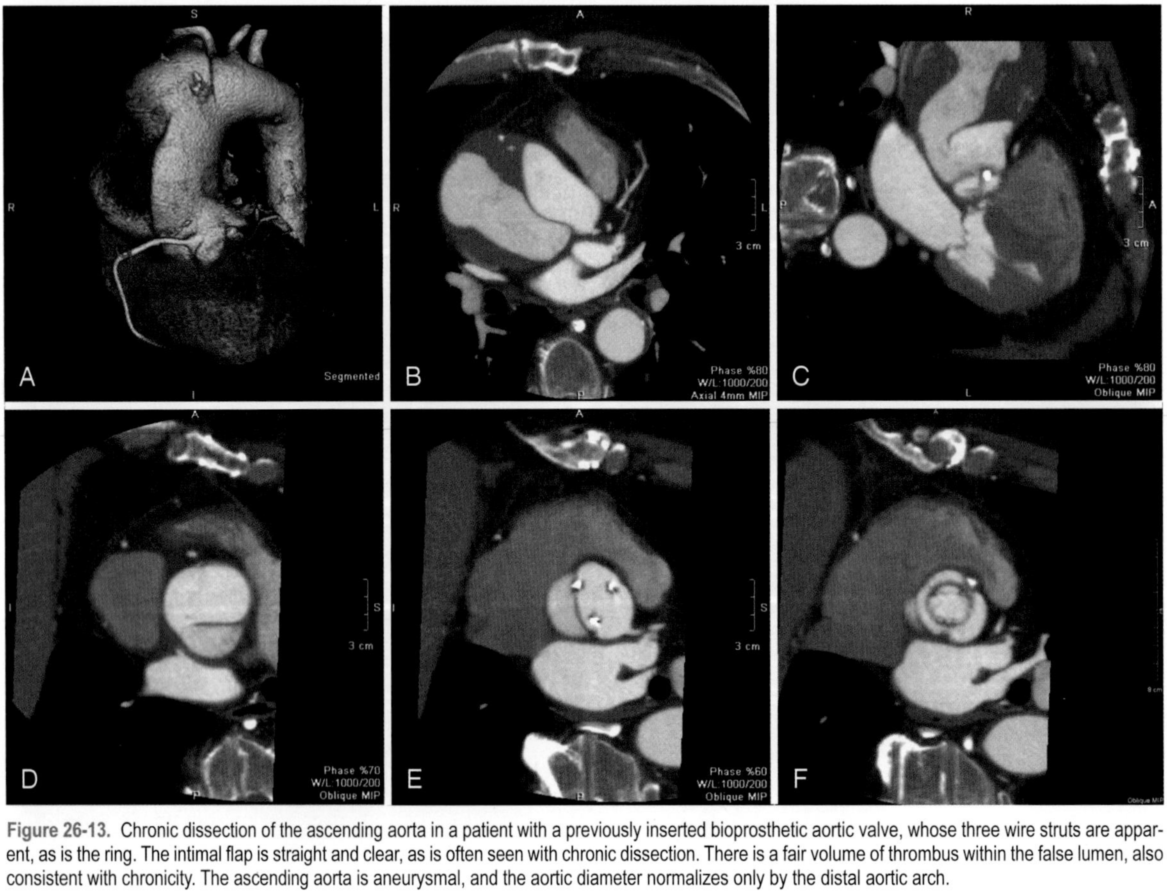

Figure 26-13. Chronic dissection of the ascending aorta in a patient with a previously inserted bioprosthetic aortic valve, whose three wire struts are apparent, as is the ring. The intimal flap is straight and clear, as is often seen with chronic dissection. There is a fair volume of thrombus within the false lumen, also consistent with chronicity. The ascending aorta is aneurysmal, and the aortic diameter normalizes only by the distal aortic arch.

Intramural Hematoma

An important variant of aortic dissection is acute intramural hematoma (IMH; Figs. 26-14 through 26-17). Approximately 10% of suspected dissection cases are IMH. Merely ruling out dissection does not achieve the diagnosis of this equally important, underrecognized pathology. There are fewer data delineating the natural history, prognostic features, and outcomes of management strategies on IMH than on AAD. To summarize what is known:

- ❐ Outcomes parallel those of AAD.
- ❐ Description of the anatomic site of involvement using "Type A/Ascending" and "Type B/ Descending/Non-Ascending") as per AAD classification is suitable. The only location of IMH and AAD that does not lend itself to description by this classification is that of isolated arch involvement.
- ❐ Both non–contrast- and contrast-enhanced views are useful to depict the mural thickening of IMH.
- ❐ The appearance usually is of a crescentic thickening of the wall. Occasionally the mural thickening is circumferential ("annular").
- ❐ The longitudinal extent of involvement is generally much less than that of AAD (8–12 cm only). Unlike AAD, most IMH do not involve the entire aorta.
- ❐ Risk appears related to:
  - Proximal location
  - Leakage
  - Greater anatomic extent of involvement
  - Association with atherosclerotic penetrating ulcer
- ❐ There is no intimal tear or connection of the false lumen to the true lumen.
- ❐ The differential is of aortic dissection with a thrombosed false lumen.
- ❐ About 5% to 10% of cases will, in time, become frank dissection with an intimal tear connecting the true and false lumens.

Management is undertaken according to the paradigm of AAD management:

- ❐ Surgery for proximal involvement
- ❐ Medical management for uncomplicated distal involvement

CT is highly accurate (100%) at identifying IMH.[6]

The aspect of surgery that is theoretically less well suited to address IMH pathology is aortic root replacement for AAD, which has a high chance of eliminating the entry tear, thus depressurizing the false lumen distal to the root replacement and facilitating its thrombosis. In IMH, there is no entry tear to eliminate. Root replacement in the context of IMH provides protection to the aortic valve and coronary artery ostia, as well as to the pericardial space.

Identification of a penetrating ulcer responsible for IMH establishes a significantly worse prognosis. Sustained or recurrent pain, increasing left pleural effusion, increasing maximal aortic diameter, and increasing penetrating ulcer depth reliably predict

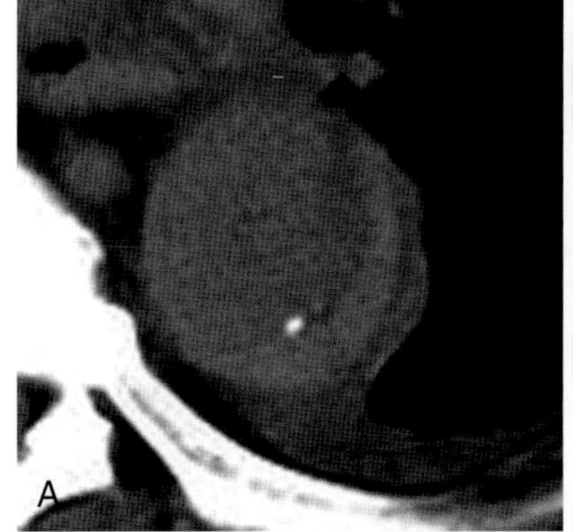

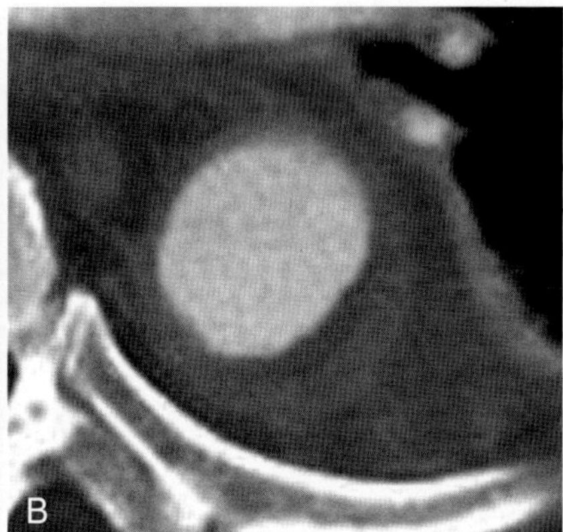

Figure 26-14. Non–contrast-enhanced (**A**) and contrast-enhanced (**B**) CT scans, at approximately the same level in a patient with intramural hematoma of the distal aorta. The noncontrast view shows posterior intimal calcification with displacement and the faint appearance of posterior crescentic wall thickening, with higher attenuation. The contrast-enhanced view effectively defines the lumen and reveals the crescentic wall thickening of the posterior aorta, but the contrast obscures visualization of the calcium.

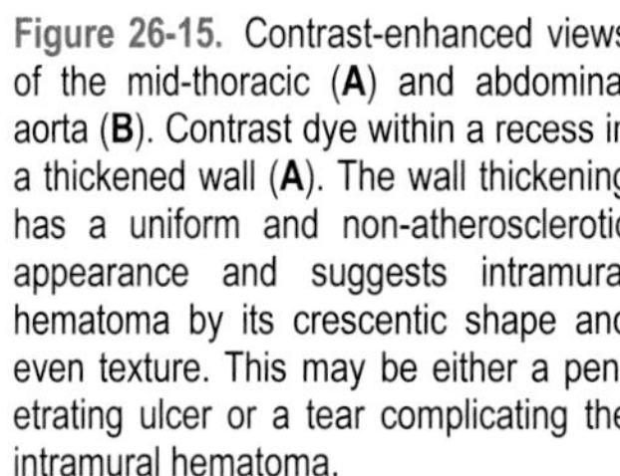

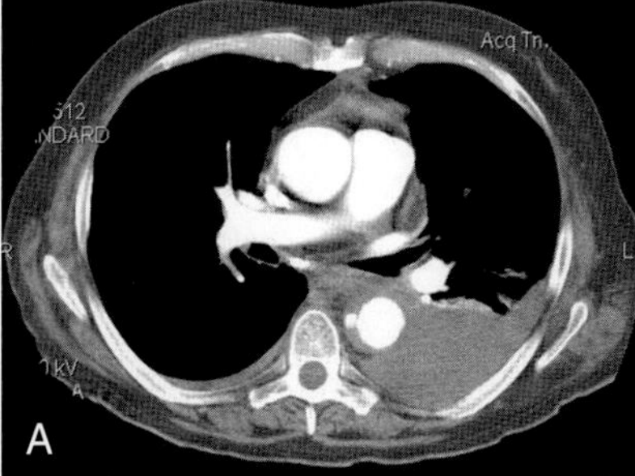

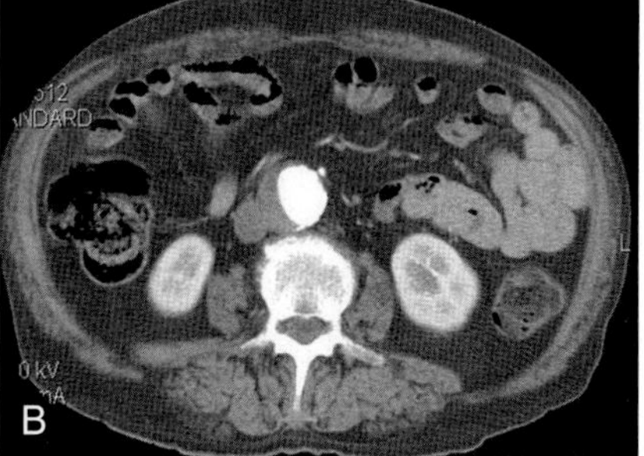

Figure 26-15. Contrast-enhanced views of the mid-thoracic (**A**) and abdominal aorta (**B**). Contrast dye within a recess in a thickened wall (**A**). The wall thickening has a uniform and non-atherosclerotic appearance and suggests intramural hematoma by its crescentic shape and even texture. This may be either a penetrating ulcer or a tear complicating the intramural hematoma.

progression and risk.[4] Development of an "ulcer-like" projection of the ascending aorta or arch is a sign of progression to overt dissection.[4]

Ulcers, Penetrating Ulcers, and Overlying Aortic Thrombus of the Aorta

The least common acute aortic syndrome is penetrating ulcer of the aorta. Atherosclerotic plaques in the aorta, as elsewhere (e.g., carotid and coronary trees), may ulcerate. Atherosclerotic plaques may eventually extend to variable depths (i.e., penetrate) within the wall of the aorta. The deeper the extent into the wall, the greater the chance of disruption of the integrity of the wall.

Weakening of the plaque that allows for communication of the lumen with deeper sections of

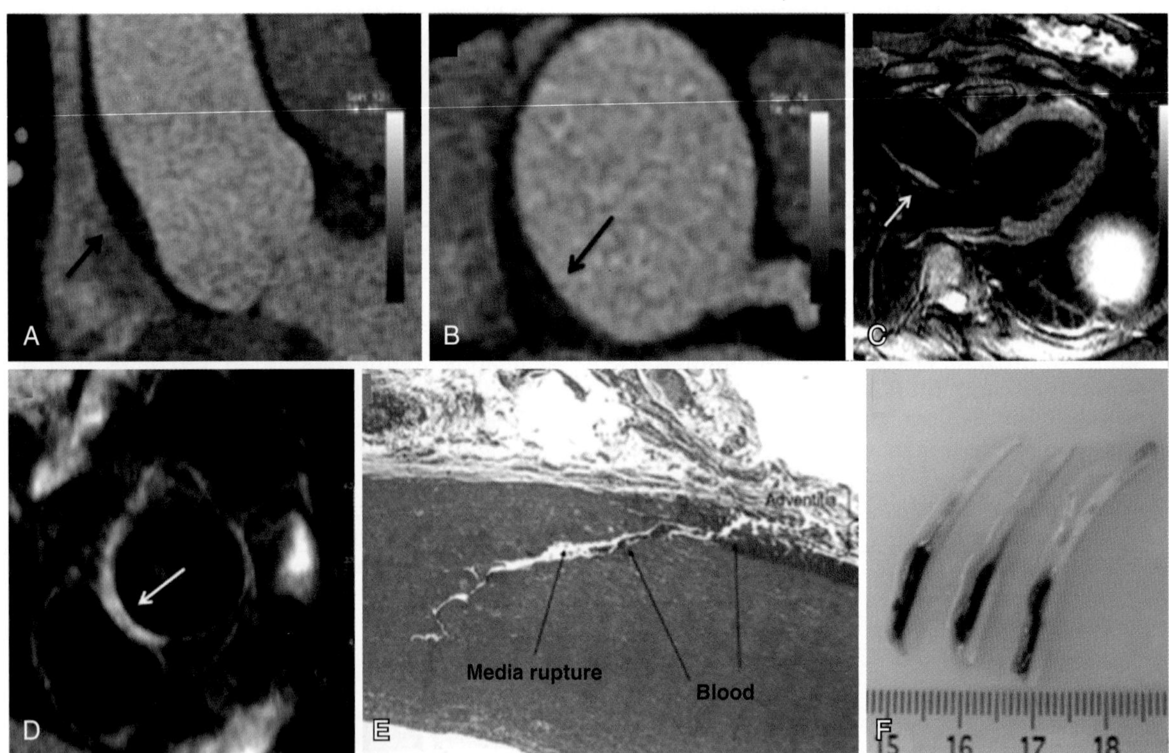

Figure 26-16. A 45-year-old woman was admitted for severe chest pain associated with sinus tachycardia. Echocardiography showed normal left ventricular function, without wall motion abnormalities, a mild aortic regurgitation, and ascending aorta dilation. Dual-source system CT showed a moderate aneurysm of the ascending aorta (46 mm) and bicuspid aortic valve. **A** and **B,** A 6-mm smooth-shaped wall thickening on the noncoronary sinus was detected, suggesting intramural aortic hematoma, without evidence of an intimal tear. **C** and **D,** MRI was performed, and the thickened aortic wall T2-weighted dark blood hypersignal confirmed the presence of fluid within the aortic wall. The patient underwent replacement of the ascending aorta and noncoronary sinus, with aortic valve sparing. **E** and **F,** Histologic examination revealed an intact intimal layer and a slender, cleftlike lesion within the outer part of the tunica media in continuous association in a larger adventitial hematoma. (Reprinted with permission from Cavarretta E, Ramadan R, Dorfmuller P, Raoux F, Paul JF. Intramural aortic hematoma definitive diagnosis combining computed tomography and magnetic resonance imaging. *J Am Coll Cardiol.* 2011;58(16):e30.)

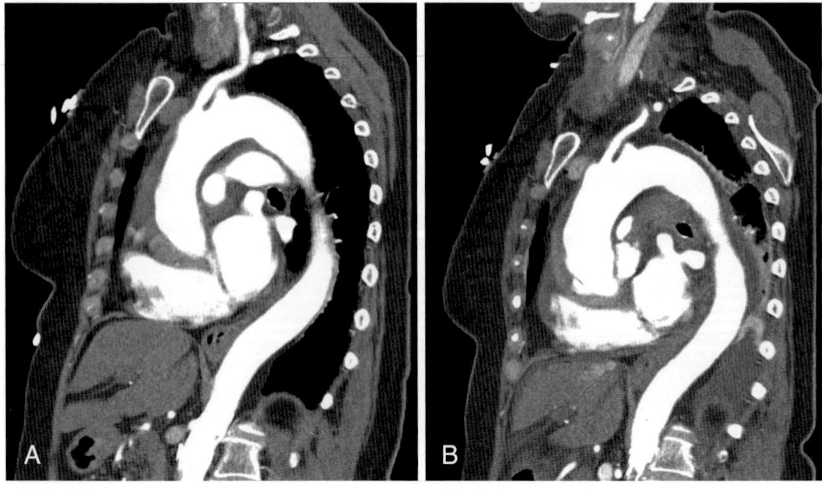

Figure 26-17. Sagittal contrast-enhanced chest CT scans of a patient with a type A intramural hematoma at presentation (**A**) and at 48 hours (**B**) with progression into a type A dissection with hemopericardium.

the wall may result in propagation of blood into the wall and formation of an intramural hematoma within the wall. It also may result in leakage of blood out of the aorta (with or without an intramural hematoma), and, rarely, rupture of the aorta may occur.

CT is able to image aortic ulcers and penetrating ulcers. The challenge for all imaging modalities, including CT, is to distinguish between the two. Ulcers are common; penetrating ulcers are not. Ulcers will not lead to disruption of the aorta, whereas penetrating ulcers may do so. Ideally, imaging modalities would have sufficient resolution to depict the layers of the wall of the aorta distinct from the plaque itself. However, this is not always the case. Depiction of a deep "button-shaped" ulcer is usually convincing evidence of penetration.

Thrombi of variable size usually form on atheromatous plaques and may embolize. They commonly coexist.

Thrombosis and thromboembolism are other complications of atherosclerotic plaques of the aorta. Thrombosis is evident only on contrast-enhanced views as contrast void. A prominent plaque usually underlies the thrombus.

For images of atherosclerosis of the aorta, see Figures 26-18 and 26-19.

For images of atherothrombosis of the aorta, see Figures 26-20 and 26-21.

OCCLUSION OF THE AORTA

Occlusion of the aorta may be acute, resulting from either LV apical or left atrial thromboembolism, from local thrombosis often seen in low flow-shock states, from intra-aortic balloon counterpulsation, or, rarely, from more proximal aortic embolization of thrombus. Occlusion will only be apparent on contrast enhancement. Chronic occlusion usually is associated with extensive collaterals, which depend on the level of occlusion and may be caused by atherosclerosis or aortitis.

For images of occlusion of the aorta, see Figure 26-22.

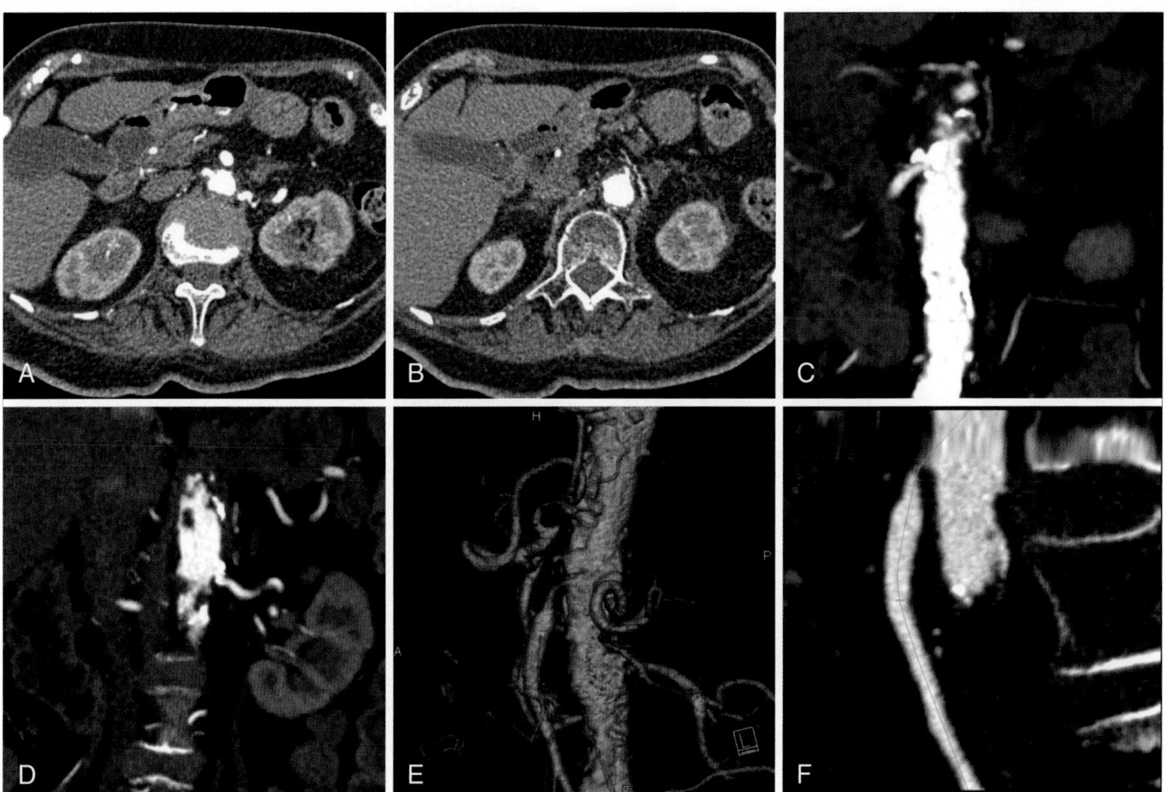

Figure 26-18. Atheromatous disease of the aorta with plaque involving the ostia to the right renal artery (**A**) and the superior mesenteric artery (**B**). Calcified plaque at the ostia to both renal arteries (**C** and **D**) and the tight stenosis of the superior mesenteric artery seen by three-dimensional reconstruction (**E**) and by "vessel extraction" (**F**).

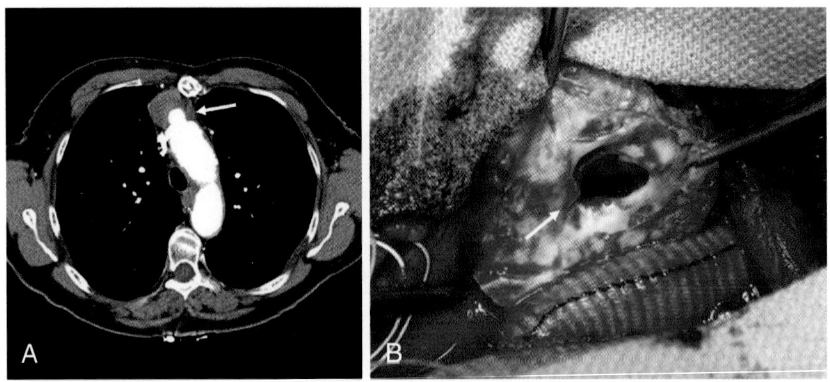

Figure 26-19. A 77-year-old woman underwent coronary artery bypass grafting in 2002. The surgeon noted a mass on the ascending aorta, adjacent to the innominate artery. He performed an off-pump coronary artery bypass grafting procedure to avoid manipulation of the aorta. The patient subsequently experienced two documented cerebral embolic events. The most recent resulted in a permanent bilateral visual field defect. Serial CT studies demonstrated progressive enlargement of a penetrating atherosclerotic ulcer of the ascending aorta adjacent to the origin of the innominate artery (**A,** *arrow*). The patient underwent excision of the penetrating ulcer (**B,** *arrow*), the ascending aorta, and the aortic arch to the level between the origins of the left carotid and innominate arteries. The ascending aorta and innominate artery were replaced with prosthetic grafts. Penetrating atherosclerotic ulcers are commonly found in the descending but rarely in the ascending thoracic aorta. Embolization from the ulcer crater was the likely cause of the cerebral embolic events. (Reprinted with permission from Stamou SC, Kouchoukos NT. Penetrating ulcer of the ascending aorta. *J Am Coll Cardiol* 2011;57(11):1327.)

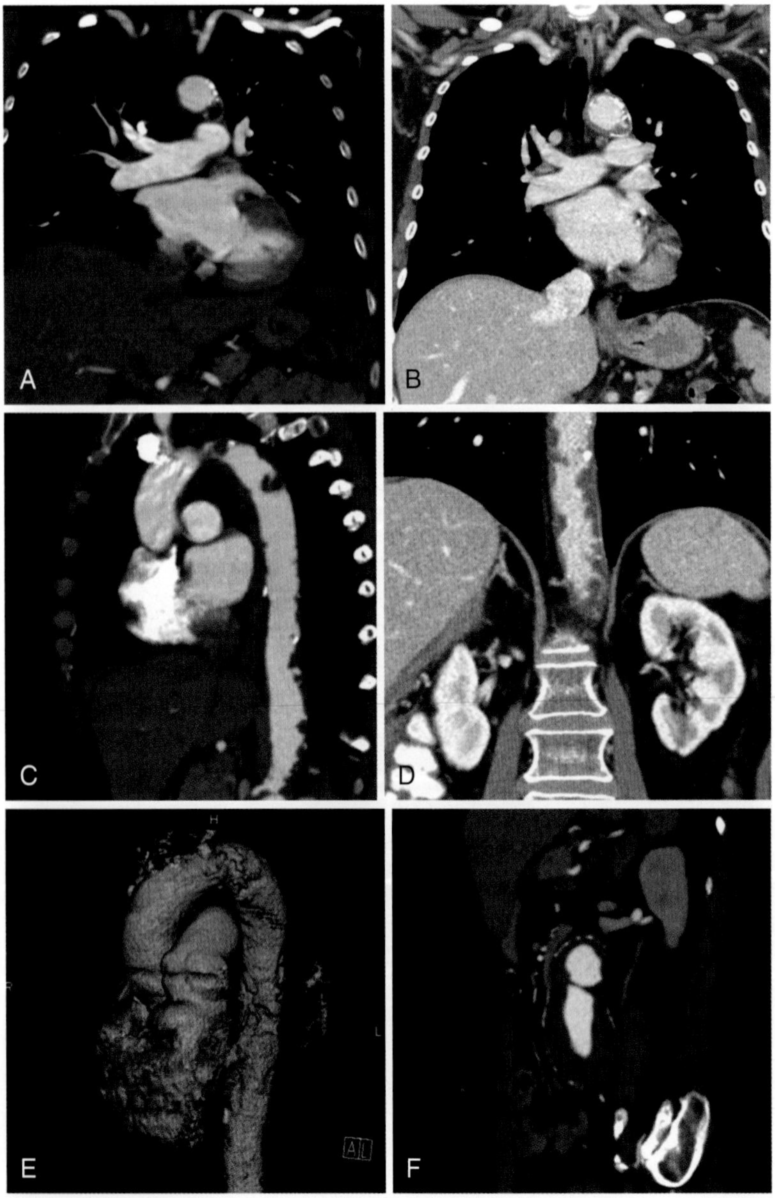

Figure 26-20. Atheromatous aorta with a penetrating ulcer of the floor of the distal arch. The upper coronal views (**A** and **B**) reveal the partially thrombus-laden penetrating ulcer extending from the floor of the distal arch. **C** and **D,** The extensive burden of protruding thrombus, and the topographically complex surface of the lumen. **E,** Three-dimensional reconstruction does provide a representation of the irregularity of the surface of the aorta, but largely fails to capture the nature of the disease as effectively as the planar views. **F,** A large abdominal aortic aneurysm in the same patient, with a large amount of mural thrombus.

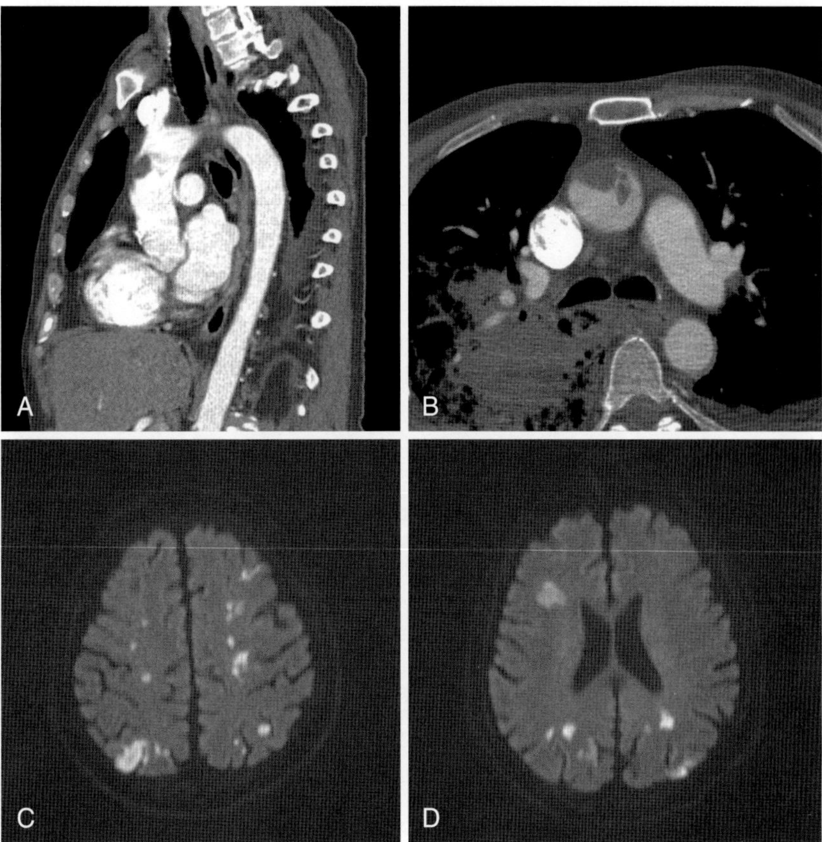

Figure 26-21. A 52-year-old man presented with strokes in dispersed territories. Diffusion-weighted MRI images (**C, D**). Chest CT (**C**) revealed a soft tissue mass in the ascending aorta, which was better imaged on an ECG-gated cardiac CT (**B**) to minimize motion artifact. The lesion was believed to be thrombus.

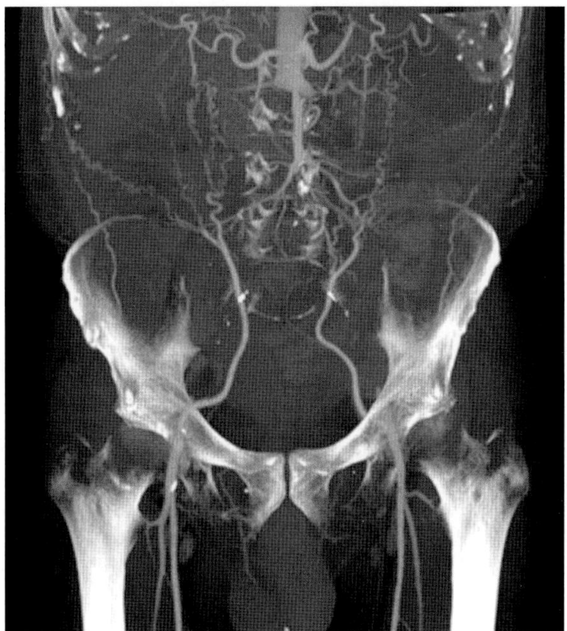

Figure 26-22. Contrast-enhanced volume intensity projection image. The complete occlusion of the aorta is evident, as are extensive collaterals and reconstitution of the femoral arteries.

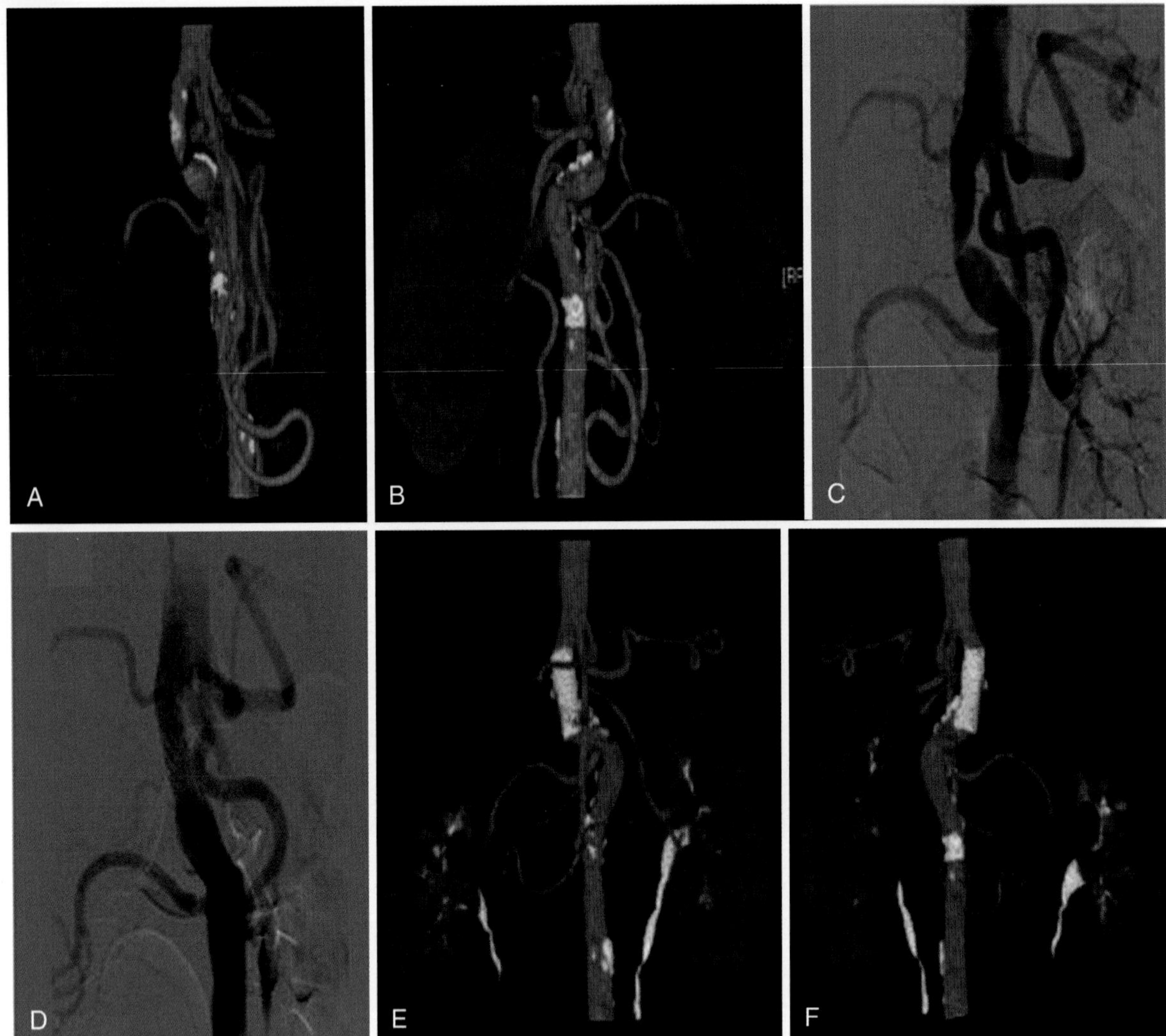

Figure 26-23. A 46-year-old woman was admitted with signs of lower limb ischemia. Her examination demonstrated a nonpalpable distal pulse. CT angiography revealed an anomalous origin of both renal arteries (**A** and **B**) and severe aortic narrowing between the renal arteries, confirmed by the angiogram (**C**). The diagnosis was middle aortic syndrome. Endovascular treatment was decided on, and a balloon-expandable covered stent (Jomed, Abbott Laboratories, Abbott Park, IL) was placed, with good stent expansion (**D**). Physical examination revealed distal pulse recovery. At 5 months, the patient remains asymptomatic. **E** and **F**, CT angiography showed stent patency. Middle aortic syndrome refers to an isolated disease of the thoracoabdominal aorta causing segmental narrowing. It often is associated with hypertension in childhood. This is a rare case of middle aortic syndrome with lower limb ischemia successfully resolved with endovascular treatment. (Reprinted with permission from Rabellino M, Garcia-Nielsen L, Gonzalez G, Baldi S, Zander T, Maynar M. Middle aortic syndrome: percutaneous treatment with a balloon-expandable covered stent. *J Am Coll Cardiol.* 2010;56(6):521.)

MIDDLE AORTIC SYNDROME

"Middle aortic syndrome" is isolated abdominal level stenosis, which has many clinical similarities with coarctation of the thoracic aorta. It may be caused by aortitis.

For images of the middle aortic syndrome, see Figure 26-23.

AORTIC ANEURYSM

CT scanning is extremely well suited to diagnosing and assessing aneurysmal disease of the aorta: thoracic, abdominal and thoracoabdominal (Figs. 26-24 through 26-30). CT scanning is able to:

- Identify aneurysms
- Establish anatomic extent
- Establish (accurately) aneurysm diameter
- Distinguish aneurysms from dissection and false aneurysm
- Identify mural thrombus within aneurysms
- Identify leakage
- Identify the relation of the aneurysm to branch vessels
- Establish interventional suitability and planning
- Establish the relation of aneurysms of the aortic root and sinuses to coronary arteries[7]

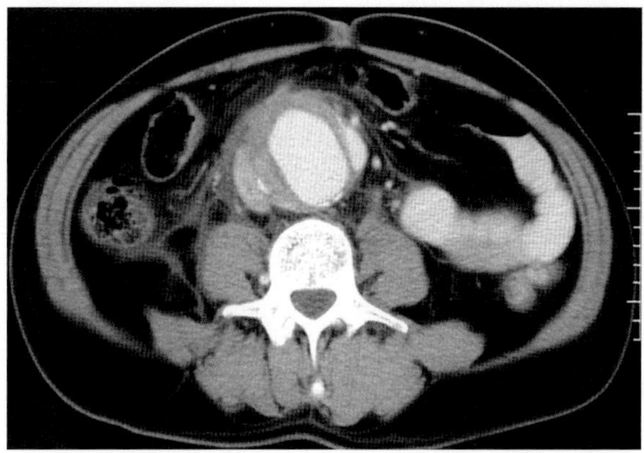

Figure 26-24. Contrast-enhanced image just below the renal arteries in a patient with a ruptured abdominal aortic aneurysm. There is a large abdominal aortic aneurysm with extensive thrombus and multiple channels through it. The hazy streaking around the abdominal aorta is consistent with extravasated blood.

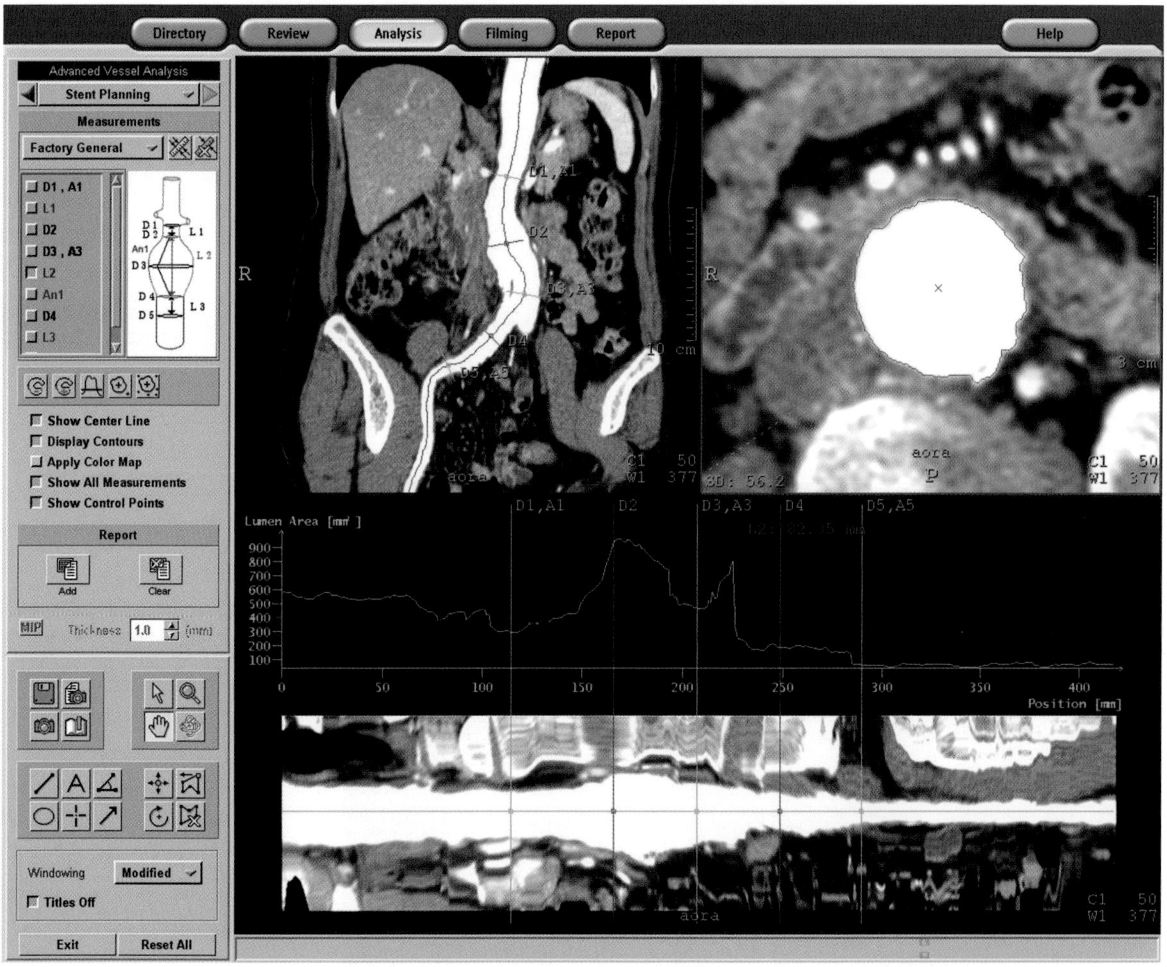

Figure 26-25. Endovascular aneurysm repair planning workstation software. The three displays—multiplanar, orthogonally oriented image to the long axis of the "seeded" vessel, and "vessel extracted" display—are integrated. Diameters for the proximal and distal landing zones of a stent, and its limbs, are being measured for planning.

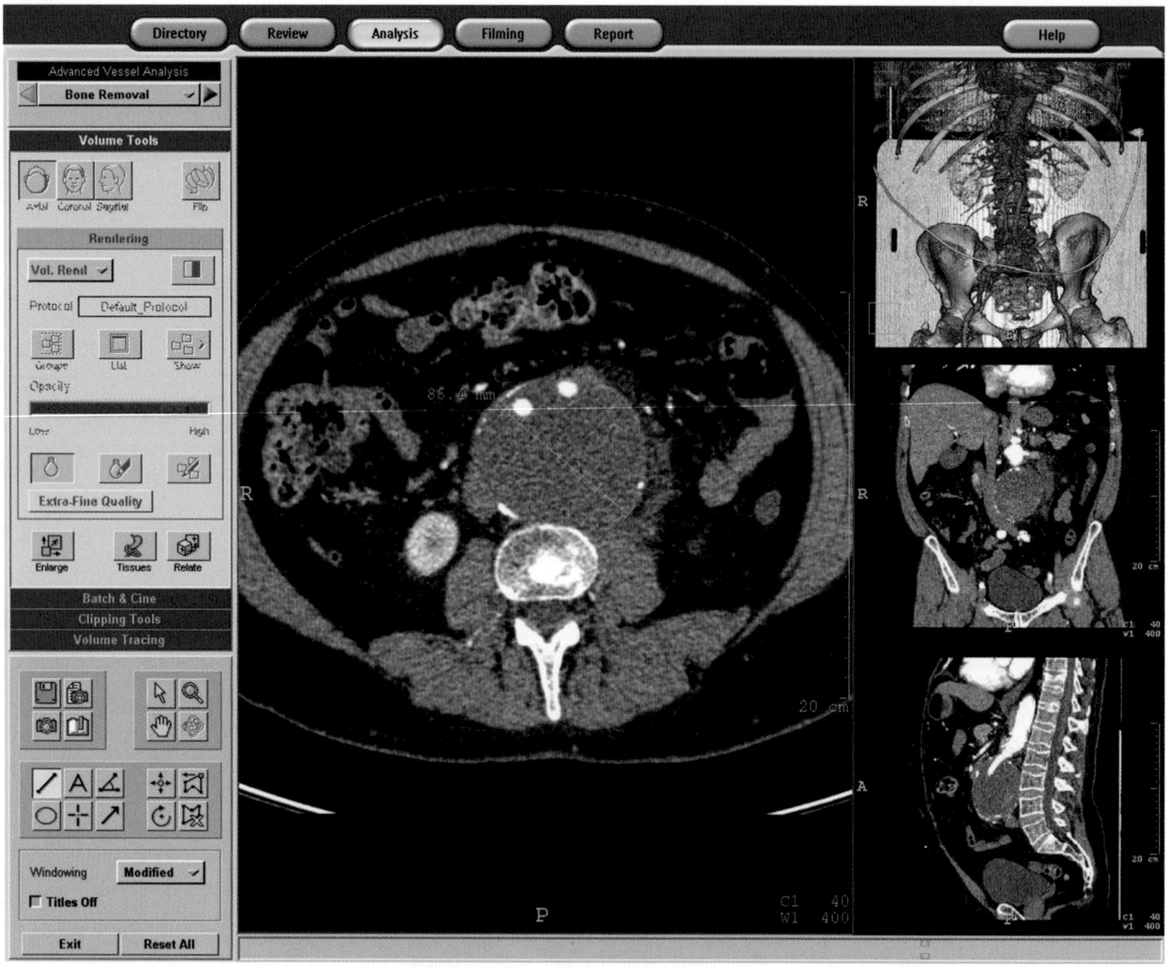

Figure 26-26. Contrast-enhanced workstation images of the abdominal aorta. The limbs of the stent are seen. There is no endoleak.

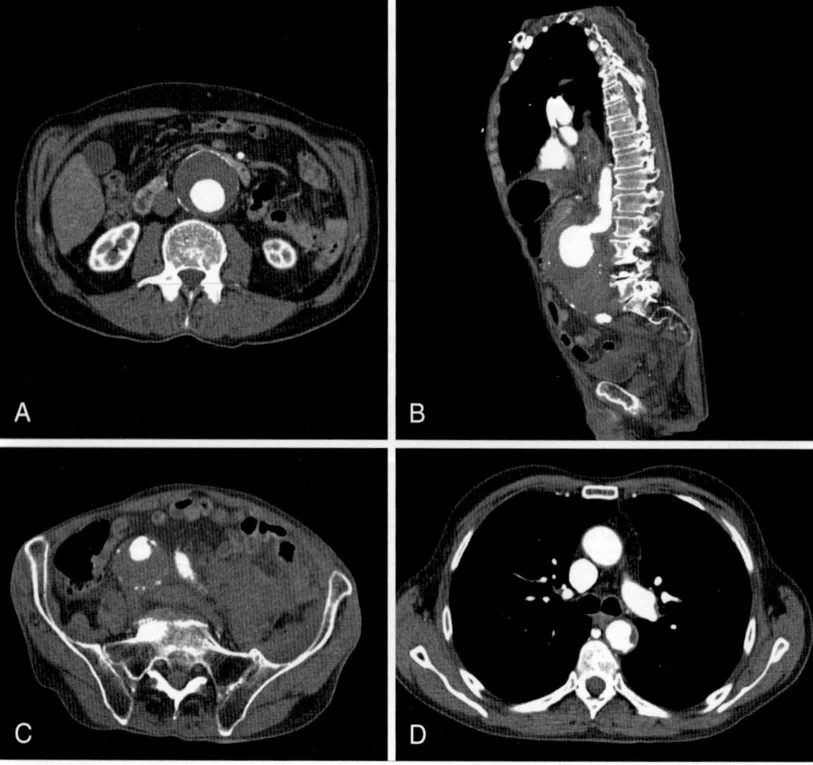

Figure 26-27. **A** and **B,** Large infrarenal abdominal aortic aneurysm with eggshell calcification and a large amount of mural thrombus. **C,** An associated large aneurysm of the right common iliac artery, also with eggshell calcification and a large amount of mural thrombus. The left common iliac artery, adjacent to it, serves as a reference standard. **D,** Associated atheromatous disease of the upper thoracic descending aorta, also with mural thrombus.

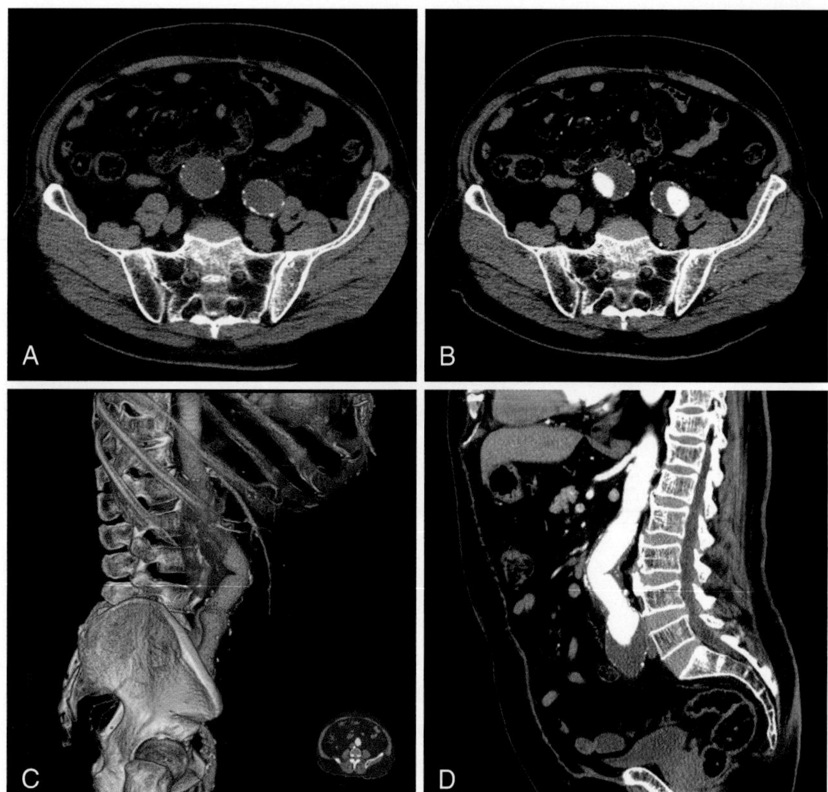

Figure 26-28. Axial CT images at the common iliac level without contrast (**A**) and with contrast (**B**). Volume-rendered reconstruction (**C**) and sagittal view (**D**). There is a small fold along the posterior wall of the graft that is more a folding than a kinking of the graft.

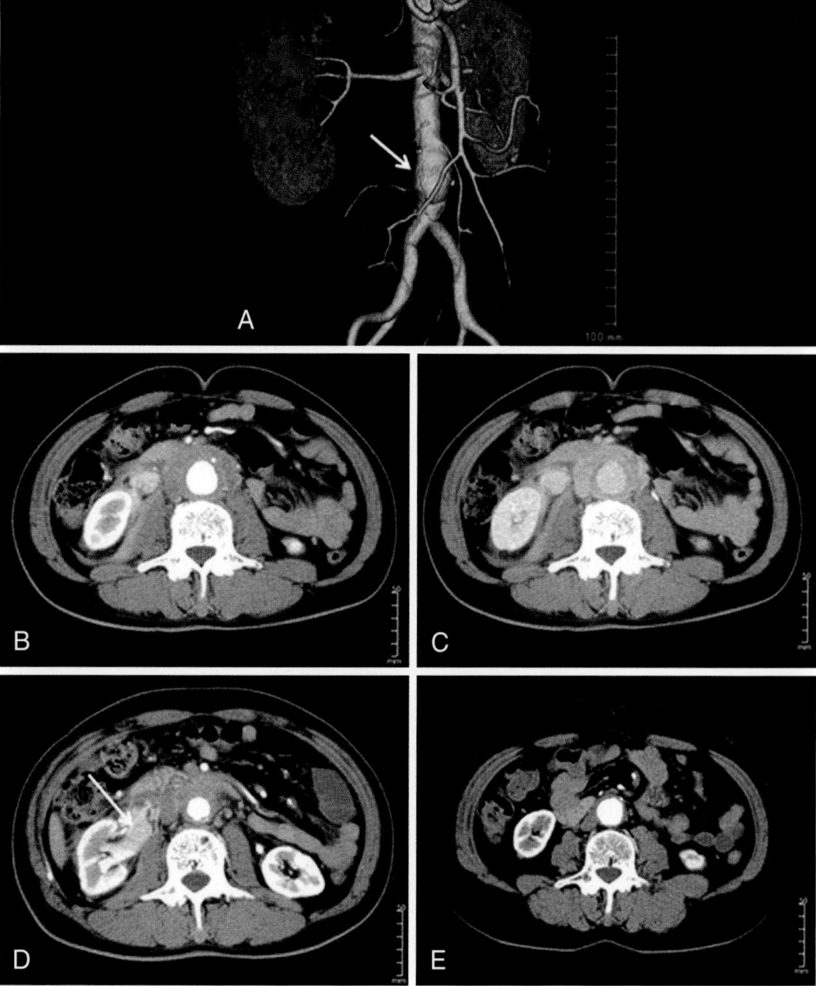

Figure 26-29. A 60-year-old man presented with low back pain. Laboratory examination revealed a raised erythrocyte sedimentation rate of 83 mm/hr, an elevated C-reactive protein of 3.9 mg/dL, and estimated glomerular filtration rate of 36 mL/min/m^2. A CT scan showed a 4.0-cm infrarenal abdominal aortic aneurysm (three-dimensional volume-rendered contrast-enhanced image [**A**]) with extremely thickened aortic wall and surrounding soft tissue mass (**B**). The periaortic mass appears as isodense to muscle and enhances circumferentially with administration of contrast medium, indicating it is in active inflammatory stage (**C**). As a result of inflammatory tissue enveloping the right ureter, the right kidney showed ureterohydronephrosis (**D**). To control the perianeurysmal inflammation, corticosteroid therapy was started with prednisolone at an initial dose of 30 mg/day, which was gradually reduced to a maintenance dose of 2.5 mg/day, based on the improvement of inflammatory signs as well as change in size of the retroperitoneal mass. Six months later, a CT scan demonstrated marked regression of the retroperitoneal mass and thickened aortic wall (**E**) and resolution of the ureteral obstruction. The patient is doing well at 4 years of follow-up. (Reprinted with permission from Yabe T, Hamada T, Kubo T, et al. Inflammatory abdominal aortic aneurysm successfully treated with steroid therapy. *J Am Coll Cardiol.* 2010;55(25):2877.)

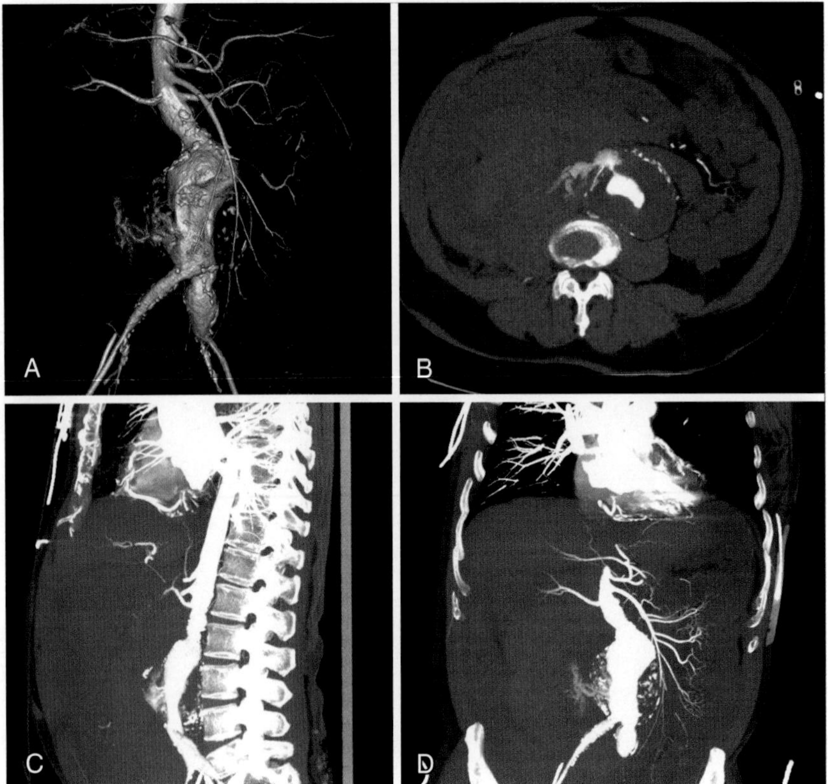

Figure 26-30. Multiple volume-rendered and maximum intensity projection images from an 82-year-old man who presented to the emergency department with abdominal pain. A large infrarenal abdominal aortic aneurysm is appreciated. These CT angiographic images demonstrate a focal area of leakage of contrast outside the confines of the abdominal aorta. Extensive retroperitoneal and intraperitoneal fluid is present. These findings are typical of acute rupture of an abdominal aortic aneurysm.

Contrast (catheter-based) aortography offers little additional information to CT scanning since CT can perform multiplanar imaging.

CCT is better suited to determining the anatomic extent of aortic aneurysm than is aortography.[8] Older studies suggest that in the claudicant patient with aortic aneurysms, aortography retains a role for determination of iliac stenosis or obstruction[5]; studies using newer systems have yet to follow up on this.

Thoracic Aortic Aneurysms

For images of thoracic aortic aneurysms, see Figures 26-31 through 26-39.

Arch Vessel Aneurysms

Arch vessel aneurysms may be congenital, may arise from an aberrant right subclavian artery (diverticulum of Kommerell), or may be associated with a thoracic outlet syndrome, post-traumatic false aneurysm, infection, atherosclerosis, or even Takayasu disease. Most arch vessel aneurysms are asymptomatic until complications arise or may be detected as an incidental finding on a plain radiograph.

Mycotic Aneurysms

Mycotic aneurysm is a rare clinical entity with an incidence of 0.8% to 3.4% of all aortic aneurysms. Virtually any artery may be involved. In the pre-antibiotic era, most mycotic aneurysms were secondary to valvular disease. Today approximately 80% result from either circulating bacteria implanting in diseased atherosclerotic or traumatized intima or secondary to direct extension or through lymphatic vessels from a nearby infection. Additionally, infection of a pre-existing aneurysm can occur. Risk factors include arterial catheterization, intravenous drug abuse, concurrent sepsis, or immunocompromised states. The mean age at presentation is the seventh decade. The predominant organisms are *Staphylococcus aureus* and *Salmonella* species. Presentation may be of pyrexia of unknown origin, and diagnosis rests on a high index of suspicion. Lobular, saccular, or eccentric aneurysms can occur, which on MRI appear as small outpouches of signal void along the lateral walls of the vessel, often accompanied by periaortic soft tissue. Enlargement of the vessel lumen eventually develops, usually in a time span between 10 days and 3 months. Progression of a normal vessel to a markedly dilated and thinned one may be very rapid.[9]

Text continued on page 457

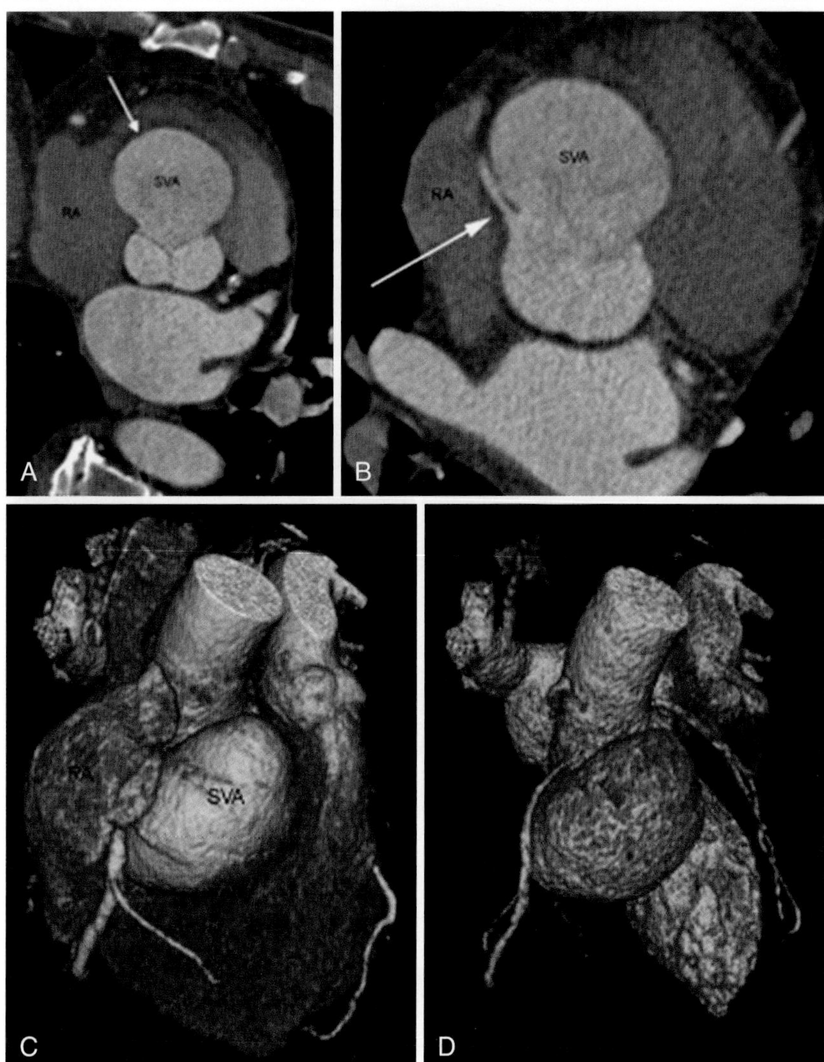

Figure 26-31. **A,** This CT axial oblique image shows a sinus of Valsalva aneurysm (*white arrow*). **B,** The CT axial image shows compression of the proximal right coronary artery (*white arrow*) between the sinus of Valsalva aneurysm (SVA) and the right atrium (RA). **C,** CT volume-rendered reconstruction again shows compression of the right coronary artery between the SVA and the RA. **D,** The CT volume-rendered reconstruction shows an SVA. (Reprinted with permission from Joines M, Barack BM, Chang DS. Right coronary sinus of Valsalva aneurysm evaluated by cardiac computed tomography angiography. *J Cardiovasc Comput Tomogr.* 2008;2(3):193-194.)

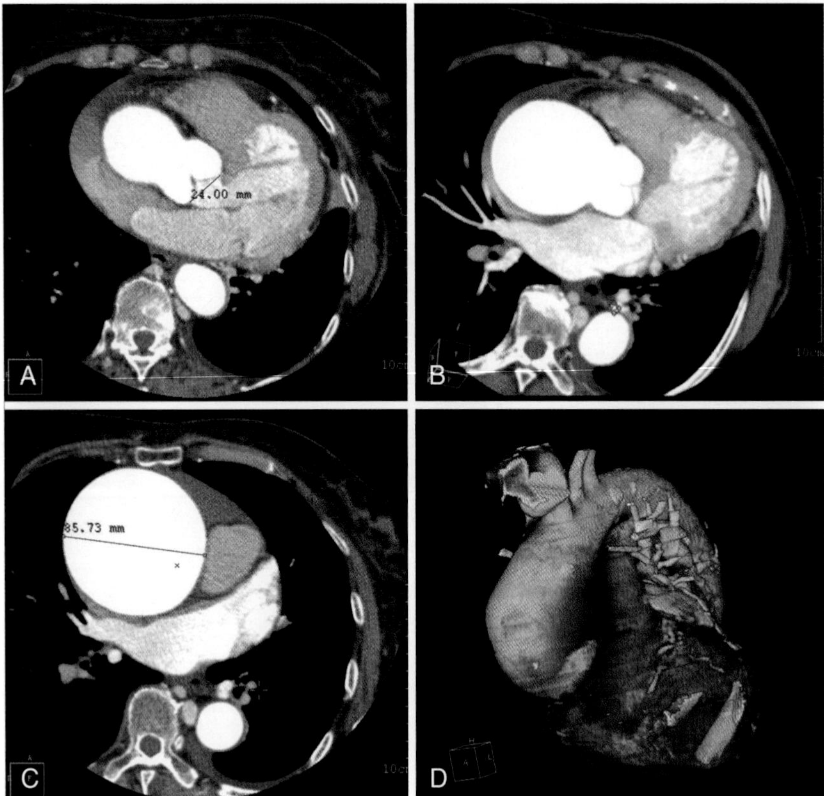

Figure 26-32. Contrast-enhanced axial and three-dimensional volume-rendered views of a large aneurysm, without dissection, involving the ascending aorta. The sinotubular junction and sinuses are normal. **A,** Aortic valve annulus. **B,** Maximal diameter of the ascending aorta.

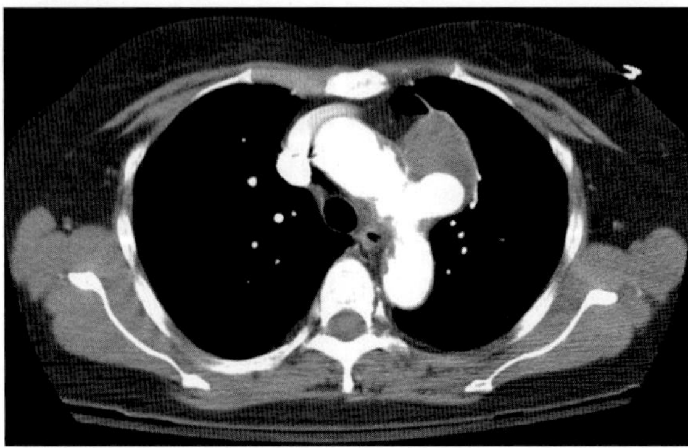

Figure 26-33. Contrast-enhanced image at the aortic arch level. There is a saccular extension of the lumen into a thrombus-filled cavity. This was a largely thrombosed false aneurysm, which subsequently ruptured.

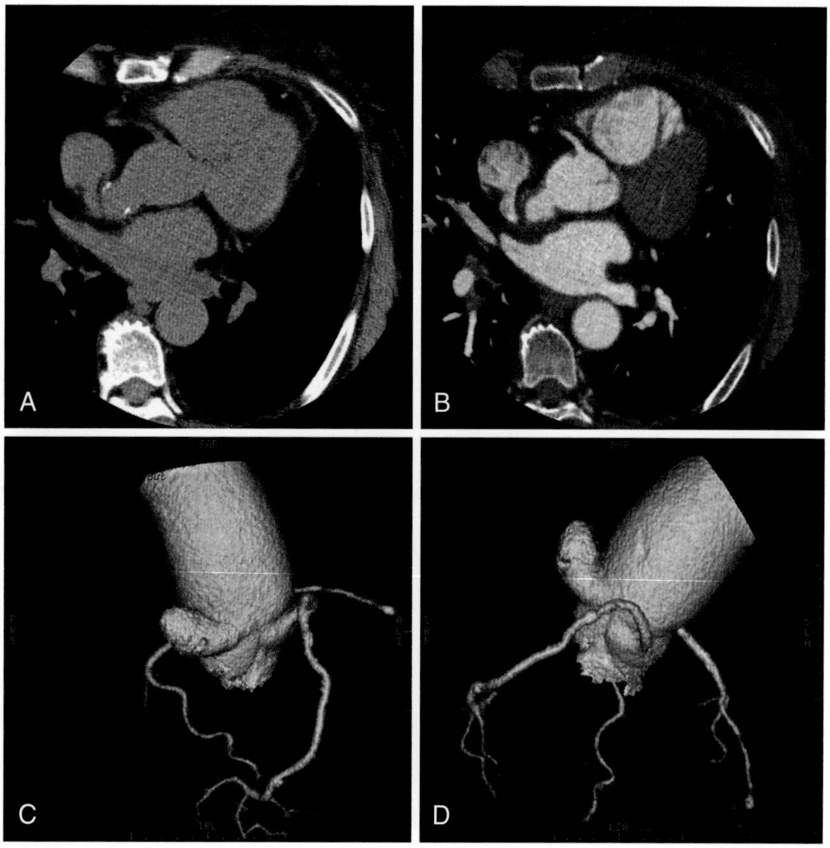

Figure 26-34. **A,** Non–contrast-enhanced axial image reveals an abnormal contour off the right posterior aortic root, with calcification. **B,** This contrast-enhanced axial source image demonstrates a small saccular aneurysm extending from the right posterior aortic root, with either a thick wall or a rind of mural thrombus. **C** and **D,** Three-dimensional volume-rendered images depict the small saccular aneurysm, the length of which is greater than its diameter, and which arises at the sinotubular junction.

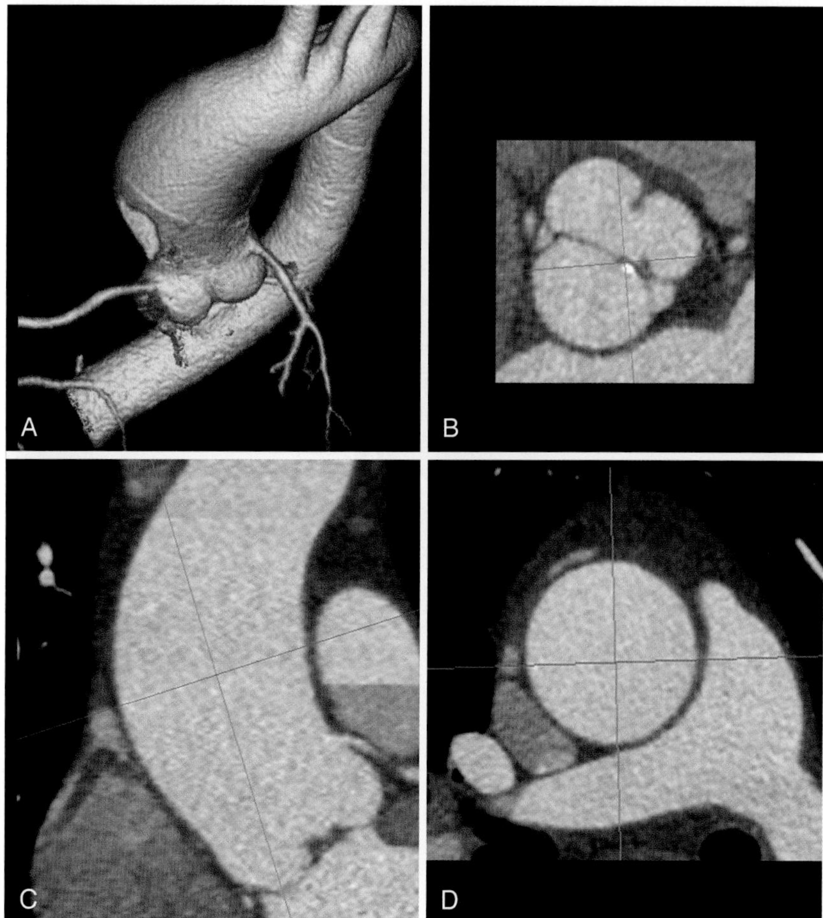

Figure 26-35. Multiple images from a cardiac CT study. A functional bicuspid aortic valve is noted with a partial raphe between the right and left coronary cusps. There is mild thickening of the aortic valve leaflets, and a small focus of calcification involving the valve leaflets. As the study was obtained prospectively, evaluation of aortic valve function is not possible. There is an associated ascending aortopathy. **C** and **D,** Double oblique evaluation of the ascending aorta demonstrated an ascending aortic aneurysm of 4.8 cm. There was no evidence of an occult dissection or of coarctation.

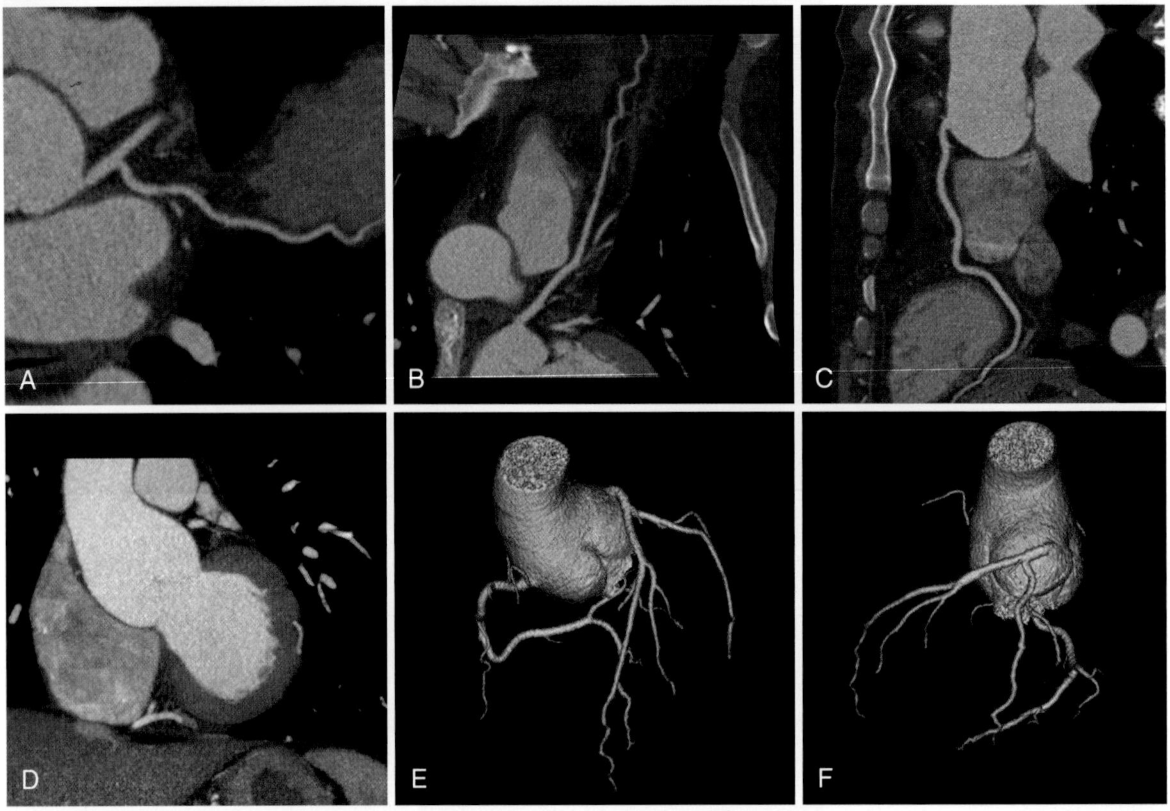

Figure 26-36. Multiple images from a cardiac CT study in a patient with known Marfan syndrome. This study was performed preoperatively to evaluate coronary arteries. The obtuse marginal/circumflex system (**A**), left anterior descending artery (**B**), and right coronary artery (**C**) are normal in appearance. The aortic root has a typical tulip bulb–like configuration as is commonly described in the setting of Marfan syndrome. The aorta at the level of the mid sinuses of Valsalva measures 5.4 cm, aneurysmal.

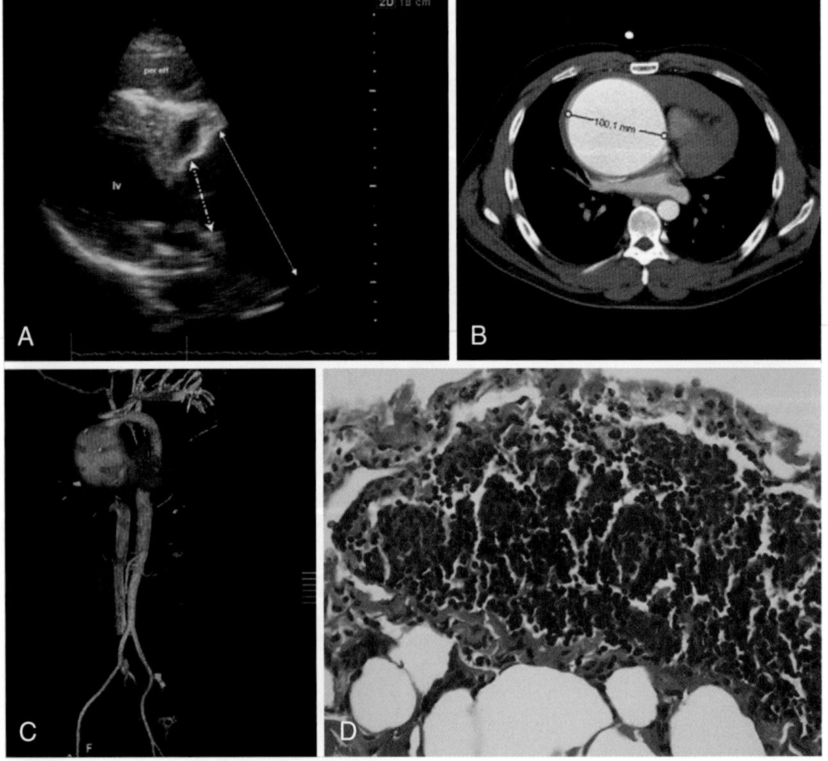

Figure 26-37. A previously healthy 38-year-old man presented with sudden-onset dyspnea, sharp, stabbing chest pain, and a clinical picture of cardiogenic shock. **A,** Echocardiography revealed a severely dilated ascending aorta beyond the sinotubular junction, with moderate aortic insufficiency. There was a large pericardial effusion with thrombus inside. CT angiography was performed, with a presumptive diagnosis of aortic dissection with rupture into the pericardium, and demonstrated a dilated ascending aorta 100 mm in diameter (**B** and **C**) compressing the right atrium, with no visible intimal tear or flap. The patient underwent an emergent Benthall procedure. Intraoperatively, no intimal tear or dissection was noted. Pathology revealed predominantly lymphoplasmacytic inflammatory cell infiltrates around the vaso vasorum of the adventitia (**D**) in the resected aortic segment, suggesting that tamponade resulted from tearing of the adventitial vessels. Blood work was positive for *Treponema pallidum* hemagglutination antibody. A diagnosis of tertiary syphilis complicated by aortic aneurysm was made. (Reprinted with permission from Acar Z, Agac MT, Demirbas M, Kurt D. Giant syphilitic aortic aneurysm presenting with pericardial tamponade as an initial sign. *J Am Coll Cardiol.* 2012;59(1):e1.)

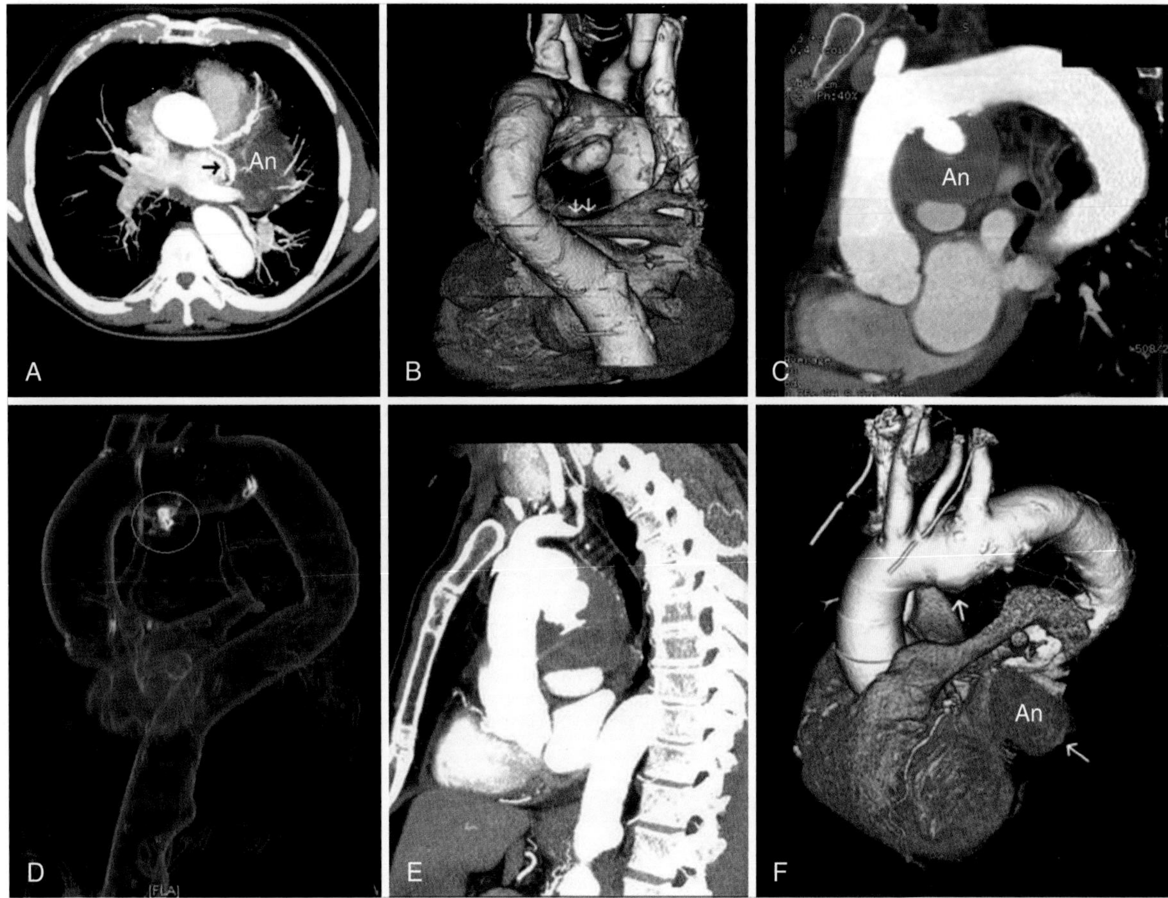

Figure 26-38. A 62-year-old man with arteriopathy and chronic obstructive pulmonary disease, coronary aneurysm, and an aortic false aneurysm. **A,** CT scan in transverse section shows a large circumflex coronary aneurysm (*arrow*) following covered stent closure of the entry. Diffuse coronary disease is apparent in the left anterior descending branch. **B,** CT reconstruction demonstrates the nonthrombosed part of a 6.5-cm saccular arch aneurysm compressing the pulmonary bifurcation (*double arrow*). **C,** A lateral view shows the partially thrombosed arch aneurysm. **D,** CT reconstruction with the Amplatzer occluder device closing the mouth of the aneurysm. **E,** A lateral view (1 year later) shows that the neck of the aneurysm has increased in size. The device has prolapsed into the sac with further pulmonary artery compression. **F,** CT reconstruction shows the repaired ascending aorta (*arrow*) and arch together with the thrombosed circumflex coronary aneurysm (*arrow*). An, aneurysm. (Reprinted with permission from Westaby W, Luthra S, Anthony S, Ormerod O, Wilson N. Amplatzer device deployment for saccular aortic arch aneurysm. A note of caution. *Circulation.* 2012;125:1318-1320.)

COARCTATION OF THE AORTA

Anatomic coarctation of the aorta is well depicted by CT scanning,[10,11] but the physiologic disturbance (gradient) is not. CT scanning is able to depict:

- The location and longitudinal extent of the coarctation
- Associated features such as:
  - Dilation or aneurysm of the ascending aorta
  - Associated bicuspid aortic valves
  - Dissection of the proximal or distal aorta
  - Patent ductus arteriosus
  - Collateral vessels
  - Intracranial "berry" aneurysms

The gradient across the coarctation can be assessed by a hybrid strategy using echocardiography, or an alternate imaging strategy using MRI to obtain the gradient.

Diameter measurements are subject to some variability, and serial comparisons should be interpreted with caution.[10] The same appears to be true for MRI measurements.[10]

Maximum intensity projection images are useful for assessing coarctation,[12,13] as are three-dimensional views.[13]

For images of coarctation of the aorta, see Figures 26-40 through 26-50 and **Video 26-2**.

ANOMALIES OF THE AORTA

CT is a superb test for imaging virtually any and all anomalies of the aorta and its branch vessels (Figs. 26-51 through 26-54), including[14]:

- Right-sided aortic arch
- Aberrant right subclavian artery (arteria lusoria)
- Aberrant left subclavian artery
- Coarctation of the aorta
- Interruption of the aorta

Text continued on page 467

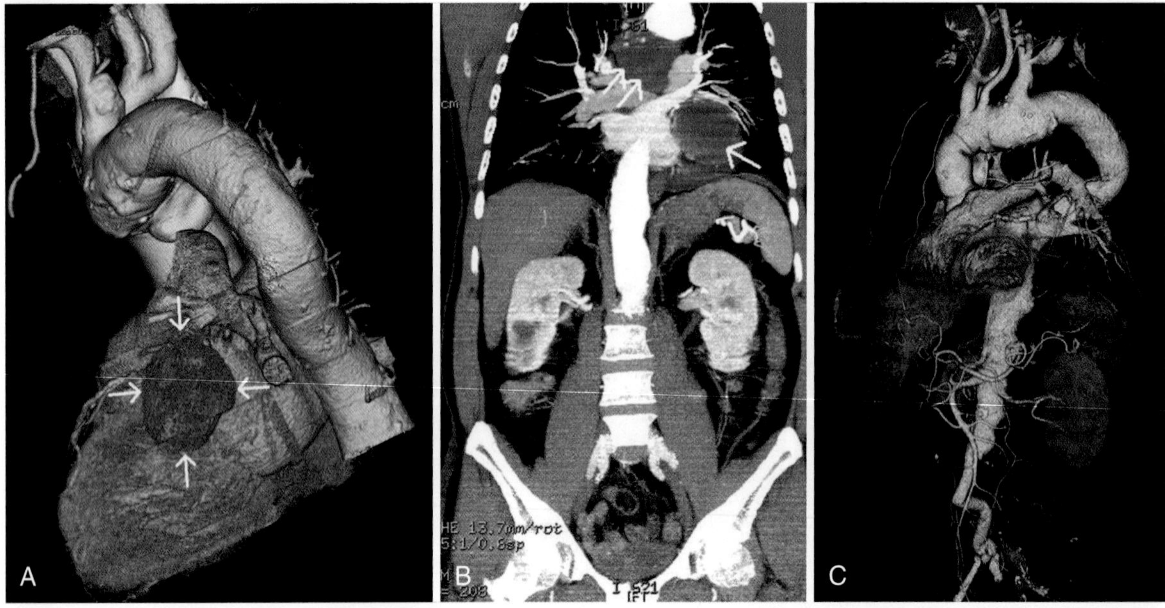

Figure 26-39. **A** and **B,** A 62-year-old man with arteriopathy and chronic obstructive pulmonary disease, coronary aneurysm, and an aortic false aneurysm. **A,** CT reconstruction, lateral view, defines the morphology of the circumflex aneurysm before intervention (*arrows*). **B,** CT scan shows both the saccular arch (*single arrow*) and the circumflex aneurysms (*double arrows*) in coronal profile. **C,** CT reconstruction of a recent follow-up scan showing the whole aorta, including the aorto-bifemoral graft with occlusion of one limb. There is no significant compression of the pulmonary artery and no flow into the excluded saccular aneurysm. (Reprinted with permission from Westaby S, Luthra S, Anthony S, Ormerod O, Wilson N. Amplatzer device deployment for saccular aortic arch aneurysm. A note of caution. *Circulation.* 2012;125:1318-1320.)

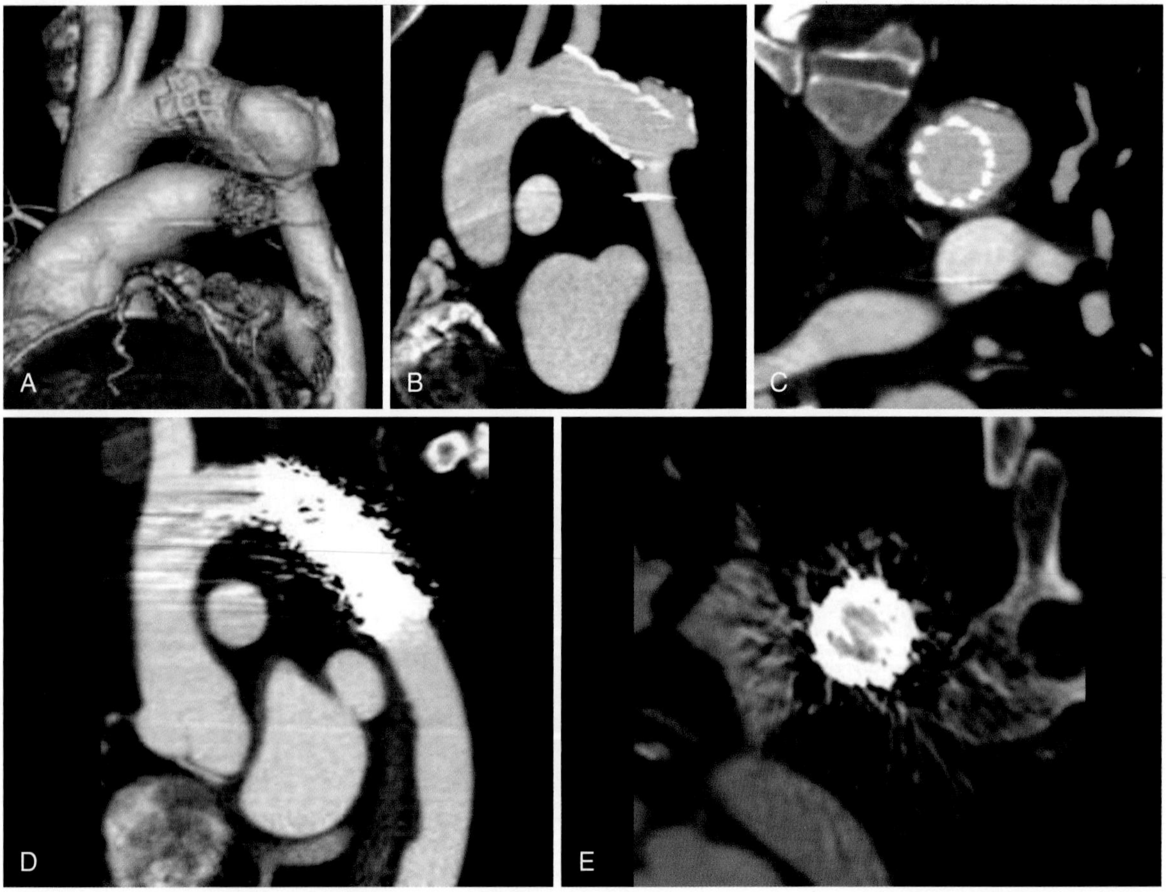

Figure 26-40. Multiple images from two separate cardiac CT studies. **B** and **C,** A cardiac CT study post–bare metal stenting for coarctation of the aorta. This study and subsequent imaging demonstrate a growing pseudoaneurysm with contrast collecting outside the confines of the stent. Repeat imaging with placement of an internal covered stent demonstrates subsequent thrombosis of the false aneurysm with no residual extravasation of contrast.

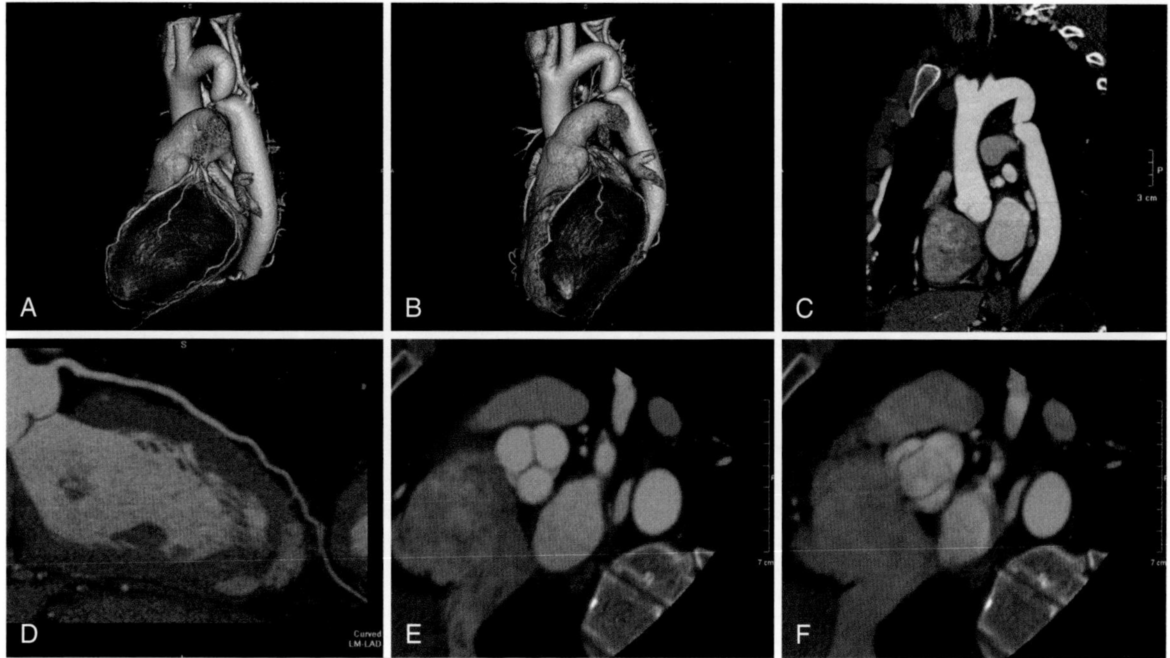

Figure 26-41. Composite images from a cardiac CT study demonstrate a tight shelf-like coarctation in the proximal descending thoracic aorta. Normal coronary arteries were identified, and a functionally bicuspid aortic valve is present.

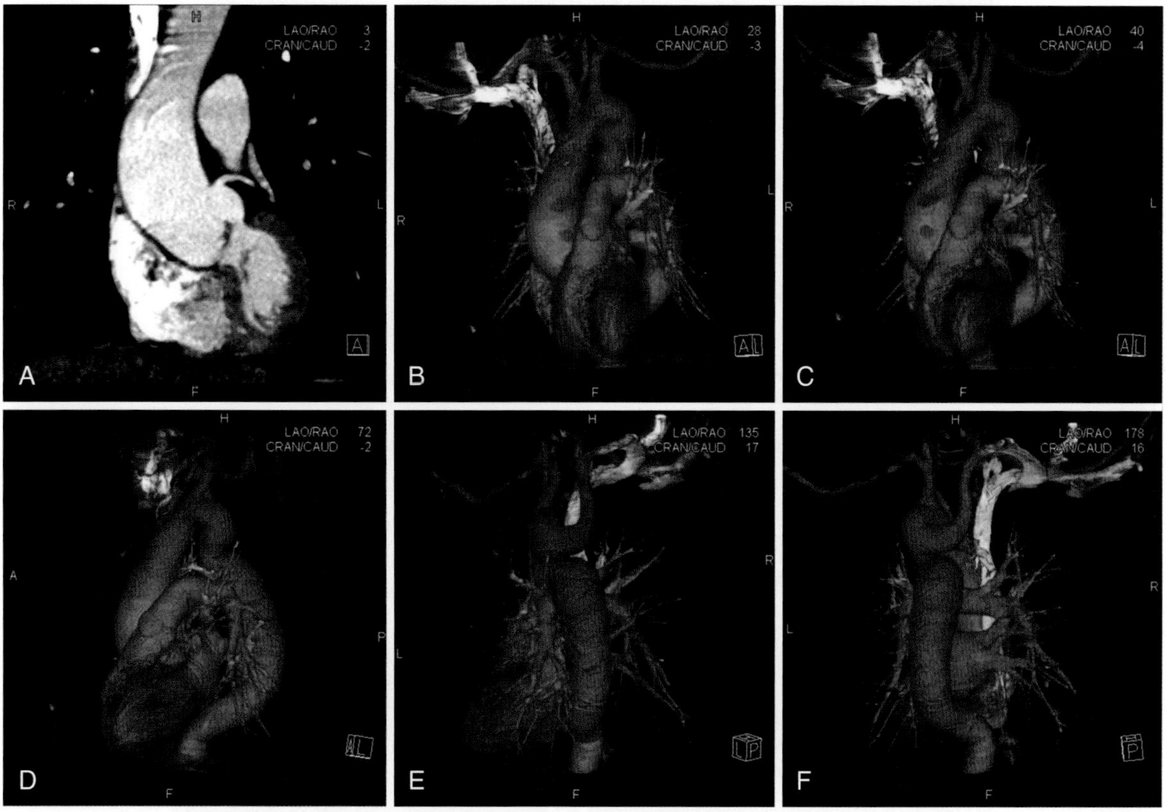

Figure 26-42. Planar and three-dimensional reconstructions (with varied projections) depict dilation of the aortic root and ascending aorta (associated with a bicuspid aortic valve), a mild narrowing (30 mm Hg gradient) at the site of a previously repaired coarctation, tortuosity at the site of repair, and dilation of the ongoing descending aorta, both before and after the repaired coarctation.

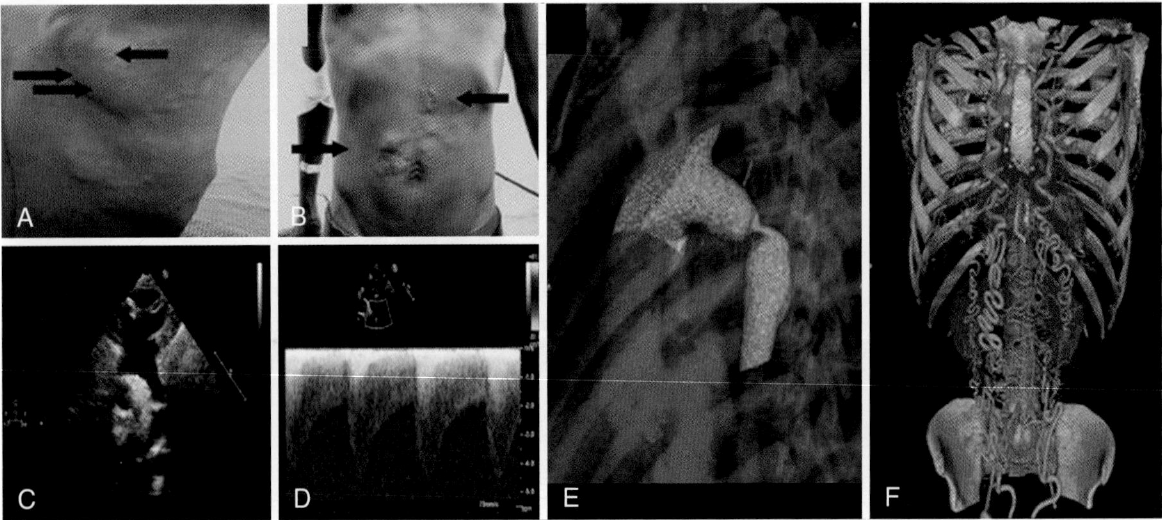

Figure 26-43. A 37-year-old man presented with resistant hypertension on four drugs. The physical examination revealed radiofemoral delay and clinical left ventricular hypertrophy. **A** and **B,** Very distinct palpable pulsatile collateral vessels were discovered over his left scapular, left chest wall, and anterior abdominal wall. Echocardiography confirmed left ventricular hypertrophy with good systolic function and a normal left ventricular outflow tract. Suprasternal echocardiography revealed a stenosis in the descending aorta (**C**) with a peak systolic gradient of 84 mm Hg and a pan-diastolic gradient (**D**). **E** and **F,** A 64-mm CT scan of the chest revealed a focal coarctation and collaterals extending over the scapular and over the anterior abdominal wall. The patient decided to consider his options of surgical correction versus an endovascular stent. (Reprinted with permission from Peters F, Essop R. Coarctation of the aorta with visible palpable collaterals over the scapular and anterior abdominal wall. *J Am Coll Cardiol.* 2010;56(5):423.)

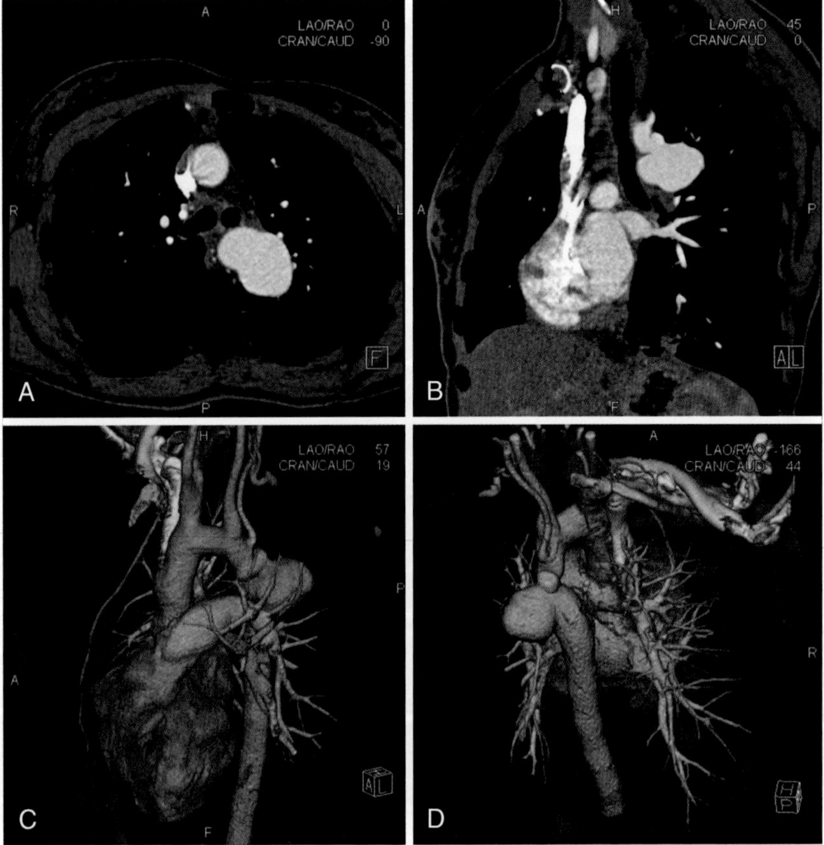

Figure 26-44. Axial, oblique, and three-dimensional reconstructions of an aneurysm/false aneurysm at the site of a remotely repaired coarctation. The absence of the proximal left subclavian artery strongly suggests that it was used to repair the coarctation.

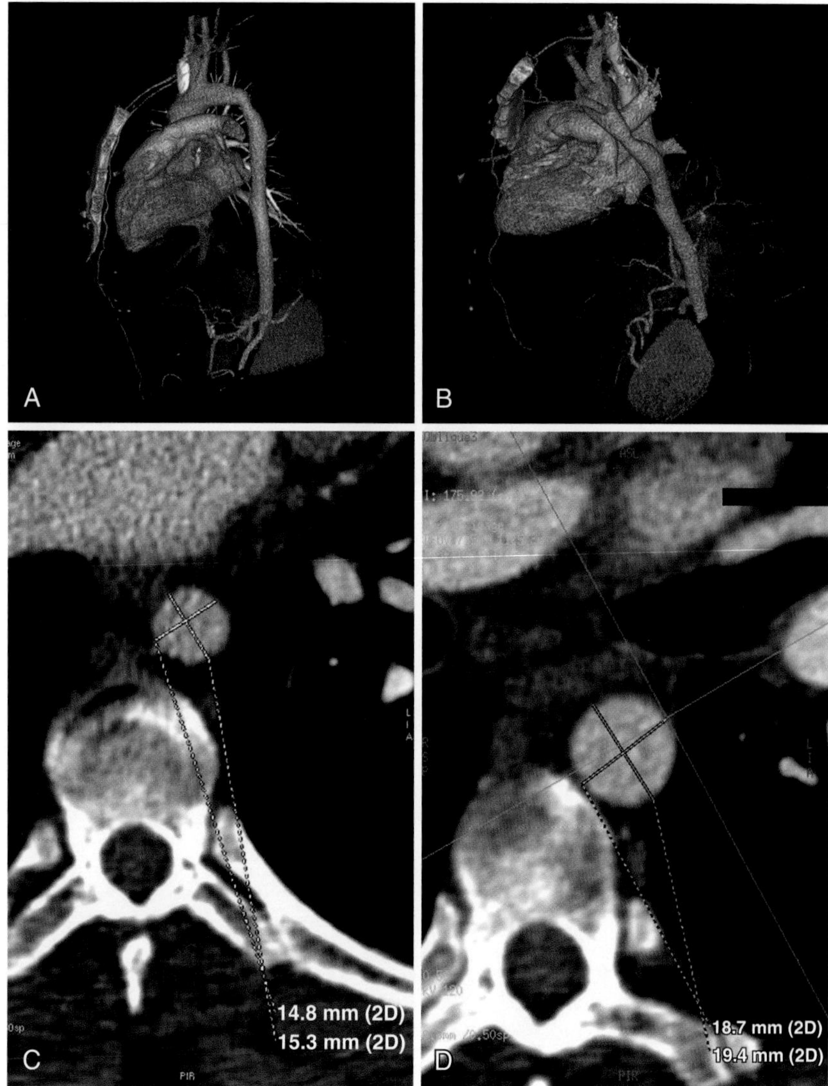

Figure 26-45. Volume-rendered (**A** and **B**) and axial source images (**C** and **D**) from a gated CT angiogram of the chest in a patient with a prior history of coarctation and previous end-to-end surgical repair. The volume-rendered images demonstrate a mild recoarctation at the surgical site. There is focal dilatation of the proximal descending aorta distal to the coarctation site, which may represent some mild poststenotic dilatation

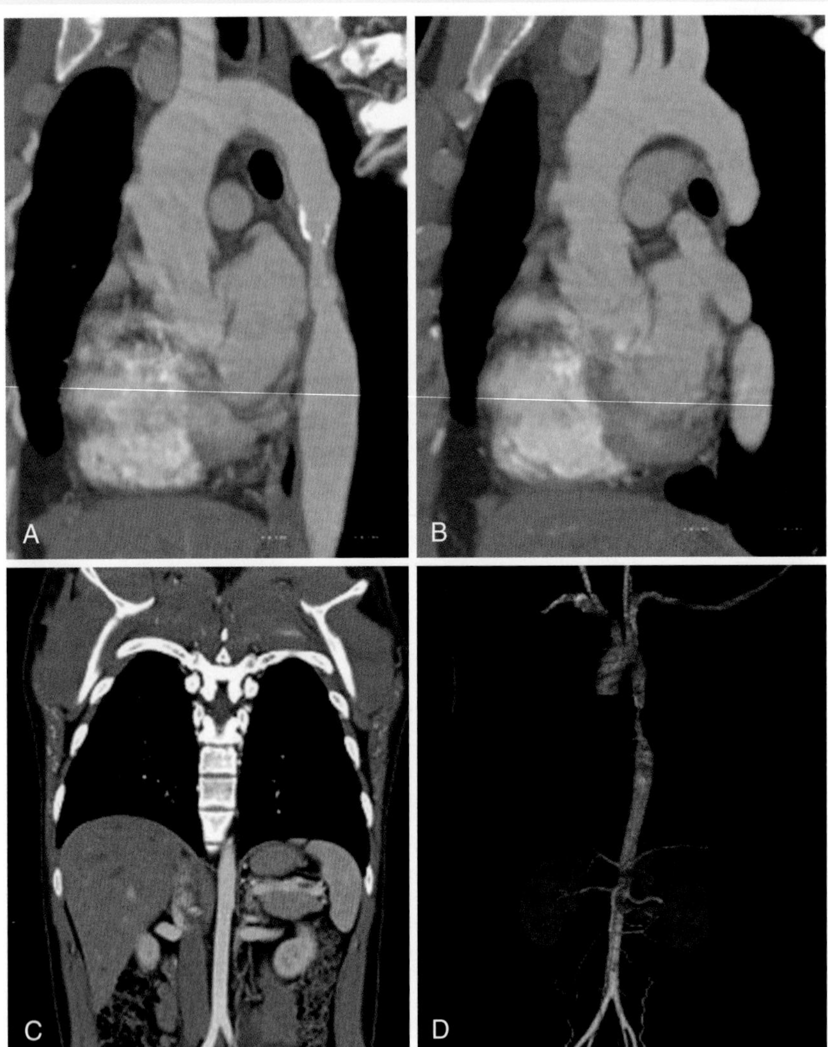

Figure 26-46. A 20-year-old man presented with hypertension resistant to antihypertensive medication. **A,** CT showed focal stenosis of the mid-portion of the descending aorta at the T4 to T5 level. **B,** The aortic arch, its branches, and the aortic isthmus showed well-developed contours without stenosis. **C** and **D,** The abdominal aorta and its major branches and aortic bifurcation also were morphologically normal. The patient was a healthy young man except for incidentally found upper body hypertension. There was no history of any inflammatory signs or symptoms suggesting a diagnosis of Takayasu arteritis. Routine laboratory work, including C-reactive protein and erythrocyte sedimentation rate, was normal. No other systemic changes, such as neurofibromatosis or chromosomal anomalies, were detected. The etiology in this patient's case is believed to be congenital, because no evidence of inflammatory arteritis or systemic disease was found and no other segment of the aorta or its branches was involved. (Reprinted with permission from Park HK, Cho SH, Park YH. Atypical coarctation of the aorta: congenital stenosis of the mid-thoracic aorta. *J Am Coll Cardiol.* 2009;53(22):2098.)

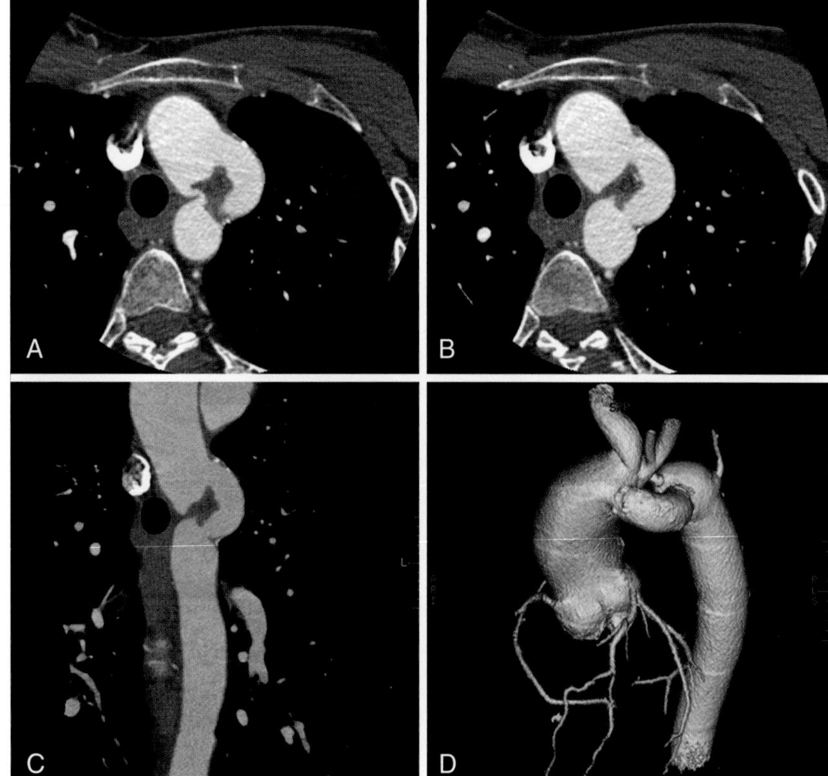

Figure 26-47. A 35-year-old man with a history of severe arch hypoplasia/coarctation. There is a marked narrowing of the midportion of the aortic arch. There has been a surgical Dacron graft bypass from the proximal portion of the aortic arch to the distal arch. The surgical bypass is intact, with no evidence of a stenosis, aneurysm, or pseudoaneurysm. A small amount of calcification within the graft is noted. The arch vessels are patent and extend from the proximal portion of the aortic arch. The ascending aorta is mildly dilated and measures 4.3 cm.

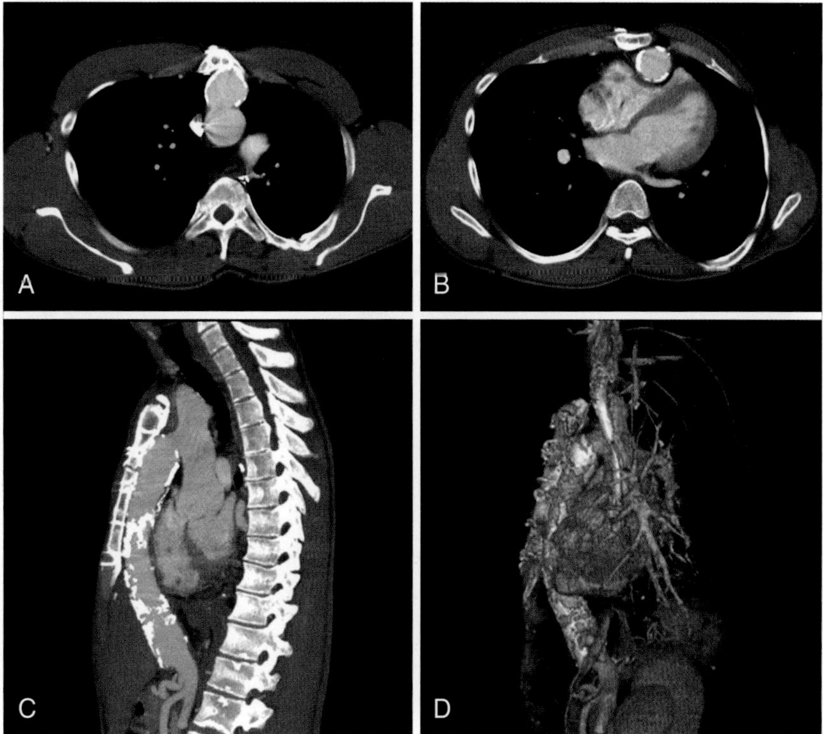

Figure 26-48. Multiple images from a gated CT angiogram of the chest and abdomen in a patient with a history of severe coarctation of the thoracic aorta with multiple failed surgeries. No evidence of a descending thoracic aorta is seen. This likely represents atresia of the descending thoracic aorta. **A** and **B,** There is a large conduit extending from the anterior aspect of the ascending aorta, which courses within the anterior mediastinum. **A** demonstrates the conduit compressing the midportion of the right ventricle. The conduit is heavily calcified, but not stenotic. **C** and **D,** Heavy calcification within the conduit, and normal distal anastomosis to the upper abdominal aorta, above the level of the celiac axis. See **Video 26-2.**

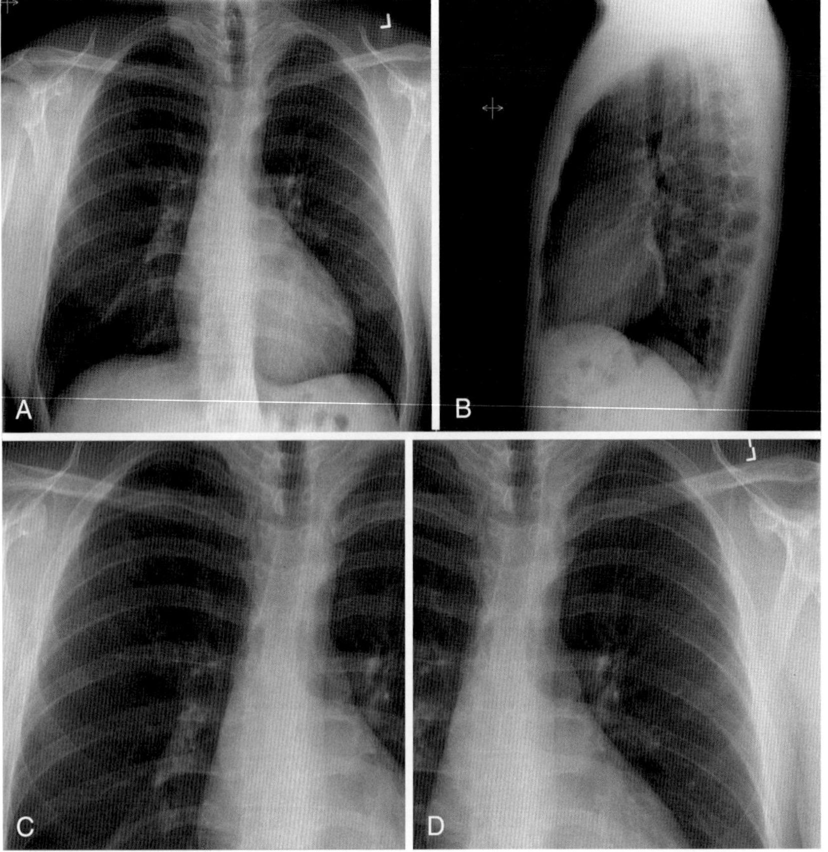

Figure 26-49. A 27-year-old man with a history of hypertension and paroxysmal atrial fibrillation. The posteroanterior (**A**) and lateral (**B**) chest radiographs demonstrate mild prominence of the left ventricular shadow as well as fullness in the anterior mediastinum on the lateral study. There is subtle prominence of the aortic arch, but a convincing "three sign" involving the aortic arch and proximal descending aorta is not appreciated. **C** and **D**, The presence of moderate bilateral rib notching is more obvious, especially on the magnified views.

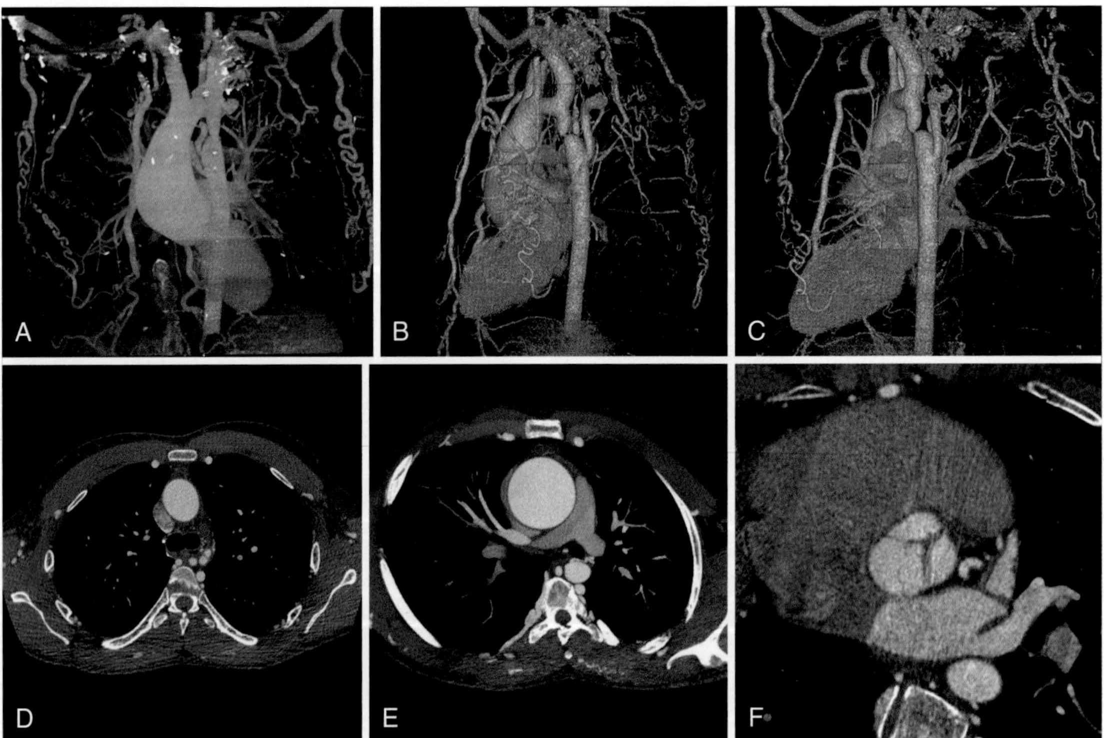

Figure 26-50. A 27-year-old man with hypertension and paroxysmal atrial fibrillation underwent ECG-gated CT angiography of the chest. The maximum intensity projection image (**A**) and the volume-rendered image (**B**) demonstrate marked collateral flow within the chest bilaterally, including massively hypertrophied internal mammary arteries as well as chest wall and intercostal arteries. **C** and **D**, Discrete focal coarctation in the proximal descending aorta with a bandlike cut-off. A short-segment aortic interruption likely is present. **E** and **F,** A large (6.2 cm) ascending aortic aneurysm is present. Aortic valve morphology is difficult to determine on prospective gated studies but suggests a "functionally bicuspid" aortic valve, confirmed on echocardiography. The aortic aneurysm therefore relates to bicuspid aortopathy.

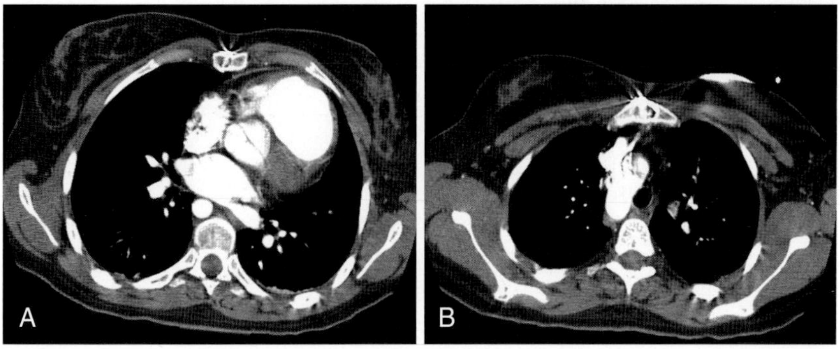

Figure 26-51. CT angiogram of the thorax in a 28-year-old woman with repaired tetralogy of Fallot. **A,** There is a moderately enlarged right ventricular outflow tract. Incidental note is made of a bicuspid aortic valve. The aortic arch is right-sided. Right-sided aortic arches are a common finding in patients with tetralogy of Fallot.

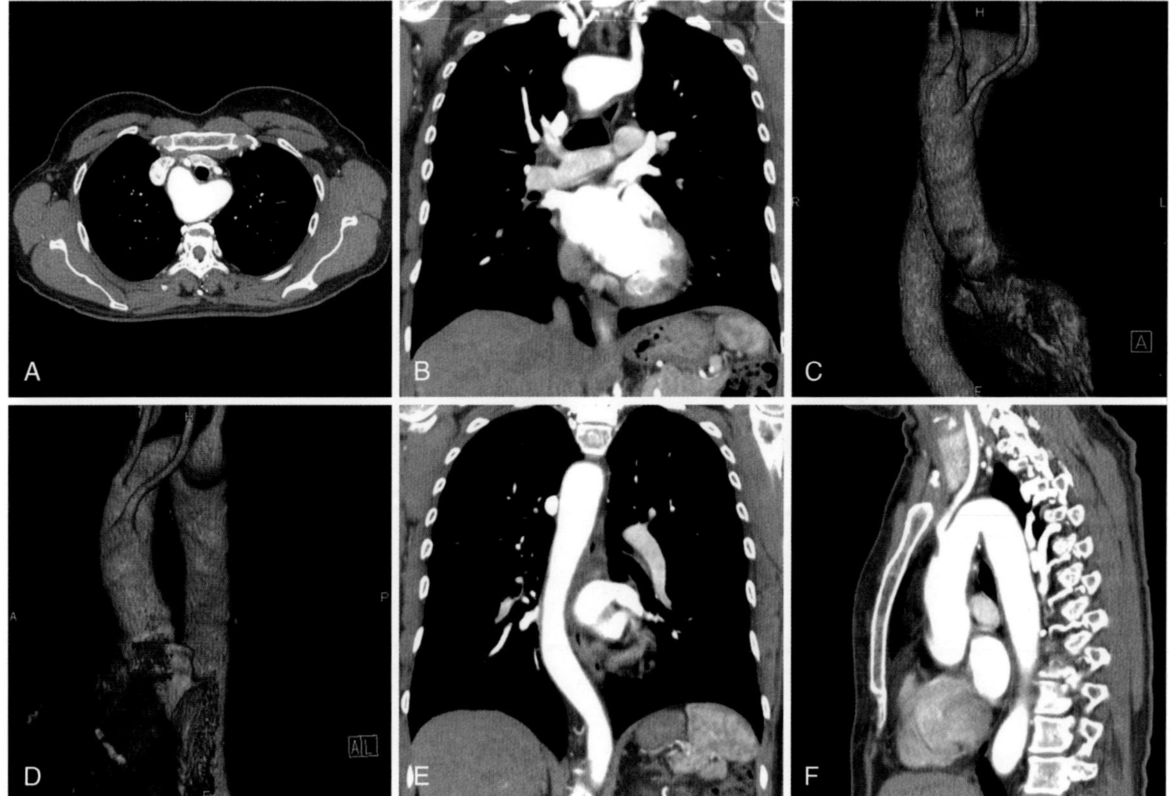

Figure 26-52. Right-sided aortic arch with arch branch vessel anomalies. A diverticulum of Kommerell is present at the origin of the left subclavian artery. The left common carotid artery arises as the first branch vessel. The arch also peaks unusually abruptly and high in the chest.

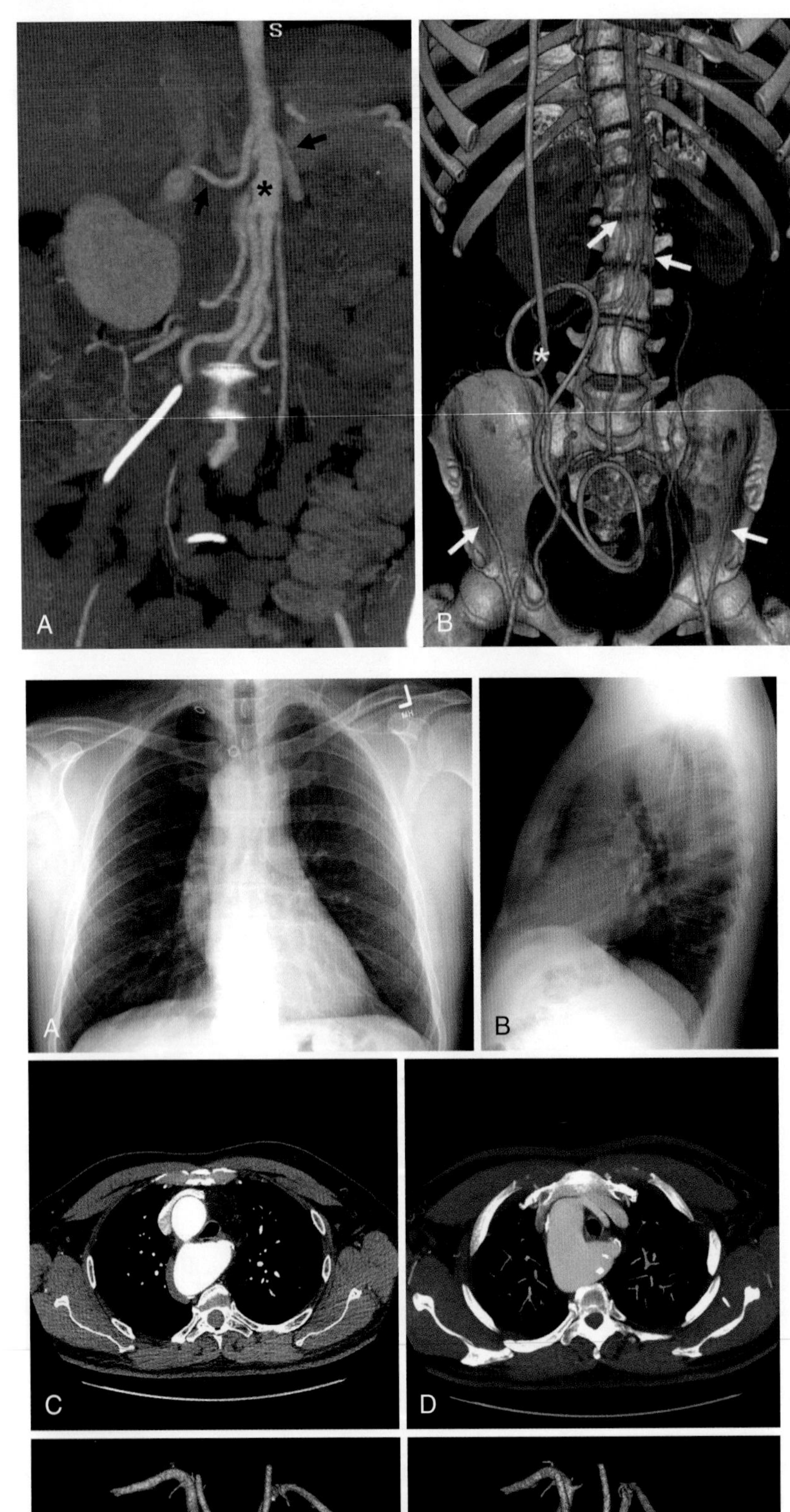

Figure 26-53. Hypoplasia of the abdominal aorta associated with hypomelanosis of Ito. **A,** Contrast-enhanced multidetector CT imaging of the thorax and abdomen on a coronal plane shows an interruption of the abdominal aorta (*) immediately distal to the origin of the renal arteries. **B,** Three-dimensional reconstruction shows hypoplasia of the abdominal aorta. Multiple small vessels arise to irrigate the lower extremities (*white arrows*), mimicking a pseudo cauda equina. The asterisk marks the ventriculoperitoneal shunt. (Reprinted with permission from Vivas D, Garcia-Guereta L, Bret M, et al. Images in cardiovascular medicine. Hypoplasia of the abdominal aorta and hypomelanosis of Ito: "Pseudo-cauda equina" imaging. *Circulation.* 2009;120(20):2025-2026.)

Figure 26-54. A 32-year-old male presenting with dysphagia. Posteroanterior (**A**) and lateral (**B**) chest radiographs demonstrate a right-sided aortic arch. The lateral study (**B**) demonstrates a large region of soft tissue posterior to the trachea. **C** and **D,** Axial images from gated CT angiography of the thorax demonstrate a right-sided aortic arch, and a large focal outpouching representing a diverticulum of coronal coursing posterior to the trachea. The esophagus is almost entirely effaced. **E** and **F,** The volume-rendered images demonstrate a large diverticulum of Kommerell from which an aberrant left subclavian artery arises. A moderate amount of calcific plaque is seen involving the diverticulum of Kommerell. Vascular compression of the esophagus resulting in dysphagia has been described as *dysphagia lusoria*.

- Diverticulum of Kommerell
- Patent ductus arteriosus
- Multiple patent ducti
- Bronchopulmonary sequestration
- Hypoplasia of the abdominal aorta

TRAUMATIC DISRUPTION OF THE AORTA

Violent deceleration injury to the body may result in traumatic disruption of the aorta (Figs. 26-55 through 26-61 and **Videos 26-3 and 26-4**).

Victims typically were not wearing seatbelts and were ejected from a vehicle moving faster than 50 km/hr. The most common sites of disruption are the isthmus (proximal descending aorta), the ascending aorta, and the supradiaphragmatic aorta.

Findings are not typically those of aortic dissection. Notably, the length of disrupted aorta is usually only a few centimeters, whereas in dissection half or more of the aorta usually is involved.Also, the principal finding is of a localized disruption/ irregularity of the intima, not of a long, obvious, and freely mobile intimal flap.

As to be expected, older studies showed that CT was of limited value to exclude aortic disruption.[15,16] However, more recent studies have demonstrated that for the evaluation of acute traumatic thoracic aortic injury, helical CT is equivalent to aortography in terms of sensitivity and negative predictive value,[17] but CT is less expensive than aortography.[17,18] The finding of mediastinal hemorrhage is sensitive for the diagnosis of traumatic aortic injury, but direct findings of aortic injury are more specific.[18]

NONINFECTIOUS AORTITIS

Several different inflammatory diseases, including Takayasu arteritis, giant cell arteritis, systemic lupus erythematosus, and others, may involve the aorta.

The cardinal feature of Takayasu arteritis is wall thickening[19,20] due to inflammation and edema. CT is as well suited as MRI/MRA to image both the thickening of the wall and the resultant narrowing of the lumen of the aorta as well as of the (arch) branch vessels. Combined positron emission tomography (PET)-CT may offer a means to show the increased metabolism of the aortic wall affected by aortitis.

Later-stage Takayasu arteritis may evolve to aneurysms, dissections, fistulas,[21] and even porcelain (diffusely calcified) aorta.[22]

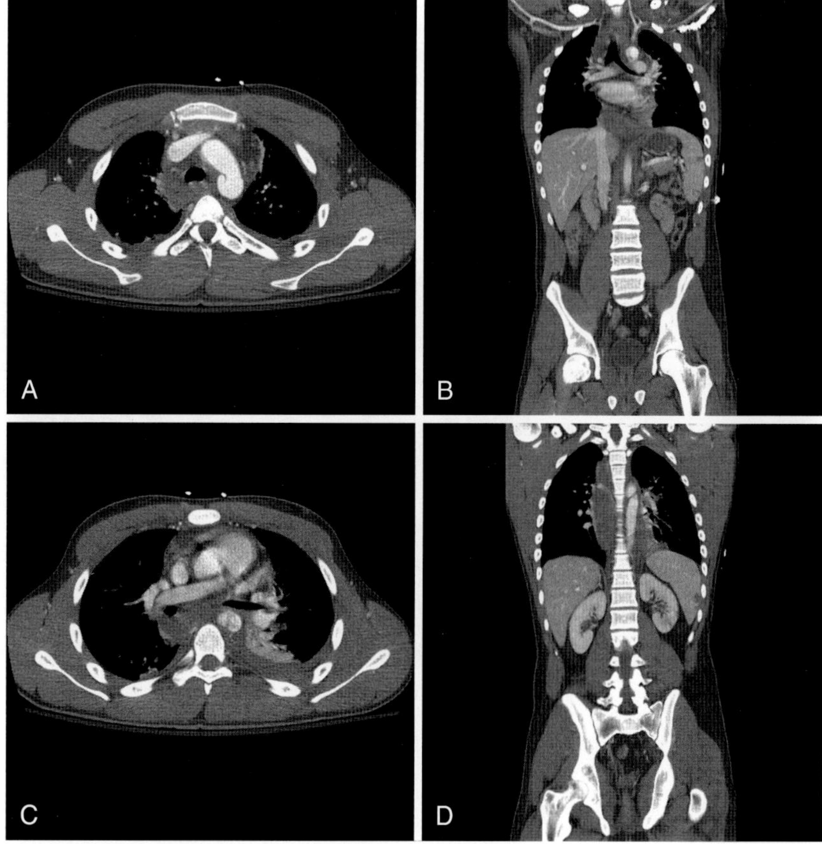

Figure 26-55. Contrast-enhanced chest and body images of a patient with a traumatic disruption of the proximal descending aorta following a motor vehicle collision. The site of disruption is short. The disruption includes a short flap and localized false lumen. There is mediastinal hematoma associated with the traumatic disruption of the aorta.

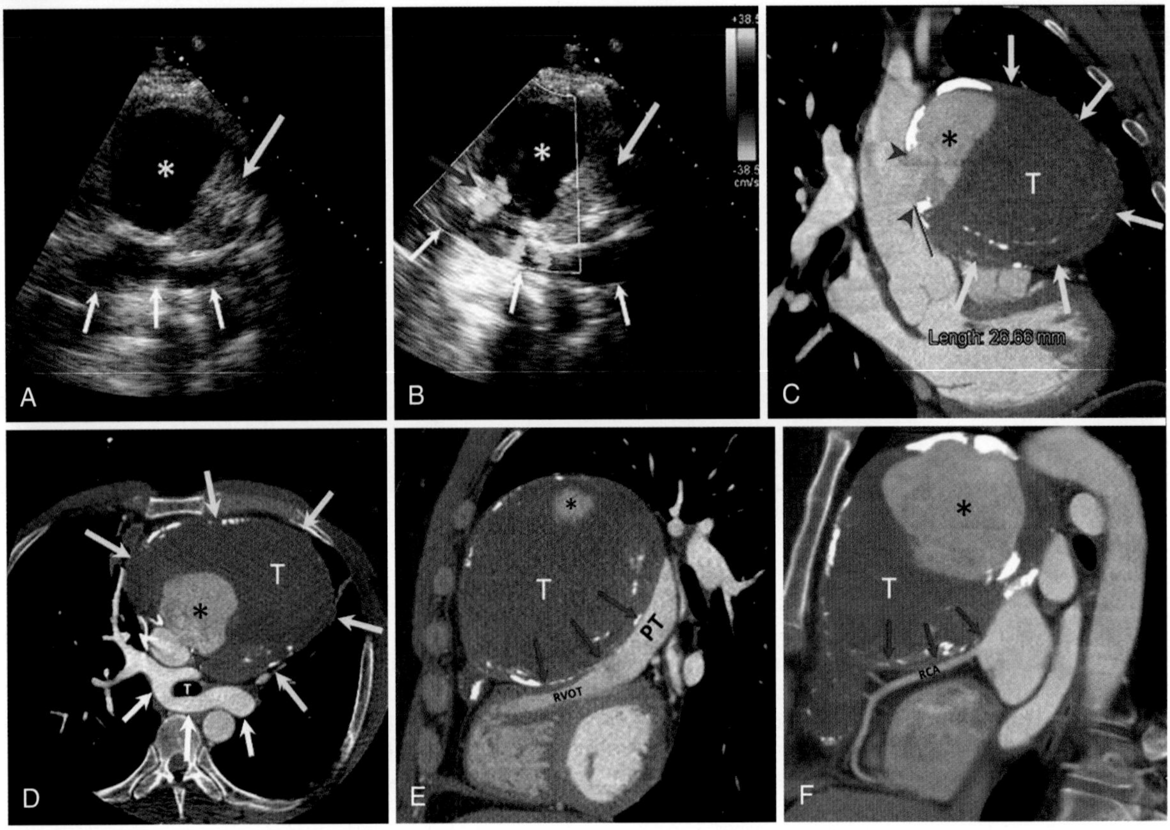

Figure 26-56. Same patient shown in Figure 26-55. Gray scale (**A**) and color Doppler (**B**) transthoracic echocardiograms (TTE) demonstrate a large, relatively anechoic lesion (*) within the mediastinum anterior to the ascending aorta (*small white arrows*). Color Doppler demonstrates communication of the anechoic lesion with the ascending aorta via a narrow neck (*red arrow*), consistent with a pseudoaneurysm. The thick peripheral rind of heterogenously echogenic material represents eccentric thrombus (*yellow arrow*). **C** through **F**, Multiplanar reformats (MPRs) from cardiac CTA demonstrate the narrow neck (*red arrowheads* in **C** and **D**) of the pseudoaneurysm that arises 2.7 cm above the sinotubular junction. Note both the patent portion (*) and extensive peripheral thrombus (label *T* and *yellow arrows*). The pseudoaneurysm markedly compresses the right ventricular outflow tract, causes the course of the pulmonic trunk to deviate, and borders the ostium and proximal right coronary artery, as indicated by red arrows in **E** and **F**. The diagnosis was chronic posttraumatic false aneurysm. (Reprinted with permission from Gupta P, Carr JJ, Kon ND, Entrikin DW. Giant pseudoaneurysm of the ascending aorta—preoperative evaluation and surgical planning facilitated by cardiac computed tomographic angiography. SCCT Case of the Month, February 2012; available at http://archive.constantcontact.com/fs027/1101901294184/archive/1109402007784.html.)

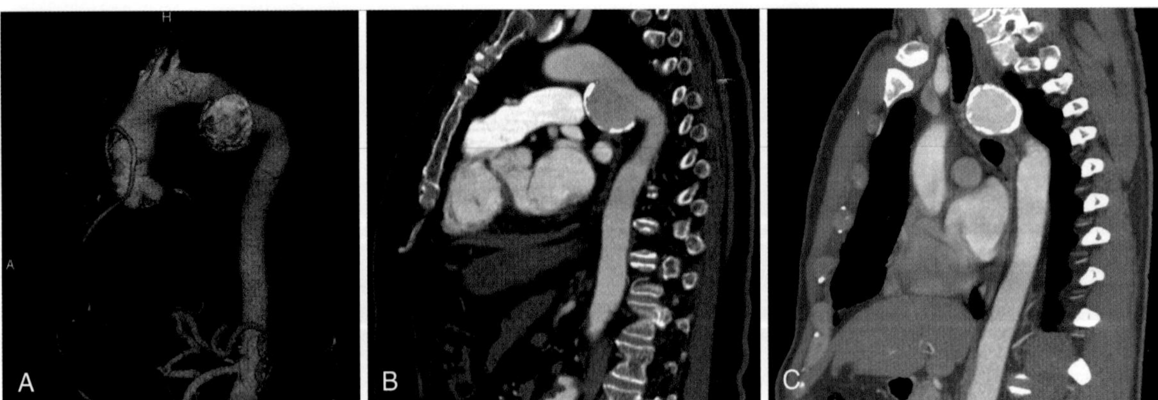

Figure 26-57. Circumferential calcification of the wall of a chronic traumatic false aneurysm.

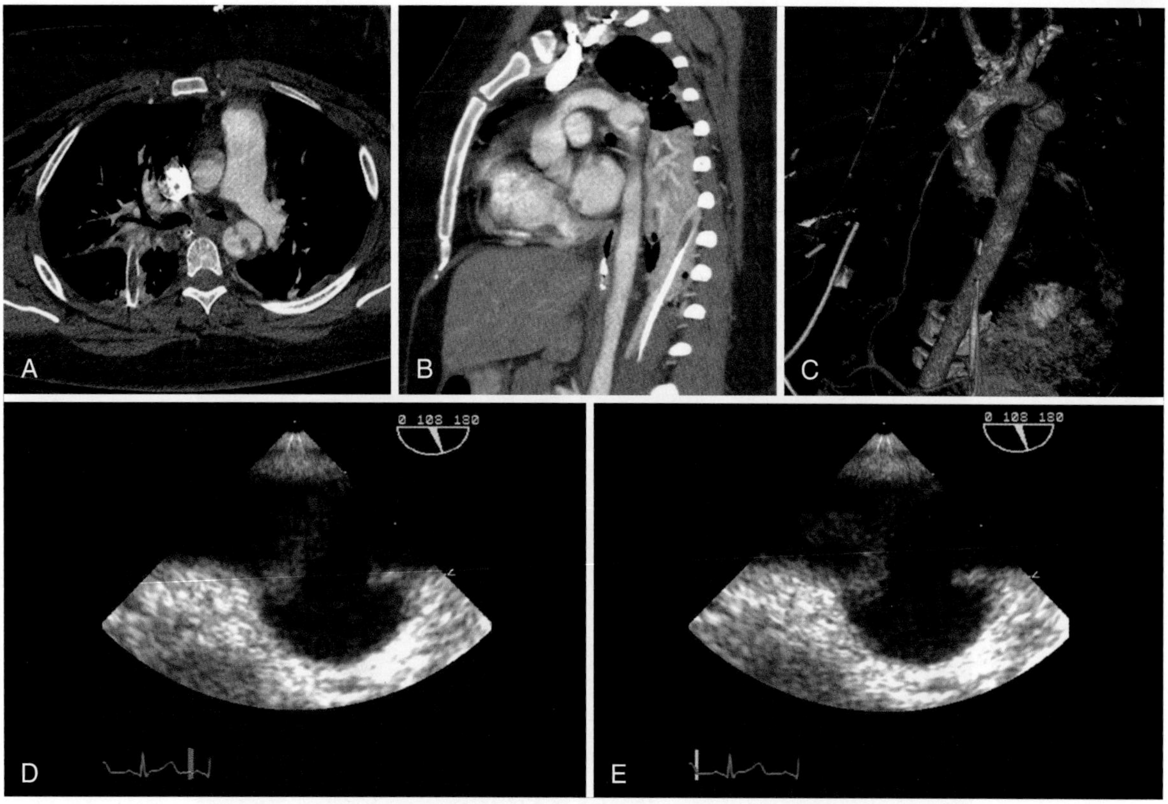

Figure 26-58. A 28-year-old woman injured in a high-speed motor vehicle accident. There is traumatic disruption of the proximal descending thoracic aorta. **A,** A linear discontinuity within the proximal descending thoracic aorta. No evidence of a mediastinal hematoma is seen on this single image. Incidental findings include extensive subcutaneous emphysema on the right and placement of a pleural drain on the right. A sagittal reconstruction (**B**) and a volume-rendered image (**C**) demonstrate a focal outpouching in the proximal descending thoracic aorta consistent with a traumatic aortic injury and development of a localized pseudoaneurysm. **D** and **E,** Transesophageal echocardiograms demonstrate focal outpouching at the level of pseudoaneurysm formation. Linear regions of intermediate echogenicity adjacent to this likely represent areas of intimal disruption, and localized clot formation. See **Videos 26-3 and 26-4.**

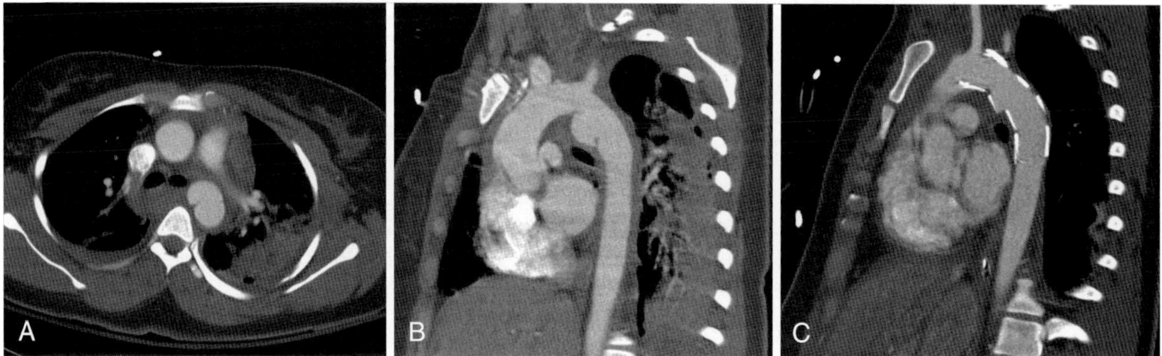

Figure 26-59. A 22-year-old female trauma patient injured in a high-velocity motor vehicle accident. **A,** Axial image demonstrates a moderate amount of mediastinal soft tissue/hemorrhage. There is an acute aortic injury, with a focal outpouching seen extending from the descending thoracic aorta anteriorly and inferiorly. This is best seen on the sagittal reconstruction "candy cane" view (**C**) and represents a focal aortic transection within the proximal descending thoracic aorta. The patient underwent stent grafting.

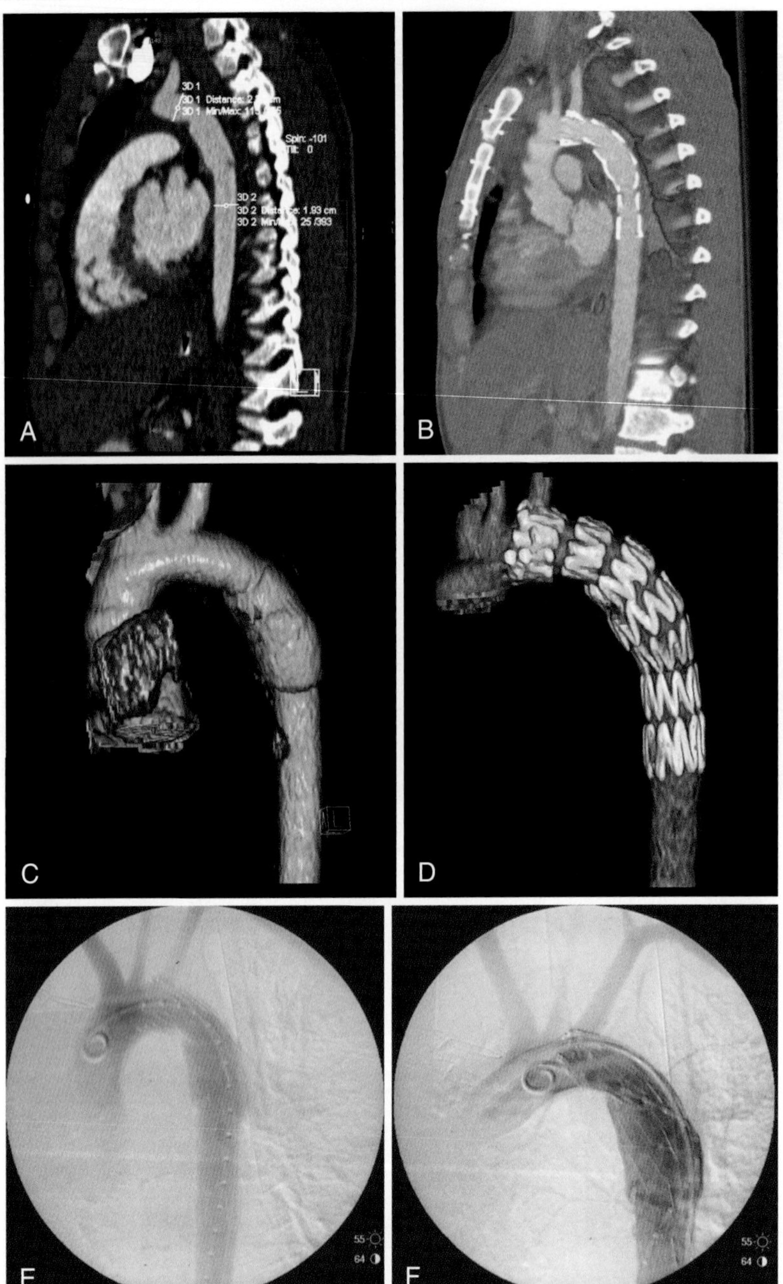

Figure 26-60. A 19-year-old man with an acute aortic injury post–motor vehicle accident. There is focal contour abnormality of the proximal descending thoracic aorta (**A, C,** and **E**). The trauma CT scan was used to plan placement of an aortic stent graft (**B, D,** and **F**).

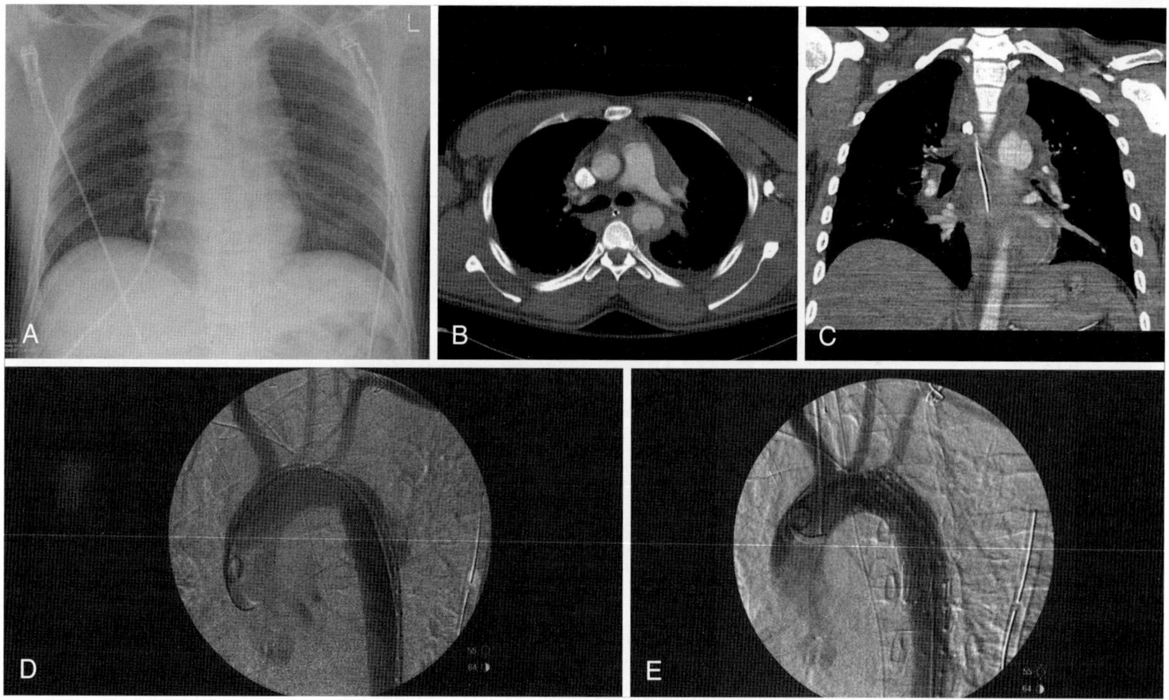

Figure 26-61. Traumatic disruption of the aorta.

For images of Takayasu arteritis, see Figures 26-62 through 26-73.

Hybrid PET-CT is able to localize increased ^{18}F-fluorodeoxyglucose (FDG) activity in the aorta and its proximal branches in cases of florid aortitis.[23]

For images of PET imaging of the aorta, see Figure 26-74.

ENDOVASCULAR TREATMENT OF THE AORTA

CT scanning is the standard imaging test to plan for endovascular therapy, and to assess for success, complications, and failures (e.g., endoleaks).

For images of endovascular treatment of the aorta, see Figures 26-75 through 26-77.

SINUS OF VALSALVA ANEURYSMS

The sinuses of Valsalva represent the potential spaces between the valve cusps and the lateral wall of the aorta. A deficiency between the aortic media and annulus fibrosus of the aortic valve results in distention and eventual aneurysmal dilatation of the sinus, which often protrudes into adjacent structures. Eventually the aneurysms may rupture. Sinus of Valsalva aneurysms usually are isolated congenital lesions; however, they can be associated with ventricular septal defects and may be seen in other conditions such as Marfan syndrome and, less commonly, as a complication of endocarditis. Acquired sinus of Valsalva aneurysms are believed to rupture with less frequency than congenital aneurysms. Aneurysms most commonly arise from the right coronary sinus, followed by the noncoronary sinus and finally the left coronary sinus. Aneurysms of the right sinus often protrude into the right ventricular outflow tract or right atrium and can rupture into these right-sided structures, creating a left-to-right shunt. The patient develops sudden onset of chest pain with rapid development of heart failure due to the left-to-right shunt.

A possible differential diagnosis for a sinus of Valsalva aneurysm is a membranous interventricular septal aneurysm (IVSA). Membranous IVSAs develop in the course of spontaneous partial or complete VSD closure, by outpouching of either the septal leaflet of the tricuspid valve or thin membranes adjacent to VSD margins. Muscular IVSAs are extremely rare; they occur mainly in children or young adults, often in association with ASD or VSD (Figs. 26-78 through 26-80; **Videos 26-5 and 26-6**).

THE POSTOPERATIVE AORTA

Complications following thoracic aortic aneurysm surgery are common. Postoperative findings that may simulate pathology or surgical complications include high-attenuation felt pledgets, native aortic wrapping around the graft, and graft kinks. Postoperative complications include perigraft

Text continued on page 485

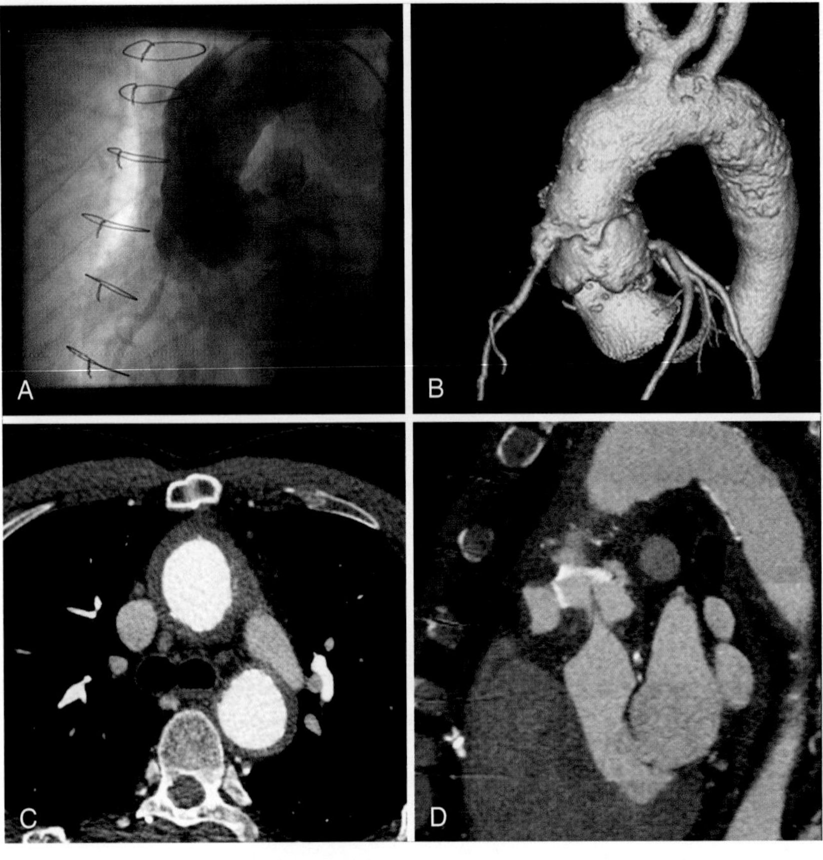

Figure 26-62. A 26-year-old man with a known history of Takayasu arteritis and prior placement of an ascending aortic graft. The patient presented with acute chest pain. **A,** Aortic root injection prior to coronary angiography. The ascending aorta is enlarged and irregular in appearance. **B,** An ECG-gated CT scan of the thorax, volume-rendered image demonstrates all irregular and diseased thoracic aorta views. Deformity of the proximal descending aorta reflects the patient's prior graft site. **C** and **D,** Extensive soft tissue thickening around the ascending and descending aorta in keeping with the patient's diagnosis of Takayasu arteritis. Multifocal areas of calcification also are seen within the thoracic aorta, likely secondary to chronic inflammation as opposed to atherosclerotic disease in this man. Small-volume lymph nodes within the mediastinum also are noted, likely reactive to the underlying inflammatory process.

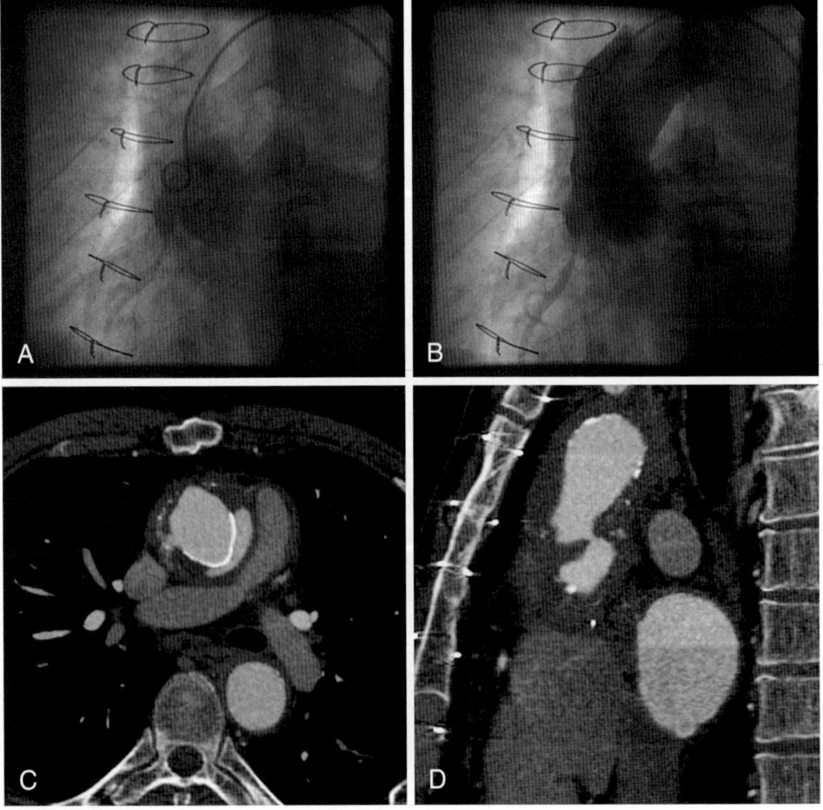

Figure 26-63. Same patient as Figure 26-62. The patient presented with acute chest pain. **A,** Initial images from an aortic root injection demonstrate ectasia of the proximal right coronary artery (RCA). **B,** Subsequent images from the aortic root injection demonstrate faint contrast outside the confines of the aortic root, best seen projecting inferior to the RCA origin and posterior to the aortic root. **C,** Peripheral high-density material seen within the aortic root demonstrates a portion of the descending aortic graft. This shows deformity and likely some compression from a collection of contrast medium, and also narrows the main and right pulmonary artery posterior to the valve aneurysm. There is suspicion of a discontinuity of the aortic graft along the right aspect of the graft. **D,** Sagittal oblique reconstruction also demonstrates communication between the aortic root and a perigraft/periaortic collection. The diagnosis was postoperative false aneurysm around the ascending aorta, potentially from breakdown of the graft anastomosis in a patient with Takayasu arteritis.

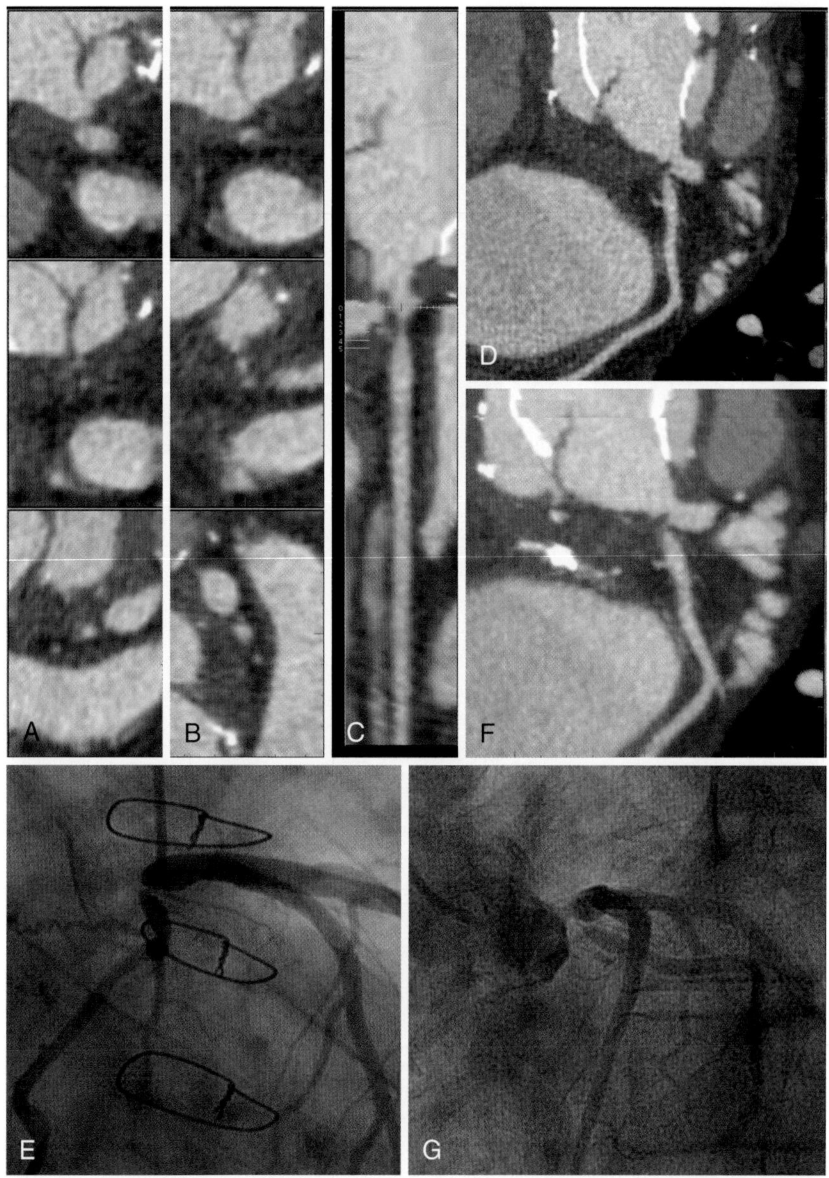

Figure 26-64. Same patient as Figure 26-62. The patient presented with acute chest pain. Multiple reconstructed images from a cardiac CT study demonstrate a severe stenosis of the proximal circumflex artery. The circumflex artery arises very proximally from a very short left main. Corresponding conventional angiography was performed. At initial evaluation of the left coronary artery (**F**) it was unclear whether the left anterior descending and circumflex arteries have separate ostia from the aortic root. **G,** A right anterior oblique projection with the catheter tip within the aortic root demonstrates the left main to be a short vessel, with a moderate left main stenosis, and suggests that the circumflex artery in fact does arise from the left main, with a severe, 90% stenosis, confirming the findings seen on the patient's cardiac CT examination.

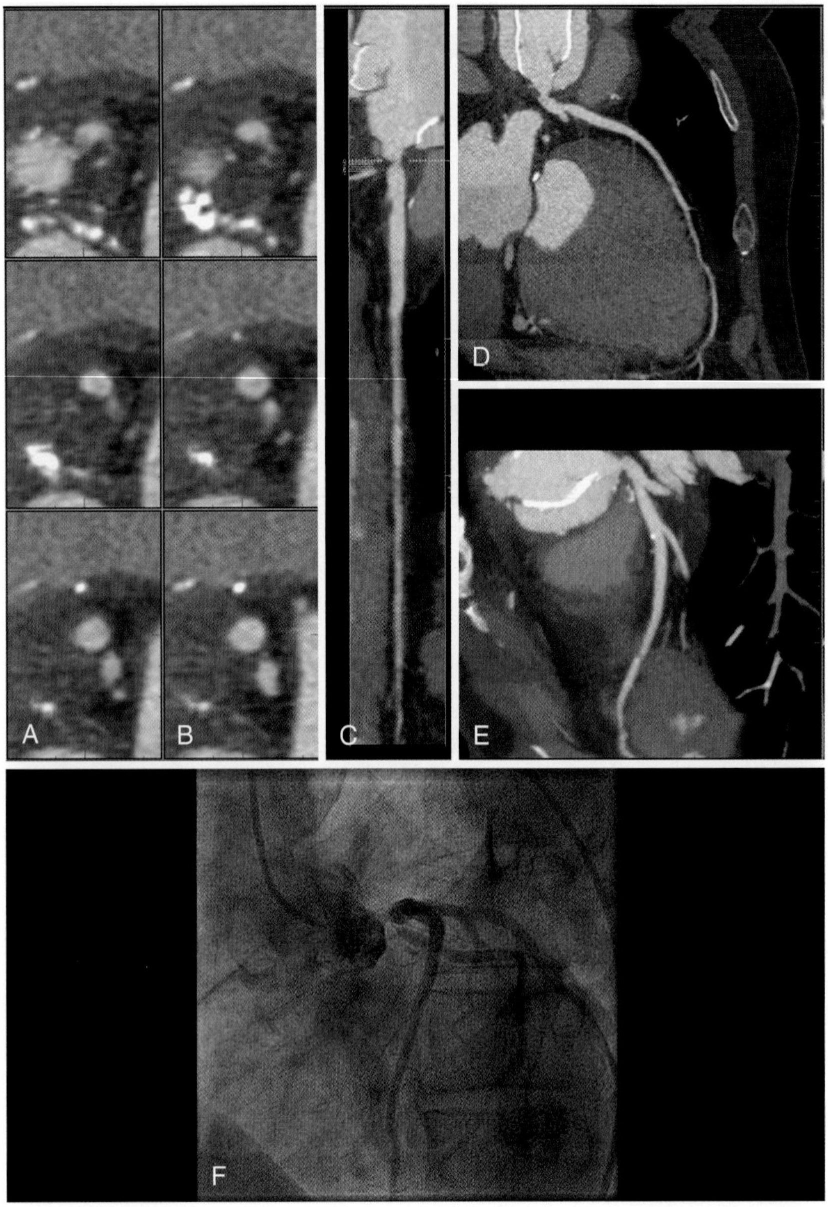

Figure 26-65. Same patient as Figure 26-62. **A** through **E,** Multiple cardiac CT images demonstrate abnormal soft tissue thickening around the aortic root, and a 50% stenosis of the left main coronary artery. This extends into the ostium of the circumflex artery (see Fig. 26-XX). This is most likely due to inflammatory process around the aortic root extending to the left main coronary artery. **F,** Conventional angiography confirms a 50% left main stenosis.

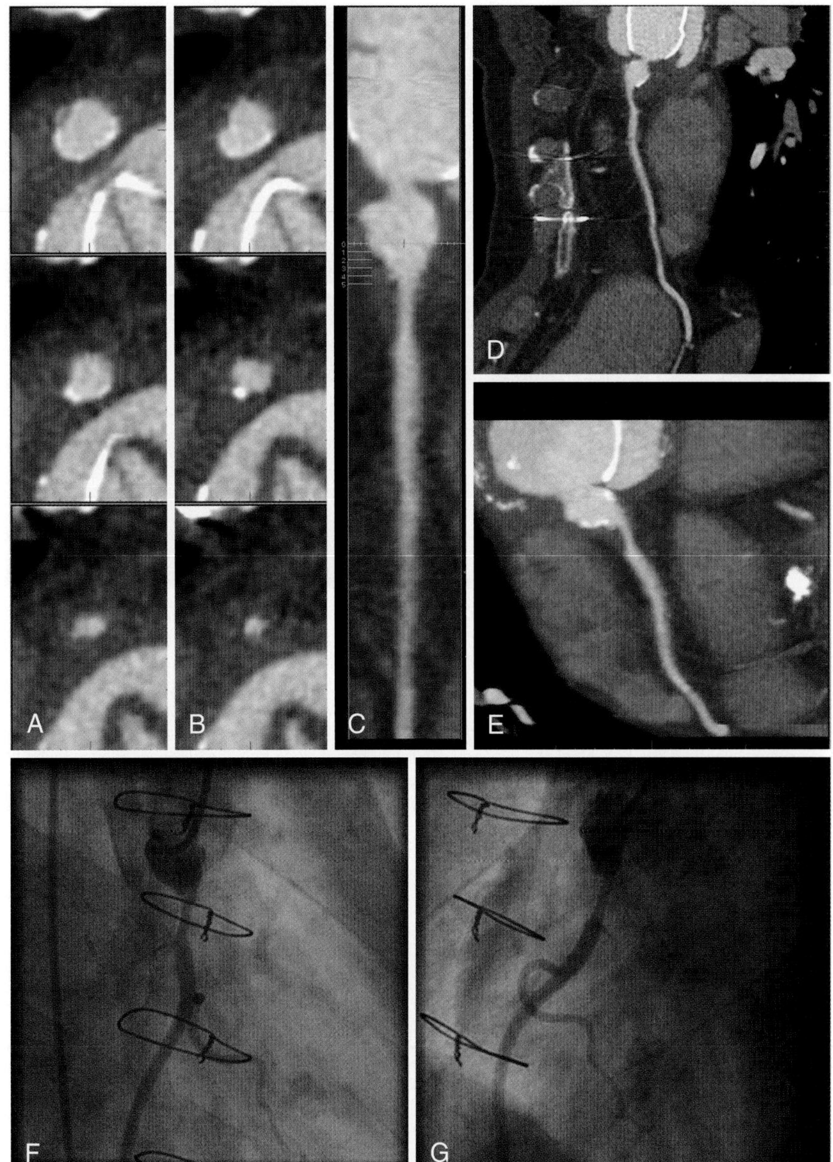

Figure 26-66. Same patient as Figure 26-62. Multiple cardiac CT images demonstrate a focal aneurysm of the proximal right coronary artery (RCA) measuring 14 mm. Cross-sectional views demonstrate moderate soft tissue extending from the ascending aorta, around the aneurysmal proximal RCA. There is a mild 30% to 40% stenosis of the RCA just distal to the aneurysm. Conventional angiography confirms the proximal RCA aneurysm, and mild narrowing of the ongoing proximal RCA.

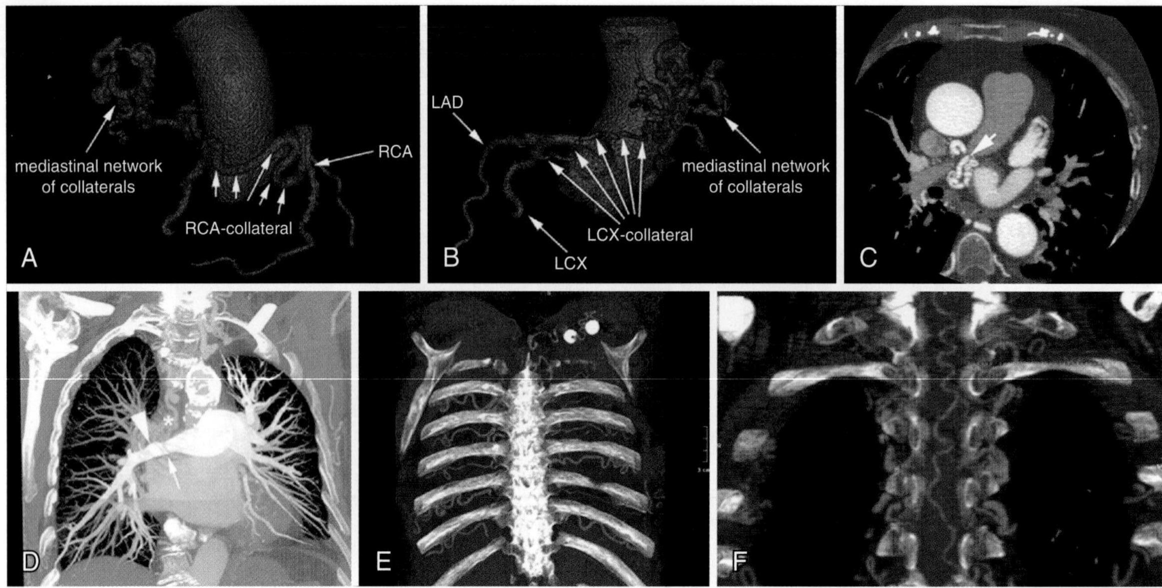

Figure 26-67. In a 78-year-old woman with chest pain and known Takayasu arteritis, prospective, electrocardiographically triggered, 320-slice cardiac CT revealed a network of arterial collateral arteries within the pericardium and mediastinum fed by the proximal right coronary artery (RCA) and proximal left circumflex coronary artery (LCX). **A** and **B,** Three-dimensional volume-rendered contrast-enhanced CT scans. **C,** Axial CT scan. Because of the patient's Takayasu arteritis, all three supra-aortal branches had progressively narrowed over decades and finally occluded. Furthermore, stenosis of the right pulmonary artery with lobar occlusion to the right upper lobe (**D**), capacious intercostal arteries with rib erosions (**E**), and a dilated spinal artery (**E**) could be identified. Other causes of chest pain, including pulmonary embolism, aortic dissection, and obstructive atherosclerotic coronary artery disease, were successfully ruled out. The patient's symptoms suggest a coronary steal phenomenon. Redistribution of blood from the coronary arteries to the depicted network leaves dependent cardiac parenchyma at increased risk for undernourishment and myocardial infarction. LAD, left anterior descending coronary artery. (Reprinted with permission from de Bucourt M, Hein PA, Patrik Rogalla P. Coronary artery proliferation and steal phenomenon in Takayasu's disease with occlusion of supra-aortal branches demonstrated by 320-slice computed tomography. *J Am Coll Cardiol.* 2010;56(12):e23.)

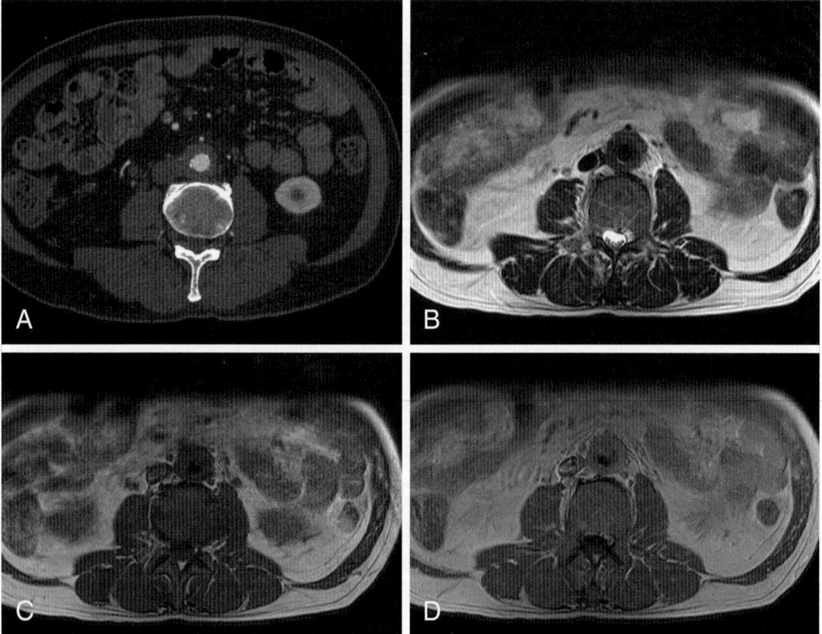

Figure 26-68. Composite images from a 28-year-old woman with Takayasu arteritis. **A,** CCT shows a moderate amount of soft tissue thickening circumferentially around the infrarenal abdominal aorta. The remainder of the images (**B–D**) are from an MRI study obtained one week later. **B,** T2-weighted image demonstrates the aortic wall thickening seen on the CT scan, but no increase in signal intensity associated with the aortic wall. The presence of aortic wall enhancement would suggest an acute inflammatory phase.

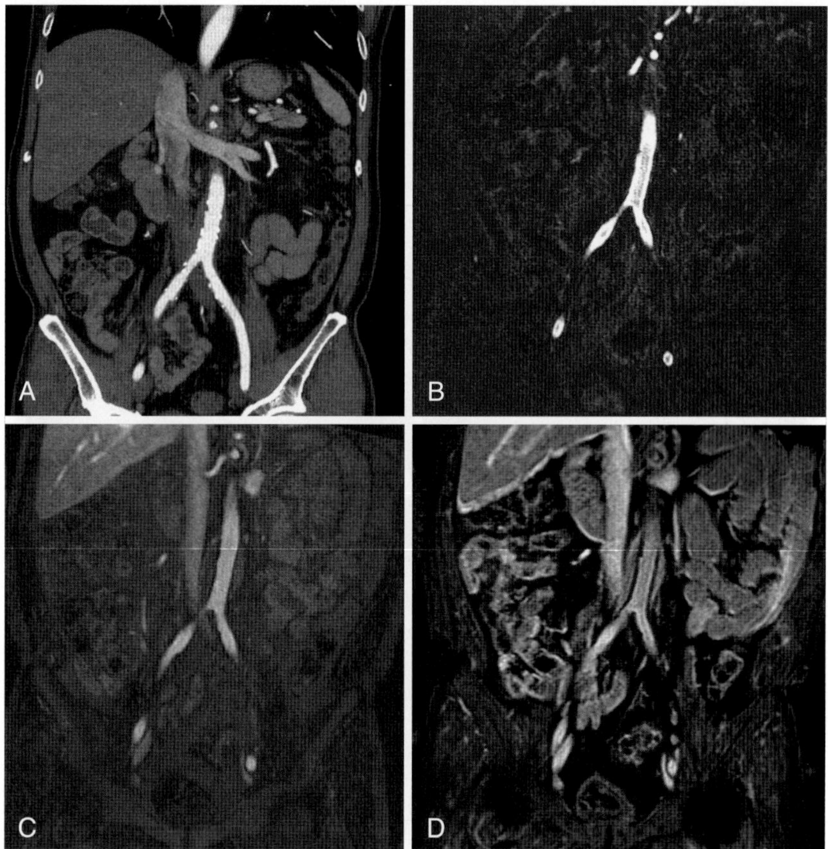

Figure 26-69. Composite images from a 28-year-old woman with Takayasu arteritis. **A,** Coronal image reformatted from an abdominal CT angiogram. There is a subtle thickening around the origins of the superior mesenteric artery and celiac axis. Also seen is soft tissue thickening around the infrarenal abdominal aorta just above the level of the bifurcation. The remaining images (**B–D**) are from an MR angiogram. **B,** MR angiogram obtained in the arterial phase immediately after administration of gadolinium. **C,** Image obtained 40 seconds later. **D,** Image obtained at 2 minutes after contrast administration. Delayed images demonstrate progressive enhancement of the soft tissue around the celiac axis and superior mesenteric artery, as well as around the infrarenal abdominal aorta. Demonstration of enhancement of the aortic wall in the setting of Takayasu arteritis is better appreciated on MR imaging than on CT imaging. This mural enhancement is suggestive of an inflammatory process.

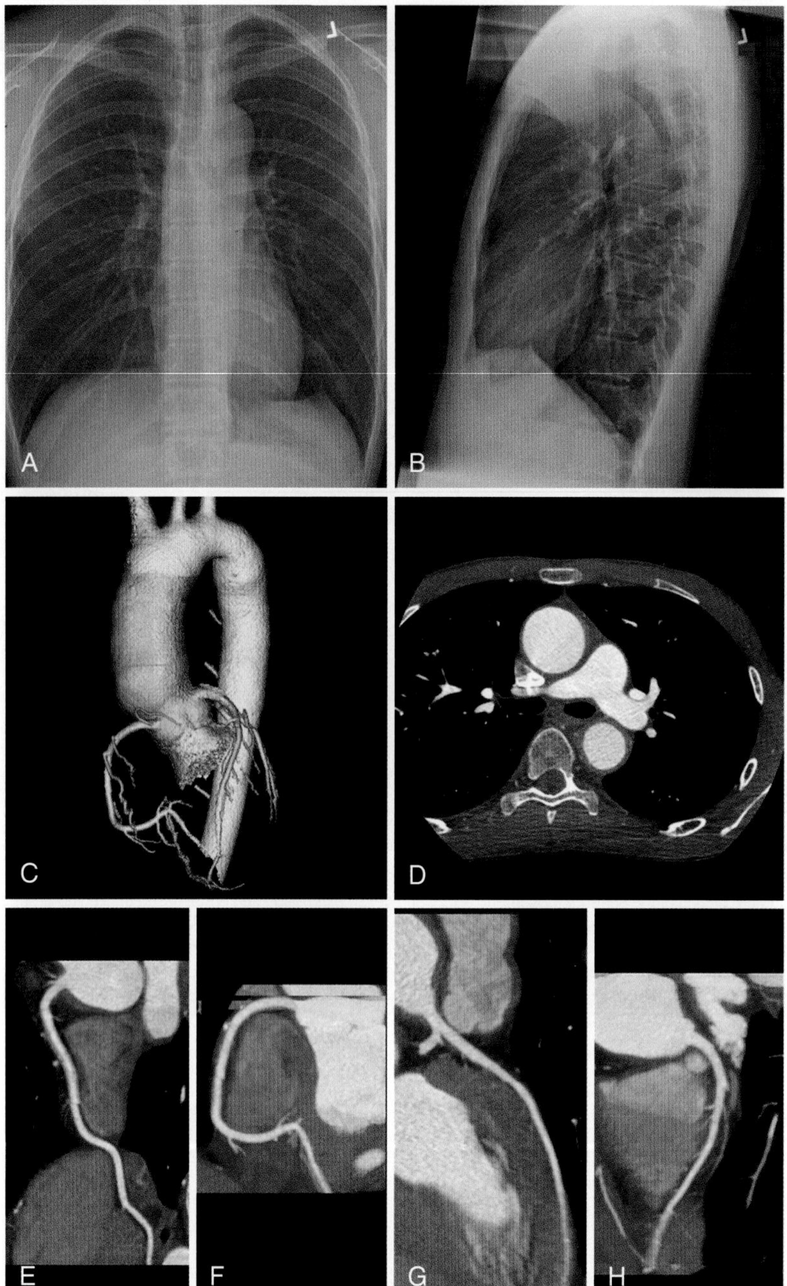

Figure 26-70. Multiple images from a 22-year-old man with Takayasu arteritis. Chest posteroanterior (**A**) and lateral (**B**) images demonstrate moderate enlargement of the aortic arch. The volume-rendered image (**C**) demonstrates moderate enlargement of the ascending aorta extending into the aortic arch, and focal dilatation of the proximal descending thoracic aorta. **D,** Mild to moderate soft tissue thickening around the ascending and descending aorta. **E** and **F,** A curved reformats and maximum intensity projection through the right coronary artery. No evidence of ostial disease or right coronary artery disease is seen. **G** and **H,** No evidence of disease extension into the left coronary artery ostium or left anterior descending artery is seen.

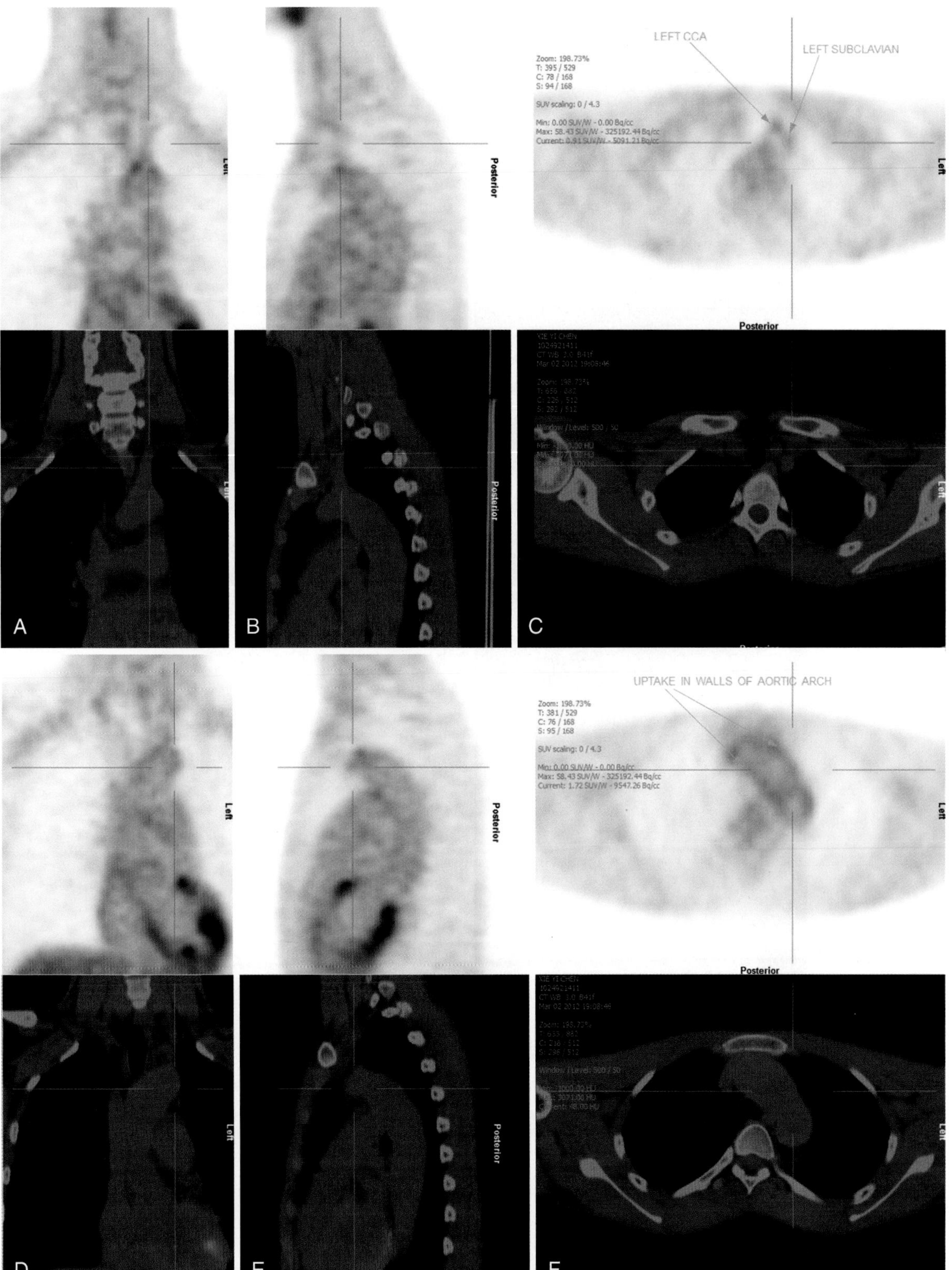

Figure 26-71. Multiple images from an 18F-fluorodeoxyglucose (FDG) CT–positron emission tomographic study on a 31-year-old man with Takayasu arteritis. **A** through **C,** A low-grade amount of increased metabolic activity within the left common carotid and left subclavian arteries. **D** through **F,** Low-grade activity within the aortic arch.

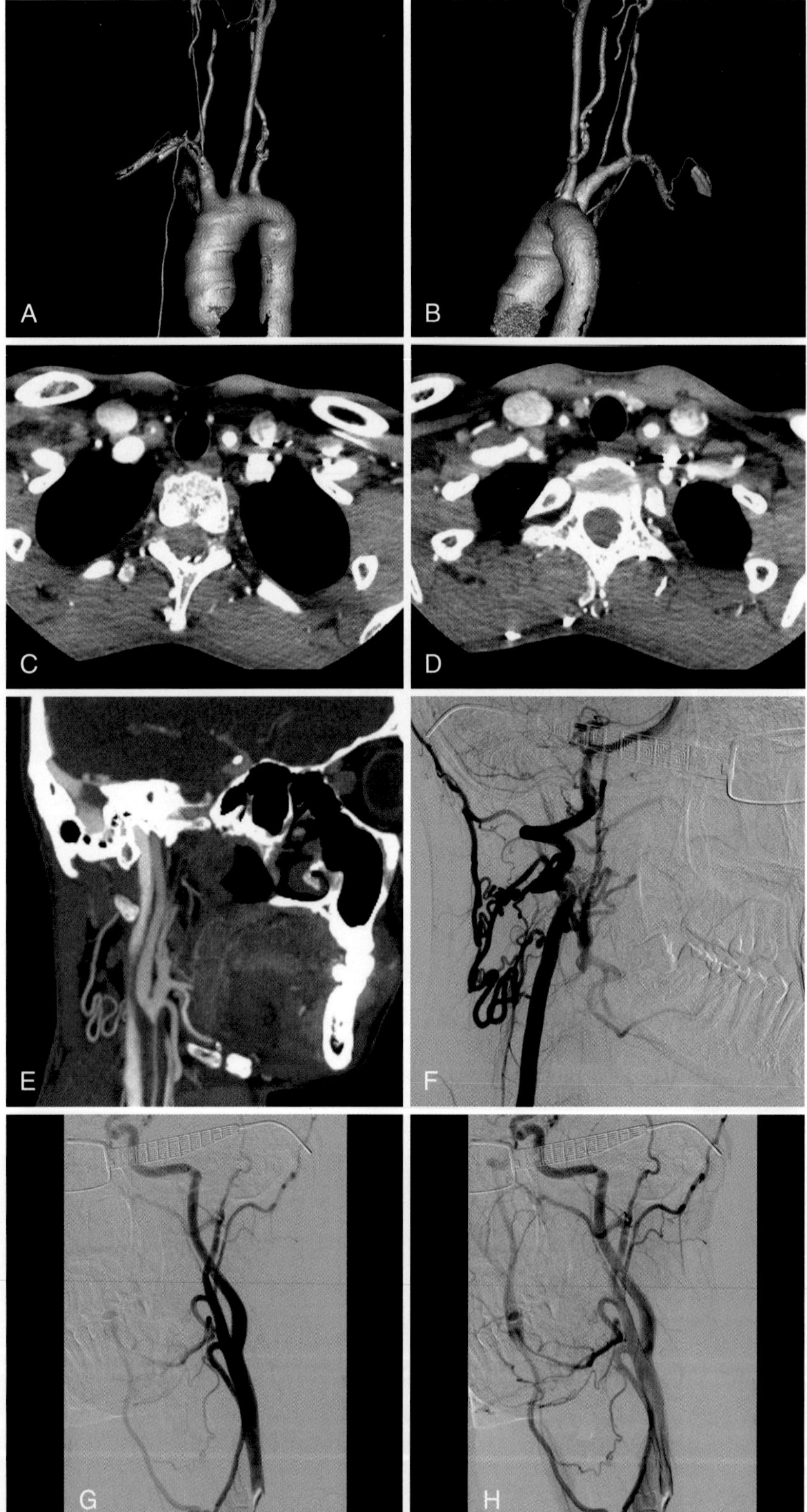

Figure 26-72. Multiple CT angiographic images of the neck in a 31-year-old man with Takayasu arteritis. **A** and **B,** The volume-rendered images demonstrate a long, string-like, attenuated right common carotid artery arising from the innominate artery. **C** and **D,** Axial source images demonstrate severe soft tissue thickening around the proximal right common carotid artery (**C**) and severe narrowing of the right common carotid artery lumen. Mild to moderate soft tissue thickening around the left common carotid artery is seen, but no significant associated stenosis is present. **E,** A sagittal maximum intensity projection image of the neck demonstrates a string-like attenuation of the right common carotid artery. The patient returned for conventional angiography 2 months later. The right common carotid artery had occluded in the interval and could not be cannulated. Cannulation of the right vertebral artery demonstrated multiple branches filling the occipital artery and external carotid branches. **G** and **H,** Injection of the left common carotid artery. A large left superior thyroid branch is seen extending across the midline to collateralize into the right superior thyroid gland and reconstitute the right internal carotid artery.

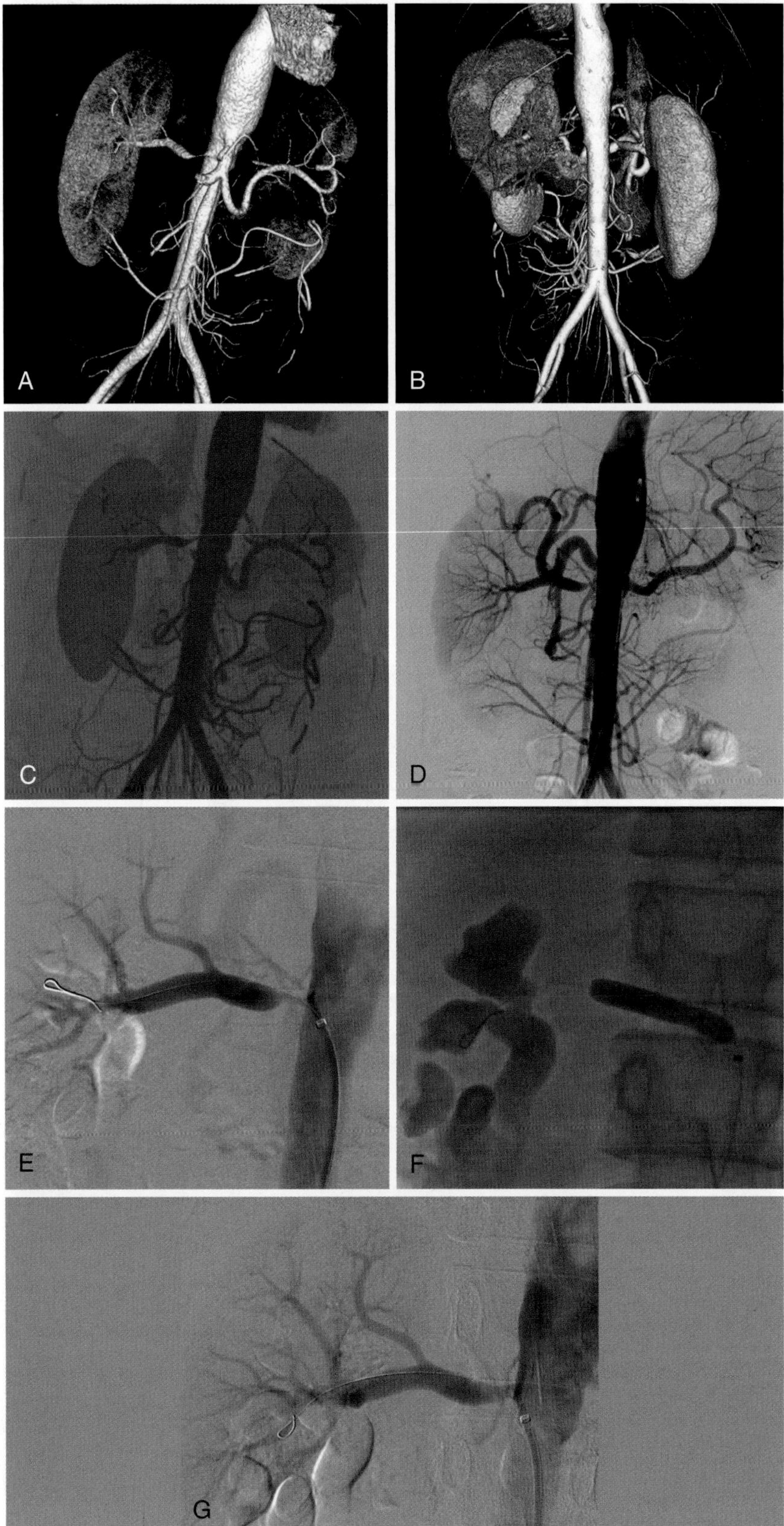

Figure 26-73. An 18-year-old woman with Takayasu arteritis and a history of hypertension. This figure describes changes involving the right renal system. **A** and **B,** Volume-rendered images from a CT angiogram demonstrate a normal right renal contour. There is ectasia of the suprarenal abdominal aorta and a severe stenosis within the proximal portion of a right renal artery that feeds the midst of the upper pole. A lower-pole accessory renal artery arises from the distal abdominal aorta. **C,** Maximum intensity projection image demonstrates the same findings. A conventional angiogram from an aortic flush on the left confirms the severe right main renal artery stenosis. Selective angiography of the right renal artery was performed with the guidewire placed beyond the stenosis (**E**). An angioplasty was subsequently performed, with a moderately successful result.

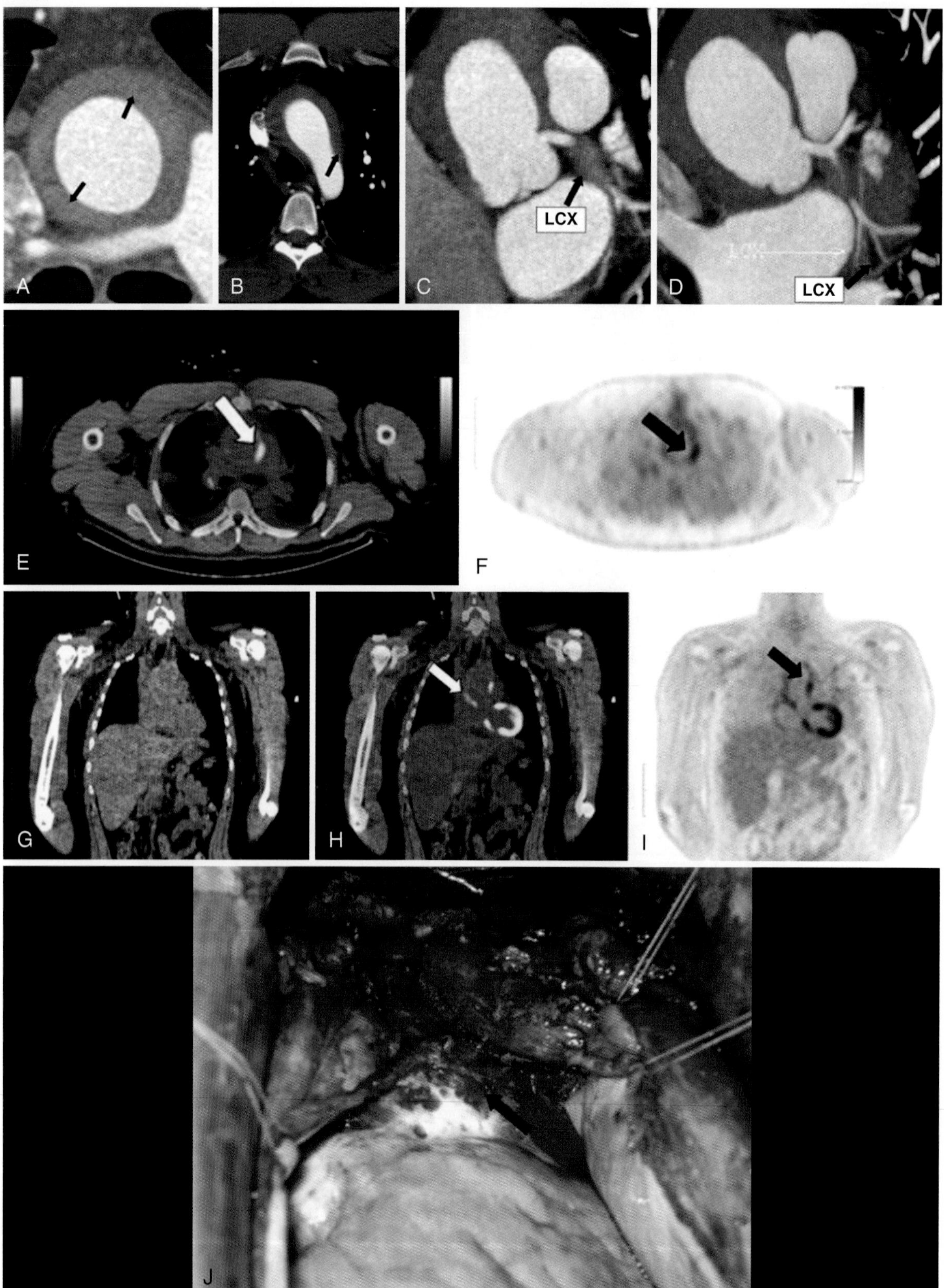

Figure 26-74. **A** and **B,** Multidirectional CT axial image of the aorta shows a smooth, contrast-filled lumen with intermediate density, extrinsic circumferential thickening of the proximal aortic wall (**A,** *black arrows*) that extends up to the aortic arch just distal to the left subclavian artery (**B,** *black arrow*). **C,** Axial CT image shows a hazy, soft tissue density over the proximal left circumflex (LCX) coronary artery with a compromised vessel lumen (*arrow*). **D,** Multiplanar reconstruction image shows proximal LCS coronary artery density with compromised contrast-filled lumen and a distal vessel that is widely patent with no atherosclerotic disease (*arrow*). **E** through **I,** Positron emission tomographic (PET) image shows areas of circumferentially increased 18F-fluorodeoxyglucose (FDG) activity of the whole proximal aortic root (*white arrows*) on a whole-body overlap noncontrast CT image. PET images show increased FDG activity in the thickened aortic wall region (*black arrows*). **J,** Intraoperative image shows a fibrotic, hardened, and inflamed proximal aorta with punctate hemorrhage that extends to the pericardium (*arrow*). (Reprinted with permission from Mahenthiran J, El Masry H, Teague SD, Shahriari AP. Inflammatory aortitis with coronary arterial involvement by multidetector cardiac computed tomography. *J Cardiovasc Comput Tomogr.* 2008;2(4):276-280.)

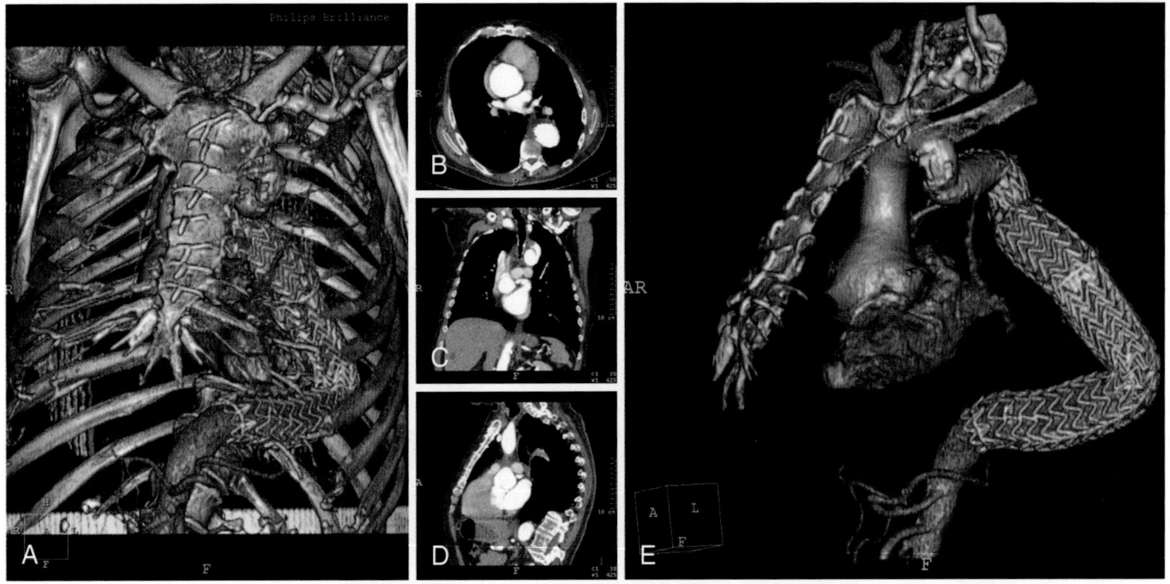

Figure 26-75. Volume-rendered images. **A,** Pre–chest cage removal function. **E,** After chest cage removal function.

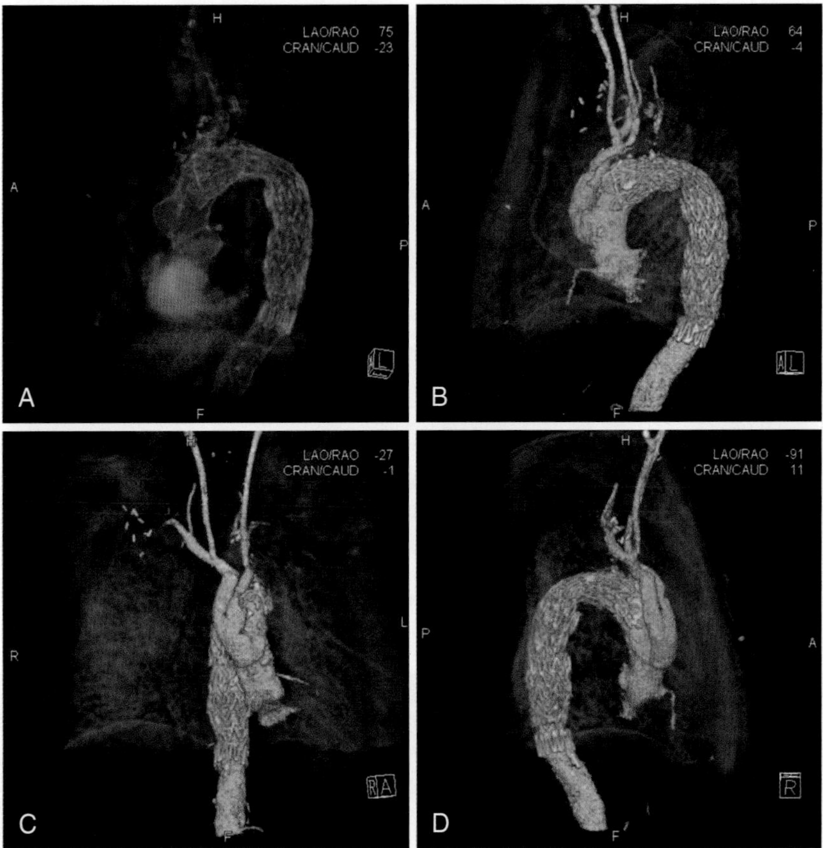

Figure 26-76. Three-dimensional volume-rendered views of the thoracic aorta following a "debranching" hybrid surgical-endovascular procedure where the arch vessels have been reimplanted onto a multiply branched graft segment anastomosed to the ascending aorta. The arch and descending aorta have been endovascularly repaired with two stent-grafts to seal off leaking penetrating ulcers. The arch vessels were moved out of the way of the stents to allow endovascular repair of the ulcer sites.

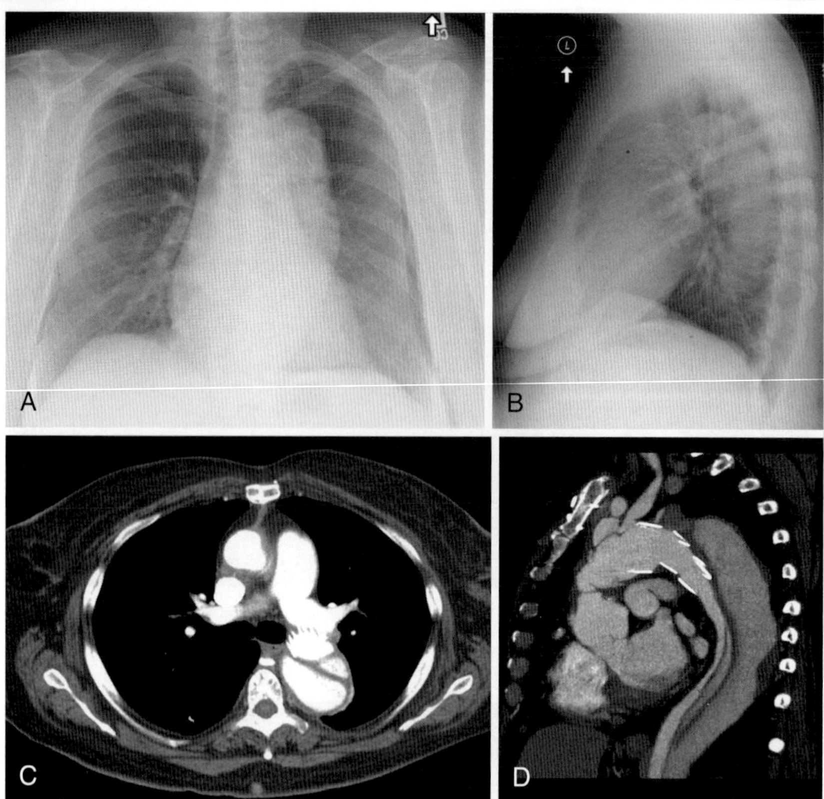

Figure 26-77. Chest radiograph and contrast-enhanced CT scan axial and sagittal views approximately matching the posteroanterior and lateral chest radiograph films. On the chest radiographs, the aortic stent is seen to be more fully deployed proximally than distally. Similarly, the posteroanterior (**A**) and lateral (**B**) chest radiographs show that the distal aspect of the stent is not deployed against the outer wall of the aorta. The CT scan images demonstrate a "triple-barreled" aorta due to recurrent dissection of the aorta. The true lumen within which the stent is deployed is clearly smaller than the false lumens, accounting for the appearance on the chest radiographs of incomplete expansion of the stents. The large false lumen posterior and lateral to the true lumen accounts for the appearance of the additional aortic tissue posterior and lateral to the stent, as seen in the chest radiographs.

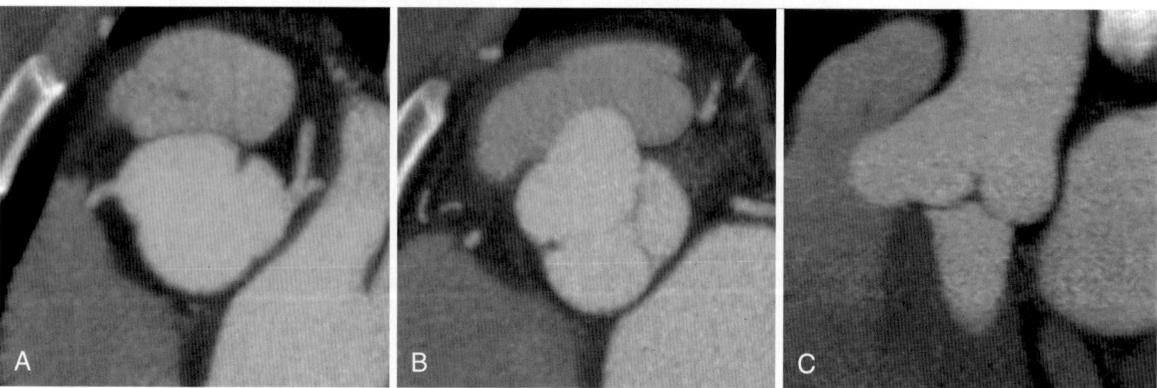

Figure 26-78. Multiple images from a cardiac CT study demonstrate a sinus of Valsalva aneurysm extending from the right coronary sinus of Valsalva. No evidence is seen of a shunt or rupture, and there is no evidence of internal thrombus or calcification.

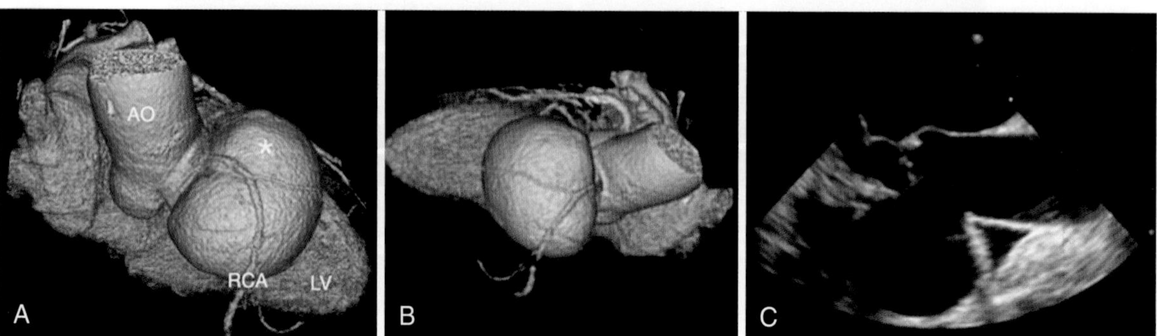

Figure 26-79. A saccular aneurysm (67 × 48 mm) of the right sinus of Valsalva protruding into the right ventricular cavity. There was no associated aortic valve insufficiency.

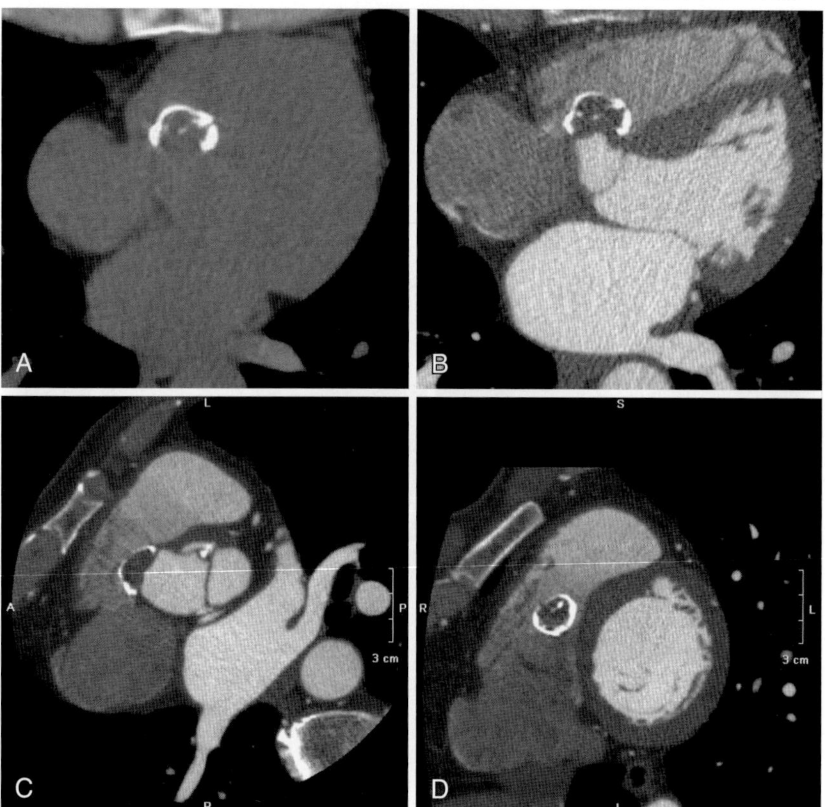

Figure 26-80. Pre- (**A**) and post-contrast (**B**) images from a cardiac CT demonstrate peripheral calcification and thrombosis of a sinus of Valsalva aneurysm. There is no sign of residual shunting. **C** and **D,** Composite centered images from a cardiac CT study in another patient demonstrate a thrombosed and calcified sinus of Valsalva aneurysm extending from the right coronary sinus of Valsalva. This projects into the right ventricular outflow tract. No associated jet or ventricular septal defect is seen. See **Videos 26-5 and 26-6.**

hematomas, false aneurysms, and infected perigraft collections. Low-attenuation material around the graft in the acute postsurgical phase likely is secondary to the postsurgical inflammatory response. This condition tends to resolve over time. An increase in the amount of low attenuation around the graft, especially in association with increased stranding of the adjacent mediastinal fat, or the development of small foci of air within the low-attenuation material increases the suspicion for an infected perigraft collection. The presence of contrast material outside the confines of the graft raises suspicion for graft dehiscence and a perigraft pseudoaneurysm (Figs. 26-81 and 26-82).

CCT PROTOCOL POINTS

- ❒ Coverage: lung apices to diaphragm
- ❒ Contrast: 90 mL at 5 mL/sec
- ❒ Automated trigger set:
    - Location: descending aorta at the level of the left atrium
    - HU: 200
- ❒ Additional scans:
    - Precontrast images are needed to identify vascular calcification and acute IMH lesions
    - Delayed scan images (1–2 min) are needed to depict chronic false lumens and endoleaks post–thoracic endovascular aortic repair.
- ❒ See Table 26-2.

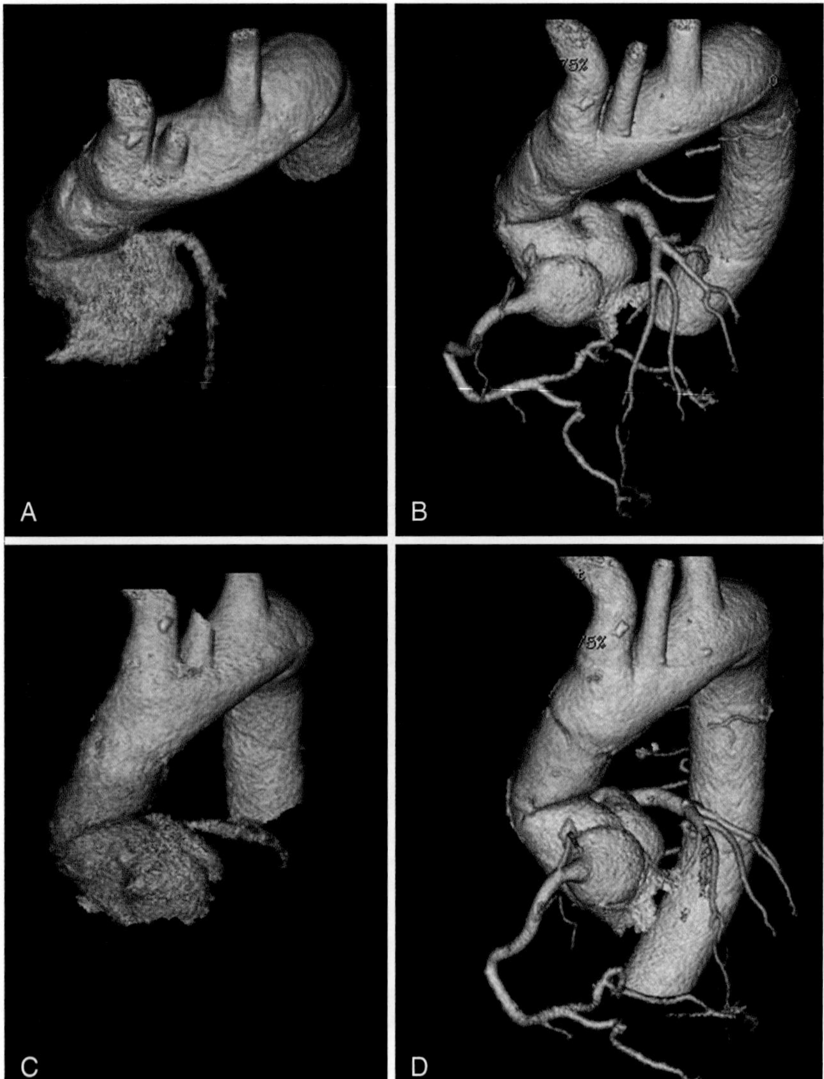

Figure 26-81. Two sets of images in a patient with prior resection of an ascending aortic aneurysm, and placement of a descending aortic tube graft. The purpose of this image set is to demonstrate image quality difference between a non-gated helical CT angiogram of the chest (**A** and **C**), and a prospectively acquired, ECG-gated CT angiogram (**B** and **D**). The ECG-gated images demonstrate much better detail of the aortic root and the coronary arteries. In this case the aortic root is negative, and will need ongoing surveillance. The proximal anastomosis above the level of the sinuses of Valsalva is kinked, but shows no evidence of any other postoperative complication. The dose of a helical non-gated study was 6.8 mSv, while the prospectively acquired gated study was done at a dose of 4.2 mSv.

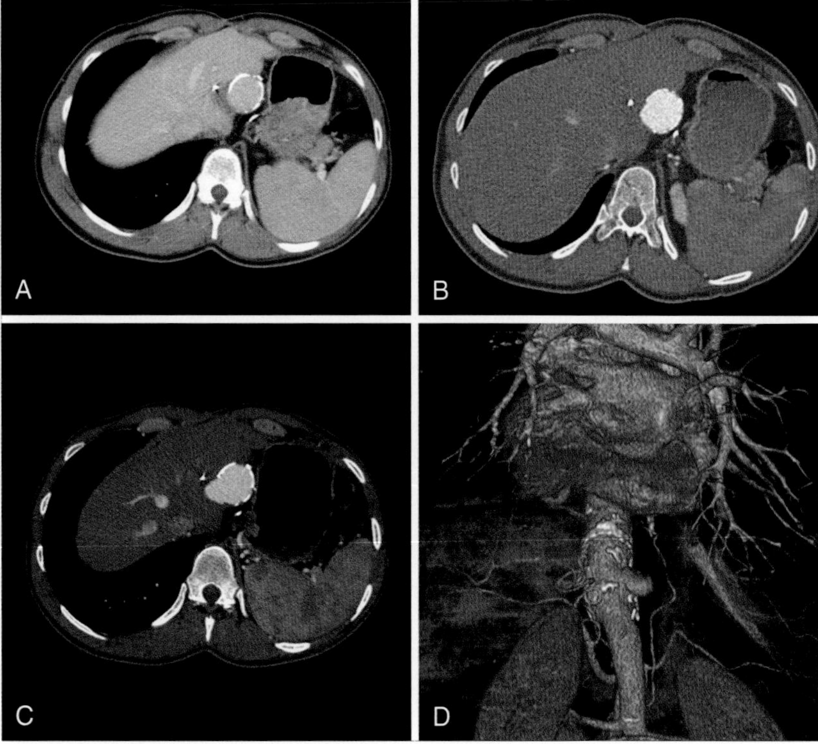

Figure 26-82. Multiple CT images in a 38-year-old man with a prior history of coarctation. He has had prior surgery to the thoracoabdominal aorta, which is more anteriorly placed than is normally seen. **A,** Obtained 1 month post-surgery when the patient presented with fever and abdominal pain. A small amount of low attenuation, possibly fluid, is seen adjacent to the right aspect of the abdominal aorta. **B,** The follow-up CT angiogram shows subtle irregularity and mild focal outpouching of the right aspect of the abdominal aorta. **C,** A further follow-up study 6 months later demonstrates a definite focal outpouching of the right side of the abdominal aorta. **D,** This is well demonstrated on the volume-rendered image (posterior projection). These images demonstrate the development of a mycotic aneurysm/pseudoaneurysm.

TABLE 26-2 ACCF 2006 Appropriateness for Use of CT Angiography for the Evaluation of Aortic Disease*

APPROPRIATENESS CRITERIA	INDICATION	MEDIAN SCORE
Appropriate	Evaluation of suspected aortic dissection or thoracic aortic aneurysm	9
Uncertain	None	
Inappropriate	None	

*No listings for aortic diseases are included in the ACCF 2010 appropriateness guidelines.

Data from Hendel RC, Manesh PR, Kramer CM, Poon M. ACCF/ACR/SCCT/SCMR/ASNC/NASCI/SCAI/SIR appropriateness criteria for cardiac computed tomography and cardiac magnetic resonance imaging. *J Am Coll Cardiol.* 2006;48(7):1475-1497.

References

1. Lin FY, Devereux RB, Roman MJ, et al. Assessment of the thoracic aorta by multidetector computed tomography: age- and sex-specific reference values in adults without evident cardiovascular disease. *J Cardiovasc Comput Tomogr.* 2008;2(5):298-308.
2. Abbara S, Kalva S, Cury RC, Isselbacher EM. Thoracic aortic disease: spectrum of multidetector computed tomography imaging findings. *J Cardiovasc Comput Tomogr.* 2007;1:40-54.
3. Hagan PG, Nienaber CA, Isselbacher EM, et al. The International Registry of Acute Aortic Dissection (IRAD): new insights into an old disease. *JAMA.* 2000;283(7):897-903.
4. Sueyoshi E, Sakamoto I, Hayashi K, Yamaguchi T, Imada T. Growth rate of aortic diameter in patients with type B aortic dissection during the chronic phase. *Circulation.* 2004;110(suppl II): II-256-II-261.
5. Yoshida S, Akiba H, Tamakawa M, et al. Thoracic involvement of type A aortic dissection and intramural hematoma: diagnostic accuracy–comparison of emergency helical CT and surgical findings. *Radiol.* 2003;228(2):430-435.
6. Ganaha F, Miller DC, Sugimoto K, et al. Prognosis of aortic intramural hematoma with and without penetrating atherosclerotic ulcer: a clinical and radiological analysis. *Circulation.* 2002;106(3):342-348.
7. Joines M, Barack BM, Chang DS. Right coronary sinus of Valsalva aneurysm evaluated by cardiac computed tomography angiography. *J Cardiovasc Comput Tomogr.* 2008;2(3):193-194.
8. Errington ML, Ferguson JM, Gillespie IN, Connell HM, Ruckley CV, Wright AR. Complete pre-operative imaging assessment of abdominal aortic aneurysm with spiral CT angiography. *Clin Radiol.* 1997;52(5):369-377.
9. Chan P, Tsai CW, Huang JJ, Chuang YC, Hung JS. Salmonellosis and mycotic aneurysm of the aorta. A report of 10 cases. *J Infect.* 1995;30(2):129-133.
10. Hager A, Kaemmerer H, Leppert A, et al. Follow-up of adults with coarctation of the aorta: comparison of helical CT and MRI, and impact on assessing diameter changes. *Chest.* 2004;126(4):1169-1176.
11. Baum U, Anders K, Ropers D, et al. Multi-slice spiral CT imaging after surgical treatment of aortic coarctation. *Eur Radiol.* 2005; 15(2):353-355.
12. Schaffler GJ, Sorantin E, Groell R, et al. Helical CT angiography with maximum intensity projection in the assessment of aortic coarctation after surgery. *AJR Am J Roentgenol.* 2000;175(4): 1041-1045.
13. Becker C, Soppa C, Fink U, et al. Spiral CT angiography and 3D reconstruction in patients with aortic coarctation. *Eur Radiol.* 1997;7(9):1473-1477.
14. Morra A, Clemente A, Del Borrello M, Berretta S, Greco P. Multidetector computed tomography and 2- and 3-dimensional postprocessing in the evaluation of congenital thoracic vascular anomalies. *J Cardiovasc Comput Tomogr.* 2008;2(4):245-255.

15. Gavant ML, Menke PG, Fabian T, Flick PA, Graney MJ, Gold RE. Blunt traumatic aortic rupture: detection with helical CT of the chest. *Radiol.* 1995;197(1):125-133.
16. Fisher RG, Chasen MH, Lamki N. Diagnosis of injuries of the aorta and brachiocephalic arteries caused by blunt chest trauma: CT vs aortography. *AJR Am J Roentgenol.* 1994;162(5):1047-1052.
17. Parker MS, Matheson TL, Rao AV, et al. Making the transition: the role of helical CT in the evaluation of potentially acute thoracic aortic injuries. *AJR Am J Roentgenol.* 2001;176(5):1267-1272.
18. Mirvis SE, Shanmuganathan K, Miller BH, White CS, Turney SZ. Traumatic aortic injury: diagnosis with contrast-enhanced thoracic CT—five-year experience at a major trauma center. *Radioly.* 1996; 200(2):413-422.
19. Matsunaga N, Hayashi K, Sakamoto I, Ogawa Y, Matsumoto T. Takayasu arteritis: protean radiologic manifestations and diagnosis. *Radiographics.* 1997;17(3):579-594.
20. Zlatkin S, Aamar S, Specter G, et al. Takayasu's arteritis identified by computerized tomography: revealing the submerged portion of the iceberg? *Isr Med Assoc J.* 1999;1(4):245-249.
21. Reddi A, Chetty R. Primary aorto-esophageal fistula due to Takayasu's aortitis. *Cardiovasc Pathol.* 2003;12(2):112-114.
22. Takahashi T, Ando M, Okita Y, Tagusari O, Hanabusa Y, Kitamura S. Redo aortic valve replacement with "porcelain" aorta in an aortitis patient. A case report. *J Cardiovasc Surg (Torino).* 2005;46(1):77-79.
23. Mahenthiran J, El Masry H, Teague SD, Shahriari AP. Inflammatory aortitis with coronary arterial involvement by multidetector cardiac computed tomography. *J Cardiovasc Comput Tomogr.* 2008; 2(4):276-280.

27 Assessment of Peripheral Vascular Diseases

Key Points

- Contrast-enhanced CT scanning has developed to afford excellent noninvasive angiography, and also affords imaging of organs and other structures, unlike conventional angiography.
- Atherosclerotic calcium can be a problem.
- Knowledge of the range of normal and collateral anatomy is critical.

Noninvasive assessment of carotid artery disease is desirable, as more than half of the permanent morbidity and mortality of the Asymptomatic Carotid Artery Surgery (ACAS) Trial was attributable to catheter-based angiography (1.3% of the 2.3% with permanent morbidity and mortality).[1]

The utility of multidirectional CT (MDCT) for the assessment of cerebrovascular, renal artery, and peripheral arterial disease is less studied and published than is its use for the assessment of coronary disease.

Cerebrovascular and peripheral arterial disease are much less subject to motion, and therefore less taxing of the limited temporal resolution of MDCT, than is coronary artery disease. However, both carotid artery disease and peripheral arterial disease are subject to at least as much calcification as is coronary artery disease. In addition, adjacent bony artifacts (to the popliteal artery from the femur and tibial head) are substantial problems for the MDCT assessment of peripheral arterial disease, and tracking a contrast bolus without getting ahead of it is a protocol challenge for the assessment of peripheral arterial disease.

The renal arteries are subject to motion due to excursion of the adjacent diaphragm, occasionally contributing motion artifacts on MDCT imaging.

RENAL ARTERY DISEASE

Assessment of the functional significance of renal artery disease is not simple, by any modality, given the complex anatomy of renal arteries, their known anatomic variants, the variability of lesion numbers and locations, and the fact that "renal artery disease" is more of a medical (over)-simplification than a single pathologic entity.

The renal arteries arise 1 cm below the origin of the superior mesenteric artery (SMA). The right renal artery is longer than the left renal artery, as the aorta lies to the left side of the spine. The main renal arteries divide into five segmental renal arteries—superior/apical, posterior, anterior superior/upper, anterior inferior/middle, and inferior/lower—which supply the kidney.

Furthermore, numerous variants or anomalies of renal arterial supply occur:

- ❒ Multiple accessory or supernumerary renal arteries
- ❒ "Polar" or "extra-hilar" renal arteries
- ❒ Accessory renal artery arising at the superior aspect of a kidney
- ❒ Accessory renal artery arising at the inferior aspect of a kidney
- ❒ Common adrenal/renal artery
- ❒ Common inferior phrenic/renal artery
- ❒ Renal branch from an adrenal artery
- ❒ Passing anterior to the inferior vena cava (IVC) (right-sided)
- ❒ Passing posterior to the IVC (right-sided)
- ❒ Proximal ramification/subdivision of a renal artery

When compared with digital subtraction angiography (DSA), neither CT angiography (CTA) nor MR angiography (MRA) appears able to reliably exclude renal artery stenosis (Table 27-1).[2]

Given the concurrent existence of renal insufficiency in renal artery disease, the nephrotoxicity of CT contrast material is a real concern for the routine use of CTA for the assessment of renal artery disease—a concern that is shared with contrast angiography, but not with MRA or ultrasound.

Approximately one third of the general population demonstrates variability in number, location, and branching patterns of the renal arteries.[3]

This is clinically important because renal artery stenosis (RAS) in an accessory renal artery can, even though rarely, be responsible for renovascular hypertension. Lesions causing stenosis of more than 50% of the diameter of the artery are considered significant. Although there are no clear-cut indications for intervention, the following criteria may be used as a guide for renal artery revascularization: recent onset of hypertension, in which the goal is to cure the hypertension; drug-refractory hypertension; intolerance to antihypertensive medications; progressive renal insufficiency/failure; and episodes of flash pulmonary edema.

In addition to atherosclerotic renal artery stenosis, another notable cause of renovascular hypertension is fibromuscualr dysplasia (FMD). FMD is a nonatherosclerotic angiopathy of unknown etiology, although a genetic association with possible autosomal dominant transmission has been suggested.[4]

FMD can involve the intima, media, and adventitia, with medial FMD representing the most common type, and is characterized by the classic "string of beads" appearance. FMD usually affects females between 15 and 50 years of age, frequently involves the mid or distal segments of the renal artery, and is bilateral in two thirds of patients.[5] It is the most common cause of renovascular hypertension in children. Renal artery stenosis secondary to FMD may affect pregnant women and thus remains an important consideration as a cause of secondary hypertension during pregnancy.

For images of renovascular disease, see Figures 27-1 to 27-3.

TABLE 27-1 Interobserver Agreement, Sensititvity, and Specificity of CTA and MRA for the Detection of Renal Vascular Disease

	CTA	MRA
Interobserver agreement	0.59–0.64	0.40–0.51
Sensitivity	64% [55–73%]	62% [54–71%]
Specificity	92% [90–95%]	84% [81–87%]

MRA, magnetic resonace angiography.
Data from Vasbinder GB, Nelemans PJ, Kessels AG, et al. Accuracy of computed tomographic angiography and magnetic resonance angiography for diagnosing renal artery stenosis. *Ann Intern Med.* 2004;141(9):674-682.

CT Protocol Points

- Coverage: arterial phase, above diaphragm to symphysis pubis
- Contrast: 80 mL at 5 mL/sec
- Automated trigger set:
  - location: upper abdominal aorta
  - HU: 180

PERIPHERAL (LOWER EXTREMITY) ARTERIAL DISEASE

Assessment of peripheral (lower extremity) artery disease by MDCT is feasible but it is challenged by:

- The huge anatomic territory to assess with thin (submillimeter) slices; hence the enormous number of images to review (~1500)
- The tendency of peripheral atherosclerosis to attract calcification and the problems inherent in luminal assessment in the presence of calcium
- The proximity of the distal femoral artery and the popliteal artery to adjacent bony structures, and the difficulties in employing "bone-removal" software features that may remove adjacent calcified vessel segments
- Accurate bolus tracking (ensuring that the acquisition speed does not exceed the contrast opacification)

Agreement of 16-slice MDCT with DSA is very good (96% sensitive), as is interobserver agreement (κ = 0.84–1.0).[6] However, agreement varies

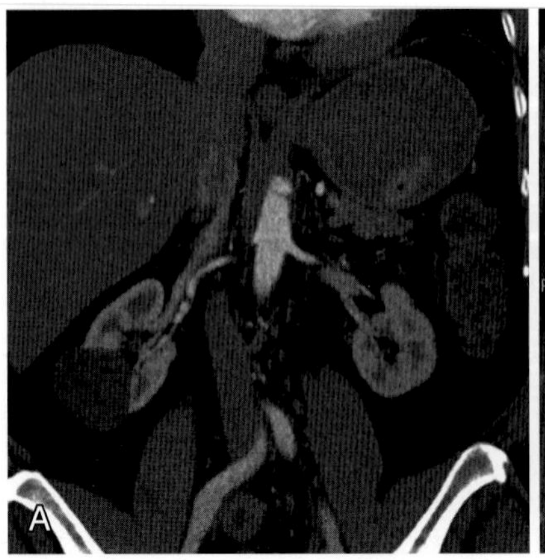

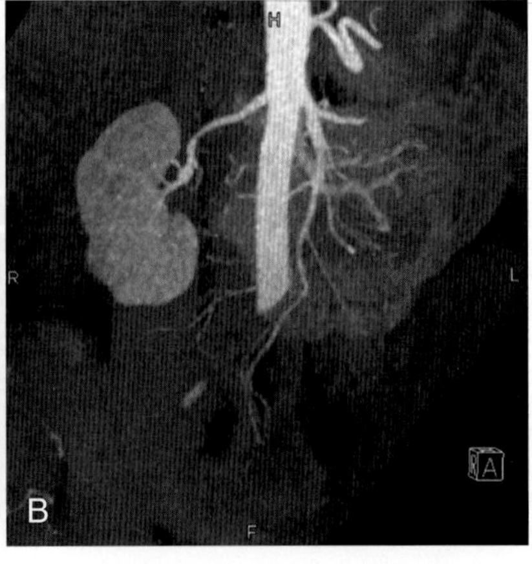

Figure 27-1. A, Renal CT angiogram. Distal "beading" is seen, consistent with renal fibromuscular disease. **B,** MRA does not depict the same findings as clearly.

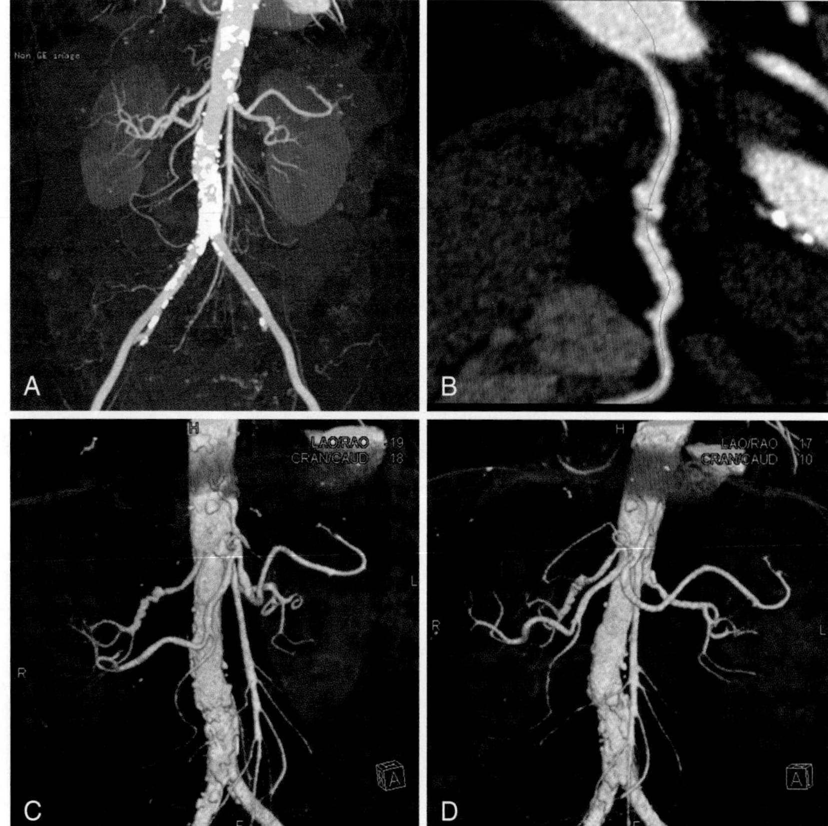

Figure 27-2. A 75-year-old woman with a history of hypertension. **A,** A heavily calcified abdominal aorta. The right renal artery demonstrates a typical corkscrew appearance, like the one seen in fibromuscular dysplasia. The right kidney is smaller than the contralateral left kidney. **B,** A curved reformatted image through the right renal artery shows multiple moderate to severe stenoses in the mid-portion of the artery. **C** and **D,** Volume-rendered images through the upper abdominal aorta demonstrate a classic beaded appearance of the right renal artery, pathognomonic for fibromuscular dysplasia.

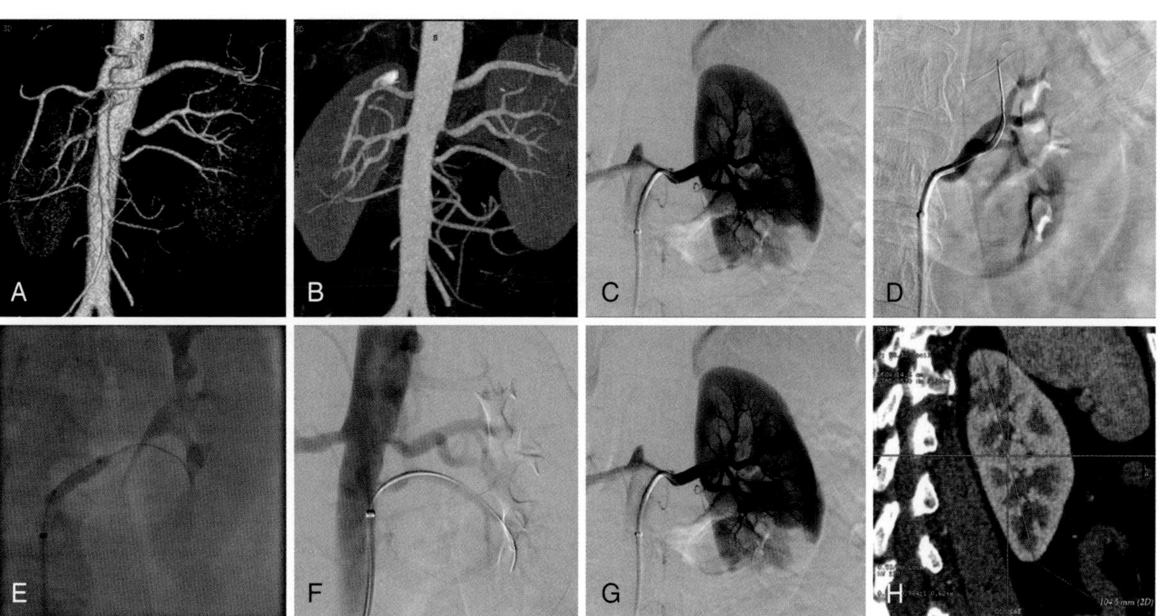

Figure 27-3. Images from a CT angiogram of the abdomen in a 38-year-old woman with hypertension. The three-dimensional CT volume-rendered view (**A**), maximum intensity projection image (**B**), and volume-rendered image demonstrate mild beading of the proximal right renal artery, with a mild focal area of ectasia. **A** and **B** also demonstrate two left-sided renal arteries. The upper, larger renal artery has a moderate to severe renal artery stenosis, which is seen at the origin of the renal artery. Similarly, the smaller, lower-pole left renal artery has a severe proximal stenosis. These findings, confirmed on the conventional angiogram (**C**), are consistent with fibromuscular dysplasia (FMD) of the renal arteries. The patient underwent conventional renal angiography and subsequent balloon angioplasty of the left upper renal artery stenosis (**D**) and the left lower renal artery stenosis (**E**, **F**). **F**, An unfortunate, but likely minor, consequence of the balloon angioplasty of the left upper renal artery was segmental renal infarction. **G,** Image obtained in a parenchymal blush prior to the angioplasty 3 months earlier shows a normal contour to the left upper pole. **H,** A follow-up CT angiogram study 3 months later demonstrates a focal area of thinning in the medial left upper pole consistent with segmental infarctions from the angioplasty.

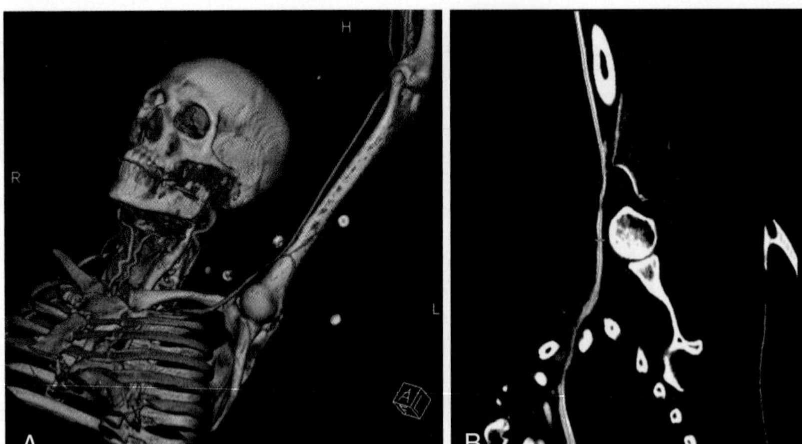

Figure 27-4. Three-dimensional reconstruction and multiplanar imaging of a patient with a thoracic outlet syndrome.

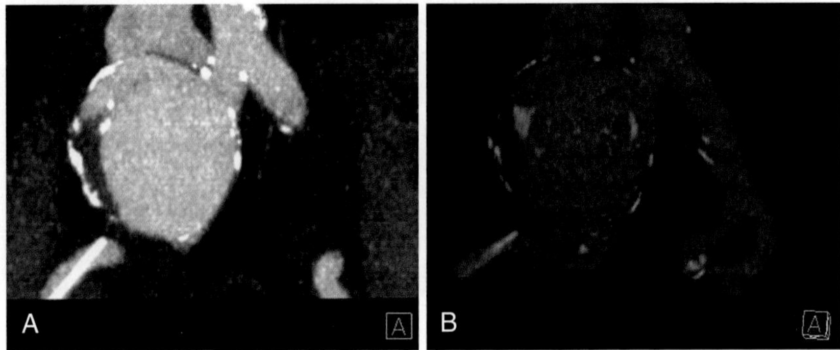

Figure 27-5. **A,** Contrast-enhanced three-dimensional coronal image of a right iliac artery aneurysm. The underlying inferior vena cava (IVC) is massively dilated due to rupture of the aneurysm into the underlying iliac vein. There is intimal calcification and mural thrombus. **B,** Contrast-enhanced three-dimensional volume-rendered depiction of a right iliac artery aneurysm. The IVC is massively dilated due to rupture of the aneurysm into the underlying iliac vein. The calcium in most sites is contiguous with the contrast-enhanced lumen. On the right side of the aneurysm, the intimal calcification is separated from the lumen by 1 cm due to mural thrombus within the aneurysm.

considerably depending on the artery in question.[7] Overestimation in a small percentage (2–3%) of cases occurs more frequently than does underestimation (1%). Anteroposteriorly directed narrowing and extensive calcification are common reasons for disagreement.[6] Older scanners (4-MDCT) were inaccurate.[8]

Confidence with MDCT is similar to that of MR angiography,[9] but is less than with DSA, leading to more testing after CT angiography (35% of cases vs. 14% of cases after DSA).[10]

More studies are needed with current scanners to understand the role of MDCT.[11]

For images of peripheral artery disease, see Figures 27-4 through 27-9.

Protocol Points

- ❒ Coverage: diaphragm to below toes
- ❒ Contrast: 25 mL at 5 mL/sec and 120 mL at 4 mL/sec
- ❒ Automated trigger set:
  - location: diaphragmatic aorta
  - HU: 180

ARTERIAL EMBOLISM

Large arterial emboli can be imaged by MDCT.

The validation comparing MDCT to other forms of imaging, including the “gold standard” of catheter-based angiography, has not been well

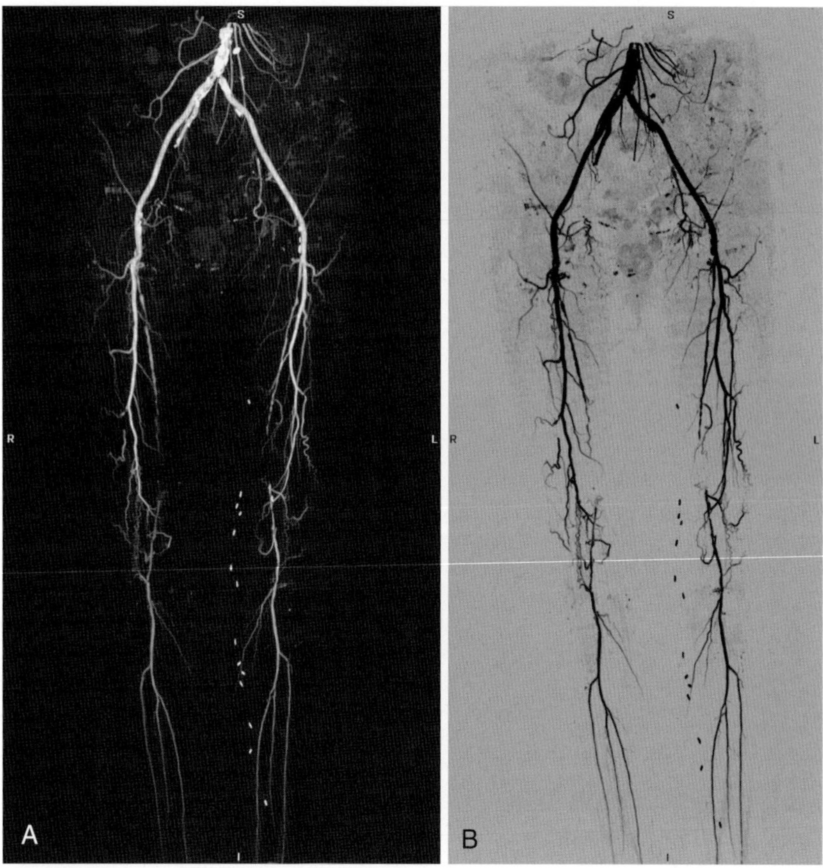

Figure 27-6. Maximum intensity projection images from a volumetrically acquired CT angiogram of the lower abdominal aorta and lower extremities in a patient with bilateral leg claudication, worse on the left. The image on the right is the same data set converted to black, to reproduce an angiographic appearance. In the right leg there is no evidence of a significant stenosis involving the common iliac or external iliac arteries. There is occlusion of the superficial femoral artery proximally, with multiple large collaterals reconstituting the distal superior femoral artery (SFA) and popliteal arteries. These collaterals extend from the profunda femoris. Ongoing runoff to the leg demonstrates good triple vessel runoff with no evidence of a distal stenosis. In the left leg, however, tight stenosis is seen at the origin of the left common iliac artery. The ongoing external iliac artery and common femoral artery show no significant stenosis. There is occlusion of the proximal superficial femoral artery, which, again, reconstitutes distally by profunda femoris collaterals. The popliteal artery and infragenicu-late vessels were normal with good three-vessel runoff to the foot. Multiple surgical clips seen in the medial aspect of the left calf and thigh represent prior saphenous vein harvesting for coronary artery bypass grafting (CABG).

established, and neither MDCT nor MRA likely has the same level of sensitivity as angiography. However, the additional information gained from CT confers a robustness to the modality.

Diagnosis of intestinal ischemia is a major clinical challenge; the diagnosis is made preoperatively in only about half of cases.[12] Average mortality is high (65%).[12] Delay in diagnosis and treatment are associated with higher mortality (71%).[12]

Intestinal ischemia is caused by venous thrombosis in only14%[12] to 28%[13] of cases. It is caused by arterial occlusive disease in 64%[14] to 86%[12] of cases. Arterial disease consists of thrombosis in about one third (30%) of cases, embolism in about one third (30%) of cases, dissection of the aorta or splanchnic artery in one sixth (15%) of cases, and nonocclusive disease or trauma in the remainder.[12]

MDCT is able to detect the presence of mesenteric ischemia and the cause (such as embolism) in over half of cases, particularly when additional findings are used, and if biphasic technique, in which arterial phase imaging is followed by a venous phase 60 to 70 seconds later, is used. A finding of (intestinal) arterial embolism, SMA occlusion, celiac and inferior mesenteric artery (IMA) occlusion with SMA disease, pneumatosis intestinalis, or venous gas has been shown to be highly (100%) specific and 73% sensitive.

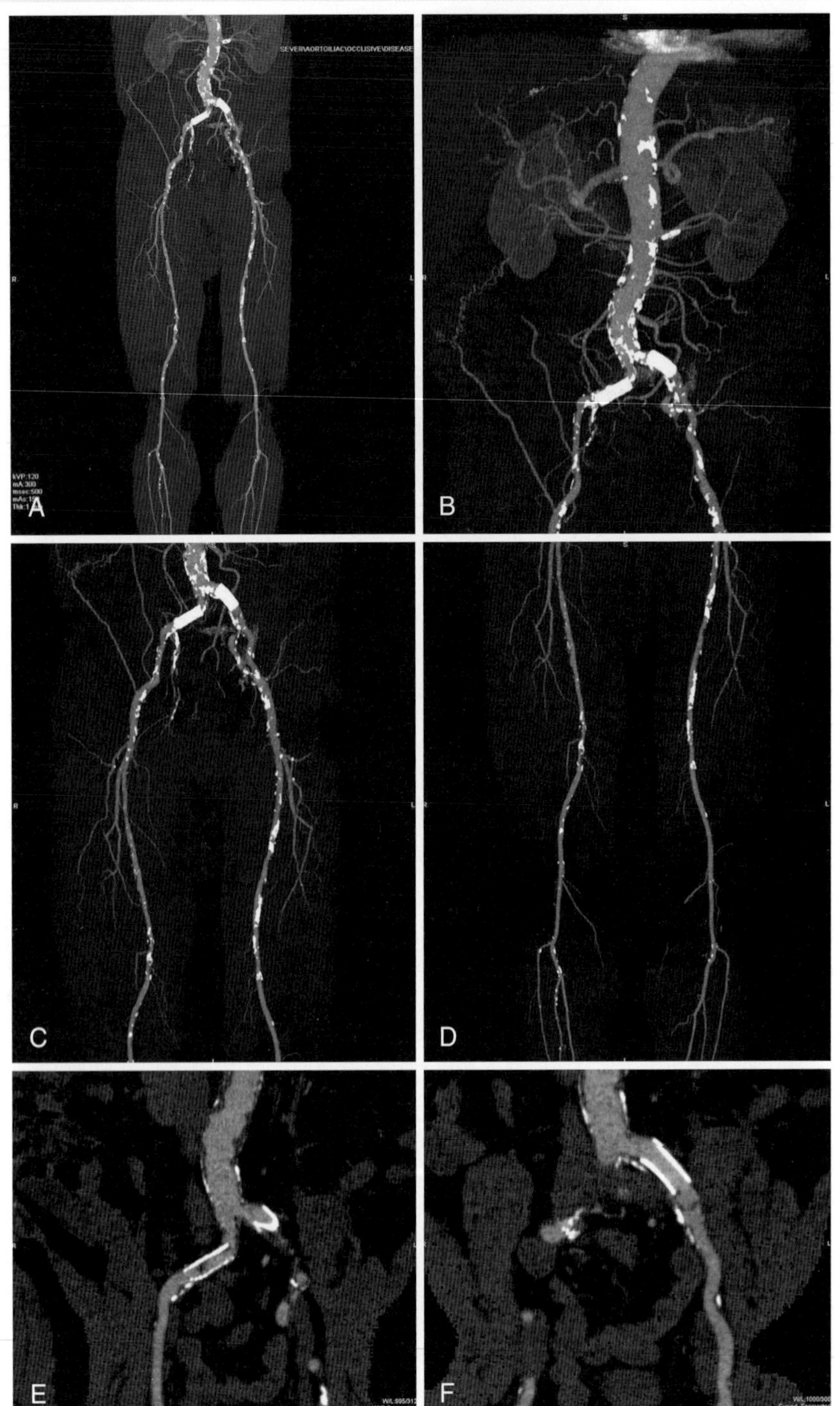

Figure 27-7. Multiple reconstructions from a helically acquired CT angiogram of the abdominal aorta and runoff vessels in a 72-year-old man with known peripheral vascular disease and prior right and left common iliac artery stenting. The patient presented with worsening right leg claudication. **A** and **B,** Multiple maximum intensity (MIP) projection images through the entire volume of acquisition (**A**) and then more segmentally through the abdominal aorta (**B**), iliac arteries (**C**) and lower extremities (**D**). The MIP images demonstrate moderate to severe diffuse calcific changes in all of the visualized major arteries. MIP images are poorly suited to evaluate extent, because only the maximum attenuation value within a pixel is demonstrated. **A** and **B** demonstrate two prominent collateral vessels, likely superior gluteal and inferior epigastric vessels acting as a collateral pathway to the distal right external iliac and common femoral arteries. **E** and **F,** Curved multiplanar reformatted images through the right and left common iliac arteries. A focus of in-stent restenosis is seen within the right common iliac artery stent; there is no evidence of in-stent restenosis on the left.

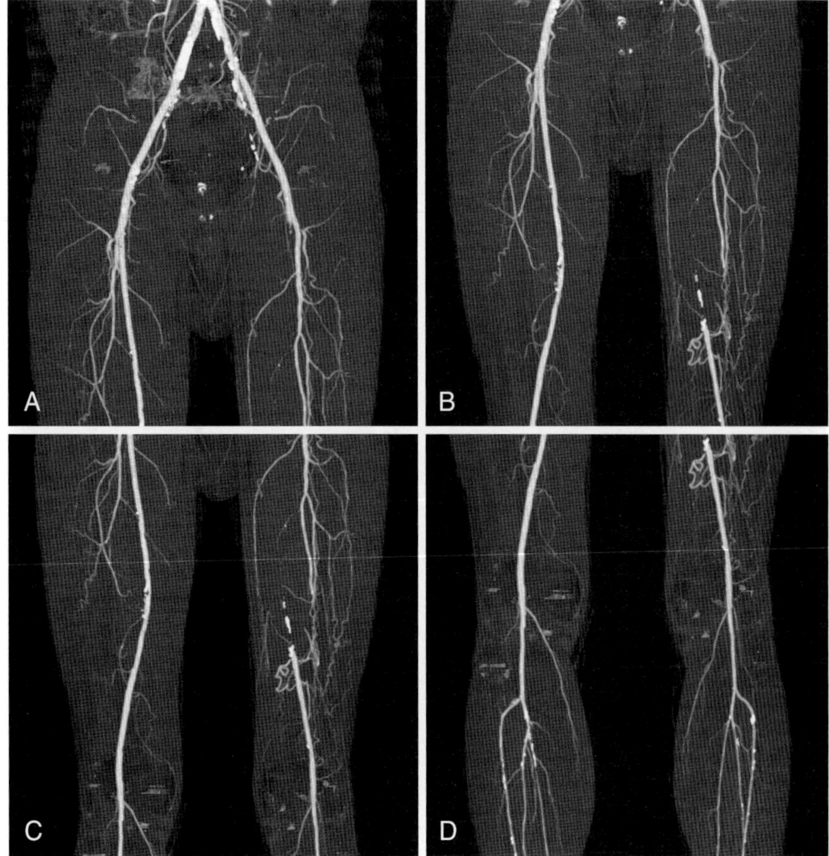

Figure 27-8. Multiple maximum intensity projection images from a CT angiogram of the lower extremities in a patient with left leg claudication demonstrate proximal occlusion of the left superficial femoral artery. There are multiple large collaterals from the profunda femoris artery reconstituting the distal left superficial femoral artery. The popliteal artery and ongoing vessel runoff to the left foot does not demonstrate a significant stenosis. No significant stenosis was identified on the right.

As a single test, catheter-based angiography has the highest diagnosis rate (92%), but even by 1997, MDCT was over 80% sensitive.[13]

For images of arterial embolism, see Figure 27-10.

VISCERAL/SPLANCHNIC ARTERIES

The visceral/splanchnic arteries can be imaged by CT angiography (Fig. 27-11). Stenoses tend to be ostial, lending themselves to recognition by CT angiography.

The sensitivity and specificity of CTA for arterial stenosis are examined in Table 27-2.

CEREBROVASCULAR DISEASE

Only limited studies have been reported to date comparing MDCT to ultrasound or contrast angiography for the assessment of extracranial carotid disease, and validating its use.

Catheter-based cerebral angiography remains the standard against which noninvasive modalities must be validated. To date duplex ultrasound has been validated, and MRA has offered less validation.

Contrast-enhanced CT scanning is able to detect carotid artery atherosclerosis. A meta-analysis of 28 publications reported[14] on a total of 864 symptomatic patients with carotid artery disease who underwent single-slice CTA and DSA,

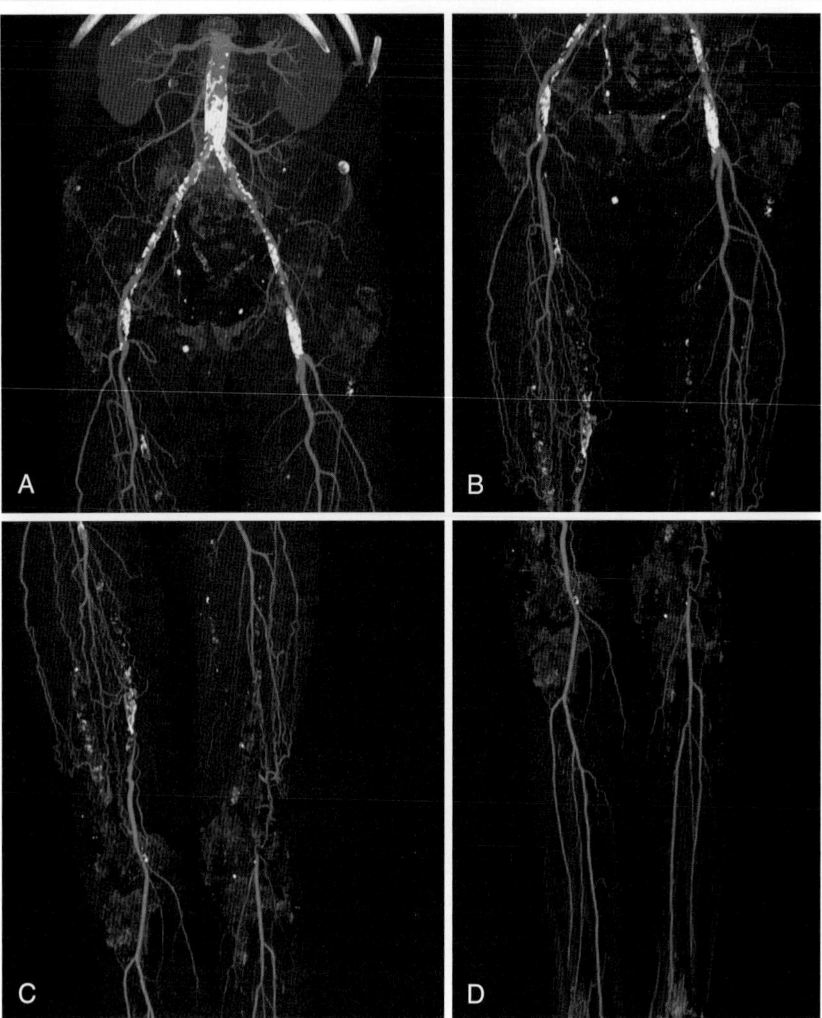

Figure 27-9. Multiple maximum intensity projection images from a CT angiogram of the lower extremities in a 77-year-old diabetic patient with leg pain and bilateral foot ulcers. There is no evidence of iliac artery stenosis. The superficial femoral and popliteal arteries are patent bilaterally, with minor disease and no significant stenosis. Minor disease is also seen within the proximal anterior tibial arteries bilaterally. The right leg demonstrates three-vessel runoff to the level of the distal calf. Distal to this point, no good runoff into the foot is identified. Similarly, the left infrageniculate runoff demonstrates a posterior tibial artery extending to the foot, but the anterior tibial and peroneal arteries are only visualized to the distal calf. A dorsalis pedis artery is not identified.

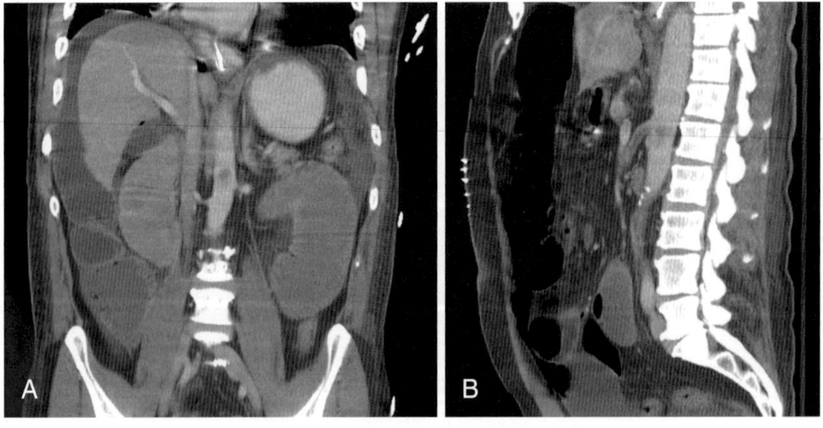

Figure 27-10. A 67-year-old man with new-onset atrial fibrillation. **A,** On the contrast-enhanced coronal view, there is a focus of low attenuation/thrombus in the mid-abdominal aorta as well the superior mesenteric artery (SMA). The bowel is severely dilated. **B,** On the contrast-enhanced sagittal view, there is a low-attenuation focus in the mid abdominal aorta, extending down the SMA. Again, the small bowel is severely dilated and fluid-filled, but without pneumatosis.

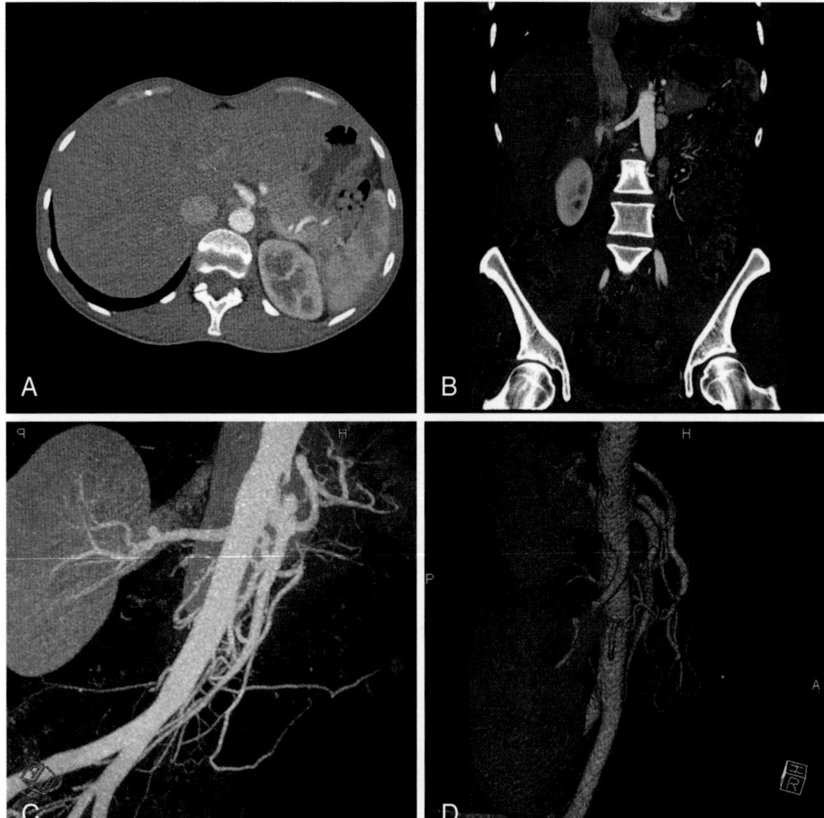

Figure 27-11. Multiple images from abdominal CT angiography in a 27-year-old woman with clinical symptoms of intestinal angina, and an unintentional 20-pound weight loss over 6 months. **A,** A significant stenosis of the celiac axis, which is also identifiable on the coronal reconstruction (**B**). Maximum intensity projection image (**C**) and volume-rendered image (**D**) demonstrate a severe stenosis of the celiac axis. The stenosis is primarily smooth, and has a somewhat bandlike configuration along the superior margin of the celiac axis. In this young patient, no evidence of atherosclerotic disease is seen, specifically no calcified or soft plaque. These findings are suggestive of median arcuate ligament syndrome.

TABLE 27-2 Accuracy of CT Angiography by Peripheral Region

PERIPHERAL VESSELS	*n*	SENSITIVITY (%)	SPECIFICITY (%)	PPV (%)	NPV (%)
Renal arteries	119	92	92	88	92
Carotid arteries	88	96	100	100	95
Total lower extremities	70	88	96	91	90
Iliac arteries	203	86	95	89	80
Femoral arteries	182	85	100	100	94
Superficial femoral arteries	193	90	90	90	84
Popliteal arteries	192	90	96	82	98

NPV, negative predictive value; PPV, positive predictive value.

Data from Fine JJ, Hall PA, Richardson JH, Butterfield LO. 64-slice peripheral computed tomography angiography: a clinical accuracy evaluation. *J Am Coll Cardiol.* 2006;47(7):1495-1496.

TABLE 27-3 Sensitivity and Specificity of CT Angiography for the Detection of Severe and Complete Carotid Artery Stenosis

	SENSITIVITY (%)	SPECIFICITY (%)
70–99% stenosis	85% [79–89%]	93% [89–96%]
Complete stenosis	97% [93–99%]	93% [98–100%]

Data from Koelemay MJ, Nederkoorn PJ, Reitsma JB, Majoie CB. Systematic review of computed tomographic angiography for assessment of carotid artery disease. *Stroke.* 2004;35(10):2306-2312.

classifying them as having (1) less than 70% stenosis, (2) 70% to 99% stenosis, or (3) complete (100% stenosis) occlusion. MDCT yielded pooled data for the detection of severe and complete carotid artery stenosis and was described as having good sensitivity and specificity (Table 27-3).

Importantly, the luminal assessment of carotid artery disease reveals that eccentricity of the lumen (length/perpendicular axis)[18] is an important clinical entity, as the ratio may be as high as 2.0.[18]

The rate of visualization of the internal carotid artery ("good" or "excellent") by routine MDCT is described as good in somewhat more than half of cases (64%)[19] as compared to 81% in cases of targeted MDCT, in comparison to a standard of contrast angiography ($P = .0005$). Agreement of CT angiography with digital subtraction angiography is high: 92%.[19]

Establishing the correlation and accuracy of current 64-MDCT to the North American Symptomatic Carotid Endarterectomy Trial's assessment of proximal internal carotid artery stenosis will be important to understanding the contribution of MDCT to carotid artery disease, especially in comparison with rival techniques such as MRA.

For images of CT angiography of the cerebral vasculature, see Figures 27-12 to 27-16.

Protocol Points

- ❒ Coverage: aortic arch to vertex
- ❒ Contrast: 50 mL at 4 mL/sec, saline push of 20 mL at 3 mL/sec
- ❒ Automated trigger set:
  - location: aortic arch
  - HU: 110

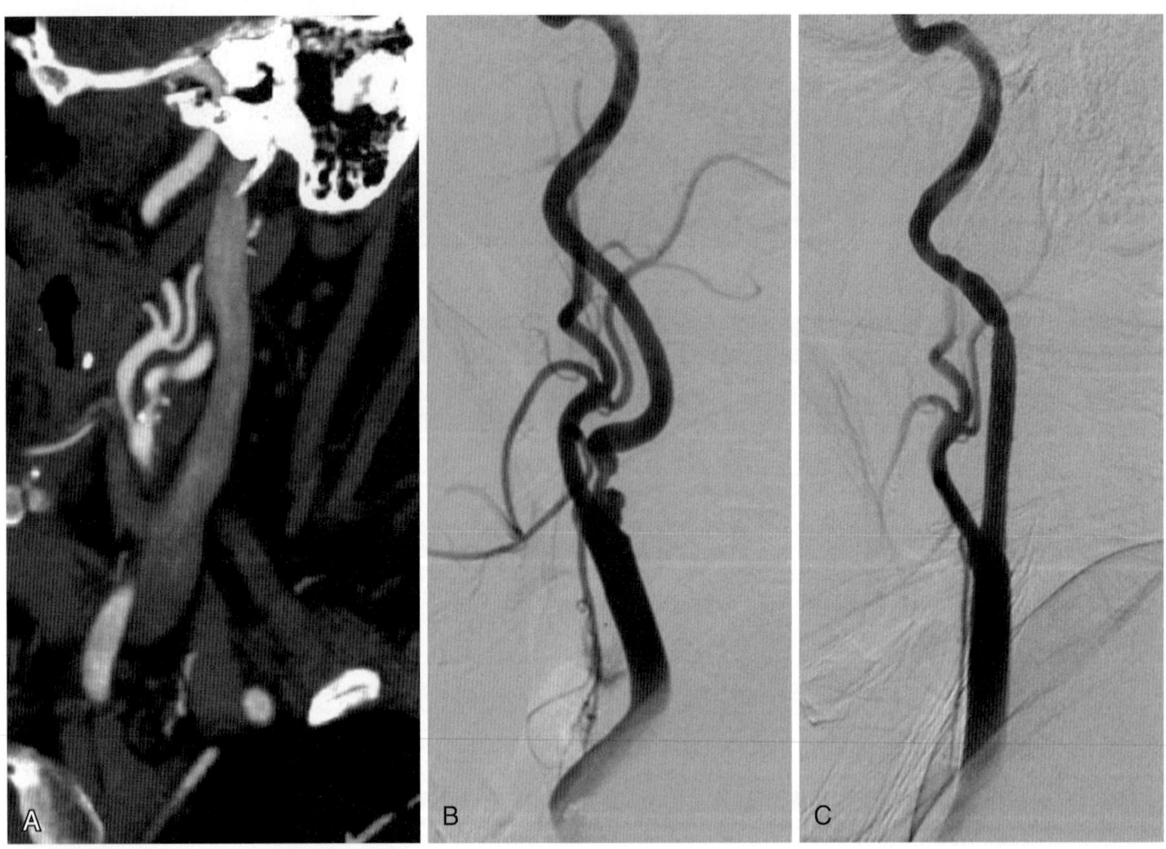

Figure 27-12. Internal carotid artery stenosis depicted by CT angiography (**A**) and confirmed by conventional angiography (**B**). Post-stenting image (**C**).

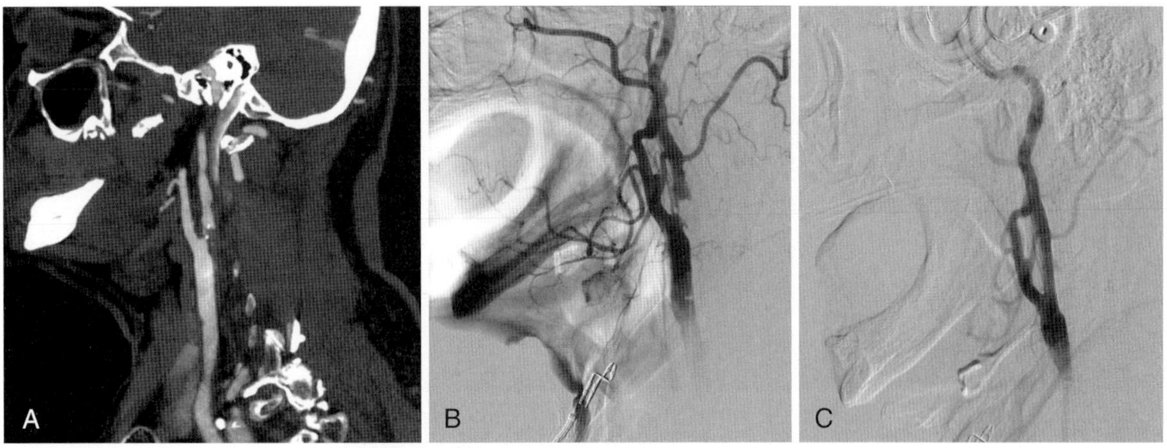

Figure 27-13. Internal carotid artery stenosis depicted by CT angiography (**A**) and confirmed by conventional angiography (**B**). Post-stenting image (**C**).

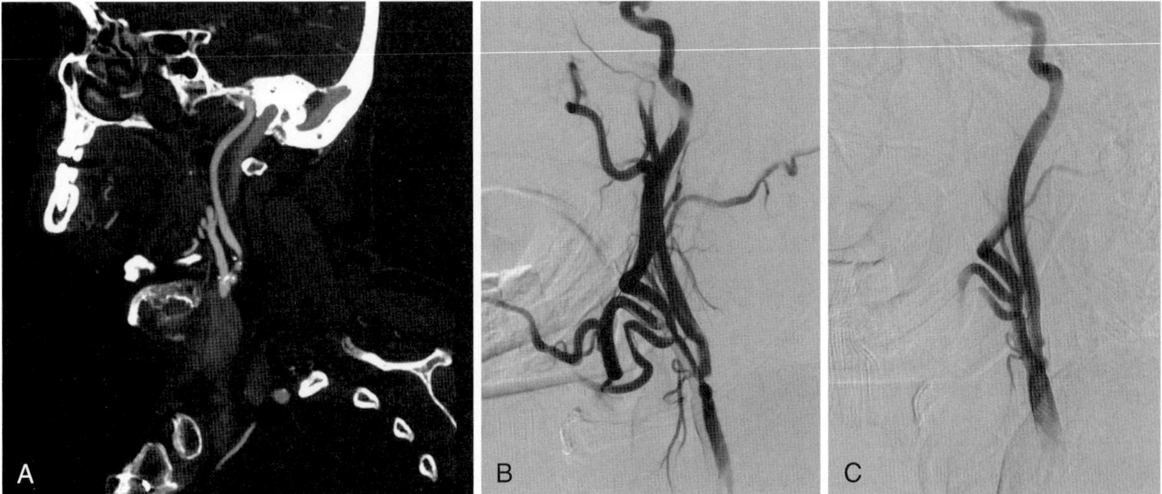

Figure 27-14. Internal carotid artery stenosis depicted by CT angiography (**A**) and confirmed by conventional angiography (**B**). Post-stenting image (**C**).

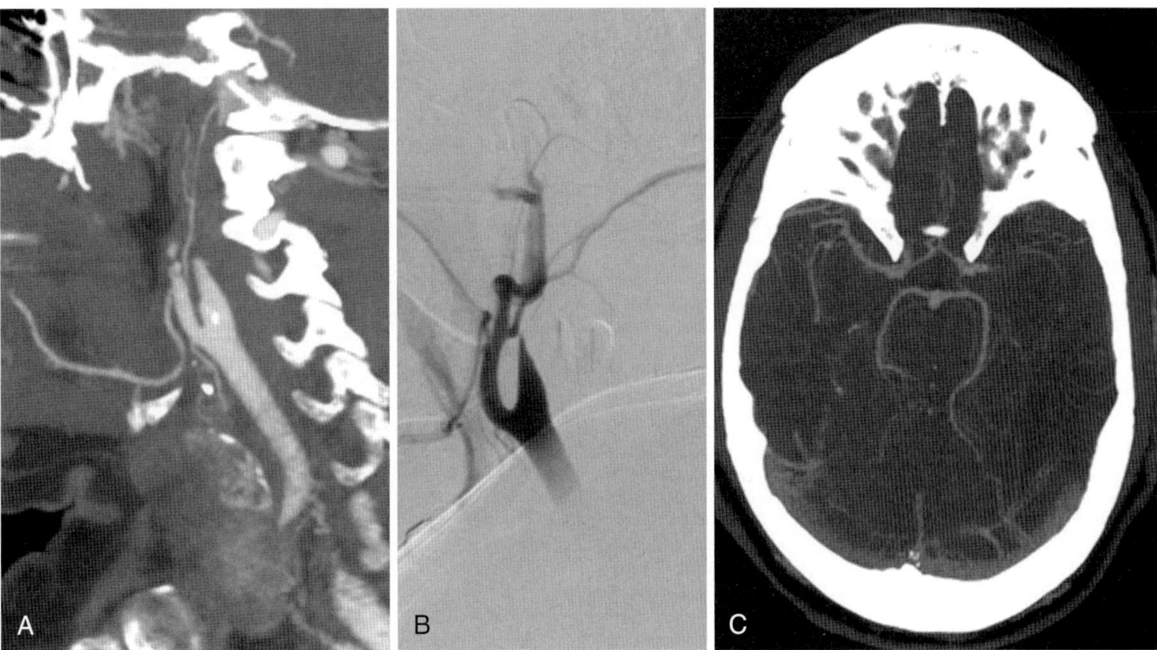

Figure 27-15. **A,** Spontaneous dissection of the internal carotid artery depicted by CTA. **B,** Tapered narrowing, confirmed by conventional angiography. **C,** Occlusion of the left middle cerebral artery.

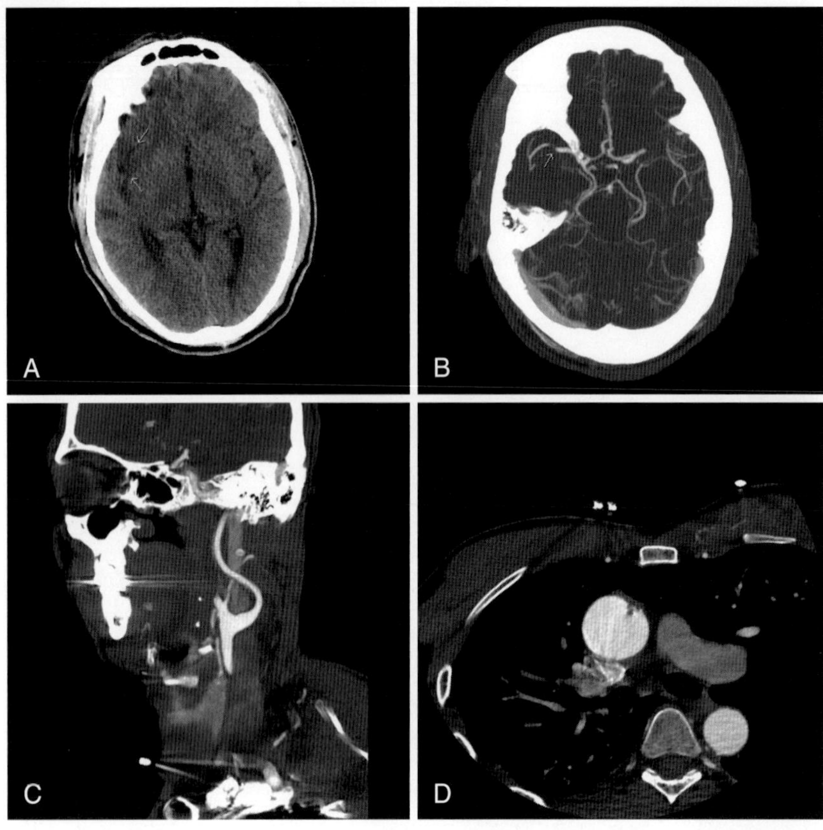

Figure 27-16. **A,** Plain (non-contrast) axial CT demonstrates an area of low attenuation of the right frontal lobe (*arrows*), consistent with infarction. **B,** Contrast-enhanced CT angiography reveals a thrombus in the right middle cerebral artery (MCA). **C,** CT angiography demonstrates a normal right extracranial internal carotid artery. **D,** ECG-gated CT angiography reveals the source of the right MCA thrombus to be thrombus arising on the ascending aorta.

References

1. Endarterectomy for asymptomatic carotid artery stenosis. Executive Committee for the Asymptomatic Carotid Atherosclerosis Study. *JAMA.* 1995;273(18):1421-1428.
2. Vasbinder GB, Nelemans PJ, Kessels AG, et al. Accuracy of computed tomographic angiography and magnetic resonance angiography for diagnosing renal artery stenosis. *Ann Intern Med.* 2004; 141(9):674-682.
3. Vasbinder GB, Nelemans PJ, Kessels AG, et al. Accuracy of computed tomographic angiography and magnetic resonance angiography for diagnosing renal artery stenosis. *Ann Intern Med.* 2004; 141(9):674-682. discussion 682.
4. Rushton AR. The genetics of fibromuscular dysplasia. *Arch Intern Med.* 1980;140(2):233-236.
5. Urban BA, Ratner LE, Fishman EK. Three-dimensional volume-rendered CT angiography of the renal arteries and veins: normal anatomy, variants, and clinical applications. *Radiographics.* 2001; 21(2):373-386. questionnaire 549–555.
6. Willmann JK, Baumert B, Schertler T, et al. Aortoiliac and lower extremity arteries assessed with 16-detector row CT angiography: prospective comparison with digital subtraction angiography. *Radiology.* 2005;236(3):1083-1093.
7. Walter F, Leyder B, Fays J, et al. [Value of arteriography scanning in lower limb artery evaluation: a preliminary study]. *J Radiol.* 2001;82(4):473-479.
8. Edwards AJ, Wells IP, Roobottom CA. Multidetector row CT angiography of the lower limb arteries: a prospective comparison of volume-rendered techniques and intra-arterial digital subtraction angiography. *Clin Radiol.* 2005;60(1):85-95.
9. Ouwendijk R, de VM, Pattynama PM, et al. Imaging peripheral arterial disease: a randomized controlled trial comparing contrast-enhanced MR angiography and multi-detector row CT angiography. *Radiology.* 2005;236(3):1094-1103.
10. Adriaensen ME, Kock MC, Stijnen T, et al. Peripheral arterial disease: therapeutic confidence of CT versus digital subtraction angiography and effects on additional imaging recommendations. *Radiology.* 2004;233(2):385-391.
11. Jakobs TF, Wintersperger BJ, Becker CR. MDCT-imaging of peripheral arterial disease. *Semin Ultrasound CT MR.* 2004; 25(2):145-155.
12. Luther B, Moussazadeh K, Muller BT, et al. [The acute mesenteric ischemia - not understood or incurable?]. *Zentralbl Chir.* 2002; 127(8):674-684.
13. Czerny M, Trubel W, Claeys L, et al. [Acute mesenteric ischemia]. *Zentralbl Chir.* 1997;122(7):538-544.
14. Koelemay MJ, Nederkoorn PJ, Reitsma JB, Majoie CB. Systematic review of computed tomographic angiography for assessment of carotid artery disease. *Stroke.* 2004;35(10):2306-2312.
15. Kirkpatrick ID, Kroeker MA, Greenberg HM. Biphasic CT with mesenteric CT angiography in the evaluation of acute mesenteric ischemia: initial experience. *Radiology.* 2003;229(1):91-98.
16. Fine JJ. 64-Slice Peripheral Computed Tomography Angiography: A Clinical Accuracy Evaluation. *J Am Coll Cardiol.* 2006;47(7): 1495-1496.
17. Koelemay MJ, Nederkoorn PJ, Reitsma JB, Majoie CB. Systematic review of computed tomographic angiography for assessment of carotid artery disease. *Stroke.* 2004;35(10):2306-2312.
18. Hirai T, Korogi Y, Ono K, et al. Maximum stenosis of extracranial internal carotid artery: effect of luminal morphology on stenosis measurement by using CT angiography and conventional DSA. *Radiology.* 2001;221(3):802-809.
19. Iwanaga S, Yoshiura T, Shrier DA, Numaguchi Y. Efficacy of targeted CT angiography in evaluation of intracranial internal carotid artery disease. *Acad Radiol.* 2000;7(5):325-334.

28 Pulmonary Embolism and Other Pulmonary Artery Lesions

Key Points

- CT scanning is currently the de facto test of choice to identify pulmonary embolism.
- CT scanning should be used within a clinically based cost-conscious algorithm to approach the diagnosis of thromboembolic disease.
- Imaging features may help distinguish acute from chronic pulmonary emboli—although patients may have both acute and chronic disease.
- Maximum intensity projection imaging should not be used to evaluate for pulmonary emboli.
- Other acquired pulmonary artery lesions do occur, such as air embolism of tumor and of medical devices, aneurysms, pseudoaneurysms, mycotic aneurysms, angioinvasion, dissections, aorticopulmonary dissection, traumatic disruptions, compression, calcification, and primary sarcomas.
- Congenital lesions of the pulmonary artery also may occur, such as central or peripheral stenosis, post-stenotic aneurysms, absence of a pulmonary artery, pulmonary artery slings, and arteriovenous malformations.
- Pulmonary embolism CT scanning may identify other lesions responsible for chest pain or acute dyspnea presentations.

PULMONARY ARTERY ANATOMY

Normally, there are 17 bronchopulmonary segments, any of which may develop an embolism. The main pulmonary artery bifurcates into the right and left main pulmonary arteries. The right main pulmonary artery then trifurcates into three lobar arteries, which divide into segmental arteries (and subsequently into subsegmental arteries, which are not precisely distinguished from the segmental arteries by tomographic imaging):

- Upper lobe
  - S1: apical segment
  - S2: posterior segment
  - S3: anterior segment
- Middle lobe
  - S4: lateral segment
  - S5: medial segment
- Lower lobe
  - S6: superior segment
  - S7: medial basal segment
  - S8: anterior basal segment
  - S9: lateral basal segment
  - S10: posterobasal segment

The left main pulmonary artery bifurcates into two lobar arteries, which divide into:

- Upper lobe
  - Superior division
    - S1, S2: apical posterior segment
    - S3: Anterior segment
  - Lingular division
    - S4: superior segment
    - S5: inferior segment
- Lower lobe
  - S6: superior segment
  - S7: anteromedial basal segment
  - S8: lateral basal segment
  - S9: posterobasal segment

Thus, the pulmonary arterial tree can be described as having:

- A main pulmonary artery (trunk)
- The left and right main pulmonary arteries
- Nine right and eight left segmental pulmonary arteries
- Subsegmental pulmonary arteries

See Figure 28-1.

PULMONARY THROMBOEMBOLISM

Approximately 700,000 persons per year in North America experience pulmonary embolism (PE). Due to protean presentations, often obfuscated by comorbidity or by surgical issues, delay or missed diagnosis occurs in most cases of PE,[1] causing or contributing to death in an estimated 120,000 patients in the United States alone.[1]

Untreated PE has a recurrence rate of approximately 33%, which entails considerable 3-month mortality: the International Cooperative Pulmonary Embolism Registry reported a rate of 15% to 17%,[2] and historically a rate of 20% to 40% has been reported.[3-5] In patients in whom PE is identified and treated appropriately, the mortality rate

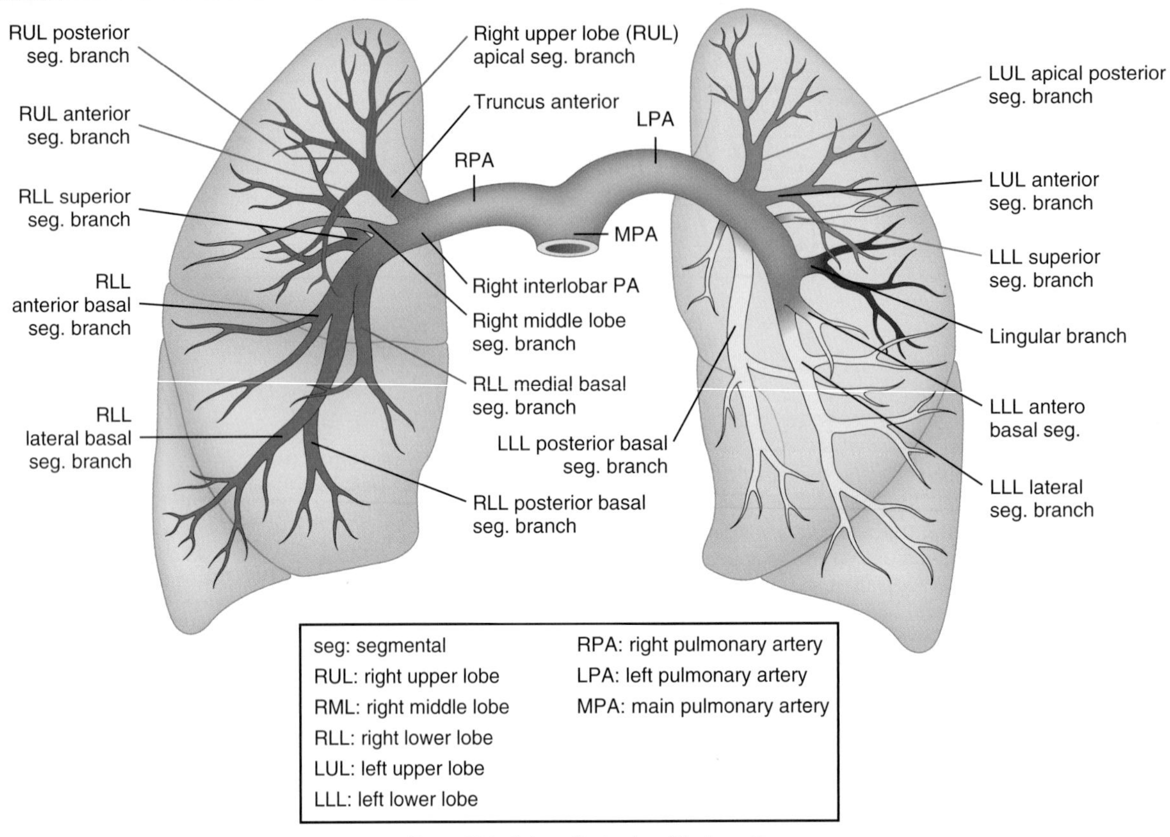

Figure 28-1. Schematic drawing of the bronchi.

is approximately 8%, versus 30% for untreated patients.[6-8] It remains strongly suspected that the antemortem detection of PE is considerably suboptimal.

The increasing use of CT scanning to detect pulmonary emboli is associated with an increased detection rate, and declining mortality from pulmonary thromboembolism,[9] although whether this is due to the increase in CT scanning or to an overall more aggressive approach to the disorder has not been determined.

The approach to suspected PE entails integration of clinical assessment with or without blood testing for D-dimers into an overall assessment to establish a pre-test probability and decision to proceed to subsequent testing. CT pulmonary angiography is the principal imaging test to assess for suspected pulmonary emboli. CT increasingly affords venography as well, but CT venography is not a proficient test, and its use in the context of suspected PE remains controversial. CT pulmonary angiography contributes to the assessment of medical in-patients and postoperative cases.

Nuclear scintigraphy is less useful in patients with comorbidities and postsurgical cases than it is in ambulatory patients. Pulmonary angiography, the historic "gold standard" examination, retains a role in assessing cases where clinical suspicion remains despite negative testing, and in evaluating cases where there is clinical suspicion and poor CT images. Although CT pulmonary angiography is a robust test, unless poor-quality scans are excluded from analysis, sensitivity and negative predictive value may not always be as strong as is assumed by its users.

For the detection of pulmonary emboli, all pulmonary artery lobar and segmental branches must be investigated. Importantly, there are many possible congenital variants to the pulmonary arterial blood supply.

Determination of the specific anatomic pulmonary artery affected is most readily done with conventional pulmonary angiography, which "lays out" the pulmonary arterial vasculature of one lung. Imaging is intentionally done early to avoid the venous (levo) phase, thereby simplifying the number of vessels depicted and minimizing overlap.

Determination of the specific pulmonary arterial anatomic segment also can be achieved with CT pulmonary angiography, especially if combinations of axial, sagittal, and coronal views are used. It is not clinically essential to pinpoint the exact pulmonary artery segment involved.

Pulmonary perfusion scanning makes the most assumptions about the particular anatomic segment involved, because actual anatomy is not visualized, but inferred by location (i.e., where,

TABLE 28-1 Risk of Fatal Pulmonary Embolism Within 3 Months in Patients with a Treatment Duration of at Least 3 Months

CASE REPORT	% RISK OF FATAL PULMONARY EMBOLISM (n = 15,520)
Patient < 75 years, deep vein thrombosis	0.23
Patient < 75 years, nonmassive symptomatic pulmonary embolism	1.24
Patient > 75 years, nonmassive symptomatic pulmonary embolism	3.42
Patient > 75 years, nonmassive symptomatic pulmonary embolism, immobilization > 4 days for neurologic disease	9.81
Patient > 75 years, massive pulmonary embolism, immobilization > 4 days for neurologic disease	24.70

Data from Laporte S, Mismetti P, Decousus H, et al. Clinical predictors for fatal pulmonary embolism in 15,520 patients with venous thromboembolism: findings from the Registro Informatizado de la Enfermedad TromboEmbolica venosa (RIETE) Registry. *Circulation.* 2008;117(13):1711-1716.

peripherally, the perfusion defect is seen and what normally perfuses that location).

Clinical parameters have some ability to predict fatality risk from PE in patients with deep venous thrombosis (Table 28-1).[10]

Screening and Supportive Diagnostic Testing for Pulmonary Embolism

Venous Doppler Examination

Venous Doppler examination is widely available and often used to assess suspected venous thromboembolic disease. Its use is widely accepted for the evaluation of *symptomatic* deep venous thrombosis (DVT) (venous Doppler is insensitive for asymptomatic DVT), but controversial for screening for PE. Older contrast venography studies established that one fifth of cases of PE had negative venograms. The number is considerably higher with venous Doppler examinations—one third to one half.[11] The greatest protocol variation is inclusion or exclusion of the distal venous circulation. The role and utility of venous Doppler scanning are variable, depending on the center where it is being done. Its contribution to the assessment of PE is limited.[12] A strategy of initial whole-leg scanning with color Doppler assessment versus two-point (i.e., superior femoral artery [SFA] and popliteal artery) serial scans (1 week apart) in patients with positive D-dimers appears to provide equivalent information.[13] Lack of familiarity with venous anatomic variants such as bifid superficial femoral veins or bifid popliteal veins, and scanning only the readily imaged portion of the popliteal vein, diminish the utility of Doppler assessment as performed in such an abbreviated fashion.

D-dimer Blood Test

The D-dimer blood test for degraded cross-linked fibrin is widely available. There is assay variation (e.g., enzyme-linked immunosorbent assay [ELISA], latex, whole agglutination), and threshold variation. The usual threshold is 500 $\mu g/L^{-1}$. In an emergency department scenario, its sensitivity for thromboembolic disease is very high (97%) and the negative predictive value is excellent (99.7%). Specificity, however, is poor, particularly among the in-patient ranks, because many pulmonary illnesses, including pneumonia and sepsis, and the postoperative state, as well as healthy pregnancy, are associated with elevated D-dimers.[11,14] Although a negative D-dimer test—in patients either with or without prior venous thromboembolism—has excellent negative predictive value (100%), a negative D-dimer test is uncommon in patients with prior venous thromboembolism.[15]

The differential diagnosis of a positive D-dimer blood test includes:

- Trauma
- Inflammation
- Liver disease
- Malignancy
- Advanced age
- Elevated rheumatoid factor
- Postoperative state
- Pneumonia
- Sepsis
- Aortic dissection
- Myocardial infarction
- Stroke
- Atrial fibrillation
- Acute limb ischemia
- Intracardiac thrombus
- Disseminated intravascular coagulation
- Preeclampsia and eclampsia
- Use of thrombolytic agents
- Sickle cell disease
- Renal disease
- Nephrotic syndrome (e,g., renal vein thrombosis)
- Oral contraceptive use
- Ovarian cyst rupture
- Venous malformations

Diagnostic Testing for Pulmonary Embolism

Contrast Catheter-Based Pulmonary Angiography

Contrast catheter-based pulmonary angiography formerly was the "gold standard" for assessment of PE, but it is invasive (which is relevant with respect to anticoagulation and thrombolysis risks) and has imperfect interobserver agreement: only 45% to 66% for subsegmental emboli.[16,17] A negative pulmonary angiogram, in the context of a suspected pulmonary embolus, using super-selective magnification, has an excellent associated 6-month death rate from thromboembolism or recurrent embolism rate of less than 1% (0/180).[18] Vessel superimposition, as occurs with severe lung volume loss, renders image analysis difficult. Catheter-based pulmonary angiography may be used to enable catheter-directed thrombolysis. Motion and other technical problems for CT angiography are less of a problem for catheter-based angiography; hence pulmonary angiography may be used to evaluate cases of suspected PE with poor-quality CT pulmonary angiograms.

Gadolinium Contrast-Enhanced MR Angiography

Gadolinium contrast-enhanced MRA lacks the spatial resolution to demonstrate peripheral emboli,[19,20] is poorly suited to the evaluation of ill patients, and lacks general availability. It cannot yet be considered a standard test, but the technology is developing.[21] A role may potentially emerge for it in the assessment of suspected PE in pregnancy with nondiagnostic CT PE studies.

Nuclear Scintigraphy

Nuclear scintigraphy studies, although they potentially offer excellent negative predictive value, now are less likely to be used[22,23] because they yield a very high proportion of nondiagnostic indeterminate studies (73% in the Prospective Investigation of Pulmonary Embolism Diagnosis [PIOPED] Study),[23] they are less suitable to in-patient and postoperative cases, and they offer limited availability and lower interobserver correlation (when compared with CTA).[11] Furthermore, in the PIOPED study, 12% of high-probability scans had normal pulmonary angiograms.[23] The utility of ventilation/perfusion testing, especially for postoperative patients, critically ill in-patients, and patients with substantial lung or cardiac disease, added impetus to development and validation of tests short of pulmonary angiography. Although safer than CT scanning, over half of test results establish intermediate probability, and there is a 10% false-positive rate with high-probability scans and a 10% false-negative rate with low-probability scans.[24] Still, a clear unmatched segmental defect is a useful finding.

CT Pulmonary Angiography

CT pulmonary angiography became the de facto test of choice for diagnosis of PE because of its ability to visualize thrombi directly,[25,26] the widespread and generally 24-hour availability of CT scanning, the suitability and track record of CT scanning in general to evaluate critically ill patients, and its robustness in its diagnostic ability in identifying other major intrathoracic pathologies[27-29] that are present in a high (often >50%) proportion of patients suspected of having PE.[27] Interobserver variability is far better by CT ($\kappa = 0.72$) than by nuclear scintigraphy ($\kappa = 0.22$).[30,31] Sensitivity for detection of emboli in the main arteries and segmental arteries is excellent, even by older-generation scanners. Older-generation scanners (single-slice CT [SSCT]) reported sensitivities of only 70% (compared with angiography), although that was for the detection of subsegmental emboli.[32-35] Current cardiovascular CT systems have greater spatial resolution, have superior isotropic resolution, are less affected by partial volume averaging effects, and appear to have superior sensitivity. Maximum intensity projection (MIP) reformatting is poorly suited to the evaluation of PE because of its tendency to maximize high attenuation, thus underrepresenting small (low-attenuation) emboli.

Approximately one third (30%[36]) of emboli are seen within vessels smaller than lobar and segmental pulmonary arteries ("subsegmental arteries") on pulmonary angiography; only about one third of these were detectable by SSCT, and the interobserver agreement of SSCT for small peripheral emboli was very poor. The clinical significance of *isolated* small peripheral pulmonary emboli is uncertain, and the issue of treatment of small isolated peripheral emboli is controversial. The clinical significance of *widespread* small peripheral emboli is less controversial. Because of the advent of and advances in multidirectional CT (MDCT), the small, isolated subsegmental pulmonary embolus is now a more common finding, but it proves to be a vexation as well. The lesion is beneath the resolution of predictive value of scintigraphy; few cases will undergo correlative pulmonary angiography, which has poor interobserver agreement for subsegmental emboli; and, furthermore, the medical literature and community are unsure of the correct management of these emboli.[37]

Earlier, CT scanning showed promise,[38] but clearly had clinically imperfect sensitivity for PE,[39,40] and concern arose about the safety of withholding anticoagulation on the basis of CT pulmonary angiography, given its imperfect sensitivity.[41] The sensitivity of MDCT for detection of pulmonary emboli is evolving, and until well tested with contemporary 64-slice detector systems and newer, wide-detector 256- and 320-slice systems, dual energy systems with lung perfusion (blood volume), and new non-gadolinium detector systems, remains unknown.

MDCT is more reliable when assessing for more central rather than far peripheral emboli.[39]

Although the mortality of untreated PE is related to how proximal the untreated PE is, small peripheral pulmonary emboli may have considerable hemodynamic consequences in critically ill patients.[42]

CT Pulmonary Angiography Image Data Set Review

- The CT scan data should be reviewed on axial images, not MIPs, because the MIP modality underrepresents low-attenuation structures such as emboli.
- Sagittal and coronary views may be helpful.
- IV contrast is obviously a prerequisite for a PE protocol study, but sometimes it is a relative contraindication due, for example, to advanced renal insufficiency.

Ancillary Findings on CT Pulmonary Angiography

- Right ventricular enlargement, in which the diameter of the right ventricle is greater than that of the left ventricle:
  - On CT, the axial four-chamber view is 83% sensitive (but only 49% specific) for major adverse clinical events and has a relative risk of 4.2 [1.06–15.19].[43] See Figure 28-2.
- Reflux of dye into the inferior vena cava (IVC):
  - Reflux of dye (injected via an arm vein) into the IVC is seen in pulmonary hypertension, right ventricular systolic dysfunction, right ventricular diastolic dysfunction (pericardial constriction), and tricuspid regurgitation.[44]
  - The length of the column of dye reflux down the IVC correlates (r = 0.84) with echocardiography-derived estimates of pulmonary hypertension.[45]

CT CRITERIA FOR THE DIAGNOSIS OF PULMONARY EMBOLISM

CT criteria for the diagnosis of PE include the following:

- Partial intraluminal filling defect
- Complete intraluminal filling defect
- Abrupt cessation of blood flow
- "Railway tracks"[46]
- Mural defects [46]

The following findings are not considered criteria of PE:

- Abrupt tapering of a pulmonary artery
- Decrease in blood flow
- Indirect signs such as a wedge-shaped pleural-based parenchymal shadow corresponding to pulmonary infarction[47]

Underlying respiratory disease does not appear to reduce the negative predictive value of MDCT.[48]

Thin collimation[48] and breath-holding improve image quality and negative predictive value. Inability to breath-hold is not an exclusion criterion for CT assessment. Images are generally assessed with lung windows (window width 1500 HU; window center 500 HU) and mediastinal windows (window width 400 HU; window center 400 HU) as well.[47] A high degree of vascular opacification (>200 HU) is desirable.[47] The figures in this chapter depict a number of variants and complications:

- PE detected on CT (Fig. 28-3)
- Cavitation of pleural-based infarcts (Fig. 28-4)
- Submassive and massive PEs (Figs. 28-5 and 28-6)
- Cases with pleural-based infarction (Hampton humps; Fig. 28-7)
- Emboli in-transit: usually, emboli stick into a patent foramen ovale (PFO) due to right heart failure and an underlying PFO that "caught" an otherwise pulmonary embolism as it was directed by hydrostatic pressures to traverse a PFO when the embolism arrived in the right atrium during systole (Figs. 28-8 and 28-9)
- Segmental oligemia (Westermark sign; Fig. 28-10)

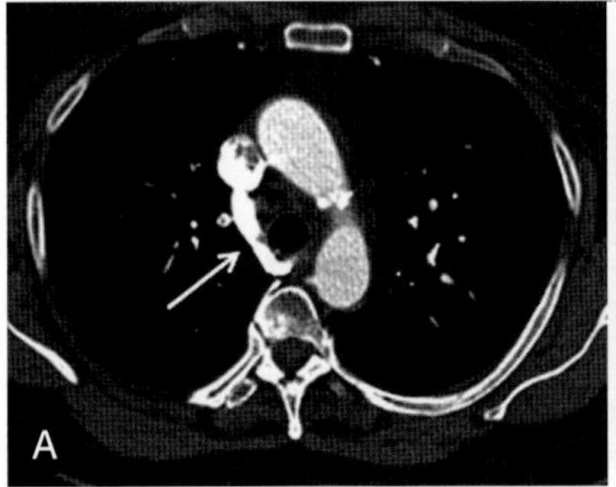

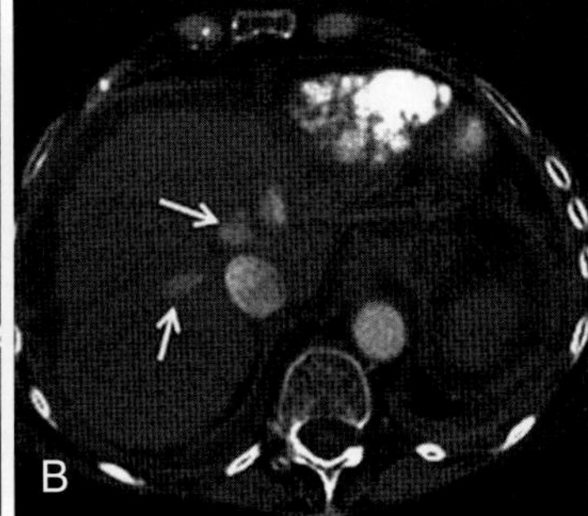

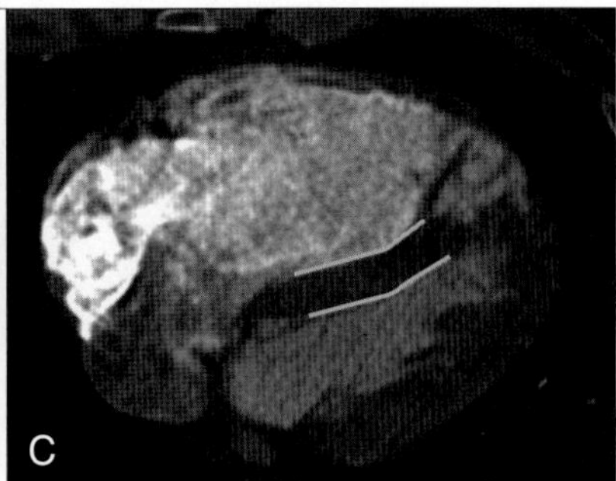

Figure 28-2. Dilatation of and reflux of contrast material into the azygous vein (**A,** *arrow*), as well as reflux of contrast material into the hepatic veins (**B,** *arrows*) in a 64-year-old man with acute pulmonary embolism. Both are nonspecific signs of right ventricular dysfunction (RVD). **C,** "Septal bowing" of the interventricular septum toward the left ventricle (*green lines*) in a 55-year-old woman with acute central pulmonary embolism and echocardiographically confirmed severe RVD. (Reprinted with permission from Henzler T, Barraza JM Jr, Nance JW Jr, et al. CT imaging of acute pulmonary embolism. *J Cardiovasc Comput Tomogr.* 2011;51:3-11.)

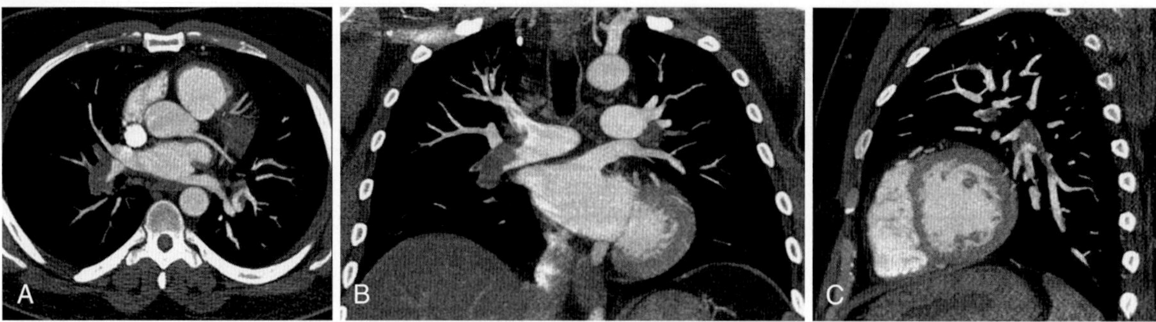

Figure 28-3. Axial, coronal, and sagittal maximum intensity projection reformations of a 34-year-old man with acute central pulmonary embolism and multiple segmental and subsegmental clots. Thin-section CT pulmonary angiography allows image reformations that improve the detection of segmental and subsegmental clots. (Reprinted with permission from Henzler T, Barraza JM Jr, Nance JW Jr, et al. CT imaging of acute pulmonary embolism. *J Cardiovasc Comput Tomogr*. 2011;51:3-11.)

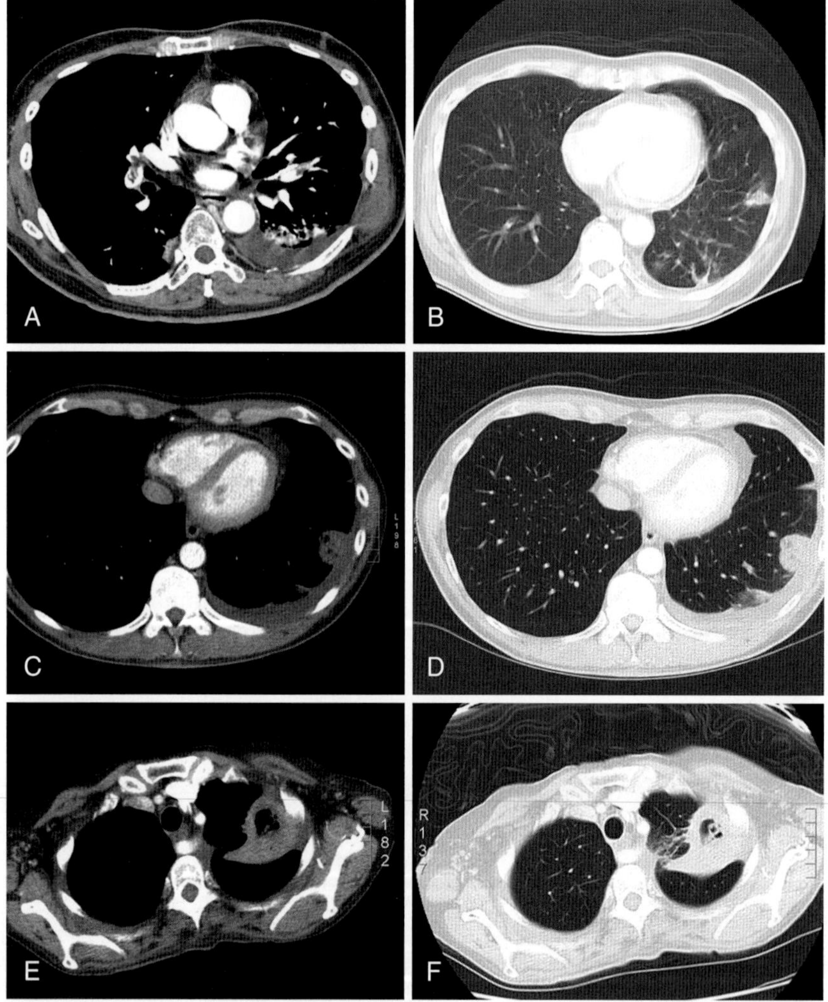

Figure 28-4. Pulmonary embolism and pulmonary infarction. **A** and **B,** Contrast-enhanced CT scans of a patient with a pulmonary embolism and a pleural-based wedge-shaped infarction of the left lower lobe. There is a pleural effusion as well. **C** and **D,** Contrast-enhanced CT scans of a patient with a pulmonary embolism and a cavitated pleural-based wedge-shaped infarction of the left lower lobe. There is a pleural effusion as well. **E** and **F,** Pulmonary embolism and infarction. Contrast-enhanced CT scans of a patient with a pulmonary embolism and a cavitated pleural-based wedge-shaped infarction of the left upper lobe.

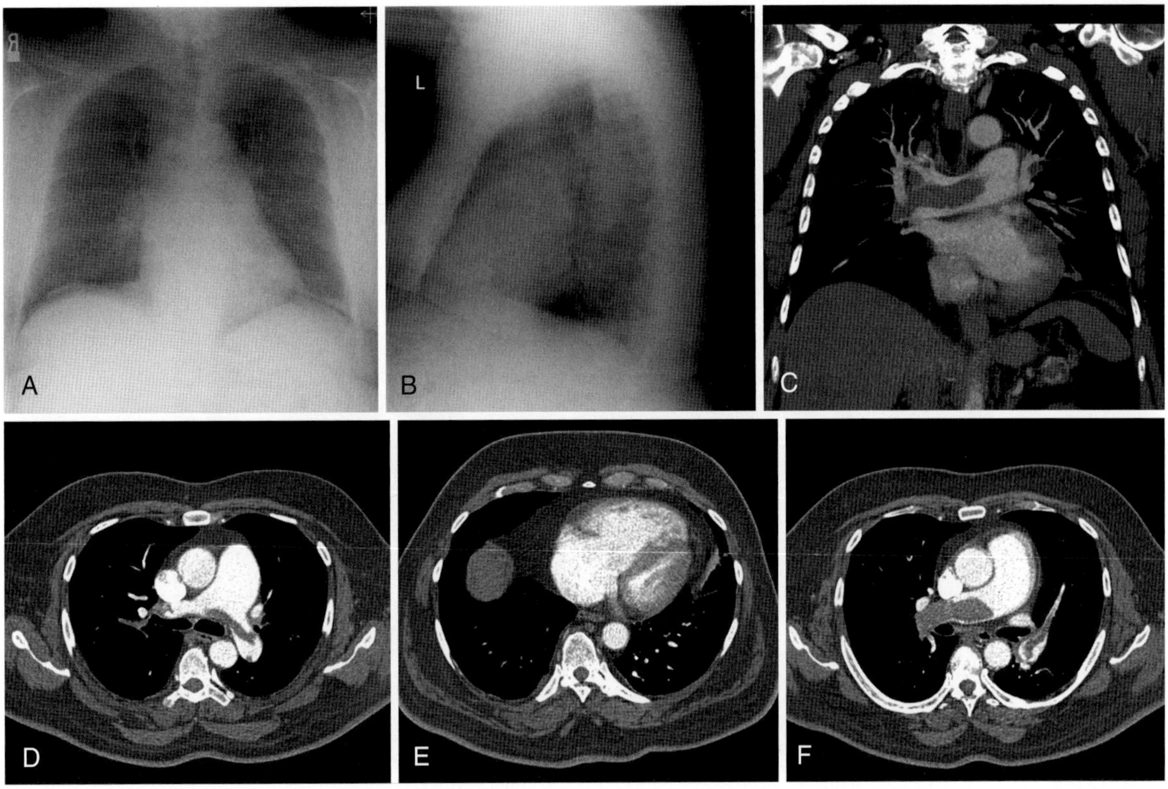

Figure 28-5. Chest radiographs and contrast-enhanced CT scan views of a patient with pulmonary hypertension from chronic recurrent pulmonary embolism. The right ventricle and the main and central pulmonary arteries are dilated. A large burden of clot is present centrally within the pulmonary arteries. The peripheral arteries are diminished in size and appear few in number.

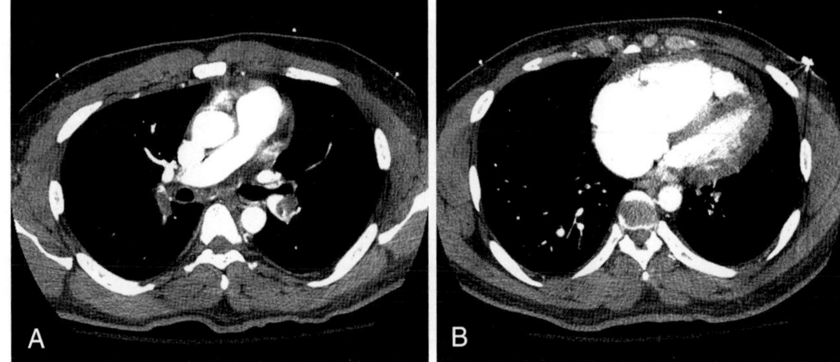

Figure 28-6. CT pulmonary angiography: note the high concentration of contrast in the right ventricle. There are bilateral pulmonary emboli, and the right heart is clearly dilated due to right heart strain from pulmonary vascular obstruction.

Although the clinical risk to patients with suspected PE and normal pulmonary angiography is small, it is measurable, and higher than that of the general hospitalized patient population,[49] which suggests that a more comprehensive assessment, such as inclusion of lower limb Doppler ultrasound studies, may be useful.

The following issues may be relevant in the assessment of patients with suspected PE:

- Pulmonary emboli tend to fragment with time, and the residua embolize more distally. Thus, the detection rate directly relates to the promptness of testing, and detection may be forfeited if unduly delayed.
- Cost
- Invasiveness of testing and the tolerability of complications
- Patient's ability to tolerate contrast dye
- Patient's ability to tolerate transport to either the CT scanner or the angiography suite
- Bleeding rates from heparin (per day):
  - Fatal: 0.05%
  - Major: 0.8%
  - Minor: 2%

It appears increasingly less likely that CVCT can ever be formally compared in a large trial to pulmonary angiography, which has been the traditional gold standard for PE diagnosis and now is the true standard.

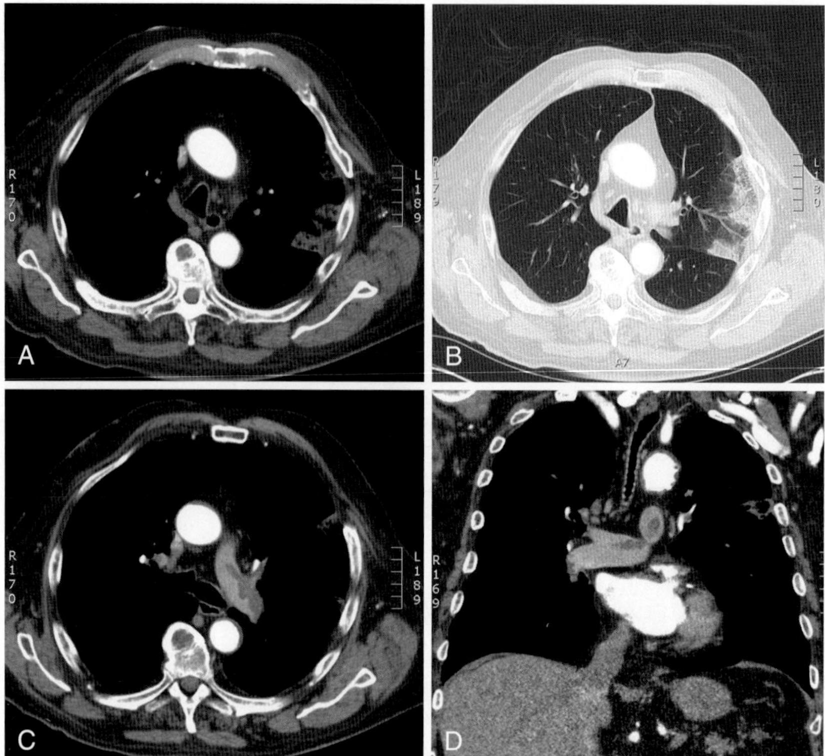

Figure 28-7. Contrast-enhanced CT scans of a patient with pulmonary embolism and infarct of the left upper lobe. The pulmonary infarction, with its characteristic pleural-based triangular or wedge shape, is seen more easily in the lung window. The aorta is mildly dilated and heavily atherosclerotic.

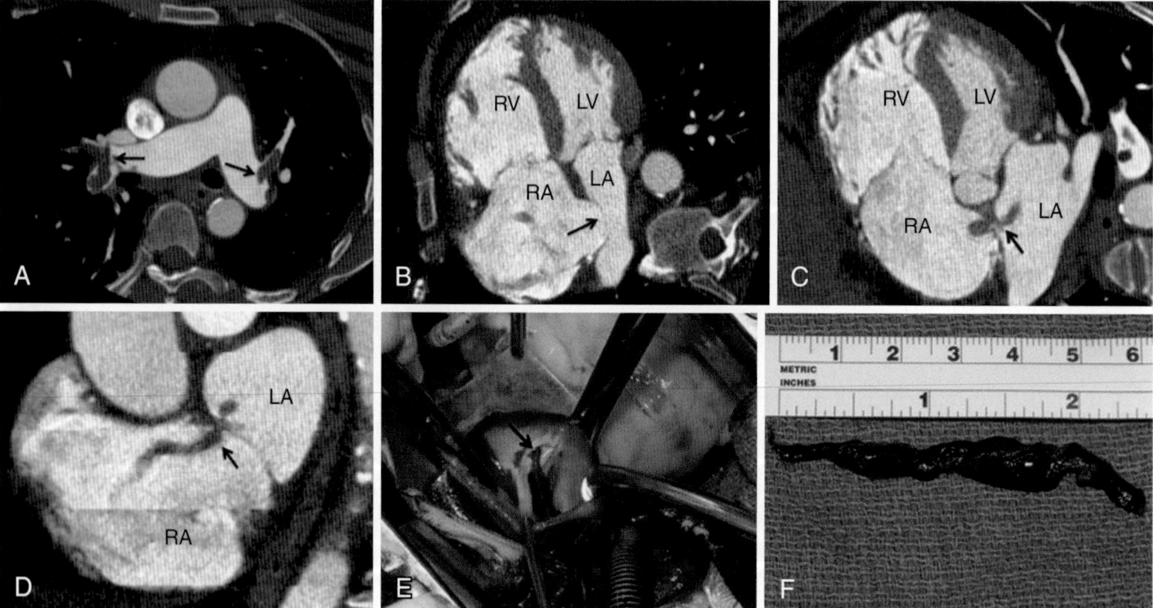

Figure 28-8. Comprehensive cardiothoracic CT examination. **A,** Axial image at the level of the pulmonary artery bifurcation shows bilateral pulmonary embolism (*arrows*). **B,** The four-chamber image shows right ventricular enlargement consistent with right ventricular strain and leftward bowing of the interatrial septum (*arrow*) consistent with elevated right-sided pressures. **C,** The modified four-chamber image shows thrombus in transit (*arrow*) straddling a patent foramen ovale. **D,** Parasagittal image at the level of the atria also shows thrombus in transit (*arrow*). **E** and **F,** Intraoperative findings. **E,** Thrombus was seen extending through the patent foramen ovale (*arrow*) at the time of surgery. **F,** Intracardiac thrombus after removal. LA, left atrium; LV, left ventricle; RA, right atrium; RV, right ventricle. (Reprinted with permission from Syed IS, Motiei A, Connolly HM, Dearani JA. Pulmonary embolism, right ventricular strain, and intracardiac thrombus-in-transit: evaluation using comprehensive cardiothoracic computed tomography. *J Cardiovasc Comput Tomogr*. 2009;33:184-186.)

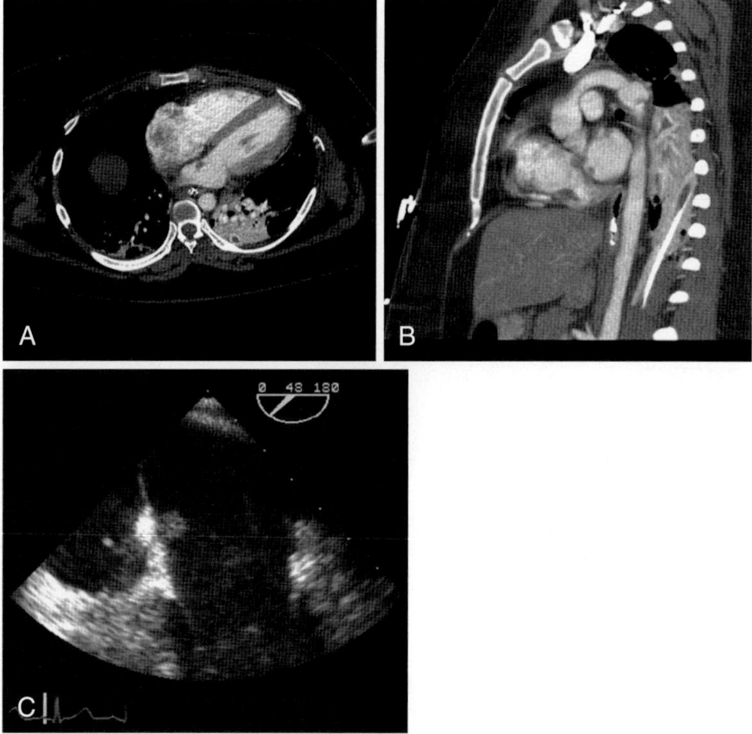

Figure 28-9. A composite image in a young woman after a high-speed motor vehicle accident. The patient incurred an acute aortic injury that is best seen on the sagittal reconstruction through the chest (**B**). An underlying left posterior pulmonary contusion is also noted (**A** and **B**). **A** and **B,** CT images also demonstrate a small soft tissue density affixed to the interatrial septum, residing within the left atrium. **C,** This was confirmed on TEE as an embolism in transit, across the foramen ovale.

Algorithms for Assessment of Pulmonary Embolism

The optimal use of CT to evaluate cases of suspected PE is still not entirely clear. The question is really in what algorithm (i.e., combination and sequence with other testing) CT scanning should be employed. The tests most commonly combined with CT scanning are D-dimer assay and venous leg Doppler examination. Increasingly, emphasis is placed on detailed clinical risk assessment (Table 28-2) in combination with testing.[50] D-dimer assays do not all appear comparable, and there is a tendency to shorten algorithms (i.e., omit lower limb Doppler ultrasound),[51] although this may simply reflect more of a drive toward expediency, away from comprehensiveness.

Bayesian theory holds true—that is, that the post-CTA probability of PE is significantly skewed by the pretest probability, which can be approximated by clinical assessment (Table 28-3).

Visualization of subsegmental pulmonary arteries is lowest with single-slice CT, significantly better with 4-slice CT, and probably slightly better yet again with 16-slice CT. It is not known whether 64-slice CT achieves better detection than does 16-slice, and what 64-, 256-, and 320-slice systems offer, as with, similarly, dual source and non-gadolinium detector systems.

The PIOPED II Study[52] investigated the accuracy of multidetector CT for the detection of pulmonary emboli (compared against a composite reference diagnosis), whether or not the addition of CT venography increases the detection or exclusion of PE, and whether clinical assessment (Wells score[53]) improves the ability to detect or exclude PE by CTA or CT venography (Table 28-4).

Clinical algorithms are numerous and variable, including or excluding venous assessment. Earlier studies favored duplex assessment, whereas later studies preferred CT venography assessment.

Series Including Venous Doppler Examinations

In a report by Perrier et al.[55] in 965 outpatients with suspected PE presenting to the emergency department, the most common presentations were chest pain and dyspnea. All patients underwent helical CT, venous duplex examination, and D-dimers (cutoff >500 μg/L). Normal D-dimers were used to exclude venous thromboembolism (29%), and venous duplex scanning identified venous thrombosis in 9.5%, leaving 61% to undergo helical CT, which identified PE in 12.8%. Only 1% of patients went on to pulmonary angiography (duplex: negative; CT: negative; high

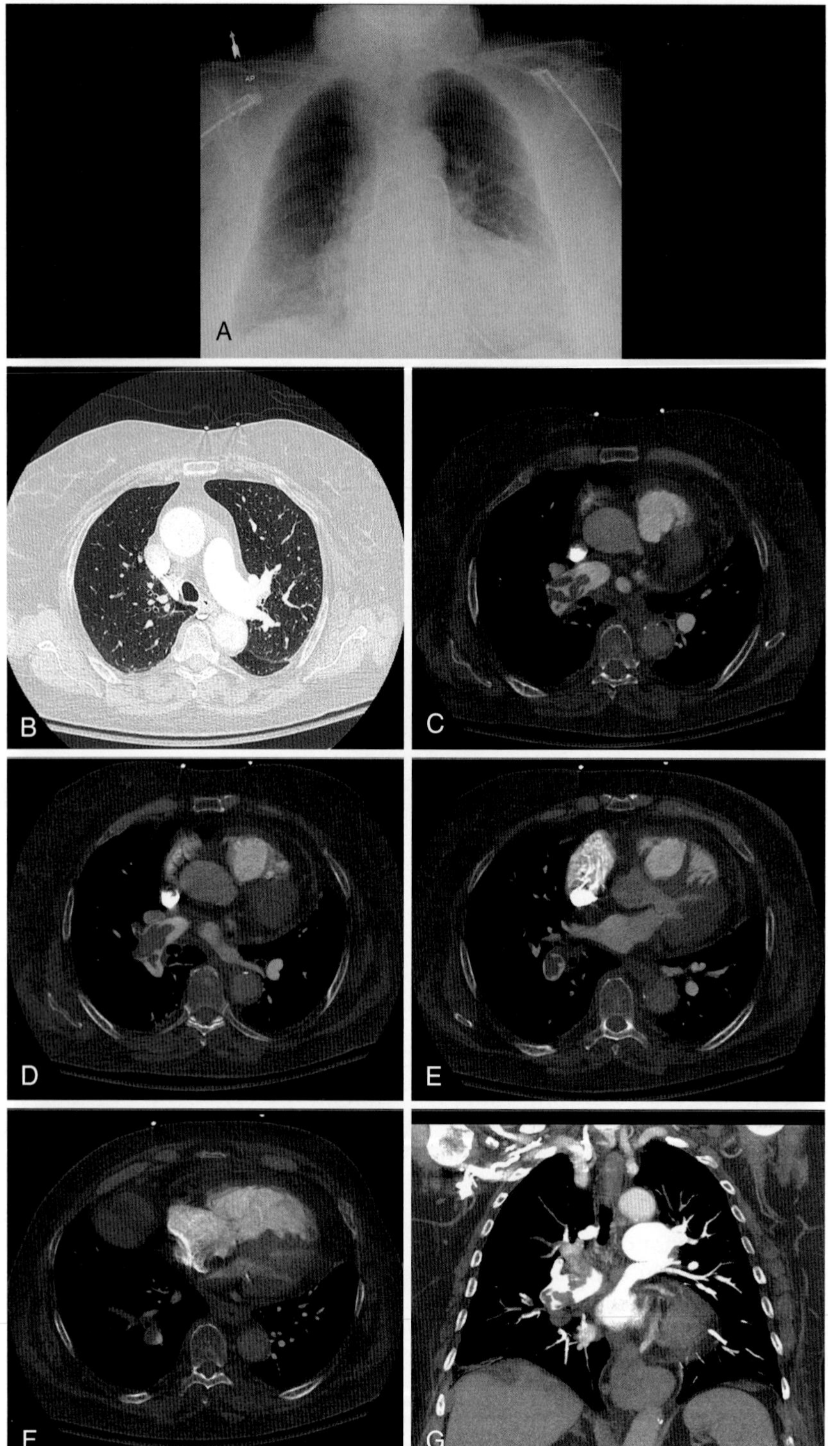

Figure 28-10. CT angiography of a 78-year-old woman with chest pain and acute shortness of breath. **A,** The anteroposterior chest radiograph demonstrates moderate enlargement of the cardiac silhouette. There is also appreciable asymmetry in pulmonary arterial vascular markings within the lungs, with the right lung demonstrating much less peripheral pulmonary arterial vasculature. This finding is known as a Westermark sign. **B,** Lung reconstruction from a CT pulmonary embolism (PE) study also demonstrates asymmetry in pulmonary arterial vasculature between the right lung (decreased on the right). The remaining CT images from the same CT PE study demonstrate a large burden of thrombus within the right pulmonary arterial tree, and no definite left-sided pulmonary embolism. **F,** Secondary signs of elevated pulmonary artery pressure are present, with an enlarged right ventricle and right atrium.

TABLE 28-2 Model for Determining the Clinical Probability of Pulmonary Embolism, According to the Wells Score*

CLINICAL FEATURE	SCORE
Clinical signs and symptoms of DVT (objectively measured leg swelling and palpation in the deep vein system)	3.0
Heart rate >100 beats/min	1.5
Immobilization for ≥3 consecutive days (bed rest except to go to bathroom) or surgery in previous 4 weeks	1.5
Previous objectively diagnosed pulmonary embolism or DVT	1.5
Hemoptysis	1.0
Cancer (with treatment within past 6 mo or palliative treatment)	1.0
Pulmonary embolism likely or more likely than alternative diagnoses (on the basis of history, physical examination, chest radiography, ECG, and blood tests)	3.0

*Scoring method indicates high probability if score is 3 or more; moderate if score is 1 or 2; and low if score is 0 or less.
DVT, deep vein thrombosis.
Data from Stein PD, Fowler SE, Goodman LR, et al. Multidetector computed tomography for acute pulmonary embolism. *N Engl J Med.* 2006;354(22):2317-2327; and Wells PS, Anderson DR, Rodger M, et al. Excluding pulmonary embolism at the bedside without diagnostic imaging: management of patients with suspected pulmonary embolism presenting to the emergency department by using a simple clinical model and d-dimer. *Ann Intern Med.* 2001;135(2):98-107.

TABLE 28-3 Positive and Negative Predictive Values of CT Angiography, as Compared with Previous Clinical Assessment*

	HIGH CLINICAL PROBABILITY		INTERMEDIATE CLINICAL PROBABILITY		LOW CLINICAL PROBABILITY	
VARIABLE	NO./ TOTAL NO.	VALUE (95% CI)	NO./ TOTAL NO.	VALUE (95% CI)	NO./ TOTAL NO.	VALUE (95% CI)
Positive predictive value of CTA	22/23	96 (78–99)	93/101	92 (84–96)	22/38	58 (40–73)
Positive predictive value of CTA or CTV	27/28	96 (81–99)	100/111	90 (82–94)	24/42	57 (40–72)
Negative predictive value of CTA	9/15	60 (32–83)	121/136	89 (82–93)	158/164†	96 (92–98)
Negative predictive value of both CTA and CTV	9/11	82 (48–97)	114/124	92 (85–96)	146/151†	97 (92–98)

*The clinical probability of pulmonary embolism was based on the Wells score: <2.0, low probability; 2.0 to 6.0, moderate probability; and >6.0, high probability.
†To avoid bias for the calculation of the negative predictive value in patients deemed to have a low probability of pulmonary embolism on previous clinical assessment, only patients with a reference test diagnosis by ventilation-perfusion scanning or conventional pulmonary DSA were included.
CI, confidence interval; CTA, computed tomographic angiography; CTV, computed tomographic venography.
Data from Stein PD, Fowler SE, Goodman LR, et al. Multidetector computed tomography for acute pulmonary embolism. *N Engl J Med.* 2006;354(22):2317-2327.

clinical probability: 2 positive, 6 negative). Patients negative for thromboembolism were not anticoagulated: the 3-month thromboembolism rate was 1% (0.5–2.1%). Overall, PE was identified in 7% of low-, 34% of intermediate-, and 85% of high-probability patients.

The authors concluded that a combined clinical and laboratory testing approach using D-dimers, duplex ultrasound, and CT excluded thromboembolism in 99% of cases.[55]

Series Not Using Venous Doppler

In a study by van Belle et al.,[56] 3306 patients were prospectively evaluated for suspected PE. Initially using the Wells' criteria, patients were classified as either unlikely or likely to have had PE. Patients "unlikely" to have had PE were tested with D-dimers, and only underwent CT scanning if the D-dimer was abnormal. All other patients underwent CT scanning as the definitive test for PE. In patients with negative D-dimers and negative CT

TABLE 28-4 Pulmonary Embolism Detection: Prospective Evaluation of Dual-Section Helical CT Versus Selective Pulmonary Arteriography in 157 Patients

	CT PULMONARY ANGIOGRAPHY	CT PULMONARY ANGIOGRAPHY AND VENOGRAPHY
Inconclusive	6%	10%
Sensitivity	83%	90%
Specificity	96%	95%
Positive predictive value		
Clinical Assessment		
High probability	96%	
Intermediate probability	92%	
Low probability	Nondiagnostic	

Data from Stein PD, Fowler SE, Goodman LR, et al. Multidetector computed tomography for acute pulmonary embolism. *N Engl J Med.* 2006;354(22):2317-2327.

scans, the 3-month incidence of nonfatal venous thromboembolism was 0.5%. Among patients with PE not imaged by CT scanning (1236 of 1505 [82%] of whom were not treated with anticoagulants), the 3-month incidence of PE was 1.3% (0.7–2.0%). Pulmonary embolism was considered as a possible cause of death in seven patients (0.5%) after a negative CT scan (0.2–1.0%).

In a recent large study by Righini et al.,[57] patients with suspected PE were randomized to D-dimer, CT, and lower extremity ultrasound (n = 916) versus D-dimer and CT. This study demonstrated a prevalence of PE of 21% in both groups, and 0.3% thromboembolic events at 3 months for both groups. The authors concluded that the diagnosis of PE and the 3-month incidence of thromboembolic events are the same regardless of which of the two testing strategies is used.

Withholding anticoagulation on basis of a negative work-up for suspected PE is a major decision. There is no basis to withhold anticoagulation on the basis of a negative venous Doppler study. Series describing the subsequent DVT and PE rate among patients with a negative CT scan have different in-patient profile, duration, and observed clinical event rates. Negative predictive values of CT scanning over 3 to 24 months of follow-up of 96% to 100% have been described.[11,58]

For the PE assessment algorithm, see Figure 28-11.

DEEP VENOUS THROMBOSIS

A small number of good comparative studies of MDCT detection of DVT versus venous sonography have been published.[59-61] In the literature, there appears little incremental yield of CT over ultrasound, or ultrasound over CT.[62] Larger reviews of CT pulmonary angiography establish an approximately 10% incidence of DVT,[63] occurring equally in the common femoral, superficial femoral, popliteal, and deep calf veins.[63]

CT contrast venography appears to provide a 20% increase in detection of thromboembolic disease compared with CT pulmonary angiography alone (95% confidence interval, 17–23%).[64]

Usually, 2 minutes after completion of the pulmonary artery portion of scanning, a series of contiguous images from the iliac crest to the popliteal fossa is acquired, with a section width of 1 cm, as most (76%) patients with PE have DVT longer than 4 cm, 18% have clots 3 to 4 cm long, and 6% have clots measuring less than 2 cm in length.[64] CT venography appears to increase the detection rate of thromboembolic disease requiring anticoagulation,[65] although not necessarily in patients with prior venous ultrasonography (Fig. 28-12).

LUNG BLOOD VOLUME TECHNIQUES

Dual-energy CT scanning enables depiction of lung blood volume. To date there is little validation, but the depiction of plausibly typical triangular areas of hypoperfusion is promising (Fig. 28-13).[66]

DISTINGUISHING ACUTE AND CHRONIC PULMONARY EMBOLISM

Commonly, the question arises whether a PE/thrombosis is an acute event or a finding of chronic thromboembolic disease. Chronic thromboembolic pulmonary hypertension (CTEPH) represents a rare but serious sequela of acute PE. In about 0.1% to 0.5% of patients with acute pulmonary thromboembolism who survive, the emboli do not resolve completely.[67] The underlying pulmonary arteries recannulate, reorganize, and develop characteristic imaging features that can help to distinguish between an acute embolism and a chronic process.

PE Assessment Algorithm (1): Perrier	PE Assessment Algorithm (2): Christopher Study
PE Symptoms ± DVT Symptoms ↓ Lower Extremity Duplex Ultrasound Positive → Treat Negative → CT CT Positive → Treat CT Negative → Poor quality CT study / Good quality CT study Poor quality CT study → Further testing- Pulm Angio? Repeat CTA? Good quality CT study → High clinical Supicion: Pulm Angio? Good quality CT study → Stop → 1% 3 month VTE rate	PE Symptoms ± DVT Symptoms ↓ Clinical Risk Model Low Probability → D-dimer D-dimer → Negative / Positive Negative → Stop → 0.5% 3-month non-fatal VTE rate Positive → CT Not Low Probability → CT CT → CT Negative / CT Positive CT Negative → Do not Treat → 1.3% 3-month VTE rate; PE a possible cause of death: 0.5% CT Positive → Treat

Figure 28-11. Assessment algorithms for pulmonary embolism. CTA, CT angiography; DVT, deep venous thrombosis; PE, pulmonary embolism; Pulm Angio, pulmonary angiography; VTE, venous thromboembolism. (Left panel reprinted with permission from Perrier A, Roy PM, Aujesky D, et al. Diagnosing pulmonary embolism in outpatients with clinical assessment, D-dimer measurement, venous ultrasound, and helical computed tomography: a multicenter management study. *Am J Med.* 2004;1165:291-299. Right panel reprinted with permission from Musset D, Parent F, Meyer G, et al. Diagnostic strategy for patients with suspected pulmonary embolism: prospective multicentre outcome study. *Lancet.* 2002;3609349:1914-1920.)

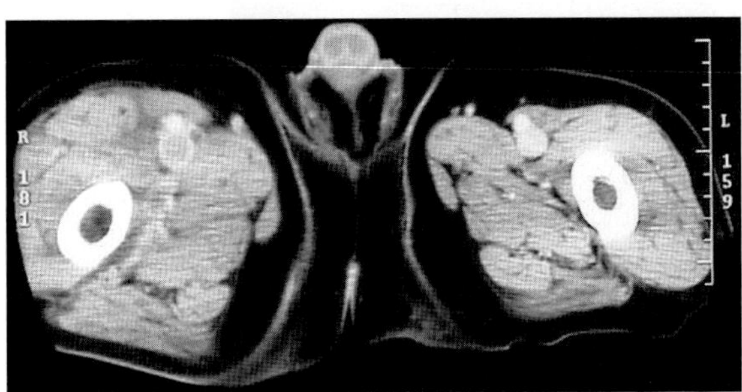

Figure 28-12. Contrast-enhanced axial view at the level of the common femoral artery and vein. There is deep venous thrombosis (low-attenuation matter) of the right femoral vein, which is dilated as a result.

Direct and indirect signs of acute and chronic PE are presented in Table 28-5[68] and Figure 28-14.

PULMONARY TUMOR EMBOLISM

Tumors that invade the large systemic veins, right heart cavities, or pulmonary artery may potentially embolize into the pulmonary arteries. The most common such tumors are:

- ❐ Renal cell adenocarcinoma
- ❐ Hepatic adenocarcinoma
- ❐ Wilms tumor
- ❐ Right atrial myxoma
- ❐ Leimyosarcoma

Features that may be detected in addition to findings positive for PE are mass invasion of the IVC, the right heart cavities, or the pulmonary arteries (Fig. 28-15).

PULMONARY EMBOLISM OF MEDICAL DEVICES AND MATERIALS

Iatrogenic embolization into the pulmonary arteries may occur from:

- ❐ Central venous catheter fragments
- ❐ Central venous guidewires
- ❐ IVC filters and filter fragments
- ❐ Bone "cement"
- ❐ Closure devices, coils

PULMONARY ARTERY ANEURYSMS

Pulmonary artery aneurysms are uncommon. Focal enlargement of a pulmonary artery may be secondary to either congenital or acquired causes.

- ❐ Congenital causes:
  - Connective tissue disorders
  - Secondary to congenital shunts such as patent ductus arteriosus, atrial septal defect, or ventricular septal defect
  - Congenital pulmonary valvular stenosis
  - Tetralogy of Fallot
- ❐ Acquired causes
  - Pulmonary arterial hypertension (primary or secondary)
  - Pulmonary emboli
  - Vasculitis, especially Behçet syndrome
  - Postsurgical, commonly seen in transannular repair of tetralogy of Fallot
  - Acquired pulmonic valvular stenosis
  - Post-traumatic (non-iatrogenic and iatrogenic) (Figs. 28-16 through 28-18; **Video 28-1**)

PULMONARY ARTERY STENOSES

Pulmonary arterial stenoses should not be confused with pulmonary valvular stenosis and may be secondary to congenital or acquired disease.

Congenital Lesions

Congenital stenosis may be focal and discrete or diffuse so that the entire vessel remains small and resembles pulmonary hypoplasia. The most common site of pulmonary arterial stenosis is around the bifurcation of the main pulmonary artery involving the distal main pulmonary artery, and occasionally extending a variable distance into

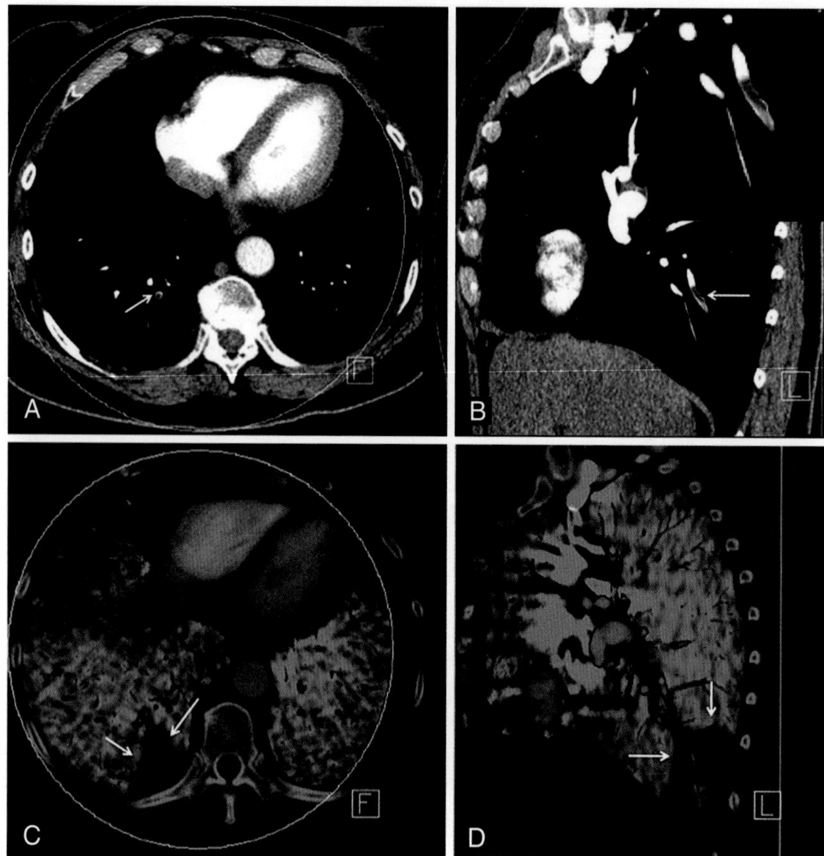

Figure 28-13. Isolated segmental pulmonary embolism (PE) of the right lower lobe in a 46-year-old man. Axial (**A**) and sagittal (**B**) dual energy CT pulmonary angiographic gray-scale images display a subtle PE in the right lower lobe (**B**, *arrow*). The resultant perfusion defect is well visualized on axial (**C**) and coronal (**D**) dual energy perfusion maps (*arrows*), showing the hemodynamic significance of the embolus in the affected segment. (Reprinted with permission from Henzler T, Barraza JM Jr, Nance JW Jr, et al. CT imaging of acute pulmonary embolism. *J Cardiovasc Comput Tomogr.* 2011;51:3-11.)

TABLE 28-5 Acute and Chronic Pulmonary Emboli: Correlation Between Angiography and CT

SIGN	ACUTE PE	CHRONIC PE
Direct Signs	***Complete Obstruction*** The trailing edge of the thrombus/contrast interface has a convex margin. At the site of thrombus, the diameter of the pulmonary artery may be increased because of impaction of the thrombus. ***Partial Filling Defect*** A well-defined central or eccentric filling defect. In acute PE the nonobstructive filling defect forms acute angles with respect to the vessel walls. Longer emboli can demonstrate a "railroad track" sign.	***Complete Obstruction*** The appearance of chronic complete obstruction differs from that of acute PE in that the trailing edge of the thrombus may have a concave margin relative to the contrast interface, with a reduction in vessel size due to contraction of the thrombus. ***Nonobstructive Filling Defects*** Residual intimal soft tissue that is broad-based with or without calcification Bands and webs: filamentous structures attach to the vessel wall at both ends with an unattached midportion. Abrupt vessel narrowing
Indirect Signs	Large central PEs can cause relative oligemia and a decrease in distal pulmonary artery vessel diameter.	Tortuous pulmonary arteries Enlargement of the main pulmonary artery Nonuniform arterial perfusion represented as mosaic attenuation on CT

PE, pulmonary embolism.

Reprinted with permission from Wittram C, Kalra MK, Maher MM, Greenfield A, McLoud TC, Shepard JA. Acute and chronic pulmonary emboli: angiography-CT correlation. *AJR Am J Roentgenol.* 2006;186(6 Suppl 2):S421-429.

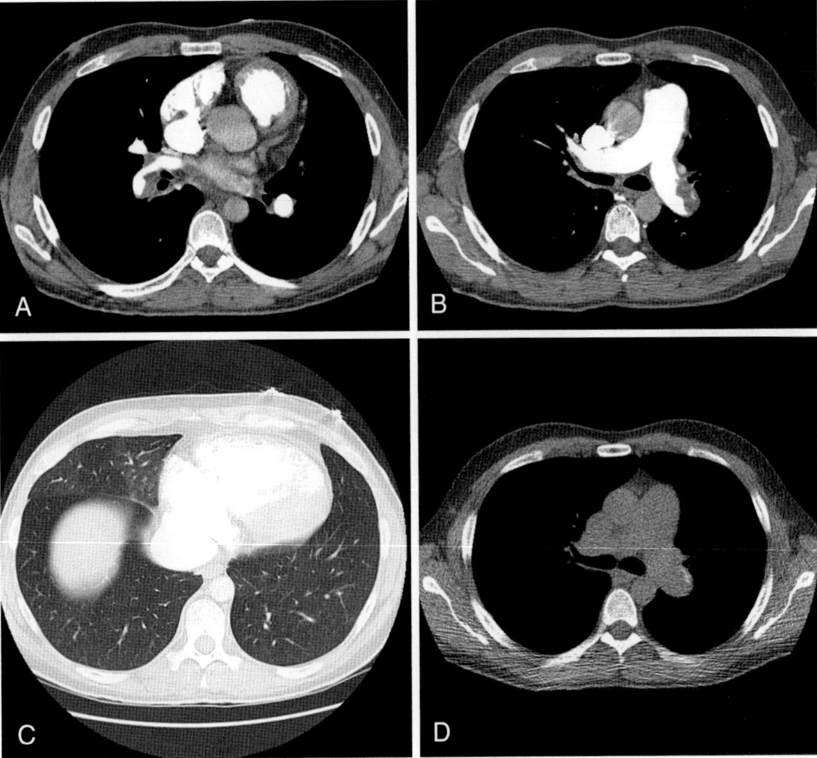

Figure 28-14. A 32-year-old woman, not on anticoagulation therapy, with documented pulmonary thromboembolic disease on four occasions, presented with a new syncopal episode. CT angiography demonstrates evidence of chronic pulmonary thromboembolic disease on this study, which is of good technical quality. Mural adherent thrombus is identified in the main pulmonary artery, the left main pulmonary artery, the right interlobar artery, the right upper lobe pulmonary artery, and the right lower lobe segmental pulmonary arteries. The thrombus in the left main pulmonary artery demonstrates calcification consistent with a chronic thromboembolus. There is evidence of mosaic attenuation of the lung parenchyma bilaterally, consistent with small vessel disease secondary to pulmonary thromboembolic disease. The right ventricular outflow tract is enlarged and hypertrophied, consistent with the right ventricular pressure overload and strain.

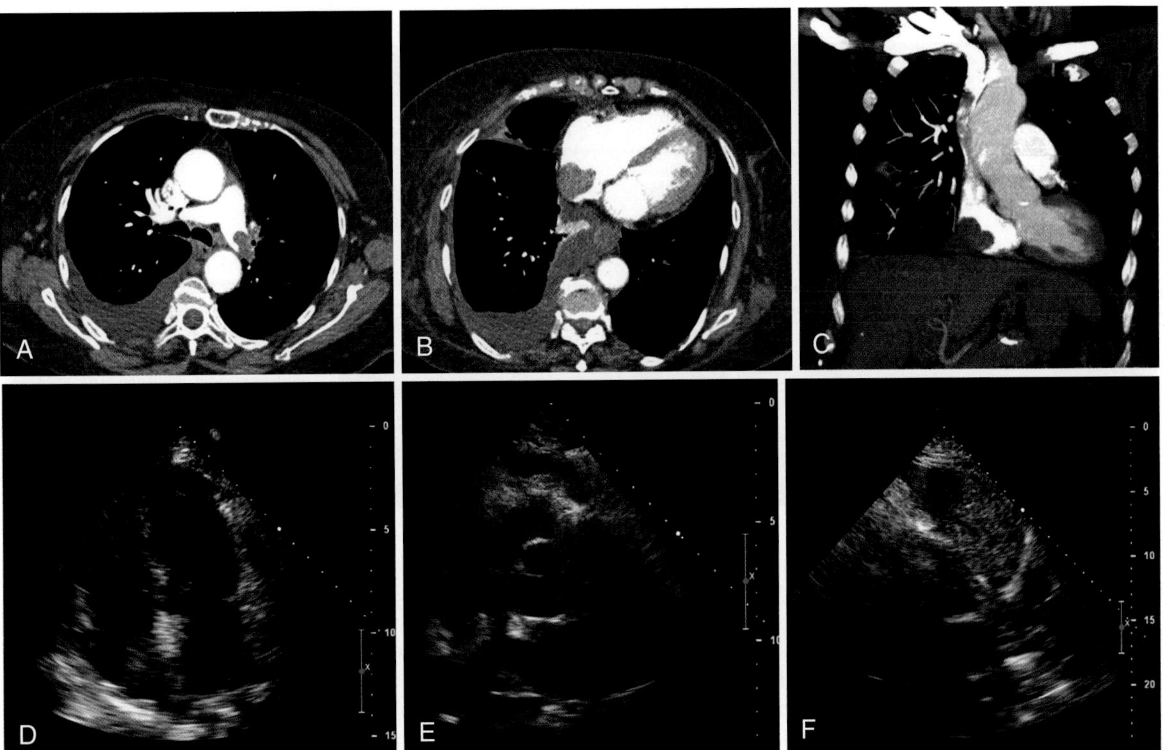

Figure 28-15. A 68-year-old woman presented with chest pain and dyspnea and elevated troponins. A chest CT detected embolism to the left main pulmonary artery, and also a large mass in the inferoposterolateral aspect of the right atrium. Transthoracic echocardiography (**D** and **F**) confirmed a soft tissue mass extending into the right atrium. The mid–inferior vena cava (IVC) was unremarkable. Soft tissue was seen extending via a hepatic vein into the very distal aspect of the IVC into the right atrium. She was determined to have hepatocellular carcinoma, with tumor embolism.

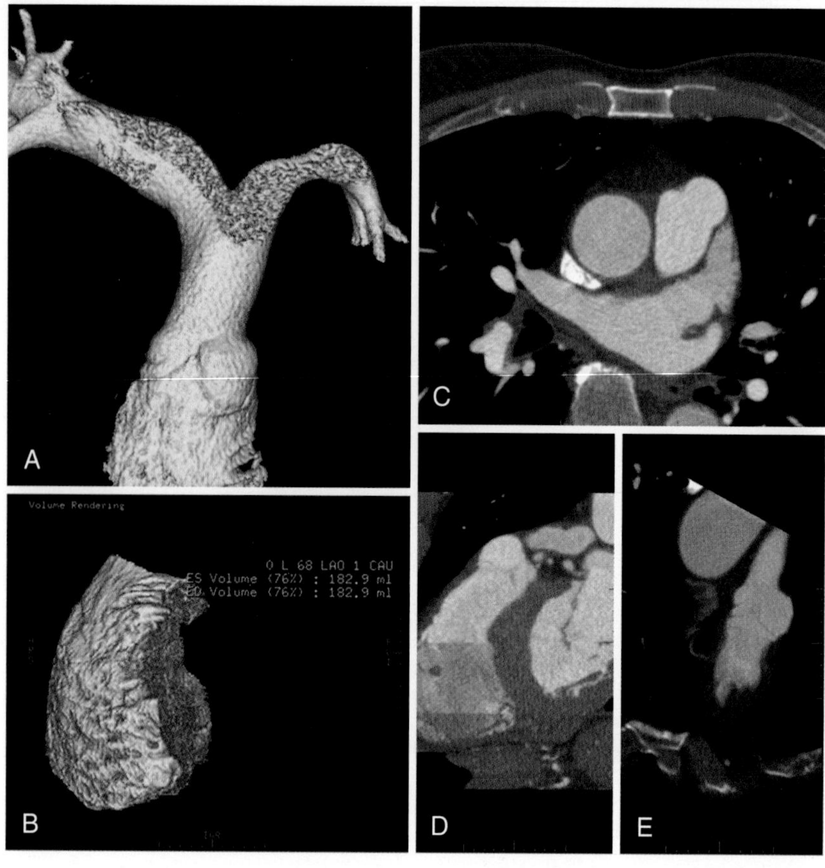

Figure 28-16. A 58-year-old man presented with shortness of breath and increased cardiac risk factors. A cardiac CT study was performed. No evidence of significant coronary artery disease was seen (images not shown). Mild prominence of the left pulmonic sinus of Valsalva is noted. The pulmonic valve leaflets on this prospectively acquired study appear to be normal (**D** and **E**). Right ventricular mid-diastolic volume (76% of the R-R interval) is mildly dilated at 107 mL/m^2. No evidence of an intracardiac shunt was seen. The diagnosis was a small pulmonary sinus of Valsalva dilatation/aneurysm, likely congenital. Mild right ventricular dilatation may be related to pulmonic insufficiency and should be correlated with echocardiography.

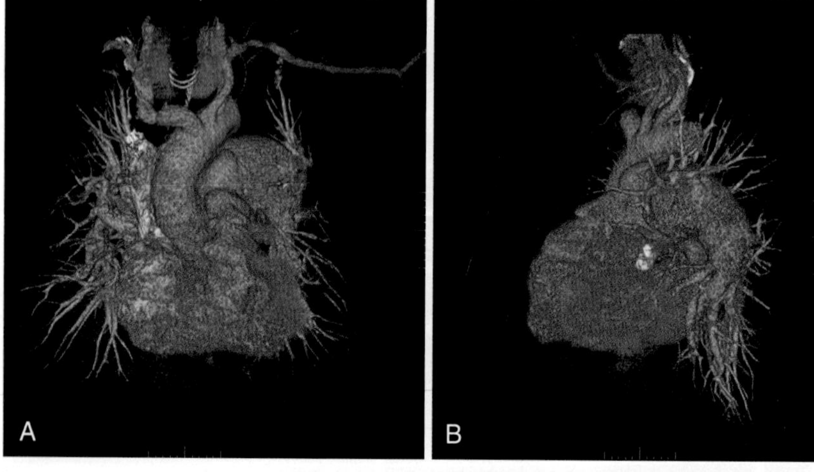

Figure 28-17. Volume-rendered CT angiography demonstrates a 5.2-cm aneurysm of the main pulmonary artery extending into the left pulmonary artery, with pruning of the peripheral pulmonary arteries in the left lung when compared with those of the right lung. The pulmonary artery systolic pressure was severely elevated: 95 mm Hg. There was no evidence of chronic thromboembolic disease or a previous surgical shunt, or pulmonic stenosis. **See Video 28-1.**

the proximal right or left central pulmonary artery. Peripheral branch stenoses may reflect an intrinsic abnormality within the pulmonary arteries, as in the setting of tetralogy of Fallot and Williams syndrome, but also have been reported as a consequence of previous systemic arterial–to–pulmonary arterial shunt surgery (e.g., Waterston or Potts shunts) or, increasingly, following the arterial switch operation for congenital transposition of the great arteries. Central and peripheral pulmonary arterial stenoses also have been described as a consequence of congenital rubella syndrome due to maternal rubella infection.[69] Stenosis may affect surgical repairs of the pulmonic valve, such as post–tetralogy of Fallot repair and post–Ross procedure (Figs. 28-19 and 28-20).

Acquired Lesions

Neoplastic processes can encase and narrow central pulmonary arteries. The most common of

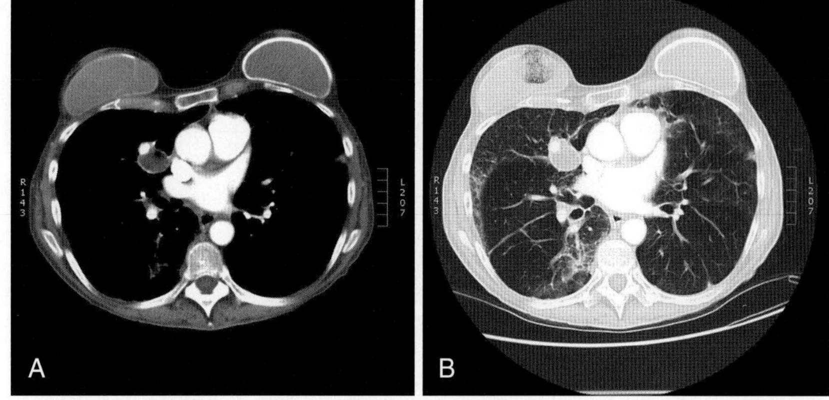

Figure 28-18. Contrast-enhanced CT scans of a patient with a mycotic aneurysm of the right pulmonary artery.

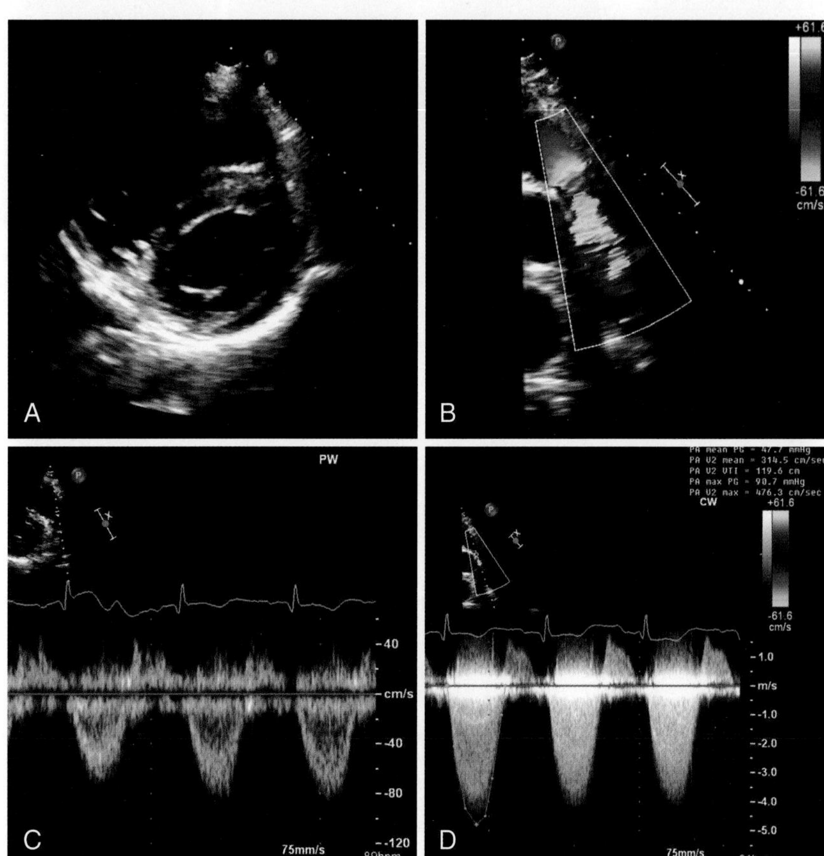

Figure 28-19. A 26-year-old man 4 years post–Ross repair presented with shortness of breath. Transthoracic echocardiography demonstrated right ventricular dilation, dysfunction, and hypertrophy (**A**), flow acceleration at the neo-pulmonic valve level (**B**), normal flow velocity beneath the neo-pulmonic valve (**C**), and severe flow acceleration across the neo-pulmonic valve and neo-ascending aorta, yielding a peak instantaneous gradient of 90 mm Hg (**D**).

these is bronchogenic carcinoma. In general, tumors that encase a central pulmonary artery, or extend around more than 180 degrees of the arterial circumference, are unlikely to be resectable. If the more distal parts of the central right and left pulmonary arteries are encased, complete resection may be possible with pneumonectomy.

Mediastinal fibrosis, an uncommon benign chronic inflammatory condition, also can cause stenosis or obstruction of the central pulmonary artery. This condition can have both focal and diffuse appearances. The focal morphology probably is the result of an intense inflammatory reaction to prior granulomatous infection, most commonly from histoplasmosis or tuberculosis.[70] The more diffuse type has the CT appearance of an infiltrative mass affecting multiple compartments of the mediastinum and often can occur in association with certain drugs, autoimmune disorders, or retroperitoneal fibrosis, or may be idiopathic.[71]

Stenosis or occlusion of segmental and subsegmental arteries, and, less commonly, lobar or central pulmonary arteries can be seen in the setting of Takayasu arteritis. Pulmonary arterial

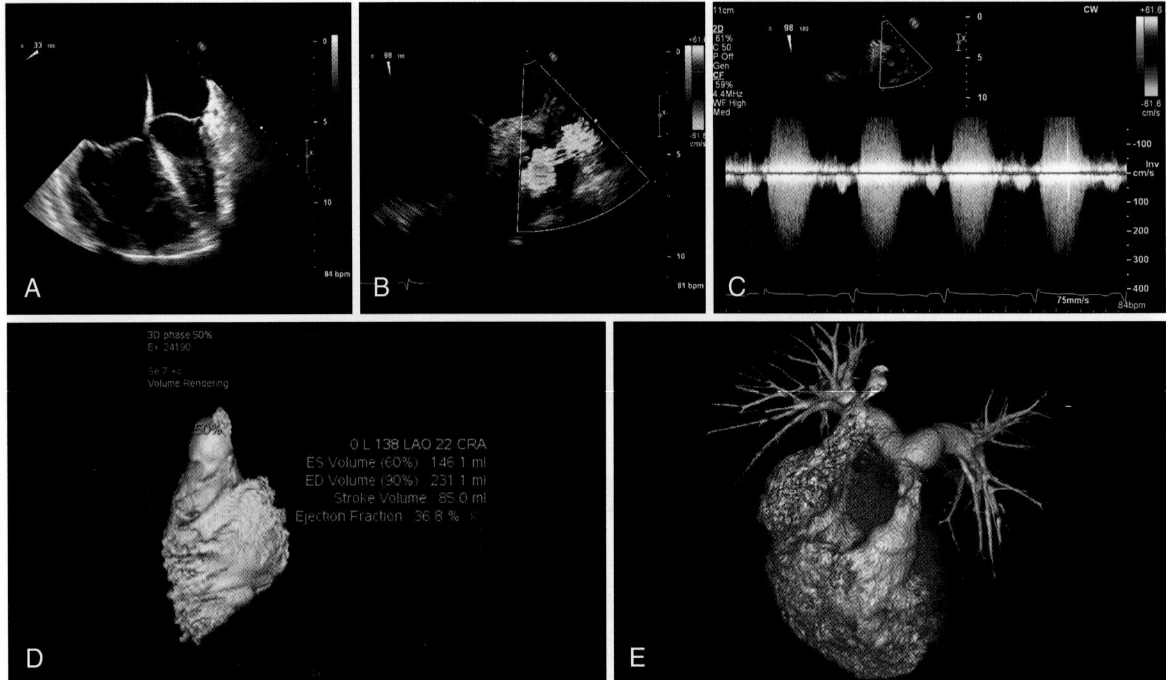

Figure 28-20. Same patient as Figure 28-19. **A,** Transesophageal echocardiography (TEE), lower esophageal view, depicts right ventricle (RV) dilation and systolic dysfunction. **B,** TEE right ventricular outflow tract (RVOT)/pulmonic valve outflow view with color Doppler. A large proximal isovelocity surface area is seen under the pulmonic valve, revealing a severe outflow gradient. **C,** TEE continuous wave Doppler spectral depiction of the flow across the outflow obstruction: at least a 40-mm Hg gradient is sampled. **D** and **E,** Contrast-enhanced, ECG-gated cardiac CT imaging. **D,** Volumetric reconstruction of the RV and its systolic dysfunction. **E,** Three-dimensional volume-rendered depiction of the RVOT and pulmonic valve, revealing a complex narrowing at the pulmonic valve level.

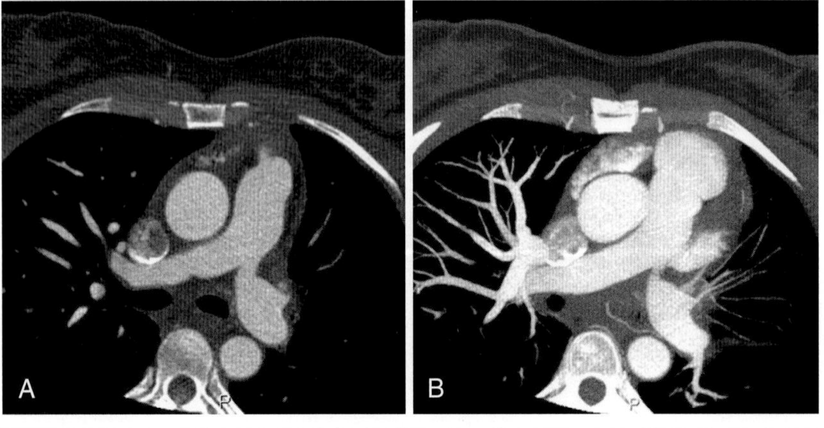

Figure 28-21. Axial cardiac CT image (**A**) and a maximum intensity projection image (**B**) at the same level demonstrate a moderate amount of soft tissue in the prevascular space extending around the left internal mammary artery. Note is also made of moderate proximal left pulmonary artery stenosis with post-stenotic dilatation. Mediastinoscopy and biopsy revealed mediastinal infiltration from a rare granular cell neoplasm.

involvement can occur in up to 80% of patients and is believed to represent a late finding in the disease process.[72]

PULMONARY ARTERY COMPRESSION

Compression of the main or central pulmonary arteries is facilitated by their thin walls and relatively low distending pressure. Common causes include

- Anterior mediastinal masses
- Middle mediastinal masses
- Aortic aneurysm
- Leaking aortic aneurysms
- Mediastinal hematoma

Pulmonary artery compression is illustrated in Figures 28-21 and 28-22.

PRIMARY SARCOMA

Primary sarcoma of the pulmonary artery is a rare lesion, but it is notable for masquerading clinically and by CT scanning as PE, and leading therefore to

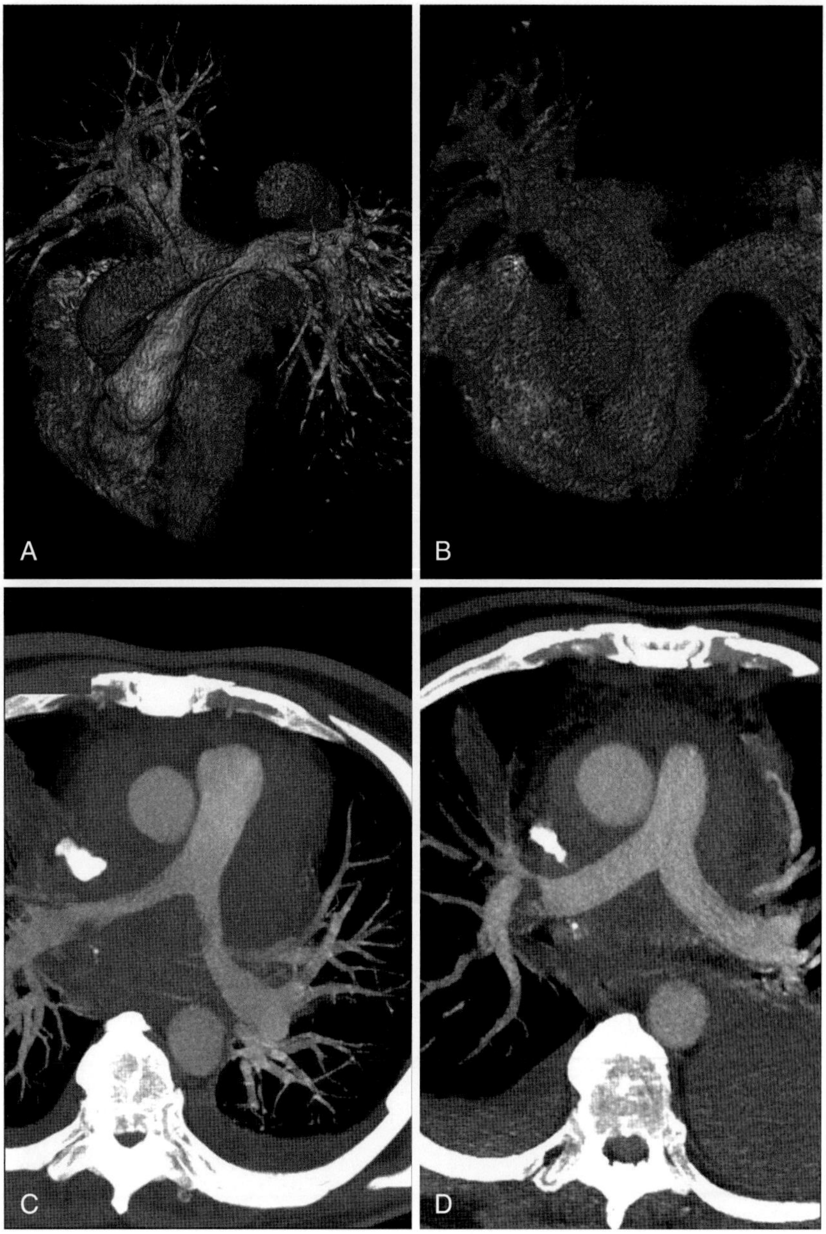

Figure 28-22. Multiple gated CT images in a 58-year-old man with metastatic small cell lung cancer. **B** and **D** were obtained 6 weeks after **A** and **C**. **A** and **C** demonstrate extensive mediastinal soft tissue mass consistent with tumor infiltration. This markedly narrows the right and left central pulmonary arteries, and causes narrowing and irregularity of the superior vena cava. This is well appreciated on both the volume-rendered image (**A**), and a short-thickness maximum intensity projection image (**C**). Six weeks later, after chemotherapy and radiation therapy, there has been significant interval reduction in the amount of mediastinal metastatic disease, although the pleural effusions bilaterally have worsened.

misdiagnosis and belated diagnosis. Most cases are unnecessarily exposed to delay in treatment and to risks of prolonged anticoagulation or thrombolysis. In a review of 110 cases of primary pulmonary sarcoma, the following symptoms were described[73]:

- Dyspnea: 67%
- Chest pain: 54%
- Cough: 43%
- Hemoptysis: 22%

Syncope also has been reported.[74]

Progression of size of a lesion within a pulmonary artery while the patient is on anticoagulation often prompts consideration of the diagnosis of pulmonary artery sarcoma. Unfortunately, the correct diagnosis rarely is made preoperatively. Surgical treatment is the standard and includes "shelling out" the tumor, thromboembolectomy, pneumonectomy, and extended resection with extensive reconstruction. Recurrences have been described. Some cases are too extensive by the time of diagnosis for surgical treatment. Median survival without surgery is 1.5 months, and with surgery is 10 months. Two thirds of cases have distant metastases by the time of diagnosis.[75-77]

Features more consistent with malignancy than with thromboembolic disease include[78]:

- Occupation of the entire luminal diameter of the main or proximal pulmonary artery
- Extraluminal expansion of the defect beyond the artery
- Expansion of the artery with the defect

See Figures 28-23 through 28-25.

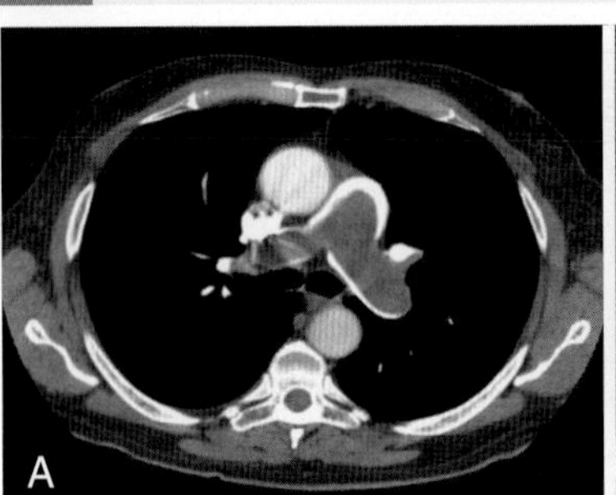

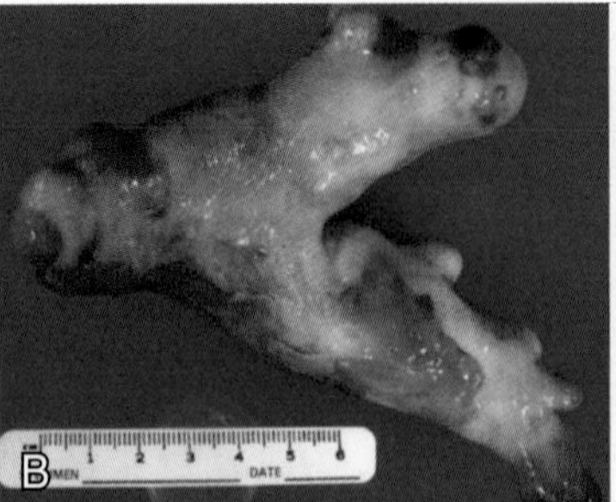

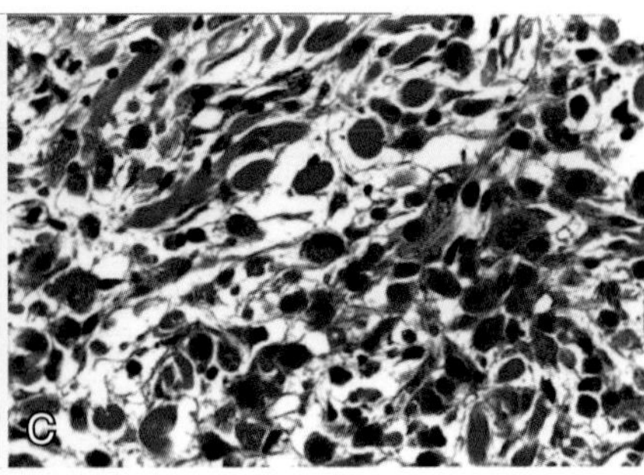

Figure 28-23. Intimal sarcomas of the pulmonary artery are rare tumors that often are difficult to distinguish from pulmonary thromboembolic disease, complicating accurate diagnosis and timely therapy. We report the case of a man with a primary pulmonary artery sarcoma who presented with a massive pulmonary embolism and complete right ventricular outflow tract obstruction. The patient's condition was successfully managed with urgent pulmonary artery thromboendarterectomy, pulmonary valve replacement, and tricuspid valve annuloplasty. **A,** The large saddle pulmonary thrombus extended into both right and left main pulmonary arteries and their segmental branches. **B,** The gross pathologic specimen, including the mass in the main pulmonary trunk and the bifurcation, as well as the distal branching into the segmental pulmonary arteries. **C,** Hematoxylin & eosin–stained sections of the tumor demonstrated a spindle cell neoplasm with moderate nuclear atypia and a patchy myxoid background. (Reprinted with permission from Alsoufi B, Slater M, Smith PP, Karamlou T, Mansoor A, Ravichandran P. Pulmonary artery sarcoma mimicking massive pulmonary embolus: a case report. *Asian Cardiovasc Thorac Ann.* 2006;14:e71-73.)

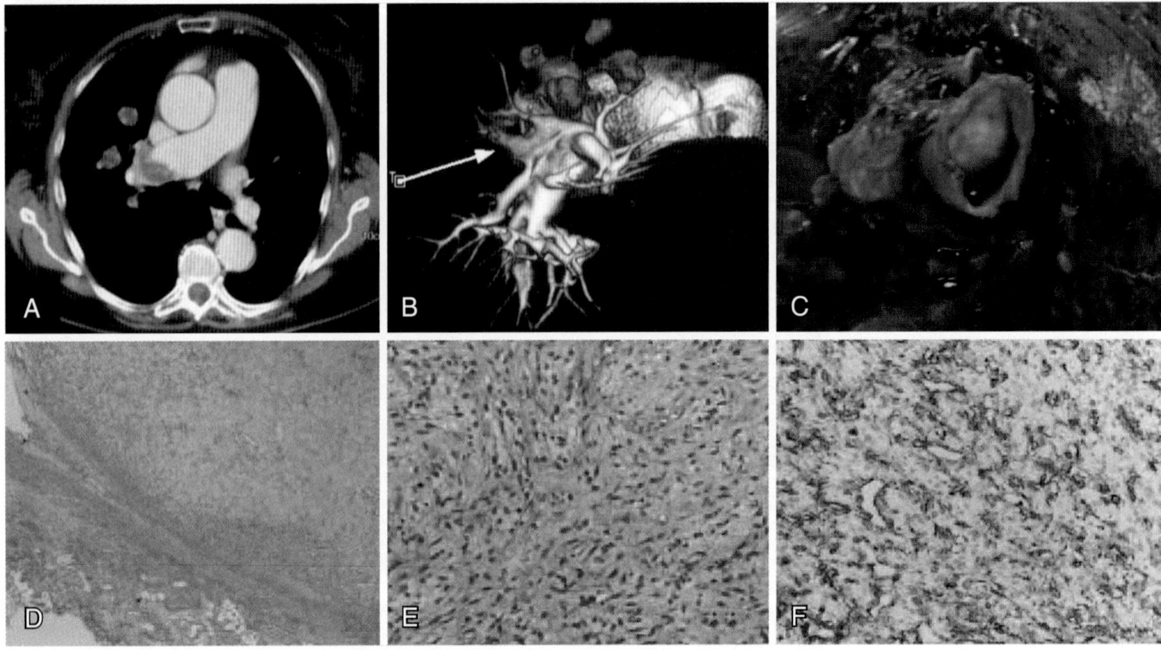

Figure 28-24. **A,** Contrast-enhanced CT study reveals a mass in the right pulmonary artery with an intraluminal filling defect and three nodular masses appearing as opacities in the right pulmonary parenchyma. **B,** Multislice CT angiography with three-dimensional reconstruction. **C,** Macroscopic specimen: the tumor appears as a yellowish endoluminal mass completely filling the arterial lumen. **D,** Pulmonary artery leiomyosarcoma: intraluminal protrusion of the tumor (hematoxylin & eosin stain, original magnification ×4). **E,** The neoplasm is characterized by pleomorphic spindle cells with a storiform growth pattern (hematoxylin & eosin stain, original magnification ×20). **F,** Leiomyosarcoma of the pulmonary artery with cells positive for smooth muscle actin (original magnification ×20). (Reprinted with permission from Stella F, Davoli F, Brandolini J, Dolci G, Sellitri F, Bini A. Pulmonary artery leiomyosarcoma successfully treated by right pneumonectomy. *Asian Cardiovasc Thorac Ann.* 2009;175:513-515.)

PULMONARY ARTERY ANGIOINVASION

Whereas tumor invasion of the central pulmonary arteries can be seen in the setting of bronchogenic carcinoma (stage IV) or mediastinal metastatic disease, infiltration of the arterial wall remains a diagnostic challenge. CT angiography can be misleading in cases of extrinsic compression and may not reliably demonstrate vascular involvement except in advanced cases when there is intraluminal extension of tumor or marked circumferential stenosis of central pulmonary arteries.

PULMONARY ARTERY SLING

Pulmonary artery sling is a rare congenital defect in which the left pulmonary artery originates anomalously from the right pulmonary artery. As the left pulmonary artery courses back toward

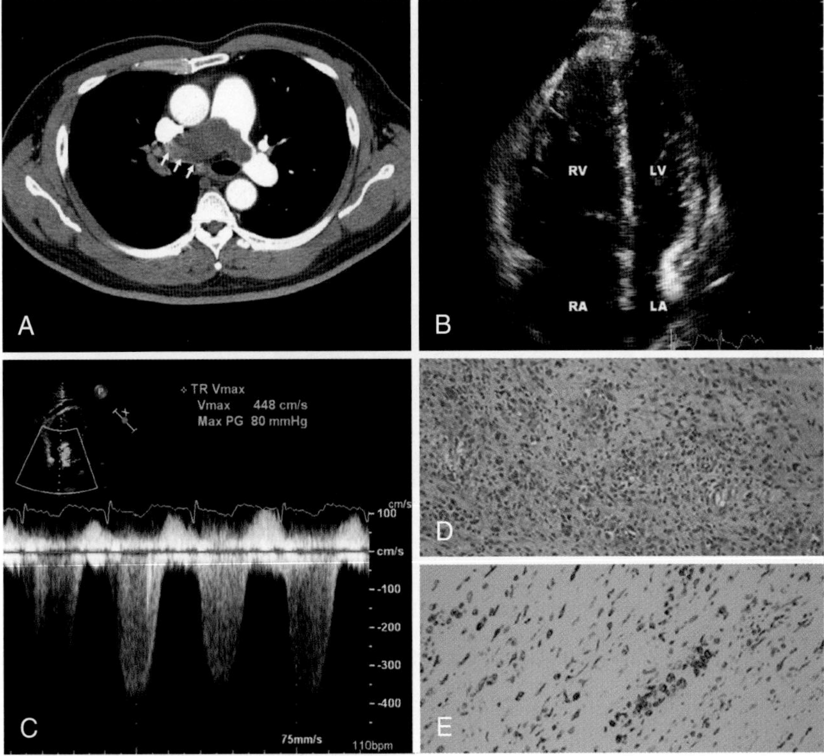

Figure 28-25. A 47-year-old previously healthy man presented with progressive dyspnea, hemoptysis, and near syncope. He had findings of cor pulmonale. **A,** Spiral chest CT scan shows massive filling defects bilaterally and almost total obliteration of right pulmonary artery flow (*arrows*). **B,** Two-dimensional transthoracic echocardiographic four-chamber view demonstrates dilation of the right atrium and right ventricle. **C,** Severe elevation of the right ventricular systolic pressure is shown from the marked elevation of the TR velocity. **D** and **E,** Histologic examination (hematoxylin & eosin stain) reveals pleomorphic tumor cells in the myxoid background (**D**) and positivity for the HHF-35 (muscle actin–specific monoclonal antibody) imunohistochemical stain (**E**). LA, left atrium; LV, left ventricle; RA,right atrium; RV, right ventricle. (Reprinted with permission from Huang SS, Huang CH, Yang AH, Yu WC. Images in cardiovascular medicine. Solitary pulmonary artery intima sarcoma manifesting as pulmonary embolism and subacute cor pulmonale. *Circulation.* 2009;12022:2269-2270.)

the left lung, it encircles the distal trachea and right mainstem bronchus, and is interposed between the trachea and esophagus. Patients with pulmonary arterial slings commonly have respiratory symptoms. These may be due to extrinsic compression of the trachea by the anomalous course of the total pulmonary artery, or due to the presence of severe tracheal stenosis associated with complete cartilaginous rings within the distal trachea. The pulmonary artery sling may be an isolated entity, but it also may be seen in association with other congenital heart abnormalities (Figs. 28-26 and 28-27).

CALCIFICATION OF THE PULMONARY ARTERY

Calcification of the pulmonary arteries is rare, but may be seen in association with syndromes of chronic systemic level pulmonary artery hypertension such as Eisenmenger syndrome, or following chest radiotherapy (Fig. 28-28).

TRAUMATIC DISRUPTION OF THE PULMONARY ARTERY

Blunt force deceleration/acceleration injury to the chest may disrupt the pulmonary artery, just as it may disrupt the aorta. Characteristics of this lesion, as with traumatic disruption of the aorta, are shorter linear intimal tears and false aneurysms (Fig. 28-29).

PULMONARY ARTERY DISSECTION AND AORTICOPULMONARY DISSECTION

Isolated pulmonary artery dissection is rare, and usually is seen in cases of longstanding severe/systemic pulmonary hypertension, such as Eisenmenger syndrome.

Aorticopulmonary dissection, which also is rare, results when the ascending aorta ruptures into the main pulmonary artery, causing dissection of the pulmonary artery[79] (Figs. 28-30 through 28-32).

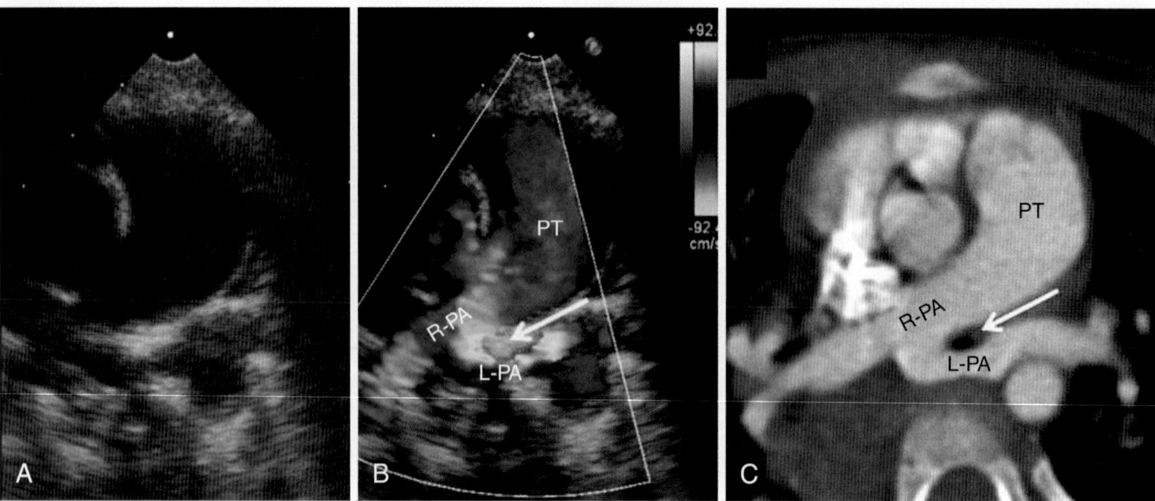

Figure 28-26. A 22-month-old child with a history of "airway noises" and congestion due to a pulmonary artery sling. Transthoracic echocardiogram (TTE) through the pulmonic trunk (PT) and main pulmonary arteries without (**A**) and with (**B**) color Doppler demonstrates no normal bifurcation of the pulmonic trunk; rather, the left main pulmonary artery (L-PA) arises directly from the distal right pulmonary artery (R-PA). **C,** On an axial image from the cardiac-gated CTA in the same patient, note how the L-PA wraps around the posterior aspect of the distal airway (in this case, referred to as the *left intermediate bronchus*) which is severely narrowed (*white arrow*). (Reprinted with permission from Entrikin DW, Otaki Y, Ungerleider R, Carr JJ. Pulmonary artery sling as demonstrated by transthoracic echocardiography and low-dose cardiac gated computed tomographic angiography in a 22 month old. Society of Cardiovascular Computed Tomography Case of the Month, July 2011. Available at http://archive.constantcontact.com/fs027/1101901294184/archive/1106802883318.html)

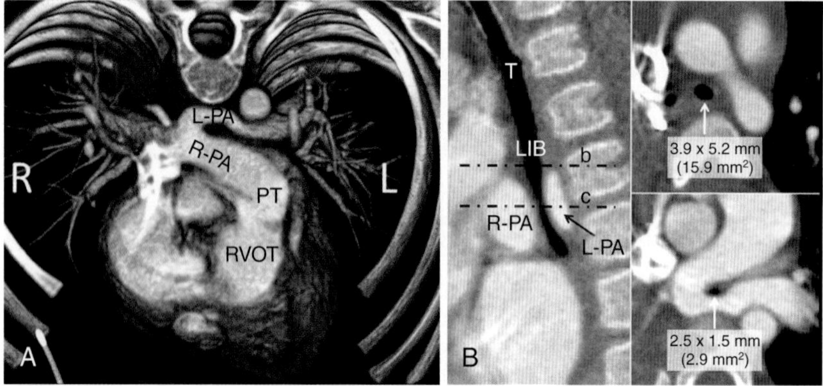

Figure 28-27. Additional images from the 22-month-old child described in Figure 28-26. **A,** Three-dimensional volumetric reconstruction from the cardiac-gated CT angiographic examination demonstrates the abnormal origin of the left main pulmonary artery (L-PA) from the distal right pulmonary artery (R-PA), rather than a typical bifurcation of the pulmonic trunk (PT). **B,** Oblique sagittal multiplanar reformat (*left image*) through the trachea (T) and left intermediate bronchus (LIB). Note how the LIB is encircled by the pulmonary artery sling with the proximal R-PA anteriorly and the L-PA posteriorly. Two dashed lines traversing the LIB correspond to the axial images at levels immediately above (*top right image*) and at (*left image*) the pulmonary artery sling demonstrating the short segment of >75% cross-sectional narrowing of the LIB. (Reprinted with permission from Entrikin DW, Otaki Y, Ungerleider R, Carr JJ. Pulmonary artery sling as demonstrated by transthoracic echocardiography and low-dose cardiac gated computed tomographic angiography in a 22 month old. Society of Cardiovascular Computed Tomography Case of the Month, July 2011. Available at http://archive.constantcontact.com/fs027/1101901294184/archive/1106802883318.html)

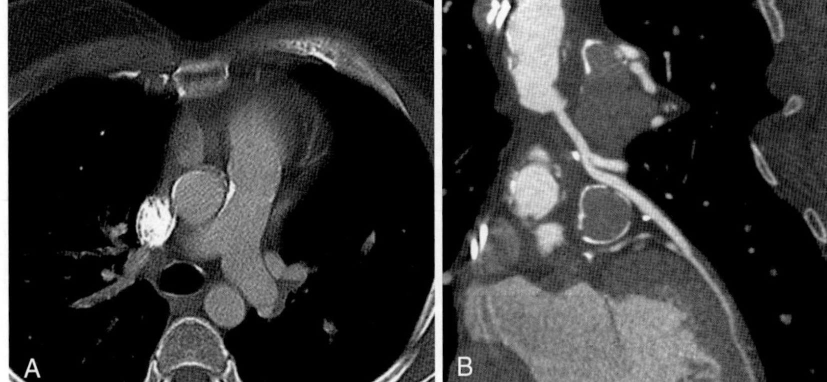

Figure 28-28. Calcification of the main pulmonary artery (and aortic) walls due to chronic radiation damage from prior radiotherapy for lymphoma treatment. The left-sided cardiac valves also were calcified and dysfunctional

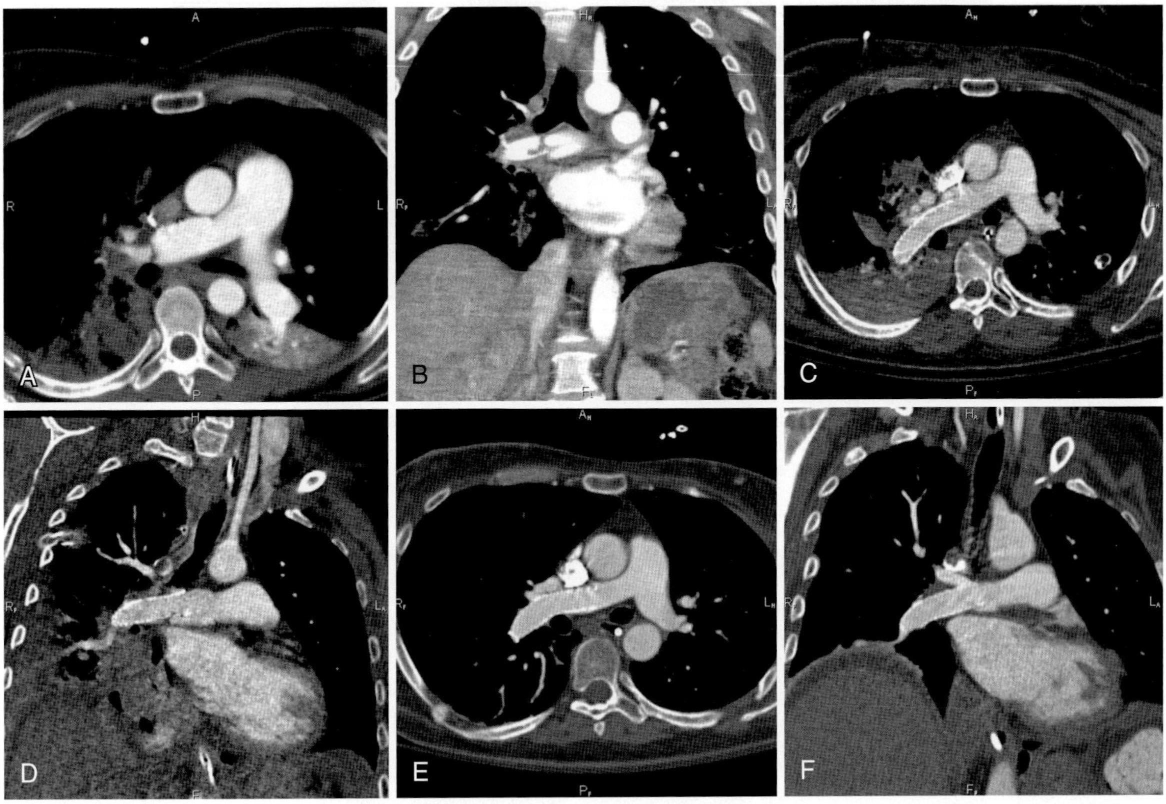

Figure 28-29. **A** and **B,** Initial CT scan at presentation demonstrates transection of the right pulmonary artery with a linear filling defect. There is concomitant airspace disease of the right lower lobe. **C** and **D,** Follow-up study 2 days later after placement of a stent demonstrates patency of the stent. **E** and **F,** The 1-month follow-up examination confirms patency of the stent with remodeling of the right pulmonary artery and interval clearing of the right lower lobe consolidation. **E,** Note the healing rib fracture. **F,** Note the small amount of ascites.

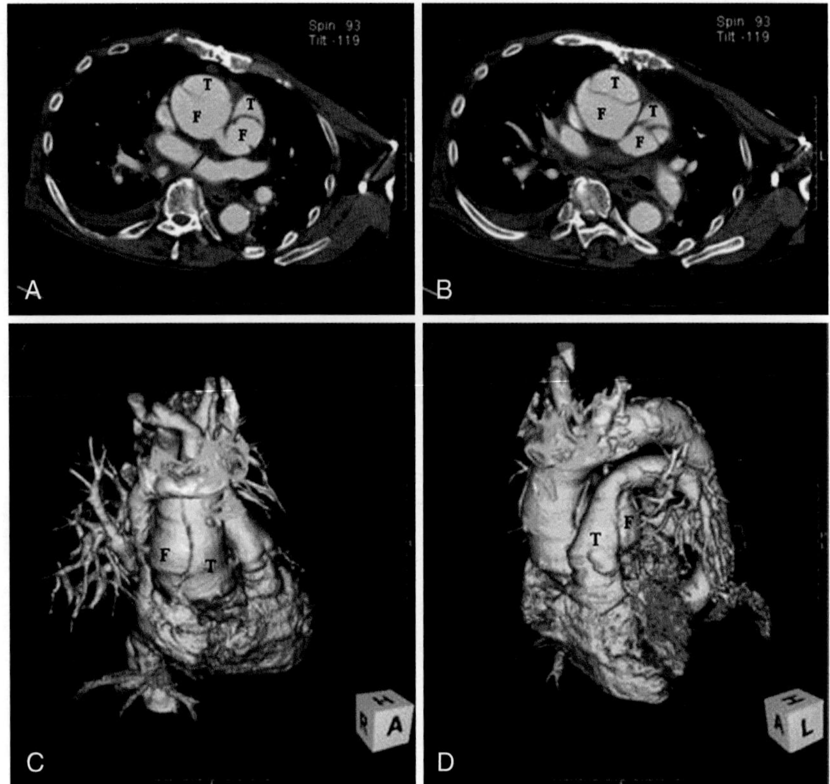

Figure 28-30. A 71-year-old man was brought to the hospital by ambulance and admitted because of intermittent back pain. Physical examination revealed continuous heart murmur. The chest radiograph showed cardiomegaly and pulmonary congestion. The patient received continuous hydration for renal dysfunction and severe metabolic acidosis (base excess of –16.5 mmol/L and pH of 7.24) and underwent enhanced chest CT. The chest CT showed not only ascending aortic dissection of Stanford type A but also pulmonary artery dissection with an aortopulmonary window (*red arrow*). An aortopulmonary shunt could not only increase pulmonary circulation and cause untreatable congestive pulmonary edema but also cause severe metabolic acidosis. Aortopulmonary artery dissection is very rare but is fatal, requiring surgical repair as rapidly as possible. F, false lumen; T, true lumen. (Reprinted with permission from Itoh H, Yamamoto T, Sugihara H, et al. Aortopulmonary artery dissection. *J Am Coll Cardiol.* 2009;5421:1990.)

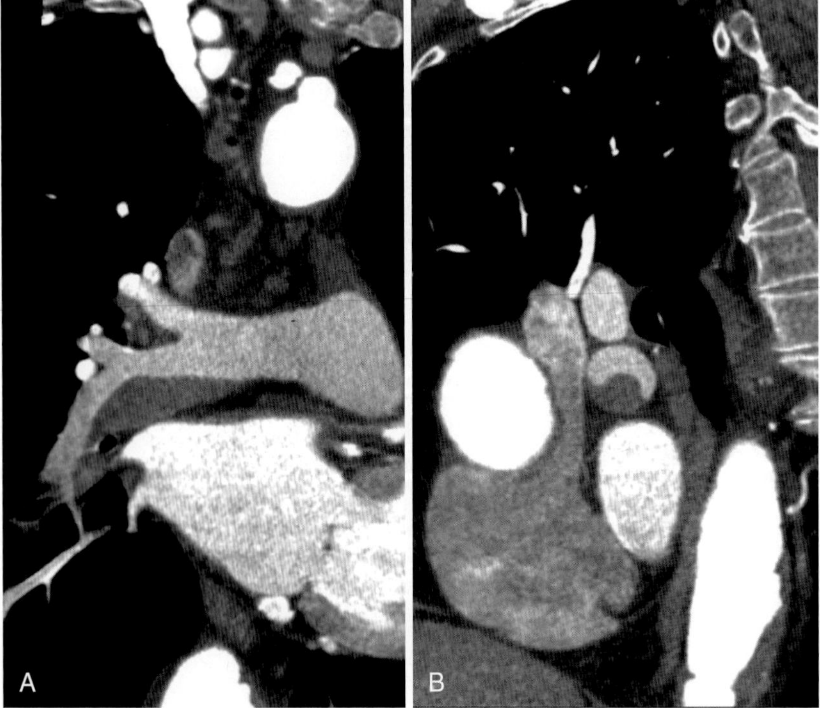

Figure 28-31. Presumed chronic pulmonary artery dissection. Note the linearity of the contour. The lesion was present on CT scans several years apart, with no evidence of pulmonary arterial filling defects within the pulmonary arterial tree seen on any of the CT scans.

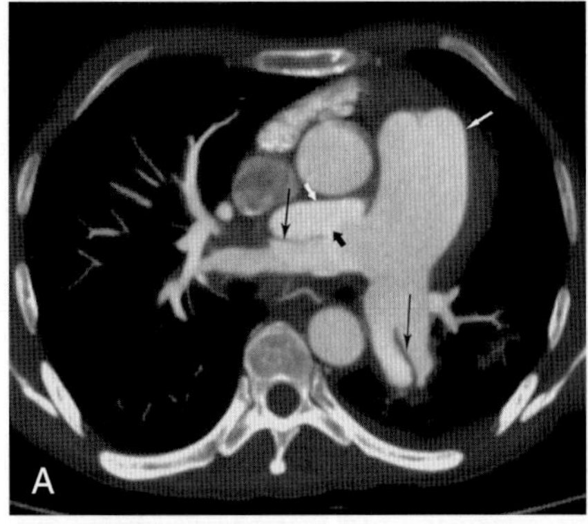

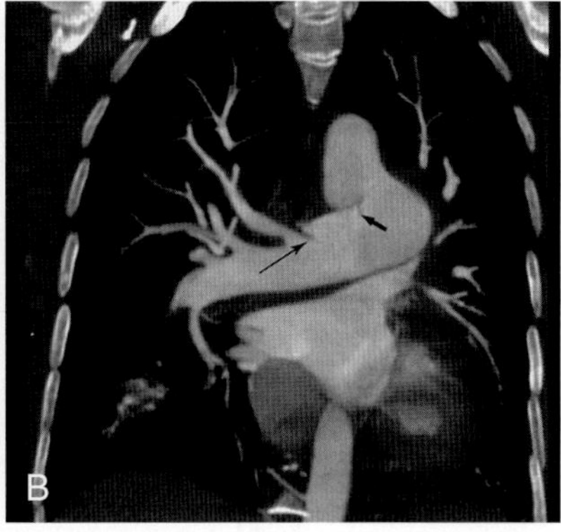

Figure 28-32. **A,** Axial image of a CT pulmonary angiogram shows a markedly dilated main pulmonary artery (*long white arrow*) with a diameter of 42 mm and bilateral pulmonary artery dissections. Note the intimal flaps (*long black arrows*), lower in attenuation than the contrast-opacified blood, originating at the proximal ends of the right and left pulmonary arteries, respectively. Note the false lumens (*short white arrow*) and tear (*short black arrow*). **B,** Multiplanar reformatted coronal image of the right pulmonary artery displays the precise extent of the dissection (*arrows*). The dissection flap does not involve the upper and lower lobe arteries (*long arrow*). (Reprinted with permission from Peng LQ, Yu JQ, Chu ZG, Yuan HM. A rare case of right and left pulmonary artery dissections on 64-slice multidetector computed tomography. *J Thorac Imaging.* 2010;254:W136-137.)

PULMONARY ARTERIOVENOUS MALFORMATIONS

Pulmonary arteriovenous malformation (AVM) is a condition in which there is an abnormal direct communication between a pulmonary artery and pulmonary vein. The most common cause of pulmonary AVM is congenital, and this is believed to result from a defect in the development of terminal capillary loops. Although pulmonary AVMs can occur in any segment of the lungs, there is a predilection for the lower lobe. Pulmonary AVMs have been described in association with a number of conditions, including hereditary hemorrhagic telangiectasia, hepatic cirrhosis, trauma, and previous cardiac surgery for congenital heart disease such as Glenn and Fontan procedures (Fig. 28-33).

PULMONARY ARTERY RUPTURE

Pulmonary arterial rupture is a rare, life-threatening condition. Causes include rupture of a pulmonary arterial aneurysm, development of a pulmonary arterial dissection, and traumatic transection of the pulmonary artery. Traumatic causes include a high-velocity deceleration injury as can be seen in a motor vehicle accident, but also may be iatrogenic, secondary to pulmonary arterial catheter misplacement or attempted interventional angioplasty of a pulmonary arterial stenosis.

ALTERNATIVE DIAGNOSES FROM CT PULMONARY EMBOLISM STUDIES

Not uncommonly, an alternative (and incorrect) diagnosis for the patient's symptoms (usually chest pain or dyspnea) is identified on a CT PE protocol type study. For example, this is manifested as subtle areas of ground-glass density with early "tree-in-bud" formation—the typical appearance of an early pneumonia, beneath the resolution of chest radiography. Uncommonly, but not rarely, a more sinister diagnosis is made, such as aortic dissection or intramural hematoma.

CT PROTOCOL POINTS

- ❒ Coverage: Above lung apices to below lung bases
- ❒ Contrast: 70 mL at 5 mL/sec
- ❒ Automated trigger set:
  - Location: MPA/RPA
  - HU: 100
- ❒ See Table 28-6.

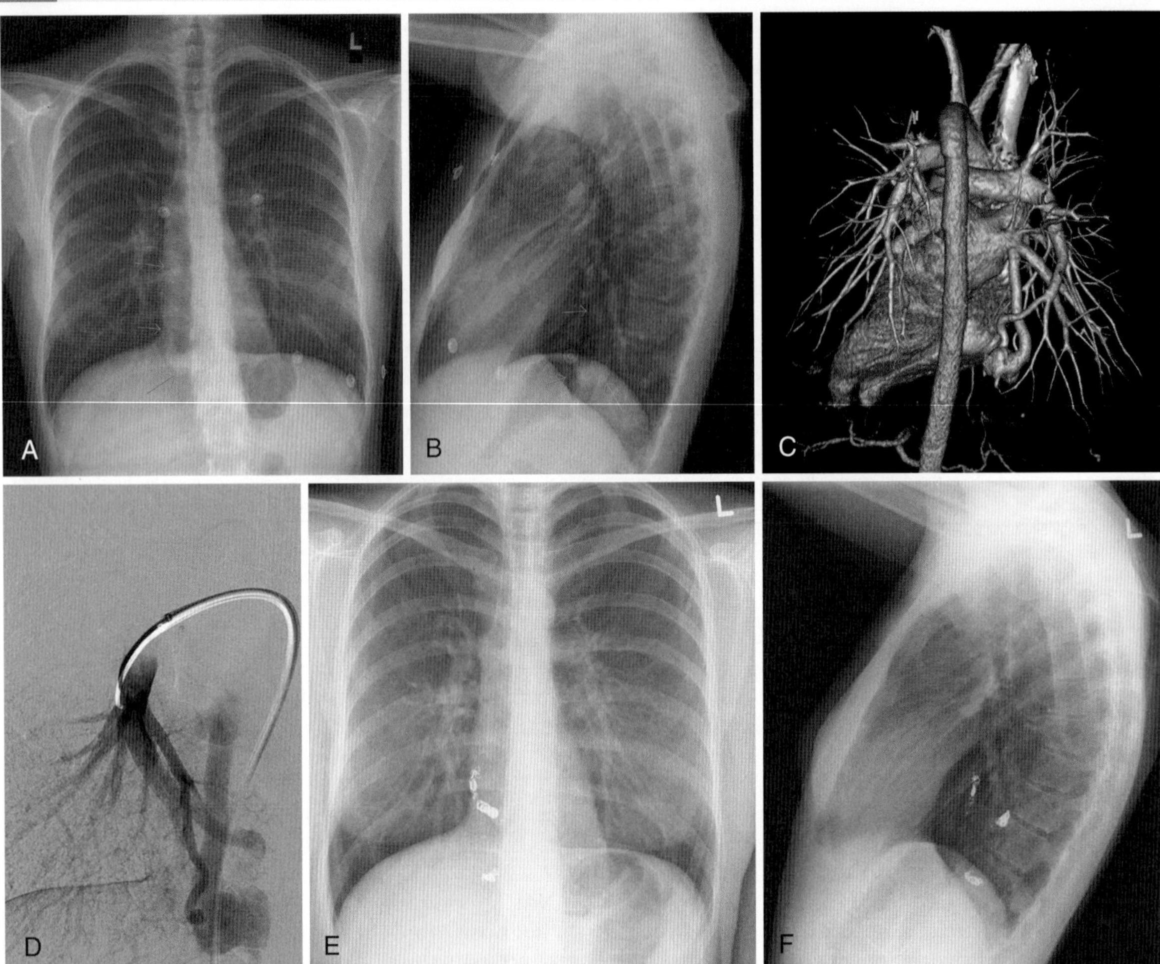

Figure 28-33. A composite image in a 28-year-old man with chest pain. At the initial presentation a chest radiograph was obtained. The posteroanterior (**A**) and lateral (**B**) studies demonstrate a retrocardiac nodular opacity with a vascular structure extending toward it. The lateral study suggests impaired vascular structures extending down to this retrocardiac nodule. **C,** A CT angiogram from a posterior view demonstrates an arterial supply to a left lower lobe nodule with a large draining vein into the left atrium. This appearance is very suggestive of a moderate-sized pulmonary arterial venous malformation (AVM). This was confirmed on the conventional angiogram (**D**), and coiling of the AVM was performed. **E** and **F,** Multiple coils within the AVM, and its vascular supply and egress.

TABLE 28-6 ACCF 2006 Appropriateness Criteria for the Use of Cardiac Computed CT for the Evaluation of Pulmonary Disease*

APPROPRIATENESS CRITERIA	INDICATION	MEDIAN SCORE
Appropriate	Evaluation of suspected pulmonary embolism	9
Uncertain	None	
Inappropriate	None	

*There is no specific entry in the ACCF 2010 Appropriateness Guidelines for cardiac CT.

Data from Hendel RC, Manesh PR, Kramer CM, Poon M. ACCF/ACR/SCCT/SCMR/ASNC/NASCI/SCAI/SIR appropriateness criteria for cardiac computed tomography and cardiac magnetic resonance imaging. *J Am Coll Cardiol.* 2006;48(7):1475-1497.

References

1. Dalen JE, Alpert JS. Natural history of pulmonary embolism. *Prog Cardiovasc Dis.* 1975;17(4):259-270.
2. Goldhaber SZ, Visani L, De RM. Acute pulmonary embolism: clinical outcomes in the International Cooperative Pulmonary Embolism Registry (ICOPER). *Lancet.* 1999;353(9162):1386-1389.
3. Barker NW. The diagnosis and treatment of pulmonary embolism. *Med Clin North Am.* 1958;42(4):1053-1063.
4. Barritt DW, Jordan SC. Anticoagulant drugs in the treatment of pulmonary embolism. A controlled trial. *Lancet.* 1960;1:1309-1312.
5. Genton E, Hirsh J. Observations in anticoagulant and thrombolytic therapy in pulmonary embolism. *Prog Cardiovasc Dis.* 1975;17(5):335-343.
6. Pollack EW, Sparks FC, Barker WF. Pulmonary embolism: an appraisal of therapy in 516 cases. *Arch Surg.* 1973;107(3):492.
7. Alpert JS, Smith R, Carlson J, Ockene IS, Dexter L, Dalen JE. Mortality in patients treated for pulmonary embolism. *JAMA.* 1976;236(13):1477-1480.
8. Carson JL, Kelley MA, Duff A, et al. The clinical course of pulmonary embolism. *N Engl J Med.* 1992;326(19):1240-1245.
9. DeMonaco NA, Dang Q, Kapoor WN, Ragni MV. Pulmonary embolism incidence is increasing with use of spiral computed tomography. *Am J Med.* 2008;121(7):611-617.
10. Laporte S, Mismetti P, Decousus H, et al. Clinical predictors for fatal pulmonary embolism in 15,520 patients with venous thromboembolism: findings from the Registro Informatizado de la Enfermedad TromboEmbolica venosa (RIETE) Registry. *Circulation.* 2008; 117(13):1711-1716.
11. Schoepf UJ, Goldhaber SZ, Costello P. Spiral computed tomography for acute pulmonary embolism. *Circulation.* 2004;109(18): 2160-2167.
12. Zierler BK. Ultrasonography and diagnosis of venous thromboembolism. *Circulation.* 2004;109(12 suppl 1):I9-I14.
13. Bernardi E, Camporese G, Buller HR, et al. Serial 2-point ultrasonography plus D-dimer vs whole-leg color-coded Doppler ultrasonography for diagnosing suspected symptomatic deep vein thrombosis: a randomized controlled trial. *JAMA.* 2008;300(14):1653-1659.
14. Guidelines on diagnosis and management of acute pulmonary embolism. Task Force on Pulmonary Embolism, European Society of Cardiology. *Eur Heart J.* 2000;21(16):1301-1336.
15. Le Gal G, Righini M, Roy PM, et al. Value of D-dimer testing for the exclusion of pulmonary embolism in patients with previous venous thromboembolism. *Arch Intern Med.* 2006;166(2):176-180.
16. Diffin DC, Leyendecker JR, Johnson SP, Zucker RJ, Grebe PJ. Effect of anatomic distribution of pulmonary emboli on interobserver agreement in the interpretation of pulmonary angiography. *AJR Am J Roentgenol.* 1998;171(4):1085-1089.
17. Stein PD, Henry JW, Gottschalk A. Reassessment of pulmonary angiography for the diagnosis of pulmonary embolism: relation of interpreter agreement to the order of the involved pulmonary arterial branch. *Radiology.* 1999;210(3):689-691.
18. Novelline RA, Baltarowich OH, Athanasoulis CA, Waltman AC, Greenfield AJ, McKusick KA. The clinical course of patients with suspected pulmonary embolism and a negative pulmonary arteriogram. *Radiology.* 1978;126(3):561-567.
19. Gupta A, Frazer CK, Ferguson JM, et al. Acute pulmonary embolism: diagnosis with MR angiography. *Radiology.* 1999;210(2):353-359.
20. Oudkerk M, van Beek EJ, Wielopolski P, et al. Comparison of contrast-enhanced magnetic resonance angiography and conventional pulmonary angiography for the diagnosis of pulmonary embolism: a prospective study. *Lancet.* 2002;359(9318):1643-1647.
21. Kanne JP, Lalani TA. Role of computed tomography and magnetic resonance imaging for deep venous thrombosis and pulmonary embolism. *Circulation.* 2004;109(12 Suppl 1):I15-I21.
22. Schibany N, Fleischmann D, Thallinger C, et al. Equipment availability and diagnostic strategies for suspected pulmonary embolism in Austria. *Eur Radiol.* 2001;11(11):2287-2294.
23. Leveau P. [Diagnostic strategy in pulmonary embolism. National French survey]. *Presse Med.* 2002;31(20):929-932.
24. Value of the ventilation/perfusion scan in acute pulmonary embolism. Results of the Prospective Investigation of Pulmonary Embolism Diagnosis (PIOPED). The PIOPED Investigators. *JAMA.* 1990;263(20):2753-2759.
25. Gurney JW. No fooling around: direct visualization of pulmonary embolism. *Radiology.* 1993;188(3):618-619.
26. Woodard PK. Pulmonary arteries must be seen before they can be assessed. *Radiology.* 1997;204(1):11-12.
27. Hull RD, Raskob GE, Ginsberg JS, et al. A noninvasive strategy for the treatment of patients with suspected pulmonary embolism. *Arch Intern Med.* 1994;154(3):289-297.
28. van Rossum AB, Pattynama PM, Mallens WM, Hermans J, Heijerman HG. Can helical CT replace scintigraphy in the diagnostic process in suspected pulmonary embolism? A retrolective-prolective cohort study focusing on total diagnostic yield. *Eur Radiology.* 1998;8(1):90-96.
29. Garg K, Welsh CH, Feyerabend AJ, et al. Pulmonary embolism: diagnosis with spiral CT and ventilation-perfusion scanning–correlation with pulmonary angiographic results or clinical outcome. *Radiology.* 1998;208(1):201-208.
30. Blachere H, Latrabe V, Montaudon M, et al. Pulmonary embolism revealed on helical CT angiography: comparison with ventilation-perfusion radionuclide lung scanning. *AJR Am J Roentgenol.* 2000;174(4):1041-1047.
31. van Rossum AB, van Erkel AR, van Persijn van Meerten EL, Ton ER, Rebergen SA, Pattynama PM. Accuracy of helical CT for acute pulmonary embolism: ROC analysis of observer performance related to clinical experience. *Eur Radiol.* 1998;8(7):1160-1164.
32. Remy-Jardin M, Remy J, Artaud D, Deschildre F, Duhamel A. Peripheral pulmonary arteries: optimization of the spiral CT acquisition protocol. *Radiology.* 1997;204(1):157-163.
33. Goodman LR, Curtin JJ, Mewissen MW, et al. Detection of pulmonary embolism in patients with unresolved clinical and scintigraphic diagnosis: helical CT versus angiography. *Am J Roentgenol.* 1995;164(6):1369-1374.
34. Qanadli SD, Hajjam ME, Mesurolle B, et al. Pulmonary embolism detection: prospective evaluation of dual-section helical CT versus selective pulmonary arteriography in 157 patients. *Radiology.* 2000;217(2):447-455.
35. Schoepf UJ, Helmberger T, Holzknecht N, et al. Segmental and subsegmental pulmonary arteries: evaluation with electron-beam versus spiral CT. *Radiology.* 2000;214(2):433-439.
36. Oser RF, Zuckerman DA, Gutierrez FR, Brink JA. Anatomic distribution of pulmonary emboli at pulmonary angiography: implications for cross-sectional imaging. *Radiology.* 1996;199(1):31-35.
37. Schoepf UJ, Costello P. CT angiography for diagnosis of pulmonary embolism: state of the art. *Radiology.* 2004;230(2):329-337.
38. Mayo JR, Remy-Jardin M, Muller NL, et al. Pulmonary embolism: prospective comparison of spiral CT with ventilation-perfusion scintigraphy. *Radiology.* 1997;205(2):447-452.
39. Mullins MD, Becker DM, Hagspiel KD, Philbrick JT. The role of spiral volumetric computed tomography in the diagnosis of pulmonary embolism. *Arch Intern Med.* 2000;160(3):293-298.
40. Velmahos GC, Vassiliu P, Wilcox A, et al. Spiral computed tomography for the diagnosis of pulmonary embolism in critically ill surgical patients: a comparison with pulmonary angiography. *Arch Surg.* 2001;136(5):505-511.
41. Rathbun SW, Raskob GE, Whitsett TL. Sensitivity and specificity of helical computed tomography in the diagnosis of pulmonary embolism: a systematic review. *Ann Intern Med.* 2000;132(3): 227-232.
42. Bates SM, Ginsberg JS. Helical computed tomography and the diagnosis of pulmonary embolism. *Ann Intern Med.* 2000;132(3): 240-242.
43. Quiroz R, Kucher N, Schoepf UJ, et al. Right ventricular enlargement on chest computed tomography: prognostic role in acute pulmonary embolism. *Circulation.* 2004;109(20):2401-2404.
44. Groves DW, Einstein AJ. A step toward hemodynamic assessment with CT angiography. *J Cardiovasc Comput Tomogr.* 2011;5(1):50-51.
45. Dusaj RS, Michelis KC, Terek M, et al. Estimation of right atrial and ventricular hemodynamics by CT coronary angiography. *J Cardiovasc Comput Tomogr.* 2011;5(1):44-49.
46. Remy-Jardin M, Remy J, Wattinne L, Giraud F. Central pulmonary thromboembolism: diagnosis with spiral volumetric CT with the single-breath-hold technique–comparison with pulmonary angiography. *Radiology.* 1992;185(2):381-387.
47. van Rossum AB, Treurniet FE, Kieft GJ, Smith SJ, Schepers-Bok R. Role of spiral volumetric computed tomographic scanning in the assessment of patients with clinical suspicion of pulmonary embolism and an abnormal ventilation/perfusion lung scan. *Thorax.* 1996;51(1):23-28.
48. Tillie-Leblond I, Mastora I, Radenne F, et al. Risk of pulmonary embolism after a negative spiral CT angiogram in patients with pulmonary disease: 1-year clinical follow-up study. *Radiology.* 2002;223(2):461-467.
49. Henry JW, Relyea B, Stein PD. Continuing risk of thromboemboli among patients with normal pulmonary angiograms. *Chest.* 1995;107(5):1375-1378.
50. Wells PS, Owen C, Doucette S, Fergusson D, Tran H. Does this patient have deep vein thrombosis? *JAMA.* 2006;295(2):199-207.
51. Hull RD. Diagnosing pulmonary embolism with improved certainty and simplicity. *JAMA.* 2006;295(2):213-215.
52. Stein PD, Fowler SE, Goodman LR, et al. Multidetector computed tomography for acute pulmonary embolism. *N Engl J Med.* 2006;354(22):2317-2327.

53. Wells PS, Anderson DR, Rodger M, et al. Excluding pulmonary embolism at the bedside without diagnostic imaging: management of patients with suspected pulmonary embolism presenting to the emergency department by using a simple clinical model and d-dimer. *Ann Intern Med.* 2001;135(2):98-107.
54. Enden T, Klow NE. CT pulmonary angiography and suspected acute pulmonary embolism. *Acta Radiol.* 2003;44(3):310-315.
55. Perrier A, Roy PM, Aujesky D, et al. Diagnosing pulmonary embolism in outpatients with clinical assessment, D-dimer measurement, venous ultrasound, and helical computed tomography: a multicenter management study. *Am.J Med.* 2004;116(5):291-299.
56. van Belle A, Buller HR, Huisman MV, et al. Effectiveness of managing suspected pulmonary embolism using an algorithm combining clinical probability, D-dimer testing, and computed tomography. *JAMA.* 2006;295(2):172-179.
57. Righini M, Le Gal G, Aujesky D, et al. Diagnosis of pulmonary embolism by multidetector CT alone or combined with venous ultrasonography of the leg: a randomised non-inferiority trial. *Lancet.* 2008;371(9621):1343-1352.
58. Musset D, Parent F, Meyer G, et al. Diagnostic strategy for patients with suspected pulmonary embolism: a prospective multicentre outcome study. *Lancet.* 2002;360(9349):1914-1920.
59. Taffoni MJ, Ravenel JG, Ackerman SJ. Prospective comparison of indirect CT venography versus venous sonography in ICU patients. *Am J Roentgenol.* 2005;185(2):457-462.
60. Kim T, Murakami T, Hori M, Kumano S, Sakon M, Nakamura H. Efficacy of multi-slice helical CT venography for the diagnosis of deep venous thrombosis: comparison with venous sonography. *Radiat Med.* 2004;22(2):77-81.
61. Lim KE, Hsu WC, Hsu YY, Chu PH, Ng CJ. Deep venous thrombosis: comparison of indirect multidetector CT venography and sonography of lower extremities in 26 patients. *Clin Imaging.* 2004;28(6):439-444.
62. van Strijen MJ, de MW, Schiereck J, et al. Single-detector helical computed tomography as the primary diagnostic test in suspected pulmonary embolism: a multicenter clinical management study of 510 patients. *Annals of Internal Medicine.* 2003;138(4):307-314.
63. Katz DS, Loud PA, Bruce D, et al. Combined CT venography and pulmonary angiography: a comprehensive review. *Radiographics.* 2002;22:S3-S19 Spec No.
64. Cham MD, Yankelevitz DF, Henschke CI. Thromboembolic disease detection at indirect CT venography versus CT pulmonary angiography. *Radiology.* 2005;234(2):591-594.
65. Richman PB, Wood J, Kasper DM, et al. Contribution of indirect computed tomography venography to computed tomography angiography of the chest for the diagnosis of thromboembolic disease in two United States emergency departments. *J Thromb Haemost.* 2003;1(4):652-657.
66. Sueyoshi E, Tsutsui S, Sakamoto I, Uetani M, Maemura K. Images in cardiovascular medicine. Lung perfusion blood volume computed tomographic images of pulmonary embolism: before and after thrombolysis. *Circulation.* 2009;119(25):3242-3243.
67. Moser KM, Auger WR, Fedullo PF. Chronic major-vessel thromboembolic pulmonary hypertension. *Circulation.* 1990;81(6):1735-1743.
68. Wittram C, Kalra MK, Maher MM, Greenfield A, McLoud TC, Shepard JA. Acute and chronic pulmonary emboli: angiography-CT correlation. *AJR Am J Roentgenol.* 2006;186(6 suppl 2):S421-S429.
69. Ellis JG, Kuzman WJ. Pulmonary artery stenosis, a frequent part of the congenital rubella syndrome. *Calif Med.* 1966;105(6):435-439.
70. Loyd JE, Tillman BF, Atkinson JB, Des Prez RM. Mediastinal fibrosis complicating histoplasmosis. *Medicine (Baltimore).* 1988;67(5):295-310.
71. Rossi SE, McAdams HP, Rosado-de-Christenson ML, Franks TJ, Galvin JR. Fibrosing mediastinitis. *Radiographics.* 2001;21(3):737-757.
72. Matsunaga N, Hayashi K, Sakamoto I, Ogawa Y, Matsumoto T. Takayasu arteritis: protean radiologic manifestations and diagnosis. *Radiographics.* 1997;17(3):579-594.
73. Nonomura A, Kurumaya H, Kono N, et al. Primary pulmonary artery sarcoma. Report of two autopsy cases studied by immunohistochemistry and electron microscopy, and review of 110 cases reported in the literature. *Acta Pathol Jpn.* 1988;38(7):883-896.
74. Kpodonu J, Cusimano RJ, Johnston MR. An unusual cause of syncope. *Asian Cardiovasc Thorac Ann.* 2005;13(4):400.
75. Alsoufi B, Slater M, Smith PP, Karamlou T, Mansoor A, Ravichandran P. Pulmonary artery sarcoma mimicking massive pulmonary embolus: a case report. *Asian Cardiovasc Thorac Ann.* 2006;14(4):e71-e73.
76. Stella F, Davoli F, Brandolini J, Dolci G, Sellitri F, Bini A. Pulmonary artery leiomyosarcoma successfully treated by right pneumonectomy. *Asian Cardiovasc Thorac Ann.* 2009;17(5):513-515.
77. Komanapalli C, Alsoufi B, Shen I, Slater M. Recurrent pulmonary artery sarcoma. *J Card Surg.* 2006;21(6):587-589.
78. Yi CA, Lee KS, Choe YH, Han D, Kwon OJ, Kim S. Computed tomography in pulmonary artery sarcoma: distinguishing features from pulmonary embolic disease. *J Comput Assist Tomogr.* 2004;28(1):34-39.
79. Itoh H, Yamamoto T, Sugihara H, et al. Aortopulmonary artery dissection. *J Am Coll Cardiol.* 2009;54(21):1990.

29 Caval Anatomy: Variants and Lesions

Key Points

- Contrast-enhanced CT scanning is well suited to imaging congenital anatomic variants of the cavae as well as caval pathologies, including caval thrombi, tumors, obstructions, and occlusions.
- Congenital variants of the cava are not uncommon and may be complex.

The cavae are large vessels with near-vertical orientation, which makes them particularly accessible for assessment by all manner of contrast-enhanced CT examinations, such as axial source imaging, as well as sagittal and coronal projections.[1]

In addition to being diseased, both the superior (SVC) and inferior (IVC) venae cavae have congenital variants that are regularly encountered and that have clinical relevance. Familiarity with the congenital variants of IVC is important so as not to misinterpret them as adenopathy or other structures on cross-sectional imaging, particularly when the degree of venous opacification is poor.[2] Venous anomalies often are dilated and may be tortuous, increasing the risk of surgical injury and bleeding. Preoperative identification of anomalies allows for better surgical planning and may avoid potentially disastrous errors.[3,4]

ANATOMY OF THE SUPERIOR VENA CAVA

The SVC (or precava) returns deoxygenated blood from the upper half of the body to the right atrium. Its proximal aspect is the union of the left and right brachiocephalic veins; its distal aspect is the union with the superomedial aspect of the right atrium (Fig. 29-1).

Branches and Tributaries of the Superior Vena Cava

- Left brachiocephalic (innominate) vein
  - Left subclavian vein
  - Left internal jugular vein
  - Left superior intercostal vein
- Right brachiocephalic (innominate) vein
  - Right subclavian vein
  - Right internal jugular vein
- Azygos vein
  - Hemiazygos vein
  - Accessory hemiazygos vein

Congenital Variants

Persistent Left Superior Vena Cava

See Figures 29-2 through 29-6; **Video 29-1.**

- Incidence:
  - Isolated: 0.3% to 0.5%[5]
  - Presence of congenital heart disease: 3% to 10%[5]
- Results from failure of involution of the left cardinal vein
- The right SVC is absent in 30% of cases.[6]
- The left SVC usually drains into the coronary sinus, which is dilated. Rarely, the left SVC may drain into the left atrium.
- Clinical relevance:
  - Association with congenital heart disease
  - May confer difficulty in catheterizing the right heart, in placement of pacemakers or implantable cardioverter defibrillators
  - Alters the technique of placing the heart on bypass

Double Superior Vena Cava

- Incidence:
  - Isolated: 0.3%[5]
  - Presence of congenital heart disease: 11%[5]

Superior Vena Cava Agenesis and Drainage into the Inferior Vena Cava via the Azygos Vein

- Total absence of the SVC
- Due to lack of development of the right anterior cardinal vein
- The azygos vein is dilated and carries blood posterior to the diaphragm to the IVC.
- Incidence: rare

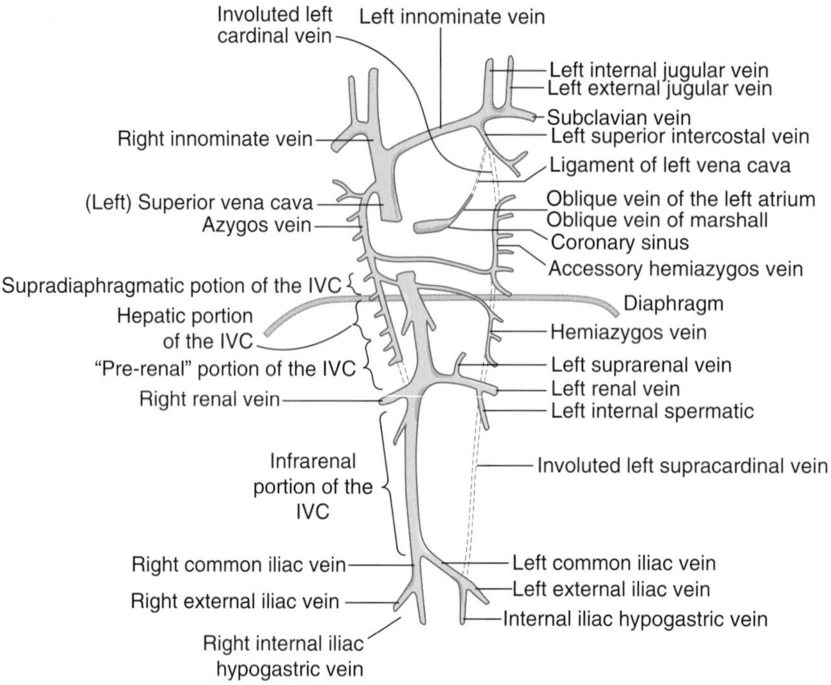

Figure 29-1. Caval anatomy. IVC, inferior vena cava.

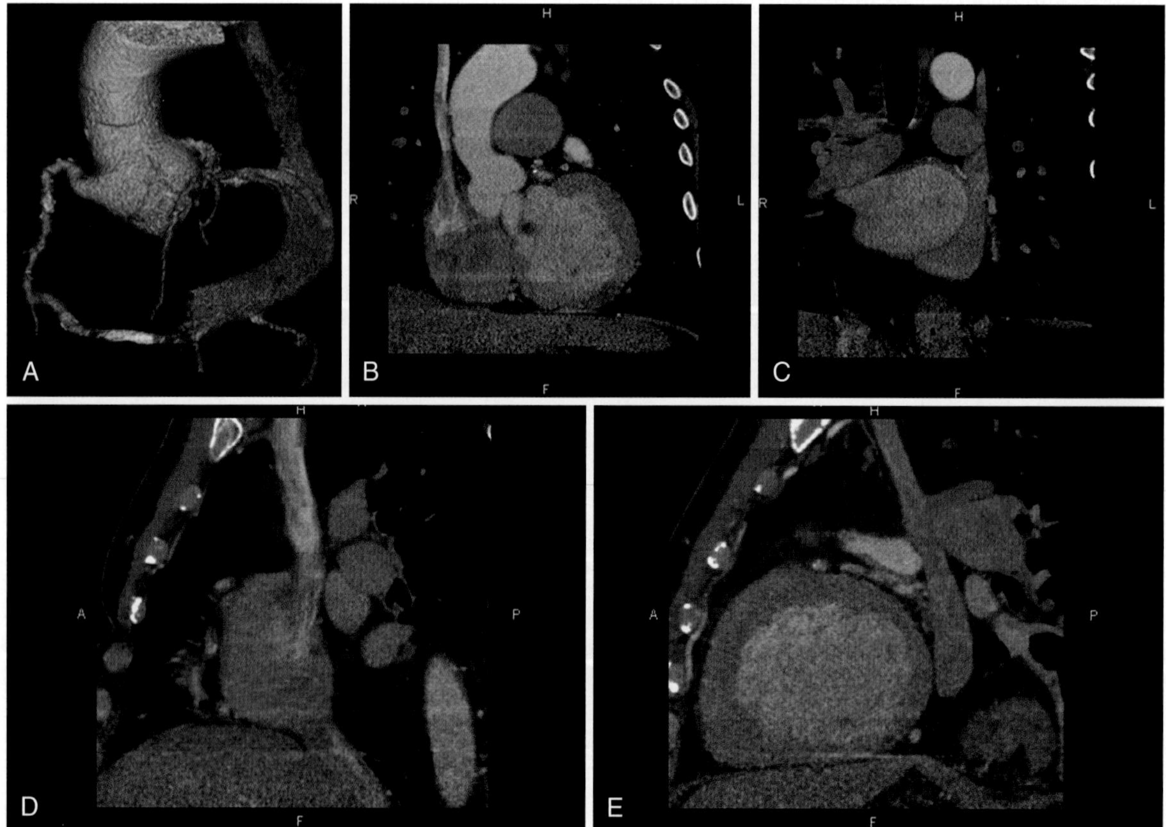

Figure 29-2. Multiple composite images from a cardiac CT study demonstrate bilateral superior venae cavae (SVC), with the right-sided SVC entering into the right atrium in a normal fashion. A left-sided SVC is seen entering into the coronary sinus, which is enlarged due to the presence of the left SVC.

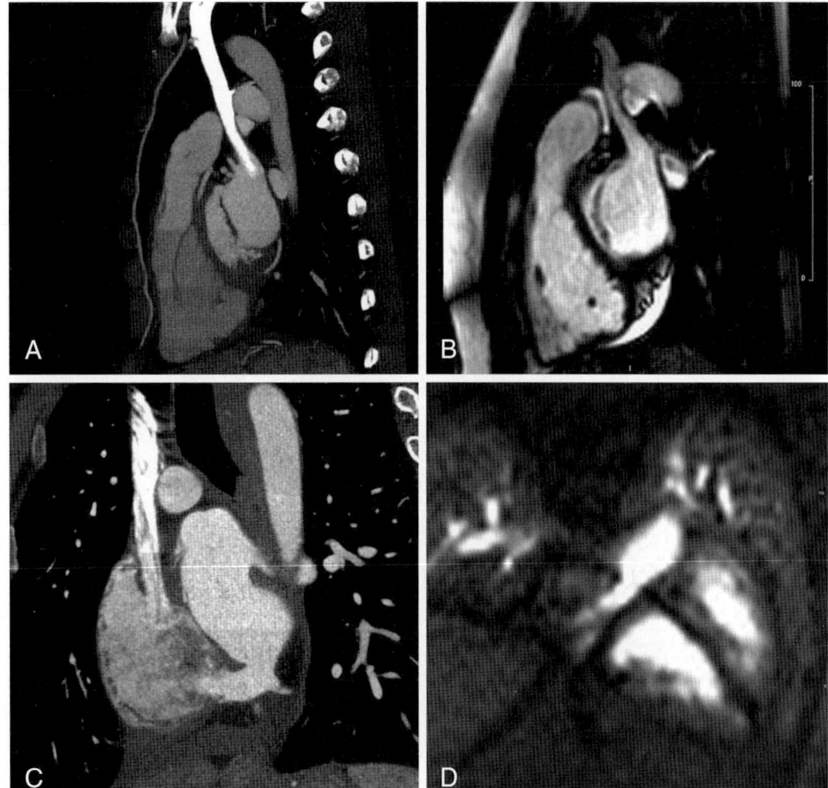

Figure 29-3. CT (**A** and **C**) and cardiac MR (**B** and **D**) images of persistence of the left superior vena cava (SVC). **A** and **B** are corresponding CT and CMR images. The left SVC in this case enters the left atrium through the left atrial appendage. The detail is better appreciated on the CT image. **C,** The right SVC entering the superior right atrium. An "unroofed" coronary sinus atrial septal defect is seen as well. **D,** CMR perfusion image demonstrating contrast returning to the right atrium via the coronary sinus.

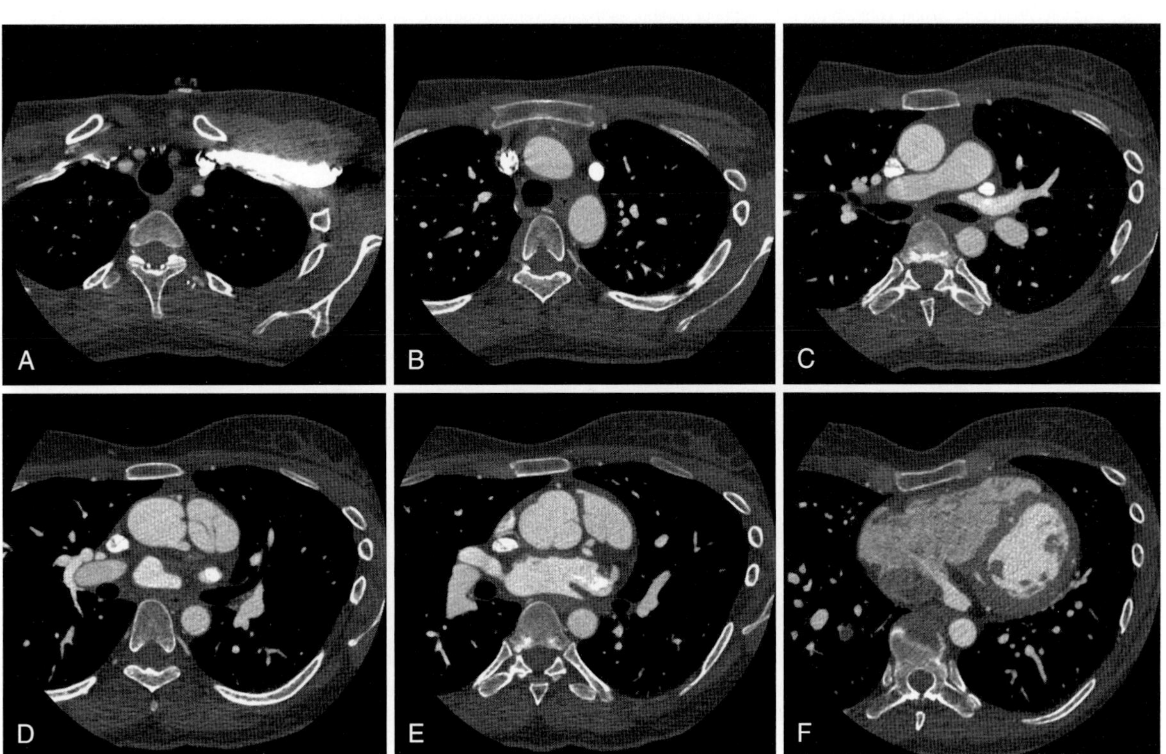

Figure 29-4. Serial axial contrast-enhanced ECG-gated CT scan images reveal the course of a persistent left superior vena cava (SVC). The left SVC has an unusual course and drains into the left atrial appendage (**D**). The coronary sinus is not dilated (**F**), because the left SVC does not drain into it. There is differential contrast density in the coronary sinus relative to the right atrium. The contrast density in the coronary sinus mirrors that of the left heart, suggesting a left-to-right shunt, in this case an unroofed coronary sinus. There is an incidental pulmonary embolus to the right lower lobe in this patient presenting with chest pain. **See Video 29-1.**

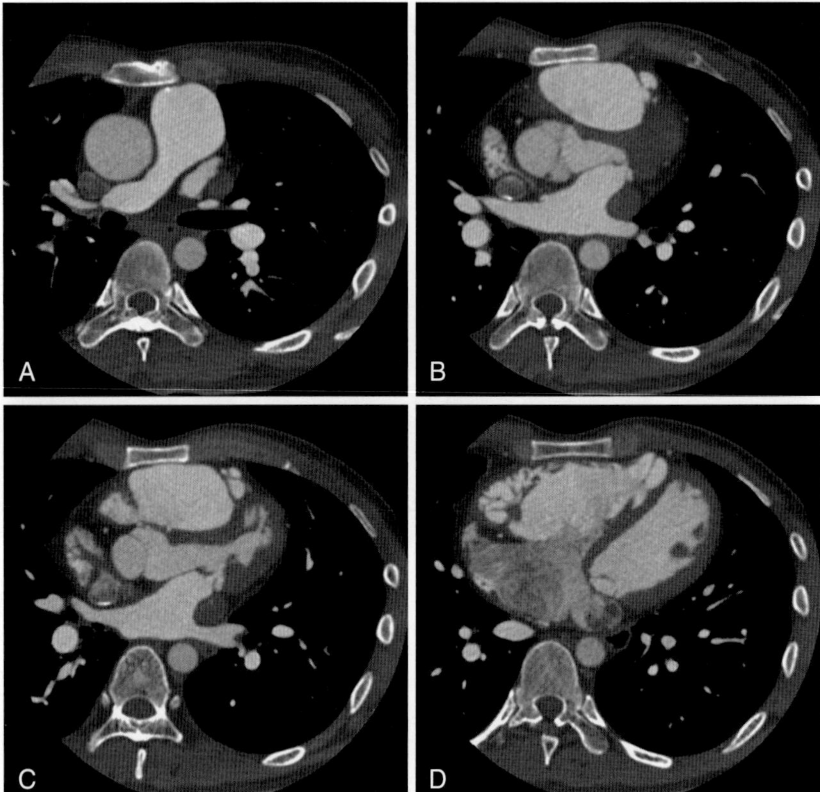

Figure 29-5. Multiple ECG-gated CT angiographic images obtained prospectively in a 32-year-old patient with repaired tetralogy of Fallot. Bilateral superior venae cavae (SVCs) are present. A right SVC contains a small amount of contrast, showing that it forms its confluence appropriately with the right atrium. The left SVC has no visible contrast within its superior portion; as the intravenous contrast was injected into the right antecubital fossa. The lower course of the left SVC forms a confluence with the coronary sinus. The coronary sinus is dilated. Contrast does reflux from the right atrium into the terminal portion of the left SVC. Evidence of this patient's previous transannular repair for tetralogy of Fallot also is seen. **A,** Dilatation of the main pulmonary artery with a small amount of pulmonary arterial calcification anteriorly. There is a right ventricular outflow tract (RVOT) patch, with prior surgical resection of RVOT muscle bundles. This is seen in close proximity to the substernal tissues. **C,** A small amount of calcification is seen within the high ventricular septal defect patch.

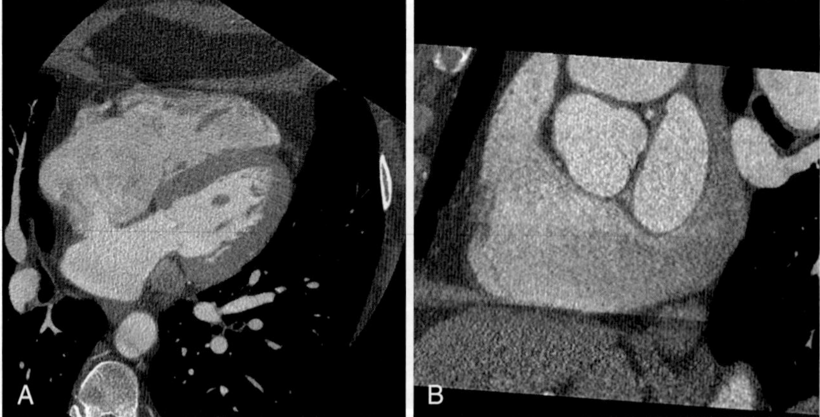

Figure 29-6. **A,** The four-chamber projection demonstrates a secundum atrial septal defect (ASD) with higher-attenuation left-sided contrast tracking into the right atrium through the ASD. Note the enlarged right-sided chambers, and the enlarged coronary sinus. **B,** Short-axis oblique projection demonstrates the superior vena cava (SVC) on the left of the image entering the right atrium, and a persistent left SVC on the right of the image and its continuity with the coronary sinus.

Superior Vena Cava Obstruction/Superior Vena Cava Syndrome

Caval obstruction may be partial or complete (occlusion) and may result from any combination of extrinsic compression, intramural scarring, and intraluminal thrombosis or other mass lesion. Etiologies are diverse and include:

- Extrinsic compression:
  - By tumor: 90% of cases of SVC syndrome are due to malignant compression of the SVC, especially by:
    - Bronchogenic carcinoma
    - Lymphomas
    - Breast carcinoma
  - By ascending aortic aneurysms
    - Syphilis
    - Tuberculosis
- Iatrogenic intraluminal thrombosis due to instrumentation of the SVC

Superior Vena Cava Stenosis

Caval stenosis is evident on contrast-enhanced CT scanning by focal narrowing and proximal venous engorgement, with or without venous collateral formation.

SVC Occlusion

SVC occlusion is evident on contrast-enhanced CT scanning[7-9] by the absence of contrast enhancement within the cava. CT is able to image structures near the cava and elsewhere inside the body that may explain or suggest the cause of the obstruction. Proximal venous distention is usual. The presence of collateral vessels indicates chronicity.

Intraluminal Thrombus Versus Tumor Mass

Distinguishing thrombosis from tumor (angio) invasion may be possible and requires finding the origin of the soft tissue caval intraluminal mass. Chronic thrombosis organizes and usually contracts the cava, whereas acute thrombosis distends the cava. Indwelling lines, pacemaker wires, and implantable cardioverter defibrillator leads that are the source of thrombosis confer artifacts. Streaming artifacts from the contralateral venous drainage, and also from the azygos vein, may make it difficult to confirm thrombosis. (Figs. 29-7 through 29-9; **Video 29-2**).

ANATOMY OF THE INFERIOR VENA CAVA

The inferior vena cava (also known as the posterior vena cava) runs posterior to the abdominal cavity and returns the deoxygenated blood to the right atrium. At its inferior aspect it is formed by the union of the right and left iliac veins; at its superior aspect is the eustachian valve (or valve of the IVC) at the inferoposterior aspect of the right atrium. It crosses the diaphragm at the T8 level. Its branches (tributaries) and their anatomic levels are as follows:

- The hepatic veins: T8
- The inferior phrenic veins: T8
- The suprarenal veins: L1
- The renal veins: L1
- The gonadal veins: L2
- The lumbar veins: L1–L5
- The common iliac veins: L5

The branches exhibit some asymmetry: the suprarenal and gonadal veins on the left side drain into the left renal vein, whereas on the right side they drain directly into the IVC.

Segments of the IVC include the:

- Supradiaphragmatic segment (crura of the diaphragm to the eustachian valve)
- Hepatic (or post-hepatic) segment

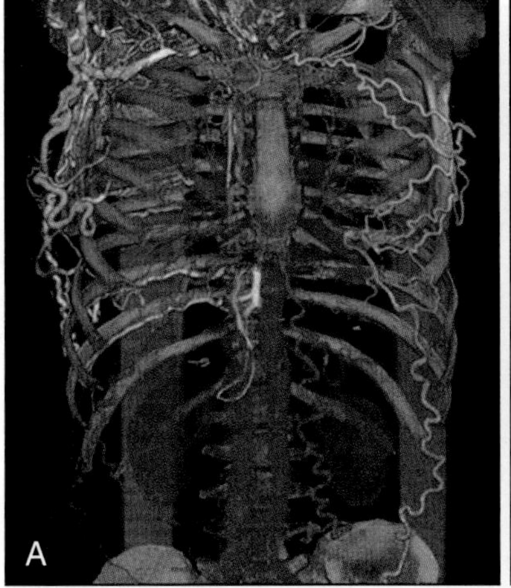

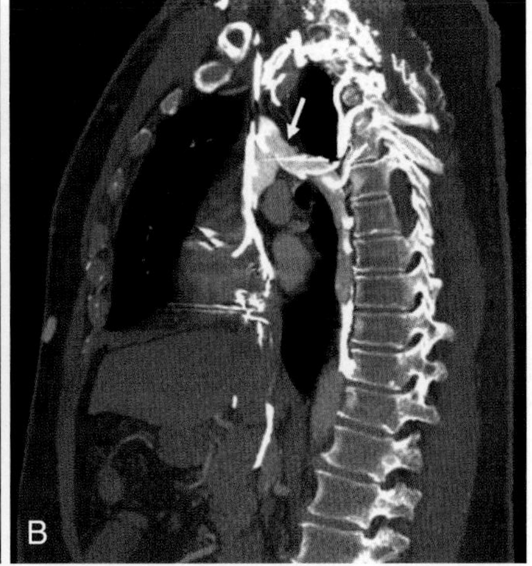

Figure 29-7. Obstruction of the superior vena cava. **A,** Volume-rendered chest CT angiogram with contrast injection via the right upper extremity. Extensive venous collaterals are evident with engorgement of the subcutaneous veins of the right and left chest and abdomen. **B,** Maximum intensity projection sagittal plane rendering of the chest CT angiogram. Contrast within the dilated azygos vein is seen emptying into the superior vena cava (*arrow*). (Reprinted with permission from Thompson RC, Thibodeau JM, Ramza BM. Computed tomography angiographic demonstration of collateral circulation in superior vena cava syndrome. *J Cardiovasc Comput Tomogr*. 2008;2:57-58.)

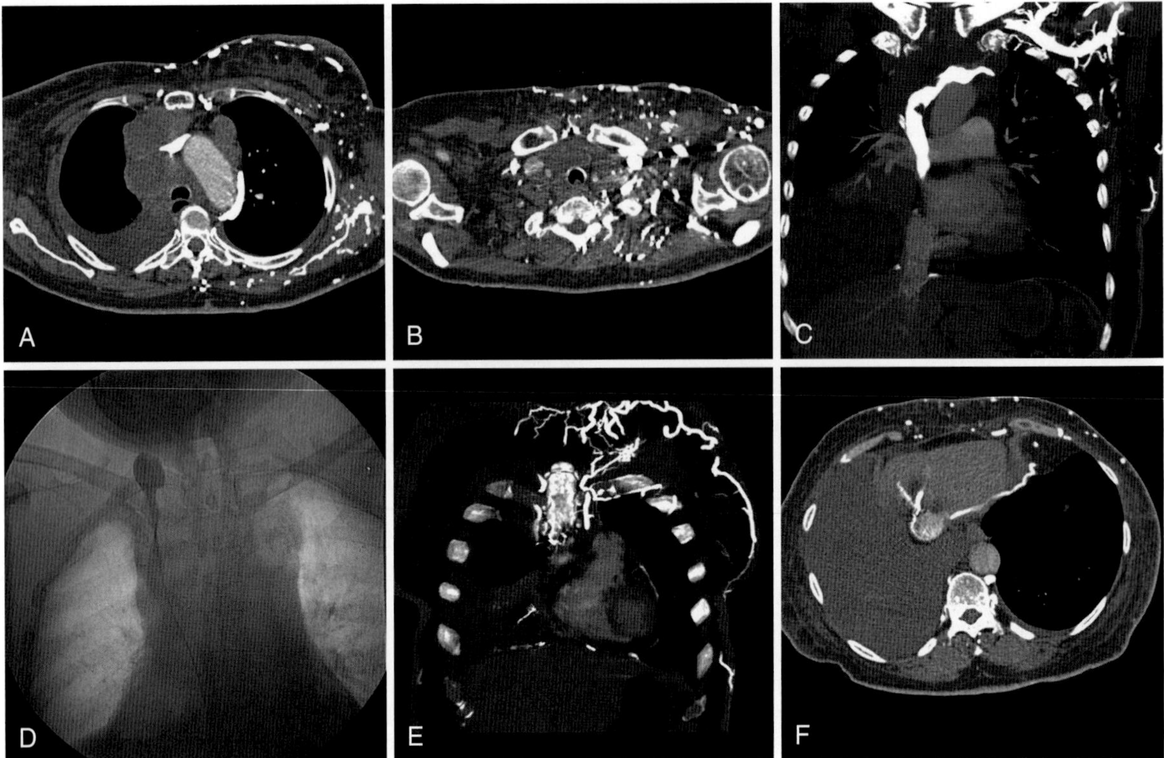

Figure 29-8. Superior vena cava (SVC) obstruction due to carcinoma. **A** and **B,** Axial contrast-enhanced CT scan images. There is extensive upper mediastinal bulky adenopathy and prominent left chest collateralization due to the SVC obstruction. **C,** Coronal plane contrast-enhanced image of the SVC. **D,** Contrast venographic image of the SVC. Note the similar SVC obstruction. **E,** Extensive left chest collateralization resulting from the SVC obstruction. **F,** Collateralization returning blood flow to the inferior vena cava, adaptive to the SVC obstruction.

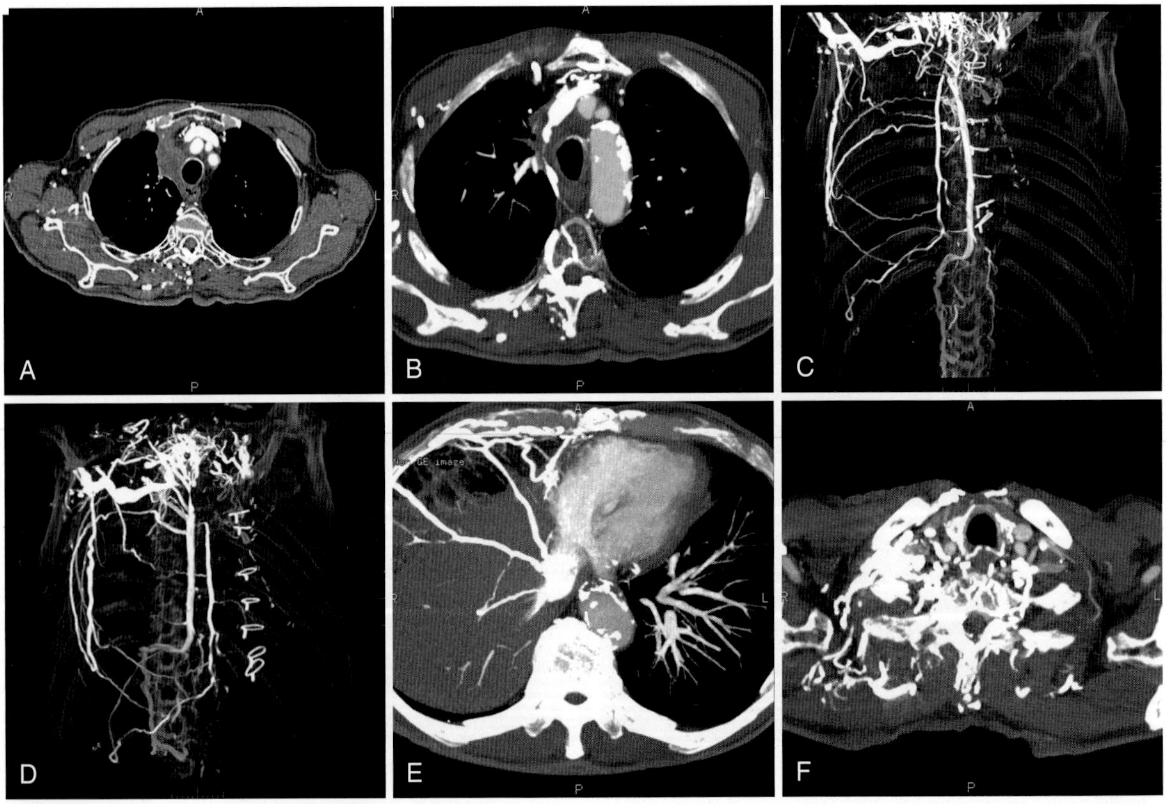

Figure 29-9. A 48-year-old man with non–small cell lung cancer with clinical presentation suspicious for superior vena cava (SVC) syndrome. **A** and **B,** CT scan demonstrates an amorphous high right paratracheal mass which sub-totally occludes the SVC as well as the confluence of the SVC and the azygos vein. **C** through **F,** Extensive collateral pathways from the supraclavicular, intercostal, and intervertebral collateral vessels which bypass the SVC and reconstitute at the level of the inferior vena cava. **See Video 29-2.**

- ❒ Renal segment
- ❒ Infrarenal segment

Congenital Variants

In 1920 Huntington and McLure[10] proposed 14 theoretical anatomic variants of the (infrarenal) IVC, most of which have been observed in humans.[2]

Left Inferior Vena Cava

- ❒ Due to involution of the right supracardinal vein, and persistence of the left suprarenal vein
- ❒ Incidence: 0.2% to 0.5%[11]
- ❒ The left IVC usually drains into the left renal vein, and usually crosses anteriorly to the aorta in its normal fashion, to join the right renal vein and continue in its usual course.
- ❒ Clinical relevance:
  - May be misdiagnosed as adenopathy
  - Rupture of an abdominal aortic aneurysm into a left IVC[12]
  - Difficulty encountered in placing IVC filters

Double Inferior Vena Cava

- ❒ Due to persistence of both the right and left supracardinal veins
- ❒ Incidence: 0.2% to 0.3%[11]
- ❒ The left IVC usually drains into the left renal vein, and usually crosses anteriorly to the aorta in is normal fashion, to join the right renal vein and continue in its usual course. Variations are encountered.
- ❒ The size of the left and right IVCs may differ.
- ❒ Clinical relevance:
  - Misdiagnosis as adenopathy
  - Recurrent pulmonary embolism may occur despite placement of an IVC filter.[11]

Azygos Continuation of the Inferior Vena Cava

- ❒ Also referred to as *absence of the hepatic segment of the IVC with azygos continuation,* although the hepatic segment is not absent, but drains directly into the right atrium
- ❒ Due to involution of the right subcardinal vein with persistence of anastomoses of the right retrocrural azygos vein
- ❒ The IVC passes posteriorly to the diaphragm as the azygos vein to enter the SVC in its usual position.
- ❒ Incidence: 0.6%[11]
- ❒ Clinical relevance:
  - The enlarged azygos vein may be misdiagnosed as mediastinal adenopathy.
  - Confers difficulty in catheterization of the heart via the groin
  - Changes the technique of placing the heart on bypass

Circumaortic Left Renal Vein Variant

- ❒ Incidence: 8.7%.[11]
- ❒ There are two left renal veins: the superior one crosses anteriorly to the aorta, and the inferior one passes posteriorly to the aorta, 1 to 2 cm inferiorly.
- ❒ Clinical relevance:
  - Misdiagnosis as adenopathy
  - Planning for renal surgery

Retroaortic Left Renal Vein

- ❒ The left renal vein passes posteriorly to the aorta.
- ❒ Incidence: 2.1%[11]

Double Inferior Vena Cava with Retroaortic Right Renal Vein and Hemiazygos Continuation of the Inferior Vena Cava

- ❒ Clinical relevance: misdiagnosis of the hemiazygos vein as a mediastinal mass

Other Variants

- ❒ Double IVC with retroaortic left renal vein and azygos continuation of the IVC
- ❒ Circumcaval ureter
- ❒ Absent IVC with preservation of the suprarenal segment

Inferior Vena Cava Obstruction

Obstruction of the IVC results in IVC syndrome. The incidence is approximately 5 to 10 per 100,000 people per year.

Caval obstruction may be partial or complete (occlusion) and may result from any combination of extrinsic compression, intramural scarring, and intraluminal thrombosis or other mass lesion. Etiologies are diverse and include:

- ❒ Extrinsic compression by:
  - The gravid uterus, commonly in the third trimester of pregnancy
  - Extrinsic tumor (discussed later)
  - Abdominal aortic aneurysm
  - Retroperitoneal fibrosis
- ❒ Tumors (Figs. 29-10 through 29-13):
  - Angioinvasion by tumor:
    - Renal cell carcinoma
    - Hepatoma
    - Wilms tumor
  - Leiomyosarcoma of the IVC
  - Compression (which may result in thrombosis) by:
    - Colorectal carcinoma
    - Renal cell carcinoma
    - Ovarian cancer
- ❒ Iatrogenic due to thrombosis or scarring induced by:
  - Catheterization
  - Filters
  - Surgery (liver transplantation)
- ❒ Intraluminal thrombus

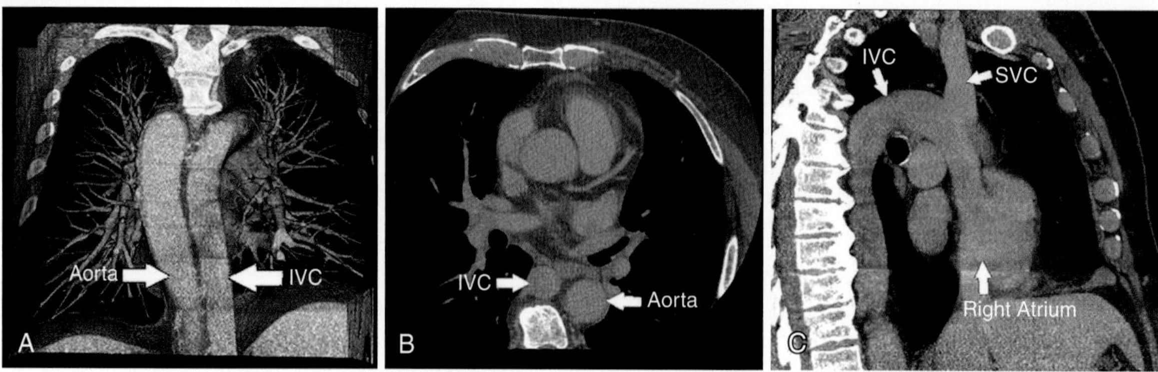

Figure 29-10. A 70-year-old man presented for typical atrial flutter ablation. Right femoral venous access was obtained, but there was difficulty in advancing the catheter into the right atrium, and the procedure was abandoned. The patient was sent for cardiac CT angiography. The images showed that the patient had azygos continuation of the inferior vena cava (IVC) running adjacent to the aorta (**A** and **B**) and merging with the superior vena cava (SVC) at the level of the aortic arch (**C**). The incidence of such an anomaly in the general population is less than 0.3%. Recognition of this unusual anomaly is important, because it can pose technical challenges during invasive procedures. The dilated azygos vein may be misinterpreted as a paracardiac or mediastinal mass on chest radiography. This anomaly is associated with recurrent deep venous thrombosis of lower extremities, sick sinus syndrome, and atrial flutter. (Reprinted with permission from Mamidipally S, Rashba E, McBrearty T, Poon M. Azygous continuation of inferior vena cava. *J Am Coll Cardiol*. 2010;56(21);e41.)

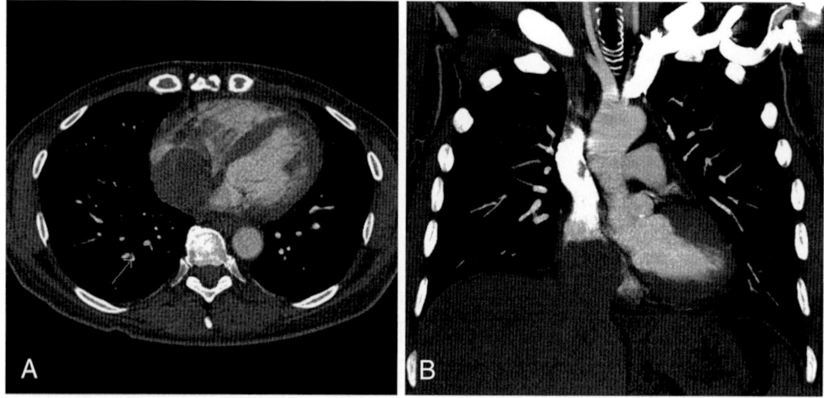

Figure 29-11. A 55-year-old man presented with chest pain and shortness of breath and underwent a CT PE protocol study which confirmed pulmonary embolism (**A,** *arrow*), but also identified a large mass in the right atrium (**B**). The patient underwent further transthoracic echocardiography, transesophageal echocardiography, and cardiac CT imaging (see Figs. 29-12 and 29-13), and subsequently underwent surgery. The source of the embolism was either thrombus or tumor.

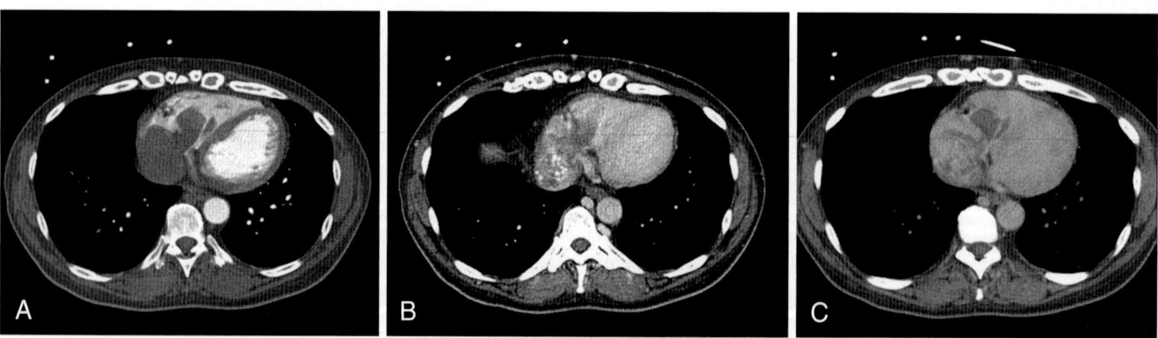

Figure 29-12. Triple-phase CT scan of the abdomen and pelvis in the same patient shown in Figure 29-11. **A,** Early arterial phase acquisition demonstrates a large soft tissue density mass within the IVC right atrial junction extending into the right atrium. Fingerlike projections extend across the tricuspid valve into the right ventricle. This demonstrates uniform attenuation on the early arterial phase image, but on the late arterial phase image (**B**), serpentine vessels are seen within the right atrial/inferior vena cava (IVC) portion of the mass. On the 1-minute delayed image (**C**), mixed attenuation within the right atrial component of the mass is seen, while no enhancement is seen within the right ventricular portion of the mass. These findings demonstrate a mass consistent with elements of tumor thrombus within the right atrium, and bland thrombus within the right ventricle. A search for an intra-abdominal cause for this would be required. The two most likely sources for tumor thrombus would be from a renal cell carcinoma extending into the IVC, or a hepatocellular carcinoma extending into the hepatic veins and also the IVC.

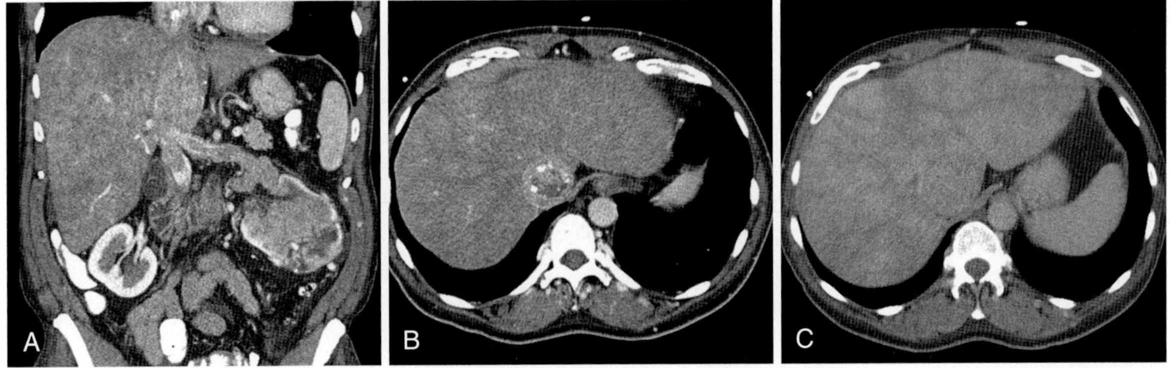

Figure 29-13. Abdominal CT scan in a patient with a suspected right atrial mass (same patient shown in Figures 29-11 and 29-12) . **A,** Coronal image in a late arterial phase. There is a large irregular mass within the left kidney. This mass extends into the left renal vein, and subsequently into the inferior vena cava (IVC). This likely extends all the way up into the right atrium. **B,** Image also acquired in the late arterial phase demonstrates arterial enhancement within the IVC. **C,** Some delayed enhancement also is noted within the IVC on this image. The image demonstrates a bizarre enhancement pattern to the liver, with irregular linear septa seen within the liver. This appearance is suggestive of underlying hepatic vein or IVC congestion and can be seen in some forms of Budd-Chiari syndrome.

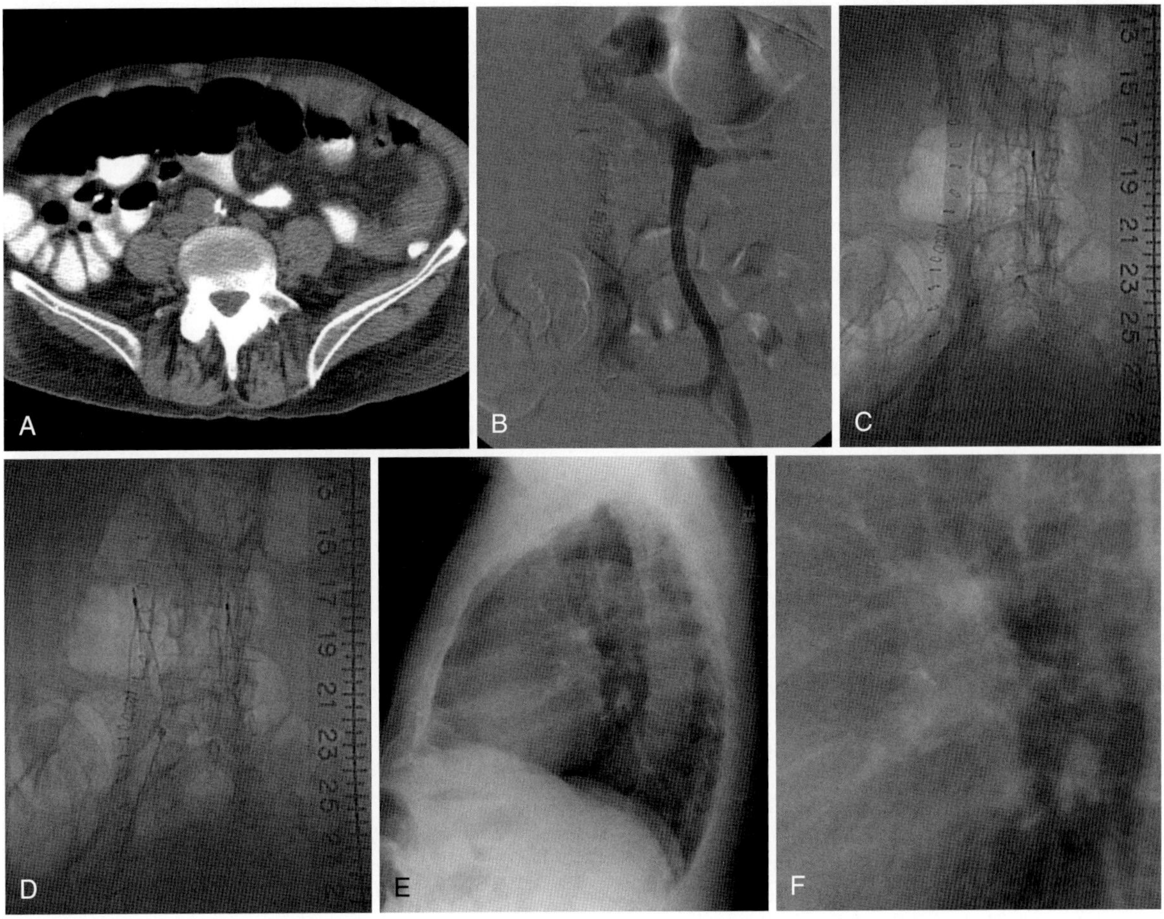

Figure 29-14. **A,** Axial CT image reveals rounded structures in cross-section on either side of the abdominal aorta. **B,** Contrast venogram delineating a left-sided inferior vena cava (IVC). **C** and **D,** Deployment of bilateral IVC filters. **E** and **F,** Lateral chest radiographs reveal embolization of a filter into the pulmonary artery.

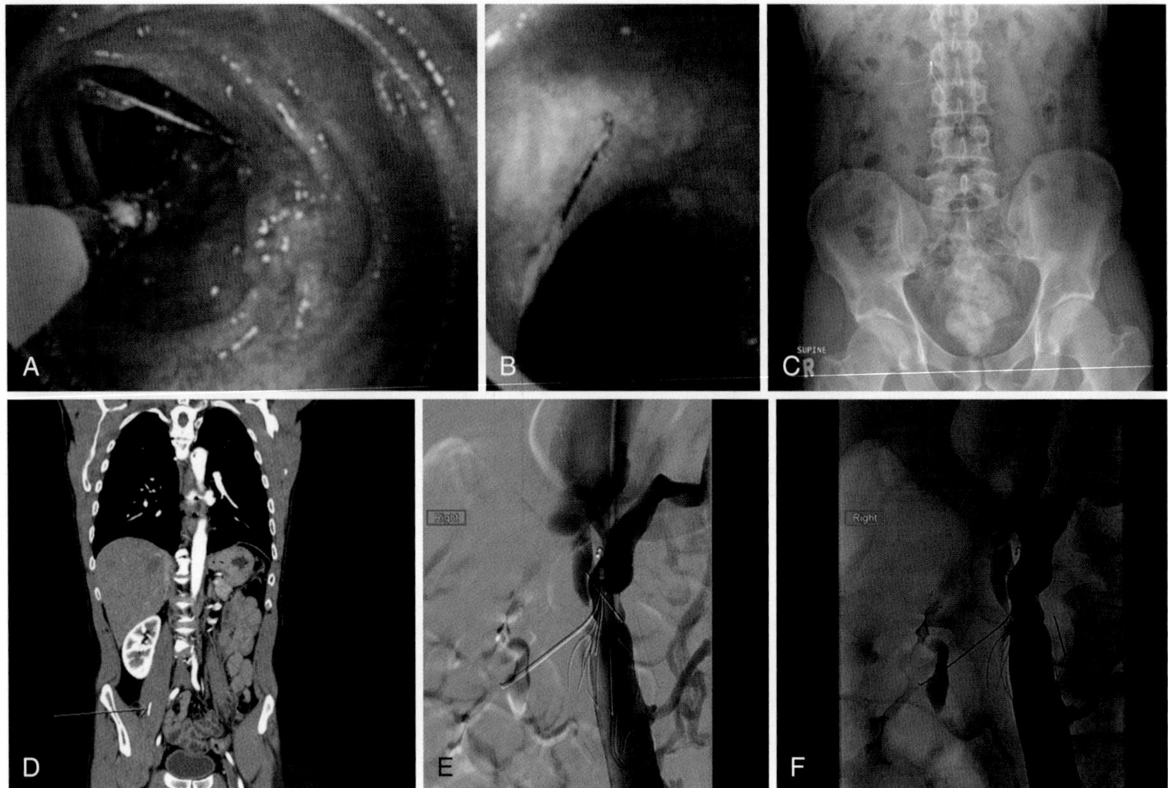

Figure 29-15. A 48-year-old man presented with abdominal pain 2 months post–insertion of an inferior vena cava (IVC) filter. **A** and **B,** Esophagogastroduodenoscopy demonstrates perforation of a tine of the filter into the duodenum. Abdominal flat plate radiography (**C**) and the corresponding coronal CT scan (**D**) reveal that a fragment of a tine of the filter also has entered into the right psoas muscle and migrated inferiorly. Repeat IVC cavogram (**E** and **F**) reveals that multiple tines have perforated the IVC locally.

Inferior Vena Cava Stenosis

IVC stenosis is indicated on contrast-enhanced CT scanning by focal narrowing and proximal venous engorgement with or without venous collateral formation.

Occlusion of the Inferior Vena Cava

IVC occlusion is evident on contrast-enhanced CT scanning by the absence of contrast enhancement within the cava. CT is able to image structures near the cava and elsewhere inside the body that may explain or suggest the cause of the obstruction. Proximal venous distention is usual. The presence of collateral vessels indicates chronicity.

Intraluminal Thrombus Versus Tumor Mass

Distinguishing thrombosis from tumor (angio) invasion may be feasible and requires attention to finding the origin of the soft tissue caval intraluminal mass. Chronic thrombosis organizes and generally contracts the cava, whereas acute thrombosis will distend the cava. Indwelling lines may confer artifacts. Streaming artifacts from the contralateral venous drainage may make it difficult to confirm thrombosis. Distinguishing thrombus complicating tumor from the tumor itself is problematic.

Inferior Vena Cava Filters

IVC filters are inserted percutaneously into the infrarenal IVC to prevent large pulmonary emboli. IVC filters reduce pulmonary embolism but increase the rate of deep vein thrombosis. The optimal indications for filters are evolving. There are numerous designs of filters. IVC filters are visible on radiography. Complications of IVC filters include embolization in part or whole into the lung, displacement superiorly, erosion of a tyne through the wall of the IVC into the aorta or the duodenum, embolization of a fragment down the aorta, and obstruction/occlusion of the aorta (Figs. 29-14 through 29-16).

CCT PROTOCOL POINTS

Inferior Vena Cava

- Coverage: diaphragm to symphysis pubis
- Contrast: 120 mL at 3 mL/sec with an 80-sec delay

Superior Vena Cava

- Coverage: above lung apices to below lungs
- Contrast: 120 mL at 3 mL/sec with a 60-sec delay

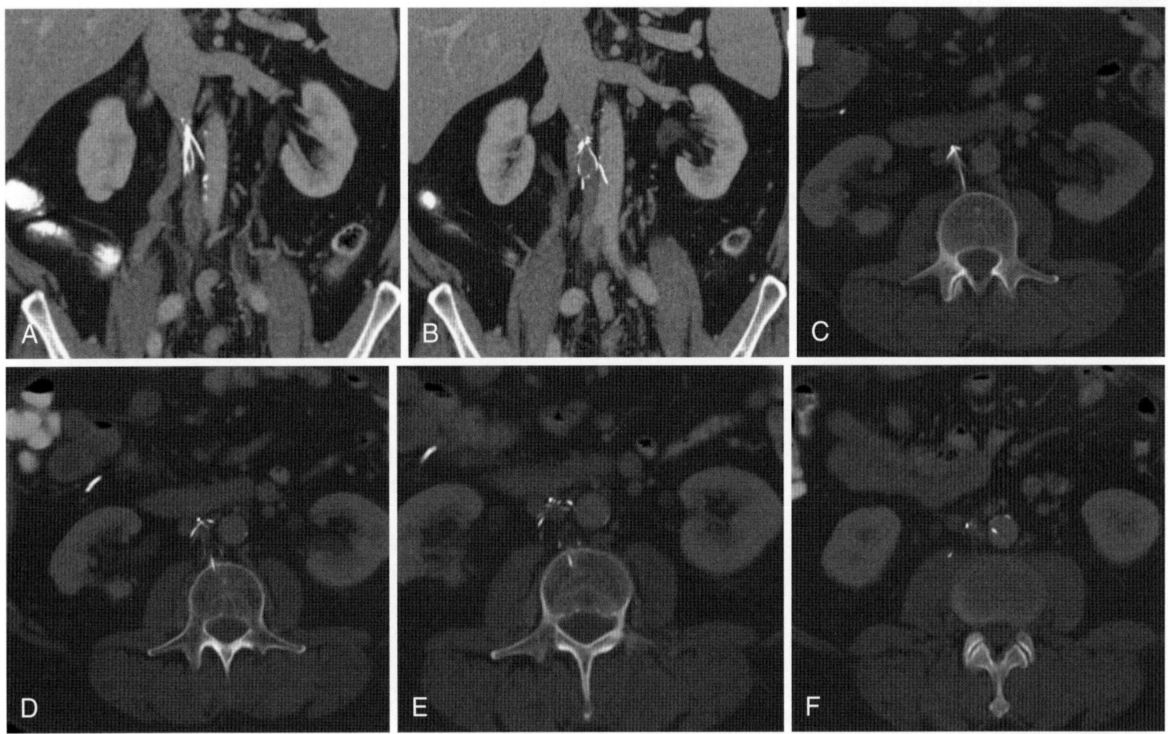

Figure 29-16. A 72-year-old patient 4 months post–inferior vena cava (IVC) filter insertion. **A** and **B,** A left-sided tine has perforated through the wall of the IVC and penetrated into the aorta. **C** through **E,** CT images reveal that a tine of the filter has perforated through the IVC wall and penetrated into the spine. **F,** A third truant tine has perforated the wall of the IVC and penetrated into the right psoas muscle.

References

1. Morra A, Clemente A, Del Borrello M, Berretta S, Greco P. Multidetector computed tomography and 2- and 3-dimensional postprocessing in the evaluation of congenital thoracic vascular anomalies. *J Cardiovasc Comput Tomogr.* 2008;2(4):245-255.
2. Bass JE, Redwine MD, Kramer LA, Huynh PT, Harris Jr JH. Spectrum of congenital anomalies of the inferior vena cava: cross-sectional imaging findings. *Radiographics.* 2000;20(3):639-652.
3. Mathews R, Smith PA, Fishman EK, Marshall FF. Anomalies of the inferior vena cava and renal veins: embryologic and surgical considerations. *Urology.* 1999;53(5):873-880.
4. Effler DB, Greer AE, Sifers EC. Anomaly of the vena cava inferior; report of fatality after ligation. *J Am Med Assoc.* 1951;146(14):1321-1322.
5. Minniti S, Visentini S, Procacci C. Congenital anomalies of the venae cavae: embryological origin, imaging features and report of three new variants. *Eur Radiol.* 2002;12(8):2040-2055.
6. Sarodia BD, Stoller JK. Persistent left superior vena cava: case report and literature review. *Respir Care.* 2000;45(4):411-416.
7. Di Giammarco G, Storto ML, Marano R, Di Mauro M. Superior vena cava syndrome: a 3D CT-scan reconstruction. *European Journal of Cardio-Thoracic Surgery.* 2006;30:384-385.
8. Thompson RC, Thibodeau JM, Ramza BM. Computed tomography angiographic demonstration of collateral circulation in superior vena cava syndrome. *J Cardiovasc Comput Tomogr.* 2008;2:57-58.
9. Aryana A, Sobota KD, Esterbrooks DJ, Gelbman AI. Superior vena cava syndrome induced by endocardial defibrillator and pacemaker leads. *Am J Cardiol.* 2007;99(12):1765-1767.
10. Huntington GS, McLure CFW. The development of veins in the domestic cat (felis domestica) with especial reference 1) to the share taken by the supracardinal vein in the development of the post-cava and azygos vein and 2) to the interpretation of the variant conditions of the postcava and its tributaries, as found in the adult. *Anat Rec.* 1920;20:1-29.
11. Philips E. Embryology, normal anatomy, and anomalies. In: Ferris EJ, Hipona FA, Kahn PC, Philips E, Shapiro JH, eds. *Venography of the Inferior Vena Cava and Its Branches.* Baltimore, MD: Williams & Wilkins; 1969:1-32.
12. Davachi AA, Thomas J, Dale WA, Perry FA, Michael OB. Acute spontaneous rupture of an arteriosclerotic aneurysm into an isolated left-sided inferior vena cava. *Am J Cardiol.* 1965;15:416-418.

30 Noncoronary/Noncardiac Lesions

Key Points

- Cardiac CT scans may encounter a wide spectrum of noncoronary/noncardiac lesions, in both the chest and upper abdomen, of widely ranging clinical relevance.
- The incidence of noncoronary/noncardiac findings is significant.
- Review of the study by a radiologist is necessary, therefore, to ensure accurate reporting of noncoronary lesions and so that an appropriate management plan can be instituted.
- Systematic scrutiny of noncardiac structures can offer alternative causes for the patient's symptoms.
- The notion that cardiac CT scanning provides a measure of noncardiac "screening" should be discouraged, because the entire chest is not imaged and the detection of noncardiac lesions by electron beam CT or coronary CT angiography is more a matter of chance than design.

DETECTION OF INCIDENTAL NONCORONARY CARDIAC AND EXTRACARDIAC LESIONS

Coronary CT angiography (CTA) may encounter both significant and nonsignificant noncoronary cardiac lesions. An overview of these lesions is presented in Table 30-1; their treatment has been reviewed in the preceding chapters of this book. An overview of significant and nonsignificant extracardiac findings is presented in Table 30-2; their treatment is discussed in this chapter. The term "incidental" for the discovery of pathology that was not within the intended purview of the coronary artery examination is, of course, of cold comfort to the patient.

Cardiac-directed CT studies detect noncardiac pathology of significance or potential relevance in 5% to18% of examinations[1-6] and nonsignificant noncardiac findings in 40% to 60%.[3,7] The range of both these potential findings is vast, as is the potential significance of both. The high incidence of detection of noncardiac pathologies is one of the principal rationales behind having a trained radiologist read, co-read, or over-read a cardiac CT (CCT) study.[8] The two large series that have been reported to date arose from calcium scoring by electron beam CT (EBCT) series. A recent large study[6] retrospectively reviewing 1764 patients who had undergone CCT studies demonstrated a significant difference in the presence of incidental and clinically significant findings in patients studied for coronary artery bypass grafting and other indications for CTA compared with patients referred only for calcium scoring, with 18% of patients in the former group having extracardiac findings that required further follow-up.

All studies to date have been observational. No study has been properly structured to address the influence on outcome according to the identification of noncoronary and noncardiac lesions.

CT scans of the aorta detect an even higher percentage of noncardiac pathologies, because in those scans the abdomen also is imaged.

The term "incidental" is regrettably used to describe noncoronary/noncardiac findings: it is hard to understand what is incidental about identifying primary or metastatic malignancies of lung, esophagus, breast, or other organs; aortic aneurysms; pulmonary emboli; or other serious disorders.

Whether or not incidental detection of noncardiac findings constitutes any real form of screening is unproven, unknown, and unlikely. Detection by CCT of noncardiac lesions fundamentally amounts to detection by accident, not methodologic screening by design.[4,8] Unless the entire lung fields are included within the field of view (a far wider field of view than is standard for non–bypass graft/coronary/cardiac studies), pulmonary imaging as a part of CCT will always be incomplete, and inappropriate to categorize as a screening examination.

The detection of noncardiac lesions by EBCT or CCT remains of unproven utility in improving clinical outcomes.

Horton et al.[4] reported on 1326 patients who had undergone EBCT (3-mm slices) and found that the incidence of noncardiac pathologies detected that required follow-up imaging or further investigation was 7.8% (Table 30-3).

TABLE 30-1 Cardiac Noncoronary Findings

Myocardium	
Left ventricular hyperplasia	Regional fatty metaplasia
Diverticula	Regional calcification
Crypts	Mural thrombus
Signs of prior infarction	
Regional thinning	
Valvular	
Aortic valve	Mitral
Bicuspid	Annular calcification
Calcification	Valvular
Stenosis	
Pericardial	
Effusion	Calcification
Simple	Trauma
Complex	Infection
Thickening	Asbestosis
Infection	Cyst
Tumor	
Congenital	
Patent foramen ovale	Ventricular septal defect
Nonadherent IAS	Ventricular septal aneurysm
Atrial septal defect	

TABLE 30-2 Noncardiac Findings

Mediastinal	
Anterior	
Thymus	Lymphoma
Thymoma	Thyroid
Teratoma	Metastasis
Middle	
Lymphoma	Vascular: aortic dissection
Infectious	IMH
Tumor	Penetrating ulcer
Sarcoid	Aneurysm
Esophageal	Aortitis
Esophagitis	Vascular: pulmonary arteries
Carcinoma	Embolism
Hiatal hernia	Aneurysm
Pericardial	Vascular: other lesions
Effusion	Patent ductus arteriosus
Thickening	PLSVC
Calcification	
Tumor	
Posterior	
Neurogenic	
Aortic aneurysm	
Lymphadenopathy	

Continued

TABLE 30-2 Noncardiac Findings—cont'd

Lungs
Nodules/Masses
Infection
Neoplasia
Non-Nodular Lesions
Consolidation
Pneumonia
Tumor
Bronchiectastsis
Infection
Congenital
Emphysema
Chest Wall
Bones
Sclerosis (degenerative, metastatic)
Fractures
Destruction (metastasis, infection)
Lymph Nodes
Internal mammary
Axillary
Supraclavicular
Breast Tissue
Nodules/masses
Calcification
Soft Tissue
Abscess
Hematoma
Tumor
Pleura
Effusion
Simple
Complex
Thickening
Infection
Tumor
Calcification
Trauma
Infection
Asbestosis
Upper Abdominal
Gastrointestinal Tract
Hiatus hernia
Tumor
Liver
Cyst
Nodule
Adrenal
Nodule

TABLE 30-3 Incidence of Noncardiac Pathologies Detected

PATHOLOGY	PATIENTS (n = 1326)
Noncalcified lung nodules < 1 cm	53
Noncalcified lung nodules ≥ 1 cm	12
Infiltrates	24
Indeterminate liver lesions	7
Sclerotic bone lesions	2
Breast abnormalities	2
Polycystic liver disease	1
Esophageal thickening	1
Ascites	1

Data from Horton KM, Post WS, Blumenthal RS, Fishman EK. Prevalence of significant noncardiac findings on electron-beam computed tomography coronary artery calcium screening examinations. *Circulation.* 2002;106(5):532-534.

TABLE 30-4 Incidence of Accidental Pathologies Detected in Electron Beam CT

PATHOLOGY	PREVALENCE (%)
Cardiac structures/pericardium	32
Pericardial	
Thickening	4.5
Effusion	1.6
Calcification	0.9
Cardiac	
Mitral calcification	7.6
Aortic valve	13
Left atrial thrombi	
Myxoma	
Aortic disease	23
Calcification	
Ectasia	0.2
Aneurysm	0.6
Type A dissection	0.06
Lung disease	20
Further diagnostic testing	11
Specific therapy initiated	1.2

Data from Hunold P, Schmermund A, Seibel RM, Gronemeyer DH, Erbel R. Prevalence and clinical significance of accidental findings in electron-beam tomographic scans for coronary artery calcification. *Eur Heart J.* 2001;22(18):1748-1758.

Hunold et al.[1] described a 53% incidence of accidental pathologies (2061 lesions) detected among 1812 patients who had undergone EBCT (Table 30-4).

Schragin et al.[5] reviewed 1356 EBCT scans over 2 years and established a 20.5% incidence of one or more noncardiac findings among a population with only a 13% incidence of smoking. Findings without follow-up recommendations (n = 221)

TABLE 30-5 Incidence of Having One or More Non-Cardiac Findings

PATHOLOGY	NO. OF PATIENTS
Findings without follow-up recommendations (n = 221)	
Pulmonary scarring	63
Granuloma	39
Emphysema/bullae	29
Nonsuspicious nodules	28
Pleural disease	21
Pulmonary fibrosis	5
Atelectasis	8
Calcified lymph nodes	6
Lung cysts	4
Bronchiectasis	2
Small infiltrate	2
Hepatomegaly	2
Dilated aorta	1
Fissure thickening	1
57 patients were recommended to have follow-up CT scans	
Pulmonary nodules	46
Consolidation and infiltrations	3
Fibrosis and interstitial disease	3
Hilar adenopathy	2
Large pulmonary mass	1
Thoracic aneurysm	1
Liver mass	1

Data from Schragin JG, Weissfeld JL, Edmundowicz D, Strollo DC, Fuhrman CR. Non-cardiac findings on coronary electron beam computed tomography scanning. *J Thorac Imaging.* 2004;19(2):82-86.

and recommendations for follow-up CTA scans are shown in Table 30-5. There was one reported death during follow-up that included a cancer identified by EBCT; that death was attributed to renal cell carcinoma.

Onuma et al.[3] reviewed noncardiac findings among 503 patients who underwent 16- or 64-slice CCT and found that

- Noncardiac findings were detected in 58% of patients (n = 292).
- A total of 346 noncardiac findings were detected in 292 patients.
- Significant noncardiac findings were noted in 23% of patients.
- Malignancies were found in 0.8% of patients (n = 4).

As with many examples of low-pretest probability imaging, the detection of noncoronary/noncardiac findings by CCT scanning leads to repeat imaging, generally with CT scanning, thereby beginning to accrue radiation exposure and risk.

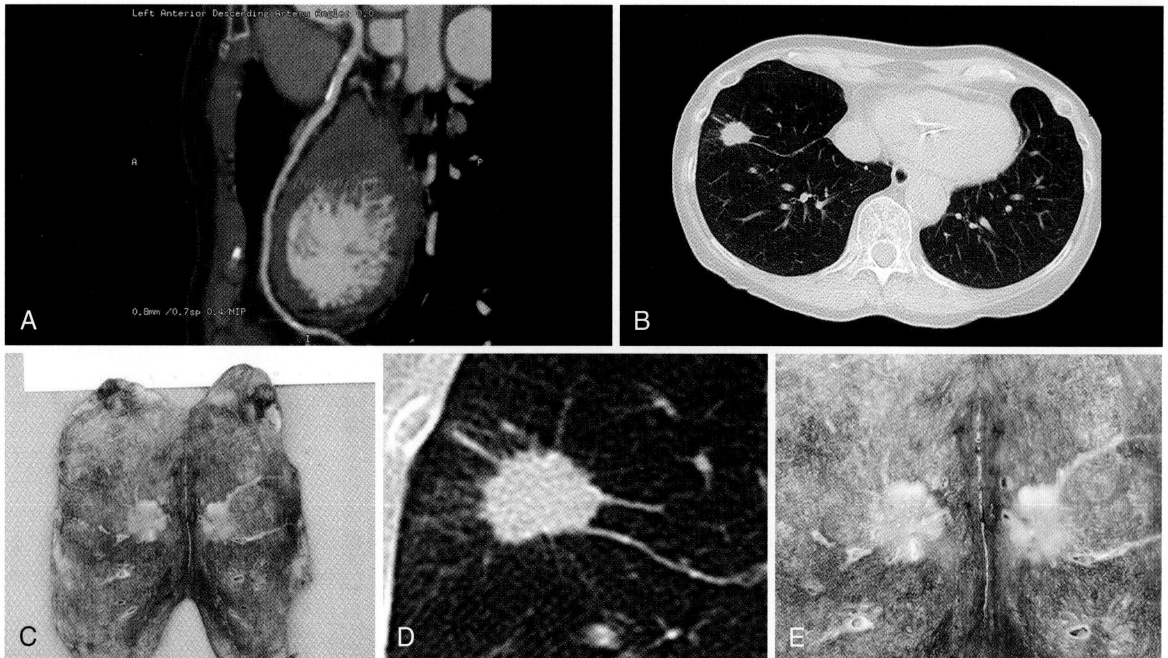

Figure 30-1. Cardiac CT scan in a 52-year-old woman being sent for valve surgery. CCT demonstrated no obstructive coronary artery disease (**A**). There is a 3-cm speculated mass in the right middle lobe laterally involving the minor fissure and with linear extension toward the lateral pleura (**B–D**). Background lung demonstrates mild emphysematous changes consistent with the prior history of smoking. **C** and **E,** The middle lobe pathology specimen showing the speculated shape and linear extensions.

Machaalany et al.[2] described a 1% incidence of clinically significant findings and a 7% incidence of "indeterminate" findings among a low-risk, largely outpatient (98%) population who were followed for 3 years. Over this short period of follow-up, noncardiac and cancer death did not differ between patients with and without "indeterminate findings." Evaluation of clinically significant findings and indeterminate findings were not standardized. One death occurred secondary to an investigation of an indeterminate finding. High costs were associated with investigating indeterminate findings (US $83,000/Canadian $57,000).[2]

The utility and appropriateness of large-field versus small-field reconstructions and over-reading is a debated topic.[9] Compared with large-field reconstruction, small-field reconstructions lead to lower detection of possibly significant findings, and a far lower rate of subsequent investigation.

LUNG LESIONS

Pulmonary Nodules and Masses

Pulmonary nodules are the most common incidental finding on CCT, reported in 10% to 12% of studies[3,6] (Figs. 30-1 through 30-3). Important features of a pulmonary nodule to evaluate include:

- **Size**: Guidelines for follow-up for small pulmonary nodules based on size have been presented and incorporated by most radiology departments.[10]
- **Margin**: The presence of an irregular or speculated margin should raise concern for an aggressive lesion.[11] Small nodules associated with ground-glass densities and a "tree-in -bud" configuration are commonly seen in infectious conditions such as pneumonia and represent impaction of the bronchiolar lumen secondary to pus, mucus, or fluid.
- **Internal characteristics**: The presence of dense central calcification is more likely to reflect a nodule secondary to prior granulomatous infection. Calcified granulomas can be multiple. One rare element in the differential diagnosis for multiple calcified nodules would be metastatic disease from primaries such as osteosarcoma. "Popcorn" type calcifications, especially in association with intralesional fat, are commonly seen in hamartomas, a benign lung lesion.

Non-nodular Lung Disease

Focal Consolidation

Focal consolidation is seen most commonly in the setting of lobar pneumonia. Other diagnostic considerations include:

- Atypical pulmonary edema, which, especially on a background of emphysematous lung disease, can mimic the appearance of pneumonia
- Pulmonary hemorrhage
- Bronchoalveolar cell carcinoma, which can present as a focus of airspace disease with air bronchograms

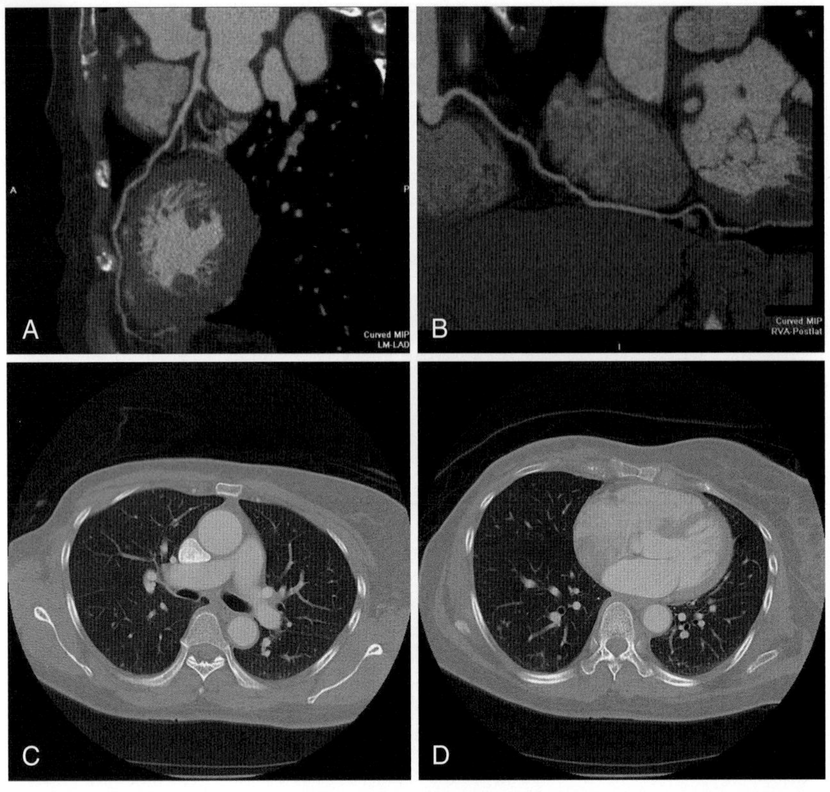

Figure 30-2. Composite images from a cardiac CT study to rule out coronary artery disease. No significant underlying coronary artery disease was noted. Multiple small pulmonary nodules are seen scattered diffusely in both lungs. A subsequent diagnosis of melanoma was obtained, with pulmonary nodules likely representing metastatic disease.

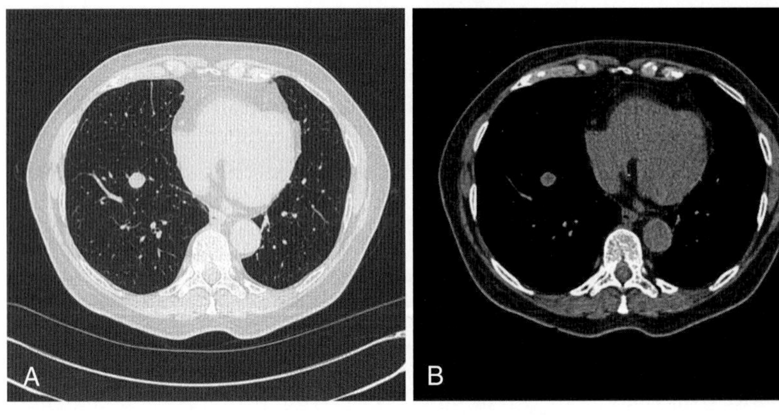

Figure 30-3. Images from a cardiac CT calcium score study. **A,** The image has been reconstructed using a lung coronal, with lung windows. A 1.1-cm nodule is seen in the left lower lobe. **B,** On the mediastinal window, an area of low attenuation is seen within the center of this nodule. No definite fatty attenuation or calcification is seen. Tissue sampling of this nodule subsequently provided the diagnosis of a benign pulmonary hamartoma.

It is important, therefore, to follow up on these findings. In most cases, follow-up chest radiographs of the opacity, until it has resolved, are sufficient.

For images of lung consolidation, see Figure 30-4.

Bronchiectasis

Bronchiectasis is defined as a localized, irreversible dilatation of part of the bronchial tree (Figs. 30-5 and 30-6). On CT imaging it appears as dilated thick-walled airways, usually extending toward the periphery of the lung. Bronchiectasis has many causes, both congenital and acquired. When it is detected on CCT in an adult patient, the presence of bronchiectasis should raise concern for an underlying infective process.

Emphysema

Because CCT scans typically include approximately 70% of lung volume, they afford some measure of detection of emphysema. A substudy of The Multi-Ethnic Study of Atherosclerosis (MESA) Lung Study, defining moderate to severe emphysema as voxel counts no greater than 910 HU, established the following[12]:

- CCT scans for coronary calcium yielded high interscan correlation of detection of emphysema ($r = 0.92$ to 0.95; mean difference –0.05% (–8.3% to 8.4%).

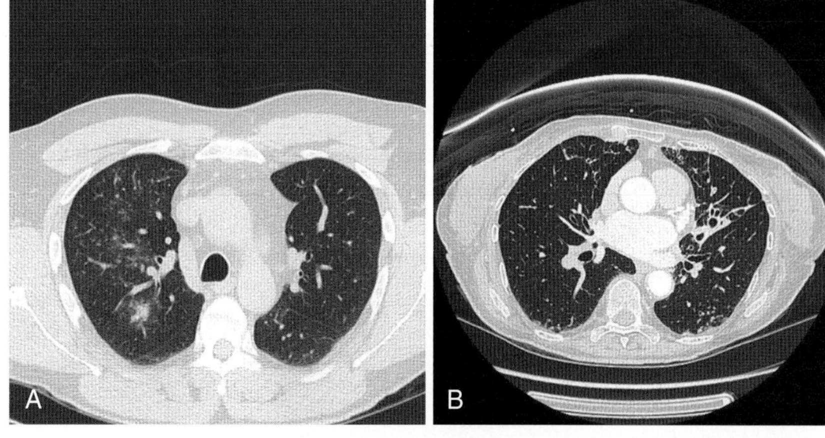

Figure 30-4. Images from two different patients who had cardiac CT studies for atypical chest pain and shortness of breath. **A,** This patient has a small focus of consolidation within the posterior segment of the right upper lobe. Ground-glass density in the right upper lobe is seen anterior to it. This was identified on follow-up chest radiography, and subsequently resolved. A presumptive diagnosis of a resolved pneumonia was given. **B,** In the second patient, mild bronchiectatic change is seen within the lingula, and small nodules are noted posteriorly in the left lower lobe. These likely reflect postinflammatory changes.

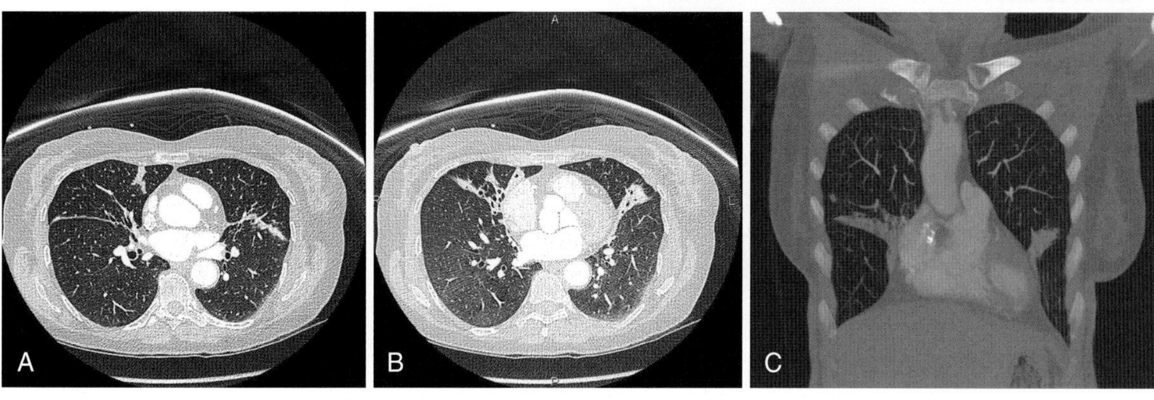

Figure 30-5. A 57-year-old woman with a history of progressive shortness of breath and prior right coronary artery stenting. A cardiac CT was performed to evaluate the status of the right coronary artery stent. An incidental finding on the cardiac CT is the presence of a moderate amount of bronchiectasis with associated segmental lung collapse within the right middle lobe and lingula. The patient subsequently was diagnosed with community-acquired mycobacterial infection. The imaging features are typical for this condition.

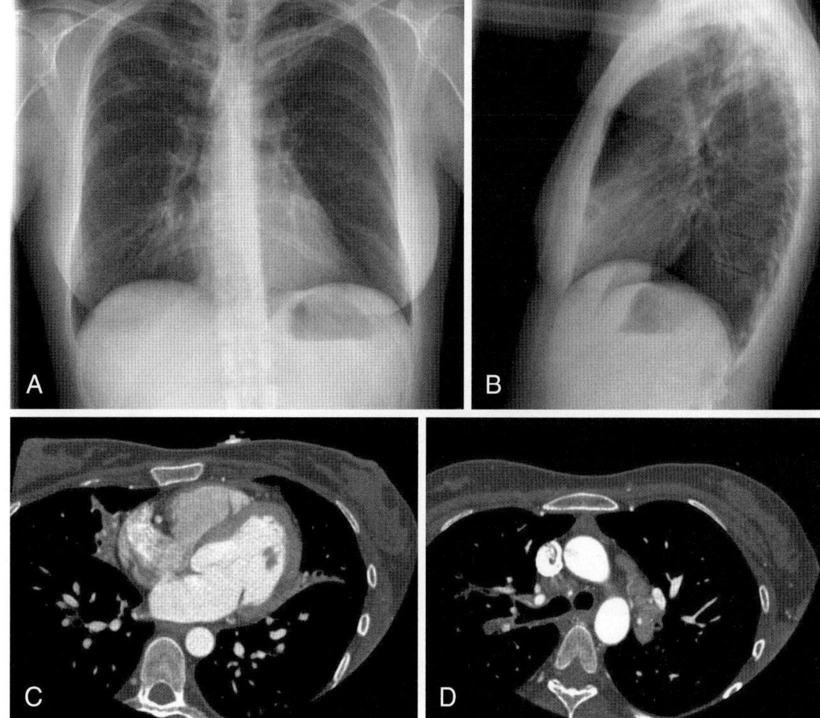

Figure 30-6. A 30-year-old woman with pregnancy-related coronary dissections underwent a CT coronary angiogram in follow-up. Her chest radiographs (**A** and **B**) had revealed bronchiectatic changes (note the dilated bronchus to the right upper lobe and cuffing of the bronchus due to mucosal edema). The CCT exam (**C** and **D**) revealed periaortic mediastinal adenopathy and bronchiectasis. Note in particular the consolidation in the medial segment of the right middle lobe against the right atrium. Investigations confirmed a cystic fibrosis variant.

- Measurements from EBCT scanners and CCT scanners yielded comparable results: mean difference –0.09% (–5.1% to 3.3%).
- Emphysema measurements were highly correlated between CCT scans and full-chest CT scans ($r = 0.93$) and demonstrated "reasonable" agreement: mean difference 2.2% (–9.2 to 13.8%).

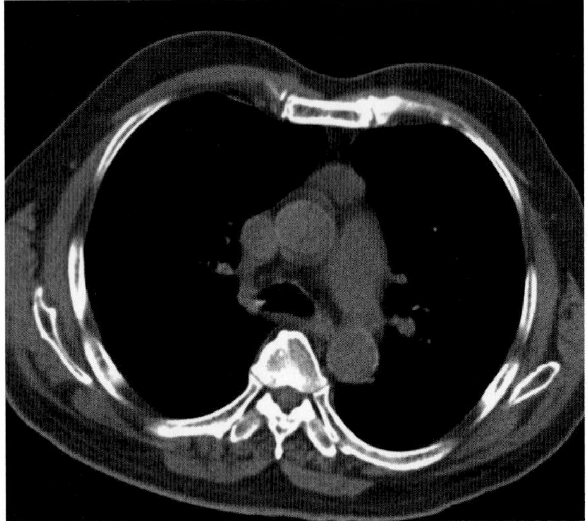

Figure 30-7. Thymoma is present anterior to the aorta and pulmonary artery.

MEDIASTINAL DISEASE

Anterior Mediastinum

Thymus

On CT, the thymus is a bilobed triangular structure (Fig. 30-7). It is located in the anterior mediastinum, anterior to the descending aorta. The size of the normal thymus gland varies with age, ranging from a mean of 1.1 ± 0.4 cm between the ages of 6 and 19 years to 0.5 ± 0.3 cm for patients over the age of 50 years. Remnant thymic tissue appears as small foci of low attenuation and soft tissue attenuation on a background of more abundant fat. A variety of diseases are associated with the thymus gland, including thymic hyperplasia, thymoma, and thyroid carcinoma. CT images of thymic hyperplasia demonstrate a diffuse, symmetrically enlarged thymus gland. If enlargement is asymmetric, the differential should include atypical thymic hyperplasia versus thymoma.

Middle Mediastinum

Lymph Nodes

Normal mediastinal lymph nodes have a smooth, ovoid contour, may have a central fatty hilum, and usually measure less than 1 cm in the short axis (Figs. 30-8 and 30-9). Mild lymphadenopathy can be seen as a reactive process to an underlying

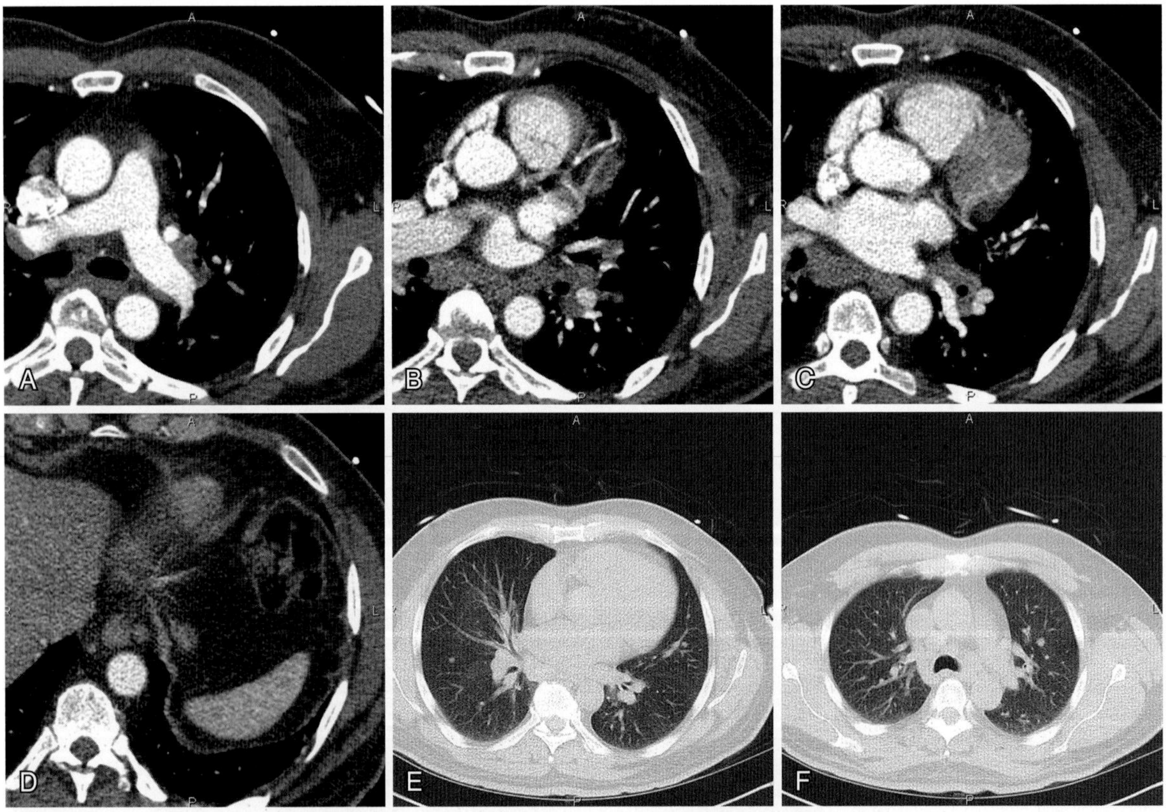

Figure 30-8. Multiple images from a cardiac CT study in a patient with atypical chest pain. Lymphadenopathy is noted in multiple stations within the thorax. Bilateral hilar and subcarinal lymphadenopathy is noted. Periesophageal lymphadenopathy is present at the level of the gastroesophageal junction. The lungs demonstrate multiple small pulmonary nodules and a mild increase in interstitial markings. The patient subsequently was diagnosed with sarcoidosis.

pneumonia and usually resolves post-treatment. Calcified lymph nodes most likely are due to a prior granulomatous infection, usually from a fungal or mycobacterial source. Other nonneoplastic causes for mediastinal lymphadenopathy include sarcoidosis, which often demonstrates bilateral hilar lymphadenopathy in conjunction with mediastinal lymphadenopathy. Bulky or low-attenuation lymph nodes should raise concern for malignancy. This may reflect metastatic disease from within the thorax, as well as remotely from other parts of the body. Lymphoma commonly involves the mediastinum as well as other node stations within the thorax, such as the internal mammary chain, retrocrural region, and axillae.

Sarcoidosis

Lymphadenopathy on CT imaging of the heart or chest most commonly is seen in the paratracheal, subcarinal, and bilateral hilar lymph node stations. When lymphadenopathy and this pattern are seen, pulmonary parenchymal disease also should be sought. Characteristic parenchymal lesions include pulmonary nodules, typically in a peribronchovascular pattern or along the fissures.

Vascular Lesions

Aortic Lesions. Aortic aneurysms are a common incidental mediastinal finding.[6] They are most commonly seen in the ascending aorta. If the patient presents with an acute chest pain syndrome, evaluation for aortic dissection, intramural hematoma, and penetrating ulcers also should be undertaken. (See Chapter 26.)

Pulmonary Arterial Lesions. Pulmonary emboli, while an uncommon incidental finding, can be identified by a partial or complete filling defect within an opacified pulmonary artery. The pulmonary arteries usually are not the target vessel for peak enhancement in a CCT study, so care must be taken not to mistake partial mixing of unopacified blood for a pulmonary embolism.

For images of pulmonary artery lesions, see Figure 30-10.

Other Lesions. For images of other vascular lesions, see Figure 30-11 and **Video 30-1.**

Esophageal Lesions

On typical CCT studies, only the mid- to distal esophagus usually is visualized. Air within the esophageal lumen is the common, normal finding on a CT study. Distinguishing between mucosal and submucosal abnormalities on the CCT, where esophageal barium paste is not routinely administered, can be difficult. Submucosal lesions such as gastrointestinal stromal tumors, leiomyomas, and lipomas usually are well defined. An irregular masslike thickening or stricture-like

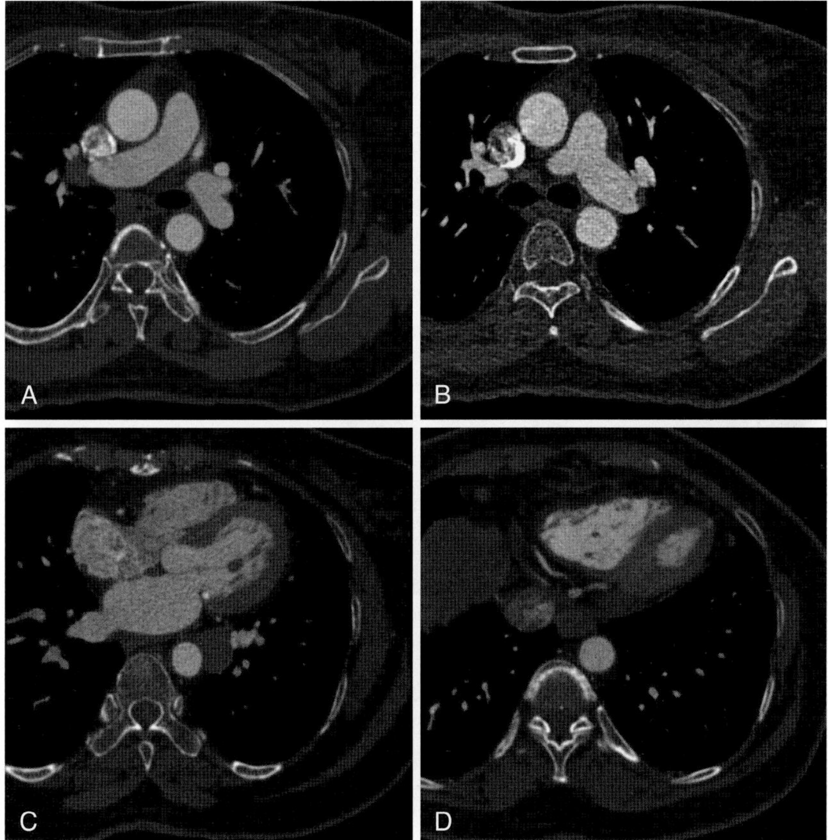

Figure 30-9. A 51-year-old woman presented with atypical chest pain and nonspecific changes on echocardiography. A cardiac CT study found no evidence of coronary artery disease. Small- to medium-volume lymph nodes were seen within the thorax. **A,** A 1-cm right hilar lymph node. **B,** A small lymph node seen through the aortico-pulmonary window. **C,** A 1.4-cm lymph node seen in a left periaortic location. **D,** A 0.8-cm right cardiophrenic angle lymph node. Tissue sampling revealed a diagnosis of lymphoma.

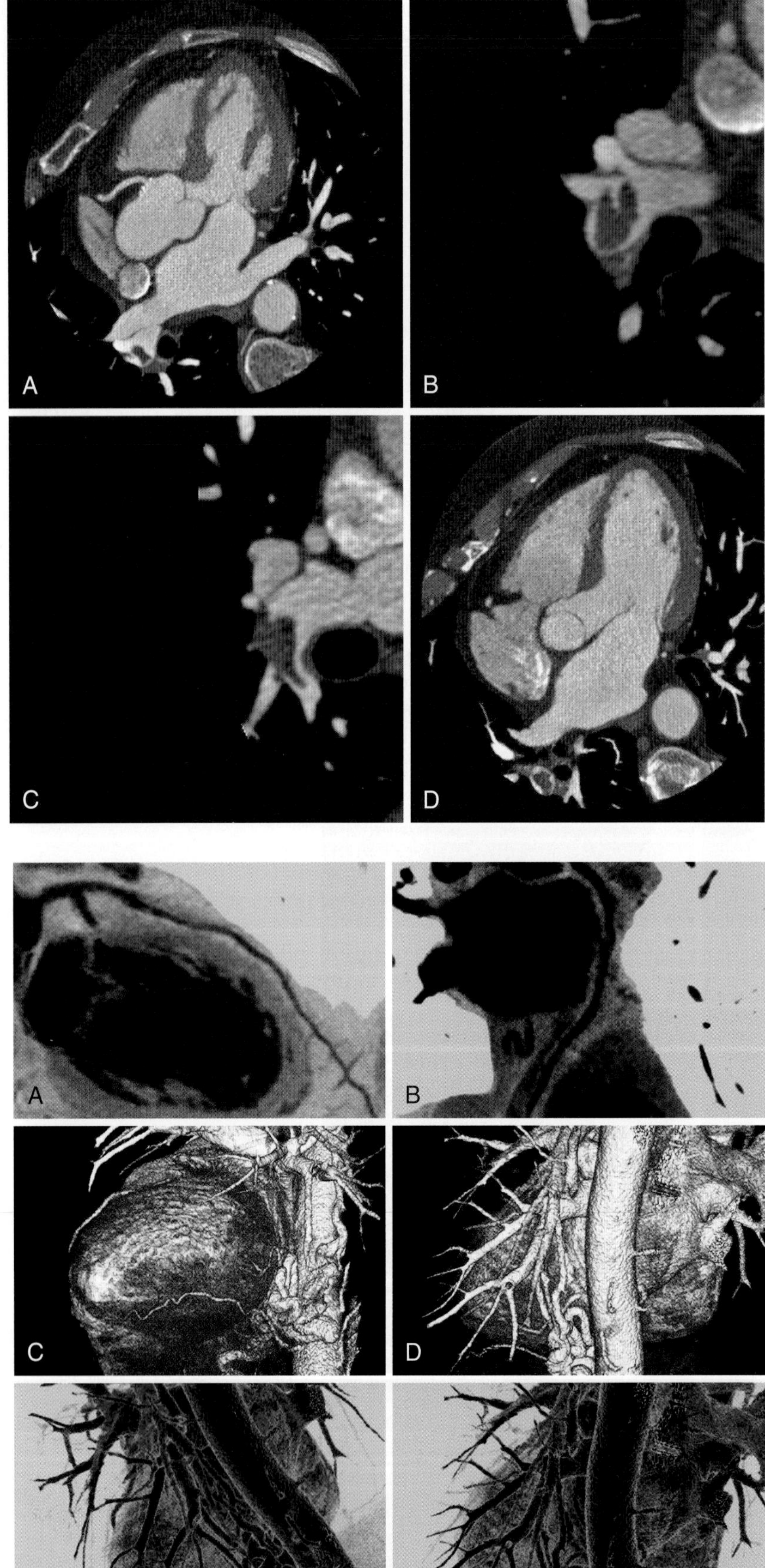

Figure 30-10. A 57-year-old patient presented with chest pain and nonspecific ECG changes. A cardiac CT study was done to rule out coronary artery disease. Composite images from the cardiac CT study demonstrate an unexpected finding of multiple filling defects within both pulmonary arteries, more so on the right. These are typical for multiple pulmonary emboli.

Figure 30-11. Composite images from a cardiac CT study in a patient with atypical chest pain. Inverted coronary CT images demonstrate normal-appearing coronary arteries. There is a mid-intramyocardial bridge in the proximal to mid–left anterior descending artery. A large aortopulmonary collateral with multiple tortuous vessels extends from the aorta to the left lower lobe pulmonary artery. No evidence of underlying pulmonary sequestration was present. The aortopulmonary collateral was believed to be an isolated congenital anomaly. See **Video 30-1.**

formation of the esophagus would raise more concern for a malignant process. Small (<1 cm) short-axis lymph nodes are nonspecific, but would be more likely to be reactive. Large irregularly shaped lymph nodes, especially when associated with irregular esophageal thickening, should raise the possibility of an underlying neoplastic process.

For images of esophageal lesions, see Figures 30-12 through 30-14.

Pericardial Lesions

See Chapter 17 for discussion and images of pericardial lesions.

PLEURA

Pleural Effusions

Pleural effusions are commonly identified on CCT. Simple transudative effusions demonstrate uniform low attenuation (<20 HU), and are commonly seen in congestive heart failure.

Pleural Thickening

Focal regions of pleural thickening or calcification can be seen from prior infection, trauma, or asbestos exposure. Pleural enhancement post–contrast administration, as well as pleural nodularity or thickening, should raise concern for possible infection or malignant involvement.

Pleural Calcification

Pleural calcification usually is related to either post-inflammatory, post-traumatic disease, or asbestos-related pleural disease. Post-inflammatory/infectious pleural calcification usually is seen as an asymmetric, occasionally diffuse, thickened peel of calcified pleura. Asbestos-related pleural disease can be focal and plaque-like, or more diffuse. Plaques can vary in thickness from several millimeters to several centimeters and may or may not be calcified. Asbestos-related calcified plaques most often affect the parietal and diaphragmatic pleura and tend to spare the costophrenic sulci and apices.

For images of pleural lesions, see Figure 30-15 and **Video 30-2.**

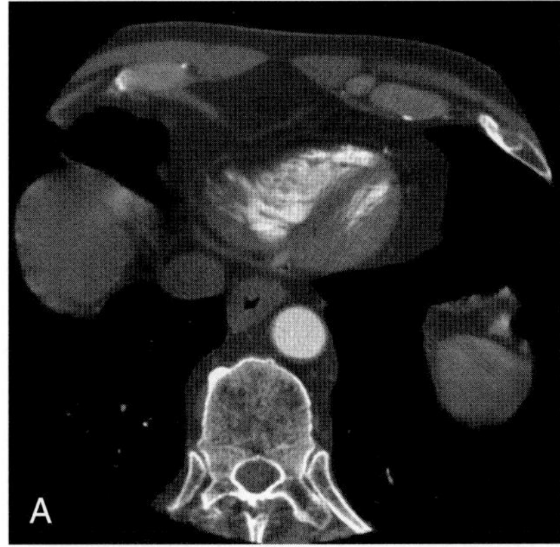

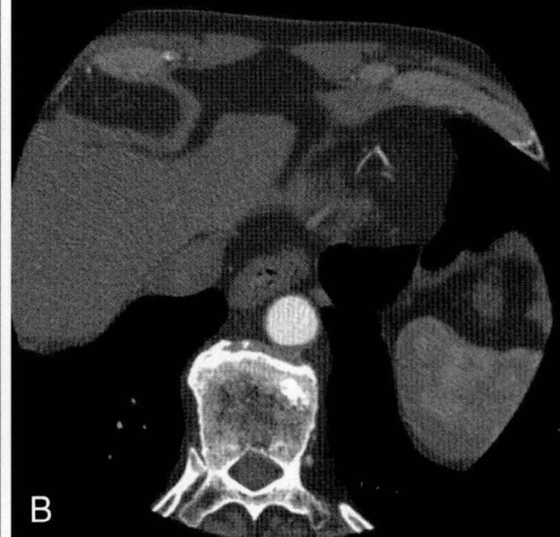

Figure 30-12. A 69-year-old male with chest pain. Circumferential distal esophageal thickening with small periesophageal lymph nodes. The diagnosis was esophageal carcinoma.

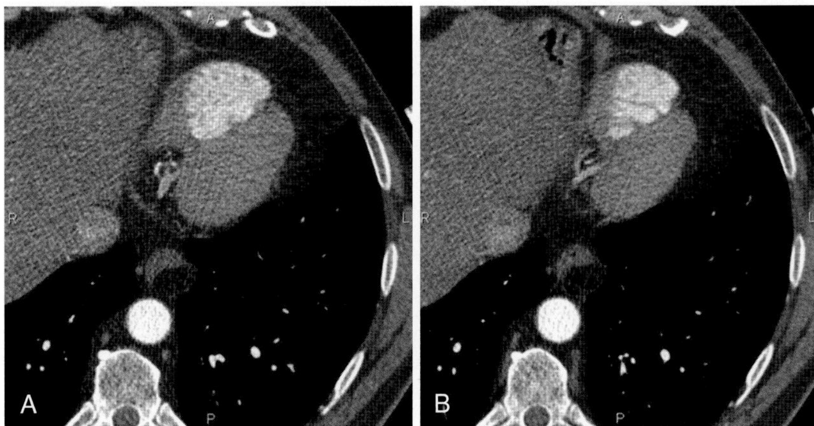

Figure 30-13. Two axial images from a cardiac CT study demonstrate an incidental finding of a small esophageal lipoma.

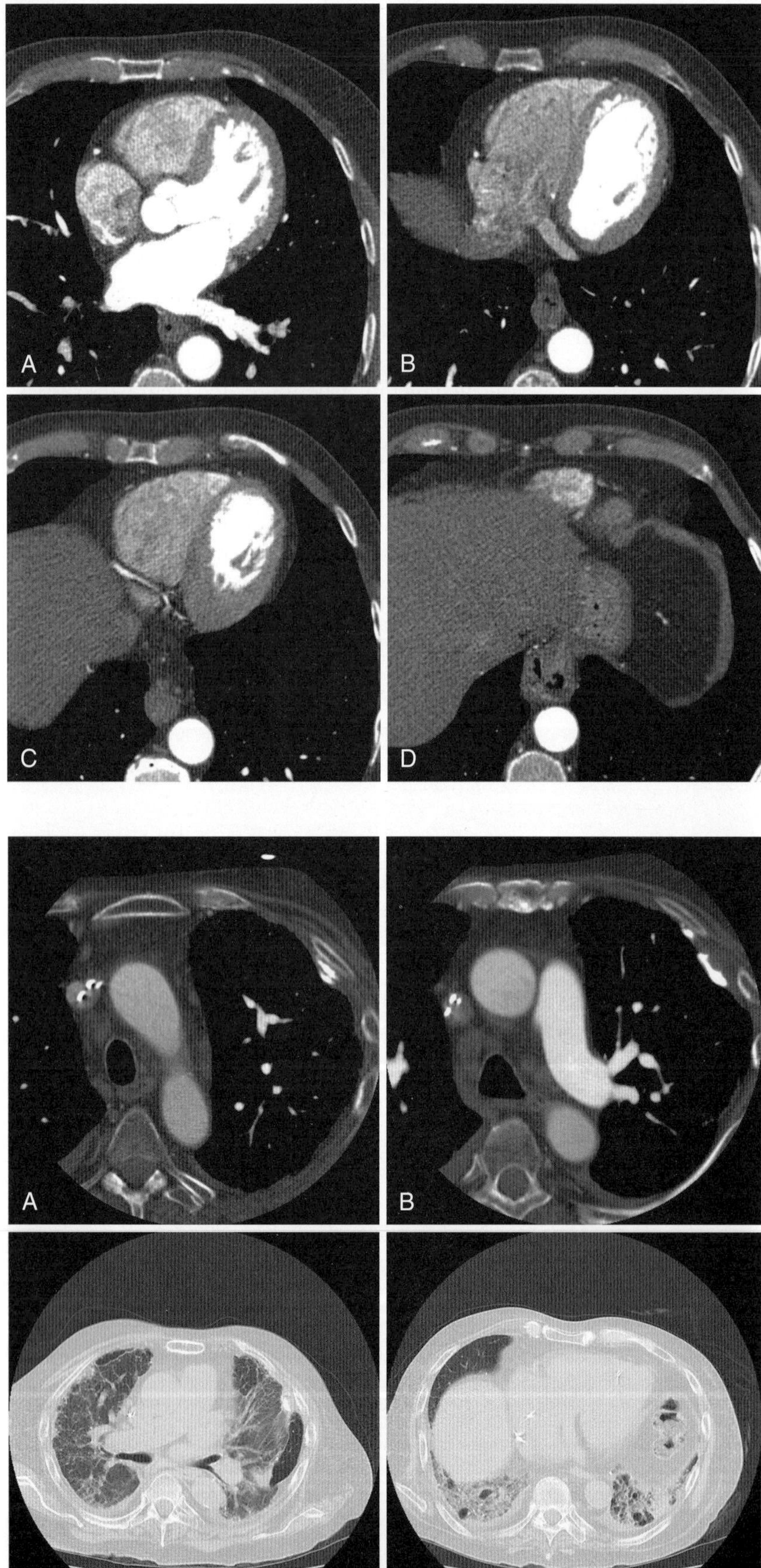

Figure 30-14. Multiple contrast-enhanced cardiac CT images in a 52-year-old male with atypical chest pain and indeterminate maximum projection intensity study. These images demonstrate moderate diffuse thickening of the esophagus. Small periesophageal lymph nodes are seen anterior to the esophagus, which are likely reactive. **D,** A moderate-sized hiatus hernia. The patient went on to have a gastroenterology evaluation. The diagnosis was reflux esophagitis.

Figure 30-15. Composite images from a cardiac CT study demonstrate calcified and noncalcified pleural plaques, in conjunction with marked areas of underlying interstitial fibrosis, worse in both lower lobes. These findings are consistent with prior asbestos exposure, and asbestos-related pleural and lung disease. See **Video 30-2.**

CHEST WALL

A wide variety of pathologic processes can involve the chest wall, including congenital, inflammatory/infectious, and neoplastic processes. The most common congenital deformity of the sternum is a pectus excavatum, where the sternum is depressed so that the ribs protrude more anteriorly on each side of the sternum than the sternum itself. A pectus carinatum deformity occurs when the sternum has an abnormal anterior extension. This deformity can be seen in patients with underlying cyanotic congenital heart disease. De novo infectious processes of the chest wall are unusual, but can be seen spontaneously, and in the setting of an immunosuppressed patient. Postoperative infections are more common, and can be seen on CCT studies in relation to a median sternotomy, where mediastinitis, osteomyelitis, and sternal dehiscence can occur. See Figure 30-16. Neoplasms of the chest wall are very uncommon. The most common soft tissue neoplasm is a lipoma. These are generally benign and do not require any treatment unless they become large. The most common malignant tumors are generally fibrosarcomas. Other soft tissue tumors involving the chest wall include neurogenic tumors and hemangiomas.

For images of chest wall lesions, see Figure 30-17.

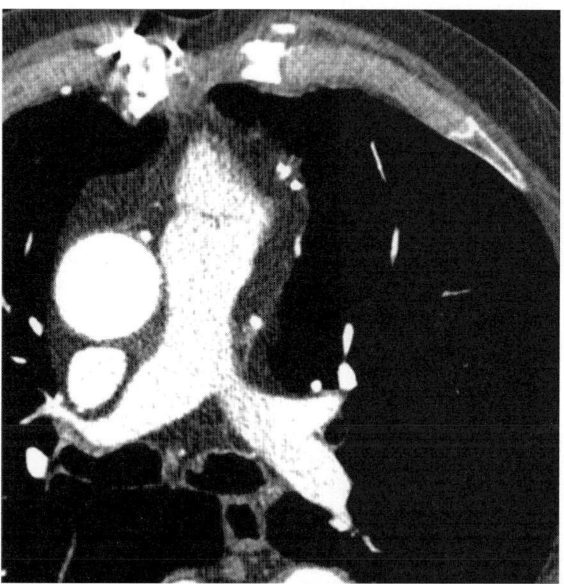

Figure 30-16. A single image from a cardiac CT study performed to evaluate bypass graft patency. On this study, dehiscence of the sternum is noted, with the lack of bony union from the patient's prior sternotomy.

UPPER ABDOMEN

Gastrointestinal Tract

More than 50% of the general population over the age of 50 have a hiatal hernia.[13] This is, therefore, a very common finding on CCT studies and may be associated with esophageal thickening in patients with gastroesophageal reflux disease. Hiatal hernias extend into the middle mediastinum, and on CT imaging often appear as a large heterogeneous mass posterior to the heart and anterior to the aorta. Pockets of air may commonly be seen within a collapsed esophageal lumen. This is a normal finding in the absence of any other associated abnormality.

For images of upper GI tract lesions, see Figures 30-18 and 30-19.

Liver Lesions

In most CCT studies, a small portion of the upper abdomen is imaged. Slice locations may change between the noncontrast calcium score study and the CTA acquisition, which precludes comparison of a liver lesion before and after contrast administration. Additionally, because the CTA is obtained in an arterial phase, it often is not possible to properly characterize a given lesion. The most common incidental liver finding is a liver cyst, which typically is circular, demonstrates a sharp margin, and is of uniform low density. An abnormal region of liver enhancement can be difficult to characterize and may require further follow-up with an ultrasound. For images of liver lesions, see Figures 30-20 through 30-24.

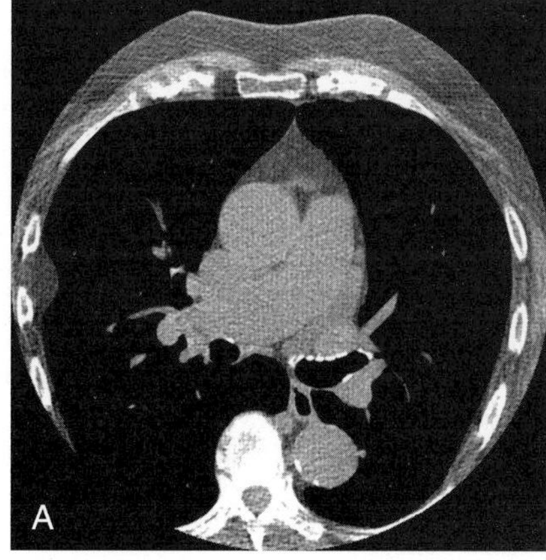

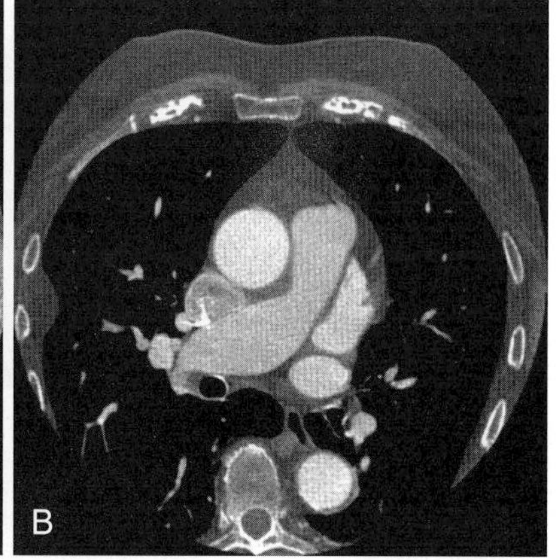

Figure 30-17. A 48-year-old woman with chest pain and an abnormal nuclear medicine study. **A,** The noncontrast calcium score study demonstrates a focal area of low attenuation within the right lateral intercostal space. The Hounsfield unit measurement of this lesion was –40. Its smooth rounded contour has a configuration more in keeping with a chest wall/extrapleural lesion. **B,** No enhancement was seen during the CT angiography study. No vessels are seen within the lesion. The diagnosis was a chest wall/extrapleural lipoma.

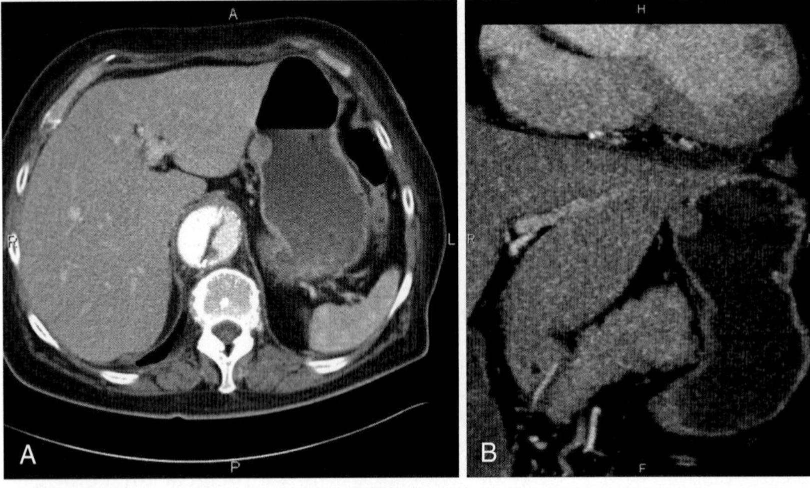

Figure 30-18. Images from a cardiac CT study for aortic dissection. These images demonstrate an aortic dissection in the upper abdominal aorta. Incidental note was made of a soft tissue nodule within the lesser curvature of gastric fundus. This was subsequently proven to be a gastrointestinal stromal tumor.

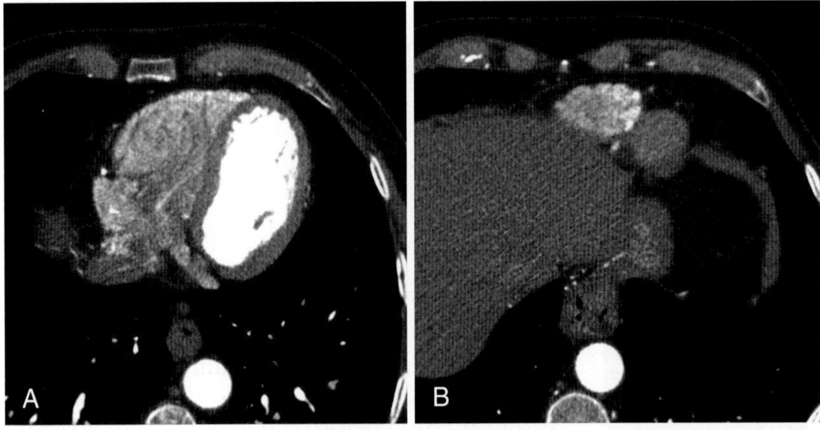

Figure 30-19. Two images from a cardiac CT study in a 52-year-old man with atypical chest pain. **A,** Moderate thickening of the lower esophagus. A small 6-mm periesophageal lymph node is noted just anterior to the esophagus. **B,** A moderate-sized hiatal hernia. Further evaluation with an upper gastrointestinal tract series and endoscopy revealed moderate reflux and esophagitis, but no evidence of malignancy.

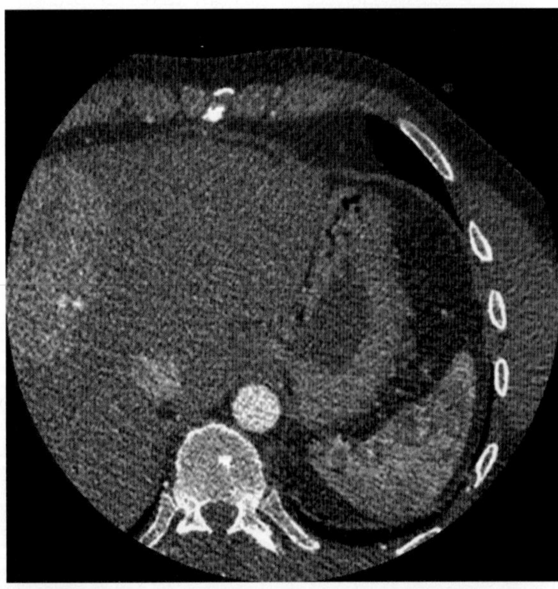

Figure 30-20. On the inferiormost slice of this cardiac CT study, a large arterially enhancing mass is seen within the liver. This likely spans segment 4A, and extends into segment 2 of the liver. Two arterial enhancing vessels are seen within the periphery of the lesion. On this single phase of enhancement, the lesion is nonspecific. Given its arterial enhancing characteristic, the differential would include focal nodular hyperplasia, atypical hepatocellular carcinoma, hepatic adenoma, and—less likely—atypical hemangioma. In this 48-year-old woman, a subsequent diagnosis of focal nodular hyperplasia was made based on imaging findings from an abdominal MRI and nuclear medicine study.

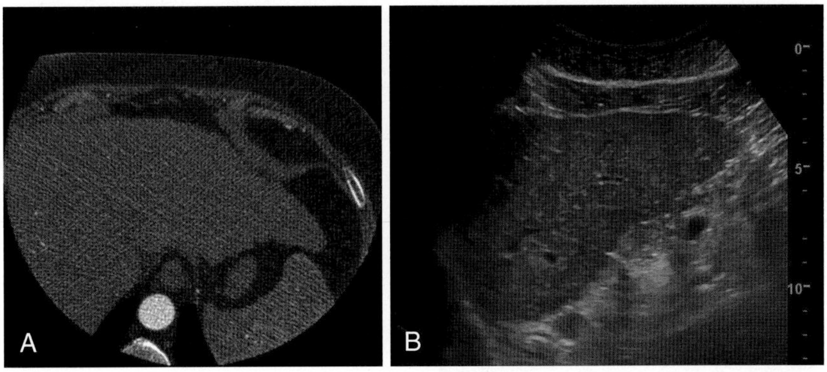

Figure 30-21. A 52-year-old man with multiple cardiac risk factors and atypical angina. **A,** This cardiac CT image was obtained in the inferiormost portion of the field of view. It demonstrates lobar redistribution of the left lobe of the liver, which is enlarged, as well as contour nodularity and irregularity of the liver. This appearance has been described in hepatic cirrhosis. **B,** An ultrasound image demonstrates marked coarseness of the underlying liver echotexture and an irregular rounded contour to the liver. Sonographic appearance is suggestive of cirrhosis. The patient was subsequently diagnosed with hepatitis C–related cirrhosis.

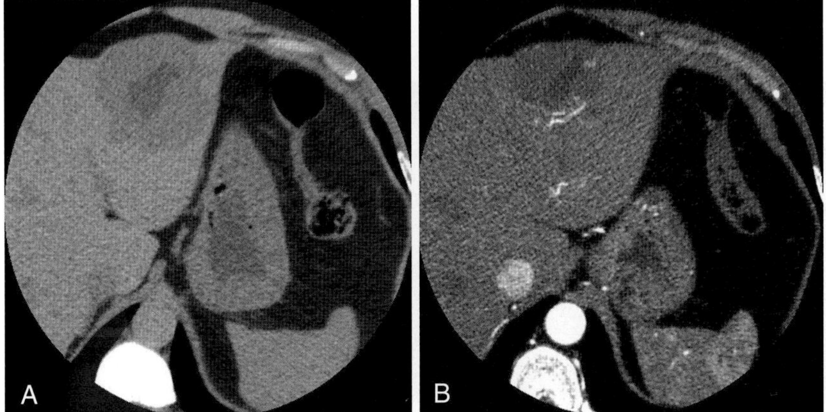

Figure 30-22. Two images from a cardiac CT study in a 38-year-old man with typical angina demonstrate a well-defined lesion within segment 2 of the liver. **A,** The noncontrast/calcium score demonstrates that this lesion is deforming the liver capsule. There is a large central area of decreased attenuation. **B,** On the arterially enhancing study, small areas of enhancement are seen within this lesion. Further work-up of this lesion included contrast-enhanced ultrasound and MRI. A final diagnosis of focal nodular hyperplasia was made, an unusual diagnosis in a 38-year-old man.

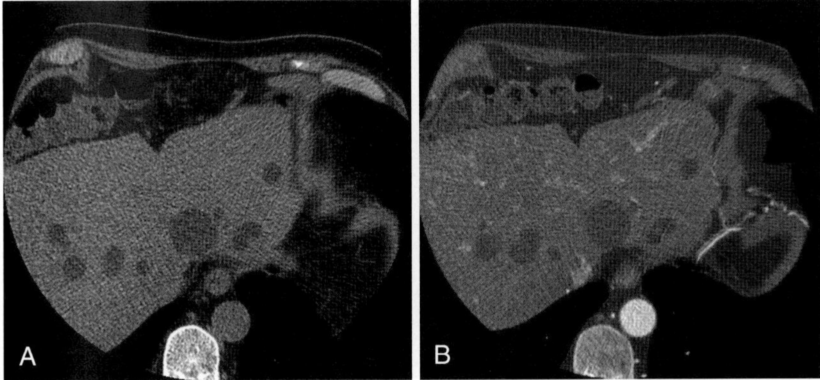

Figure 30-23. Two images from a cardiac CTA study, with the noncontrast calcium score on (**A**) and arterially enhanced (**B**). Multiple well-circumscribed hypodense lesions are seen scattered throughout the liver. These do not have any calcification associated with them, and demonstrate no arterial enhancement. Precontrast Hounsfield unit measurement within the larger lesions ranged from −2 to14 HU, consistent with simple fluid. These most likely represent simple hepatic cysts. If clinical concern for hepatic disease is present, or if the patient has other risk factors such as an underlying known malignancy, further evaluation of these hypodensities can be obtained, initially with abdominal ultrasound.

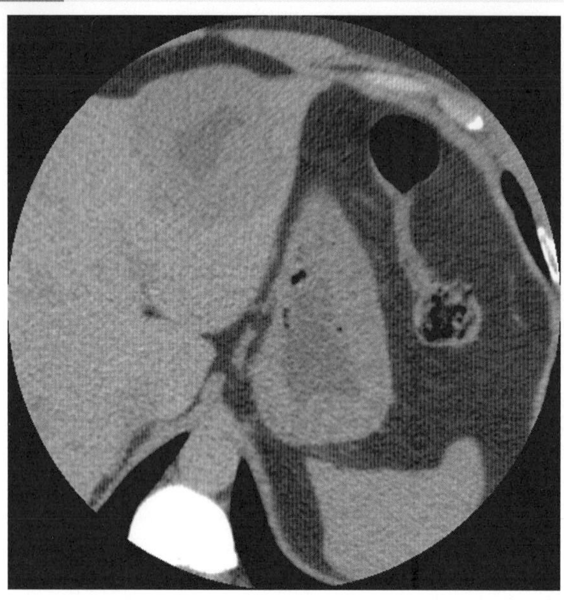

Figure 30-24. Calcium scoring study (no contrast) demonstrates a 5-cm mass that is subcapsular in location within segment 2 of the liver. There is a linear area of decreased attenuation within this mass. In the absence of IV contrast, the appearance of the mass is nonspecific, but possibilities include focal nodular hyperplasia with a possible central scar, an atypical hemangioma, and—less likely given the central hypodensity—a fibrolamellar variant of heptocellular carcinoma.

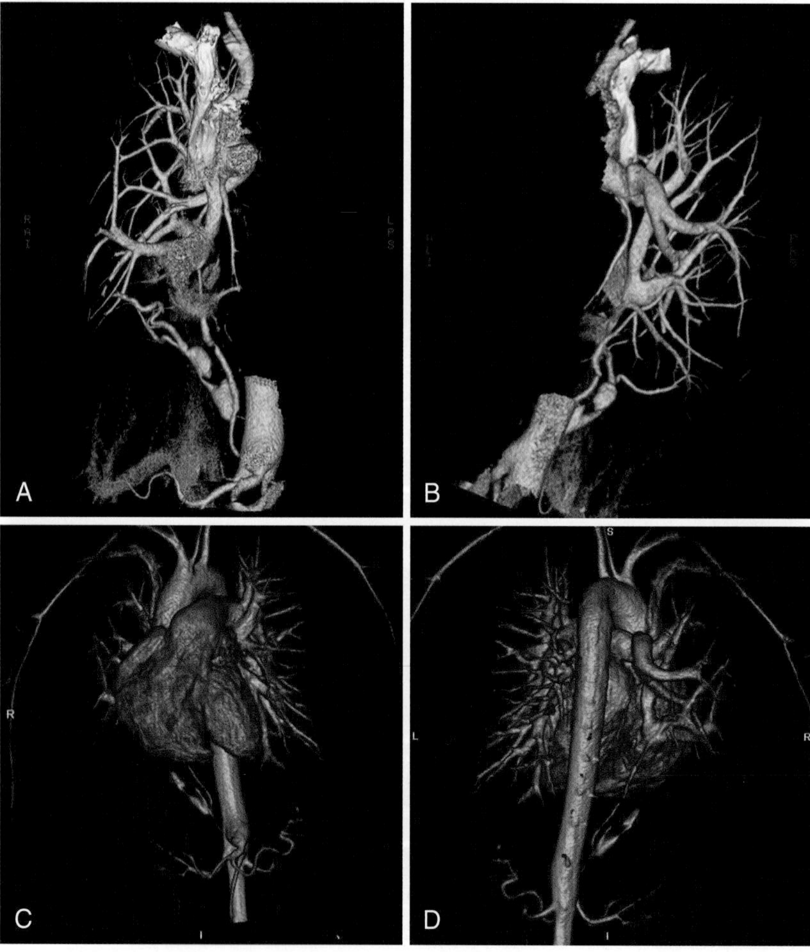

Figure 30-25. **A** and **B,** Three-dimensional volume-rendered contrast-enhanced CT images. **C** and **D,** Three-dimensional volume-rendered gadolinium-enhanced CMR images depicting an arterial anomaly arising from the celiac axis and supplying the sequestered right lower lobe.

Other Upper Abdominal Lesions

See Figure 30-25.

FOREIGN BODIES

In adults, metallic foreign bodies within the chest usually are related to penetrating injury such as stabbings, gunshot wounds, and the sequelae of high-velocity motor vehicle accidents. In the setting of a CCT study, shrapnel and other metallic foreign bodies can cause extensive beam-hardening artifact, significantly degrading image quality.

CCT PROTOCOL POINTS

Post-processing: includes "lung windowing" to depict pulmonary parenchymal detail and pathologies.

References

1. Hunold P, Schmermund A, Seibel RM, Gronemeyer DH, Erbel R. Prevalence and clinical significance of accidental findings in electron-beam tomographic scans for coronary artery calcification. *Eur. Heart J.* 2001;22(18):1748-1758.
2. Machaalany J, Yam Y, Ruddy TD, et al. Potential clinical and economic consequences of noncardiac incidental findings on cardiac computed tomography. *J Am Coll Cardiol.* 2009;54(16):1533-1541.
3. Onuma Y, Tanabe K, Nakazawa G, et al. Noncardiac findings in cardiac imaging with multidetector computed tomography. *J Am Coll Cardiol.* 2006;48(2):402-406.
4. Horton KM, Post WS, Blumenthal RS, Fishman EK. Prevalence of significant noncardiac findings on electron-beam computed tomography coronary artery calcium screening examinations. *Circulation.* 2002;106(5):532-534.
5. Schragin JG, Weissfeld JL, Edmundowicz D, Strollo DC, Fuhrman CR. Non-cardiac findings on coronary electron beam computed tomography scanning. *J Thorac Imaging.* 2004;19(2):82-86.
6. Koonce J, Schoepf JU, Nguyen SA, Northam MC, Ravenel JG. Extra-cardiac findings at cardiac CT: experience with 1,764 patients. *Eur Radiol.* 2009;19(3):570-576.
7. Jacobs PC, Mali WP, Grobbee DE, van der Graaf Y. Prevalence of incidental findings in computed tomographic screening of the chest: a systematic review. *J Comput Assist Tomogr.* 2008;32(2): 214-221.
8. Bolger AP. When does serendipity become screening? The deliberate search for noncardiac pathology on electron-beam computed tomography. *Circulation.* 2003;107(7):e54.
9. Budoff MJ, Gopal A. Incidental findings on cardiac computed tomography. Should we look? *J Cardiovasc Comput Tomogr.* 2007; 1(2):97-105.
10. MacMahon H, Austin JH, Gamsu G, et al. Guidelines for management of small pulmonary nodules detected on CT scans: a statement from the Fleischner Society. *Radiology.* 2005;237(2): 395-400.
11. Lindell RM, Hartman TE, Swensen SJ, et al. Five-year lung cancer screening experience: CT appearance, growth rate, location, and histologic features of 61 lung cancers. *Radiology.* 2007;242(2): 555-562.
12. Hoffman EA, Jiang R, Baumhauer H, et al. Reproducibility and validity of lung density measures from cardiac CT scans–the Multi-Ethnic Study of Atherosclerosis (MESA) Lung Study. *Acad Radiol.* 2009;16(6):689-699.
13. Goyal R. Diseases of the Esophagus. In: Fauci AS, Braunwald E, Kasper DL, et al., eds. *Harrison's Principles of Internal Medicine.* New York: McGraw-Hill; 2008.

INDEX

A

Page numbers followed by f refer to figures; page numbers followed by t refer to tables; page numbers followed by b refer to boxes,

B

C

D

E

F

G

H

I

J

K

L

M

S

T

U

V

W

X

Z